AF715998

Handbook of Burns Volume 1

Marc G. Jeschke • Lars-Peter Kamolz
Folke Sjöberg • Steven E. Wolf
Editors

Handbook of Burns Volume 1

Acute Burn Care

Second Edition 2020

Springer

Editors
Marc G. Jeschke
Ross Tilley Burn Centre Sunnybrook Health Sciences Centre
Toronto
ON, Canada

Folke Sjöberg
Department of Clinical and Experimental Medicine
Linköping University
Linköping
Sweden

Lars-Peter Kamolz
Division of Plastic
Aesthetic and Reconstructive Surgery
Department of Surgery
Medical University of Graz
Graz
Austria

COREMED- Centre for Regenerative Medcine
Joanneum Research Forschungsgesellschaft mbH
Graz
Austria

Steven E. Wolf
Department of Surgery
University of Texas Health Science Center
San Antonio, TX
USA

ISBN 978-3-030-18942-6 ISBN 978-3-030-18940-2 (eBook)
https://doi.org/10.1007/978-3-030-18940-2

This Springer imprint is published by the registered company Springer Nature Switzerland AG
The registered company address is: Gewerbestrasse 11, 6330 Cham, Switzerland

Preface

Severe burn injuries are maybe not the most common injuries occurring on a daily basis; however, it is estimated that within North America approximately 300,000–500,000 patients are hospitalized annually due to a burn-related injury and that worldwide approximately 500,000–1,000,000 people die due to a burn-related injury. Once a burn injury has occurred, it is one of the most severe forms of any injury, inducing a complex cascade of various responses including inflammatory, hypermetabolic, immune, as well as infectious responses. These responses interact with each other and are extremely complex and difficult to treat. Specialized centers, protocolized treatment, multicenter trials, and close collaborations improved morbidity and mortality after severe burn injury over the last two decades. However, a vast morbidity and mortality postburn still occurs and represent one of the major problems in burn treatment.

One of the major characteristics of burn injury that has been evolving over the last decade is that a burn injury is not treated and healed once the wounds are healed. This used to be a landmark that no longer exists. Various studies have indicated that a burn injury and its pathophysiologic sequelae persist for at least 5–10 years, not only in terms of scarring, infection, metabolism, and various other responses. Therefore, this leads to the importance of the current two volumes of these burn books. It has been speculated and hypothesized that early intervention and alleviation of these detrimental responses benefit in terms of clinical outcomes; therefore, the individual book chapters focus on the treatment and complexity of each of these responses to improve outcomes.

We reedited and worked over the two books to include novel aspects of burn. We now focus more on quality of life, on mental health, and on novel technologies. The up-to-date chapters provide evidence-based medicine and current state-of-the-art treatments for any practitioner dealing with acute burn wounds, chronic burn wounds, and all other types of burn wounds. The second volume will then delineate the importance for long-term treatment as it describes the reconstructive and alternative approaches of long-term treatment postburn.

This is unique and therefore will hopefully improve the outcome of burn patients by guiding various kinds of burn practitioners from nursing, physicians, occupational therapy, physical therapy, pharmacy, and so forth. The focus of each chapter is not only to give an overview but also to "summarize" current best treatments and to make it easy for each reader to easily access the treatment options and knowledge.

We hope that these books will raise as much enthusiasm as it has for its contributors.

Toronto, ON, Canada	Marc G. Jeschke
Graz, Austria	Lars-Peter Kamolz
Linköping, Sweden	Folke Sjöberg
San Antonio, TX, USA	Steven E. Wolf

Contents

Part I

History, Prevention, Education, Quality, and Team Building

A History of Burn Care

1

Leopoldo C. Cancio and Steven E. Wolf

1.1 "Black Sheep in the Surgical Wards"

If one uses the incontrovertible index of postburn mortality, it is evident that our ability to care for burn patients has improved markedly since World War II. This can be quantified by the lethal area 50% (that burn size which is lethal for 50% of a population), which in the immediate postwar era was approximately 40% of the total body surface area (TBSA) for young adults, whereas it increased to approximately 80% TBSA by the 1990s in the USA [1]. Furthermore, the mortality rate at the Galveston Shrine for children with 80% TBSA burns or greater (mean 70% full-thickness burn size) during 1982–1996 was only 33% [2]. What has been responsible for these improved outcomes in burn care? What practices were essential to this growth, and what are the major problems that remain unsolved? In this chapter, we will take as our focal point the fire disaster at the Cocoanut Grove Night Club which took place in Boston in 1942, less than a year after Pearl Harbor. The response to that disaster, and the monograph written in its aftermath, serves as a useful benchmark for the burn care advances which followed. To fully appreciate those advances, however, we must go back in time to an earlier era.

A wide variety of therapies for burns have been described since ancient times [3], but the idea of collecting burn patients in a special place is relatively new and emerged in Scotland during the nineteenth century. James Syme established the first burn unit in Edinburgh in 1843. He argued that mixing burn patients with postoperative patients would make him "chargeable with the highest degree of culpable recklessness." This logic motivated the Edinburgh Royal Infirmary leadership to set aside the former High School Janitor's House for burn patients. This experiment was relatively short-lived, however, since burn patients were transferred to one of the "Sheds" in 1848 to make way for an increased number of mechanical trauma casualties from railway accidents [4].

Another Scottish hospital, the Glasgow Royal Infirmary, had by 1933 accumulated 100 years of experience with over 10,000 burn patients, having established a separate burn ward midway through that period in 1883. In Dunbar's report on these patients, he commented:

> Burn cases have until recently been looked upon as black sheep in surgical wards, and have been almost entirely treated by junior members of the staff, who have not had any great clinical experience from which to judge their results (…) In the pre-antiseptic era only the worst burns would come to the hospital. The state of the hospitals was well known to the public, who also knew that a burn of slight or moderate severity had a better chance of recovery at home.

He documented the steady rise in the number of admissions to this hospital, a biphasic mortality pattern (with the highest number of deaths between postburn hours 12 and 24), the high incidence of streptococcal wound infection, the infrequency of skin grafting, and a frustratingly high mortality rate of 20–30% despite the introduction of antisepsis [5].

1.2 Toxemia, Plasmarrhea, or Infection?

Against this background, the founders of modern burn care must be credited with considerable clinical courage and intellectual foresight. Although the era of growth which they introduced is often dated to World War II, its roots were in earlier fire disasters and in World War I. This period featured a debate about the cause of postburn death and accordingly the appropriate treatment. A prevailing theory attributed

The opinions or assertions contained herein are the private views of the authors, and are not to be construed as official or as reflecting the views of the Department of the Army or the Department of Defense.

L. C. Cancio (✉)
U.S. Army Institute of Surgical Research,
Fort Sam Houston, TX, USA

S. E. Wolf
Shriners Hospitals for Children - Galveston,
University of Texas Medical Branch, Galveston, TX, USA
e-mail: steven.wolf@utmb.edu

M. G. Jeschke et al. (eds.), *Handbook of Burns Volume 1*, https://doi.org/10.1007/978-3-030-18940-2_1

death to the release of toxic substances from the burn wound: "The reaction of the body to a burn strongly resembles the clinical state described by the term 'toxaemia,' which implies the presence in the circulation of some toxic agent. The more serious cases usually present early in the course a clinical picture commonly described by such terms as shock or exhaustion" [6]. Treatments were widely employed to prevent this from happening. The most important such treatment was tannic acid, popularized by Davidson in 1925 [6]. Tanning of eschar, or of animal leather, involves collagen cross-linking and the formation of lipid-protein complexes in the remaining dermis. This generates a brown, supple, leather-like eschar [7]. Davidson asserted ambitiously that tannic acid not only lessens toxemia but also provides analgesia, prevents loss of body fluid, limits infection, decreases scar formation, and generates a scaffold for healing [6].

By contrast, in 1930 Frank Underhill published seminal observations on the pathophysiology of burn shock based on experience gained following the Rialto Theater fire of 1921 in New Haven, CN. These included the concepts of "anhydremia" and "hemoconcentration." Here is his description:

> When loss of water from the blood becomes great, the circulatory deficiency becomes magnified. The thick, sticky blood… finds great difficulty in passing through the capillaries…the blood is quickly robbed of its oxygen by the tissues…the tissues in general suffer from inadequate oxygenation…the heart pumps only a portion of its normal volume at each stroke [8].

Underhill then points out that his thinking on this process began during World War I, when he noted that inhalation of chemical warfare agents (chlorine, phosgene, and chloropicrin) produced both massive pulmonary edema and hemoconcentration. Applying this concept to thermally injured skin led to our basic understanding of burn shock: "fluid rushes to the burned skin with great rapidity and is lost to the body… or the part affected becomes edematous with great celerity." The fluid lost is similar to plasma—implying increased capillary permeability—whereas in cholera it is a dilute salt solution. Measurement of the blood hemoglobin percentage is proposed as an index of resuscitation, and resuscitation aimed at preventing hemoconcentration is required for 24–36 h postburn. Intravenous sodium chloride solutions should be used, supplemented by oral, rectal, and subdermal solutions [8].

In 1931, Alfred Blalock reported laboratory confirmation of Underhill's theory. Dogs underwent burns to one third of the body surface area, limited to one side of the body. After death, animals were sagittally bisected, and the difference in weight between the halves was estimated to be the amount of fluid lost into the tissues as a consequence of injury. This weight difference was on average 3.34% of the initial total body weight, indicating a loss of approximately one half of the circulating plasma volume. He also noted that the fluids collected in the subcutaneous tissues had a protein concentration similar to that of plasma and that the blood hemoglobin content increased markedly [9].

But plasma loss was an incomplete description of the biphasic death pattern documented for burn patients. Shortly thereafter, Aldrich introduced the treatment of burn wounds with gentian violet, a coal-tar derivative which kills Gram-positive organisms. He argued against the toxemia theory and attributed postburn toxic symptoms not to the eschar but to streptococcal wound infection. Early use of gentian violet would prevent this, whereas tannic acid did not. He distinguished this delayed infectious process from "primary shock," downplaying the latter's importance: "it is sufficient to say that if it is combated early and adequately, with heat, rest, fluids, and stimulants, it can be overcome in the majority" [10].

1.3 The Guinea Pig Club

The transformation of burn care required not only the above observations but also an institutional commitment. In 1916, Sir Harold Gillies returned from service in France to lead the first plastic and oral-maxillofacial surgery service in the UK at Cambridge Military Hospital, Aldershot, later moving to Queen's Hospital in Sidcup, Kent. Gillies and team treated over 11,000 casualties with facial injuries by the end of the war, including burns [11, 12]. The Spanish Civil War (1936–1939) convinced the British leadership that the next war would involve air combat and asked Gillies to establish plastic surgery units around London [12]. At that time, there were only four plastic surgeons in the country, including Gillies' cousin, Sir Archibald McIndoe, who had joined Gillies in 1930 after training at the Mayo Clinic [13]. During 1939, McIndoe established the burn unit for the Royal Air Force at East Grinstead, UK, which persists to this day. Beginning in summer 1940, approximately 400 RAF personnel (mainly fighter pilots) were seriously burned during the Battle of Britain, revealing both aircraft design limitations and the intensity of aerial combat. The focus of the new unit was on the reconstruction and rehabilitation of these patients. McIndoe assembled a team of nurses, anesthetists, microbiologists, orderlies, and others to undertake this journey into the unknown:

> Historically there was little to guide one in this field apart from the general principles of repair perfected by British, Continental and American surgeons. There had until then been no substantial series of cases published and none in which a rational plan of repair had been proposed. At most, individual cases appeared… in which only too often the end result seemed to convert the pathetic into the ridiculous [13]

Soon, four more units were established in the UK, which together with East Grinstead served the hundreds of casualties who followed from operations such as Royal Air Force's strategic bombing campaign.

McIndoe's work underscores several important points about burn care. First, the impetus for a breakthrough in the organization and delivery of burn care was the catastrophic nature of modern warfare, the large number of casualties therefrom, and both a national and an individual commitment to care for these casualties. Second, the experimental nature of burn care was recognized, and a scientific approach based on clinical evidence was espoused. Among the East Grinstead unit's contributions were the condemnation of tannic acid as coagulation therapy for acute burn wounds; perfection and description of a methodology for burn wound reconstruction; and, in collaboration with Leonard Colebrook (see below), early experience with penicillin therapy for Gram-positive infections. Third, the East Grinstead unit became a hub for new UK burn units, as well as a training center for scores of surgeons and nurses in the principles of the emerging specialty. Fourth, the psychological and social needs of the patients were highlighted. At East Grinstead, this was embodied in the "Guinea Pig Club," a social network for burn survivors whose membership totaled 649 people (Fig. 1.1). The longevity of both the needs of burn survivors, and the strength of this network, is exemplified that the last issue of *The Guinea Pig* magazine was published in 2003 [13]. Clearly, none of these steps—the scientific approach to improving burn care, the emphasis on clinical expertise on the part of all members of the multidisciplinary team, and the creation of a mechanism for effective psychosocial support—would have been possible without the concentration of patients at a center dedicated to overcoming a seemingly insurmountable problem.

The origin of infection control in burn patients, however, belongs not to McIndoe but to Leonard Colebrook, a physician, bacteriologist, and colleague of Alexander Fleming [14]. In an era dominated by multidrug-resistant Gram-negative and methicillin-resistant *Staphylococcus aureus* infections, it is important to recall the major role played by *Streptococcus pyogenes* infections before the introduction of antibiotics. Colebrook confirmed Domagk's 1935 "startling

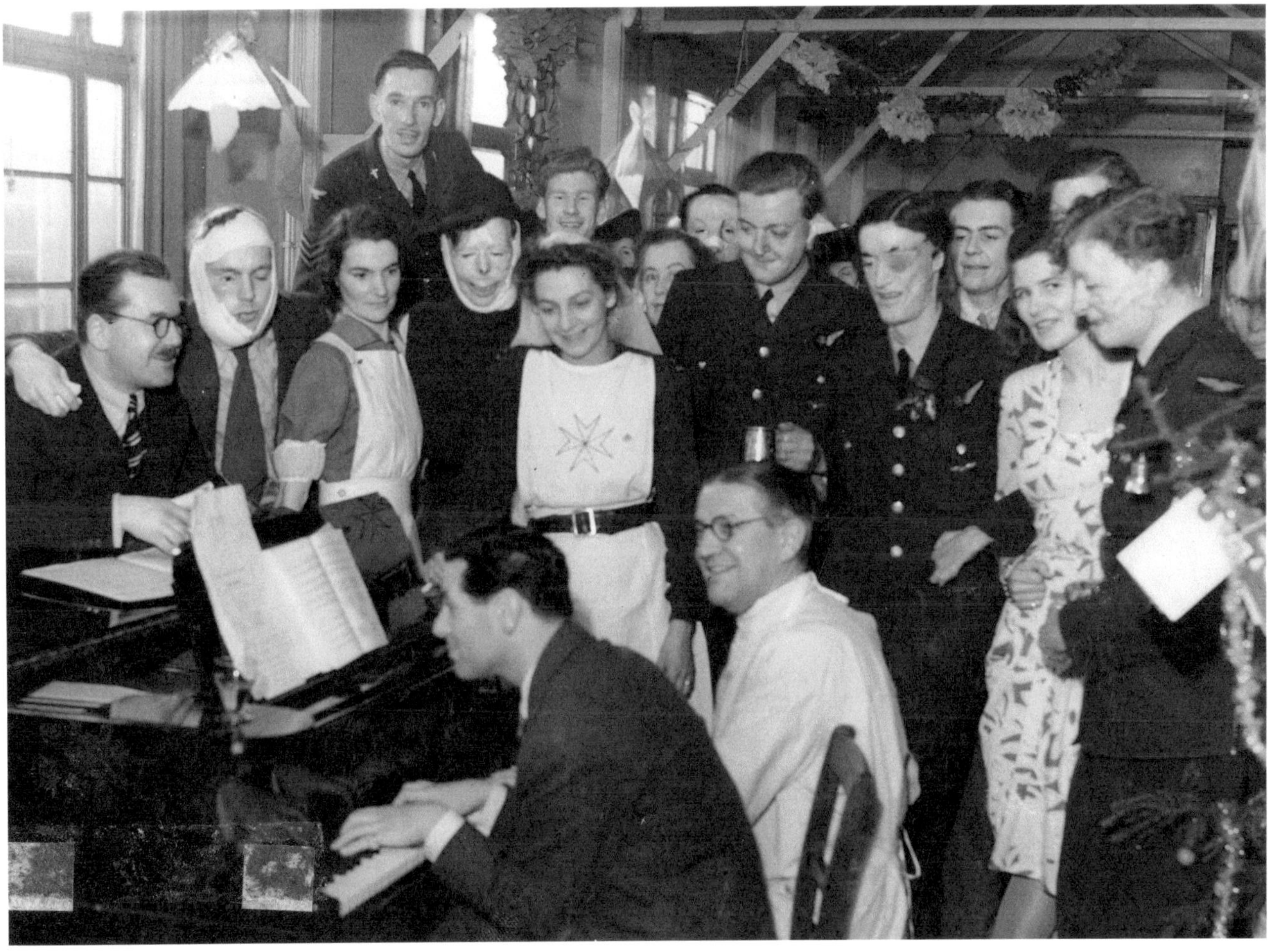

Fig. 1.1 Members of the "Guinea Pig Club" of war-injured burn survivors, nurses from the burn unit at East Grinstead, UK, and Sir Archibald McIndoe celebrating around the piano. This photograph graphically depicts the value of peer support in the recovery of the whole patient. Source: East Grinstead Museum, East Grinstead, UK

success" on the efficacy of the sulfanilamide parent drug, Prontosil, using a murine model of streptococcal peritonitis, and reported lifesaving treatment of 38 patients with puerperal fever [15, 16]. Turning his attention to burns at the Glasgow Royal Infirmary, he studied dressings impregnated with sulfanilamide and penicillin creams [14, 17] and the use of serum and plasma for burn shock resuscitation [18]. (The problem of Gram-negative burn wound infection remained to be recognized and solved at another time, since "coliform bacilli, *B. proteus* and *Ps. pyocyanea*, when present in the wounds, were apparently not affected" by these drugs.) [17]. He then established a new burn unit at the Birmingham Accident Hospital [19]. In contrast to the toxemia theory, Colebrook and others proposed that burn wounds became infected with bacteria and that strict infection control practices could prevent infection by reducing transfer of these organisms; these concepts were incorporated into both the design and practices of the new burn unit [20, 21].

1.4 Burns and Sulfa Drugs at Pearl Harbor

In the USA, the attack on Pearl Harbor on December 7, 1941 served a function similar to that of the Battle of Britain by energizing burn care research. Fortuitously, the USA, anticipating the likelihood of war, had already made two major national commitments to supporting medical research of military relevance. The first such effort was the creation, by the National Research Council's (NRC) Division of Medical Sciences, of Advisory Committees to the Surgeons General in April 1940 [22]. Critical among these for the burn care in the USA were the Committee on Chemotherapeutic and Other Agents and the Committee on Surgery (which included, among others, Subcommittees on Surgical Infections and on Burns).

The second such effort was the creation by the federal government of the Committee on Medical Research (CMR) of the Office of Scientific Research and Development (OSRD) in June 1941 [23, 24]. The purpose of the CMR was to identify problems of military medical importance and to fund university research to solve these problems. These two activities (the NRC Advisory Committees and the CMR) were collocated at NRC headquarters, and the NRC advised the CMR on how best to expend federal funds [22]. In brief, by the time of Pearl Harbor, the USA had the framework in place for academic, military, and federal collaboration in pursuit of solutions for combat casualty care.

For the NRC and the CMR, Pearl Harbor highlighted the importance of burns in modern warfare. About 60% of over 500 casualties admitted to the Pearl Harbor Naval Hospital were thermally injured (Fig. 1.2). Many of these wounds were contaminated by fuel oil or complicated by fragment injuries. Care was variable and included some sort of topical tanning agent, delayed debridement, infusion of available intravenous fluids, and treatment of fractures [25]. "At the Naval Hospital, ordinary flit guns were used to spray tannic acid solution upon the burned surfaces," indicating the persistence of the toxemia theory in clinical care. On the other hand, both plasma and saline solution were used for fluid resuscitation, and sulfa drugs were given to patients with infected wounds—indicating a conglomeration of the competing theories of burn pathophysiology. In response to Pearl Harbor, the NRC rapidly dispatched Perrin Long, the chairman of the Committee on Chemotherapeutic and Other Agents, and surgeon I.S. Ravdin to Hawaii, in order to evaluate the use of sulfa drugs and other aspects of care.

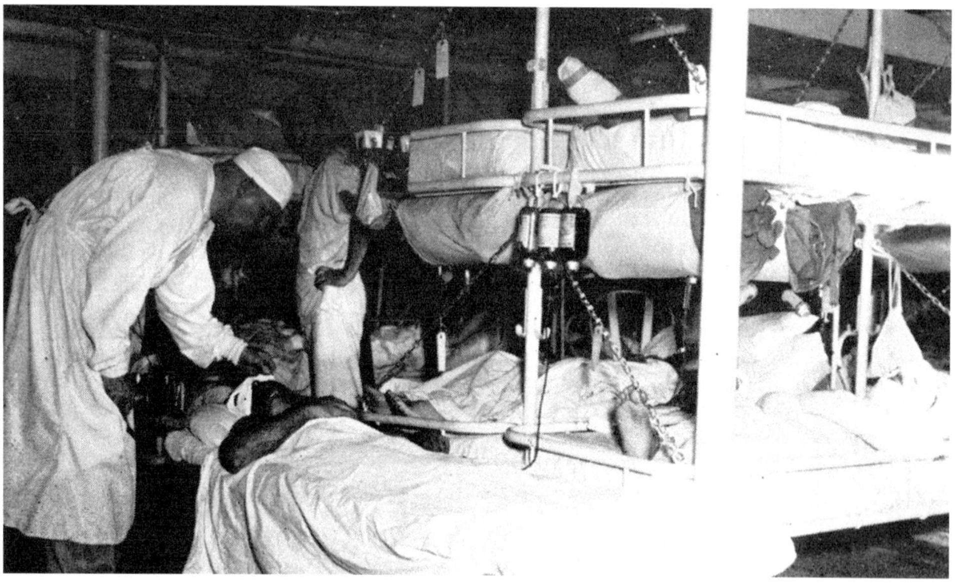

Fig. 1.2 Aboard the USS Solace hospital ship, caring for wounded from the attack on Pearl Harbor, December 7, 1941. The Solace dispatched small boat crews to rescue casualties: "they boarded the burning Arizona, while its crew was abandoning ship, and they rescued the burned and injured casualties found on its deck, some very close to the flames" [131]. Pearl Harbor alerted the US Government of the urgent need for burn research. Source: US Navy [132]

They submitted their report to the War Department on January 18, 1942, emphasizing the lifesaving characteristics of sulfa drug use and the value of plasma for resuscitation:

> We have been impressed again and again with the incalculable value of sulfonamide therapy in the care of many of the casualties…We believe that it is highly important that physicians—both civilian and military—become familiar with the general and specific considerations which govern the oral and local use of the sulfonamides in the treatment of wounds and burns…. [25, 26]

Despite this impression and the fact that the sulfa drugs were the only antibiotics available in significant quantities in 1941, their indications and limitations were unknown. Accordingly, the Subcommittee on Surgical Infections, chaired by Frank Meleney, defined this question as a major objective at its initial meeting in June 1940 [22]. Wound study units were set up at eight US hospitals, and a multicenter trial was conducted of both local and systemic sulfa use. Meleney, in his report on this study, lamented that

> The original plan was altered to a considerable extent by the reports which came back from Pearl Harbor. Observers who saw the casualties there were profoundly impressed by the low incidence of wound infection, which they believed to be due to the copious application of sulfanilamide to the wounds. Our original plan called for observation on control cases without drugs and other controls receiving treatment with local bacteriostatic agents other than the sulfonamides. But, said the Pearl Harbor observers: "You cannot withhold from these patients the benefit of the sulfonamide drugs." [27]

By the end of 1942, 1500 patients (with soft tissue injuries, fractures, and burns) had been enrolled. In his report on this study, Meleney concluded that neither local nor systemic sulfonamides were effective at controlling local wound infection and that inadequate surgical treatment predisposed to infection. The antibiotics were effective at preventing systemic sepsis, but were not a panacea [27]. An awareness of these limitations and emerging experience with *Staphylococcus* and *Clostridium* resistance to sulfa drugs [22] set the stage for research on penicillin.

1.5 Penicillin and the Burn Projects

Although Alexander Fleming discovered penicillin in 1929, its clinical utility was not appreciated until 10 years later, when Howard W. Florey, Ernest Chain, and others (the "Oxford Team") performed murine and human experiments demonstrating the new drug's lifesaving potential against *Streptococcus*, *Staphylococcus*, and *Clostridium* infections [28, 29]. Since British pharmaceutical firms were overwhelmed with wartime production of other drugs, Florey went to the USA in summer 1941 to obtain support for large-scale manufacturing, ultimately meeting with and convincing the chairman of the CMR, Alfred N. Richards [24]. Once a method of mass-production of the drug had been developed, the CMR turned in January 1942 to the Committee on Chemotherapeutic and Other Agents, headed by Perrin Long, for help in organizing clinical trials [30]. Long appointed Champ Lyons at the Massachusetts General Hospital (MGH), Chester Keefer, and colleagues to accomplish this [30]. This was the origin of one of the two burn-related research programs in place at the MGH at the time of the Cocoanut Grove fire in 1942 [31].

The second MGH research program dealt specifically with thermal injury [31]. On January 7, 1942, the NRC sponsored a pivotal conference on burns, chaired by I.S. Ravdin [32, 33]. The conference proceedings recommended plasma, topical tannic acid, and oral sulfadiazine. Henry Harkins presented the available formulas for resuscitation of burn patients. His own method (the "Method of Harkins") was based on hemoconcentration: give 100 cc of plasma for each point that the hematocrit exceeds 45. For wartime, when lab facilities are unavailable, he recommended the "First Aid Method": slowly give 500 cc of plasma for each 10% of the total body surface area (TBSA) burned [34, 35]. The latter is the first formula based on TBSA. The NRC report from the conference advocated 1000 cc of plasma for each 10% TBSA over the first 24 h, in divided doses [32].

The Subcommittee on Burns was organized under Allen Whipple in July 1942 [22] and was charged with determining the best therapies for acute burns and whether tanning was appropriate. The wound study units of the Subcommittee on Surgical Infections found that tanned burns had a high wound infection rate, and the Subcommittee on Burns soon recommended against use or further procurement of tannic acid in October 1942—less than 1 year after it was liberally used at Pearl Harbor. Nevertheless, "it cannot be said that unanimous agreement was ever attained on the choice of the best local agent" [22]. Another early contribution by Whipple was stating for the first time the importance of well-organized "burn teams":

> By burn team we mean a group made up of a general surgeon, interested in problems of infection and wound healing, a physician or technician, thoroughly trained in problems of fluid, protein and electrolyte imbalance, a general plastic surgeon…with experience in skin grafting large granulating areas, a group of trained nurses and orderlies, able and willing to stand the stress and strain of caring for severely burned patients. [36]

1.6 The Cocoanut Grove Fire of 1942 and Beyond

The fire at the Cocoanut Grove (CG) nightclub in Boston, MA on November 28, 1942 was one of the worst civilian fire disasters in the US history, killing 492 of the estimated 1000 occupants [37]. Oliver Cope, editing the monograph published on the MGH's response, felt that they were well prepared in large part because of the war:

> Had such a catastrophe taken place before Pearl Harbor, the hospital would have been swamped. As it was, the injured found the staff prepared, for the war had made us catastrophe minded. (…) A plan of therapy for burns, suited to use in a catastrophe, was developed and decided upon. When the victims of the Cocoanut Grove fire arrived, the treatment was ready and it was applied to all. [31]

Specific preparations for war that were already in place at the time of this fire included organization of personnel, publication of a disaster manual, preparation of sterile supplies for 200 operations, acquisition of wooden i.v. poles and of sawhorses to support stretchers, establishment of a blood bank, and training of Red Cross volunteers and of Harvard students as orderlies [38].

The CG monograph contains the first detailed description of a scientific approach to multidisciplinary burn care [37]. As such, it serves as an invaluable point of departure for understanding subsequent changes and current practice.

1.6.1 Burn Center Concept

Although the MGH did not have a dedicated burn unit in 1942, the 39 CG patients were all hospitalized on a single ward. "In a disaster of this type, where the injuries were all of the same kind, the importance of concentration of casualties in one group in one ward or floor where they can be under concentrated medical treatment and where isolation procedures can be set up if needed, was clearly demonstrated" [39]. The first permanent unit in the USA was established in Richmond, VA by Everett Evans, who had become chairman of the NRC Committee on Burns [40]. In 1947, the Army Wound Study Unit was moved from Halloran General Hospital to Fort Sam Houston, Texas by Edwin Pulaski—an Army surgeon who had trained under Meleney—and was renamed the Surgical Research Unit (SRU) [41]. At that unit, patients with infected burns and other wounds were treated on a special ward at the US Army's Brooke General Hospital. Two years later, growing concerns about the possibility of nuclear war with the Soviet Union, and recognition that such a war would generate thousands of burn survivors, refocused the SRU on the treatment of burns, and the second US burn unit was formally established [40].

The US Army Burn Center at the SRU (later renamed as the US Army Institute of Surgical Research, USAISR) was at the forefront of many of the advances in burn care described below. Also critical for improving care in the US was the unit's commitment to training surgeons, many of whom became directors of civilian burn centers [42–44]. Designation of the unit as the single destination for all the US military burn casualties, as well as for civilians in the region, provided the number of patients needed both to maintain clinical competence and to support the research mission during war and peace. Another major factor in the development of burn care in the USA was the decision in 1962 by the Shriners Hospitals for Crippled Children privately to fund the construction and operation of three pediatric burn units—in Cincinnati, Ohio; Boston, Massachusetts; and Galveston, Texas. These units opened during 1966–1968, and like the US Army Burn Center, became centers of excellence in care, teaching, and research [45, 46].

1.6.2 Shock and Resuscitation

The MGH used a version of the NRC First Aid Formula for resuscitation of the CG casualties. All but 10 patients were given plasma intravenously (Fig. 1.3):

> The initial dosage of plasma was determined on the basis of the surface area of the burns. For each 10 percent of the body surface involved, it was planned to give 500 cc in the first 24 hours. Because the plasma delivered by the Blood Bank during the first 36 hours was diluted with an equal volume of physiologic saline solution, the patient was to receive 1000 cc of fluid for each 10 percent burned. The plasma dosage was modified subsequently on the basis of repeated hematocrit and serum protein determinations. [47]

Cope and Moore, in a follow-on paper in 1947, described a refinement of the NRC formula called the Surface Area Formula: 75 mL of plasma and 75 mL of isotonic crystalloid solution per TBSA, with one-half given over the first 8 h and one-half over the second 16 h. The urine output was to be used as the primary index of resuscitation [33].

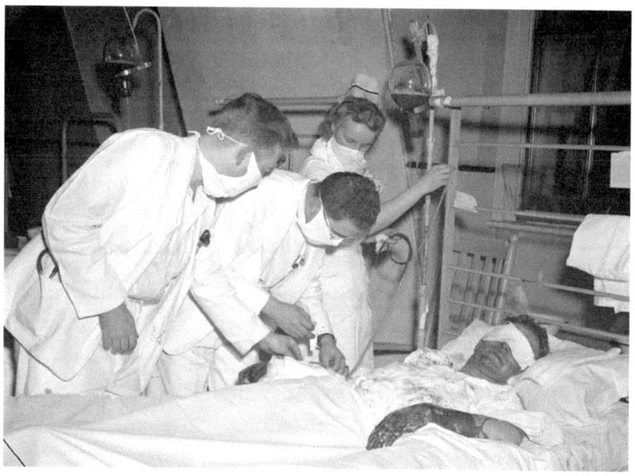

Fig. 1.3 A survivor of the Cocoanut Grove nightclub fire in November 1942 receives an infusion of plasma. Ongoing preparations for war enabled Boston hospitals to respond more effectively to this civilian disaster. Source: Boston Public Library, Leslie Jones Collection [133]

Subsequent revisions of this basic concept included the following formulas:

- *Evans Formula*: incorporation of body weight; colloid 1 mL/kg/TBSA and crystalloid 1 mL/kg/TBSA [48]
- *Brooke Formula*: decrease in colloid content to 0.5 mL/kg/TBSA, with crystalloid 1.5 ml/kg/TBSA; replacement of plasma with 5% albumin because of hepatitis risk [49]
- *Parkland Formula*: elimination of colloid during the first 24 h; increase in crystalloid to 4 mL/kg/TBSA [50]
- *Modified Brooke Formula*: elimination of colloid during first 24 h; crystalloid 2 mL/kg/TBSA [51]

Despite their differences, employment of these formulas reduced early deaths due to burn shock to about 13% of postburn deaths, and made acute renal failure due to burn shock distinctly unusual. Today, the hazards of "fluid creep" mandate a continued search for an approach to resuscitation that decreases the rate of edema formation [52, 53].

1.6.3 Wound Care and Infection

By the time of the CG fire, tannic acid had fallen into disfavor: "A bland, protective ointment dressing is indicated in the treatment of skin burns since the chemical agents currently recommended are believed to be injurious to otherwise viable epithelium and delay wound healing" [54]. Attention turned to use of i.v. antibiotics for the prevention of infection. Hemolytic streptococcal infection responded to sulfa drugs: "an effective blood level of sulfonamide offers the most certain control of systemic infection due to the hemolytic streptococcus" [55]. Meanwhile, Champ Lyons, the surgeon in charge of penicillin research at MGH, received enough of the experimental drug from Chester Keefer to treat 13 CG patients. The doses given were too low and the experience was inconclusive, although he did not observe toxic side effects [55]. From there, Lyons undertook larger studies of penicillin at Bushnell General Hospital, Brigham City, Utah (April 1943) and at the new Wound Study Unit at Halloran General Hospital, Staten Island, New York (June 1943) [56, 57]; the latter was the forerunner of the US Army SRU. These studies constituted the first large-scale studies of penicillin, documented efficacy against staphylococcal and streptococcal combat wound infections [57], and convinced the Army of the need for large-scale production of the drug [24]. Lyons next obtained a commission as an Army Major in August 1943, deploying to the North African theater to facilitate the introduction of penicillin into battlefield care under Edward Churchill [56].

Penicillin, however, was only a partial answer to the problem of late postburn death. In 1954, the SRU noted that effective fluid resuscitation now kept many patients with greater than 50% TBSA burns alive past the 2-day mark, only to succumb at a later date [58]. The conquest of hemolytic *Streptococcus* now revealed the role of Gram-negative organisms, and the presence of positive blood cultures, particularly in patients with large full-thickness burns, pointed at bacteremia of burn wound origin [58]. The natural history of this "burn wound sepsis" was not clear, however, until a model of invasive *Pseudomonas* burn wound infection in rats was conceived and characterized by Walker and Mason at the SRU [59–61]. At that time, however, no effective topic or intravenous therapy had been identified.

Pruitt and colleagues at the SRU achieved a dramatic improvement in postburn mortality in 1964, with the introduction into clinical care of a topical antimicrobial effective against Gram-negative burn wound infection, mafenide acetate (Sulfamylon) cream (Fig. 1.4) [62]. This drug had been first synthesized in the 1930s and evaluated by Domagk, but abandoned, interestingly, because of lack of efficacy against *Streptococcus* [63]. It was rediscovered by US Army researchers at Edgewood Arsenal, who demonstrated efficacy in an otherwise lethal caprine model of *Clostridium perfringens* infection following extremity blast injury [64]. Because it penetrates deeply, it appeared particularly effective in wounds with devitalized tissue, a feature which also made it attractive for the treatment of full-thickness burns. Lindberg and colleagues at the SRU had similar success in the Walker–Mason *Pseudomonas* model [65]. In thermally injured patients, death from invasive burn wound infection declined from 59% (pre-mafenide) to 10% (post-mafenide) [62]. Meanwhile, Moyer and Monafo confirmed the effectiveness of 0.5% silver nitrate soaks in preventing burn wound infection [66]. Charles Fox subsequently developed silver sulfadiazine to combine the advantages of a sulfonamide with the silver ion [67]. Silver sulfadiazine, the recently developed silver-impregnated fabrics [68], and mafenide acetate are the commonly employed antimicrobials used in burn care today.

1.6.4 Burn Surgery

Surgeons accustomed to early excision of the burn wound should bear in mind that at the time of the CG fire, burn surgery was performed after the separation of eschar: "The first graft was applied on the twenty-third day…and the last at four months to several small areas" [69]. Originally, the surgical treatment of burn wounds, if performed, was limited to contracture release and reconstruction after the wound had healed by scar formation. In patients with larger wounds or burns of functional areas, this was wholly unsatisfactory. The creation of burn units committed to care for these patients led to the development of more effective techniques for wound closure. Artz noted that one should "wait until natural

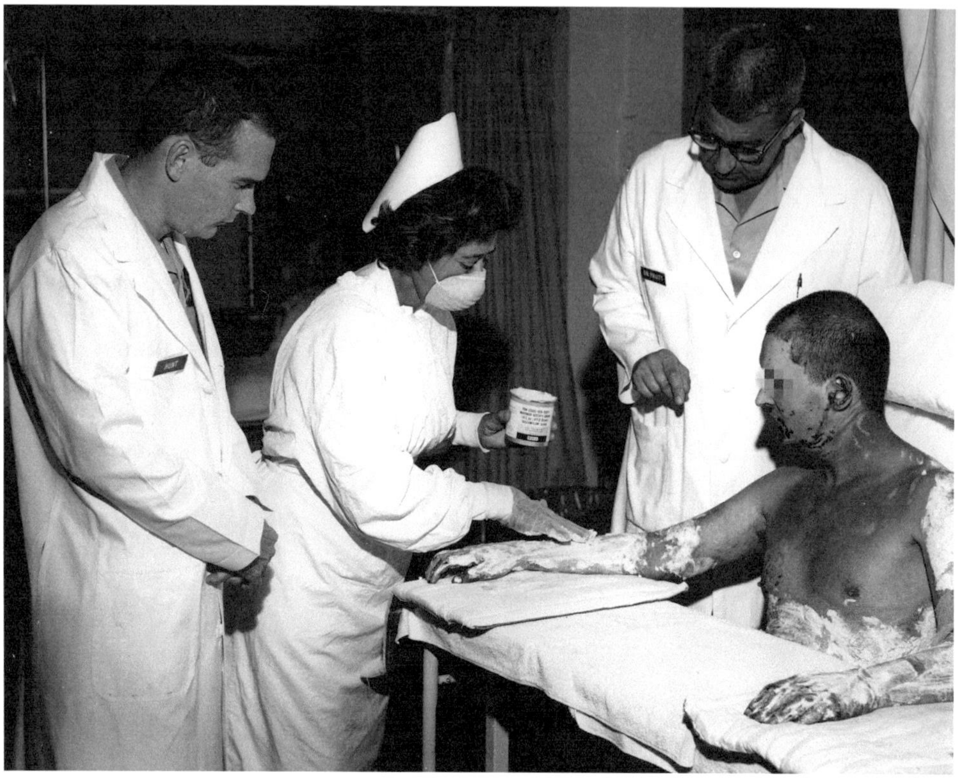

Fig. 1.4 Application of mafenide acetate cream (Sulfamylon) to a thermally injured patient at the US Army Surgical Research Unit in 1964. At the left, Dr. John L. Hunt; at the right, Dr. Basil A. Pruitt, Jr. The dramatic decrease in invasive Gram-negative burn wound infection, that followed the introduction of Sulfamylon, was the epitome of integrated laboratory and clinical research championed by Dr. Pruitt. Source: Collection of the US Army Institute of Surgical Research, Courtesy Mr. Glen Gueller

sequestration has occurred and a good granulating barrier has formed beneath the eschar…After removing the eschar… skin grafting should be performed as soon as the granulating surface is properly prepared" [70]. Debridement to the point of bleeding or pain during daily immersion hydrotherapy (Hubbard tanks) was used to facilitate separation of the eschar [71]. Then, cadaver cutaneous allografts (homografts) were often used to prepare the granulating wound bed for autografting [72].

In patients with larger (>50% TBSA) burns and in the absence of topical antimicrobials, this cautious approach did not prevent death from invasive burn wound infection, leading some to propose a more radical solution: that of primary excision of the burn wound. Surgeons at the SRU suggested that a "heroic" practice of early excision, starting postburn day 4, should be considered for patients with large burns. This would reduce the "large pabulum" of dead tissue available for microbial proliferation; immediate coverage with a combination of autograft and cadaver allograft would further protect the wound [61]. Several authors during the 1950s and 1960s demonstrated the feasibility of this approach, but not an improvement in mortality [73].

In 1968, Janzekovic described the technique of tangential primary excision of the burn wound with immediate grafting; operating in postwar Yugoslavia, she recalled that "a barber's razor sharpened on a strap was the pearl among our instruments" [74, 75]. In a retrospective study, Tompkins et al. reported an improvement in mortality over the course of 1974–1984 which they attributed to excision [76]. William F. McManus and colleagues at the Army Burn Center compared patients who underwent excision with those who did not during 1983–1985, noting that an improvement in mortality could not be attributed to excision because preexisting organ failure precluded surgery in many unexcised patients. However, only six of the 93 patients (6.5%) who died in this study had invasive bacterial burn wound infection, whereas 54 of the 93 (58%) had pneumonia—indicating a shift from wound to non-wound infections [77].

In McManus' study, excision was performed in a mean of 13 days postburn. By contrast, David Herndon et al. at Galveston implemented a method of excision within 48–72 h of admission, which relied on widely meshed (4:1) autograft covered by allograft. In a small study of children during 1977–1981, these authors noted a decrease in length of stay but not in mortality with this technique [78]. During 1982–1985, adults were randomized to undergo early excision vs. excision after eschar separation 3 weeks later. Young adults without inhalation injury and with burns >30% TBSA showed an improvement in mortality [79]. A recent meta-analysis found a decrease in mortality but an increase in blood use in early excision patients without inhalation injury [80].

Despite the limitations of the early studies, early excision is today performed in most of the US burn centers—controversy remains about the definition of "early" and the feasibility of performing radical, total excision at one operation, especially in adults. We now understand excision and definitive closure of the burn wound as fundamental for patients with massive injuries; the "race" to achieve this before sepsis and other causes of organ failure supervene is the main effort; patients whose grafts fail repeatedly ("wound failure") will not, in the authors' experience, survive. To facilitate massive excision for patients with the largest wounds and limited donor sites, new methods of temporary and permanent closure have been sought. Burke and Yannas developed the first successful dermal regeneration template (Integra®), composed of a dermal analog (collagen and chondroitin-6-sulfate) and a temporary epidermal analog (Silastic) [81]. Cultured epidermal autografts provide material for wound closure for patients with the most extensive burns, although the cost is high and final take rates are variable [82–84]. The ultimate goal of an off-the-shelf bilaminar product for permanent wound closure, with a take rate similar to that of cutaneous autografts, has not yet been achieved.

1.6.5 Inhalation Injury and Pulmonary Care

Pulmonary problems were a significant cause of mortality after the CG fire, and options for diagnosis and treatment were limited. About 114 patients were brought to the MGH, some alive, some dead; it is clear that many of these casualties died of carbon monoxide poisoning or early airway obstruction. Of the 39 patients who survived long enough to be admitted, seven died, all of whom had evidence of inhalation injury. The authors noted: "Although intubation and tracheotomy were not highly successful in our cases, we believe that they fulfill a definite function in relieving labored breathing and in facilitating the delivery of oxygen, and should be resorted to in patients with acute cyanosis and in those with severe upper respiratory lesions." On the other hand, "the resuscitation of patients in acute attacks of edema was difficult and unsatisfactory" and "the pulmonary complications were bizarre and characterized by extreme variability, with areas of lung collapse and emphysema…" [85].

Subsequent improvements in inhalation injury care required the development of positive-pressure mechanical ventilators. Forrest Bird, V.R. Bennett, and J. Emerson built mechanical positive-pressure ventilators toward the end of WWII, all inspired by technology developed during the war to deliver oxygen to pilots flying at high altitudes [86]. The availability of these and similar machines, and the Scandinavian polio epidemic of 1952, spurred the creation of separate intensive care units (ICUs) within hospitals [87]. Today, in one model of burn care, burn units are separate from ICUs, and the two types of units are run by different personnel. At the US Army Burn Center and several other centers, by contrast, ICU beds have been located within the burn unit and have been directed by surgeon-intensivists—ensuring continuity of multidisciplinary care and clinical research.

Once accurate diagnosis of inhalation injury by bronchoscopy and xenon-133 lung scanning became available, it was apparent that smoke-injured patients had greatly increased risk of pneumonia and death [88]. Large animal models were developed, and the pathophysiology of the injury was defined [89, 90]. Unlike ARDS due to mechanical trauma or alveolar injury due to inhalation of chemical warfare agents, smoke inhalation injury was found to damage the small airways, with resultant ventilation–perfusion mismatch, bronchiolar obstruction, and pneumonia [91]. This process featured activation of the inflammatory cascade, which in animal models was amenable to modulation by various anti-inflammatory agents [92]. Practically, however, the most effective interventions to date have been those directly aimed at maintaining small airway patency and at avoiding injurious forms of mechanical ventilation. These include high-frequency percussive ventilation with the Volumetric Diffusive Respiration ventilator developed by Bird [93] and delivery of heparin by nebulization [94].

1.6.6 Nutrition and the "Universal Trauma Model"

Bradford Cannon described the nutritional management of the survivors of the Cocoanut Grove fire: "All patients were given a high protein and high vitamin diet…it was necessary to feed [one patient] by stomach tube with supplemental daily intravenous amogen, glucose, and vitamins" [69]. But it soon became apparent that survivors of major thermal injury evidenced a hypermetabolic, hypercatabolic state which lasted at least until the wounds were closed, and often resulted in severe loss of lean body mass. Burns thus epitomize what David Cuthbertson, summarizing work done with orthopedic injuries, identified as the biphasic response to injury: an initial "ebb" period (shock) was followed by a longer "flow" period (inflammation) [95]. Thus, burns constitute "the universal trauma model," as described by Dr. Pruitt in the 1984 Scudder Oration on Trauma:

> The burn patient in whom a local injury (the severity of which can be readily and reproducibly quantified) evokes a global systemic response (the magnitude and duration of which are proportional to the extent of injury) meets the criteria for a useful clinical model (…) Among all trauma patients, the burn patient should perhaps be regarded as a metabolic caricature, since the metabolic rate in patients with burns of more than 50 percent of the body surface exceeds that encountered in any other group of patients.

Cope and colleagues reported measurements of metabolic rate of up to 180% of normal in the early postburn period, ruled out thyrotoxicosis as an etiology, and recognized a relationship between wound size and metabolic rate [96]. Wilmore and colleagues identified the role of catecholamines

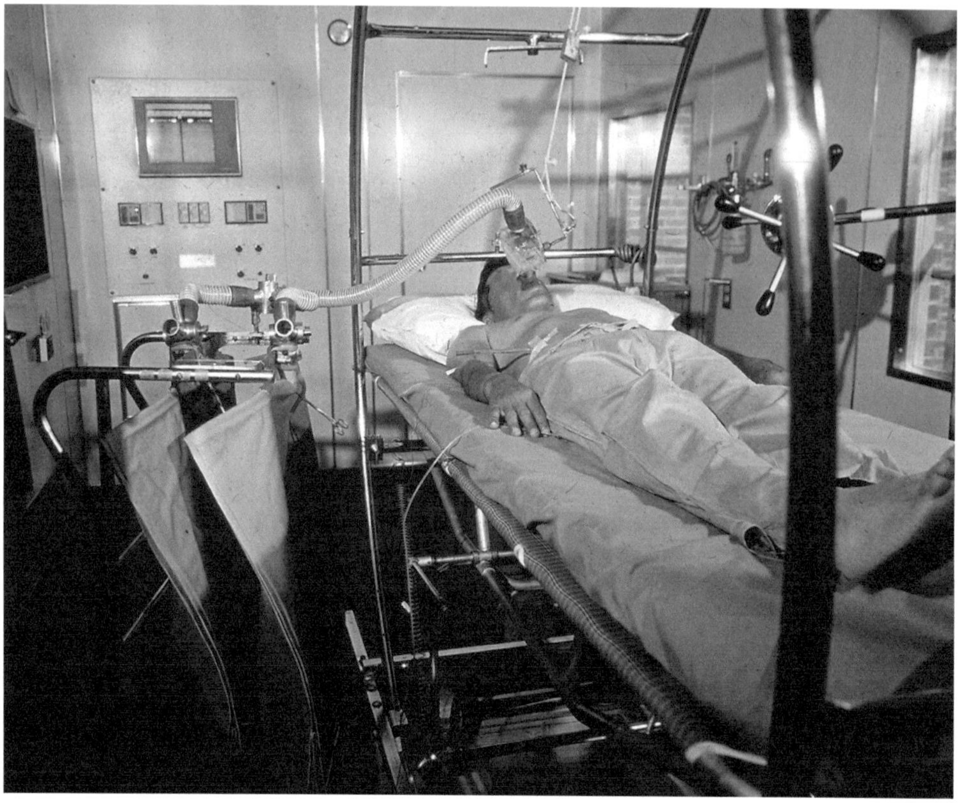

Fig. 1.5 Measurement of metabolic rate in an environmental chamber constructed inside the US Army Burn Center. Studies such as these permitted the precise determination of the nutritional needs of burn patients, and the elucidation of the underlying mechanisms of postburn hypermetabolism. Source: Collection of the US Army Institute of Surgical Research, Courtesy Mr. Glen Gueller

as mediators of the postburn hypermetabolic state (Fig. 1.5) [97]. Wilmore et al. also demonstrated the feasibility of providing massive amounts of calories by a combination of intravenous and enteral alimentation [98]. Curreri published the first burn-specific formula for estimating caloric requirements: calories/day = 25 (wt in kg) + 40 (TBSA) [99]. Provision of adequate calories and nitrogen failed to arrest hypermetabolism and reduced, but did not eliminate, erosion of lean body mass in these patients. Three approaches have recently been taken to address this problem with modest success: use of anabolic steroids such as oxandrolone [100]; blockade of catecholamines with propranolol [101]; and insulin [102], insulin-like growth factor [103, 104], or human growth hormone [105, 106].

1.6.7 Rehabilitation

As postburn mortality decreased, the problems of burn survivors, particularly those with deep and extensive injuries, became paramount [107–109]. The scientific study of rehabilitation of the thermally injured patient is a relatively young field. The CG monograph briefly states:

> Six patients who received severe burns to the dorsum of the hands and wrists were referred to the Physical Therapy Department either while in the hospital or at the time of discharge to be treated as out-patients…In all cases surface healing was complete before beginning treatment…The first patient…was referred to this department 51 days after the fire…. [110]

This method, which conceives of rehabilitation as a "phase" which begins after resuscitation and reconstructive surgery phases, may be acceptable in patients with minor injuries. But it soon became apparent that wound healing is so prolonged in patients with major thermal injuries that these three phases must be conducted concurrently rather than sequentially, to avoid the catastrophic effects of chronic bed rest, extremity immobilization, and contracture formation [108]. In the 1950s, Moncrief began rehabilitation soon after admission and resumed it 8–10 days after skin grafting [111, 112]. The advent of heat-malleable plastic (thermoplastic) material made it possible to fabricate increasingly complex and effective positioning devices [113]. This was followed by the introduction of pressure to treat hypertrophic scars and the development of customized pressure garments [114]. Others reduced or eliminated the delay between skin grafting and ambulation, without deleterious effects on graft take [115, 116]. New frontiers for physical, occupational, and neuropsychiatric rehabilitation of burn patients include the following:

- Optimizing pain control; use of novel techniques such as virtual reality [117]
- Documentation of long-term outcomes [118, 119]
- Definition of barriers of return to work and community [120, 121]
- Diagnosis and treatment of posttraumatic stress disorder [122]
- Management of scar formation [123]

1.7 Conclusions

This review indicates that the advances in burn care achieved since WWII were not accidental, but depended on integrated laboratory and clinical research; generous national funding; centers of excellence focused on comprehensive burn care; highly skilled multidisciplinary clinical teams; and committed leadership. Reflecting on recent progress in the 1976 American Burn Association presidential address, Colonel Basil Pruitt noted the importance of a tight working relationship between clinicians and basic scientists, working together to solve problems of clinical significance [124]. This paradigm should be strengthened and expanded, since we have entered an era in which the number of large burns has declined nationwide [125]. As a result, we are challenged with the need for multicenter trials if we are to continue to make progress. Fortunately, the creation of the American Burn Association (ABA) Multicenter Trials Group and federal funding have created the framework and the opportunity for such collaboration. In a manner reminiscent of events in the UK and the USA during WWII, the recent conflicts in Iraq and Afghanistan [126] and the attacks of September 11, 2001 [127] have highlighted the importance of thermal injury as a national problem. The following multicenter trials have been funded by the Department of Defense (at a total cost to date of US $25.7 million) and carried out by the ABA research network during 2008–18 (ABA, personal communication, February 1, 2018):

1.7.1 Completed Studies

- Scar contractures and rehabilitation treatment time [128]
- Restrictive vs. traditional transfusion triggers [129]
- Military and civilian outcomes [130]

1.7.2 Ongoing Studies

- High-volume hemofiltration in burn patients with septic shock and mild acute kidney injury
- Rapid polymerase chain reaction (PCR) test for *Staphylococcus aureus* infection
- Community-based exercise for adults
- Enteral glutamine effect on infections and mortality
- Inhalation injury scoring
- Effects of propranolol in adults
- Resuscitation of burn shock with albumin
- Resuscitation of burn shock with the Burn Navigator decision support system

The spirit of collaboration and inquiry embodied by these projects is the surest guarantee that they will continue to bear fruit in the years to come.

Summary Box

- There has been a doubling in burn survival since World War II in young persons, measured as the lethal dose 50% (LA50%).
- Integrated laboratory and clinical research and multidisciplinary teamwork have been the foundations of improved outcomes.
- Advances in care responsible for this improvement in survival included these areas: fluid resuscitation, infection control, topical and surgical wound care, inhalation injury care, and nutritional and metabolic support.
- In addition to continued research in these areas, new frontiers are being addressed in wound healing, rehabilitation, and psychosocial recovery.
- We are now challenged by a decrease in the number of patients with big burns in most developed countries. Thus, further progress in burn care will depend in part on multicenter trials.
- The American Burn Association (ABA), for example, has built a successful framework for multicenter burn research.

References

1. Pruitt BA, Goodwin CW, Mason AD Jr. Epidemiological, demographic, and outcome characteristics of burn injury. In: Herndon DN, editor. Total burn care. London: W.B. Saunders; 2002. p. 16–30.
2. Wolf SE, Rose JK, Desai MH, Mileski JP, Barrow RE, Herndon DN. Mortality determinants in massive pediatric burns. An analysis of 103 children with > or = 80% TBSA burns (> or = 70% full-thickness). Ann Surg. 1997;225(5):554–65.
3. Artz CP. Historical aspects of burn management. Surg Clin North Am. 1970;50(6):1193–200.
4. Wallace AF. Recent advances in the treatment of burns—1843-1858. Br J Plast Surg. 1987;40(2):193–200.
5. Dunbar J. Burn cases treated in Glasgow Royal Infirmary. Glasgow Med J. 1934;122:239–55.
6. Davidson EC. Tannic acid in the treatment of burns. Surg Gynecol Obstet. 1925;41:202–21.
7. Hupkens P, Boxma H, Dokter J. Tannic acid as a topical agent in burns: historical considerations and implications for new developments. Burns. 1995;21(1):57–61.
8. Underhill FP. The significance of anhydremia in extensive superficial burns. JAMA. 1930;95:852–7.
9. Blalock A. Experimental shock. VII. The importance of the local loss of fluid in the production of the low blood pressure after burns. Arch Surg. 1931;22:610–6.
10. Aldrich RH. The role of infection in burns: the theory and treatment with special reference to gentian violet. N Engl J Med. 1933;208:299–309.
11. Battle R. Plastic surgery in the two world wars and in the years between. J R Soc Med. 1978;71(11):844–8.
12. Mills SMH. Burns down under: lessons lost, lessons learned. J Burn Care Rehabil. 2005;26(1):42–52.

13. Mayhew ER. The reconstruction of warriors: Archibald McIndoe, the Royal air Force and the Guinea pig Club. London: Greenhill Books; 2004.
14. Jackson D. Thirty years of burn treatment in Britain—where now? Injury. 1978;10(1):40–5.
15. Colebrook L. Treatment of human puerperal infections, and of experimental infections in mice, with prontosil. Lancet. 1936;1:1279–86.
16. Lerner BH. Scientific evidence versus therapeutic demand: the introduction of the sulfonamides revisited. Ann Intern Med. 1991;115(4):315–20.
17. Clark AM, Gibson T, Colebrook L, Thomson ML, Foster A. Penicillin and propamide in burns: elimination of haemolytic streptococci and staphylococci. Lancet. 1943;241:605–9.
18. Colebrook L, Gibson T, Todd JP, Clark AM, Brown A, Anderson AB. Studies of burns and scalds. (Reports of the burns unit, Royal Infirmary, Glasgow, 1942–43). Medical Research Council special report series no. 249. London: His Majesty's Stationery Office; 1944.
19. Lawrence JC. Some aspects of burns and burns research at Birmingham Accident Hospital 1944-93: A.B. Wallace Memorial lecture, 1994. Burns. 1995;21(6):403–13.
20. Colebrook L. A burns unit at the Birmingham Accident Hospital and Rehabilitation Centre. Nurs Times. 1945;6:4–6.
21. Turk JL. Leonard Colebrook: the chemotherapy and control of streptococcal infections. J R Soc Med. 1994;87(12):727–8.
22. Lockwood JS. War-time activities of the National Research Council and the Committee on Medical Research; with particular reference to team-work on studies of wounds and burns. Ann Surg. 1946;124:314–27.
23. Stewart IP. Organizing Scientific Research for War: the Administrative History of the Office of Scientific Research and Development. Boston: Little, Brown; 1948.
24. Neushul P. Science, government, and the mass production of penicillin. J Hist Med Allied Sci. 1993;48(4):371–95.
25. Administrative History Section, Administrative Division, Bureau of Medicine and Surgery. Pearl Harbor Navy Medical Activities in "The United States Navy Medical Department at War, 1941–1945," vol. 1, parts 1–2. Washington: The Bureau, 1946. p. 1–31. http://www.ibiblio.org/hyperwar/USN/rep/Pearl/Medical.html. Accessed 30 Mar 2018.
26. Lesch JE. The first miracle drugs: how the sulfa drugs transformed medicine. Oxford: Oxford University Press; 2007.
27. Meleney FL. The study of the prevention of infection in contaminated accidental wounds, compound fractures and burns. Ann Surg. 1943;118:171–83.
28. Chain E, Florey HW, Gardner AD, Heatley NG, Jennings MA, Orr-Ewing J, et al. Penicillin as a chemotherapeutic agent. Lancet. 1940;2:226–8.
29. Ligon BL. Penicillin: its discovery and early development. Semin Pediatr Infect Dis. 2004;15(1):52–7.
30. Richards AN. Production of penicillin in the United States (1941-46). Nature. 1964;4918:441–5.
31. Forward CO. In: Aub JC, Beecher HK, Cannon B, Cobb S, Cope O, Faxon NW, et al., editors. Management of the Cocoanut Grove burns at the Massachusetts General Hospital. Philadelphia: J.B. Lippincott; 1943. p. 1–2.
32. National Research Council, Division of Medical Sciences. Treatment of burns. War Med. 1942;2:334–9.
33. Cope O, Moore FD. The redistribution of body water and the fluid therapy of the burned patient. Ann Surg. 1947;126:1010–45.
34. Harkins HN. The treatment of burns in wartime. JAMA. 1942;119:385–90.
35. Harkins HN. The treatment of burns. London: Baillere, Tindall and Cox; 1942.
36. Whipple AO. Basic principles in the treatment of thermal burns. Ann Surg. 1943;118:187–91.
37. Saffle JR. The 1942 fire at Boston's Cocoanut Grove nightclub. Am J Surg. 1993;166(6):581–91.
38. Follett GP. The Boston fire: a challenge to our disaster service. Am J Nurs. 1943;43:4–8.
39. Faxson NW. The problems of the hospital administration. In: Aub JC, Beecher HK, Cannon B, Cobb S, Cope O, Faxon NW, et al., editors. Management of the Cocoanut Grove Burns at the Massachusetts General Hospital. Philadelphia: J.B. Lippincott; 1943. p. 3–8.
40. Artz CP. Burns in my lifetime. J Trauma. 1969;9(10):827–33.
41. Pruitt BA Jr. Forces and factors influencing trauma care: 1983 A.A.S.T. (American Association for the Surgery of Trauma) Presidential address. J Trauma. 1984;24(6):463–70.
42. Heimbach DM. American Burn Association 1988 presidential address "We can see so far because...". J Burn Care Rehabil. 1988;9(4):340–6.
43. Pruitt BA Jr. The integration of clinical care and laboratory research. A model for medical progress. Arch Surg. 1995;130(5):461–71.
44. Pruitt BA Jr. Centennial changes in surgical care and research. Ann Surg. 2000;232(3):287–301.
45. Artz CP. History of burns. In: Artz CP, Moncrief JA, Pruitt Jr BA, editors. Burns: a team approach. Philadelphia: W.B. Saunders; 1979. p. 3–16.
46. Dimick AR, Brigham PA, Sheehy EM. The development of burn centers in North America. J Burn Care Rehabil. 1993;14(2 Pt 2):284–99.
47. Cope O. Rhinelander FW. The problem of burn shock complicated by pulmonary damage. In: Aub JC, Beecher HK, Cannon B, Cobb S, Cope O, Faxon NW, et al., editors. Management of the Cocoanut Grove Burns at the Massachusetts General Hospital. Philadelphia, PA: J.B. Lippincott; 1943. p. 115–28.
48. Evans IE, Purnell OJ, Robinett PW, Batchelor A, Martin M. Fluid and electrolyte requirements in severe burns. Ann Surg. 1952;135:804–17.
49. Reiss E, Stirman JA, Artz CP, Davis JH, Amspacher WH. Fluid and electrolyte balance in burns. JAMA. 1953;152:1309–13.
50. Baxter CR, Shires T. Physiological response to crystalloid resuscitation of severe burns. Ann N Y Acad Sci. 1968;150(3):874–94.
51. Pruitt BA Jr, Mason AD Jr, Moncrief JA. Hemodynamic changes in the early postburn patient: the influence of fluid administration and of a vasodilator (hydralazine). J Trauma. 1971;11(1):36–46.
52. Saffle JR. The phenomenon of "fluid creep" in acute burn resuscitation. J Burn Care Res. 2007;28(3):382–95.
53. Pruitt BA Jr. Protection from excessive resuscitation: "pushing the pendulum back". J Trauma. 2000;49(3):567–8.
54. Cope O. The treatment of the surface burns. In: Aub JC, Beecher HK, Cannon B, Cobb S, Cope O, Faxon NW, et al., editors. Management of the Cocoanut Grove burns at the Massachusetts General Hospital. Philadelphia: J.B. Lippincott; 1943. p. 85–93.
55. Lyons C. Problems of infection and chemotherapy. In: Aub JC, Beecher HK, Cannon B, Cobb S, Cope O, Faxon NW, et al., editors. Management of the Cocoanut Grove burns at the Massachusetts General Hospital. Philadelphia: J.B. Lippincott; 1943. p. 94–102.
56. Dalton ML. Champ Lyons: an incomplete life. Ann Surg. 2003;237(5):694–703.
57. Lyons C. Penicillin therapy of surgical infections in the U.S. Army: a report. JAMA. 1943;123:1007–18.
58. Liedberg NC, Reiss E, Artz CP. Infection in burns. III. Septicemia, a common cause of death. Surg Gynecol Obstet. 1954;99:151–8.
59. Teplitz C, Davis D, Mason AD Jr, Moncrief JA. Pseudomonas burn wound sepsis. I. Pathogenesis of experimental pseudomonas burn wound sepsis. J Surg Res. 1964;4:200–16.
60. Teplitz C, Davis D, Walker HL, Raulston GL, Mason AD Jr, Moncrief JA. Pseudomonas burn wound sepsis: II. Hematogenous infection at the junction of the burn wound and the unburned hypodermis. J Surg Res. 1964;4:217–22.

61. Walker HL, Mason AD Jr, Raulston GL. Surface infection with Pseudomonas aeruginosa. Ann Surg. 1964;160:297–305.
62. Pruitt BA Jr, O'Neill JA Jr, Moncrief JA, Lindberg RB. Successful control of burn-wound sepsis. JAMA. 1968;203(12):1054–6.
63. Jelenko CD, Jelenko JM, Mendelson JA, Buxton RW. The marfanil mystery. Surg Gynecol Obstet. 1966;122(1):121–7.
64. Mendelson JA, Lindsey D. Sulfamylon (mafenide) and penicillin as expedient treatment of experimental massive open wounds with C. perfringens infection. J Trauma. 1962;2:239–61.
65. Lindberg RB, Moncrief JA, Mason AD Jr. Control of experimental and clinical burn wound sepsis by topical application of sulfamylon compounds. Ann N Y Acad Sci. 1968;150(3):950–60.
66. Moyer CA, Brentano L, Gravens DL, Margraf HW, Monafo WW Jr. Treatment of large burns with 0.5% silver nitrate solution. Arch Surg. 1965;90:812–67.
67. Fox CL Jr. Silver sulfadiazine--a new topical therapy for Pseudomonas in burns. Therapy of Pseudomonas infection in burns. Arch Surg. 1968;96(2):184–8.
68. Tredget EE, Shankowsky HA, Groeneveld A, Burrell R. A matched-pair, randomized study evaluating the efficacy and safety of Acticoat silver coated dressing for the treatment of burn wounds. J Burn Care Rehabil. 1998;19(6):531–7.
69. Cannon B. Procedures in rehabilitation of the severely burned. In: Aub JC, Beecher HK, Cannon B, Cobb S, Cope O, Faxon NW, et al., editors. Management of the Cocoanut Grove burns at the Massachusetts General Hospital. Philadelphia: J.B. Lippincott; 1943. p. 103–10.
70. Artz CP, Soroff HS. Modern concepts in the treatment of burns. JAMA. 1955;159:411–7.
71. Dobbs ER. Burn therapy of years ago. J Burn Care Rehabil. 1999;20(1 Pt 1):62–6.
72. Jackson D. A clinical study of the use of skin homografts for burns. Br J Plast Surg. 1954;7:26–43.
73. Jackson D, Topley E, Cason JS, Lowbury EJL. Primary excision and grafting of large burns. Ann Surg. 1960;152:167–89.
74. Janzekovic Z. Once upon a time...how West discovered East. J Plast Reconstr Aesthet Surg. 2008;61:240–4.
75. Janzekovic Z. Early surgical treatment of the burned surface. Panminerva Med. 1972;14(7–8):228–32.
76. Tompkins RG, Burke JF, Schoenfeld DA, Bondoc CC, Quinby WC Jr, Behringer GC, et al. Prompt eschar excision: a treatment system contributing to reduced burn mortality. A statistical evaluation of burn care at the Massachusetts General Hospital (1974-1984). Ann Surg. 1986;204(3):272–81.
77. McManus WF, Mason AD Jr, Pruitt BA Jr. Excision of the burn wound in patients with large burns. Arch Surg. 1989;124(6):718–20.
78. Herndon DN, Parks DH. Comparison of serial debridement and autografting and early massive excision with cadaver skin overlay in the treatment of large burns in children. J Trauma. 1986;26(2):149–52.
79. Herndon DN, Barrow RE, Rutan RL, Rutan TC, Desai MH, Abston S. A comparison of conservative versus early excision. Therapies in severely burned patients. Ann Surg. 1989;209(5):547–52.
80. Ong YS, Samuel M, Song C. Meta-analysis of early excision of burns. Burns. 2006;32(2):145–50.
81. Burke JF, Yannas IV, Quinby WC Jr, Bondoc CC, Jung WK. Successful use of a physiologically acceptable artificial skin in the treatment of extensive burn injury. Ann Surg. 1981;194(4):413–28.
82. Gallico GG, O'Connor NE, Compton CC, Kehinde O, Green H. Permanent coverage of large burn wounds with autologous cultured human epithelium. N Engl J Med. 1984;311(7):448–51.
83. Rue LW III, Cioffi WG, McManus WF, Pruitt BA Jr. Wound closure and outcome in extensively burned patients treated with cultured autologous keratinocytes. J Trauma. 1993;34(5):662–7.
84. Barret JP, Wolf SE, Desai MH, Herndon DN. Cost-efficacy of cultured epidermal autografts in massive pediatric burns. Ann Surg. 2000;231(6):869–76.
85. Aub JC, Pittman H, Brues AM. The pulmonary complications: a clinical description. In: Aub JC, Beecher HK, Cannon B, Cobb S, Cope O, Faxon NW, et al., editors. Management of the Cocoanut Grove burns at the Massachusetts General Hospital. Philadelphia: J.B. Lippincott; 1943. p. 34–40.
86. Morris MJ. Acute respiratory distress syndrome in combat casualties: military medicine and advances in mechanical ventilation. Mil Med. 2006;171:1039–44.
87. Rosengart MR. Critical care medicine: landmarks and legends. Surg Clin North Am. 2006;86:1305–21.
88. Shirani KZ, Pruitt BA Jr, Mason AD Jr. The influence of inhalation injury and pneumonia on burn mortality. Ann Surg. 1987;205(1):82–7.
89. Shimazu T, Yukioka T, Hubbard GB, Langlinais PC, Mason AD Jr, Pruitt BA Jr. A dose-responsive model of smoke inhalation injury. Severity-related alteration in cardiopulmonary function. Ann Surg. 1987;206(1):89–98.
90. Herndon DN, Traber DL, Niehaus GD, Linares HA, Traber LD. The pathophysiology of smoke inhalation injury in a sheep model. J Trauma. 1984;24(12):1044–51.
91. Shimazu T, Yukioka T, Ikeuchi H, Mason AD Jr, Wagner PD, Pruitt BA Jr. Ventilation-perfusion alterations after smoke inhalation injury in an ovine model. J Appl Physiol. 1996;81(5):2250–9.
92. Traber DL, Hawkins HK, Enkhbaatar P, Cox RA, Schmalstieg FC, Zwischenberger JB, et al. The role of the bronchial circulation in the acute lung injury resulting from burn and smoke inhalation. Pulm Pharmacol Ther. 2007;20(2):163–6.
93. Cioffi WG Jr, Rue LW III, Graves TA, McManus WF, Mason AD Jr, Pruitt BA Jr. Prophylactic use of high-frequency percussive ventilation in patients with inhalation injury. Ann Surg. 1991;213(6):575–82.
94. Enkhbaatar P, Herndon DN, Traber DL. Use of nebulized heparin in the treatment of smoke inhalation injury. J Burn Care Res. 2009;30(1):159–62.
95. Cuthbertson DP. Post-shock metabolic response. Lancet. 1942;1:433–7.
96. Cope O, Nardi GL, Quijano M, Rovit RL, Stanbury JB, Wight A. Metabolic rate and thyroid function following acute thermal trauma in man. Ann Surg. 1953;137:165–74.
97. Wilmore DW, Long JM, Mason AD Jr, Skreen RW, Pruitt BA Jr. Catecholamines: mediator of the hypermetabolic response to thermal injury. Ann Surg. 1974;180(4):653–69.
98. Wilmore DW, Curreri PW, Spitzer KW, Spitzer ME, Pruitt BA Jr. Supranormal dietary intake in thermally injured hypermetabolic patients. Surg Gynecol Obstet. 1971;132(5):881–6.
99. Curreri PW, Richmond D, Marvin J, Baxter CR. Dietary requirements of patients with major burns. J Am Diet Assoc. 1974;65(4):415–7.
100. Wolf SE, Edelman LS, Kemalyan N, Donison L, Cross J, Underwood M, et al. Effects of oxandrolone on outcome measures in the severely burned: a multicenter prospective randomized double-blind trial. J Burn Care Res. 2006;27(2):131–9.
101. Herndon DN, Hart DW, Wolf SE, Chinkes DL, Wolfe RR. Reversal of catabolism by beta-blockade after severe burns. N Engl J Med. 2001;345(17):1223–9.
102. Sakurai Y, Aarsland A, Herndon DN, Chinkes DL, Pierre E, Nguyen TT, et al. Stimulation of muscle protein synthesis by long-term insulin infusion in severely burned patients. Ann Surg. 1995;222(3):283–94; 94-7.
103. Cioffi WG, Gore DC, Rue LW 3rd, Carrougher G, Guler HP, McManus WF, et al. Insulin-like growth factor-1 lowers protein oxidation in patients with thermal injury. Ann Surg. 1994;220(3):310–9.

104. Spies M, Wolf SE, Barrow RE, Jeschke MG, Herndon DN. Modulation of types I and II acute phase reactants with insulin-like growth factor-1/binding protein-3 complex in severely burned children. Crit Care Med. 2002;30(1):83–8.
105. Wilmore DW, Moylan JA Jr, Bristow BF, Mason AD Jr, Pruitt BA Jr. Anabolic effects of human growth hormone and high caloric feedings following thermal injury. Surg Gynecol Obstet. 1974;138(6):875–84.
106. Hart DW, Wolf SE, Chinkes DL, Lal SO, Ramzy PI, Herndon DN. Beta-blockade and growth hormone after burn. Ann Surg. 2002;236(4):450–6.
107. Pereira C, Murphy K, Herndon D. Outcome measures in burn care. Is mortality dead? Burns. 2004;30:761–71.
108. Richard RL, Hedman TL, Quick CD, Barillo DJ, Cancio LC, Renz EM, et al. A clarion to recommit and reaffirm burn rehabilitation. J Burn Care Res. 2008;29(3):425–32.
109. Esselman PC, Thombs BD, Magyar-Russell G, Fauerbach JA. Burn rehabilitation: state of the science. Am J Phys Med Rehabil. 2006;85(4):383–413.
110. Watkins AL. A note on physical therapy. In: Aub JC, Beecher HK, Cannon B, Cobb S, Cope O, Faxon NW, et al., editors. Management of the Cocoanut Grove burns at the Massachusetts General Hospital. Philadelphia: J.B. Lippincott; 1943. p. 111–4.
111. Moncrief JA. Complications of burns. Ann Surg. 1958;147:443–75.
112. Moncrief JA. Third degree burns of the dorsum of the hand. Am J Surg. 1958;96:535–44.
113. Willis B. The use of orthoplast isoprene splints in the treatment of the acutely burned child: preliminary report. Am J Occup Ther. 1969;23(1):57–61.
114. Larson DL, Abston S, Evans EB, Dobrkovsky M, Linares HA. Techniques for decreasing scar formation and contractures in the burned patient. J Trauma. 1971;11(10):807–23.
115. Schmitt MA, French L, Kalil ET. How soon is safe? Ambulation of the patient with burns after lower-extremity skin grafting. J Burn Care Rehabil. 1991;12(1):33–7.
116. Burnsworth B, Krob MJ, Langer-Schnepp M. Immediate ambulation of patients with lower-extremity grafts. J Burn Care Rehabil. 1992;13(1):89–92.
117. Carrougher GJ, Hoffman HG, Nakamura D, Lezotte D, Soltani M, Leahy L, et al. The effect of virtual reality on pain and range of motion in adults with burn injuries. J Burn Care Res. 2009;30(5):785–91.
118. Yoder LH, McFall DC, Glaser DN. Quality of life of burn survivors treated in the military burn center. Nurs Outlook. 2017;65(5):S81–9.
119. Klein MB, Lezotte DL, Fauerbach JA, Herndon DN, Kowalske KJ, Carrougher GJ, et al. The National Institute on Disability and Rehabilitation Research burn model system database: a tool for the multicenter study of the outcome of burn injury. J Burn Care Res. 2007;28(1):84–96.
120. Esselman PC, Askay SW, Carrougher GJ, Lezotte DC, Holavanahalli RK, Magyar-Russell G, et al. Barriers to return to work after burn injuries. Arch Phys Med Rehabil. 2007;88(12 Suppl 2):S50–6.
121. Esselman PC, Ptacek JT, Kowalske K, Cromes GF, de Lateur BJ, Engrav LH. Community integration after burn injuries. J Burn Care Rehabil. 2001;22(3):221–7.
122. Gaylord KM, Holcomb JB, Zolezzi ME. A comparison of posttraumatic stress disorder between combat casualties and civilians treated at a military burn center. J Trauma. 2009;66(4 Suppl):S191–5.
123. Kwan P, Hori K, Ding J, Tredget EE. Scar and contracture: biological principles. Hand Clin. 2009;25(4):511–28.
124. Pruitt BA Jr. Multidisciplinary care and research for burn injury: 1976 presidential address, American Burn Association meeting. J Trauma. 1977;17(4):263–9.
125. Latenser BA, Miller SF, Bessey PQ, Browning SM, Caruso DM, Gomez M, et al. National Burn Repository 2006: a ten-year review. J Burn Care Res. 2007;28(5):635–58.
126. Kauvar DS, Cancio LC, Wolf SE, Wade CE, Holcomb JB. Comparison of combat and non-combat burns from ongoing U.S. military operations. J Surg Res. 2006;132(2):195–200.
127. Anonymous. Rapid assessment of injuries among survivors of the terrorist attack on the World Trade Center—New York City, September 2001. Morb Mortal Wkly Rep. 2002;51(1):1–5.
128. Richard R, Santos-Lozada AR. Burn patient acuity demographics, scar contractures, and rehabilitation treatment time related to patient outcomes: the ACT study. J Burn Care Res. 2017;38(4):230–42.
129. Palmieri TL, Holmes JH IV, Arnoldo B, Peck M, Potenza B, Cochran A, et al. Transfusion requirement in burn care evaluation (TRIBE): a multicenter randomized prospective trial of blood transfusion in major burn injury. Ann Surg. 2017;266(4):595–602.
130. Taylor S, Jeng J, Saffle JR, Sen S, Greenhalgh DG, Palmieri TL. Redefining the outcomes to resources ratio for burn patient triage in a mass casualty. J Burn Care Res. 2014;35(1):41–5.
131. Anonymous. USS Solace, Report of Pearl Harbor Attack. Pearl Harbor, Territory of Hawaii: 12 Dec 1941. https://www.history.navy.mil/research/archives/digitized-collections/action-reports/wwii-pearl-harbor-attack/ships-s-z/uss-solace-ah-5-action-report.html. Accessed 30 Mar 2018.
132. Anonymous. 1941. http://navymedicine.navylive.dodlive.mil/archives/3809/uss-solace-patients. Accessed 30 Mar 2018.
133. Boston Public Library, Leslie Jones Collection. 1942. https://www.digitalcommonwealth.org/search/commonwealth:5h73wj30v. Accessed 30 Mar 2018.

2 Epidemiology and Prevention of Burns Throughout the World

Michael D. Peck and Jason Thomas Toppi

2.1 Introduction

Injury is the physical damage that results when a human body is suddenly subjected to energy in amounts that exceed the threshold of physiologic tolerance [1]. Injury is a significant public health problem—injuries caused 8.5% of all deaths worldwide in 2015 [2]. Injuries are the fourth leading cause of death in men throughout the world (11% of total deaths) after cardiovascular, infectious, and neoplastic diseases. Although progress is being made against many illnesses, the incidence of injuries is decreasing at a rate slower than the reduction in illness in high-income countries (HIC). In low- and middle-income countries (LMIC), both death and disability from injuries are increasing very rapidly. In LMIC of the Americas, Europe, and the Eastern Mediterranean Region, the cause of more than 30% of disability-adjusted life years (DALYs, the loss due to either death or disability of the equivalent of 1 year of good health) among men aged 15–44 years in 2004 was from injury [3].[1]

Injury is a burden on the young, taking more productive life-years than cancer or heart disease. Road traffic collisions are among the leading causes of DALYs lost in LMIC [3, 4]. In 2004, burns under 20% were approximately 6% of all unintentional injuries in children less than 15 years of age [3]. A community-based cross-sectional survey in Egypt found that burn injuries were the second most common type of injury (after falls) in children less than the age of 18 years [5].

Injuries are also the most common cause of DALYs lost worldwide: in 2004, injuries accounted for 17% of DALYs lost in adults aged 15–59 years [3].

Burns are an important mechanism of injury. Unintentional injuries include not only burns but traffic collisions, drownings, poisonings, and falls. Intentional injuries result from homicide, suicide, legal interventions, and conflicts; burns and fires can be the mechanism for assault or self-harm. Without question, burns contribute a significant proportion of the morbidity and mortality attributed to injuries throughout the world.

A burn is an injury to the skin or other organic tissue primarily caused by thermal or other acute trauma, according to the International Society of Burn Injuries. A burn occurs when some or all of the cells in the skin or other tissues are destroyed by hot liquids (scalds), hot solids (contact burns), or flames (flame burns). Injuries to the skin or other organic tissues due to radiation, radioactivity, electricity, friction, or contact with chemicals are also identified as burns.

In 2015, incidence of burns severe enough to require hospital outpatient presentation or an admission to hospital was 31 million people [6, 7]. Burns covering less than 20% of the body surface area occur to 153 per 100,000 population of children aged 0–15 years, making these burns the fifth most

[1]Income categories for 2004 as defined by the World Bank by 2004 gross national income per capita. Low, US$285 or less; lower middle, US$285–3255; upper middle, US$3256–10,065; high, US$10,066 or more.

M. D. Peck (✉)
Arizona Burn Center, Maricopa Medical Center, Phoenix, AZ, USA

University of Arizona College of Medicine-Phoenix, Phoenix, AZ, USA

Division of Community, Environment and Policy, Mel and Enid Zuckerman College of Public Health, University of Arizona Health Sciences Center, Tucson, AZ, USA
e-mail: michael_peck@dmgaz.org

J. T. Toppi
Department of Epidemiology and Preventive Medicine, The Alfred Centre, Monash University, Melbourne, VIC, Australia

M. G. Jeschke et al. (eds.), *Handbook of Burns Volume 1*, https://doi.org/10.1007/978-3-030-18940-2_2

common cause of nonfatal childhood injuries after intracranial injury, open wounds, poisoning, and forearm fractures [3]. Five percent of disabilities at all ages in Nepal are due to burns and scalds [8].

Low- and middle-income countries represent a disproportionately high level of burn injury incidence and mortality. Data from WHO estimates that 265,000 deaths result from fire-related incidents per year globally [4]. This burden of disease is significantly higher in LMIC, with over 96% of fatal fire-related burn injuries occurring in these countries [4]. High-income countries have made significant progress in reducing the incidence of burn injuries and burn severity, lowering rates of burn deaths, and length of hospital stay through a combination of prevention and care strategies [9–13]. However, many of these improvements have been incompletely applied in LMIC [4].

When confronted with the narrative of a burn survivor, one first pictures agonizing open wounds, followed by resolution into undeniably obvious burn scars. But the thickened, noncompliant skin tells only part of the story. Much of the impact of burns is emotional, psychological, and spiritual. Studies of recovery from burn injury in the United States show clearly that the ability to adjust following injury is less dependent on the physical characteristics of the burn (such as burn size, burn depth, or location) and more on preinjury adjustment. Coping skills, family and community support, and general psychological health have more impact on recovery from burns than the nature of the burn itself [14].

In HIC, this means that burn survivors from struggling family backgrounds are likely to have problems reassimilating into school and community life. In LMIC, the consequences are direr, with isolation from or even abandonment by the family, social segregation, unemployment, and extreme poverty. Although burn victims from affluent families in LIC have a chance of recuperation, the vast majority of burn survivors will start from living situations that deny them the opportunity to recover from even a small burn.

Additionally, the sequelae of nonfatal burn injuries are often severe enough to cause permanent disability. In the Global Childhood Unintentional Injury Surveillance pilot study conducted among children (0–12 years of age) in Bangladesh, Colombia, Egypt, and Pakistan, 17% of survivors had long-term (greater than 6 weeks) temporary disability and 8% had permanent disability [15]. The incidence of long-term temporary disability was highest in children surviving burns and traffic injuries. Only near-drowning victims had a higher rate of permanent disability. Permanent disability was eight times more common in burn survivors than in those children recovering from falls.

Thus the wisdom of one of the founding fathers of burn care in India, Dr. M.H. Keswani: "The challenge of burns lies not in the successful treatment of a 100% burn, but in the 100% prevention of all burn injuries" [16].

2.2 Epidemiology

Collection of data specific to burn etiologies has been challenging. The most efficient approach is to join modules specific for injury causation with existing data collection systems. As an example, software was developed to employ the comprehensive categorization of multiple facets of injury events as described by the International Classification of External Causes of Injury (ICECI). This software was then used by registrars collecting and entering data into the National Burn Repository (NBR) of the American Burn Association (ABA). Use of this tool significantly augmented the quality and quantity of etiologic data entered into the existing data repository [17]. A global registry has recently been developed through collaboration among the World Health Organization (WHO), Global Alliance for Clean Cookstoves, and United States Centers for Disease Control (CDC). A process evaluation performed in 30 countries showed good user acceptance and the potential to prioritize the selection, development, and testing of primary prevention interventions throughout the world [18]. Fortunately, although burns and fires throughout the world in 2015 accounted for 238,000 deaths, the vast majority of burn injuries are not fatal [19]. Globally, 2016 data show 337 burns per 100,000 outpatient presentations and 32 burns per 100,000 inpatient admissions [19]. In 2008 there were 410,149 nonfatal burn injuries in the United States, giving an age-adjusted rate of 136 per 100,000 each year [20]. A higher estimate comes from data collected from the National Hospital Ambulatory Medical Care Survey during the period of 1993 to 2004 in the United States, in which the average annual emergency department visit rate for treatment of burns was 220 per 100,000 population [21]. The vast majority of these burn patients were treated and released from the emergency department; only 5% were hospitalized or transferred. In comparison, only 45% of those with nonfatal firearm injuries and near-drowning effects were treated and released, suggesting that the severity of most burns requiring medical treatment is low compared to other types of injury [22].

More severe burns also tend to be less common among hospitalized patients. A European study by Brusselaers et al., which reviewed 76 papers encompassing data on a total of 186,500 patients, found an annual incidence of 0.2–2.9 per 10,000 inhabitants for burn injuries requiring admission to a specialized burn service [23]. Dokter and associates reported an incidence approaching 1 per 100,000 person-years in the Netherlands for burns of 20% total body surface area (TBSA) or greater [24]. Other studies from high-income regions, including Australia, Singapore, and the United States, have reported rates of severe burn injuries (20% TBSA or greater) of less than 20% of burn injuries admitted to hospital [25–27].

Epidemiologic studies from LIC lend insight into the true impact burns have in communities. A cross-sectional survey of nearly 1400 households in Tigray, Ethiopia, revealed that 1.2% of the population is burned each year. Over 80% of these burns occurred at home, and 90% healed without any complications. Only 1% of the burn victims died [28]. A population-based survey of over 170,000 households representing nearly 350,000 children and 470,000 adults during 2003 in Bangladesh showed that the overall incidence of nonfatal burn injuries was 166 per 100,000 and that about 173,000 Bangladeshi children suffer moderate to severe burns each year; this calculates to an annual rate of 288 burns per 100,000 children. Similar to the study results from Ethiopia, 90% of the burns occurred at home. The rate of permanent disability due to burns in childhood was 5.7 per 100,000, and the mortality rate was 0.6 per 100,000 [29–31].

Other studies confirm the relative infrequency with which burn patients require hospitalization. In a study of patients treated for burns at emergency departments in North Carolina, 4% were admitted and only 4% were transferred to burn centers [32]. Based on the incidence of burns treated at emergency departments, and the proportion of those patients requiring admission, it appears that anywhere from 5 to 16 burn patients per 100,000 population require admission for the treatment of their injuries. In Pennsylvania in 1994, hospital discharge records showed the rate of hospitalizations for the treatment of burn injuries was 26.3 per 100,000 [33].

Global data are even more elusive, but an estimate of the frequency with which children are hospitalized throughout the world for treatment of burns is a rate of 8 per 100,000 [34]. In a rural community survey in Ethiopia, burns were the second most common injury to children under 15 years of age. The annual incidence of burns severe enough to restrict activity for one or more days was 80 per 1000 children [35]. Burns were therefore the leading cause of admission for injury to pediatric hospitals in Ethiopia and ranked third as a source of outpatient visits [36, 37].

In the United States, emergency department visits for burn injury decreased between 1993 and 2004 [20]. The absolute number of burn injuries in the United States may be declining, or the severity of those injuries decreasing, or both [38]. Fortunately, a similar trend is being observed overseas. For example, the number of burn patients admitted annually to the Burn Unit of Lok Nayak Hospital and Maulana Azad Medical College, New Delhi, India, from 1993 to 2007 has declined from 1276 to 724 [39].

In parallel with the decline in emergency department visits and hospitalizations for burns, mortality due to fire and flames has declined across the world. The Global Burden of Disease (GBD) 2015 project showed nearly a 10% decline in burn deaths over the previous decade [2]. The two decades from 1982 to 2002 have witnessed a decrease in fire and burn mortality in many countries. During this period of time, for instance, fire and burn mortality in Australian men declined from 1.5 to 0.7 per 100,000. Similarly the fire death rate in Brazilian women went from 1.1 to 0.5 per 100,000. Other countries observing reduction in fire and burn mortality from 1982 to 2002 include Canada, France, Mexico, Panama, Thailand, the United Kingdom, and Venezuela. In the United States, the age-adjusted death rate from fire and burns has dropped from 2.99 per 100,000 in 1981 to 1.2 per 100,000 in 2006 [22].

Yet not all countries have experienced a simple linear decline in the incidence of burn deaths during the last three decades. Significant political and economic upheaval in the nations that used to belong to the Union of Soviet Socialist Republics (USSR) has left its mark on trends in fire and burn deaths. Following a gentle decline through the early 1980s, fire and burn deaths began to rise before and just after the dissolution of the USSR in 1991. By the late 1990s, as capitalism and democracy began to replace communism, death rates again began to decline [40]. National variations in injury-related mortality may be related to individual factors, such as alcohol consumption and risk-taking behavior, as well as alterations in social, political, and environmental factors [41].

2.2.1 The Inequitable Distribution of Burns

As noted by Mock and associates in an editorial in the Bulletin of the World Health Organization, injuries and violence cause disability and death to tens of millions of people across the globe each year, and this burden is unfairly borne primarily by those in LMIC where prevention programs are uncommon and the quality of acute care is inconsistent [42, 43]. Burn injuries are dramatic examples of the inequity of injury.

The majority of burn deaths (90%) occur in lower middle- or low-income countries. Slightly more than 7% occur in HMIC. Only 3% of burn deaths across the world occur in HIC (Fig. 2.1). The rate of child injury death from fire and flames is nearly 2 1/3 times higher in low SDI (sociodemographic index) countries than in high SDI (Table 2.1; Global Health Data Exchange, http://ghdx.healthdata.org/gbd-results-tool, Accessed 12 Sept 2017). In absolute numbers, the proportion of childhood deaths due to fire and flames in LIC is four times that in HIC (Table 2.2; WHO Health Statistics and Information Systems, http://www.who.int/healthinfo/global_burden_disease/estimates/en/index2.html, Accessed 12 Sept 2017). In HIC, although the death rate in children from fire and flames is only 4% of the overall rate of death from unintentional injuries of all kinds, it is over 9% the death rate of all unintentional injuries in LIC.

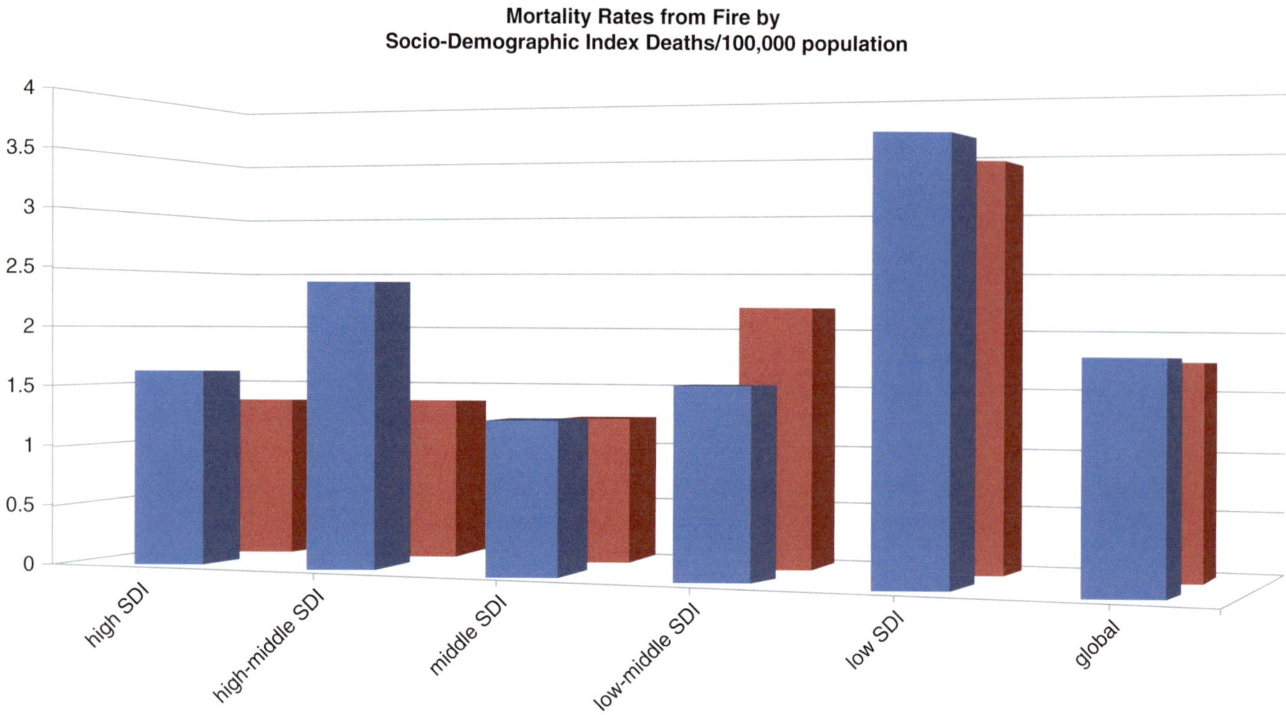

Fig. 2.1 Low sociodemographic index (SDI) countries disproportionately suffer the impact of fire deaths and burn injuries throughout the world, according to statistics from the Global Health Data Exchange project. (Blue bars represent data about men and red bars about women.) (Global Health Data Exchange. Accessed 12 Sept 2017, at http://ghdx.healthdata.org/gbd-results-tool)

Table 2.1 Global Burden of Disease Study 2015 (GBD 2015) Results

	All causes	Drowning	Fire and burns	Falls	Poisoning
HIC	3.1	1.1	0.4	0.4	0.2
LIC	27.4	7.5	3.5	2.7	2.0
World	15.7	5.5	1.7	1.7	0.9

Seattle, USA: Institute for Health Metrics and Evaluation (IHME); 2016. http://ghdx.healthdata.org/gbd-results-tool. Accessed 12 Sept 2017

Even in HIC, burn injuries disproportionately occur to racial and ethnic minorities in which socioeconomic status—more than cultural or educational factors—account for most of the increased susceptibility to burns. In the Republic of Korea (South Korea), for instance, the severity of burn injury is highest in the lowest socioeconomic groups [44]. As another example, the proportion of African-American infants requiring hospitalization at US burn centers for treatment is double the proportion of African Americans in the general population [45]. Similarly, the standardized mortality ratio for fire deaths in 1981–1982 among aboriginals in Manitoba was 4.3 times that of the population of the entire province [46]. Indeed, in many aboriginal communities in North America and Greenland, the third most common cause of unintentional fatal injury is house fires [47, 48].

At the time of burn injury, all patients—young and old—experience shock, horror, pain, and anxiety. The events that follow the injury may confuse the victims and lead them to believe (sometimes correctly) that their death is imminent. Because few burn victims in LMIC receive appropriate first aid or immediate acute care, the medical mismanagement of the burn is likely to lead the survivor to the hopeless conclusion that little or nothing can be done to soothe the pain and relieve the suffering. As a result, burn survivors become emotionally overwhelmed and typically withdraw. They lose interest in food and activity and retreat to dark corners where they may lay motionless for hours. Unfortunately, this lack of activity compounds the speed with which the healing burn wound causes wound contractures to occur, and heightens the survivor's disability. For these reasons, the distribution of burn morbidity is also imbalanced. The prevalence of moderate and severe disability due to unintentional injuries in people under age 60 is 35.4 million in LMIC, 12.5 times higher than in HIC [3].

Differences in burn mechanism are also noted across income distributions. Flame burns are the most frequent cause of burn injury in adults in HIC, with a higher %TBSA associated with this type of burn. Over 80% of cases in the United States are caused by flame (43%), scald (35%), or contact injuries (8.9%) [25]. Scald injuries are more common in elderly patients; this is consistent with data from Australia, New Zealand, England, Wales, South Asia, and the East Mediterranean [26, 49, 50]. In LMIC however, the incidence of workplace burns, particularly those involving electricity, is higher than in other regions, likely due to differences in safety regulations and poorer infrastructure.

Table 2.2 Disability-adjusted life years (DALYs) lost (in thousands) in 2015 by cause and country income level (WHO Health Statistics and Information Systems)

	Road traffic	Drowning	Fire and burns	Falls	Poisoning	All unintentional injuries
HIC	5690	770	613	5583	367	18,610
UMIC	27,631	5873	2408	8703	1683	61,774
LMIC	31,670	11,862	6579	14,241	3080	98,103
LIC	11,030	4150	2441	2982	1428	33,720

http://www.who.int/healthinfo/global_burden_disease/estimates/en/index2.html. Accessed 12 Sept 2017

2.3 Cost of Fires and Burns

Those costs that result as a consequence of fires and burns are incurred as a result of the fire exposure to property, individuals, and/or environment. Approximately 15–34% of the total fire expenditures are associated with cost as a consequence for HIC such as the United States, Canada, the United Kingdom, Australia, and Denmark [51]. These estimated costs include the following [51]:

- Property loss
- Fatalities and injuries
- Health care costs
- Loss of business (e.g., production, market share, public goodwill)
- Loss of wages/employment
- Environmental costs
- Heritage and cultural costs
- Removal of debris

Direct medical costs include costs associated with emergency department care, inpatient admissions, rehabilitation, medications, and investigative tests. Also included in direct costs are outpatient visits, medical home health care, medical devices, and ambulance transfers. Most of these costs are borne either by the patient's health care insurance plan or by the regional or federal authority, although the amount of reimbursement allowed according to government fee schedules is often less than the cost of treatment for major burns [52].

On the other hand, indirect costs are almost always paid by the patients and their families and can accumulate significantly over time. In Spain, direct health care costs of burn patients represent only 20% of the total cost of care [53]. Indirect medical costs include time spent by family members or other caregivers providing nonmedical care, either in the hospital or at home. Additionally, reduction of working time by both the patient and caregivers results in cumulative lost income. Temporary disability of the patient can evolve into permanent disability, which is particularly disabling for families without provisional plans for short- or long-term disability. Finally, mortality, particularly in the young, leads to a loss of many productive working years, which impacts not only the family but the community as a whole.

In 2015 in the United States, a country with a relatively low incidence of burns, $14.3 billion in property damage was reported, an increase of 23% over the previous year. There were 3280 civilian deaths and 15,700 injuries from residential fires (National Fire Protection Association, NFPA [54]). In England and Wales in 2004, the economic burden of fires was estimated at £2.5 billion and included property damage, casualties (395 deaths and 12,300 injuries), and business disruptions [55]. In Australia, the estimated cost of fires in 2005 was AUD$12.5 million, with an estimate of 100 deaths and 3000 injuries annually [51].

Survivors of moderate to severe burn injuries may suffer a disability that will prevent or diminish employment and income. In 2015, 40,867 total years of potential life were lost in the United States alone because of burn fatalities, including 3483 by suicide and 2699 by homicide [56]. Cost-utility analysis of 898 patients treated at the Burn Center of Valencia, Spain, from 1997 to 2001 revealed that the mean cost per quality-adjusted life-year was US$686.

A mass casualty incident with a large number of patients with burn injuries will create a significant financial hardship for those hospitals assigned to treat the multiple patients with injuries because a significant proportion of these patients will be under- or uninsured. Typical routes of financial support for the care of these disaster victims may be insufficient to cover the cost of care [57]. Expected sources of cost include the additional burden of care of patients in excess of usual operating census. Most burn centers run at a capacity of around 80%, which means that sudden expansion to surge capacity (150% of designated burn beds) would tax human resources and significantly expand expenditures on personnel. Additionally, it may be difficult if not impossible to offload the burden of mass casualty victims to other hospitals because transportation resources may be compromised by the disaster. Moreover, out-of-state hospitals are reluctant to accept the care of patients in the absence of guarantees by federal or state medical reimbursement programs [58].

A variety of features characteristic of burns lead to prolonged and expensive hospital stays. In addition to pain management and wound care, burn patients require attention to nutritional deficiencies, to the consequences of suppression of the immune system, and to rehabilitation therapy. In the United States, the average hospital charge for care of a child (age 5–16 years) with extensive third-degree burns requiring skin grafting is over US$140,000 [45]. In one state alone in 1994, hospital charges for the treatment of burn injuries totaled over $93 million [33]. Yet in spite of this lavish medical care, many burned children leave hospitals in the United States with permanent physical and psychological scars.

During the decade from 1999 to 2008, patients at burn centers in the United States stayed a mean of 10 days in the hospital. The dominant predictors of hospital stay in burn patients are burn size and burn depth [59, 60]. In the time period 2006–2015 involving 69,015 survivors and 2421 nonsurvivors in the 2016 National Burn Repository of the American Burn Association, mean total charges for survivors were $94,130; for patients with burns smaller than 20% TBSA (whose survival rate is >99%), the mean total charges were $60,505. In contrast, mean total charges were $309,656 for nonsurvivors. Mean daily charges for survivors were $8179. In contrast, mean daily charges for nonsurvivors were $24,809. The mean daily hospital charges ranged by age from $7402/day for children under 5 years to $9938/day for the elderly over 60 years (ABA NBR [61]). In the last decade, charges for hospitalization have changed. Compared with data from the 2006 ABA National Burn Repository (ABA NBR [62]), mean charges for survivors rose from $57,575, an increase of 35% when adjusted for inflation. This may be because hospital charges per day for survivors increased from $4336 to $8179, a rise of 56% when adjusted for inflation.

Loss from burns and fires includes not only health care expenditures and property damage, but destruction of human resources as well. In 2006, nearly 70,000 years of potential life were lost in the United States because of burn fatalities [20]. The indirect costs of such loss of productive years of life arise from the absence of useful employees from the workplace and lack of wage earners in families.

2.3.1 Cost by Age

In some cases, where charges may be viewed as a surrogate for intensity of care, certain trends are apparent. The presence of comorbid medical conditions typical in the elderly increases the need for more complex services and longer hospitalizations. Whereas the mean hospital charge per day for survivors was only $2900 for children aged 1–5 years, it was $4700 for elderly adults 60 years of age or older. Elderly patients admitted to a New York City burn center from 2000 to 2004 for the treatment of scald burns incurred mean hospital charges of $113,000 per patient, even though the burns were relatively small (mean 7% TBSA) [63]. In contrast, mean hospital charges per day for fatal cases in US burn centers from 1999 to 2008 were $8850 for children aged 1–5 years, compared to only $9400 for elderly adults, suggesting that more intense utilization of resources used in attempts to salvage dying children [45].

At hospitals contributing to the ABA National Burn Repository, charges for survivors ranged from a mean of $60,505 for patients with burns less than 20% TBSA to $845,616 for patients with burns greater than 80% TBSA. For nonsurvivors, charges ranged from $224,807 for patients with less than 20% TBSA burns to $182,428 for patients with greater than 80% TBSA burns. In general, hospital charges are less for nonsurvivors than for survivors, for all burn sizes greater than 30% TBSA, because the shortened hospital stay of nonsurvivors reduces cost of care [61].

The majority of patients who seek medical care for their burn injuries can be treated and released from emergency departments. For example, in 2010 only 6.4% of burn patients in the United States were hospitalized [56]. The average cost (medical cost and work loss) of treating outpatients is much less ($5394) than that for treating inpatients ($65,022), but because of the vast difference in patient numbers (380,397 vs. 25,823, respectively), the total cost of treating outpatients each year in the United States is more than the total cost of treating inpatients ($2.1 Bn vs. $1.7 Bn). In addition, the proportion of total cost as work loss is far greater in outpatients ($1.4 Bn vs. $761 Mn).

As the proportion of the US population above 60 years of age grows, shifts in expenditures for burn care will occur. From 1999 to 2008 in the United States, the percentage of patients admitted to burn centers who used Medicaid for health insurance stayed the same at nearly 13% of all patients. However, with the aging of the population, the percentage of Medicare-insured patients rose in the sa me time period from 9 to 12%. During that time period, the proportion of Workers Compensation patients sank from 13 to 8%, reflecting the departure of working adults into retirement [45].

Children are also particularly impacted by thermal injuries and smoke inhalation. Fire and burn injuries resulted in the deaths of 1461 children in the United States in 1985. Children treated for burns totaled 440,000, of which nearly 24,000 were hospitalized. The society losses from these childhood burn injuries and deaths were estimated at approximately $3.5 billion [64]. The Multicenter Benchmarking Study at the Shriners Hospitals for Children-Boston estimated the cost of hospitalization for a cohort of 230 pediatric burn patients from between 2001 and 2009 [65]. The average number of hospitalizations was two per patient, typically over a 3- to 4-year period of time. The median cost of hospitalization in 2006 USD was $16,331.

Fortunately, the majority of young children have small burns requiring short hospitalizations. Seventy-five percent of children between the ages of 1 and 5 years in the United States from 1999 to 2008 were burned over less than 10% of their body surface area. These young children with small burns spent an average of only 3.6 days in the hospital [45]. In addition to children being healthier than their older counterparts prior to injury, children are more likely to be injured by hot liquids than by flames, and there are significant cost differences between the two burn mechanisms.

Using the Healthcare Cost and Utilization Project Kids' Inpatient Database for 2000 in the United States, retrospective data analysis of pediatric burn–associated hospitalizations was performed.[2] This analysis permitted an estimate that 10,000 children younger than 18 years were hospitalized for burn injuries during that year and that the charges for these hospitalizations totaled over $211 million. The mean length of stay was 6.6 days, and only 10% of admissions lasted longer than 14 days. Because of the predominance of short lengths of stay, mean charges were only $21,840 per patient, and only 10% of patients accumulated charges in excess of $47,000. More than half of admissions were children younger than 2 years, and males outnumbered females at all ages. Children under 2 years were more likely to suffer from scald burns, whereas older children were more likely burned by fire or flame [60].

2.3.2 Cost by Mechanism

Fire and flames are responsible for the bulk of the cost of burns. In 2008, fire departments in the United States responded to nearly 1.5 million fires. There were 16,705 fire injuries, 3320 fire deaths, and nearly $15.5 billion direct property losses. A fire death occurred every 158 min in the United States in 2008 [66]. The majority of the lost years of life are due to fire and flames (68,272), with only 1218 years of life lost due to scalds or contact burns [20]. In 2010, the combined costs (medical costs and work loss) of burn care for all fatal burns approached $26 Bn. Of those costs, nearly 99% were attributed to deaths by fire and flames, compared with only $36 Mn for scald and contact burns [56].

The hospital charges per day in Pennsylvania in 1994 for the treatment of flame burns from conflagrations were $4102, compared to $2187 for scald burns. This difference reflects the difference in depth of burn (flame burns are more likely to be third degree in depth than are scald burns) and the subsequent additional intensity of resources needed to treat third-degree flame burns and smoke inhalation injury, which include intensive care, surgery, blood transfusions, and antibiotics [33].

[2]The Healthcare Cost and Utilization Project (HCUP) is a family of health care databases and related tools for research and decision-making sponsored by the Agency for Healthcare Research and Quality. The four Shriners hospitals for burned children do not generally contribute data to their respective states' HCUP databases, and thus approximately 10% of the estimated 10,000 children admitted for burn care in the United States each year were not included in this study. Therefore, the collective incidence and related charges of pediatric burn admissions may be underestimated by approximately 10% in this study [60].

Data from LMIC regarding cost of burn treatment are scarce, but there are studies that corroborate the US experience that flame burns are expensive. For example, the cost of care for patients injured by kerosene stoves is high in LMIC. In 2003 in Cape Town, South Africa, the mean total cost per patient was US$6410. Extrapolating these costs to South Africa nationwide gives an estimated annual expense of US$26,250,000, which is more than 50 times the amount expended annually for kerosene in South Africa [67].

Nonetheless, because of the frequency with which scald burns occur, the cost of care for scalds is significant. Annual charges for treatment of scald burns in US children less than 14 years old is approximately $2.1 billion. Sixty percent of these charges are for children under the age of 5 years [68]. Again, indirect costs are difficult to quantify, but are no doubt significant because each day a child is hospitalized or home ill with burn injuries, is a day that one of the parents or caregivers has to miss work. In addition, the cost of burn wound dressings is frequently not covered by most insurance policies, leaving the parents responsible for purchasing supplies out-of-pocket.

The cost of care for electrical injuries is typically much higher than the cost of care for flame or scald burns. In Ankara, Turkey, the mean total cost of electrical burns between 2005 and 2008 was US$22,501, compared with US$15,250 for other types of burn injury [69].

2.4 Limitations of Data

The majority of uncertainty in estimates of death in the Global Burden of Disease reports is associated with the assessment of systematic errors in primary data. That is, information about prevalence, incidence, and mortality from injuries is generally fragmented, partial, incomparable, and diagnostically uncertain [70]. To estimate uncertainly for regional mortality, a simulation approach was used to create uncertainty ranges that take into account uncertainty in the expected number of total deaths, uncertainty in the diagnosis of underlying cause of injury, and uncertainty arising from miscoding of cause, among others. Based on these estimates, the range of uncertainty for fire deaths is 3000 to 5000 deaths lower or higher than the estimates for fire deaths in East Asia, the Pacific, Europe, and Central Asia. Even more uncertain are the estimates in South Asia and sub-Saharan Africa, where the range of uncertainty surrounding the stated estimates is 10,000 to 14,000 deaths lower or higher. Thus the real number of fire deaths each year may be almost 30,000 higher than the estimate of 310,000. Sources of uncertainty for estimating burden of injury in the GBD reports include [70]:

- Incomplete information
- Biases in information

- Disagreement among heterogeneous information sources
- Model uncertainty
- The data generation process itself

The foundation for assigning disability weights to specific sequelae rests on an agreed-upon definition and on an accepted method for measuring disability. First required is delineation of the health states among those living with the particular sequelae (such as burn scars), where a health state is determined by the levels on the various dimensions that constitute health. Second, a valuation function is needed to provide a systematic way to aggregate across multiple dimensions of health in order to arrive at a single index value that captures the overall level of health associated with a given health state [71]. Clearly the challenge is to find universal definitions for disability and tools for disability assessment. Accordingly, as many as half a million more DALYs may be lost each year to fires [70].

Routine reporting of fatal burns may be poor in LMIC. Special surveys or demographic surveillance by verbal autopsy and lay reporting may be needed to obtain trustworthy information. Community surveys, such as performed by Mashreky and associates [30] in Bangladesh, will determine the incidence, circumstances, agent and mechanism, and severity and consequences of burns, both fatal and nonfatal. The prevalence of disability and disfigurement, as well as the economic impact on the household, probably cannot be obtained except from comprehensive and thorough community surveys [72].

Much of the published literature on burn epidemiology characterizing etiology, severity, and outcomes arises from studies of populations of patients treated at burn centers. Because of their design, these studies cannot enumerate the incidence and prevalence of important factors and variables that typify the burns that are commonly treated either at home or in primary care settings. Community surveys and emergency room or clinic data are preferable sources used to establish the magnitude of the burden of burn injuries throughout a district or region.

Other limitations arise in the interpretation of data from the United States. Although race is often studied as a variable, the limitations of racial and ethnic designations commonly used are subject to misinterpretation [73]. Other pitfalls are associated with using length of stay as an outcome variable [74]. In one retrospective study of length of stay in burn patients, the variance unexplained by the studied variables was very high, with a coefficient of variance of nearly 100% [59]. Patients admitted on Fridays may have longer lengths of stay for the same severity of injury than those admitted early in the week because of limited resources for discharge planning over weekends. Excision and grafting of even small burns will lead to longer length of stay for pain control, immobilization, rehabilitation therapy, and assistance with activities of daily living than treatment of burns with topical antimicrobials only. Administration of intravenous medications, especially antibiotics and narcotics, will increase length of stay. Smoke inhalation injury and high-voltage electrical injury will also increase length of stay beyond the range noted for any given burn size. Lack of social support systems leads to longer hospital stays in the absence of medical factors necessitating continued inpatient care.

2.5 Risk Factors

2.5.1 Socioeconomic Factors

Household income and home value are correlated with fire deaths and burn injuries. In metropolitan Oklahoma City in 1987–1990, the fire-related hospitalization and death rate was 3.6/100,000 [75]. However, when the examination of data from Oklahoma City was focused on an area characterized by a lower median household income, lower property values, and poorer quality of housing, the fire injury rate was much higher, 15.3/100,000 [76]. In addition, census tracts with low median incomes in Dallas, Texas, had the highest rates of injury related to house fires, over eight times that in tracts with high incomes [77]. Although in low-income neighborhoods a multitude of risk behaviors, such as alcohol and drug abuse, put those communities at risk for residential fires, clearly one important factor is the frequent absence of functioning smoke detectors. From 1991 through 1997 in Dallas, the prevalence of operational smoke detectors was lowest in houses in the census tracts with the lowest median incomes [77].

Fire injuries also show the steepest social class gradient among all childhood injuries in England and Wales, with a 16-fold increase in death from fire and flames in the lowest socioeconomic class compared to the highest [78]. Nonfatal smoke inhalation injuries in an impoverished, multiethnic area of inner-city London in 1996–1997 occurred at an incidence of 25/100,000 persons per year, over 30 times higher than the mortality from smoke inhalation in this series [79]. In this same quarter of London, the hospitalization rate for unintentional fire and flame injuries (8.2 per 100,000) was 1.75 times that in the southeastern United Kingdom, which includes urban, suburban, and rural neighborhoods [79]. A more recent study from Wales confirms that children under 16 years of age in poorer socioeconomic areas are at exceptionally high risk of burn injuries [80].

Longitudinal observations of patients admitted to a single burn center in New Delhi suggest that overall socioeconomic improvements lead to a reduction in the frequency of injuries severe enough to require admission to a burn center. In 1993, the per capita income in Delhi was US$450/year and 1276 patients were admitted that year; by 2005 the per capita

Table 2.3 Summary of Data from the National Burn Repository of the American Burn Association, 2006–2015

Age in years	White	Hispanic	Black	Scald	Flame	Contact	Electrical	Chemical	Burns <10% TBSA	Mortality
0–0.9 *N* = 4083	44%	17%	26%	53%	4%	21%	0.3%	0.8%	64%	0%
1–1.9 *N* = 15,547	38%	21%	26%	67%	5%	23%	0.7%	1.1%	78%	0.1%
2–4.9 *N* = 13,957	41%	21%	27%	58%	15%	17%	2%	1.3%	73%	0.6%
5–15.9 *N* = 13,457	50%	16%	26%	39%	40%	9%	2.2%	1.3%	70%	<1%
16–19.9 *N* = 8334	65%	12%	17%	27%	52%	6%	2.1%	2.8%	59%	1%
20–29.9 *N* = 26,349	62%	14%	17%	28%	47%	5%	4.3%	4.3%	65%	1.3%
30–39.9 *N* = 22,281	60%	14%	19%	27%	47%	5%	6%	6%	63%	1.9%
40–49.9 *N* = 24,132	63%	11%	20%	25%	49%	6%	5%	5%	63%	2.7%
50–59.9 *N* = 21,892	65%	8%	20%	24%	51%	6%	4%	4%	63%	4.5%
60–69.9 *N* = 12,872	68%	6%	19%	23%	55%	6%	2%	3%	63%	7.4%
70–79.9 *N* = 7061	70%	6%	18%	21%	60%	6%	0.8%	1.8%	61%	12.8%
80+ *N* = 4639	72%	5%	16%	25%	53%	8%	0.4%	1.5%	56%	21.5%
(Census 2010)	(72%)	(16%)	(13%)							

income in Delhi had risen to US$1542 and the number of admissions declined to 695 [39]. Although unproven, the hypothesis is compelling that the gradual decline in fire and burn deaths across the world is following improvements in living conditions and income.

2.5.2 Race and Ethnicity

In the United States, there are striking differences in susceptibility to burn injury by race. From 1991 through 1997, African Americans in Dallas were 2.8 times more likely to be injured in house fires than whites [77]. In 2008 in the United States, the rate of nonfatal burns was 161 per 100,000 African Americans, much higher than the observed rate of 109 per 100,000 in white non-Hispanics. In fact, in black Americans aged 35–39 years, the rate was 221 per 100,000, remarkably higher than was the rate in whites in the same age group, which was 135 per 100,000 [20]. The emergency department visit rate for burn injuries from 1993 to 2004 in the United States was 62% greater among black subjects than white subjects (340 vs. 210 per 100,000, respectively) [21].

The age-adjusted death rate from burns of all causes in the United States in 2006 was highest in blacks (2.43 per 100,000) and lowest in Asians (0.44 per 100,000) [20]. Intermediate rates were noted among Native Americans (1.45), white non-Hispanics (1.11), and Hispanics (0.77 per 100,000). Among children, a striking disparity in fire death rates exists between black and white children under the age of 15 years, with African-American children dying in residential fires at a rate nearly three times that of white children. However, by the teenage years of 15–19, this difference between the races is no longer present [20]. However, older African Americans had 4.6 times the death rates of white seniors [81]. In Alabama from 1992 to 1997, the fire fatality rate was highest among older African Americans [82]. An intriguing finding is that as household income increases, differences in fire death rates between blacks and whites diminish [83].

In data collected by the American Burn Association for the National Burn Repository, racial differences in burn admissions occur by age group.[3] Whereas for children under 5 years of age, 26% of admissions to burn centers were black children and 40% were white children, only 18% of seniors aged 60 years or older were black and nearly 70% were white (Table 2.3). In parallel with the decline of prevalence of blacks in the hospitalized burn population as age increases, Hispanic representation at burn centers was only 6% of the

[3]The 2016 report of the National Burn Repository reviews the combined data set of acute burn admissions for the period 2006–2015. Ninety-six hospitals (including 65 verified by the ABA as centers of excellence) from 36 states plus the District of Columbia contributed to this report, totaling 205,033 records. Data were not dominated by any single center and appeared to represent a reasonable cross section of the US hospitals.

elderly, compared to nearly 33% of children under 5 (Table 2.3). Hospital discharge rates for treatment of burns in Pennsylvania in 1994 showed that blacks were hospitalized for burns more than twice as frequently as whites (46.6 vs. 20.6 per 100,000, respectively) [33].

2.5.3 Age-Related Factors: Children

Important risk factors for burn injuries include lack of supervision of children, frailty, and comorbid illnesses of older adults, clothing made of flammable materials, parental illiteracy, congested housing, preexisting impairment of a child, and low socioeconomic status [84, 85]. Despite their remarkable resilience, children across the world are commonly seriously injured, with pain and suffering, disability, and occasionally death as the outcome. The highest fire-related death rates in children across the world occur in infants and children under 4 years of age. After age 15, death rates begin to climb again, presumably because of greater exposure to hazards, experimentation, and risk-taking, as well as employment [3]. Similarly, age distributions among HIC European countries, the United States, Australia, and New Zealand are highest among adults, with 40–50% of burn injuries seen in these patients [23, 25, 26]. In the United States, patients aged between 20 and 30 years are the most prevalent age group, representing 15% of cases [25]. Fires and burns were the third leading cause of unintentional injury death in the United States in 2006 for children 1–9 years of age [22].

Nonfatal burns in children are extremely common as well. In 2008 in the United States, the crude rate of nonfatal burns was 156 per 100,000 in those under the age of 18 [22]. Strikingly, the rate for children up to 3 years of age was a staggering 358 per 100,000, and the fifth leading cause of unintentional nonfatal injury in US infants is burns [22]. The fact that 93% of these young children were treated and released from emergency departments suggests that the burns were probably minor scald and contact burns. In fact, in the US, 67% of the children hospitalized for burn injuries sustained burns of less than 10% TBSA [60].

Compared to children in HIC, children under age 5 in LMIC have a disproportionately higher rate of burns [15]. For example, in Brazil, Côte d'Ivoire, and India, nearly half of all childhood burns occur in infants [86–88]. Even in HIC, children who live in poor districts are at high risk of residential fire-related injuries [89].

Various issues impact the likelihood that a child will be burned. These include literacy among mothers, knowledge of the risk of burns and of the means to secure health care, ownership of the house, kitchens separated from other living areas, use of fire-retardant chemicals in fabrics and upholstery, installation of smoke alarms and residential water sprinklers, appropriate first-aid and emergency response systems, and the existence of quality health care services [15]. Compared with children in the state of Tennessee (1980–1995) whose mothers had a college education, children whose mothers had less than a high school education had nearly 20 times greater risk of dying in a fire. Similarly, children whose mothers had three or more other children had over six times greater risk of dying in a fire when matched with children whose mothers had no other children. Likewise, when contrasted with children whose mothers were 30 years or older, children whose mothers were younger than 20 years of age had almost four times increased risk of dying in a fire. Fortunately, children thus characterized comprise only 1.5% of the population. Nonetheless, the fatal fire rate for this high-risk group was 28.6 per 100,000, far exceeding the national norms for fire fatalities [90].

Children are more susceptible to burns than adults; the curiosity and desire to experiment is matched neither by their capacity to understand the potential of danger nor by their ability to respond to it [91]. Beginning at 6 months of age, children start reaching for objects and crawling, and are fully mobile by 18 months. This escalation in motor skills and activity increases the chance that children will encounter hot liquids and solids, electrical cords, candles, fireplaces, microwaves, treadmills, hair curlers and curling irons, ovens and stoves, chemicals, and other harmful agents. For instance, the majority of scald burns in children between the ages of 6 and 36 months come from hot foods and liquids spilled in the kitchen or dining room [68].

Hot liquid and vapor injuries were the leading specific causes for children 12–17 months in a review of injuries in Californian children under the age of 4 years (Fig. 2.2). This age coincides with developmental achievements such as independent mobility, exploratory behavior, and hand-to-mouth activity. Although the child is able to gain access to hazards, he or she has not yet developed cognitive hazard awareness and avoidance skills [92]. Just as poisoning is linked to grasping and drinking behavior of children 1–3 years of age, scald burns are more common in children between 1 and 5 years of age than in any other age group [45].

Once risks are encountered, the child may lack the ability to escape danger. And because their cognitive development is not as advanced as their motor development, they are not aware of the potentially damaging consequences of their behavior. For example, fires resulting from children's play are the leading cause of residential fire deaths in children under 10 years [68]. Therefore, developmental stage becomes a risk factor for burn injuries [60].

Although the home is full of hazards, the young child views his or her dwelling as the centerpiece of their physical existence, in which they must eat, sleep, play, and resolve conflicts. Most home environments were not configured by architects to minimize the risk of injury to children. The

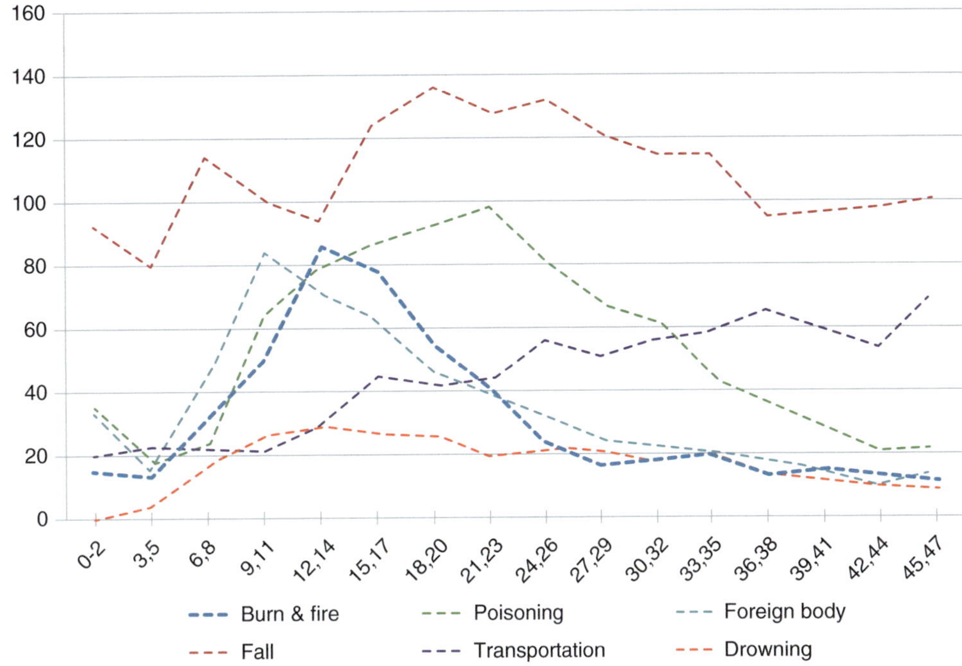

Fig. 2.2 Rates of injury, hospitalization, and death per 100,000 for children under 4 years of age in California 1996–1998 [92]. Rates are illustrated by 3-month intervals for the major categories of injury. The rate of burn and fire injuries peak between 12 and 18 months, similar to the pattern seen with foreign bodies in the airway and gastrointestinal tract. Rates of poisoning begin to rise at the same period of childhood as burns but do not decrease until after 27 months of age, nearly ¾ year later than the onset of the decrease in burns

space set aside for preparing and consuming food is such an example. Most women (mothers, grandmothers, aunts, nieces, and older female children) find themselves involved in multiple tasks while preparing meals, including caring for the younger children. It is not surprising that low-income families are functioning in overcrowded conditions with only basic utilities and utensils, throughout which they are stressed by hunger, fatigue, frustration, and fear. The prevention of scald or flame burns may be the last item on the agenda of the teenage sister charged with making dinner and caring for her younger siblings while her parents are away at work. In this regard, there is little difference between impoverished families in LMIC and HIC, thus explaining why scald burns in young children are universally common.

However, the presence of adults does not eliminate risk to children. In Greece the incidence of burns from contact with hot exhaust pipes while riding motorcycles is 17 per 100,000 per year; many of these burns occur in children, who are passengers on the rear of the motorcycle. The responsibility of assuring safety to the child passenger rests with the motorcycle operator; the presence of contact burns from the exhaust pipe suggests negligence of this responsibility [93]. Similarly, review of childhood injuries treated at a large urban hospital in the United States from 1972 through 1993 showed that adults were present 54% of the time that children were injured by fireworks; for whatever reason, the presence of adults did not protect the children from harm [94]. Nonetheless, parents are aware of the importance of their responsibility to protect children from the risk of burns, and consider risk around the home to be negligence, as noted in a survey of parents, students and teachers in rural Bangladesh [95].

2.5.4 Age-Related Factors: The Elderly

The elderly are at higher risk of injury than the younger age groups because they are more prone to injury due to deterioration of judgment and coordination as well as to the alterations in cognition and balance secondary to medications and are more susceptible to the pathophysiologic consequences of the physical insults of injury. Deaths from fires are the fourth leading cause of unintentional injury death (behind falls, motor vehicle incidents, and suffocation) among people aged 65 years or older in 2006 [20]. The elderly are at higher risk of dying in a residential fire than any other age group except for the very young [96]. Mortality data from 1984 collected by the National Center for Health Statistics showed that 29% of the residential fire deaths were victims older than 65 years, although older people only represented 12% of the US population at this time [81].

Even small, shallow burns are poorly tolerated by seniors. Elderly burn patients treated for scald burns had relatively small burns (mean 7% TBSA) but high mortality (22%). In addition, two thirds who were living independently before the burn injury were forced into skilled nursing facilities after hospitalization for burn care [63].

Behavior patterns exacerbate the risk to the elderly. Seniors who smoke are more likely to die in residential fires than younger people who smoke [97]. Smoke detectors were absent in 75% of the fatal fires involving the urban African-American elderly in Alabama from 1992 to 1997 and were completely absent in all of the fires leading to the deaths of the rural African-American seniors. The cause of fire ignition was most often heating devices, which are used more commonly by the elderly and often with inadequate attention to the safe functioning of the device. Interestingly, alcohol was a factor in only 29% of deaths of the elderly, compared with 74% of the middle-aged [82].

Not only are the elderly more likely to die in residential fires, they are also more likely to succumb to complications following thermal injury. In US burn centers during the decade 2006–2015, in-hospital mortality was 7.4% for the seventh decade of life, 12.8% for the eighth, and 21.5% for those over 80 years. These rates are even more striking when compared to the mortality rates for adults from 20 to 50 years (2%) and especially to those for children under 16 years (less than 1%) (Table 2.3).

In addition to their increased susceptibility to infectious and metabolic complications, the elderly are also at higher risk for death after burns because the burns for which they are admitted are larger in area. For example, although only 25% of children under 2 years of age who hospitalized for treatment of burns have burns greater than 10% of their body surface area, nearly 40% of the elderly over 60 years of age who are hospitalized for burns have burns greater than 10% BSA (Table 2.3). One study in Pennsylvania noted that patients 75 years and older had significantly more severe fire and burn injuries than did younger patients (using the MedisGroups™ morbidity score assigned during hospital stay) [33].

Indeed, age (along with burn size and presence of smoke inhalation injury) is one of the three most powerful predictors of outcome following thermal injury. Whereas the percentage of body surface area burned at which 50% of cases will be fatal (LA_{50}) is over 90% in children under 2 years of age, the LA_{50} for the elderly in the seventh decade of life is under 40% TBSA, and is under only 20% TBSA for those 80 years and older [45].

2.5.5 Regional Factors

The burden of burns is also unevenly distributed throughout the regions of the world. For instance, the incidence of burn injuries severe enough to require medical care is nearly 20 times higher in the Western Pacific (including China) than in the Americas [3]. (Note: WHO regions of the world are graphically depicted in Fig. 2.3; specific lists of countries within each region can be found at http://www.who.int/about/regions/en/index.html.)

Burn fatalities are more likely to occur in certain regions of the world, even when gender and national income status are considered. Infants in Africa also have an incidence of

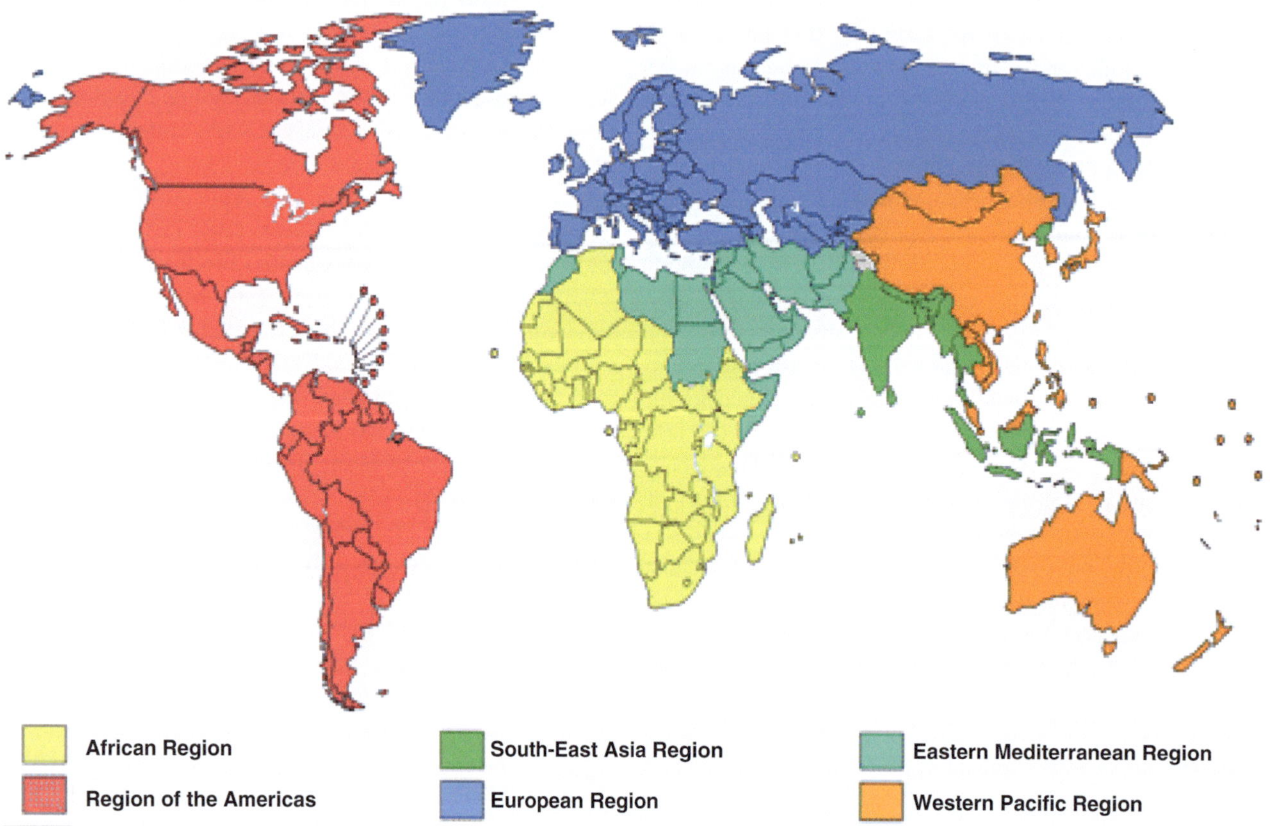

Fig. 2.3 WHO Member States are grouped into six regions. Each region is further subdivided into low-income (LIC), middle-income (MIC), and high-income (HIC) countries. Both Africa and South-East Asia have no high-income countries. Listings of the countries in each region can be found at http://www.who.int/about/regions/en/index.html

fire-related burns which is three times the world average for this age group [98]. Specifically, the 2004 fire mortality rate in infant girls in Africa was 35 per 100,000, considerably higher than that in LMIC in Europe (3.5/100,000), the Americas (2.2/100,000), or the Western Pacific (0.4/100,000) [15]. Similarly, fire death rates in boys 1–4 years in the Eastern Mediterranean LMIC were nearly twice that of boys 1–4 years in European LMIC. Moreover, fire mortality in South-East Asia was nearly six times that in the Western Pacific LMIC for boys under the age of 4 years.

In a Shanghai cohort of patients aged over 64 years, the majority had mostly flame injuries (73%) related to domestic tasks [99]. Of Chinese adults, the majority had flame-type burns (41% and 46% of patients admitted to regional burn services in Hong Kong and Shanghai, respectively) [99, 100]. The highest rate of flame injuries in China was seen in northeastern China (51% of patients admitted to a number of regional burn services) and was thought to be related to firework injuries during the Spring Festival [101]. Flame was also identified as a major cause of severe burn injury in a number of LMIC in South Asia [49]. For example, Ahuja et al. reported that in India, an average %TBSA of 42% among flame burns caused by liquid petroleum gas. The authors identified constrained living conditions in single room dwellings and preventable gas leaks from faulty rubber tubing or gas stoves as contributing factors [49, 102]. As more households in resource-limited settings move away from kerosene as a fuel source for domestic stoves and heaters, a subsequent increase is being seen in the number of injuries sustained from the use of natural gas and propane. In the decade 2005–2014 in Ecuador, domestic methane gas was the most frequent agent causing thermal burns in patients admitted to the specialized public hospital in Quito [103].

In sub-Saharan Africa, among burn injuries in the total population, scald burns predominated (59% of cases), as compared with flame burns, which accounted for 33% [104]. Among adults with severe burn injuries (20% TBSA or greater) reported in one South African study, flame was the most common cause [105]. Rates of flame injury approached 75% for adults with a %TBSA of 20% or greater, while scald, electrical and chemical causes accounted for less than 25% of such cases. Flame burns also accounted for 81% of adult fatal burns, with most occurring in patients with a %TBSA of 30% or greater [105]. A large number of injuries related to petroleum products involved illegal petrol siphoning and accidents from kerosene lamps and stoves [104]. Othman et al. identified intentional self-harm burns as corresponding with a greater %TBSA and resulting in higher rates of mortality. These injuries tended to be flame burns in young (mean age range 17–27 years) female victims (74–99%) [50]. The most common motives cited were marital problems or quarrels with husbands or other family members [50, 85].

Cold climates may be associated with a higher incidence of burn injury. Fatal residential fires in rural North Carolina that were not associated with smoking materials were caused primarily by heating appliances [106]. Lack of electricity mandates the use of hazardous flammable fuels, including open wood fires and kerosene heaters. In Nepal, because children spend a great deal of time huddled together to keep warm around open fires, flame burns are common in Nepalese children. Older children are often responsible for lighting and tending fires, stoves, and lamps, thus increasing their vulnerability to burns [107, 108].

On the other hand, the colder Northeastern region of the United States had a lower fire and burn mortality rate in 2006 (0.97 per 100,000) than the more temperate South (1.49 per 100,000). In fact, the fire and burn mortality rate in some of the coldest states in the United States were lower than the average national fire and burn mortality rate (1.23 per 100,000). For instance, the fire and burn mortality rate in New Hampshire and Vermont was 0.5 per 100,000, and in Minnesota it was 0.7 per 100,000. Nonetheless, Alaska had the highest fire and burn mortality rate in the United States, 2.72 per 100,000. Although temperate climates are not protective, warmer climates in the United States seem to have lower fire and burn death rates, as noted in Arizona with 0.87 and Florida with 0.84 per 100,000 [20]. Even though it is tempting to associate fire and death mortality rates with alcohol use, data from the Substance Abuse and Mental Health Services Administration (SAMHSA) do not suggest any correlation between the two variables at a state level [109]. More discerning inspection of data from districts, cities, and neighborhoods will be necessary to establish the association between burns and environmental or behavioral variables.

2.5.6 Gender-Related Factors

Gender differences in injury rates begin to appear within the first year of life for many injuries. Sex differences in behavior appear about the same time as differences in injury rate and correlate with injury type. Boys are 70% more likely to die by injury than girls in OECD[4] countries [110]. For children under 15 years of age, 24% more injury deaths occur among boys than among girls [3].

[4]The Organization for Economic Cooperation and Development (OECD) includes 29 countries which produce two thirds of the world's goods and services. The OECD member countries, as of December 2000, are Australia, Austria, Belgium, Canada, the Czech Republic, Denmark, Finland, France, Germany, Greece, Hungary, Iceland, Ireland, Italy, Japan, the Republic of Korea, Luxembourg, Mexico, the Netherlands, New Zealand, Norway, Poland, Portugal, Spain, Sweden, Switzerland, Turkey, the United Kingdom of Great Britain and Northern Ireland, and the United States of America [110].

Burn death patterns follow a slightly different pattern. In the United States in 2006, the mortality rates for burn deaths for children under 20 years of age was nearly identical (0.7 per 100,000 for boys and 0.65 per 100,000 for girls). However, in the youngest age group (infancy through 4 years), the fire death rate for boys was 1.24 that of girls [22].

Several theories suggest why boys are more likely to be injured than girls. Boys are socialized differently: parents are more likely to allow boys to roam further with fewer limits and to play alone [111–113]. Boys are also engaged in more risk taking and higher activity levels and behave more impulsively than girls [114, 115]. However, in a 1978 study of injuries in children reported to the Consumer Product Safety Commission, the gender differences were not explained by exposure to risk [116].

The gender difference is observed in adults as well. The emergency department visit rate for burn injuries from 1993 to 2004 in the United States was 50% greater among men than women (270 vs. 180 per 100,000, respectively) [21]. In Pennsylvania in 1994, t he overall hospital discharge rate for men who had been treated for burns was over twice that for women (37 vs. 16.5 per 100,000, respectively) [33]. The age-adjusted rate of nonfatal burns in the United States in 2008 was 143 per 100,000 in men, higher than the rate of 128 per 100,000 seen in women [20]. However, in the United States from 2001 to 2006, nonfatal scald burns were more common among elderly women than elderly men (age 65 years or older) [22].

Nonetheless, in the United States, a higher fire death rate is seen for elderly males than for elderly females [81]. Yet the difference is most prominent in the 20–44 age group, in which the ratio of fire mortality in men is nearly twice that in women [20].

Additionally, males shoulder a higher proportion of the disability associated with injury. Men account for 78% of the DALYs lost from injuries to adults 15–44 years of age in Australia [117].

Occupational activities put people at risk for work-related injuries. During the time period 1993 to 2004 in the United States, 23% of emergency department visits for burn injury were work-related [21]. From 1999 to 2008, 11% of admissions to US burn centers were for occupational injuries [45]. US workers in the mining, transportation, and public utility industries had the highest rate of death from thermal injury in 1992 to 1999. Perhaps because of rapid economic growth, an increase has occurred in occupational injuries in China (Smolle 2016, [118]). Occupations with the highest risk of death by fire include truck drivers, firefighters, miners, airline pilots, and operators of ovens, furnaces, and kilns [119]. Because the majority of these high-risk occupations are held by men, adult males will have higher rates of burn injuries in countries that offer them these roles. Men were seen nearly twice as often as women for work-related burns in the US emergency departments between 1993 and 2004 [21].

Gender differences in burn incidence may vary by age, region, and national income categories. For instance, in rural Ethiopia burns occur more often to boys than girls, but it is women who are more frequently burned than men [120]. Unfortunately, pregnancy increases the risk of mortality both to the mother and the fetus [121].

In HIC and LIC, gender differences in fire deaths are polar opposites. Rates of death by fire in HIC are twice as high in males as in females in the 15–59 year age group. However, in this same age group in LIC, female deaths from burns occur at a rate 2.3 times that in males. The discrepancy is greatest in WHO South-East Asia and Eastern Mediterranean Regions [3]. Nine percent of all deaths among Egyptian women of reproductive age were caused by burns [122].

However, the gender distribution of nonfatal burns differs between countries. Although some countries such as Egypt and India have a greater proportion of burns among girls, a higher number of cases in boys has been reported in Angola, Bangladesh, China, Côte d'Ivoire, Kenya, and Nigeria [29, 88, 123–129].

The gender discrepancy in LMIC fire death rates is present but less pronounced in young children. However, between the ages of 15 and 19, women begin to suffer a disproportionate share of fire deaths. Women between the ages of 15 and 59 in LIC have an astonishingly high fire death rate of 15.6 per 100,000 [3]. In India, approximately 65% of burn deaths occur to women, most often caused by kitchen accidents, self-immolation, and domestic violence [130].

The increasing proportion of burns among girls as they enter adolescence can be explained in some cases by the changing activities as they approach the responsibilities of adulthood. In the Ardabil province of Iran in 2006, teenage girls were three times as likely to be burned in the kitchen as teenage boys. In Ardabil, 21%–37% of children are involved in kitchen jobs such as lighting the oven, preparing tea, and carrying hot food; the mean age for starting to help in the kitchen is approximately 8 years old [131].

Among burns in South Asian LMIC, including India, Pakistan, Sri Lanka, and Bangladesh, gender trends closely follow age patterns. Burns in younger patients tend to be associated with male gender, but burns in females predominate during adolescence and adulthood [49]. This same trend is also demonstrated in a number of Iranian studies [50]. This is contrasted by populations in Australia, the United States, Europe, China, and South America where males tend to predominate across most age groups [23, 25, 26, 99, 100, 103, 132]. Golshan et al. postulate the reason for this shift in gender distribution in some South Asian countries is related to young women being brought into the kitchen to help their mothers cook. In doing so they are exposed to faulty appliances, kerosene stoves, and hot liquids while wearing loosely fitting and flammable garments. Of 16 studies included in the review by Golshan et al., five implicated loose/flammable clothing and a further 12 identified kitchen cooking as a separate contributing factor [49]. In Nepal, cooking, heating, and lighting—using kerosene and biomass as the major fuels—were the main activities associated with burn injury in women [133].

2.5.7 Intent

The vast majority of burn injuries in the world are unintentional. In US burn centers from 1999 to 2008, 2% of admissions were for assault-by-burning (including child abuse), and less than 1% were for self-harm or attempted suicide [45]. Similarly, in 1994 in Pennsylvania, 2% of burn admissions were for self-inflicted injuries, and another 2% were for assault-by-burning; 95% were unintentional [33]. Only 2.4% of admissions to burn centers in Taiwan, ROC, from 1997 to 2003 were for self-inflicted injuries [134].

India has the highest number of cases in the world of intentional self-harm by burning. The majority of victims are young women, as opposed to Europe, where they are more often men in their fourth or fifth decade of life [135, 136].

Self-immolation is also more common in a number of other areas, including the Middle East, Africa, and South Asia. Self-immolation was found to account for 7–9% of suicides in India, and 71% in some regions of Iran [137]. In Europe and North America, rates of between 2 and 14% have been reported [138]. Self-harm burns are mostly flame injuries that tend to be more severe in nature and have higher mortality rates when compared with accidental burns [139]. Self-inflicted burns have a significantly higher %TBSA, burn depth, inhalation injury and mortality when compared with accidental flame burns [138–140]. Dousing and setting alight an accelerant is the most common method of self-immolation and is the main contributor to increased size and depth of burn, and thus is a significant contributor to the higher mortality rates seen in this patient population [140].

Studies investigating self-inflicted burn injury characteristics and outcomes, such as mortality, generally consist of small sample sizes (<50 patients) from single burn centers. This has resulted in contradictory descriptions of the characteristics and outcomes in these patients [138]. Although self-immolation results in increased mortality, few studies have evaluated mortality after adjusting for important confounders such as comorbidities, %TBSA, and burn depth.

Duarte et al. investigated a cohort of 114 self-inflicted burn injuries admitted to a regional burn service in Porto Alegre, Brazil, between 2003 and 2012. Intentional self-inflicted burns were associated with a 59% higher risk of inpatient death when compared with accidental injuries after adjusting for burn severity, comorbidities, inhalation injury, age, and previous psychiatric disorders. Duarte et al. recognized the challenge of discerning why this phenomenon arises, and speculated that changes in biologic and social interactions may occur after self-immolation. Higher rates of posttraumatic stress disorder, depression, and self-injurious behavior are found in these patients, which can worsen the course of mood disorders and hamper patient recovery. These factors can also contribute to poor motivation, noncompliance with treatment, and ongoing self-harm which may also contribute to poorer outcomes independently of injury severity [138]. Negative attitudes expressed by medical staff toward patients with self-inflicted injuries, including irritation, a diminished willingness to help, and ambivalence, have been documented previously [138, 141, 142]. However, the role these attitudes and behaviors play in mortality outcomes is unknown [138].

Thombs and Bresnick [138] reported on an adult population of 593 self-inflicted burns across 70 burn centers in the United States using data from the NBR. They found no increased risk of mortality among patients with self-inflicted burns when compared with patients with similar demographic, health, and injury characteristics (including %TBSA) [138]. The notion that self-inflicted injury is not an independent predictor of death has been reported elsewhere [140]. Duarte et al. studied a smaller patient population from one burn service; these results may have reflected the characteristics of one practice rather than a definitive phenomenon. Nevertheless, other studies have demonstrated an association between self-harm and death independent of other mortality risk factors [143, 144]. These contradictory results were most likely related to the heterogeneous nature of burn injuries, the relatively small sample sizes of studies investigating self-immolation, and differences in how papers define a self-immolation injury.

2.5.8 Comorbidity

Because epilepsy is often untreated in LMIC, it is a frequent initiating factor in many severe burns [145]. During a seizure, the epileptic may fall into an open fire or onto a stove. The severity of injury is sometimes and unfortunately exacerbated by traditional beliefs that epilepsy is contagious; victims in Ethiopia are often left to burn because of fear by potential rescuers of contacting the disease by touching the victim [146]. Burns precipitated by epileptic seizures represented 44% of adult burn injuries in a community survey in rural Ethiopia, and 29% of adult hospital admissions for burns were precipitated by epileptic seizures [120]. Epilepsy was the most common personal risk factor, other than age, in a remote subsistence village of the highlands of Papua New

Guinea during 1971–1986, where the mortality rates from fire and flames were nearly 15 per 100,000, many times higher than reported rates from other countries [147]. In rural Bangladesh, 0.7% of all deaths to women (15–44 years of age) were caused by falls into fires during seizure activity; this is an annual rate of approximately 2 per 100,000 [148].

Many Muslim epileptics insist on fasting during the holy month of Ramadan and hence miss their antiepileptic medications. Therefore, burns in epileptics are commonly seen during Ramadan in Islamic populations. These burns are typically sustained during seizures while in the kitchen or falling on the hot ground (which can reach temperatures over 115 ° F). In a prospective study of burns in epileptics in Saudi Arabia, 40% of injured patients sustained the burn while fasting because they did not take their antiepileptic medications [149, 150].

Peripheral neuropathy is a disorder commonly caused by leprosy and diabetes mellitus, and results in sensory loss of the extremities. People with sensory peripheral neuropathy are vulnerable to burn injuries, especially hot water scalds [151]. Handling hot cooking utensils or warming neuropathic feet too close to a fire can also cause deep burns.

One of the reasons that the elderly are at higher risk of sustaining injuries is because of coexisting medical conditions. Seventy-seven percent of burn center patients aged 59 years or older in a single-center study had one or more preexisting medical conditions at the time of injury; and in 57% of patients' judgment, mobility or both were impaired [152]. In another study, 50% of octogenarians admitted for burn treatment sustained injury because of a cerebrovascular accident [153]. Physical and mental comorbid illnesses including blindness, deafness, arthritis, and diabetes are associated with burns, particularly in older adults [154]. In addition, being alone not only increases the risk of injury in the elderly but also increases the likelihood of mortality [155].

Physical or cognitive disabilities are distinct risk factors for burns, especially for scald burns or for death from residential fires. Of the 37 patients with disabilities who were admitted to a burn center in Toronto between 1984 and 1992, the majority (84%) were admitted for scald burns suffered at home. Although some were elderly as well (median age, 58 years), the extent of disability was significant in all cases, including spinal cord disorders or injuries, epilepsy or other neurologic disorders. Given the relatively small size of burn (mean: 10% TBSA), the mortality rate was 22%, which is high compared to 4% in the general burn population. The average length of stay for disabled burn patients was 2.8 days per %BSA burned, in comparison to that of the general population of burn patients in whom length of stay is approximately one day per percent burn [45, 156]. Although the relative risk of burns in the elderly with dementia has not yet been established, expert opinion among burn centers suggests that dementia is a significant risk factor for burns. Indeed, elderly patients with dementia tend to have poorer outcomes from burn injuries, and rehabilitation outcomes are ineffective at returning patients to prior levels of independence [157].

2.5.9 Agents

Flame burns and scalds occur at approximately the same frequency in children under the age of 18 years in some LMIC, including China and Iran [129, 158]. In general, however, and particularly in younger children, scald burns are more common than flame burns in children. For example, three pediatric hospitals in Mexico noted that the majority of emergency department visits for burns in children under 10 years of age was due to exposure to boiling liquids, most commonly overly hot bath water [159]. Over 75% of children under the age of 18 hospitalized for the treatment of burns in Taiwan, Republic of China, had been injured by scalding liquids [134]. The most common cause of burn injuries in infants hospitalized for burn care in Eastern Saudi Arabia is scald burns (87% of all burns) [160]. In burn centers in the United States, scald burns account for nearly half the admissions of children under 5 years of age. For very young children under 2 years, flame burns cause less than 5% of admissions; contact burns are more common in this age group, involving over 20% of admissions (Table 2.3). Unfortunately, many children who suffer scald burns in LMIC do not receive appropriate first aid; in Delhi, India, for instance, 37% of children with scald burns arrive at the hospital without having received any first aid [161].

Even when older children up to the age of 18 years are included in analysis, scald burns still outnumber fire and flame injuries by a ratio of 5:1 in all the US hospitals [60]. Nonetheless, older children and young teenagers between 5 and 16 years of age experience fewer scald burns than their younger siblings: only 39% of admissions are for scalds, compared to 69% of admissions of children under 5 years of age (Table 2.3).

Scald burns are very common in adults as well. A study of all hospital discharges in Pennsylvania in 1994 (including from hospitals without burn centers as well as the six hospitals with burn centers) showed that 56% of admissions were for treatment of scald burns [33].

Overall, flame burns still cause more admissions to US burn centers than any other single cause of thermal injury. Through the adult decades, flame burns continue to be the cause for 47–60% of admissions and scalds for 25–28% (Table 2.3).

Fortunately, the majority of burns of any etiology are small to moderate in size: 86% of patients admitted to US burn centers in 1999–2008 had burns involving less than 20% of the BSA [45].

Clothing ignition is a common cause of severe flame burns. Although conflagrations caused 78% of the deaths in the elderly in the United States in 1984, 11% of fatalities were from clothing ignitions [81]. Women of the Indian subcontinent wearing loose flammable saris (made of cotton or synthetic textiles) are vulnerable to fire deaths when their clothing is ignited while cooking near open flames, particularly if the cooking source is an open fire pit or a small kerosene stove on the ground [162]. Ninety-three percent of burn injuries in rural Ethiopia occurred inside the home where open fires are used in the common room and often ignite clothing [35]. Likewise, ignition of grass skirts in warm coastal areas of Papua New Guinea account for nearly half of hospitalizations for burns [163].

Flammable fuels are often the agents of fire acceleration or heat production in incidents that result in flame burns. In a retrospective study of burn patients admitted to a single site from 1978 to 1996 in the United Stats, the unsafe use of gasoline was implicated in 87% of burns where the cause could be identified [164]. Liquefied petroleum gas (LPG) has replaced kerosene in many households in LMIC as per capita income has risen and availability of smaller and more affordable LPG cylinders has improved. In Delhi, LPG-related burns were responsible for over 10% of admissions from 2001 to 2007 [39].

Electrical and chemical burns are rarely reasons for admission in children, occurring less than 2% of the time; but these burns account for 4–5% of admissions of adults from 20 to 60 years of age (Table 2.3). The frequency of admissions for contact burns declines precipitously with age: although over one fifth of admissions of children less than 2 years are for contact burns, only about 6% of adult admissions are for contact burns (Table 2.3).

2.5.9.1 Residential Fires

The products of combustion include fire gases, heat, visible smoke, and toxicants. The hazards created by these products of combustion include effects of heat on the upper airway, toxicant damage to the subglottic respiratory system, impaired vision due to smoke density or eye irritation, and narcosis from inhalation of asphyxiants. These effects lead or contribute to restricted vision, loss of motor coordination, impaired judgment, disorientation, physical incapacitation, and panic. The resultant delay or prevention of escape from the burning structure leads to injury and death from inhalation of toxic gases and from thermal burns. Extricated survivors may go on to die later in the hospital from complications such as respiratory failure, septic shock, and multiple organ system failure, all of which are rooted in the initial exposure to products of combustion [165].

Smoke is defined as the airborne solid and liquid particulates and fire gases created during combustion and when materials undergo decomposition or transformation by heat [166]. Pyrolysis is the decomposition of a material from heat, and because this decomposition does not require the normal atmospheric level of oxygen, the result is incomplete combustion. The toxicant gases produced in a fire can be categorized into separate classes: the asphyxiants which induce unconsciousness, and the irritants which inflame the eyes and respiratory tract. The major threat in most fire atmospheres is carbon monoxide, an asphyxiant produced by incomplete combustion.

The vast majority of deaths due to fires in the United States each year occur because of exposure to products of combustion in structure conflagrations. From 1992 to 2001, two thirds of fire deaths in the United States occurred in residential fires (Federal Emergency Management Agency, FEMA [167]). (Although residential fires are the primary cause of fire mortalities, they account for only half of structure fire injuries and less than one third of the dollar loss for fires.) Residential fires accounted for 76% of the years of life lost in 2006 in the United States due to flame burns [20].

Although most victims of fatal fires die from smoke inhalation, a few will die of thermal injury directly. Temperatures higher than 300 °F are reached within 5–10 min in building fires, and in an aircraft cabin the temperatures near 500 °F in just 5–6 min [168, 169]. Flashover[5] can occur in less than 10 min in even a slowly progressing residential fire, at which time temperatures soar from 1100 °F to over 2000 °F in seconds, creating an environment in which survival is unprecedented. In the absence of inhalation of products of combustion and pyrolysis, death can be caused by heat-induced laryngospasm or by vagal-reflex-mediated cardiac arrest [170].

Although a well-burning fire produces much more carbon dioxide than carbon monoxide (CO), materials in most structure fires smolder because of rapid depletion of oxygen in the interior of the building. Although the pathophysiology of CO poisoning is well understood, there remains no readily apparent explanation for the observation that the range of carboxyhemoglobin (COHb) tolerated is very wide. Although COHb saturation greater than 35% can cause death in some people, others have survived COHb saturations as high as 64% [165]. The average COHb level in fire fatalities is 60%, with a range of 25–85% [170]. About 10–15% of CO binds to myoglobin and cytochrome a3, blocking the production of adenosine triphosphate (ATP) and causing muscular weakness, thus

[5]Flashover is defined as a transitional phase in the development of a compartment fire in which surfaces exposed to thermal radiation reach ignition temperature more or less simultaneously and fire spreads rapidly throughout the space resulting in full room involvement or total involvement of the compartment or enclosed area [306].

exacerbating the difficulties the victim encounters during escape maneuvers [171].

Unfortunately, COHb levels rise rapidly in house fires. When the CO level in inspired, air reaches 5%, COHb rises to 10% in 10 s and to 40% (a fatal level in some people) in only 30 s [172]. A study in East Denmark from 1982 to 1986 demonstrated that the blood alcohol concentration averaged about 190–200 mg/dL in fatalities from residential fires, and the mean COHb was about 60% [173]. However, it is clear that some people with preexisting functional impairments are at risk for increased CO toxicity at lower COHb levels, including children and the elderly, the physically disabled, and those impaired by alcohol, drug, or medication intoxication [77, 174]. Largely for this reason, children under age 5 years and the elderly over 65 years account for 45% of home fire deaths [175]. Patients with coronary artery disease cannot increase coronary blood flow when COHb rises above 10% [176]. In addition to inhibiting cognitive responses, ethanol also potentiates the effects of CO such that lower levels of COHb are associated with fatality [177].

Although hydrogen cyanide (HCN), which is produced by the combustion of materials that contain nitrogen (such as wool, silk, acrylonitrile polymers, nylons, and polyurethanes), is 20 times more toxic than CO, its role as a causative agent in human fire fatalities is less clear than that of CO. For example, in many fire deaths, COHb is in the toxic range, but cyanide levels are not toxic [178]. Nonetheless, low levels of COHb in other fire fatalities suggest that other toxic gases such as HCN may play a role in causing death [179].

Because oxygen (O_2) is consumed during combustion, the oxygen level in the inspired air can drop from 21% to levels that affect coordination, mentation, and consciousness. When O_2 drops to 17%, coordination is impaired; when it drops to 14%, judgment becomes faulty; and below 6%, unconsciousness occurs [165].

Acrolein is formed from the smoldering of all plant materials (including wood and the natural fibers used in decorations and furnishings) and is a potent sensory and pulmonary irritant. It is extremely irritating to the eyes at concentrations as low as a few parts per million [180].

Level of consciousness and thus ability to escape fire are affected by drugs and alcohol [179]. One third to one half of victims of fatal fires have ingested alcohol [82, 181, 182]. Ethanol intoxication significantly impairs the ability to escape from fire and smoke and is a contributory factor in smoke-related mortality. Whereas victims found near escape exits had blood alcohol levels averaging 88 mg/dL, the mean blood alcohol level was 268 mg/dL in those found dead in bed, presumably having made no attempt to escape [183]. Moreover, if even one person in the house is impaired by alcohol or drug usage, others in the dwelling are at increased risk of death from fire as well [106].

Perhaps the most deadly combination leading to fatal fires is alcohol and cigarettes. Not only in higher socioeconomic neighborhoods is smoking in bed while inebriated one of the most common causes of death by fire, but also in indigenous communities in North America. About 76% and 90% of the adult victims of residential fires in Canadian Indians in Manitoba and Alberta, respectively, were under the influence of alcohol at the time of death [46, 184].

Risk factors for fatal and nonfatal house fire injuries include young or old age, male gender, nonwhite race, low income, disability, smoking, and alcohol use [185]. Single, detached mobile homes had the highest rate of fire deaths of all types of residences [185]. In rural areas, risk of death from a residential fire in a mobile (manufactured) home is 1.7 times the risk of that in a single- or multiple-family home [106]. In addition, the presence of an able-bodied adult who is not impaired by alcohol or drugs will significantly increase the odds of survival in a house fire [96]. Burn injuries and fire fatalities are more common in older homes and from fires started in the bedroom or living room from heating equipment, smoking or children playing with fire [77].

2.5.9.2 Non-Electric Domestic Appliances

In many households in LMIC, especially in rural areas lacking electrification, open flames are common and include floors of huts with open hearths which are used for cooking and warmth, candles, and small kerosene and naphtha stoves and lanterns. The fire risk from these sources is contributed to by a lack of enclosure for open fires, floor-level location of fires and stoves, instability of appliances, nearby storage of volatile and flammable fuels, flammable clothing and housing materials, and lack of exits [72].

A large number of burn injuries and fire deaths in LMIC are related to the nature of nonelectric domestic appliances that are used for cooking, heating, lighting, or all three. The incidence of injuries is largely associated with the use of stoves and lamps and with kerosene (termed paraffin in some countries) and petroleum as well as butane, LPG, and alcohol. Associated problems include appliance design and construction, fuel combustion and instability, and mechanical inefficiency. Ignorance of safe usage techniques is also contributory. Industry and government regulations and standards are either nonexistent or not adequately enforced [186].

Informal settlements in densely populated urban areas are often scenes for fires that lead to incalculable property damage and horrific loss of life. From 2002 to 2004, approximately 12% of households in South Africa were "shacks," living quarters assembled from highly combustible and toxic materials and usually assembled close to one another on uneven ground. Kerosene is used as fuel for small stoves; the more inexpensive the stove, the more likely it is to tip over or malfunction. During a simulated shack fire triggered by a kerosene stove that was knocked over while burning, the temperature in the shack reached an excess of 1670 °F in less than 4 min [187]. Shack-fire burns are the second most common reason for admission to burn centers in Cape Town, and the most common cause of shack fires in these cases is the use of kerosene stoves [188].

Serious injuries from kerosene stoves have been documented in Egypt, Ethiopia, India, Nigeria, Pakistan, and other LMIC [189–194]. The underlying problem of kerosene stove–related fires often lies with design issues. Poor design allows for fuel leakage, which is especially common when stove reservoirs are being filled. Kerosene can leak onto clothing, or if heat or flames are present nearby during fueling, vapors can ignite. Ignorance of safe techniques in using fuel and appliances will also lead to catastrophic explosions if gasoline contaminates or is substituted for kerosene. In addition, these small, portable stoves are often very unstable, easily tipping over while being moved or even when resting in place. On occasion, the small stove is used as a weapon, thrown by the assailant at the victim, igniting his or her clothing on fire [108].

The essential issue is that families at greatest risk because of poverty, ignorance, and overcrowding lack the resources needed to purchase stoves of safe and dependable design. The most affordable stoves in South Africa are little over US$3 each, but these flame or wick stoves are notorious for rapidly fluctuating flame size, instability, and explosions. In addition, the impoverished housing conditions lead to poor air circulation, and incomplete combustion of kerosene in flame stoves produces significant levels of toxicants such as carbon monoxide. Even in dwellings supplied with electricity, low-income families will often choose to use kerosene stoves for cooking because of cost savings.

2.5.9.3 War, Mass Casualties, and Terrorism

Military personnel are at high risk for burn injury in wartime. In general, however, the distribution of burn size in combat is similar to that observed in the US community: 80% of burns are less than 20% TBSA in size [195]. Many burn casualties occur during combat at sea. In the Falkland Islands campaign (1982), for instance, 34% of all British Navy casualties were burns [196]. Personnel in armored fighting vehicles are also at relatively high risk for burn injuries and fire deaths. For example, the proportion of burn casualties during the Yom Kippur War (1973) was nearly 11%, higher than that of the less than 5% seen during the Israeli Six-Day War (1967), because of a greater saturation of the battlefield with tanks and anti-tank weaponry [197]. Subsequent to the Yom Kippur War, the Israeli army enforced the use of flame-retardant garments and installed automatic fire extinguishing systems within tanks. These changes led to a decrease in incidence to less than 9% of military burn casualties during the Lebanon War (1982). Those modifications have also been credited with reduction of burn size in those who were injured [198].

Fire, flames, and explosions have caused mass burn casualties over the centuries. In 1190, a fire in Clifford's Tower, York, UK, took the lives of 150 Jews who had been besieged by an anti-Semitic mob [199]. A theater fire in Canton, China, claimed the lives of 1670 in 1845. In Santiago, Chile (1863), between 2000 and 3000 lives were lost when a gas lamp near the main altar ignited veils on the walls of la Iglesia de la Compañía de Jesús (the Church of the Company of Jesus) [200]. On April 27, 1865, *USS Sultana*, a steamboat returning Union prisoners-of-war to their homes in the North, caught fire when one of its boilers exploded on the Mississippi River near Memphis and sank, taking with her approximately 1800 casualties from burns and drowning [201].

Throughout the twentieth century in the US, several fire or burn disasters occurred in which more than 100 people were killed, including the Iroquois Theater fire in Chicago (1903) with 602 fatalities and 220–250 injuries, forest fires near Cloquet and Moose Lakes in Minnesota (1918) with 800 fatalities and 85 injuries, and the Cocoanut Grove Nightclub fire in Boston (1942) with 492 fatalities and 166 injuries [202]. More recent examples include fire disasters at the Beverly Hills Supper Club in Kentucky (1977) with 165 fatalities, the MGM Grand Hotel in Las Vegas (1980) with 84 fatalities, the Alfred P. Murrah Federal Building explosion in Oklahoma City (1995) with 168 fatalities, and the attacks on the Pentagon Building and the World Trade Center (2001) with 189 and 2750 deaths, respectively. These last three mass-casualty incidents were the result of terrorism, and casualties were caused not only by smoke inhalation and thermal injuries but by blast, crush, and fall injuries.

Indeed, most of the mass-casualty terrorist attacks in the United States have employed conventional explosives or incendiary agents (such as jet fuel). A bomb placed under the staircase in the 16th Street Baptist Church in Birmingham, Alabama, in 1963 caused the death of four young girls; the motivation was anger over public integration of the races [203]. The first attack by foreign terrorists on American soil came in 1993 when a truck bomb with conventional explosives was detonated in the underground parking garage of the World Trade Center, taking the lives of six persons. The use of ammonium nitrate and fuel oil in Oklahoma City and of jet fuel delivered by commercial airliners at the Pentagon and World Trade Center (2001) has escalated the toll from such deadly terrorist attacks.

Terrorist attacks have dominated regions of religious, cultural, and political conflicts since the later half of the twentieth century. Sectarian violence in Northern Ireland has resulted in nearly 3000 deaths since 1968, many of them from explosions. Progress in peace negotiations between Israelis and Palestinians has been hampered by the frequency of terrorist incidents; between 2000 and 2002, Israel sustained two bombings per month. From the late 1980s until they were neutralized in Sri Lanka in

2009, the Liberation Tigers of Tamil Eelam conducted approximately 200 suicide bombings. The armed conflicts in Iraq, Afghanistan, and Pakistan have all been marked by frequent suicide bombings. Clearly, preparation for any terrorist event in the future must take into account the inevitability of burn injuries as a result of explosive devices [204].

2.6 Interventions

A priority in LMIC must be to improve the provision of health care for burns to all in the population so that inequity in acute treatment is eliminated. This improvement includes the training of doctors and nurses in acute burn care management as well as those in the allied services (such as physiotherapists, nutritionists, occupational therapists, psychologists, and social workers). However, the reality is that social, political, and fiscal challenges drive this goal into the distant future.

Thus the conclusion to be drawn is that prevention is the key to alleviation of suffering from burns. Truly the best way to treat a burn is to prevent it from happening in the first place. In reality, effective prevention programs will face similar barriers to implementation as those faced by efforts to improve acute care, but in many ways prevention is much more cost-effective and will clearly affect vastly greater numbers of people. Expanding the global effort to eliminate burns will best protect the people of LMIC from the horrors of burn injuries.

Prevention works. The number of child deaths by injury in Organization for Economic Co-operation and Development (OECD) nations fell by about 50% between 1970 and 1995 [110].

According to research in Israel during 1998–2000, injury prevention programs were effective in reducing burn-related hospitalizations among infants and toddlers, especially from more affluent communities [205]. In Harstad, Norway, in 1987, a comprehensive community-based injury prevention program characterized by strengthening of public participation and the enhancement of community empowerment achieved by recording and actively using the local burn injury data, resulted in a reduction in burn injuries in children [206].

Aside from the reduction in pain and suffering, prevention efforts are cost-effective as well. It has been estimated that for every dollar spent on smoke alarms, USD$69 in fire-related costs are saved [207].

The traditional approach to injury prevention involves the three E's: education, engineering, and enforcement. Education is an active process that requires behavior modification. There are very few data on the effectiveness of fire prevention educational programs. Passive measures, such as engineering or product design and legislation, have been more effective [208].

Clearly, a void in understanding regarding risk and prevention of injuries exists in the community. A report from South Africa shows that people living in environments in which burns are likely to occur (such as informal settlements) are not well educated about burn prevention and treatment [209]. Parents and other caregivers of children in Thailand were surveyed for their knowledge of injury prevention awareness in the home. Although 90% of respondents recognized the need to ensure inaccessibility to matches and lighters, only 60% saw the need to restrict access to the kitchen stove and to cover unused electrical outlets [210]. Traditional approaches to educational intervention have had limited success. Evaluation of a burn prevention program for children in a rural area of Zambia demonstrated some improvement in burn knowledge, but also an unfortunately large residual deficit after education [211].

Although many resources are expended on community education, the beneficial effects are not clear. Two reviews have not identified evidence of beneficial effects from community-, school-, or clinic-based fire safety education on fire injuries [212]. Counseling and educational interventions had only a modest effect on the likelihood of owning a smoke alarm (odds ratio [OR] 1.3) or having a functional alarm (OR 1.2), but these effects were enhanced in the setting of primary child health care surveillance (OR 1.9 and 1.7, respectively) [79, 213]. Similarly, review of the effectiveness of school education programs in reducing the incidence of burns in Israel noted a lack of efficacy [205]. However, studies in LMIC show that educational programs effectively reduce hazardous behaviors, incidence of burns, morbidity, and mortality [214].

A review of 30 pediatric burn prevention strategies from 16 developing/developed countries found only two papers that evaluated the effectiveness of the intervention [205, 206, 215]. It appears, based on limited data, that multipronged community-based interventions were most effective to reduce the risk of burn injuries. The likely explanation is that these multifaceted community approaches typically focus on effective prevention communication, which has been documented to improve outcomes such as the adoption and maintenance of healthy behaviors [216].

Injury prevention programs conducted in Israel between 1998 and 2000 were effective in reducing pediatric burn-related hospitalizations from 1.39 to 1.05 per 1000 infants, in contrast to areas where the program did not exist [205]. The effect was greatest among infants and toddlers from affluent areas; no significant change in burn-related hospitalizations occurred among school-aged children.

A comprehensive community-based injury prevention program in Harstad, Norway, resulted in a 52.9% reduction in burn injuries in children [206]. This educational program strengthened public participation and enhanced community empowerment by recording and using the local burn injury data.

Although many resources are expended on community education, the beneficial effects are not clear. Two previous publications reviewing the literature to 1999 did not identify evidence of beneficial effects from community, school, or clinic-based fire safety education on fire injuries [185]. Counseling and educational interventions had only a modest effect on the likelihood of owning a smoke alarm or having a functional alarm, but these effects were enhanced in the setting of primary child health care surveillance [174, 213].

The effectiveness of education programs for burn prevention may be enhanced by targeting specific at-risk groups with culturally appropriate teaching tools. Based on research conducted in Amish communities, school-based tools, including storyboards, safety curricula, and test questions, were provided to private schools in Amish communities in eight US states. Burn prevention knowledge was significantly improved by use of this tool [217, 218].

In the rapidly evolving environment of social media, novel opportunities are available to help prevent burn injuries. In 2013, 21 videos were posted on YouTube with technically accurate content covering prevention and first-aid treatment of pediatric burns [219]. Due to the ease of access and wide audience (over six billion hours of video are watched each month on YouTube), exciting opportunities exist to use these platforms to raise public awareness of burn prevention and treatment, although validation of content by qualified health care professionals is still a challenge.

Engineering (modification of agents or environment) and enforcement (creation and implementation of guidelines, codes, and laws) require more resources but are also more effective. Several examples of successful approaches to reduce the incidence or severity of burns can serve as interventions.

2.6.1 Smoke Detectors

During combustion, the combined hazards of heat and smoke intensify over time to a point at which environmental conditions are incompatible with life. Between the time at which the fire is discovered and the critical point at which escape is impossible is a period during which actions can be taken to minimize or prevent injury. The role of early detection systems is to lengthen this interval. (In some cases, when victims are overcome by hypoxia and CO poisoning while asleep or intoxicated, there is effectively no interval time period for action.) Data from the United Kingdom, which tracks the interval between the time of ignition and the time of discovery, confirm that smoke alarms result in quicker fire discovery. Sixty-three percent of the home fires in which the alert was set off by the smoke alarm were discovered within 5 min of ignition, and the fire was confined to the item of origin in 62% of these incidents (Department for Communities and Local Government [220]).

Early detection systems include different types of fire warning equipment such as sprinklers and devices that detect heat or smoke.[6] From 1977 to 1982, a rapid increase in the number of homes protected by smoke alarms was followed by a slower but continual rise in installation, through 1993. Although the prevalence of usage has leveled since then, 96% of homes surveyed by telephone reported having at least one working smoke alarm (US Fire Administration [221, 222]). The death rate per 100 reported home structure fires from 2003 to 2006 in the United States was twice as high when no working smoke alarm was operative (i.e., either no smoke alarm was present or an alarm was present but did not operate) compared to the rate with working smoke alarms (1.16 vs. 0.59). Having a working smoke alarm cuts the chances of dying in a residential fire in half [223]. The effectiveness of smoke alarm distribution projects can be greatly enhanced by community canvassing programs that involve both the local fire departments and community health workers [224].

Inversely correlating with the rise in the usage of smoke detectors has been the decline in residential fire and flame deaths. The age-adjusted death rate in 1981 from residential fires was 2.28; by 1997 that rate was reduced by almost 50% (Fig. 2.4; [20]). Although smoke alarms have contributed significantly to this reduction in mortality, other factors have been beneficial as well, including safer heating and cooking appliances; child-resistant lighters; flame-resistant mattresses, furniture, and clothing; and improvement in acute care of burn victims.

Laws in many US states and the District of Columbia require smoke alarms to be installed in both new and existing buildings. Other states have laws governing specific conditions, such as new home construction, multifamily dwellings, or rental properties. As a result, burn injuries have decreased by 26% and deaths decreased by 31% [68].

These efforts to promote smoke detectors are best combined with accompanying educational efforts so that build-

[6]Photoelectric detectors pass a beam of light above a sensor. Under normal conditions, the light beam passes above the sensor with no deflection of light to the sensor, which is positioned at 90 degrees from the light beam. However, when smoke particles in the air cause some of the light to scatter, some of the light is dispersed to the sensor, which then triggers the alarm. Photoelectric alarms respond sooner to fires that begin with a long period of smoldering without flames. Ionizing detectors contain a small amount of Americium-241, which emits *alpha* particles. The Americium ionizes the oxygen and nitrogen in the air of the ionization chamber, causing a small current to flow between the two plates in the chamber. The presence of smoke in the chamber disrupts this current flow, which is then detected and triggers the alarm. Ionizing detectors respond quickly in flaming fires.

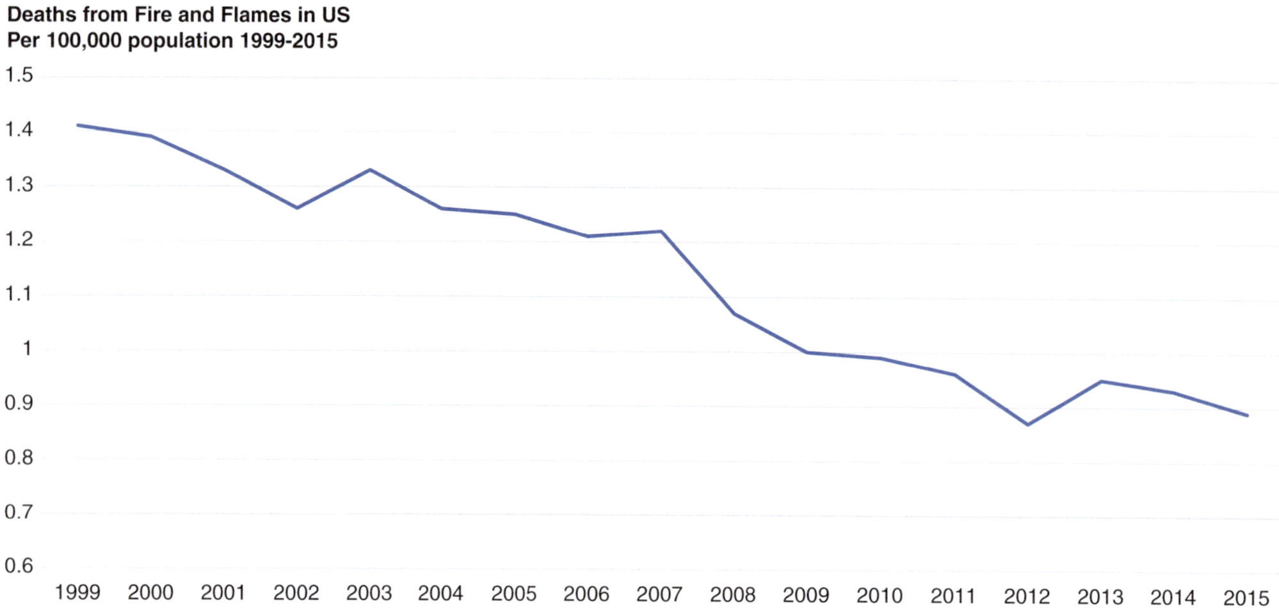

Fig. 2.4 Deaths from fire and burns in the United States have declined from a rate of 1.41 per 100,000 in 1999 to 0.89 per 100,000 in 2015, according to the Web-based Injury Statistics Query and Reporting System of the Centers for Disease Control and Prevention (http://webappa.cdc.gov/sasweb/ncipc/mortrate.html). (CDC accessed on 18 Sept 2017) Residential fire deaths cause the majority of deaths due to fire and burns in the United States, ranging from 70 to 80% each year. Age-adjusted death rates from residential fires declined an average of 20% every 5 years from 1981 to 1991. The decrease in residential fire death rates recently has been less remarkable, with only a 12% decrease from 2010 to 2015

ing occupants develop and rehearse escape plans in advance. Likewise, plans should be made as to whether ancillary devices, such as escape ladders might be necessary [225]. Installing, testing, and maintaining smoke alarms are critical for protection from a residential fire, but these actions are not enough. A smoke alarm merely sounds the warning but it cannot by itself remove people from harm. Unfortunately, many households have not developed the escape plans that would allow them to use to best advantage the extra warning time smoke alarms provide. Escape plans should identify obstacles to secondary exits if the main door is blocked, establish a meeting place outside the home for household members to gather, and make provisions for disabled, young or old household members [223].

In one US study, almost two thirds of home fire deaths resulted from fires in properties without sounding smoke alarms. In 2003–2006, smoke alarms were present in roughly two-thirds (69%) of reported home fires and sounded alerts in roughly half (47%) of the home fires reported to US fire departments. Forty percent of home fire deaths resulted from fires in which no smoke alarms were present at all. Twenty-three percent of the deaths were caused by fires in properties in which smoke alarms were present but failed to operate [223].

Despite the dissemination of smoke detectors into homes, 2704 people died in 2006 from residential fires [20]. Although the death rate in residential fires is doubled if smoke alarms are either not installed or not functional, the presence of functional alarms does not eliminate the risk of death. Functional smoke alarms were found in 34% of residential fire deaths from 2000 to 2004, and the mortality rate in residences with functional smoke alarms was 0.55 per 100,000 [221]. The households with smoke alarms that do not work now outnumber the households with no alarms by a substantial margin [223]. Any program established to ensure adequate protection must include smoke alarm maintenance. In one fifth of all homes with smoke alarms, none were working [223].

In reality, people do not always evacuate when fire alarms sound. Fire alarms are intended to meet four objectives: (1) warn occupants, (2) stimulate them to respond immediately, (3) initiate the evacuation process, and thus (4) provide enough time to escape. In truth, however, rather than assuming that a fire is occurring, people who hear a fire alarm tend to seek the reason for the alarm, such as the smell of smoke. Once they do recognize a fire, instead of calling the fire department and evacuating, they may engage in other activities such as fighting the fire or collecting belongings. People often fail to respond for a variety of reasons: (1) the signal is sometimes not recognized as a fire alarm, being misinterpreted as a burglar, elevator, or security door alarm; (2) sometimes people do not know what they should do, particularly if they are outside the home environment such as in a commercial space; (3) because of nuisance alarms, people may not believe the smoke alarm signals are a real danger; and (4) because of distance from the alarm, background noise, or individual characteristics, they may not hear the signal [226].

Studies of unwanted alarms have consistently shown that smoke alarms produce far more nuisance activations than real alarms. A study of Veterans Administration hospitals found one unwanted activation for every six devices per year and 15.8 unwanted activations for every real alarm [227]. The 2000 New Zealand smoke alarm installation follow-up study found that smoke alarms provided warnings of actual fires in 7% of the households, but 38% of the households reported problems with nuisance alarms [228].

Regrettably, for some people, the stress of nuisance alarms outweighs the benefit of smoke alarm protection. A study in the United Kingdom during 1999–2002 conducted group and individual interviews with adults and children to explore the perceptions of fire risk, the benefits and problems associated with smoke alarms, and whether they would recommend smoke alarms to others. Some adults described feeling very stressed by false alarms and expressed resentment about the smoke alarm going off during what was perceived as normal cooking. The perception of some children was that smoke alarms activated any time someone was cooking. As a consequence, smoke alarm activations were not viewed as emergencies. The authors remarked, "In a population already managing a range of health risks, a public health intervention that makes mealtime more, rather than less, stressful, and where noise can threaten leisure or relationships with fellow occupants, alarms could pose a threat to immediate wellbeing" [229].

A Cochrane review of interventions to promote residential smoke alarms, assess their effect on the prevalence of owned and working smoke alarms, and assess the incidence of fires and burns was performed with controlled (randomized or nonrandomized) trials published between 1969 and 2007 [230]. Of 26 completed trials, 17 were randomized. Counseling and educational interventions, with or without allocation of free or discounted smoke alarms, only modestly increased the likelihood of owning an alarm (OR 1.36) and having an installed, functional alarm (OR 1.29). Only one randomized controlled trial reported injury outcomes, and no effect was found on injuries, hospitalizations, or deaths from a smoke alarm donation program. Two trials showed that smoke alarm installation programs increase the likelihood of having a working smoke alarm, and one of these studies also noted a reduction in fire-related injuries. The reviewers concluded that (1) programs to promote smoke alarms have only a modest beneficial effect on ownership and function, (2) programs to promote smoke alarms have no demonstrated beneficial effects on fires or fire-related injuries, (3) community smoke alarm donation programs neither increase smoke alarm prevalence or reduce fires and injuries, and (4) community smoke alarm installation programs increase the prevalence of functional alarms and decrease injuries [213]. A paucity of the type of data needed by practitioners and policymakers who are seeking to implement smoke alarm promotion interventions challenges their work [231].

In 2003–2006, smoke alarms were present but did not sound in 23% of the home fire deaths [223]. When smoke alarms were not present on all floors of the residence, they sounded in only 4% of the fires and alerted occupants in only 2% of the fires [223]. On the other hand, when interconnected smoke alarms are present on all floors, they sounded in half the fires and alerted occupants 26% of the time [223]. Whereas hardwired alarms operated 91% of the time, battery-powered alarms sound in only 75% of fires [223]. Of the alarms that failed to operate, 75% had missing, disconnected or dead batteries [223].

In a study in Dallas from 1991 to 1998, smoke alarms showed no protective efficacy in preventing burn injuries or fire deaths in fires started by arson or by children playing with matches or lighters, although alarms conferred protection against injuries and deaths from all other causes [89]. In rural North Carolina in 1988, the absence of a smoke alarm was relatively more lethal in the case of fires in which children were present, and when no one in the house was impaired by alcohol or drug use. Moreover, the presence or absence of a smoke alarm had no correlation with the risk of death when a person with either a cognitive impairment or physical disability was present [106].

In 1998 the Centers for Disease Control and Prevention, the US Fire Administration, the Consumer Product Safety Commission, and several other national organizations combined efforts to develop the Smoke Alarm Installation and Fire Education (SAIFE) Program. The plan includes recruiting local communities and community partners, hiring a local coordinator, canvassing neighborhood homes, installing long-lasting lithium-powered smoke alarms, and providing general fire safety education and 6-month follow-up to determine alarm functionality. This program has demonstrated 90% functional alarms in follow-up surveys (of those the program installed), potentially saving 610 lives in the 16 states involved [232].

Unfortunately, LMIC provide only scarce data on utilization of smoke alarms. In Mexico, only 9% of homes in the upper socioeconomic stratum had smoke alarms, and none of the homes in the poorest stratum had alarms. An injury prevention educational campaign that included promotion of smoke alarm installation and use had no effect on the use of smoke alarms. This was not surprising, however, considering that smoke alarms could not be purchased in any of the nearby retail stores [233]. Clearly, more work is needed in LMIC, starting with an analysis of the impact of residential fires on injury and mortality.

An Alaskan study compared photoelectric and ionization smoke alarms in rural Eskimo Inupiat villages and ionization smoke alarms where the home area averaged roughly 1000 square feet or less. At the time of follow-up after installation, 81% of the ionization homes had working smoke alarms compared to 96% of the homes with photoelectric devices. Ninety-two percent of the ionization homes but only 11% of the photoelectric homes had experienced at least one false alarm. Ninety-three percent of the 69 ionization false alarms were due to cooking as were four of the six of the photoelectric false alarms. False alarms were more common in homes that were smaller, that used wood fuel for heat, and in which the smoke alarms were located near the cooking areas. Thus photoelectric alarms may be the preferred choice for homes with limited living space, an observation that is relevant as smoke alarm installation programs are advanced in LMIC.

The following are recommendations for use of smoke alarms from the National Fire Protection Association (www.nfpa.org/smokealarms):

- Ensure that smoke alarms are working by testing monthly, replacing batteries at least yearly, and performing maintenance as instructed by the manufacturer. (Use of lithium batteries ensures that the alarm will function for several years. All alarms should be replaced every 8–10 years, because of dust and moisture accumulation, clouding of the receptor and lens of photoelectric devices, and degradation of Americium-421 in ionization alarms.)
- Smoke alarms should be installed on every level of the home, outside each sleeping area, and inside each bedroom.
- Smoke alarms should be interconnected, so that a fire detected by any of them will trigger the other alarms to sound.
- Develop an escape plan, so that all occupants know what to do when a smoke alarm sounds.
- Use both ionization and photoelectric alarms because their effectiveness varies with how much flame is present in the fire.
- Install smoke alarms at a safe distance from nuisance sources, such as kitchen stoves, to minimize the number of nuisance alarms. Under no circumstances should an alarm be disabled because of repeated nuisance alarms—it should be replaced or repositioned.

2.6.2 Residential Sprinklers

Prevention of burn injuries and fire deaths, as well as amelioration of fire damages, is effectively and efficiently accomplished through the combined use of smoke detectors and sprinkler systems [234]. Smoke detectors are triggered in the initial moments of the fire event; sprinklers act throughout the event to minimize spread of the fire and in some cases extinguish it. The National Fire Protection Association estimates that the fire death rate in 2003–2006 was 80% lower in structures protected by sprinklers. In homes with both smoke detectors and sprinklers, the chance of surviving a residential fire is nearly 97% [235].

However, neither smoke detectors nor sprinklers nor a combination of the two will work effectively to protect certain individuals, including victims

- Who act irrationally, return to the fire after safely escaping, or are unable to act to save themselves, such as people who are physically disabled, bedridden or under restraint
- Whose clothing is on fire and sustain fatal fire injuries from fires too small to activate smoke detectors or sprinklers
- Who are unusually vulnerable to fire effects, such as older adults, and those impaired by alcohol or drugs

Unfortunately, fewer than 2% of US single-family dwellings are fitted with sprinkler systems [236]. San Clemente, California, was the first US jurisdiction to mandate installation of sprinklers in all new residential structures. The cost of installation of sprinkler systems in new houses is approximately \$1–\$2 per square foot; retrofitting sprinklers in existing buildings is somewhat more expensive but is comparable to the cost of purchasing and installing new carpeting.

2.6.3 Hot Water Temperature Regulation

Although scald burns are nearly as common as flame burns, particularly in children, across the globe in 2002 only 5.4% of all burn deaths were attributed to scalds; 93% of deaths were fire-related [15]. Hot tap water causes nearly one-quarter of all pediatric scald burns, and most of these occur in the bathroom. The damage caused by hot tap water burns tends to be more severe than that by other types of scald burns [68]. Experiments on human subjects have shown that partial- or full-thickness burns occur only after 6 h of exposure if water is at 111 °F (44 °C). Yet if the temperature of the water is increased to 140 °F (60 °C), burns occur within 3 s of exposure [237]. Because water at 120 °F (49 °C) takes 10 min to cause significant thermal injury to the skin, hot water heaters are ideally set at this temperature to allow people to escape the damaging effects in time.

In HIC among all childhood age groups, those under age 5 years are at highest risk for hospitalization for burns, and nearly 75% of these burns are from hot liquid, hot tap water or steam [15]. For instance, 100% of burns to children admitted from 1994 through 2004 to two burn centers in Finland resulted from hot water scalds [238]. A hospital-based survey in France during 1991–1992 noted that 17% of childhood burn injuries were due to scalds [239]. However, a large proportion of scald burns in children are treated in clinics and emergency rooms without requiring hospitalization.

In 1977 in Washington State, 80% of homes had tap water temperatures greater than 129 °F (54 °C). In 1983 a Washington State law was passed, requiring new water heaters to be preset at 120 °F (49 °C). Five years later, 77% of homes (84% of homes with postlaw and 70% of homes with prelaw water heaters) had tap water temperatures of less than 129 °F (54 °C). Mean temperature in 1988 was 122 °F (50 °C) compared with 142 °F (61 °C) in 1977. Few people increased their heater temperature after installation. Compared with the 1970s, numbers of patients admitted for treatment of scald burns, as well as TBSA burned, mortality, grafting, scarring, and length of hospital stay for scald burns, were all reduced. The combination of education and legislation seems to have resulted in a reduction in frequency, morbidity, and mortality of tap water burn injuries in children [240].

In the mid-1980s in Wisconsin, an educational campaign, which included free thermometers mailed with utility bills, resulted in the reduction in the temperature of an estimated 20,000 hot water heaters [241]. A similar study in Dunedin, New Zealand, of a national media campaign combined with educational interventions to households with young children noted a reduction of 50% in the number of homes with hot water heater temperatures over 158 °F (70 °C). However, the majority of households still maintained temperatures above 131 °F (55 °C) at the end of the intervention [242].

The first state legislation regulating water temperatures was a bill passed in Florida in May 1980, which mandated preset water heater temperatures to no higher than 125 °F (52 °C). Legislation now exists within the administrative code concerning the regulation of tap water temperature for the District of Columbia and 47 states. In addition, hospitals and related health care facilities often have building codes that limit the temperature of hot water supplied to the patients. A majority of states has also adopted a model plumbing code developed by a standards organization, such as the International Code Council (ICC) or International Association of Plumbing and Mechanical Officials (IAPMO), and amend the code to fit their regional needs. These codes not only differ in their individual content but by their differing editions as well. Different editions of each code can be adopted by different jurisdictions, making plumbing legislation even less uniform across the United States. Besides having several different codes to choose from, the application of the code differs from state to state. Some states enforce a state-wide code, while others allow the code to be amended by individual counties. Moreover, different states may apply the code toward only certain buildings. Thus there is no uniform national standard for tap water temperature regulation. Instead, the US system comprises state and local jurisdictions adopting a variety of codes and applying them inconsistently across counties and cities. These codes and regulations attempt to reduce scald burns, but because of the lack of uniformity, tap water scalds still remain a serious issue.

Building service engineers are directed to store and operate hot water systems at a temperature of 140 °F (60 °C) to prevent outbreaks of Legionnaires' disease. To prevent scald burns from direct exposure to water at this temperature, mixing valves can be installed in the hot water supply pipework to provide hot water at safe temperatures for bathing, showering and washing. Thermoscopic or thermostatic mixing valves were developed and first marketed in 1979. Thereafter, the UK Department of Health and Social Security issued a recommendation that the suitable reduction in water temperature from the heating source (recommended 60 °C) to the tap (recommended 52 °C) should be achieved by a "suitable mixing arrangement" [243]. In the United Kingdom, Electricity Association Technology Ltd. (EATL) investigated the performance of automatic mixing valves in 1992. EATL found that although the valves studied all performed equally well at mixing hot and cold water when the supply was constant, clear differences in function among the valves occurred during a loss of cold water supply (as might happen in the household during bathing or showering when another water appliance is activated, such as when a toilet is flushed or a washing machine is turned on) [244].

2.6.4 Lamps and Stoves

Although there is slow progress in providing electricity to residences, less than one quarter of Africans had access to electricity in 2005 [245]. The global use of kerosene in lamps and stoves will no doubt continue for years to come. Unfortunately, many low-income families use makeshift lamps from wicks placed in discarded beverage or medicine bottles, and even from burned-out light bulbs [15]. Burns caused by homemade bottle lamps or commercial wick lamps are common in LMIC [246, 247].

Prevention of lamp burns in LMIC includes three approaches. The first is educational campaigns that promulgate safe behavior with kerosene lamps, including avoiding replenishment of the fuel reservoir while the wick is lit, and placing the lamps on stable surfaces. One study in low-income South African communities demonstrated limited but demonstrable success in educating those at highest risk [248]. Another approach is to use safer oil, such as vegetable oils (i.e., coconut and sesame oils). Unfortunately, these oils are too heavy to rise to the top of the wick and do not perform well.

The third option is to provide impoverished families with an inexpensive lamp that is designed with safety in mind. Such a lamp is currently being produced and marketed in Sri Lanka. This lamp is short and heavy so that it does not easily tip over, and has two flat sides that prevent it from rolling if it does tip over. The screw-top lid averts fuel spillage, and the thick glass with which it is made prevents breakage if the lamp falls. This lamp is produced from recycled glass at the low cost of only US$ 0.35 each, and its production pro-

Table 2.4 Haddon Matrix applied to the problem of residential fires in LMIC due to non-electric domestic appliances

	Host/human factors	Object/substance	Physical environment	Sociocultural environment
Pre-event	• Wear tight clothing • Keep water and dry sand at hand • Teach consumers safe techniques for use	• Identify safer fuels • Change appliance design • Provide pictograms with operating instructions • Safer containers for kerosene • Teach safe fuel use techniques	• Store fuels in clearly marked, red containers • Teach consumers how to assess kerosene for quality before purchase • Place stoves on stable surfaces, away from flammable substances and out of reach of children	• Prevent kerosene contamination • Create political or economic leverage for adoption of design improvement • Legislate for design regulations and enforcement • Use evidence-based research to support advocacy and programs • Implement building codes • Develop safety curricula in schools • Train caregivers and health workers • Train volunteers to observe risky behaviors and unsafe practices
Event	• "Stop, drop and roll" when clothing catch fire • Use blankets to smother clothing flames • Use water or sand to extinguish structure fires	• Turn off device if possible when fire starts	• Have emergency contact information nearby	• Prepare neighbors to intervene in putting out fires and assisting victims
Post-event	• Appropriate first aid • Acute care for burns • Rehabilitation for injuries	• Discard faulty equipment	• Clean and retrofit environment with regard to future prevention	• Educate community using event as an example

vides a boost to the local economy. Its use has been credited with a significant reduction in burn injuries and fires in Sri Lanka [249].

The use of kerosene stoves is even more widespread than that of homemade lamps, and the magnitude of injury, death, and destruction that accompanies kerosene stoves places a tremendous burden on low-income communities. The conceptual framework the for prevention of these injuries lends itself to the Haddon Matrix [250]. Table 2.4 is an inventory of options for interventions in all three time dimensions (pre-event, event, and post-event) including education programs, environmental modifications, and enforcement of existing or creation of new legislation.

Multiple options outlined in this table appear to be suitable for application in many LMIC. Clearly much could be accomplished by addressing issues of verification of fuel quality, safety of fuel storage and usage, and dispersion of appropriately designed appliances. Compulsory standards covering the performance, safety, and homologation requirements for nonpressure paraffin-fueled cooking stoves and heaters intended primarily for domestic use were put into effect by the South African government on January 1, 2007 [251]. These standards were developed after the evaluation of nine commonly used stove designs in 2003 showed that not one of the designs met the current national standards. Currently, the South African National Standard (SANS) 1906:2006 standard for nonpressure stoves and heaters is the only compulsory standard in place. Only one heater has a license to trade under this standard—the Goldair Heater model RD85A. The new PANDA stove holds a temporary license under this standard. The standard for pressurized kerosene-fueled appliances (SANS 1243:2007) is currently voluntary and none of the pressure appliances on the market have applied for approval from the South Africa Bureau of Standards Commercial against this standard [252].

Feasibility and cost of implementation of such regulations are often the final barriers to improvements in burn prevention. Enforcement of regulations and codes depends not only upon government commitment but also upon consumer investment in the plan. It is essential that consumers are informed and use their purchasing power to insist that manufacturers, distributors, and suppliers of appliances adhere to existing safety standards. Local and regional government health departments should use their influence to support the standards and their enforcement. The public and government should insist on appropriate standards approval before purchasing appliances destined for domestic use regardless of whether the relevant applicable standard is voluntary or compulsory. Such an approach requires intensive educational campaigns both for the community and for relevant government agencies.

2.6.5 Fireworks Legislation

Nearly 10,000 people were treated for firework-related injuries in the US emergency departments in 2007 [68, 253]. Boys between the ages of 5 and 15 years have the highest injury rates. Nearly 4200 children under the age of 15 years were admitted to emergency departments in the US in 2002 for treatment of firework-related injuries. Similarly, the association between boys and fireworks injuries has been noted in other countries, such as Australia and Greece [254, 255]. Almost 33,000 fires were started by fireworks in 2006 in the United States, resulting in six deaths, 70 injuries, and $34 million in property damages [97].

The injuries caused by fireworks can be very severe because of heat production (temperatures of ignited devices may exceed 1200 °F) and blast effect. Only approximately 50% of treated fireworks injuries in the United States are burns; approximately one third are contusions or lacerations, and one quarter affect the eyes [94, 97]. In Northern Ireland, over half of the patients with fireworks injuries present with blast injuries to the hand [256]. The use of illegal fireworks accounts for only 8% of the injuries; most injuries in the United States occur while using fireworks approved by Federal regulations. Sparklers and small firecrackers cause 40% of fireworks injuries. The risk of fire death relative to exposure makes fireworks one of the riskiest consumer products available in the United States [97].

Fireworks are associated with national and cultural celebrations throughout the world [150]. On Independence Day in the United States each year, more fires are reported than on any other day of the year [97]. As a prelude to the arrival of spring, Persians since at least 1700 BCE have celebrated Chahārshanbe-Sūri on the last Wednesday night of each year. The festivities include participants jumping over bonfires in the streets and setting off fireworks, both hazardous activities. Despite the ubiquity of these practices in Iran and their persistence since ancient times, in 2007 in Tehran only 1% of surveyed families acknowledged having any education on the safe use of fireworks; over 98% of families were ignorant of fireworks safety standards [257].

Fireworks have been regulated in the United Kingdom since 1875, starting with laws covering the manufacture, storage, supply, and behavior in the presence of gunpowder. In particular, the last decade has seen the passage of several pieces of fireworks legislation in the United Kingdom [258]. The US Consumer Product Safety Commission (CPSC) has regulated consumer fireworks safety since the 1970s. Current regulations prohibit the sale of the most dangerous types of fireworks, including large reloadable shells, "cherry bombs," aerial bombs, M-80s, "silver salutes," and aerial fireworks containing more than two grains (130 mg) of powder. Other firecrackers and ground devices are limited to only 50 mg of powder, which is the pyrotechnic composition designed to produce an audible effect ("bang"). Also regulated are the composition of the materials (hazardous materials such as arsenic and mercury are proscribed), the length of time fuses must burn (at least three but no more than 9 s), and the stability of the bases [259].

Access to all fireworks is banned in the US states of Delaware, Massachusetts, New Jersey, New York, and Rhode Island. Arizona allows the exclusive use of novelty fireworks, and only sparklers are permitted in Illinois, Iowa, Maine, Ohio, and Vermont [260]. The impact of legislation on the incidence of firework-related injuries is unclear. In the United Kingdom, presumably because of the proliferation of fireworks legislation, the number of fireworks injuries dropped from 707 in 2001 to 494 in 2005 [258]. Another opportunity for studying the efficacy of fireworks legislation occurs when restrictions are neutralized. After repeal of a law banning private fireworks in Minnesota, the number of children suffering firework-related burns increased [261]. However, this increase was not observed after liberalization of fireworks laws in Northern Ireland [256].

Reduction in firework-related injuries has been observed elsewhere as a result of focused campaigns. In Denmark, where fireworks are commonly used at New Year's celebrations, prohibition of the sale of firecrackers coupled with school education programs led to a reduction in the number of children treated for fireworks injuries at two Danish burn centers: from 17 in 1991–1992 to only three children in 1993–1994 [262].

Passage and enforcement of legislation in LMIC is often challenging, and education programs may currently be the only option for injury prevention in some cases. In India firework injury commonly occur during Diwali (Festival of Lights). One hospital in Mumbai observed that the prevalence of fireworks injuries decreased from 1997 through 2006; the decrease was attributed to aggressive education campaigns by government and nongovernment organizations. Forty-one injuries were treated at the beginning of the study period; only three injuries were treated in 2006 [263].

2.6.6 Fire-Safe Cigarettes

In the United States in 2006, over 140,000 smoking-material (lighted tobacco products) fires led to 780 deaths, 1600 injuries, and $606 million in property damage. The global costs of fires related to cigarette smoking alone are estimated at US$27 Bn [264]. One fourth of all structure fire deaths in the United States involved smoking materials in 2006 [265]. Most fire deaths are associated with the ignition of upholstered furniture, mattresses, and bedding by dropped cigarettes. Sadly, in one-quarter of fatalities from smoking-material fires, it was not the smokers whose cigarettes started the fires. Smoking-material fires were reduced by 57% in the United

States between 1980 and 2006. Both the decline in cigarette consumption as well as standards and regulations that have made mattresses and upholstered furniture more resistant to ignition have contributed to this trend [265].

Smoking-material fires result from the intersection of human behavior, a source of ignition, and a supply of fuel. Prevention of such fires requires modifications of one or more of these factors. Fortunately, cigarette consumption has decreased over 40% since 1980. Modification of smoking behavior includes emphasis on smoking out-of-doors, but efforts to modify smoking behavior are hampered by the relatively high prevalence of alcohol use among those at highest risk for death from residential fires. Newer furniture, mattresses, and bedclothes are more fire resistant, but older models will be more prevalent in low-income housing where the risk of fire is greater. Because cigarettes are the most common source of ignition in fatal residential fires, US consumer safety movements since the 1970s have focused on legislating mandatory production of fire-safe cigarettes [266].

The first bill to address this issue was introduced in 1978 by Rep. Joseph Moakley (D-Mass.), who continued his efforts in this regard in the US House of Representatives for another two decades. By the end of the twentieth century, it was clear that passage of federal laws was progressing too slowly, so the emphasis was redirected toward state laws. In 2003, the first state law requiring all cigarettes to be low-ignition was passed in the state of New York. By the end of 2009, all states except Wyoming had either passed or enacted fire-safe cigarette legislation [267].

A fire-safe cigarette is less likely to burn when left unattended. To achieve this effect, most manufacturers wrap cigarettes with two or three thin bands of less-porous paper. These bands act as "speed bumps" to slow down the rate at which the cigarette burns. If a fire-safe cigarette is left unattended, the burning tobacco will reach one of these speed bumps and extinguish itself. Fire-safe cigarettes meet an established cigarette fire safety performance standard (based on ASTM E2187, Standard Test Method for Measuring the Ignition Strength of Cigarettes) [265].

One year after the New York State law went into effect, researchers from the Harvard School of Public Health compared the physical properties of cigarettes sold in New York with cigarettes sold in Massachusetts and California. Although nearly 100% of cigarettes purchased in those two states burned to the end, only 10% of cigarettes from New York fully burned. The quantity and quality of toxins present in cigarette smoke was not different among the products. Consumer acceptance was acceptable, as evidenced by the observation that tobacco tax income in New York State did not change after the implementation of the law [268].

2.6.7 Children's Sleepwear

Regulation of the manufacture of children's sleepwear exemplify the power of coalitions—including health care experts, safety advocacy groups, technical experts, and government agencies—in responding to the needs of the public. An all-too common cause of severe burn injury in children in the 1960s was ignition of sleepwear[7] (most often by stoves and matches), leaving the young survivors with the scars and complications of third-degree burns. One study found that the average sleepwear fire caused burns over nearly one third of the child's body surface, two thirds of which was third-degree in depth [269].

In 1971, the US Secretary of Commerce delivered a flammability standard for children's sleepwear in the Flammable Fabrics Act. In 1973 the responsibility for administration and enforcement of this act was passed to the US Consumer Product Safety Commission. The primary aim of the standard was to minimize the risk of ignition of children's sleepwear; the secondary aim was to diminish the extent of injury by reducing the speed at which fire would spread after ignition occurred. The mandatory resistance to flammability was applied to all children's sleepwear garments, sizes 0–6x and 7–14. To meet the children's sleepwear standard, the dry garment had to char fewer than 7 in. on its bottom edge after exposed to flame for 3 s [270].

By requiring that children's sleepwear be flame-resistant, these standards helped protect children from burns. A retrospective study of children admitted to the Shriners Burns Institute of Boston during the 8-year period 1969 through 1976 showed that the promulgation of flammability standards reduced the incidence of flame burns from the ignition of sleepwear (Fig. 2.5; [269]). The National Fire Protection Association estimated that the enactment of the flammability standards for sleepwear in 1971 resulted in a tenfold decrease in childhood deaths caused by ignition of sleepwear [271].

However in 1996, amendments to these standards allowed exemption of tight-fitting children's sleepwear and infant garments sized 9 months or smaller.[8] The rationale for relaxation of the standards was that there were decreased sales of sleepwear because daywear was being used for night clothes.[9] CPSC was subsequently challenged by an alliance of stake-

[7]"Sleepwear" is defined as any article of clothing intended to be worn primarily for sleeping or activities related to sleeping. "Daywear" is defined as clothing designed to be worn during the day. However, it is now common to see daywear used at night in place of pajamas, nightgowns, or other traditional night clothes.

[8]Current requirements are published in the Code of Federal Regulations, Title 16, Parts 1615 and 1616.

[9]Although difficult to quantify, the clothing industry's perception of consumers was that sleepwear treated for reduction in flammability was less comfortable (and therefore less popular) than untreated cotton, such as that found in T-shirts.

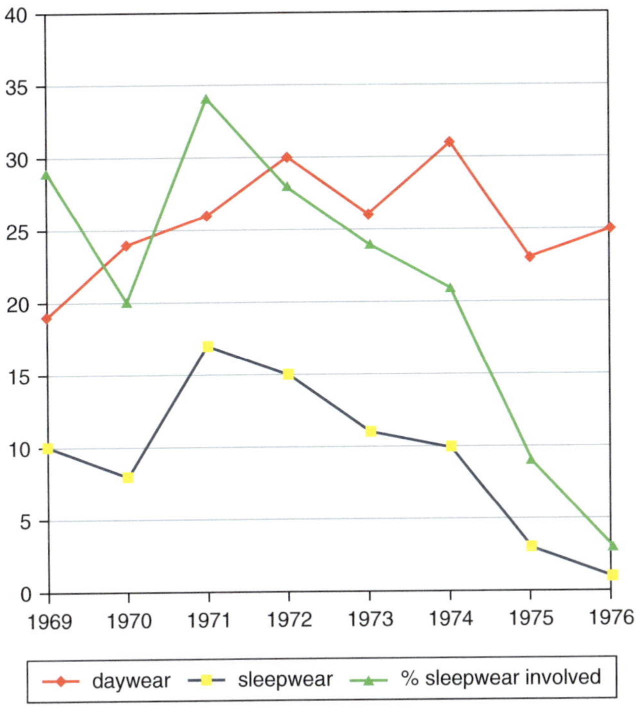

Fig. 2.5 Sleepwear involvement in flame burns at the Boston Shriners Burns Institute 1969–1976 [269]

holders (Safe Children's Sleepwear Coalition) with a mutual interest in the health and safety of children, including the NFPA's Center for High-Risk Outreach, the American Burn Association, and the Shriners Hospitals for Children [272]. In response to this challenge, the CPSC resolved to collect data prospectively using a National Burn Center Reporting System (NBCRS) starting in 2003. The NBCRS was a surveillance system focused on clothing-related burn injuries to children treated in the United States in which children were injured by the ignition, melting or smoldering of clothing. Ninety-two burn centers in the United States participated.

The first report was issued in September 2004 [273]. This analysis scrutinized the cases of 213 victims of 209 incidents, which were submitted by 44 burn centers. Of the 209 reported incidents, only 36 involved clothing worn for sleeping, most of which was daywear.[10] Of those incidents involving sleepwear, none involved tight-fitting sleepwear or infant garments sized 9 months or smaller.

Results from the second report were distributed in a memo dated January 12, 2007. These data were provided by 33 burns centers about 261 children injured in 253 incidents. In only 33 of these incidents were the children injured while wearing clothing that at some point was worn for sleeping. Nineteen of these 33 incidents involved daywear which was being worn for sleeping. Only 14 incidents involved sleepwear subject to the Standards for the Flammability of Children's Sleepwear. As in the first report, there were no incidents involving tight-fitting sleepwear or infant garments sized 9 months or smaller.

The conclusion reached by the author of this memo, Patricia K. Adair, in the Directorate for Engineering Sciences for CPSC, was that the analysis of data from March 2003 through December 2005 revealed no deaths or injuries attributable to the exempted infant size and tight-fitting sleepwear.

Thus the CPSC allowed remain the modifications to the standards. However, there are marketing responsibilities for retailers, distributors, and wholesalers who sell children's sleepwear [259, 274]. They should

1. Not advertise, promote, or sell as children's sleepwear any garment which another party has indicated does not meet the requirements of the children's sleepwear flammability standards and/or are not intended or suitable for use as sleepwear.
2. Place or advertise fabrics and garments covered by the children's sleepwear standards in different parts of a department, store, catalog, or website, from those in which fabrics and garments which may resemble but are not children's sleepwear are sold or marketed.
3. Use store display signs and/or catalog or website notations that point out the difference between different types of fabrics and garments, for example, by indicating which are sleepwear items and which are not.
4. Avoid advertising or promoting garments or fabrics that do not comply with the children's sleepwear standards in a manner that may cause consumers to view those items as children's sleepwear or as being suitable for making such sleepwear.

In a letter dated January 4, 2007, Dr. Russell Roegner, Associate Executive Director of Epidemiology at the US Consumer Product Safety Commission, noted that the study on clothing-related burn injuries to children had ended. The result of data analysis led the CPSC staff to conclude that because more than half of children's clothing fires involved flammable liquids, they had initiated a new project on flammable liquids. To date, the results of the new project on flammable liquids have not been distributed, aside from the publication on September 20, 2008, of a public information safety alert on the dangers of flammable liquids (USCPSC [275]).

In summary, the chronicle of Standards for the Flammability of Children's Sleepwear has ups and downs. Clearly, the institution of these standards back in the early 1970s led to a dramatic reduction in a devastating form of childhood injury. The relaxation of these standards 20 years later shows the effects of the erosion of consumer support as

[10]Daywear is subject to the Standard for the Flammability of Clothing Textiles, but is not subject to the flame-resistant requirements of the Standards for the Flammability of Children's Sleepwear.

well as the power of industry pressure. The inability of the US burn care community to demonstrate convincingly that the relaxation of standards left no mark on the incidence of childhood burns was indeed an illustration of the need for comprehensive, accurate national databases.

2.6.8 Acid Assaults

Although most burns are unintentional injuries, a small proportion occur because of assaults [276]. Chemical attacks have been reported in several countries, including Bangladesh, Cambodia, China, India, Jamaica, Nepal, Nigeria, Pakistan, Saudi Arabia, South Africa, Uganda, the United Kingdom, and the United States. Across the world, male victims are more commonly reported; many of these are associated with robbery or violent crime. Alkali is the agent most commonly used in the United States, but elsewhere the injuries sustained are due to acids [277].

The highest incidence of chemical burns in the world is in Bangladesh [278]. The perpetrators are often scorned suitors, but disagreements over property boundaries and animal ownership are also common instigations. Acids are favored over alkalis because they can be easily obtained from car batteries, jewelry workshops, and leather tanneries [279]. The face and eyes are the usual targets, with the intent being to disfigure or blind or both. Because of the scarcity of treatment options available to the victims, they often unfortunately suffer permanent mutilation, physical disability, psychological devastation, abandonment, and destitution. In the districts wherein such attacks occur, disempowerment of women and gender discrimination are common. Sadly, few perpetrators are punished for their crimes.

One shining light of an effective prevention program for these horrifying injuries is the Acid Survivors Foundation (ASF) of Bangladesh which has been working to reduce acid attacks on children and women since 1999. ASF has been raising public awareness, building institutional capacity and lobbying, and working with other nongovernmental organizations, the media, celebrities, and student groups to elevate community consciousness. ASF has also fostered advocacy and lobbying efforts with the government to ensure the passage and enforcement of laws and to create systems to provide service to acid survivors. As a result, the number of victims has dropped from 490 in 2002 to 171 in 2008 (Fig. 2.6). Based on the success of ASF, similar organizations have been formed in Cambodia, India, Pakistan, and Uganda.

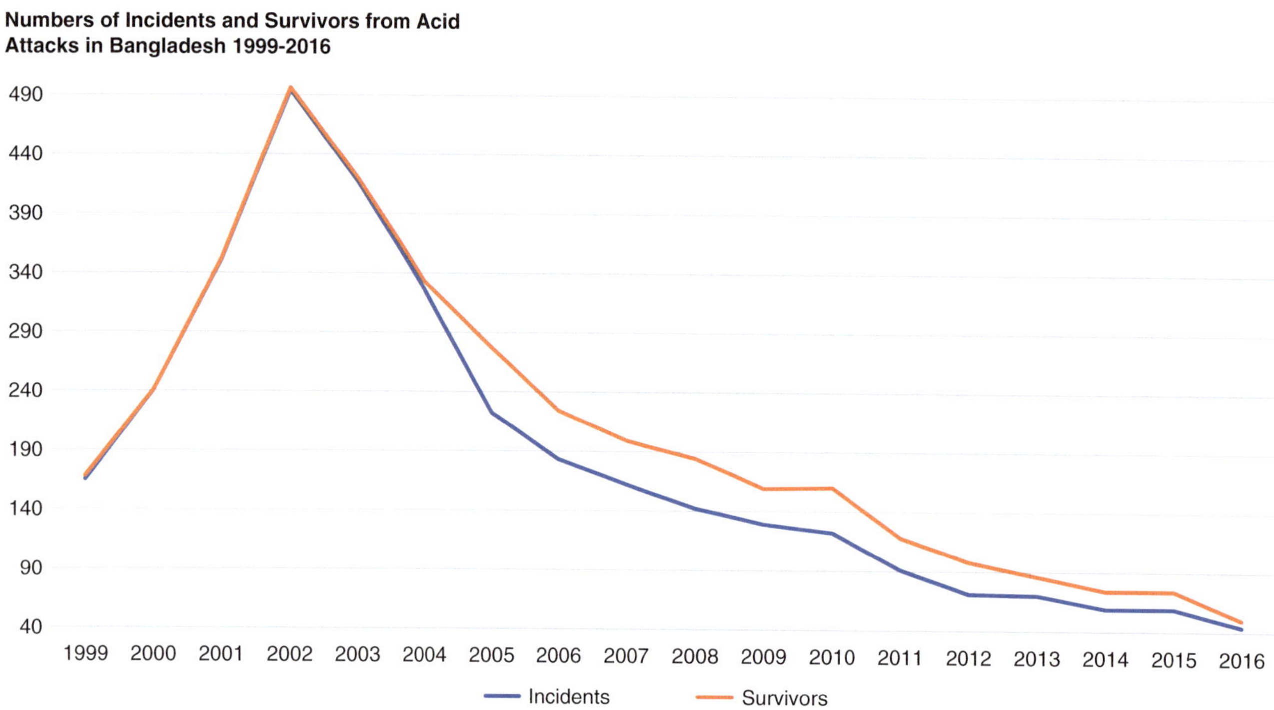

Fig. 2.6 The Acid Survivors Foundation (ASF) of Bangladesh has involved all sectors of society, including students, media, celebrity groups, and nongovernmental organizations, to address the root cause of acid violence, which is gender discrimination and disempowerment of women. ASF and its partners have successfully worked to develop and enforce laws, policies and procedures for combating acid violence. As a result, Bangladesh has seen a decrease in the incidence of acid attacks (http://www.acidsurvivors.org/index.html)

2.6.9 Burns First-Aid Treatment

The goal of injury prevention is to reduce the burden of injuries upon a community. Primary prevention seeks to do this by preventing the injuries from occurring in the first place. However, even with the most effective primary prevention programs in place, burn injuries will continue to occur. Secondary prevention, therefore, is designed to minimize the damage done when a burn occurs.

Appropriate first-aid treatment of burns plays a role in determining outcome by limiting tissue damage and therefore curtailing the depth of the burn. In some cases, particularly with scald burns, appropriate first aid may avert the need for surgical excision and grafting [280–282]. Appropriate first-aid treatment of burns is to apply cool, running water within the temperature range of 50–60 °F as soon as possible after the injury has occurred. Colder water, particularly in victims with larger body surface area burns, may induce hypothermia. Application of ice causes vasoconstriction of the dermal plexus and exacerbates the depth of thermal injury [283–288].

However, the knowledge of appropriate first-aid treatment of burns is widespread neither in the community nor among health care workers. Fewer than 40% of admissions to a regional burn center in Western Australia were treated appropriately following the burn injuries. Twenty percent used no first-aid techniques, and the remainder applied substances such as honey and toothpaste [289]. Similar surveys in Hungary and Vietnam revealed that only approximately one quarter of patients had received appropriate burns first aid [290]. A survey of understanding of appropriate burn first-aid treatment among health care workers showed even more disheartening results, with fewer than 20% of those surveyed able to answer correctly all questions put to them about burn first aid [289].

Nonetheless, appropriate burn first aid can be successfully taught. Public information campaigns in Vorarlberg, Austria, and Jamshedpur, India, have led to an improved understanding of appropriate burns first aid in the community [126, 291]. A multimedia educational campaign about burn first aid in Auckland, New Zealand, resulted in a reduction of inpatient admissions and surgical procedures [292]. Although such public education campaigns are at least temporarily effective, their long-term results are not yet known.

2.6.9.1 Burn Care Systems

Systems for care of injuries within communities is yet another component of secondary prevention. For example, establishment of trauma care systems in the United States has successfully reduced mortality from blunt and penetrating injuries [293]. Although burn centers have been functioning for nearly six decades, a dearth of evidence unfortunately supports their effectiveness at reducing morbidity and mortality. Nonetheless, the bulk of expert opinion defends the need to establish within each region a tertiary care center that can provide acute and rehabilitative care for burn victims, as well as interaction with community and prehospital primary care systems that are responsible for prevention and first aid [294].

Nearly a half million burns are treated by licensed health care providers each year in the United States [295]. Approximately 4000 deaths a year in the United States result from the combination of residential fires (3500) and other causes (500 from motor vehicle and aircraft crashes, scalds, chemical, and electrical injuries). The majority of deaths (75%) occur at the scene, typically from smoke inhalation; however, 40,000 burn patients are admitted to hospitals in the United States each year. These injured patients live within a population of over 300 million people scattered over more than 3.5 million square miles. A system must be put in place to provide regional care for burn injuries throughout the United States, whether that be with numerous small burn units that are geographically close to the patients they serve, or with large regional centers that function efficiently and effectively because of economy of scale [296].

Although emergency care for serious burns is available to most residents of the United States, the care of minor burns is often provided at primary care facilities. In North Carolina in a recent study, 92% of burn injuries were treated by emergency physicians; 4% were admitted and only 4% were transferred to burn centers [32]. Alternatively, specialty hospitals that lack burn centers may provide care to burn patients in consultation with the nearest burn center [297].

In 2008, there were 128 burn centers in the United States, including 51 centers verified by the American Burn Association. Over 45% of the US population lives within 2 h by ground transport from a verified burn center. Nearly 80% of the population lives within 2 h by air transport from a verified center. Regional variation in access to verified burn centers by both ground and rotary air transport was significant. The greatest proportion of the population with access to burn centers was lowest in the southern United States and highest in the northeast region [298].

Fortunately, even at US burn centers the proportion of patients with life-threatening burns is relatively low. The average mortality rate throughout the 62 US burn centers contributing to the ABA NBR was only 4% during the decade 1999–2008 [45]. Seventy-seven percent of patients at burn centers were hospitalized for care of burns to less than 10% of their BSA; the mortality in this subset of patients was only 0.6% [45]. This is true in other HIC, such as Taiwan, ROC, where the overall mortality rate among hospitalized burn patients from 1997 to 2003 was only 3% and the LA50 was 80% TBSA [134].

However, the profile of injury severity and mortality is distinctly different in LMIC. For instance, during the years 1992 to 2000, the mean burn size of over 11,000 patients admitted to a single burn center in Delhi was 50% TBSA, much greater than the 12% TBSA mean burn size of patients whose records were recorded in the ABA NBR during a similar period. Additionally, mortality was also 50% during this period of time in Delhi, compared to only 5% at US burn centers [39, 299]. Such contrasts reflect more on the socioeconomic differences between LMIC and HIC, as well as on the limitation of resources available to burn centers in developing countries. Nonetheless, it is notable that this same burn center in Delhi has reduced the mortality rate down from 50 to 40% during the subsequent time period 2001–2007 [39]. Although the improvement in survival may be related to the rising economic status of India, it is also a tribute to the devotion and dedication of doctors and nurses at resource-restricted burn centers.

The ability of health care systems to provide burn care to a region depends on the availability of human resources (staff and training) and physical resources (infrastructure, supplies and equipment). Resources essential for burn services at all facilities (including outpatient clinics and care provided by nonmedical providers) include training necessary to assess burn wound depth and capability (training and supplies) to apply clean or sterile dressings. Other resources essential for higher levels of facilities (such as specialist or tertiary care centers), involve the capacity for debridement and skin grafting (Table 2.5; [300]).

Table 2.5 Burns and wounds [300]

Resources	Basic	GP	Specialist	Tertiary
Burn depth assessment	E	E	E	E
Sterile dressings	D	E	E	E
Topical antimicrobials	D	E	E	E
Physiotherapy	I	E	E	E
Debridement	I	PR	E	E
Escharotomy	I	PR	E	E
Skin graft	I	PR	E	E
Reconstructive surgery	I	I	D	E
Early excision and grafting	I	I	D	D

Designation of priorities: "E"—essential; "D"—desirable; "PR"—possibly required; "I"—irrelevant

Range of health facilities: "Basic"—outpatient clinics and non-medical providers; "GP"—district hospitals and primary health centers without specialty care; "Specialist"—hospitals with operating rooms and limited surgical personnel; "Tertiary"—hospitals with broad range of subspecialists

2.7 Role of the World Health Organization

This review of burn injuries has made a number of points very clear. A large burden of burn injury-related morbidity and mortality exist in the world; this burden is disproportionately experienced within LMIC; and finally, a number of interventions can be put in place to prevent burns.

However, a deeper look at the facts presented here reveals some other aspects. Although the burden of burn injury and death is experienced primarily in LMIC, the overwhelming majority of scientific papers that underlie the evidence base on interventions to prevent burns come from HIC. Furthermore, the epidemiologic picture of the circumstances giving rise to burns comes almost entirely from HIC, and the papers that provide insight into the etiology of burns in LMIC come from relatively few papers, which have relied on disparate approaches to categorizing all epidemiologic data presented. This fragmented and relatively superficial examination of burn injury in low-income settings means that it is difficult for WHO to be confident in promoting any one course of action as a priority for LMIC to prevent burns. The initial first priority in confronting any public health problem has always been to establish the epidemiologic profile of the problem and elucidate its risk factors.

Accordingly, WHO has been working with a global network of burn experts from the clinical, epidemiologic and research sectors in an effort to improve data collection regarding burns. A first priority has been the Global Burn Registry (GBR). This is a simple, standardized form to gather information about burns; it can be administered easily in health facilities for patients admitted with burn injuries. The data give health facilities a clear picture of the major risk factors and populations at risk for burns in their setting, as well as how these compare and contrast with other settings. This information is key to identify and prioritize programs to prevent burn injuries. Data can be viewed online or exported for further analysis. More information about the GBR, as well as directions to participate in it or access its data, is available on the WHO website (http://www.who.int/en).

Whereas the GBR provides a standardized platform for gathering health-facility-based data, this is insufficient. Many important aspects of burn injuries are best understood with community-based surveys, since these can capture important information about long-term sequelae and can also provide estimates of the burn burden relative to other health conditions. Community-based surveys also provide information on burn injuries that may have been deemed as not requiring health-facility care, or not resulting in facility care because this was too expensive or the injury was so severe that health-facility care could not be provided prior to the patient dying.

Accordingly, WHO has also worked with global burn injury experts and epidemiologists to develop a modular battery of questions for burn injury. These have been developed within the context of an instrument that probes all injury outcomes and then provides more comprehensive information about burns. The community survey module has been pilot tested in LMIC and found to yield valid and relevant information about burns and their sequelae.

Improving, and in particular, developing standardized platforms for data collection on burns is but a first step. Once the global community working on burn care and burn prevention is equipped with and using these tools widely the major etiologic factors that give rise to burns will become clearer, as will the priority risk factors that need to be targeted in order to prevent burns. These steps will require governments and donors to invest in funding operational research, and will require epidemiologists and scholars to set up methodologically rigorous studies to examine burn injuries and how they may be prevented in LMIC.

2.8 Conclusions and Recommendations

2.8.1 Surveillance

The optimal approach to injury prevention includes four stages: surveillance, analysis, intervention, and evaluation. Precise description of the problem(s) is the basis to planning effective interventions, yet in many LMIC, data on burns are scarce, inaccurate, or both. In some countries, a lack of reliable data on risk factors further hampers the development and enactment of effective burn prevention strategies, while in others, incomplete description of burn incidents leads to underassessment of the magnitude of the public health problem. Better surveillance with formal epidemiologic studies, which will more accurately assess the true incidence in vulnerable populations, is needed. A model for such a system can be found in Taiwan, ROC, where the support of the Childhood Burn Foundation provides resources to all 43 hospitals in the country to collect data on hospitalized burn patients. This comprehensive database, which utilizes the Internet for data entry, captured information on over 12,000 patients from 1997 to 2003 [134].

2.8.2 Smoke Alarms

The effectiveness and reliability of smoke alarms can be improved through improvements in technology, including (1) greater waking effectiveness for certain populations, (2) quicker, more certain responses to the range of fire types coupled with reduced nuisance alarms, and (3) more cost-effective ways to interconnect alarms in existing homes. In addition, continued research is needed to improve measurement and performance of smoke alarms. Improvements must be made in educational approaches that change behavior in regard to home escape planning, inspection, and maintenance of smoke alarms, and in developing safe options for dealing with nuisance alarms. Research into human behavior in residential fires is required to determine effective cues, increase the perception of the value of immediate escape, and develop exit skills under stress and strategies to reduce the learned irrelevance of alarms [301].

2.8.3 Transition Away from Open Fires and Kerosene Appliances

An assumption held by some is that the inevitable transition from open fires and kerosene appliances toward more sophisticated devices for cooking, heating, and lighting will result in a diminution of burn injuries in LMIC. However, the current experience suggests that this transition period is not without hazard. In Delhi, for example, LPG-related burns accounted for less than 1% of admissions to a single burn center from 1993 to 2000, but from 2001 to 2007, LPG-related burns were responsible for over 10% of admissions [39]. Electrification can certainly reduce the risk of disasters caused by malfunctioning kerosene stoves but can also lead to a whole new set of hazards from electrical injury because of substandard wiring techniques, unsafe practices, illegal poaching of power and scavenging copper from overhead lines, and inadequate barriers around high-voltage poles and towers. Thus, as developing communities convert to more common use of LPG and electricity, steps must be taken to ensure the safety of the residents.

2.8.4 Gender Inequality

In LIC the burden of burns falls mostly on women and girls, who are at risk of "occupational" injuries while they tend fires and prepare food. Sadly, they are also selected as victims of horrific assaults, such as acid throwing or "bride burning" [276]. The latter is a phenomenon often related to the dissatisfaction of the husband with the wife's dowry and may occur either as self-immolation or as assault by the husband's family [302]. Clearly these particularly tragic events deserve focus above and beyond usual burn prevention efforts. Elimination of acid attacks and bride burning require a multitude of coordinated actions involving passage and enforcement of protective legislation, education of men and boys about appropriate behavior toward women, and resources for women in need of shelter or care.

2.8.5 Community Surveys

Community surveys are needed in the United States to establish the degree to which Hispanics utilize the health care system for treatment of burns. The very low incidence of nonfatal burns in Hispanics treated at US hospital emergency departments suggests that many burns are being treated by families with home remedies. WHO has established guidelines for conducting community surveys on injuries and violence [303].

The few population-based surveys conducted in Bangladesh have demonstrated the tremendous utility of this approach, clearly outlining not only the true incidence of burns within the community, but also the extent of disability and death that accompany burns. A national injury survey administered in Bangladesh [29–31, 95] generated comprehensive burns data, and district-level injury surveys in Vietnam [304] and Nepal [305] reported burns incidence rates. The Global Alliance for Clean Cookstoves (GACC), advised by a panel of burns experts, has supported the development of a burns survey module which was field-tested in two districts of Nepal in 2016 (H. Wallace, personal communication). Only with an accurate appreciation of the burden of burn injuries within a region can effective lobbying efforts move forward in funding agencies and government health departments. The integration of key questions on burns into recurring national household surveys (i.e., the Demographic and Health Survey [DHS] and the Multiple Indicator Cluster Survey [MICS]), to understand trends in the incidence of burns, health-seeking behavior, and outcomes, is the next step to ensure feasibility of data collection. Another application of burns surveillance is to evaluate the impact of potential burn prevention interventions, for example, clean/fuel-efficient cookstoves. The GACC burns survey module is being developed into a user-friendly tool for this purpose (H. Wallace, personal communication).

Summary Box

Burns contribute a significant proportion of the morbidity and mortality attributed to injuries throughout the world. In 2015, incidence of burns severe enough to require hospital outpatient presentation or an admission to hospital was 31 million people. Low- and middle-income countries represent a disproportionately high level of burn injury incidence and mortality. Differences in burn mechanism are also noted across income distributions. Although the vast majority of burn injuries are not fatal, much of the impact of burns is emotional, psychological and spiritual. Data collection specific to burn etiologies has been challenging. Risk factors for injury include socioeconomic, race and ethnicity, age-related factors (children and the elderly), regional factors, gender related factors, intent, comorbidity. Responsible agents include flame burns and scalds from residential fires, non-domestic electric appliances, and the results of war, mass casualties, and terrorism. Prevention is the key to alleviation of pain and suffering as well as mitigation of costs, and multiple interventions have been initiated. The effectiveness of education programs may be enhanced by targeting specific at-risk groups with culturally appropriate teaching tools, including social media. Engineering (modification of agents or environment) and enforcement (creation and implementation of guidelines, codes and laws) require more resources, but are also more effective. The optimal approach to injury prevention includes four stages: surveillance, analysis, intervention and evaluation. Establishment of burn care systems such as trauma centers is an important component of secondary prevention. The ability of health care systems to provide burn care to a region depends on the availability of human and physical (infrastructure, supplies and equipment) resources. The World Health Organization in concert with international burn experts from the clinical, epidemiologic and research sectors has developed the Global Burn Registry (GBR) as a first priority. Improving, and in particular, developing standardized platforms for data collection on burns is but a first step. Once the global community working on burn care and prevention is equipped with and using these tools widely, the major etiologic factors that give rise to burns will become clearer, as will the priority risk factors that need to be targeted in order to better prevent burns.

Acknowledgments The authors wish to express their gratitude to Belinda Gabbe, David Meddings, Andrea Sattinger, and Hilary Wallace for their assistance.

References

1. Baker SP, O'Neill B, Ginsburg MJ, Guohua L. The injury fact book. 2nd ed. Lexington, MA: Lexington Books; 1992.
2. GBD 2015 Mortality and Causes of Death Collaborators. Global, regional, and national life expectancy, all-cause mortality, and cause-specific mortality for 249 causes of death, 1980-2015: a systematic analysis for the Global Burden of Disease Study 2015. Lancet. 2016;388:1459–544.
3. World Health Organization. The global burden of disease: 2004 update. Geneva: World Health Organization; 2008. http://www.who.int/healthinfo/global_burden_disease/GBD_report_2004update_full.pdf. Accessed 20 Sept 2017.
4. World Health Organization. Global Health Estimates 2000–2015. 2015a. http://www.who.int/healthinfo/global_burden_disease/en/. Accessed 22 Sept 2017.
5. Halawa EF, Barakat A, Rizk HI, Moawad EM. Epidemiology of non-fatal injuries among Egyptian children: a community-based cross-sectional survey. BMC Public Health. 2015;15:1248.
6. World Health Organization. Burns. 2015b. http://www.who.int/violence_injury_prevention/other_injury/burns/en/. Accessed 29 Nov 2015.

7. World Health Organization. Global health estimates 2015: disease burden by cause, age, sex, by Country and by Region, 2000–2015. Geneva, World Health Organization. 2015c. http://www.who.int/healthinfo/global_burden_disease/estimates/en/index2.html. Accessed 8 Aug 2017.
8. Thapa NB. Report of injury survey in Bhumisthan Village Panchayat Dhadhing and in Bir Hospital Kathmandu. National Programmes on Accident and Injury Prevention. Stockholm: National Board of Health and Welfare; 1989.
9. Aldana MC, Navarrete N. Epidemiology of a decade of pediatric fatal burns in Colombia, South America. Burns. 2015;41:1587–92.
10. Hwee J, Song C, Tan KC, Tan BK, Chong SJ. The trends of burns epidemiology in a tropical regional burns centre. Burns. 2016;42:682–6.
11. Saeman MR, Hodgman EI, Burris A, Wolf SE, Arnoldo BD, Kowalske KJ, et al. Epidemiology and outcomes of pediatric burns over 35 years at Parkland Hospital. Burns. 2016;42:202–8.
12. Santos JV, Oliveira A, Costa-Pereira A, Amarante J, Freitas A. Burden of burns in Portugal, 2000–2013: a clinical and economic analysis of 26,447 hospitalisations. Burns. 2016;42:891–900.
13. Smolle C, Cambiaso-Daniel J, Forbes AA, Wurzer P, Hundeshagen G, Branski LK, et al. Recent trends in burn epidemiology worldwide: a systematic review. Burns. 2017;43:249–57.
14. Blakeney P, Meyer W, Moore P, Broemeling L, Hunt R, Robson M, et al. Social competence and behavioral problems of pediatric survivors of burns. J Burn Care Rehabil. 1993;14:65–72.
15. Peden M, Oyegbite K, Ozanne-Smith J, Hyder AA, Branche C, Rahman AKMF, et al., editors. World report on child injury prevention. Geneva: World Health Organization; 2008. p. 78–98. http://whqlibdoc.who.int/publications/2008/9789241563574_eng.pdf. Accessed 20 Sept 2017.
16. Keswani MH. The prevention of burning injury. Burns Incl Therm Inj. 1986;12:533–9.
17. Villaveces A, Peck M, Faraklas I, Hsu-Chang N, Joe V, Wibbenmeyer L. Process evaluation of software using the international classification of external causes of injuries for collecting burn injury data at burn centers in the United States. J Burn Care Res. 2014;35:28.
18. Peck M, Falk H, Meddings D, Sugerman D, Mehta S, Sage M. The design and evaluation of a system for improved surveillance and prevention programmes in resource-limited settings using a hospital-based burn injury questionnaire. Inj Prev. 2016;22(suppl 1):i56–62.
19. Haagsma JA, Graetz N, Bolliger I, Naghavi M, Higashi H, Mullany EC, et al. The global burden of injury: incidence, mortality, disability-adjusted life years and time trends from the Global Burden of Disease study 2013. Inj Prev. 2016;22:3–18.
20. Centers for Disease Control and Prevention. Fatal Injury Reports 1981–1998. Web-based injury and statistics query and reporting system (WISQARS™) 2009. http://webappa.cdc.gov/sasweb/ncipc/mortrate9.html. Accessed 19 Sept 2017.
21. Fagenholz PJ, Sheridan RL, Harris NS, Pelletier AJ, Camargo CA Jr. National study of emergency department visits for burn injuries, 1993 to 2004. J Burn Care Res. 2007;28:681–90.
22. Centers for Disease Control and Prevention. Nonfatal scald-related burns among adults aged ≥65 years—United States, 2001-2006. Morb Mortal Wkly Rep. 2009a;58:993–6.
23. Brusselaers N, Monstrey S, Vogelaers D, Hoste E, Blot S. Severe burn injury in Europe: a systematic review of the incidence, etiology, morbidity, and mortality. Crit Care. 2010;14(5):R188.
24. Dokter J, Vloemans AF, Beerthuizen GI, Van der Vlies CH, Boxma H, Breederveld R, Tuinebreijer WE, Middelkoop E, van Baar ME. Epidemiology and trends in severe burns in the Netherlands. Burns. 2014;40(7):1406–14.
25. American Burn Association National Burn Repository. v. 11.0. 2015. http://www.ameriburn.org/2015NBRAnnualReport.pdf. Accessed 11 Apr 2017.
26. Australia and New Zealand Burns Association (ANZBA). Burns Registry of Australia and New Zealand. BRANZ 1st through 6th Annual Reports 2009–2015. 2016. https://www.branz.org/node/4.
27. Song C, Chua A. Epidemiology of burn injuries in Singapore from 1997 to 2003. Burns. 2005;32(supp 1):S18–26.
28. Nega KE, Lindtjørn B. Epidemiology of burn injuries in Mekele Town, Northern Ethiopia: a community based study. Ethiop J Health Dev. 2002;16:1–7.
29. Mashreky SR, Rahman A, Chowdhury SM, Giashuddin S, SvanstrOm L, Linnan M, et al. Epidemiology of childhood burn: yield of largest community based injury survey in Bangladesh. Burns. 2008;34:856–62.
30. Mashreky SR, Rahman A, Chowdhury SM, Giashuddin S, Svanström L, Linnan M, et al. Consequences of childhood burn: findings from the largest community-based injury survey in Bangladesh. Burns. 2008a;34:912–8.
31. Mashreky SR, Rahman A, Chowdhury SM, Khan TF, Svanström L, Rahman F. Non-fatal burn is a major cause of illness: findings from the largest community-based national survey in Bangladesh. Inj Prev. 2009a;15:397–402.
32. DeKoning EP, Hakenewerth A, Platts-Mills TF, Tintinalli JE. Epidemiology of burn injuries presenting to North Carolina emergency departments in 2006-2007. Burns. 2009;35:776–82.
33. Forjuoh SN. The mechanisms, intensity of treatment, and outcomes of hospitalized burns: issues for prevention. J Burn Care Rehabil. 1998;19:456–60.
34. Burd A, Yuen C. A global study of hospitalized paediatric burn patients. Burns. 2005;31:432–8.
35. Demamu S. Community-based study of childhood injuries in Adamitulu District, Ethiopia (thesis). Addis Ababa University, Department of Community Health; 1991.
36. Tamrat A. Accidents and poisoning in children. Ethiop Med J. 1981;24:39–40.
37. Tekle Wold F. Accidents in childhood. Ethiop Med J. 1973;11:41–6.
38. Brigham PA, McLoughlin E. Burn incidence and medical care use in the United States: estimates, trends, and data sources. J Burn Care Rehabil. 1996;17:95–107.
39. Ahuja RB, Bhattacharya S, Rai A. Changing trends of an endemic trauma. Burns. 2009;35:650–6.
40. Peck MD, Shankar V, Bangdiwala SI. Trends in injury-related deaths before and after dissolution of the Union of Soviet Socialist Republics. Int J Inj Control Saf Promot. 2007a;14:139–51.
41. Notzon FC, Komarov YM, Ermakov SP, Sempos CT, Marks JS, Sempos EV. Causes of declining life expectancy in Russia. JAMA. 1998;279:793–800.
42. Mock C, Peden M, Hyder AA, Butchart A, Krug E. Child injuries and violence: the new challenge for child health. Bull World Health Organ. 2008;86:420.
43. Mock C, Peck M, Peden M, Krug E, editors. A WHO plan for burn prevention and care. Geneva: World Health Organization; 2008a. whqlibdoc.who.int/publications/2008/9789241596299_eng.pdf.
44. Park JO, Shin SD, Kim J, Song KJ, Peck MD. Association between socioeconomic status and burn injury severity. Burns. 2009;35:482–90.
45. American Burn Association. National Burn Repository, v. 5.0. 2009. http://www.ameriburn.org/2009NBRAnnualReport.pdf. Accessed 11 Apr 2017.
46. Friesen B. Haddon's strategy for prevention: application to Native house fires. Circumpolar Health, vol. 84. Seattle, WA: University of Washington Press; 1985. p. 105–9.
47. Bjerregaard P. Fatal non-intentional injuries in Greenland. Artic Med Res. 1992;51(suppl 7):22–6.
48. Muir BL. Health status of Canadian Indians and Inuit—1990. Ottawa: Indian and Northern Health Services, Medical Services Branch, Health and Welfare Canada; 1991. p. 1–58.

49. Golshan A, Patel C, Hyder AA. A systematic review of the epidemiology of unintentional burn injuries in South Asia. J Public Health. 2013;35:384–96.
50. Othman N, Kendrick D. Epidemiology of burn injuries in the East Mediterranean Region: a systematic review. BMC Public Health. 2010;10:83.
51. Ashe B, McAneney J, Pitman AJ. Total cost of fire in Australia. J Risk Res. 2009;12:121–36.
52. Takayanagi K, Kawai S, Aoki R. The cost of burn care and implication for efficient care. Clin Perform Qual Health Care. 1999;7:70–3.
53. Sanchez JL, Bastida JL, Martínez MM, Moreno JM, Chamorro JJ. Socio-economic cost and health-related quality of life of burn victims in Spain. Burns. 2008;34:975–81.
54. National Fire Protection Association (NFPA). 2017. http://www.nfpa.org/news-and-research/fire-statistics-and-reports/fire-statistics/fires-in-the-us/overall-fire-problem/fire-loss-in-the-united-states. Accessed 7 Apr 2017.
55. Office of the Deputy Prime Minister. The economic costs of fire: estimates for 2004. 2006. www.communities.gov.uk/documents/fire/pdf/144524.pdf. Accessed 19 Sept 2017.
56. Centers for Disease Control and Prevention. 2017. https://wisqars.cdc.gov:8443/costT/ProcessPart1FinishOutServlet. Accessed 9 May 2017.
57. Cancio LC, Barillo DJ, Kearns RD, Holmes JH IV, Conlon KM, Matherly AF, et al. Guidelines for burn care under austere conditions. J Burn Care Res. 2017;38:203–14.
58. Peck MD, Pressman MA, Caruso DM, Edelman LS, Holmes JH IV, Hughes WB, et al. Reimbursement for out-of-state burn patients is not always lower than that for in-state patients at regional burn centers. J Burn Care Res. 2010;31:603–9.
59. Peck MD, Mantelle L, Ward CG. Comparison of length of hospital stay with mortality rate in a regional burn center. J Burn Care Rehabil. 1996;17:39–44.
60. Shields BJ, Comstock RD, Fernandez SA, Xiang H, Smith GA. Healthcare resource utilization and epidemiology of pediatric burn-associated hospitalizations, United States, 2000. J Burn Care Res. 2007;28:811–26.
61. American Burn Association. National Burn Repository. 2016. http://www.ameriburn.org/2016ABANBR_FINAL_42816.pdf. Accessed 11 Apr 2017.
62. American Burn Association. National Burn Repository. 2006. v. 2.0. http://www.ameriburn.org/NBR2005.pdf. Accessed 14 Apr 2017.
63. Alden NE, Bessey PQ, Rabbitts A, Hyden PJ, Yurt RW. Tap water scalds among seniors and the elderly: socio-economics and implications for prevention. Burns. 2007;33:666–9.
64. McLoughlin E, McGuire A. The causes, cost, and prevention of childhood burn injuries. Am J Dis Child. 1990;144:677–83.
65. Carey K, Kazis LE, Lee AF, Liang MH, Li NC, Hinson MI, et al. Measuring the cost of care for children with acute burn injury. J Trauma. 2012;73(3 Suppl 2):S229–33.
66. Karter MJ. Fire loss in the United States 2008. National Fire Protection Association (NFPA). Quincy, MA: Fire Analysis and Research Division; 2009.
67. Thorpe T. Critical cost based analysis of inclusive expense to the South African Government of patients with burn injuries sustained from non-pressurised paraffin stoves. Emalahleni: Fincore Financial; 2004.
68. National SAFE KIDS Campaign (NSKC). Burn injury fact sheet. Washington, DC: NSKC; 2004.
69. Sahin I, Ozturk S, Alhan D, Açikel C, Isik S. Cost analysis of acute burn patients treated in a burn centre: the Gulhane experience. Ann Burns Fire Disasters. 2011;24:9–13.
70. Mathers CD, Salomon JA, Ezzati M, Begg S, Vander Hoorn S, Lopez AD. Sensitivity and uncertainty analyses for burden of disease and risk factor estimates. In: Lopez AD, Mathers CD, Ezzati M, Jamison DT, Murray CJL, editors. Global burden of disease and risk factors. The International Bank for reconstruction and development/The World Bank. New York: Oxford University Press; 2006. p. 399–426.
71. Salomon JA, Murray CJL, Üstün TB, Chatterji S. Health state valuations in summary measures of population health. In: Murray CJL, Evans DB, editors. Health systems performance assessment: debate, methods, and empiricism. Geneva: World Health Organization; 2003. p. 409–36.
72. Barss P, Smith G, Baker SP, Mohan D. Injury prevention: an International Perspective. Epidemiology, surveillance, and policy. New York: Oxford University Press; 1998. p. 375.
73. Peck MD, Brigham P, Patterson D. Invited critique: National study of emergency department visits for burn injuries, 1993-2004. J Burn Care Res. 2007;28:691–3.
74. Pereira C, Murphy K, Herndon D. Outcome measures in burn care: is mortality dead? Burns. 2004;30:761–71.
75. Barillo DJ, Goode R. Fire fatality study: demographics of fire victims. Burns. 1996;22:85–8.
76. Mallonee S, Istre GR, Rosenberg M, Reddish-Douglas M, Jordan F, Silverstein P, et al. Surveillance and prevention of residential-fire injuries. N Engl J Med. 1996;335:27–31.
77. Istre GR, McCoy MA, Osborn L, Barnard JJ, Bolton A. Deaths and injuries from house fires. N Engl J Med. 2001;344:1911–6.
78. Roberts I. Cause specific social class mortality differentials for child injury and poisoning in England and Wales. J Epidemiol Community Health. 1997;51:334–5.
79. DiGuiseppi C, Edwards P, Godward C, Roberts I, Wade A. Urban residential fire and flame injuries: a population based study. Inj Prev. 2000;6:250–4.
80. Marsden NJ, Battle CE, Combellack EJ, Sabra A, Morris K, Dickson WA, et al. The impact of socio-economic deprivation on burn injury: A nine-year retrospective study of 6441 patients. Burns. 2016;42:446–52.
81. Gulaid JA, Sacks JJ, Sattin RW. Deaths from residential fires among older people, United States, 1984. J Am Geriatr Soc. 1989;37:331–4.
82. McGwin G Jr, Chapman V, Rousculp M, Robison J, Fine P. The epidemiology of fire-related deaths in Alabama, 1992-1997. J Burn Care Rehabil. 2000;21(1 pt 1):75–83.
83. Mierley MC, Baker SP. Fatal house fires in an urban population. JAMA. 1983;249:1466–8.
84. Alnababtah K, Khan S, Ashford R. Socio-demographic factors and the prevalence of burns in children: an overview of the literature. Paediatr Int Child Health. 2016;36:45–51.
85. Forjuoh SN. Burns in low- and middle-income countries: a review of available literature on descriptive epidemiology, risk factors, treatment, and prevention. Burns. 2006;32:529–37.
86. Gupta M, Gupta OK, Goil P. Paediatric burns in Jaipur, India: an epidemiological study. Burns. 1992;18:63–7.
87. Rossi LA, Braga EC, Barruffini RC, Carvalho EC. Childhood burn injuries: circumstances of occurrences and their prevention in Ribeirão Preto, Brazil. Burns. 1998;24:416–9.
88. Vilasco B, Bondurand A. Burns in Adidjan, Côte d'Ivoire. Burns. 1995;21:291–6.
89. Istre GR, McCoy M, Carlin DK, McClain J. Residential fire related deaths and injuries among children: fireplay, smoke alarms, and prevention. Inj Prev. 2002;8:128–32.
90. Scholer SJ, Hickson GB, Mitchel EF Jr, Ray WA. Predictors of mortality from fires in young children. Pediatrics. 1998;101:E12.
91. Rivara F. Developmental and behavioral issues in childhood injury prevention. J Dev Behav Pediatr. 1995;16:362–70.
92. Agran PF, Anderson C, Winn D, Trent R, Walton-Haynes L, Thayer S. Rates of pediatric injuries by 3-month intervals for children 0 to 3 years of age. Pediatrics. 2003;111:e683–92.

93. Matzavakis I, Frangakis CE, Charalampopoulou A, Petridou E. Burn injuries related to motorcycle exhaust pipes: a study in Greece. Burns. 2005;31:372–4.
94. Smith GA, Knapp JF, Barnett TM, Shields BJ. The rockets' red glare, the bombs bursting in air: fireworks-related injuries to children. Pediatrics. 1996;98:1–9.
95. Mashreky SR, Rahman A, Chowdhury SM, Svanström L, Linnan M, Shafinaz S, et al. Perceptions of rural people about childhood burns and their prevention: a basis for developing a childhood burn prevention programme in Bangladesh. Public Health. 2009;123:568–72.
96. Marshall SW, Runyan CW, Bangdiwala SI, Linzer MA, Sacks JJ, Butts JD. Fatal residential fires: who dies and who survives? JAMA. 1998;279:1633–7.
97. Hall JR. Fireworks. Quincy, MA: National Fire Protection Association Fire Analysis and Research Division. National Fire Protection Association; 2009. http://www.nfpa.org/news-and-research/fire-statistics-and-reports/fire-statistics/fire-causes/fireworks. Accessed 19 Sept 2017.
98. Hyder AA, Kashyap KS, Fishman S, Wali SA. Review of childhood burn injuries in sub-Saharan Africa: a forgotten public health challenge: literature review. Afr Saf Promot. 2004;2:43–58.
99. Tang K, Jian L, Qin Z, Zhenjiang L, Gomez M, Beveridge M. Characteristics of burn patients at a major burn center in Shanghai. Burns. 2006;32:1037–43.
100. Ho W, Ying S. An epidemiological study of 1063 hospitalized burn patients in a tertiary burns centre in Hong Kong. Burns. 2001;27:119–23.
101. Jie X, Ren CB. Burn injuries in the Dong Bei area of China: a study of 12,606 cases. Burns. 1992;18:222–32.
102. Ahuja RB, Dash JK, Shrivastava P. A comparative analysis of liquefied petroleum gas (LPG) and kerosene related burns. Burns. 2011;37:1403–10.
103. Ortiz-Prado E, Armijos L, Iturralde AL. A population-based study of the epidemiology of acute adult burns in Ecuador from 2005 to 2014. Burns. 2015;41:582–9.
104. Nthumba PM. Burns in sub-Saharan Africa: A review. Burns. 2016;42:258–66.
105. den Hollander D, Albert M, Strand A, Hardcastle TC. Epidemiology and referral patterns of burns admitted to the Burns Centre at Inkosi Albert Luthuli Central Hospital, Durban. Burns. 2014;40:1201–8.
106. Runyan CW, Bangdiwala SI, Linzer MA, Sacks JJ, Butts J. Risk factors for fatal residential fires. N Engl J Med. 1992;327:859–63.
107. Laditan AA. Accidental scalds and burns in infancy and childhood. J Trop Pediatr. 1987;33:199–202.
108. Peck MD, Kruger GE, van der Merwe AE, Godakumbura W, Ahuja RB. Burns and fires from non-electric domestic appliances in low and middle income countries. Part I. The scope of the problem. Burns. 2008;34:303–11.
109. Hughes A, et al. State estimates of substance use from the 2005–2006 National Surveys on Drug Use and Health. Rockville, MD: Substance Abuse and Mental Health Services Administration, Office of Applied Studies; 2008. http://downloads.newsok.com/documents/Substance-Use-Estimates-2005-2006.pdf Accessed 19 Sept 2017.
110. UNICEF. A league table of child deaths by injury in rich nations. Innocenti Report Care No. 2, UNICEF. Florence: Innocenti Research Centre; 2001. p. 29. http://www.unicef-irc.org/publications/pdf/repcard2e.pdf
111. Block JH. Differential premises arising from differential socialization of the sexes: some conjectures. Child Dev. 1983;54:1335–54.
112. Fagot BI. The influence of sex of child on parental reactions to toddler children. Child Dev. 1978;49:459–65.
113. Saegert S, Hart R. The development of sex differences in the environmental confidence of children. In: Burnett P, editor. Women in society. Chicago: Maaroufa Press; 1990. p. 157–75.
114. Eaton WO, Yu AP. Are sex differences in child motor activity level a function of sex differences in maturational status? Child Dev. 1989;60:1005–11.
115. Rosen BN, Peterson L. Gender differences in children's outdoor play injuries: a review and an integration. Clin Psychol Rev. 1990;10:187–205.
116. Rivara FP, Bergman AB, LoGerfo JP, Weiss NS. Epidemiology of childhood injuries: II. Sex difference in injury rates. Am J Dis Child. 1982;136:502–6.
117. Begg S, Vos T, Barker B, Stevenson C, Stanley L, Lopez AD. The burden of disease and injury in Australia 2003. PHE 82. Canberra: Australian Institute of Health and Welfare; 2007.
118. Ye C, Wang X, Zhang Y, Ni L, Jiang R, Liu L, et al. Ten-year epidemiology of chemical burns in western Zhejiang Province, China. Burns. 2016;42:668–74.
119. Quinney B, McGwin G Jr, Cross JM, Valent F, Taylor AJ, Rue LW III. Thermal burn fatalities in the workplace, United States, 1992 to 1999. J Burn Care Rehabil. 2002;23:305–10.
120. Courtright P, Haile D, Kohls E. The epidemiology of burns in rural Ethiopia. J Epidemiol Community Health. 1993;47:19–22.
121. Vaghardoost R, Kazemzadeh J, Rabieepoor S. Epidemiology of burns during pregnancy in Tehran, Iran. Burns. 2016;42:663–7.
122. Saleh S, Gadalla S, Fortney JA, Rogers SM, Potts DM. Accidental burn deaths to Egyptian women of reproductive age. Burns. 1986;12:241–5.
123. Adamo C, Esposito G, Lissia M, Vonella M, Zagaria N, Scuderi N. Epidemiological data on burn injuries in Angola: a retrospective study of 7230 patients. Burns. 1995;21:536–8.
124. Bhalla SB, Kale SR, Mohan D. Burn properties of fabrics and garments worn in India. Accid Anal Prev. 2000;32:407–20.
125. Gali BM, Madziga AG, Naaya HU. Epidemiology of childhood burns in Maiduguri, north-eastern Nigeria. Niger J Med. 2004;13:144–7.
126. Ghosh A, Bharat R. Domestic burns prevention and first aid awareness in and around Jamshedpur, India: strategies and impact. Burns. 2000;26:605–8.
127. Hemeda M, Maher A, Mabrouk A. Epidemiology of burns admitted to Ain Shams University Burns Unit, Cairo, Egypt. Burns. 2003;29:353–8.
128. Ndiritu S, Ngumi ZW, Nyaim O. Burns: the epidemiological pattern, risk and safety awareness at Kenyatta National Hospital, Nairobi. East Afr Med J. 2006;83:455–60.
129. Yongqiang F, Yibing W, Dechang W, Baohua L, Mingqing W, Ran H. Epidemiology of hospitalized burn patients in Shandong Province, 2001-2005. J Burn Care Res. 2007;28:468–73.
130. Sanghavi P, Bhalla K, Das V. Fire-related deaths in India in 2001: a retrospective analysis of data. Lancet. 2009;373:1282–8.
131. Arshi S, Sadeghi-Bazargani H, Mohammadi R, Ekman R, Hudson D, Djafarzadeh H, et al. Prevention oriented epidemiologic study of accidental burns in rural areas of Ardabil, Iran. Burns. 2006;32:366–71.
132. De-Souza D, Marchesan WG, Greene LJ. Epidemiological data and mortality rate of patients hospitalized with burns in Brazil. Burns. 1998;24:433–8.
133. Sharma NP, Duke JM, Lama BB, Thapa B, Dahal P, Bariya ND, et al. Descriptive epidemiology of unintentional burn injuries admitted to a tertiary-level government hospital in Nepal: gender-specific patterns. Asia Pac J Public Health. 2015;27:551–60.
134. Tung KY, Chen ML, Wang HJ, Chen GS, Peck M, Yang J, et al. A seven-year epidemiology study of 12,381 admitted burn patients in Taiwan—using the Internet registration system of the Childhood Burn Foundation. Burns. 2005;31(suppl 1):S12–7.
135. Gupta RK, Srivastava AK. Study of fatal burn cases in Kanpur (India). Forensic Sci Int. 1988;37:81–9.
136. Laloë V. Patterns of deliberate self-burning in various parts of the world. A review Burns. 2004;30:207–15.

137. Gauthier ST, Reisch T, Bartsch CH. Self-burning—a rare suicide method in Switzerland and other industrialised nations—a review. Burns. 2014;40:1720–6.
138. Thombs BD, Bresnick MG. Mortality risk and length of stay associated with self-inflicted burn injury: evidence from a national sample of 30,382 adult patients. Crit Care Med. 2008;36:118–25.
139. Nakae H, Zheng YJ, Wada H, Tajimi K, Endo S. Characteristics of self-immolation attempts in Akita Prefecture, Japan. Burns. 2003;29:691–6.
140. Rashid A, Gower JP. A review of the trends of self-inflicted burns. Burns. 2004;30:573–6.
141. Mackay N, Barrowclough C. Accident and emergency staff's perceptions of deliberate self-harm: attributions, emotions and willingness to help. Br J Clin Psychol. 2005;44(Pt 2):255–67.
142. McAllister M, Creedy D, Moyle W, Farrugia C. Nurses' attitudes towards clients who self-harm. J Adv Nurs. 2002;40:578–86.
143. Forster NA, Nuñez DG, Zingg M, Haile SR, Künzi W, Giovanoli P, et al. Attempted suicide by self-immolation is a powerful predictive variable for survival of burn injuries. J Burn Care Res. 2012;33:642–8.
144. Varley J, Pilcher D, Butt W, Cameron P. Self harm is an independent predictor of mortality in trauma and burns patients admitted to ICU. Injury. 2012;43:1562–5.
145. Minn YK. Who burned and how to prevent? Identification of risk for and prevention of burns among epileptic patients. Burns. 2007;33:127–8.
146. Tekle-Haimanot R. Neurological disorders. In: Kloos H, Zein ZA, editors. The ecology of health and disease in Ethiopia. Boulder, CO: Westview Press; 1993. p. 483–91.
147. Barss P. Health impact of injuries in the highlands of Papua New Guinea: a verbal autopsy study (dissertation). Baltimore, MD: Johns Hopkins School of Hygiene and Public Health; 1991.
148. Fauveau U, Blanchet T. Deaths from injuries and induced abortion among rural Bangladeshi women. Soc Sci Med. 1989;29:1121–7.
149. Al-Qattan MM. Burns in epileptics in Saudi Arabia. Burns. 2000;26:561–3.
150. Al-Qattan MM, Al-Zahrani K. A review of burns related to traditions, social habits, religious activities, festivals and traditional medical practices. Burns. 2009;35:476–81.
151. Katcher ML. Prevention of tap water scald burns: evaluation of a multi-media injury control program. Am J Public Health. 1987;77:1195–7.
152. McGill V, Kowal-Vern A, Gamelli RL. Outcome for older burn patients. Arch Surg. 2000;135:320–5.
153. Cadier MA, Shakespeare PG. Burns in octogenarians. Burns. 1995;21:200–4.
154. Ryan CM, Thorpe W, Mullin P, Roberts W, Tompkins D, Kelleher P. A persistent fire hazard for older adults: cooking-related clothing ignition. J Am Geriatr Soc. 1997;45:1283–5.
155. Emami SA, Motevalian SA, Momeni M, Karimi H. The epidemiology of geriatric burns in Iran: a national burn registry-based study. Burns. 2016;42:1128–32.
156. Backstein R, Peters W, Neligan P. Burns in the disabled. Burns. 1993;19:192–7.
157. Alden NE, Rabbitts A, Yurt RW. Burn injury in patients with dementia: an impetus for prevention. J Burn Care Rehabil. 2005;26:267–71.
158. Lari AR, Panjeshahin MR, Talei AR, Rossignol AM, Alaghehbandan R. Epidemiology of childhood burns in Fars province, Iran. J Burn Care Rehabil. 2002;23:39–45.
159. Híjar-Medina MC, Tapia-Yáñez JR, Lozano-Ascencio R, López-López MV. Home accidents in children less than 10 years of age: causes and consequences. Salud Pública Méx. 1992;34: 615–25.
160. Alsalman AK, Algadiem EA, Alalwan MA, Farag TS. Epidemiology of infant burn in Eastern Saudi Arabia. Saudi Med J. 2015;36:324–7.
161. Sahu SA, Agrawal K, Patel PK. Scald burn, a preventable injury: analysis of 4306 patients from a major tertiary care center. Burns. 2016;42:1844–9.
162. Durrani KM, Raza SK. Studies on flammability of clothing of burn victims, changes therein, and their wearability after a borax rinse. J Pak Med Assoc. 1975;25:99–102.
163. Barss P, Wallace K. Grass-skirt burns in Papua New Guinea. Lancet. 1983;1:733–4.
164. Barillo DJ, Stetz CK, Zak AL, Shirani KZ, Goodwin CW. Preventable burns associated with a misuse of gasoline. Burns. 1998;24:439–43.
165. Hartzell GE. Combustion products and their effects on life safety. Fire protection handbook. Quincy, MA: National Fire Protection Association; 1991. p. 3-3–3-14.
166. American Society for Testing and Materials (ASTM). Standard terminology relating to fire standards. Philadelphia, PA; 1982. p. E176–82.
167. Federal Emergency Management Agency (FEMA). Fire in the United States 1992–2001. 13th ed. Emmitsburg, MD: National Fire Data Center; 2004. https://www.usfa.fema.gov/downloads/pdf/publications/fa-286.pdf. Accessed 19 Sept 2017.
168. Einhorn IN. Physiological and toxicological aspects of smoke produced during the combustion of polymeric materials. Environ Health Perspect. 1975;11:163–89.
169. Hill IR. An analysis of factors impeding passenger escape from aircraft fires. Aviat Space Environ Med. 1990;61:261–5.
170. Shkrum MJ, Ramsay DA. Forensic pathology of trauma. Totowa, NJ: Humana Press; 2007. p. 646.
171. Weaver LK. Carbon monoxide poisoning. Crit Care Clin. 1999;15:297–317.
172. Stewart RD, Stewart RS, Stamm W, Seelen RP. Rapid estimation of carboxyhemoglobin level in fire fighters. JAMA. 1976;235:390–2.
173. Theilade P. Carbon monoxide poisoning. Five years' experience in a defined population. Am J Forensic Med Pathol. 1990;11:219–25.
174. DiGuiseppi C, Higgins JP. Systematic review of controlled trials of interventions to promote smoke alarms. Arch Dis Child. 2000;82:341–8.
175. Karter MJ, Miller AL. Patterns of fire casualties in home fires by age and sex, 1983–1987. Quincy, MA: National Fire Protection Association (NFPA). Fire Analysis and Research Division; 1990. p. 46.
176. Balraj EK. Atherosclerotic coronary artery disease and "low" levels of carboxyhemoglobin; report of fatalities and discussion of pathophysiologic mechanisms of death. J Forensic Sci. 1984;29:1150–9.
177. Caplan YH, Thompson BC, Levine B, Masemore W. Accidental poisonings involving carbon monoxide, heating systems, and confined spaces. J Forensic Sci. 1986;31:117–21.
178. Lundquist P, Rammer L, Sörbo B. The role of hydrogen cyanide and carbon monoxide in fire casualties: a prospective study. Forensic Sci Int. 1989;43:9–14.
179. Alarie Y. Toxicity of fire smoke. Crit Rev Toxicol. 2002;32:259–89.
180. Potts WJ, Lederer TS, Quast JF. A study of the inhalation toxicityof smoke produced upon pyrolysis and combustion of polyethylene foams. Part I. Laboratory studies. J Combust Toxicol. 1978;5:408–33.
181. Gerson L, Wingard D. Fire deaths and drinking: data from the Ontario fire reporting system. Am J Drug Alcohol Abuse. 1979;6:125–33.
182. Squires T, Busuttil A. Alcohol and house fire fatalities in Scotland, 1980-1990. Med Sci Law. 1997;37:321–5.
183. Barillo DJ, Rush BF Jr, Goode R, Lin RL, Freda A, Anderson EJ Jr. Is ethanol the unknown toxin in smoke inhalation injury? Am Surg. 1986;52:641–5.
184. Jarvis GK, Boldt M. Death styles among Canada's Indians. Soc Sci Med. 1982;16:1345–52.

185. Warda L, Tenenbein M, Moffatt ME. House fire injury prevention update. Part I. A review of risk factors for fatal and non-fatal house fire injury. Inj Prev. 1999;5:145–50.
186. Peck MD, Kruger GE, van der Merwe AE, Godakumbura W, Oen IM, Swart D. Burns and fires from non-electric domestic appliances in low and middle income countries. Part II. A strategy for intervention using the Haddon matrix. Burns. 2008a;34:312–9.
187. Paraffin Safety Association of Southern Africa. 2003 SABS stove test report. 2003. www.psasa.org. Accessed 20 Sept 2017.
188. Godwin Y, Hudson DA, Bloch CE. Shack fires: a consequence of urban migration. Burns. 1997;23:151–3.
189. El-Badawy A, Mabrouk AR. Epidemiology of childhood burns in the burn unit of Ain Shams University in Cairo, Egypt. Burns. 1998;24:728–32.
190. Grange AO, Akinsulie AO, Sowemimo GO. Flame burns disasters from kerosene appliance explosions in Lagos. Nigeria Burns Incl Therm Inj. 1988;14:147–50.
191. Gupta M, Bansal M, Gupta A, Goil P. The kerosene tragedy of 1994, an unusual epidemic of burns: epidemiological aspects and management of patients. Burns. 1996;22:3–9.
192. Mabrouk A, El Badawy A, Sherif M. Kerosene stove as a cause of burns admitted to the Ain Shams burn unit. Burns. 2000;26:474–7.
193. Marsh D, Sheikh A, Khalil A, Kamil S, Jaffer-uz-Zaman QI, et al. Epidemiology of adults hospitalized with burns in Karachi, Pakistan. Burns. 1996;22:225–9.
194. Sawhney CP. Flame burns involving kerosene pressure stoves in India. Burns. 1989;15:362–4.
195. Pruitt BA Jr, Wolf SE, Mason AD Jr. Epidemiological, demographic, and outcome characteristics of burn injury. In: Herndon DN, editor. Total burn care. 3rd ed. Philadelphia, PA: Saunders Elsevier; 2007. p. 14–32.
196. Chapman CW. Burns and plastic surgery in the South Atlantic campaign 1982. J R Nav Med Serv. 1983;69:71–9.
197. Owen-Smith MS. Armoured fighting vehicle casualties. J R Army Med Corps. 1977;153:210–5.
198. Eldad A, Torem M. Burns in the Lebanon War 1982: 'the Blow and the Cure'. Mil Med. 1990;155:130–2.
199. Dobson RB. Clifford's Tower and the Jews of Medieval York. London: English Heritage; 1995.
200. New York Times. Terrific tragedy in Chili: two thousand five hundred persons roasted to death in a church. Dec 14, 1863.
201. Huffman A. Sultana: surviving the civil war, prison, and the worst maritime disaster in American history. New York: Harper Collins; 2010. p. 320.
202. Barillo DJ, Wolf S. Planning for burn disasters: lessons learned from one hundred years of history. J Burn Care Res. 2006;27:622–34.
203. Sikora F. Until justice rolls down: the Birmingham Church bombing case. Tuscaloosa, AL: University of Alabama Press; 1991.
204. Crabtree J. Terrorist homicide bombings: a primer for preparation. J Burn Care Res. 2006;27:576–88.
205. Peleg K, Goldman S, Sikron F. Burn prevention programs for children: do they reduce burn-related hospitalizations? Burns. 2005;31:347–50.
206. Ytterstad B, Søgaard AJ. The Harstad injury prevention study: prevention of burns in small children by a community-based intervention. Burns. 1995;21:259–66.
207. National Center for Injury Prevention and Control. Injury fact book 2001–2002. Atlanta, GA: Centers for Disease Control and Prevention; 2001.
208. Linares AZ, Linares HA. Burn prevention: the need for a comprehensive approach. Burns. 1990;16:281–5.
209. Cox SG, Burahee A, Albertyn R, Makahabane J, Rode H. Parent knowledge on paediatric burn prevention related to the home environment. Burns. 2016;42:1854–60.
210. Sutchritpongsa S, Sangwisit S, Sonjaipanich S. Parental awareness of household injury prevention: adequacy of anticipatory guidance for well childcare. J Med Assoc Thail. 2013;96:1531–5.
211. Heard JP, Latenser BA, Liao J. Burn prevention in Zambia: a work in progress. J Burn Care Res. 2013;34:598–606.
212. Warda L, Tenenbein M, Moffatt ME. House fire injury prevention update. Part II. A review of the effectiveness of preventive interventions. Inj Prev. 1999a;5:217–25.
213. DiGuiseppi C, Higgins JP. Interventions for promoting smoke alarm ownership and function. Cochrane Database Syst Rev. 2001;(2):CD002246.
214. Rybarczyk MM, Schafer JM, Elm CM, Sarvepalli S, Vaswani PA, Balhara KS, et al. Prevention of burn injuries in low- and middle-income countries: a systematic review. Burns. 2016;42:1183–92.
215. Parbhoo A, Louw QA, Grimmer-Somers K. Burn prevention programs for children in developing countries require urgent attention: a targeted literature review. Burns. 2010;36:164–75.
216. Lehna C, Carver E. Teachable moments for burn injury prevention. Burns. 2014;40:362–3.
217. Rieman MT, Kagan RJ. Development of a burn prevention teaching tool for Amish Children. J Burn Care Res. 2012;33:259–64.
218. Rieman MT, Kagan RJ. Multicenter testing of a burn prevention teaching tool for Amish children. J Burn Care Res. 2013;34:58–64.
219. Oomman A, Sarwar U, Javed M, Hemington-Gorse S. YouTube as a potential online source of information in the prevention and management of paediatric burn injuries. Burns. 2013;39:1652.
220. Department for Communities and Local Government. Fire Statistics, United Kingdom. 2006, London, UK; 2008. p. 35–42. https://www.gov.uk/government/statistics/fire-statistics-england-april-2015-to-march-2016 Accessed 19 Sept 2017.
221. Ahrens M. Home smoke alarms: the data as context for decision. Fire Technol. 2008;44:313–27.
222. U. S. Fire Administration. Residential Smoke and Fire Detector Coverage in the United States: Findings from a 1982 Survey. Washington, DC: Federal Emergency Management Agency; 1983.
223. Ahrens M. Smoke alarms in US home fires. Quincy, MA: National Fire Protection Association, Fire Analysis and Research Division; 2009.
224. Gielen AC, Shields W, Frattaroli S, McDonald E, Jones V, Bishai D, et al. Enhancing fire department home visiting programs: results of a community intervention trial. J Burn Care Res. 2013;34:e250–6.
225. Kim CT, Bryant P. Complex regional pain syndrome (type 1) after electrical injury: a case report of treatment with continuous epidural block. Arch Phys Med Rehabil. 2001;82:993–5.
226. Proulx G. Response to fire alarms. NRCC 49272. Fire Protection Engineering, Winter; 2007. p. 8–15.
227. Dubivsky PM, Bukowski RW. False Alarm Study of Smoke Detectors in Department of Veterans Affairs Medical Centers (VAMCS), NISTIR 89–4077, Gaithersburg, MD: National Institute of Standards and Technology; 1989. p. 45. http://fire.nist.gov/bfrlpubs/fire89/art012.html. Accessed 19 Sept 2017.
228. Duncanson M, Lawrence K, Simpson J, Woodward A. Follow-up survey of Auahi Whakatupato smoke alarm installation project in the Eastern Bay of Plenty. New Zealand Fire Service Commission Research Report Number Seven. Otago, NZ: University of Otago. 2000. https://fireandemergency.nz/assets/Documents/Research-and-reports/Report-7-Follow-up-survey-of-Auahi-Whakatupato-smoke-alarm-installation-project-in-the-Bay-of-Plenty.pdf. Accessed 19 Sept 2017.
229. Roberts H, Curtis K, Liabo K, Rowland D, DiGuiseppi C, Roberts I. Putting public health evidence into practice: increasing the prevalence of working smoke alarms in disadvantaged inner city housing. J Epidemiol Community Health. 2004;58:280–5.
230. Rodgers M, Sowden A, Petticrew M, Arai L, Roberts H, Britten N, Popay J. Testing methodological guidance on the conduct of narrative synthesis in systematic reviews: effectiveness of interventions to promote smoke alarm ownership and function. Evaluation. 2009;15(1):49–73.
231. Arai L, Roen K, Roberts H, Popay J. It might work in Oklahoma but will it work in Oakhampton? Context and implementation in

the effectiveness literature on domestic smoke detectors. Inj Prev. 2005;11:148–51.
232. Ballesteros MF, Jackson ML, Martin MW. Working toward the elimination of residential fire deaths: the Centers for Disease Control and Prevention's Smoke Alarm Installation and Fire Safety Education (SAIFE) Program. J Burn Care Rehab. 2005;26:434–9.
233. Mock C, Arreola-Risa C, Trevino-Perez R, Almazan-Saavedra V, Zozaya-Paz JE, Gonzalez-Solis R, et al. Injury prevention counseling to improve safety practices by parents in Mexico. Bull World Health Organ. 2003;81:591–8.
234. Council on Scientific Affairs. Preventing death and injury from fires with automatic sprinklers and smoke detectors. JAMA. 1987;257:1618–20.
235. Hall JR. U.S. experience with sprinklers and other fire extinguishing equipment. Quincy, MA: National Fire Protection Association Fire Analysis and Research Division. National Fire Protection Association; 2009a. http://www.nfpa.org/~/media/files/news-and-research/fire-statistics/fire-protection-systems/ossprinklers.pdf. Accessed 19 Sept 2017.
236. U.S. Census Bureau. Currents Housing Reports. Series H150/07, American Housing Survey for the United States: 2007. U.S. Government Printing Office, Washington, DC. Table 1C-4, 2–4, and 2–25. 2008.
237. Moritz AR, Henriques FC. Studies of thermal injury II: The relative importance of time and surface temperature in the causation of cutaneous burns. Am J Pathol. 1947;23:695–720.
238. Papp A, Rytkönen T, Koljonen V, Vuola J. Paediatric ICU burns in Finland 1994-2004. Burns. 2008;34:339–44.
239. Mercier C, Blond MH. Epidemiological survey of childhood burn injuries in France. Burns. 1996;22:29–34.
240. Erdmann TC, Feldman KW, Rivara FP, Heimbach DM, Wall HA. Tap water burn prevention: the effect of legislation. Pediatrics. 1991;88:572–7.
241. Katcher ML, Shapiro MM. Lower extremity burns related to sensory loss in diabetes mellitus. J Fam Pract. 1987;24:149–51.
242. Waller AE, Clarke JA, Langley JD. An evaluation of a program to reduce home hot tap water temperatures. Aust J Public Health. 1993;17:116–23.
243. Murray JP. A study of the prevention of hot tapwater burns. Burns Incl Therm Inj. 1988;14:185–93.
244. Stephen FR, Murray JP. Prevention of hot tap water burns—a comparative study of three types of automatic mixing valves. Burns. 1993;19:56–62.
245. World Bank. Africa results and monitoring system: improve access to and the reliability of clean energy. 2009. http://web.worldbank.org/WBSITE/EXTERNAL/COUNTRIES/AFRICAEXT/EXTAFRRES/0,,menuPK:3506948~pagePK:64168427~piPK:64168435~theSitePK:3506896,00.html. Accessed 20 Sept 2017.
246. Ahuja RB, Bhattacharya S. An analysis of 11,196 burn admissions and evaluation of conservative management techniques. Burns. 2002;28:555–61.
247. Laloë V. Epidemiology and mortality of burns in a general hospital of Eastern Sri Lanka. Burns. 2002;28:778–81.
248. Schwebel DC, Swart D, Simpson J, Hobe P, Hui SK. An intervention to reduce kerosene-related burns and poisonings in low-income South African communities. Health Psychol. 2009;28:493–500.
249. Safe Bottle Lamp Foundation. 2009. http://www.safebottlelamp.org. Accessed 13 Sept 2017.
250. Runyan CW. Introduction: back to the future-revisiting Haddon's conceptualization of injury epidemiology and prevention. Epidemiol Rev. 2003;25:60–4.
251. Government Gazette. Compulsory specification for non-pressurized paraffin stoves and heaters. Government Notice No. R 1091; 2006.
252. Paraffin Safety Association of Southern Africa. The status of paraffin appliances in South Africa—October, 2008. Cape Town, SA: Paraffin Safety Association of Southern Africa; 2008. http://www.pasasa.org/files/documents/programmes/safer-systems/20081112-The_status_of_paraffin_appliances_in_South_Africa.pdf.
253. Witsaman RJ, Comstock RD, Smith GA. Pediatric fireworks-related injuries in the United States: 1990-2003. Pediatrics. 2006;118:296–303.
254. Abdulwadud O, Ozanne-Smith J. Injuries associated with fireworks in Victoria: an epidemiological review. Inj Prev. 1998;4:272–5.
255. Vassilia K, Eleni P, Dimitrios T. Firework-related childhood injuries in Greece: a national problem. Burns. 2004;30:151–3.
256. Fogarty BJ, Gordon DJ. Firework related injury and legislation: the epidemiology of firework injuries and the effect of legislation in Northern Ireland. Burns. 1999;25:53–6.
257. Saadat S, Naseripour M, Rahimi B. Safety preparedness of urban community for New Year fireworks in Tehran. Burns. 2009;35:719–22.
258. Edwin AF, Cubison TC, Pape SA. The impact of recent legislation on paediatric fireworks injuries in the Newcastle upon Tyne region. Burns. 2008;34:953–64.
259. U. S. Consumer Product Safety Commission Office of Compliance. Summary of Children's Sleepwear Regulations, 16 C.F.R. Parts 1615 & 1616. 2001a. https://www.cpsc.gov/s3fs-public/pdfs/blk_pdf_regsumsleepwear.pdf.
260. U. S. Consumer Product Safety Commission. Fireworks. Publication #12; 2009. https://www.devens.army.mil/devens_staff/Safety/Fireworks%20safety%20tips.pdf.
261. Roesler JS, Day H. Sparklers, smoke bombs, and snakes, oh my! Effect of legislation on fireworks-related injuries in Minnesota, 1999-2005. Minn Med. 2007;90:46–7.
262. Sheller JP, Muchardt O, Jønsson B, Mikkelsen MB. Burn injuries caused by fireworks: effect of prophylaxis. Burns. 1995;21:50–3.
263. Puri V, Mahendru S, Rana R, Deshpande M. Fireworks injuries: a ten-year study. J Plast Reconstr Aesthet Surg. 2009;62:1103–11.
264. Leistikow BN, Martin DC, Milano CE. Fire injuries, disasters, and costs from cigarettes and cigarette lights: a global overview. Prev Med. 2000;31(2 Pt 1):91–9.
265. Hall JR. The smoking-material fire problem. Quincy, MA: National Fire Protection Association Fire Analysis and Research Division. National Fire Protection Association; 2008. http://www.nfpa.org/news-and-research/fire-statistics-and-reports/fire-statistics/fire-causes/smoking-materials. Accessed 19 Sept 2017.
266. Barillo DJ, Brigham PA, Kayden DA, Heck RT, McManus AT. The fire-safe cigarette: a burn prevention tool. J Burn Care Rehabil. 2000;21:162–70.
267. National Fire Protection Association (NFPA). Coalition for Fire-Safe Cigarettes™. State-by-state efforts. 2009. http://www.firesafecigarettes.org/itemDetail.asp?categoryID=93&itemID=1295&URL=Legislative%20updates/State-by-state%20efforts#oregon.
268. Connolly GN, Alpert HR, Rees V, Carpenter C, Wayne GF, Vallone D, et al. Effect of the New York State cigarette fire safety standard on ignition propensity, smoke constituents, and the consumer market. Tob Control. 2005;14:321–7.
269. McLoughlin E, Clarke N, Stahl K, Crawford JD. One pediatric burn unit's experience with sleepwear-related injuries. Pediatrics. 1977;60:405–9.
270. Liao CC, Rossignol AM. Landmarks in burn prevention. Burns. 2000;26:422–34.
271. Sleet DA, Schieber RA, Gilchrist J. Health promotion policy and politics: lessons from childhood injury prevention. Health Promot Pract. 2003;4(2):103–8.
272. Cusick JM, Grant EJ, Kucan JO. Children's sleepwear: relaxation of the Consumer Product Safety Commission's flammability standards. J Burn Care Res. 1997;18:469–76.

273. U.S. Consumer Product Safety Commission. National Burn Center Reporting System. Debra S. Ascone, Division of Hazard Analysis; 2004. http://www.cpsc.gov/CPSCPUB/PREREL/prhtml05/05028.pdf.
274. U. S. Consumer Product Safety Commission Office of Compliance. Summary of Fireworks Regulations, 16 C.F.R. Parts 1500 & 1507. 2001b. https://www.cpsc.gov/Business%2D%2DManufacturing/Business-Education/Business-Guidance/Fireworks.
275. U. S. Consumer Product Safety Commission. Flammable Liquids Safety Alert, CPSC Publication 5140. 2008. https://www.cpsc.gov/s3fs-public/5140.pdf.
276. Greenbaum AR, Donne J, Wilson D, Dunn KW. Intentional burn injury: an evidence-based, clinical and forensic review. Burns. 2004;30:628–42.
277. Mannan A, Ghani S, Clarke A, Butler PE. Cases of chemical assault worldwide: a literature review. Burns. 2007;33:149–54.
278. Bari SM, Choudhury M, Mahmud I. Acid burns in Bangladesh. Ann Burns Fire Disasters. 2002;14:115–8.
279. Shahidul B, Choudhury I. Acid burns in Bangladesh. Ann Burns Fire Disasters. 2001;14:1–8.
280. Lam NN, Dung NT. First aid and initial management for childhood burns in Vietnam—an appeal for public and continuing medical education. Burns. 2008;34:67–70.
281. Nguyen NL, Gun RT, Sparnon AL, Ryan P. The importance of immediate cooling—a case series of childhood burns in Vietnam. Burns. 2002;28:173–6.
282. Skinner A, Peat B. Burns treatment for children and adults: a study of initial burns first aid and hospital care. NZ Med J. 2002;115:U199.
283. Blomgren I, Eriksson E, Bagge U. Effect of cold water immersion on oedema formation in the scalded mouse ear. Burns Incl Therm Inj. 1982;9:17–20.
284. Boykin JV Jr, Eriksson E, Sholley MM, Pittman RN. Histamine-mediated delayed permeability response after scald burn inhibited by cimetidine or cold-water treatment. Science. 1980;209:815–7.
285. Hudspith J, Rayatt S. First aid and treatment of minor burns. BMJ. 2004;328:1487–9.
286. Ofeigsson OJ, Mitchell R, Patrick RS. Observations on the cold water treatment of cutaneous burns. J Pathol. 1972;108:145–50.
287. Raghupati N. First-aid treatment of burns: efficacy of water cooling. Br J Plast Surg. 1968;21:68–72.
288. Raine TJ, Heggers JP, Robson MC, London MD, Johns L. Cooling the burn wound to maintain microcirculation. J Trauma. 1981;21:394–7.
289. Rea S, Kuthubutheen J, Fowler B, Wood F. Burn first aid in Western Australia—do healthcare workers have the knowledge? Burns. 2005;31:1029–34.
290. Papp T, Abude E, Brindza E, Ferenczi K, Kincs M, Lipcsei E. The health education of inpatients on the prevention and first aid of burns. Burns. 1978;5:92–3.
291. Beer GM, Kompatscher P. Standardization of the first aid treatment of burn injuries in Vorarlberg, Austria. Burns. 1996;22:130–4.
292. Skinner A, Brown TL, Peat BG, Muller MJ. Reduced hospitalization of burns patients following a multi-media campaign that increased adequacy of first aid treatment. Burns. 2004;30:82–5.
293. MacKenzie EJ, Rivara FP, Jurkovich GJ, Nathens AB, Frey KP, Egleston BL, et al. A national evaluation of the effect of trauma-center care on mortality. N Engl J Med. 2006;354:366–78.
294. Saffle JA. Organization and delivery of burn care. In: Practice guidelines for burn care. Chicago: American Burn Association; 2001. p. 18–57.
295. American Burn Association. Burn incidence and treatment in the US: 2007 fact sheet. 2007. http://www.ameriburn.org/resources_factsheet.php.
296. Warden GD, Heimbach DM. Regionalization of burn care—a concept whose time has come. J Burn Care Rehabil. 2003;24:173–4.
297. Sagraves SG, Phade SV, Spain T, Bard MR, Goettler CE, Schenarts PJ, et al. A collaborative systems approach to rural burn care. J Burn Care Res. 2007;28:111–4.
298. Klein M, Kramer CB, Nelson J, Rivara FP, Gibran NS, Concannon T. Geographic access to burn center hospitals. JAMA. 2009;302:1774–81.
299. American Burn Association National Burn Repository. 2006. http://www.ameriburn.org/2006NBR.pdf. Accessed 14 Apr 2017.
300. Mock C, Lormand JD, Goosen J, Joshipura M, Peden M. Guidelines for essential trauma care. Geneva: World Health Organization; 2004. http://whqlibdoc.who.int/publications/2004/9241546409.pdf. Accessed 19 Sept 2017.
301. Public/Private Safety Council. White paper: home smoke alarms and other fire detection and alarm equipment. 2006 . www.hvfd6.org/files/news/1218/White%20Paper%20Smoke%20Alarms.pdf. Accessed 20 Sept 2017.
302. Jutla RK, Heimbach D. Love burns: an essay about bride burning in India. J Burn Care Rehabil. 2004;25:165–70.
303. Sethi D, Habibula S, McGee K, Peden M, Bennett S, Hyder AA, et al. WHO Guidelines for conducting community surveys on injuries and violence. Geneva: World Health Organization; 2004.
304. Hang HM, Bach TT, Byass P. Unintentional injuries over a 1-year period in a rural Vietnamese community: describing an iceberg. Public Health. 2005;119:466–73.
305. Pant PR, Towner E, Ellis M, Manandhar D, Pilkington P, Mytton J. Epidemiology of unintentional child injuries in the Makwanpur District of Nepal: a household survey. Int J Environ Res Public Health. 2015;12:15118–28.
306. National Fire Protection Association (NFPA). 921, Guide for fire and explosion investigations. Quincy, MA: National Fire Protection Association; 1992. http://www.nfpa.org/codes-and-standards/all-codes-and-standards/list-of-codes-and-standards/detail?code=921. Accessed 19 Sept 2017.

Bibliography

Atiyeh BS, Costagliola M, Hayek SN. Burn prevention mechanisms and outcomes: pitfalls, failures and successes. Burns. 2009;35:181–93.

Barss P, Smith G, Baker SP, Mohan D. Injury prevention: an international perspective. Epidemiology, surveillance, and policy. New York: Oxford University Press; 1998. p. 375.

Greenbaum AR, Donne J, Wilson D, Dunn KW. Intentional burn injury: an evidence-based, clinical and forensic review. Burns. 2004;30:628–42.

Horrocks AR, Nazare S, Kandola B. The particular flammability hazards of nightwear. Fire Saf J. 2004;39:259–76.

Liao CC, Rossignol AM. Landmarks in burn prevention. Burns. 2000;26:422–34.

Mock C, Peck M, Peden M, Krug E, editors. A WHO plan for burn prevention and care. Geneva: World Health Organization; 2008a. whqlibdoc.who.int/publications/2008/9789241596299_eng.pdf.

Public/Private Safety Council. White paper: home smoke alarms and other fire detection and alarm equipment. 2006 . www.hvfd6.org/files/news/1218/White%20Paper%20Smoke%20Alarms.pdf. Accessed 20 Sept 2017.

3 Prevention of Burn Injuries

Joanne Banfield

3.1 Introduction

Burns are preventable, and yet they are responsible for significant morbidity and mortality worldwide with approximately 90% occurring in low- to middle-income countries [1]. Injuries are a public health issue, and burn injuries remain the fourth most common type of trauma globally, followed by road traffic injuries, falls and interpersonal violence [2]. As a result, burn prevention is particularly important and must be a major focus of attention.

It has been shown that prevention is key for maintaining health and having the highest quality of life, despite increasing age. Injuries are like other conditions and illnesses that occur with distinct patterns and are therefore considered to be a disease. Furthermore, prevention is the more efficient way to treat an illness since it reduces not only hospital stay but also drug use, cost of complications and long-term chronic conditions. In the past, injuries were regarded as random, unavoidable accidents. In recent decades, due to a better understanding of underlying mechanisms, injuries are now regarded as largely predictable and preventable [3].

Behavioural, psychosocial, and sociocultural factors associated with lifestyle behaviours are known contributors to injury morbidity and mortality, along with characteristics of products and environments.

Like other injury mechanisms, the prevention of burns requires epidemiology and risk factors studies. In fact, the complete care of any illness or injury implies epidemiology (measurement of risk factors, frequency, and distribution of the injury), prevention, injury biomechanics (physical and functional responses of the victim to the energy), treatment and rehabilitation.

3.2 Global Impact of Burn Injuries

The World Health Organization (WHO) broadly defines a burn as an injury caused by heat (hot objects, gases, or flames), chemicals, electricity and lightning, friction or radiation [4]. Annually, burns result in more than 7.1 million injuries, the loss of almost 18 million disability adjusted life years (DALYs) and more than 250,000 deaths worldwide. More than 90% of the burden of burn injury is borne by low- and middle-income countries (LMICs). The three WHO regions with the greatest burden of injury are the Eastern Mediterranean Region, the South East Asian Region and the African Region, with the African Region bearing nearly two thirds of the total burden [5].

3.2.1 Some Country Data

- In India, over 1,000,000 people are moderately or severely burnt every year.
- Nearly 173,000 Bangladeshi children are moderately or severely burnt every year.
- In Bangladesh, Colombia, Egypt and Pakistan, 17% of children with burns have a temporary disability and 18% have a permanent disability.
- Burns are the second most common injury in rural Nepal, accounting for 5% of disabilities.
- In 2008, over 410,000 burn injuries occurred in the United States of America, with approximately 40,000 requiring hospitalization.
- In 2015, fire and heat resulted in 67 million injuries [6]. This resulted in about 2.9 million hospitalizations and 176,000 deaths [7, 8]. Most deaths due to burns occur in the developing world, particularly in Southeast Asia [9].

J. Banfield (✉)
Office for Injury Prevention, Sunnybrook Health Sciences Centre, Toronto, ON, Canada
e-mail: Joanne.Banfield@sunnybrook.ca

M. G. Jeschke et al. (eds.), *Handbook of Burns Volume 1*, https://doi.org/10.1007/978-3-030-18940-2_3

3.3 Burn Risk Factors and the Social Determinants of Injury

We know more about injury risk and those we see most frequently in emergency departments and burn units. Injury risk is disproportionate. We all do not face equal risk of injury. Injury is a lot more than an individual making a poor choice. We know some populations are at higher risk for injury than other such as Aboriginals, young males, seniors, those living in lower socioeconomic status and underdeveloped countries, and young children. As frontline practitioners and those in positions of influence, we need to understand the risk that certain populations face and advocate for changes in our communities to reduce the burden of injury to them and to our healthcare system.

3.3.1 Burn Injury Risk Factors

Burn risk is linked with poverty, lack of running water, overcrowding, illiteracy, unemployment, lapses in child supervision—mostly in large and single-parent families, occupations that increase exposure to fire, lack of proper safety measures, placement of young girls in household roles such as cooking and care of small children; underlying medical conditions, including epilepsy, peripheral neuropathy, and physical and cognitive disabilities; medications, such as sleeping pills, narcotics, and synthetic stimulant drugs, such as methamphetamines; alcohol abuse and smoking; easy access to chemicals used for assault (such as in acid violence attacks); use of kerosene (paraffin) as a fuel source for non-electric domestic appliances; and inadequate safety measures for liquefied petroleum gas and electricity.

With these risk factors in mind, one can ascertain why burns are more common in the developing world and how low socioeconomic status has been linked to increased risk of unintentional injury and mortality.

Children under 5 years of age comprise the highest risk group for burn injuries. Causative factors in all incidents involving babies are a mixture of imprudence, impulsiveness, curiosity, lack of experience and a desire to imitate adults. Furthermore, this age group lacks a sense of danger and awareness as they hardly understand cause-and-effect relationships.

At the other end of the age continuum, elderly people over 64 years are also a high-risk population. Their risk of dying in a fire is 2.5 times greater than the general population. The main causes of burn injuries in the elderly are flame burns

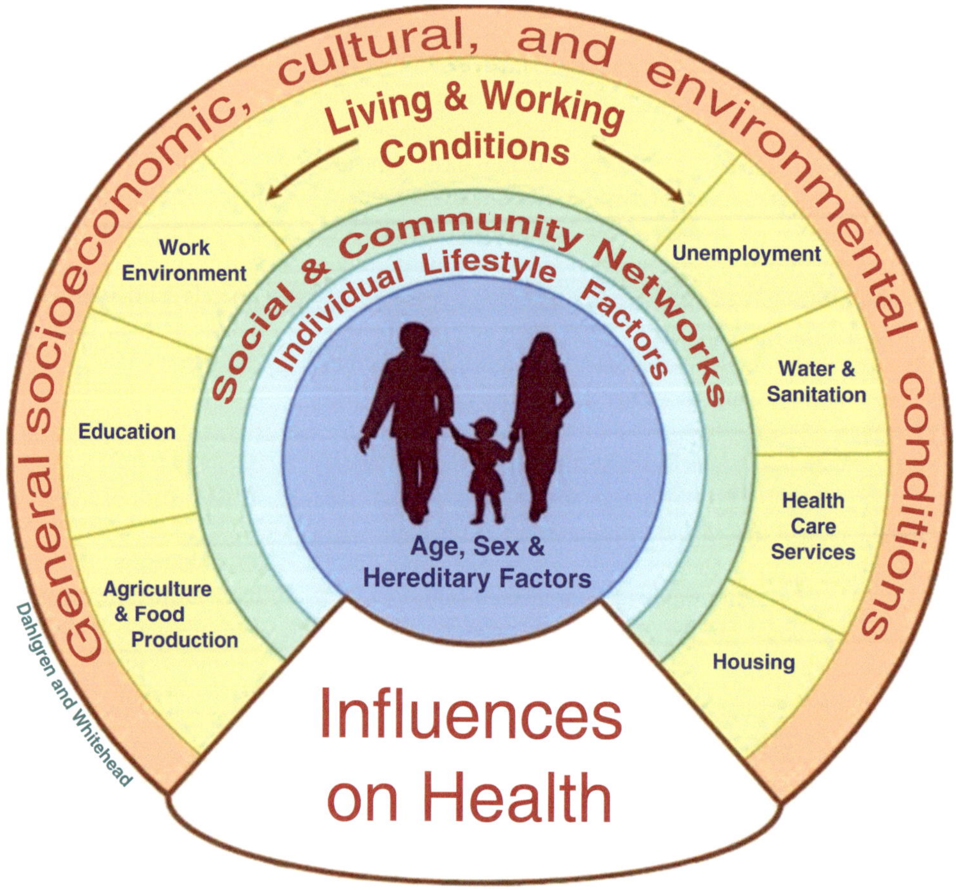

Fig. 3.1 Influences on health

due to smoking and cooking (see Table 3.1). Additional risk factors include medical conditions associated with physical or mental impairment: stroke, poor eyesight, decreased hearing and mobility, diabetes (peripheral neuropathy with decreased or no lower extremity pain perception), dementia (such as Alzheimer's, with confusion and forgetfulness), depression, and suicide.

There is no vaccine, pill or quick fix for injury prevention. Preventing injury requires a comprehensive ecological approach that extends far beyond the individual to organizations, community and government. Humans are fallible. We believe we are at lower risk for injuries and capable in avoiding circumstances that will injure us. It is part of our design, we are hardwired this way and that makes the business of reducing injury all the more challenging. We need to take what is known as an 'upstream' approach.

The Spectrum of Prevention (Fig. 3.2) is a framework for developing multifaceted approaches to injury prevention. The value of this tool is that it can help practitioners develop and structure comprehensive initiatives. Additionally, it can

Table 3.1 Elderly burn prevention tips

Flame burns	1. Ask a relative or neighbour to routinely check for gas leak odour
	2. Use large ashtrays. Smoke only while upright. Never smoke in bed or when drowsy
	3. Never use flammable liquids to start a fire or prime a carburettor or as a cleaning solvent
	4. Never store flammable liquids near a pilot light or other heat source
	5. Check the smoke detector battery once a month. Use a broom handle to perform the check or ask a friend to do so
	6. Have a flashlight, keys, eyeglasses and whistle at the bedside to summon help if needed
	7. Wear close-fitting clothes while cooking or near any potentially dangerous heat source (fireplace, campfire, wood-burning stove). Garments that are flame-resistant are recommended
	8. Use the back burners of the stove and turn handles inward
	9. Avoid throw rugs in the kitchen area and keep the floor clean to avoid falls
	10. Use a cooking timer with an audible alarm
	11. If using a space heater, ensure that the automatic shut off is in working order should the heater accidentally tip over
	12. Never lay anything on or near a heating device (e.g. space heater, wood-burning stove, kitchen stove and baseboard heater)
Contact burns	1. Use all heating devices that are placed on or near the skin with caution (e.g. heating pad, hot water bottles and space heaters)
Scald burns	1. Place a non-skid mat and handrails in the bathtub or shower to prevent accidental falls and to allow easy access in and out of the area
	2. Check the temperature on the hot water heater; the recommended setting is 120 °F (48.8 °C). Install anti-scald devices in bathroom plumbing

From: Hunt JL, Arnoldo BD, Purdue GF. Prevention of burn injuries. In: Herndon DN, editor. Total burn care. Galveston: Saunders Elsevier; 2007. p. 33–9

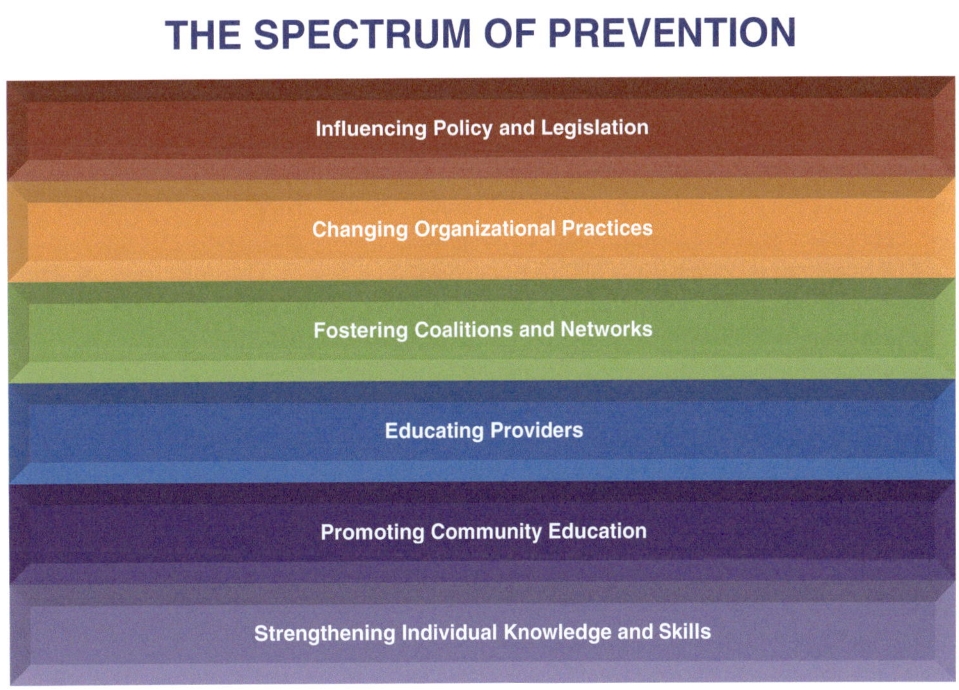

Fig. 3.2 The Spectrum of Prevention

Fig. 3.3 The Haddon matrix applied to the risk factors for burns

PHASES	FACTORS			
	HOST (PERSON)	AGENT	PHYSICAL ENVIRONMENT	SOCIOECONOMIC ENVIRONMENT
PRE-EVENT	Use of fireworks Smoking in the home or in bed Lack of knowledge about risks of fire in the home	Storage of flammable substances in the house Combustibles, matches or lighters accessible to children Unsafe stoves or lamps	Housing in slums or congested areas Overcrowded households No separation between cooking area and other areas Unsafe electrical wiring High (unsafe) temperatures of hot water heaters	Poverty, unemployment, illiteracy Lack of fire-related building codes and their enforcement Societal attitudes on acceptability of acid-throwing
EVENT	Poorly maintained smoke alarms and sprinkler systems Child not wearing flame-retardant sleepwear Poor knowledge about evacuation procedures	Lack of sprinkler systems Lack of fire hydrants or other access to water supply	Lack of functioning smoke alarms Lack of clear and easily accessible escape routes Lack of access to phones to call for help	Lack of policies or laws on smoke alarms Inadequate communications infrastructure for calling emergency services
POST-EVENT	Lack of knowledge of first aid	Flammability of household materials and children's clothing Toxicity of smoke and burning household materials	Low level of first aid, emergency medical services, and hospital burn care	Inadequate access to burn centres and rehabilitation services Insufficient community support for those who have suffered burns

help policy leaders move beyond a primarily educational approach to achieve broad community goals through injury prevention strategies that include policy development.

The Spectrum is comprised of six interrelated action levels: (1) strengthening individual knowledge and skills (enhancing an individual's capability of preventing injury or illness and promoting safety), (2) promoting community education (reaching groups of people with information and resources to promote health and safety), (3) educating providers (informing providers who will transmit skills and knowledge to others), (4) fostering coalitions and networks (bringing together groups and individuals for broader goals and greater impact), (5) changing organizational practices (adopting regulations and shaping norms to improve health and safety) and (6) influencing policy and legislation (developing strategies to change laws and policies to influence outcomes). Activities at each of these levels have the potential to support each other and promote overall community health and safety.

The Spectrum of Prevention developed in 1983 by Larry Cohen and based upon the clinical work of Dr. Marshall Swift from Hahnemann College emerged from the conviction that preventive practice was too frequently trivialized and misunderstood as simply an educational practice [10].

Perhaps the most important tool in the injury prevention field is the Haddon Matrix. Dr. William Haddon contributed immensely by distinguishing between prevention efforts that take place before an injury occurs from those that are implemented after the injury that serve only to reduce the severity of trauma. The Spectrum supplements the Haddon Matrix as it helps practitioners to specify the array of activities necessary for an effective prevention campaign. By using the two tools together, practitioners can devise a multifactored intervention that simultaneously addresses the temporal issues highlighted by the Haddon matrix (i.e. multiple strategies for before, during, and after an injury event) [11]. The Spectrum emphasizes the importance of influencing policy and legislation, an area that Haddon's approach does not specifically address.

Prevention is more than education and goes beyond the individual.

There is a commonly held misconception that individual behaviours are solely responsible for health outcomes, and therefore, individual health education is an adequate solution. Effective prevention is not that simple. The Spectrum shifts attention from being individually focused to a systems approach. One important note to keep in mind is that prevention efforts and campaigns must target the population groups most at risk and should aim at minimizing the effects of specific risk factors and harmful actions [12]. In other words, every burn prevention program has to be population-specific and different, depending on the country/individual characteristics (education, socioeconomic status, geography, traditions, cultural or religious beliefs, and social habits). Preventive interventions should be designed so that they effectively counteract the underlying mechanisms of injury, which can be different in each social group. Policies and interventions addressing unintentional injuries must be implemented with a clear view to have at least as much (if not more impact) on vulnerable groups compared with the rest of the population, in order to close the gap [13]. Knowing the general risk factors—the vector or energy source, the host or victim and the environment— is essential for preventing and controlling any injury. Finally, any injury prevention plan is not valid until the results of its application are evaluated [14]. If a prevention plan fails to have success, possible solutions may be to change the technique to measure the burn incidence reduction or modify the prevention program design to a more appropriate one.

3.4 Classifications and Strategies for Prevention

The key approach to burn injury prevention involves the three E's: education, engineering (built environment) and enforcement (legislation). Most recently added to the three E's is technology.

Injury prevention is classified as primary, secondary, and tertiary which is similar to the Haddon Matrix with the phases pre-event (primary prevention), event (secondary prevention) and post-event (tertiary prevention) while active and passive strategies focus on the three aspects of injury prevention—agent, environment and host.

Primary burn prevention aims to avoid the injury from occurring at all. Primary burn prevention strategies include automatic protection, legislation/regulation and education.

1. Automatic protection represents the most effective primary preventive strategy. It involves elimination of environmental hazards or more accurate product design.
2. Legislation/regulation: Community, state, national or international governmental regulations and laws are in place to reduce injury. For instance, local ordinances that require apartment buildings to have working smoke detectors or installation of anti-scald devices; regulation of exits and fire escapes from buildings where people work or congregate, as well as laws, not only for the installation, but more importantly for the maintenance of equipment for fire control; regulations of fire drills in educational institutions; regulations of handling and disposition of any kind of flammable materials, etc.
3. Education: Educational programs focus on providing information about an identified area of concern and seek to make the public aware of the dangers and to teach appropriate preventive strategies. They also inform people about the medical and social consequences of burn injuries; that is, parents are taught to insert plastic plugs to cover the electrical outlets to prevent electrical burns in small children.

While burn prevention educational campaigns have reduced the incidence of burn injuries, they have not eliminated the injuries entirely. Education may increase knowledge, but does not always lead to behavioural and/or lifestyle change needed to diminish or eliminate incidence or severity of burn injuries.

Probable causes of failure of burn education primary prevention programs may be the brevity of the campaign, multiplicity of messages and separation of the interventions. It has been postulated that the prevention program needs to be repeated several times to be effective. Posters, mass media and multimedia strategies are effective means of disseminating the burn prevention message in general. Social media is a great vehicle to provide burn prevention education. In 2013, there were 21 videos posted on YouTube with technically accurate content covering prevention and first aid treatment of paediatric burns [15]. Due to the ease of access and wide audience (over six billion hours of video are watched each month on YouTube), there are exciting opportunities to use these platforms to raise public awareness of burn prevention and treatment, although validation of content by qualified health care professionals is still a challenge.

Secondary burn prevention seeks to minimize the already-produced injury and consists of teaching early injury detection and treatment. For example, an individual whose shirt catches fire is taught to *Stop, Drop* to the ground and *Roll* to extinguish

Fig. 3.4 First aid counselling after a burn (secondary prevention)

> ≻ **If your clothing catches fires:**
> **STOP (don't run!) ⇨ DROP to the ground ⇨ ROLL to put the fire out.**
>
> ≻ **If a burns occur: COOL**
> **Immediately pour cool water – not ice - on the burn.**
> **Cover burn with a clean sheet and seek medical attention.**

Fig. 3.5 Strategies to reduce severity injury and parameters of injury occurrence

> **ACTIVE (Education)** ⇨ **Agent + Host + Environment**
> ⇓
> **PASSIVE**
> **(Product engineering + Environmental change + Legislation)** ⇨ **Agent + Environment**

the flames; other examples include 'apply cool water to a burn' or 'crawl under smoke' (see Fig. 3.4).

Tertiary burn prevention involves avoiding impairment and maximizing functionality during the phase of rehabilitation after a burn. Indeed, not only secondary but also tertiary burn prevention strategies aim at limiting the already-produced damage.

Active burn prevention: Active prevention requires individual effort. Education is the only active primary burn prevention strategy. For instance, teaching people to lower their tap water temperature through educational campaigns. Active prevention is the least effective and most difficult strategy to maintain, especially over a long period of time.

Passive burn prevention includes legislation/regulation and product design/environmental change. Passive prevention strategies do not require 'correct behaviour' by the individual and appear to be more successful than active prevention strategies. However, many of the more effective burn prevention programs contain both active and passive measures. Among the passive prevention methods, legislation appears to play a major role.

To sum up (see Fig. 3.5), burn prevention involves not only physicians, nurses and other health care providers but also engineers, legislators and inspectors.

3.5 Causes/Types of Burns

Burns are classified in the following four categories: thermal, chemical, electrical and radiation.

3.5.1 Thermal Burns

3.5.1.1 Burns from Residential Fires

The use of smoke alarms (with the purpose of alerting occupants of a fire) has had the greatest impact in decreasing fire deaths in the USA, but to be effective they must be maintained—not only installed. Overall, working smoke alarms reduce fatalities by about half. However, smoke alarms are limited by factors such as battery life, an inadequate power source and incorrect placement in the home and can fail to alert sleeping residents. Despite this popular early smoke detection system, individuals may still not escape because of physical or mental impairments or other frailties associated with children and the elderly.

On the other hand, fire sprinklers complement smoke detectors and are the most effective tool to prevent the spread of fires in their early stages. In 1993, the National Fire Protection Association (NFPA) estimated smoke alarms alone could reduce fire deaths by 52%; sprinklers alone could decrease fire deaths by 69% and the combined use of them by 82% [16, 17].

House fires account for most of the major burn injuries. Causes of injuries and burn prevention tips include:

(a) Careless cigarette smoking: Canada was the first country to pass fire-safe cigarette legislation in 2004. People must be aware of practicing safe behaviour while using flammable materials. It is also recommended that all occupants practice EDITH (Exit Drills in the Home), so that everyone will know the meeting place and how to escape in case of a fire. A cigarette left unattended can burn for as long as 30 min. Most smoking fires start in the bedroom or living room. Some severe COPD (chronic obstructive lung disease) patients use home oxygen and then, at the same time, light a cigarette, leading to facial burns. Furthermore, alcohol is often combined with cigarette smoking or other substance abuse, with the victim falling asleep. In fact, statistics have shown that it is quite common for burn patients to have higher blood alcohol levels.

(b) Heating equipment: Never leave small children unattended next to a heat source. Also do not leave candles unattended. In middle Asia, the 'sandal' is an ancient heating device responsible for a high number of third-degree foot burns in small children in Uzbekistan. The 'sandal' is a table, around which people sit which has a hole in the floor underneath, where lit coals are placed. Unsupervised toddlers crawl and fall into the coals leading to severe burns. During winters in Kashmir, people place charcoal braziers, known as 'kangari', between their legs to keeps warm. Repeated exposure results in erythema to the inner thighs and lower abdomen and may also promote skin cancer.

(c) Electrical equipment malfunction: You should install not only smoke but also CO (carbon monoxide) detectors. Whereas smoke alarms are now present in almost 100% of homes, CO detectors are largely absent, but they should also be present. CO inhalation is the main cause of fatal poisoning in the industrialized world and CO intoxication is present in flame injuries, especially those sustained indoors. CO is produced by open flames, whenever a carbon-based fuel, gas, oil, wood or charcoal is burned. Products include charcoal grills, gas water heaters, stoves and lanterns. Carbon monoxide-generating appliances, such as stoves, are often used during power outages or for financial reasons in low-income households. If the heating source is either used improperly or ventilation is inadequate, CO levels can become toxic and have fatal consequences.

(d) Cooking: You should be very careful when cooking, avoid wearing loose clothing that could catch fire. In many developing countries, cooking is still done using primus stoves, which are an important cause of burns, due to the presence of kerosene. Apart from the kitchen, kerosene is also used as a nightly light source and contained in home-made chimneys, located in the living rooms and bedrooms in houses in the developing world.

(e) Children playing with matches and lighters: Matches and lighters must be kept out of the reach of children. Children should be taught, at an early age, that matches and lighters are tools and not toys.

3.5.1.2 Outdoor Flame Burns

In many dry and warm climate countries, especially during the summer, forest fires are caused by unattended fallen cigarettes or intentionally by individuals with psychiatric disorders who enjoy provoking fires. In some rural areas of Spain, farmers burn olive trees or timber to produce embers or 'brasas' which leave incandescent residue. These residues remain alight and undergo slow combustion and hence are used for heating, but they may also produce flame burns.

Outdoor barbecues are commonly held in many countries during summer months. Instead of using an authorized carbon source of heat, some people use gasoline or alcohol to make the flames grow, causing flame burns. Other cooking-related burns involve the making of fondues flambeed food.

Outdoor, recreational fires are also a normal practice during the warmer months of the year and may cause severe burns. They involve mostly the hands, with a mean TBSA (total body surface area) of 3.5%, and the main mechanism is falling into the fire. Parents can play an important role in educating their children about campfire safety and the hazards of both active and extinguished fires.

In India, marital traditions are associated with 'dowry' and 'sati' burns, which both have high mortality rates. After marriage, if the gifts (known as 'dowry') are not considered enough, the wife is put on fire (usually after pouring kerosene on her body), and this is known as 'dowry burns'. In 'sati burns', the wife throws herself on the burning body of the deceased husband. Although the government has made efforts to prevent these burns by writing legislation and including it under the Penal Code, these type of injuries still occur and some families lie and report 'dowry burns' as kitchen 'accidents'.

In a similar manner, in the developing world, some religious activities involve self-inflicted ritual burns (especially in the Buddhist community) or promote unintentional burning (e.g. foot burns in Muslims who leave mosques barefoot where temperatures exceed 50 °C).

Also in India, a special type of fire-related burn (jaggery) causes severe and deadly paediatric burns. Jaggery is the non-industrial refinement of sugar cane into a sugar product and represents an important source of income and significant role in cooking and cultural rituals in rural India. Legislation aimed at improving dangerous work environments, establishing minimum age requirements and maximum hours of work, as well as with engineering or product design safety improvements, would be effective in reducing these types of injuries.

Fireworks are an important cause of burns in many countries around the world, due to its use during national holidays, traditional festivals or special events, such as New Year's Eve or other celebrations, such as the Olympic games, Independence day (US), Guy Fawkes Night (Commonwealth), Fallas (Valencia, Spain), Hari Raya (Malaysia), Mawlid and Eid al-Adha (Muslim countries), Chaharshanbe-Soori (Iran) or Purim (Jewish festivity). Contact hand burns from holding the fireworks are most frequently seen accounted for largely by boys 10–14 years of age. However, in approximately 50% of the cases bystanders are injured. Eyes are affected in 18% of cases. Flame burns may also occur when the clothes catch fire. Complete firework bans are found in Hungary, Ireland, Australia and the northeast USA, at the present time.

A specific type of outdoor burn is seen during war. Combat-related thermal injuries generally affect the hands and head, mainly through improvised explosive devices, causing blast injuries and polytrauma. They generally involve less than 20% TBSA and have relatively low mortality rates (4% of all war deaths and 5–20% of all war injuries). Preventive measures against war-related burn injuries

Table 3.2 Burn prevention tips for people with impairments

Flame burns	1. Use extreme caution when cooking. Wear close-fitting and flame-resistant clothes while cooking or near any heat source
	2. Avoid throw rugs in the kitchen area and keep the floor clean to avoid falls
	3. Use larger ashtrays. Smoke only while upright. Never smoke in bed or when drowsy
	4. Maintain smoke detectors, alarms and sprinkler systems in good working order. Check the smoke detector battery once a month
	5. Determine emergency exit plans. Practice them routinely with household members. Keep all exit routes clear
	6. Have a flashlight, keys, eyeglasses and whistle at the bedside to summon help if needed
	7. Ensure that the local fire department is aware of any household members with special needs
Contact burns	1. With individuals with decreased sensation, use all heating devices that are placed on or near the skin with caution (e.g. heating pad, hot water bottles and space heaters)
Scald burns	1. For people cooking from a wheelchair, a mirror positioned over the stovetop allows one to see the contents of a pot during cooking. Avoid using heavy, large plans that may be awkward to use especially when filled with hot food
	2. Check the temperature on the hot water heater; the recommended setting is 120 °F (48.8 °C)
	3. Install anti-scald devices in bathroom plumbing

From: Hunt JL, Arnoldo BD, Purdue GF. Prevention of burn injuries. In: Herndon DN, editor. Total burn care. Galveston: Saunders Elsevier; 2007. p. 33–9

include improvement in pre-deployment education to reduce noncombat injuries, flame retardant military clothing and decreased combat episodes.

Scald Burns

Scald burns are responsible for the majority of non-fatal burn injuries in the world. Furthermore, scald burns are the main cause of burn injury in toddlers, involving mostly splash burns from spilled liquids. Other populations at high risk for scale burns, while bathing, are the elderly and people with epilepsy, where there is a heightened risk of seizures and falls and, in the elderly, thinner skin.

Preventative strategies include reducing the temperature of hot water heaters to a maximum of 49–54 °C (see Table 3.3), installing anti-scald devices to shower heads and faucets or inserting shut-off valves in the water circuit to detect temperatures over a certain level, using large round handles or push-and-turn type handles to prevent young children from turning on the hot water or using liquid-crystal thermometers in bathtubs to alert the caregiver to the water temperature. In some US states, it is imperative, by law, to install appropriate temperature valves in all new domestic dwellings, and water from shower heads and bathtubs inlets cannot exceed 46 °C. Small children and disabled people should be constantly supervised when close to hot water.

Table 3.3 Time/temperature relationships in scalds

Temperature	Time to produce full-thickness burn
48.8 °C = 120 °F	5 min
51.6 °C = 125 °F	1.5–2 min
54.4 °C = 130 °F	30 s
57.2 °C = 135 °F	10 s
60 °C = 140 °F	5 s
62.9 °C = 145 °F	3 s
65.5 °C = 150 °F	1.5 s
68.3 °C = 155 °F	1 s

Special caution should also be paid when removing warmed foods—especially liquids—from the microwave oven to avoid steam and scald burns.

3.6 Child Burns and Scald Prevention Tips

Childproof Your Electrical Outlets and Appliances

- Keep appliance cords out of children's reach, especially if the appliances produce a lot of heat.
- Cover electrical outlets so that children are unable to insert metal objects, such as forks or keys.
- Keep an eye on appliances such as irons, curling irons or hair dryers that can heat up quickly or stay warm after use. Unplug these items after you are done.
- Do not carry or hold a child while cooking on the stove. Instead, move a high chair in the kitchen within reach or sight before you start. Then talk to your children so they know what is going on. It is a great way to spend time together.

Check to Make Sure the Water Temperature Is Just Right

- With everything going on, we know the water heater is the last thing on your mind. But a small change can give you one less thing to worry about. To prevent accidental scalding, set your water heater to 120 °F or the manufacturer's recommended setting.
- Consider installing anti-scald devices in water faucets and showerheads to avoid potential burns.
- Check the water with your wrist or elbow before giving your baby a bath.

Use the Back Burner and Oven Mitts

- Kids love to reach, so to prevent hot food or liquid spills, simply use the back burner of your stove and turn pot handles away from the edge. Keep hot foods away from the edge of your counters.
- Use oven mitts or potholders and keep hot foods and liquids away from table and counter edges. Be careful if your oven mitt is wet; when combined with heat, the moisture can cause scalds.
- Slowly open containers that have been in the microwave, as steam can burn little fingers and faces.

Engage Older Kids in Cooking

- Teach older responsible kids how to cook safely. It will make your life easier if your kids can cook some of their own meals (and maybe yours, too). Teach them never to leave the kitchen while they are using the stove or oven. Do not forget that the number one cause of home fires is unattended cooking.
- Do not allow children to use a microwave by themselves until they are tall enough to reach it safely and are able to understand that steam can cause burns.
- Instruct older kids to use oven mitts or potholders to remove items from the oven or stove and teach them how to use a microwave safely.

Be Careful with the Microwave

- Microwaves can heat unevenly and create hot spots, so avoid using them to heat baby formula or baby milk.
- Heat bottles by placing them in warm water, and make sure they have cooled to the appropriate temperature before feeding your baby.

Install Smoke Alarms and Carbon Monoxide Alarms

- Fire and burns go together. Prevent them both by installing smoke alarms and carbon monoxide alarms.

Keep Flammable Materials Away from Space Heaters

- Remember to keep space heaters at least 3 ft away from anything that can burn or catch fire.
- Make sure you turn them off when you leave the room.

Install Barriers Such as Safety Gates Around Fireplaces, Ovens and Furnaces

- Make sure your fireplace is protected by a sturdy screen. Remember that glass screens can take a long time to cool down.
- If you are using a fireplace or wood stove, burn only seasoned hardwood such as oak, ash or maple.
- If small children live in or visit your home, use a safety gate around your fireplace or wood stove.

Blow Out Candles and Store Matches Out of Reach

- Keep candles at least 12 inches away from anything that can burn and always blow them out when you leave the room or before you go to sleep.
- Make a habit of placing matches, gasoline and lighters in a safe place, out of children's reach. Avoid novelty lighters or lighters that look like toys.
- Teach kids never to play with matches, lighters or fireworks. Depending on the age and maturity level of your child, it may be reasonable to use the items with the supervision of an adult. Just be sure that a fire extinguisher and a phone are close by in case of an emergency.
- Unplug and safely store irons, flatirons and other appliances that might be hot to the touch.
- https://www.safekids.org/tip/burn-and-scald-prevention-tips-pdf. Accessed 5 Sept 2017.

3.6.1 Contact Burns

Contact burns can be avoided by adopting appropriate preventative measures. In developed countries, contact burns from the use of gas fireplaces, domestic central heating radiators, irons and ovens have been identified. The surface temperature of the glass front on gas fireplace units can reach 200 °C, on average 6.5 min after ignition. A full-thickness burn may occur in less than 1 s with this temperature, and these contact burns can occur in both adults and children. In toddlers and preschool children, domestic heating devices located too close to their beds have been found to be responsible for many hand contact burns.

3.6.2 Chemical Burns

Chemicals, used in the home, should be locked away and rendered inaccessible to children. All chemicals should be stored in their original containers as the list of ingredients are provided on the warning label. The Occupational Safety and Health Administration (OSHA) regulations require eyewash stations and showers in all facilities that use potentially injurious chemical products to allow for instant and copious irrigation following exposure. It is important for all employees who work with chemicals to undergo workplace training and to remember to transfer this educational training into their home life.

3.6.3 Electrical Burns

Electrical injuries can be prevented by strict adherence to safety rules regarding household wiring, electrical outlets and appliance cords. The majority of high-voltage electrical injuries occur at work and may be fatal or lead to devastating sequelae such as amputations. In addition, bystanders are at risk of injury and should never touch someone, who is in direct contact with electricity until the current has been shut off.

In some developing and western-world countries, thieves can also suffer electrical burns during their attempt to steal the copper wire.

In Korea, people eat using steel—not plastic or wood chopsticks; children may insert the steel chopsticks into the wall socket, producing severe paediatric electrical burns. To prevent such injuries, they could be encouraged to use wooden chopsticks and install outlet covers.

Lightning is a form of direct electrical current that kills approximately 100 people each year in the USA. Lightning injuries can be avoided by leaving the area or seeking shelter when a storm approaches.

3.6.4 Radiation Burns

Radiation burns can be caused by exposure to ultraviolet light, most often the sun, tanning booths, sunlamps, exposure to high frequency microwaves or radio waves, exposure to nuclear energy, X-rays, or radiation therapy for cancer treatment.

3.6.5 Newest Trending Causes of Burn Injuries

Lithium ion batteries supply power to many kinds of devices including smartphones, laptops, scooters, e-cigarettes, smoke alarms, toys and even cars. Take care when using them. In rare cases, they can cause a fire or explosion. These batteries store a large amount of energy in a small amount of space. Like any product, a small number of these batteries are defective. They can overheat, catch fire or explode.

Safety Tips

- Purchase and use devices that are listed by a qualified testing laboratory.
- Always follow the manufacturer's instructions.
- Only use the battery that is designed for the device.
- Put batteries in the device the right way.
- Only use the charging cord that came with the device.
- Do not charge a device under your pillow, on your bed or on a couch.
- Keep batteries at room temperature.
- Do not place batteries in direct sunlight or keep them in hot vehicles.
- Store batteries away from anything that can catch fire.

http://www.nfpa.org/public-education/resources/safety-tip-sheets

You may have heard that e-cigarettes, or 'vapes', can explode and seriously injure people. Although they appear rare, these explosions are dangerous. The exact causes of such incidents are not yet clear, but some evidence suggests that battery-related issues may lead to vape explosions.

Safety Tips

- Consider using vape devices with safety features such as firing button locks, vent hole and protection against overcharging that are designed to prevent battery overheating and explosions.
- Keep loose batteries in a case to prevent contact with metal objects such as coins, keys or other metals in your pocket.
- Never charge your vape device with a phone or tablet charger. Always use the charger it came with and only use batteries recommended for your device.
- Do not charge your vape overnight or leave it charging unattended. Charge on a clean, flat surface, away from anything that can easily catch fire and someplace you can clearly see it—not a couch or pillow where it is more prone to overheat or get turned on accidentally.
- Replace the batteries if they get damaged or wet.
- Protect your vape from extreme temperatures by not leaving it in direct sunlight or in your car on a freezing cold night.https://www.fda.gov/TobaccoProducts/Labeling/ProductsIngredientsComponents/ucm539362.htm

Hoverboard—part toy, part transportation. These self-balancing scooters have quickly become the latest fad. However, many hoverboards have been linked to fires. NFPA urges you to be fire safe when using these devices.

Safety Tips

- Choose a device with the seal of an independent testing laboratory.
- Read and follow all manufacturer directions. If you do not understand the directions, ask for help.
- An adult should be responsible for charging the hoverboard.
- Do not leave a charging hoverboard unattended.
- Never leave the hoverboard plugged in overnight.
- Only use the charging cord that came with the hoverboard.
- Stop using your hoverboard if it overheats.
- Extreme hot or cold temperature can hurt the battery.
- nfpa.org/education ©NFPA 2017.

3.7 Conclusion

Burn injuries are one of the most catastrophic and devastating injuries. While considerable progress has been made in high-income countries through proven prevention efforts such as fire sprinklers, regulations of hot water heaters and improvements in burn care, burn injuries remain a serious public health problem globally, specifically in low- and middle-income countries. For those who survive, their lives and the lives of their families are left with physical, mental, psychological and social sequelae. There is also the stigma and discrimination related to the disability and disfigurement, not to mention the extreme pain and suffering and often a decreased quality of life. From a societal perspective, the costs are enormous, from medical treatment, property damage and environmental toxins which overtime can contribute to chronic conditions.

Summary Box

Moving forward, we can and we must close the gap on these preventable injuries. To begin, we need to develop a global burn registry to harmonize data collection, increase collaboration between global and national networks and increase the number of effective programs for burn prevention. Since the vast majority of burns occur in the developing world, where resources are limited, we need to access international support such as that developed by the WHO (World Health Organization) and ISBI (International Society of Burn Injuries).

Today we know more about the causes and consequences of burn injuries and the effectiveness of burn prevention strategies, than ever before. While the rationale for using structural or environmental interventions to change injury patterns might seem straightforward, there is rarely an environmental change that does not require behavioural adaptation.

Burn prevention campaigns should include active as well as passive tools, including education (with a focus on behavioural changes to be truly effective), product safety improvements and legislation. Prevention programs should be population-specific and address the different risk factors, including age, gender, geography, comorbidities, culture and traditions. There are numerous resources and fact sheets available online which have been developed and researched from burn prevention experts in the field which can be utilized.

For those of us who are in a position to affect change, we must be seen as role models and advocates and be knowledgeable of injury prevention fundamentals to better understand the root problems. This requires us to be current in our theoretical knowledge so we can apply it to our clinical practice. This also means being aware of societal, environmental and legislative changes and practices which contribute to the injuries we see.

References

1. World Health Organization. 2017. http://www.who.int/violence_injury_prevention/other_injury/burns/en/. Accessed 30 Aug 2017.
2. World Health Organization. 2010. http://www.who.int/healthinfo/global_burden_disease/GBD_report_2004update_full.pdf. Accessed 2 Apr 2010.
3. Davis RM, Pless B. BMJ bans "accidents". Accidents are not unpredictable. BMJ. 2001;322:1320.
4. ICD-10: World Health Organization. 2015. http://apps.who.int/classifications/ icd10/browse/2010/en. Accessed 1 Mar 2015.
5. WHO Health Estimates 2014 Summary Tables: Deaths and Global Burden of Disease. 2015. http://www.who.int/healthinfo/global_burden_disease/en/. Accessed 1 Mar 2015.
6. GBD 2015 Mortality and Causes of Death, Collaborators. Global, regional, and national life expectancy, all-cause mortality, and cause-specific mortality for 249 causes of death, 1980–2015: a systematic analysis for the Global Burden of Disease Study 2015. Lancet. 2015;388(10053):1459–544. PMID 27733281.
7. Haagsma JA, Graetz N, Bolliger I. The global burden of injury: incidence, mortality, disability-adjusted life years and time trends from the Global Burden of Disease study 2013. Injury Prevention. 2016;22(1):3–18 . PMC 4752630 . PMID 26635210. https://doi.org/10.1136/injuryprev-2015-041616.
8. GBD 2015 Disease and Injury Incidence and Prevalence, Collaborators. Global, regional, and national incidence, prevalence, and years lived with disability for 310 diseases and injuries, 1990–2015: a systematic analysis for the Global Burden of Disease Study 2015. Lancet. 2016;388(10053):1545–602. PMID 27733282.
9. World Health Organization. September 2016. Archived from the original on 21 July 2017. Accessed 1 Aug 2017.
10. Injury Prevention (1999;5:203–207), a publication of the BMJ Publishing Group. www.preventioninstitute.org.
11. Haddon W. Escape of tigers: an ecologic note. Am J Public Health. 1970;60:2229–34.
12. Rivara FP, Mueller BA. The epidemiology and causes of childhood injuries. J Soc Issues. 1987;43:13–31.
13. Swift MS. Alternative teaching strategies, helping behaviourally troubled children achieve: a guide for teachers and psychologists. Champaign, IL: Research Press; 1975.
14. Albee GW. Psychopathology, prevention, and the just society. J Prim Prev. 1983;4:5–40.
15. Oomman A, Sarwar U, Javed M, Hemington-Gorse S. YouTube as a potential online source of information in the prevention and management of paediatric burn injuries. Burns. 2013;39:1652.
16. J Burn Care Res. 2015; 36(1): 213–217.doi: https://doi.org/10.1097/BCR.0000000000000194.
17. Atiyeh BS, Costagliola M, Hayek SN. Burn prevention mechanisms and outcomes: pitfalls, failures and successes. Burns. 2009;35:181–93. http://www.nfpa.org/news-and-research/fire-statistics-and-reports/fire-statistics/fire-safety-equipment/smoke-alarms-in-us-home-fires.

Bibliography

Mohammad M, Al-Qattan A-ZK. A review of burns related to traditions, social habits, religious activities, festivals and traditional medicinal practices. Burns. 2009;35:476–81.

Prasad Sarma B. Prevention of burns: 13 years' experience in northeastern India. Burns. 2011;37:257–64.

Patil SB, Anil Kahre N, Jaiswal S, et al. Changing patterns in electrical burn injuries in a developing country: should prevention programs focus on the rural population? J Burn Care Res. 2010;31:931–4.

Taira BR, Cassara GPA, Meng H, et al. Predictors of sustaining burn injury: does the use of common prevention strategies matter? J Burn Care Res. 2011;32:20–5.

Crickelair GF, Dhaliwal AS. The cause and prevention of electrical burns of the mouth in children: a protective cuff. PRS. 1976;58(2):206–9.

Rimmer RB, Weigand S, Foster KN, et al. Scald burns in young children: a review of Arizona burn center pediatric patients and a proposal for prevention in the Hispanic community. J Burn Care Res. 2008;29:595–605.

Kendrick D, Smith S, Sutton AG, et al. The effect of education and home safety equipment on childhood thermal injury prevention: meta-analysis and meta-regression. Inj Prev. 2009;15:197–204.

Abeyasundara SL, Rajan V, Lam L, et al. The changing pattern of pediatric burns. J Burn Care Res. 2011;32:178–84.
Parbhoo A, Louw QA, Grimmer-Somers K. Burn prevention programs for children in developing countries require urgent attention: a targeted literature review. Burns. 2010;36:164–75.
ABA. Fire and burn prevention news. 2011;6(1):1–5.
Hunt JL, Arnoldo BD, Purdue GF. Prevention of burn injuries. In: Herndon DN, editor. Total burn care. Galveston: Saunders Elsevier; 2007. p. 33–9.
Light TD, Latenser BA, Heinle JA, et al. Jaggery: an avoidable cause of severe, deadly pediatric burns. Burns. 2009;35:430–2.
Roeder RA, Schulman CI. An overview of war-related thermal injuries. J Craniofac Surg. 2010;21(4):971–5.
Brussselaers, et al. Severe burn injury in Europe: a systematic review of the incidence, etiology, morbidity and mortality. Crit Care. 2010;14:R188.
Wisee RPL, Bijlsma WE, Stilma JS. Ocular firework trauma: a systematic review on incidence,severity, outcome and prevention. Br J Ophthalmol. 2010;94:1586–91.
Thompson RM, Carrougher GJ. Burn prevention. In: Carrougher GJ, editor. Burn care and therapy. St. Louis: Mosby; 1998. p. 497–524.
Neaman KC, DO VH, Olenzek EK, et al. Outdoor recreational fires: a review of 329 adult and pediatric patients. J Burn Care Res. 2010;31:926–30.

Online Safety Tip Resources (Accessed Online 12 Sept 2017)

http://www.nfpa.org/public-education/resources/safety-tip-sheets
http://ameriburn.org/prevention/prevention-resources/
https://www.cdc.gov/masstrauma/factsheets/public/burns.pdf
https://www.cdc.gov/safechild/burns/index.html
https://www.safekids.org/fire
http://www.who.int/mediacentre/factsheets/fs365/en/
http://www.parachutecanada.org/child-injury-prevention/item/burns-and-scalds-prevention
http://www.preventable.ca/do-you-know-about-co/
https://www.phoenix-society.org/resources/prevention

Burns Associated with Wars and Disasters

4

Leopoldo C. Cancio and Jonathan B. Lundy

4.1 Introduction

Military operations and civilian mass casualty disasters provide among the most difficult scenarios in burn-patient management. At the same time, they historically have also led to advancements in care. The purpose of this chapter is to review experience with burn care during current combat operations and to highlight the lessons learned from major peacetime fire disasters.

4.2 Wartime Burns

The historical incidence of thermal injury during conventional (non-nuclear) warfare ranges from 5 to 20% [1, 2]. As with casualties from fire disasters, approximately 20% of thermally injured combat casualties have burns of 20% of the total body surface area (TBSA) or greater [2]. During recent operations in Iraq and Afghanistan, common causes of thermal injury in military personnel include incendiary devices, improvized explosive devices, or ignition of combustible material in armored personnel carriers or aboard ship [3]. Military personnel are also at risk of non-combat-related burns due to mishandling of munitions or carelessness during burning of waste material [4].

Unlike typical civilian care, military care uniquely requires transport of patients along multiple medical treatment facilities termed "echelons" or "roles"; the capabilities of these facilities increase as the casualty moves further from the battlefield. During recent operations, US military casualties have received rapid initial care at the point of injury from nonmedical personnel who receive additional first-aid training (Combat Lifesavers) and/or from combat medics (U.S. Army Healthcare Specialists, U.S. Navy Hospital Corpsmen). These interventions include movement away from the source of injury, intravenous (IV) or intraosseous line placement, initiation of fluid infusion, and pain management. This emergency, prehospital echelon is referred to as Role I care.

Initial burn care to include fluid resuscitation, emergency procedures, and surgical management of concomitant traumatic injuries is currently performed in the Combat Zone by small, austere, highly mobile teams termed Role II-b units (U.S. Army Forward Surgical Team or Forward Resuscitative Surgical Team, U.S. Navy Forward Resuscitative Surgical System). These teams consist of surgeons, emergency physicians, anesthetists, nurses, and medics. They are capable of damage-control surgery but have very limited infrastructure and holding capability. From there, casualties go to Role III facilities (U.S. Army Combat Support Hospital, U.S. Air Force Theater Hospital, U.S. Navy Fleet Hospital or Hospital Ship). (Alternatively, patients may be transported directly from the point of injury to a Role III facility, bypassing the Role II-b unit, depending on location.) Role III is the first echelon at which definitive surgical care, to include some surgical sub-specialties and brief hospitalization, is available. Long-term management of thermally injured US combat casualties requires evacuation, via a Role IV general hospital outside the combat zone, to the continental United States (CONUS). The Role IV hospital for the recent conflicts has been Landstuhl Regional Medical Center in Germany. Upon arrival in CONUS, most thermally injured casualties are cared for at the U.S. Army Burn Center (U.S. Army Institute of Surgical Research, USAISR), Fort Sam Houston, TX. This is the only burn center in the U.S. Department of Defense [5].

The purpose of this section is to review recent US military experience with care of thermally injured combat casualties. Topics pertinent to combat burn care include epidemiology,

Note: The opinions or assertions contained herein are the private views of the authors and are not to be construed as official or as reflecting the views of the Department of the Army or the Department of Defense.

L. C. Cancio (✉)
U.S. Army Institute of Surgical Research,
Fort Sam Houston, TX, USA

J. B. Lundy
LTC, MC, U.S. Army, Carl R. Darnall Army Medical Center,
Fort Hood, TX, USA

© Springer Nature Switzerland AG 2020
M. G. Jeschke et al. (eds.), *Handbook of Burns Volume 1*, https://doi.org/10.1007/978-3-030-18940-2_4

fluid resuscitation, evacuation, lessons learned from combat operations (e.g., recent wars in Iraq and Afghanistan), and definitive care of both injured combatants and host-nation civilians.

4.2.1 Epidemiology of Burns Sustained During Combat Operations

Between 2001 and 2017, during combat operations in Iraq, Syria, and Afghanistan, 10.1% of all US military casualties sustained thermal injury, alone or in combination with other injuries of varying severity (Table 4.1). A distinguishing feature of these conflicts has been the large number of injuries suffered as a result of improvised explosive devices (IEDs) [4]. These devices can be constructed from almost any material that can house an explosive charge. Kauvar and colleagues found that of 273 thermally injured US military personnel injured in Iraq and Afghanistan and admitted to the U.S. Army Burn Center between March 2003 and May 2005, 62% were wounded as a direct result of hostile activity. Of these, 52% sustained thermal injury as a result of the ignition of an explosive device. Over 70% of these explosive devices were IEDs or vehicle-borne IEDs. The remaining explosion-related burns were the result of landmines, mortars, or rocket-propelled grenades [3].

Explosions may cause thermal injury by one of two mechanisms: as a result of contact with the heat generated by the explosion itself (also known as "quaternary blast injury"), or as a result of the ignition of fuel or other combustible materials in close proximity to the explosion. The larger body surface area burns typically include burns to the lower extremities and trunk, and are seen more commonly in casualties confined to a burning vehicle [3, 6]. The smaller burns localized to the face and hands are seen more commonly in casualties injured by the explosion itself [3].

Burns to the hands and face comprise a significant portion of burned casualties. In Kauvar's study, the hands were burned in 80% of patients; the head (predominantly the face) was burned in 77%. Only 15% of casualties had burns isolated to the hands and head; 6% to the hands only. Burns to the hands and face require extensive treatment typically out of proportion to the TBSA burned, which impacts the return to duty rate [3].

Noncombat burns are also common during military operations, accounting for over half of the burns seen during the Vietnam War [6]. Of 102 noncombat burns sustained in the current theaters of operations by May 2005, burning waste (24.5%), ammunition and gunpowder mishaps (20.2%), mishandling of gasoline (17.3%), electrical injuries (8.2%), and scald burns (6.4%) were the leading causes. Combat burns had higher injury severity scores, a higher incidence of other injuries, and a higher incidence of inhalation injury. Despite lower severity, noncombat burns still lead to evacuation of personnel from the theater of operations and a reduction in military readiness. Kauvar noted over 30% of noncombat burned patients and over 40% of combat burned patients were unable to return to full military duty [4].

Preventive measures may be effective on the battlefield. For example, the use of fire-retardant gloves by tank crew members during the 1982 Israeli war in Lebanon decreased the incidence of hand burns from 75 to 7% in the personnel who sustained burns [7]. Fire-retardant flight suits have been reported to decrease both the incidence and severity of thermal injury suffered after military helicopter accidents [8].

4.2.2 Fluid Resuscitation and Initial Burn Care in the Combat Zone

Thermal injury results in fluid shifts from the intravascular space into the interstitium in both burned and (in larger burns) unburned tissue. The goal of burn resuscitation is to replace these intravascular volume losses and to prevent end-organ hypoperfusion and damage, at the lowest possible physiologic cost. Fluid resuscitation of burned soldiers may be complicated by problems which are less frequently present in the civilian setting. Inhalation injury increases fluid resuscitation requirements and is present more frequently in combat casualties (approximately 15% in the recent conflicts) [9]. In addition, the burned combat casualty may have multiple traumatic injuries in addition to burns, increasing the volume and complexity of fluid resuscitation. Meanwhile, lack of burn-specific experience on the part of many deployed

Table 4.1 US Military Service Members with Burns in CENTCOM AOR 11 Sept 2001 to 31 Dec 2017

Burns	Dominant MOI		Not dominant MOI		Total		Denominator (all injured)
Battle	448	2.4%	1470	7.8%	1918	10.1%	18,932
Non-battle	543	4.9%	85	0.8%	628	5.6%	11176
Unknown	0	0.0%	0	0.0%	0	0.0%	54
Total	991	3.3%	1555	5.2%	2546	8.4%	30,162

The population consists of all US military service members injured in the Central Command (CENTCOM) area of responsibility (AOR) between 11 September 2001 and 31 December 2017 whose injuries are documented in the Department of Defense Trauma Registry. Burns were identified based on ICD9 or ICD10 injury codes. The dominant mechanism of injury (MOI) was identified based on the injury with the highest Abbreviated Injury Score (AIS). Does not include killed in action (KIA) or dead on arrival (DOA) data. Courtesy of Greg Dokken, Joint Trauma System, 25 Jan 2018 providers; relatively austere field hospitals; and the diminution in care which necessarily occurs when casualties are placed aboard evacuation aircraft all compound the difficulty of initial resuscitation.

Early experience during current combat operations revealed a trend towards over-resuscitation of thermally injured casualties [9, 10]. Over-resuscitation may cause abdominal compartment syndrome, extremity compartment syndrome, pulmonary edema, airway obstruction, and/or progression of wound depth [11]. Together, these complications have been termed "resuscitation morbidity" [12]. As a result, a burn resuscitation guideline was developed and disseminated to all deployed US medical treatment facilities [10]. The guidelines included a 24-h burn resuscitation flow sheet (Fig. 4.1), as well as recommendations for the management of casualties with difficult burn resuscitations. After the implementation of the guideline, US casualties experienced a significant decrease in the combined endpoint of abdominal compartment syndrome and mortality [10].

Other steps taken by the USAISR to improve care of the burned casualty on the battlefield include pre-deployment training of providers in wartime burn care, the stationing of a burn surgeon at the busiest Combat Support Hospital in Iraq, and a weekly theater-wide video teleconference to communicate patient outcomes and provide feedback [1, 13]. A burn Clinical Practice Guideline was published on the Internet and includes instructions on the management of the difficult resuscitation, indications for and technique of escharotomy, initial wound care, and USAISR contact information [14].

The USAISR pioneered the modified Brooke formula for fluid resuscitation, which predicts the fluid requirements for the first 24 h postburn as lactated Ringer's solution, 2 mL/kg/% TBSA burned, with half of this volume programmed for delivery over the first 8 h and half over the following 16 h. Chung and colleagues, in an attempt to simplify fluid calculations for adults, developed the ISR Rule of 10s [15]. This rule initiates fluid resuscitation at a rate in mL/h equal to TBSA X 10 for patients weighing 40–80 kg. Regardless of how the initial fluid infusion rate is determined, it must be adjusted during the first 48 h postburn based on the patient's physiologic response.

Initial burn wound care in the combat zone includes debridement and dressing of burn wounds in the operating room under sterile conditions. This is typically carried out at a Role III facility. US military Role II and III facilities have wound care materials to include mafenide acetate, silver sulfadiazine, and silver-impregnated dressings [16]. Classically, burn wounds have been treated at the USAISR by alternating mafenide acetate cream in the morning, with silver sulfadiazine cream in the evening. During transport, silver-impregnated dressings offer the advantage of less frequent wound care, but this supposes that the wounds are clean and that burned extremities are well perfused, thus decreasing the need for frequent dressing changes and wound inspection.

The usual indication for escharotomy of an extremity is the loss or progressive diminution of arterial pulsatile flow as determined by Doppler flowmetry. In the deployed setting, it may be prudent to perform escharotomies in patients with large burn size and circumferential (or nearly so) full-thickness burns of an extremity since monitoring in flight is nearly impossible. This concern should be balanced by the need to obtain good hemostasis before flight, and the potential for escharotomy sites to bleed in flight.

4.2.3 Evacuation of Thermally Injured Combat Casualties

During the Vietnam War, thermally injured military personnel were evacuated to a U.S. Army General Hospital in Japan and remained at that facility for variable amounts of time (up to several weeks) before evacuation to the USA [6, 17]. Injuries sustained during current operations have been evacuated more rapidly. Evacuation out of the theater of operations to the Role IV hospital in Germany takes about 8 h and is carried out by a U.S. Air Force Air Evacuation (AE) crew for stable patients, or by an AE crew augmented by a U.S. Air Force Critical Care Air Transport Team (CCATT) for critically ill patients [18].

The flight from LRMC to CONUS requires an AE crew, often augmented by a CCATT or by the USAISR Burn Flight Team. The flight from LRMC to the USAISR is over 5300 miles (8600 km) and takes approximately 12–13 h [19]. In sum, it is now feasible for a severely burned casualty to arrive at the Army Burn Center within 3–4 days of injury on the battlefield.

The USAISR Burn Flight Team pioneered the air evacuation/transportation of critically ill burn patients in 1951. Guidelines for Burn Flight Team utilization are listed in Table 4.2 [19]. BFT crews are equipped and experienced in the management of severely burned, critically ill casualties and are ideally suited to evacuate multiple casualties during a single mission (Fig. 4.2). Flights staffed by BFTs have carried as many as 13 burned casualties on a single mission during the recent conflicts. BFTs bring specialized equipment to perform emergency procedures en route such as fiberoptic bronchoscopy, escharotomy, resuscitation, management of septic shock, emergency airway procedures, and tube thoracostomy.

Renz and colleagues conducted a retrospective analysis of the evacuation of war-related burn casualties that were treated at the USAISR [19]. The study encompassed a four-year period from March 2003 to February 2007 and included 540 burned US military casualties. The mean TBSA involved was 16.7% (range 0.1–95%) and 342 (63.3%) of casualties

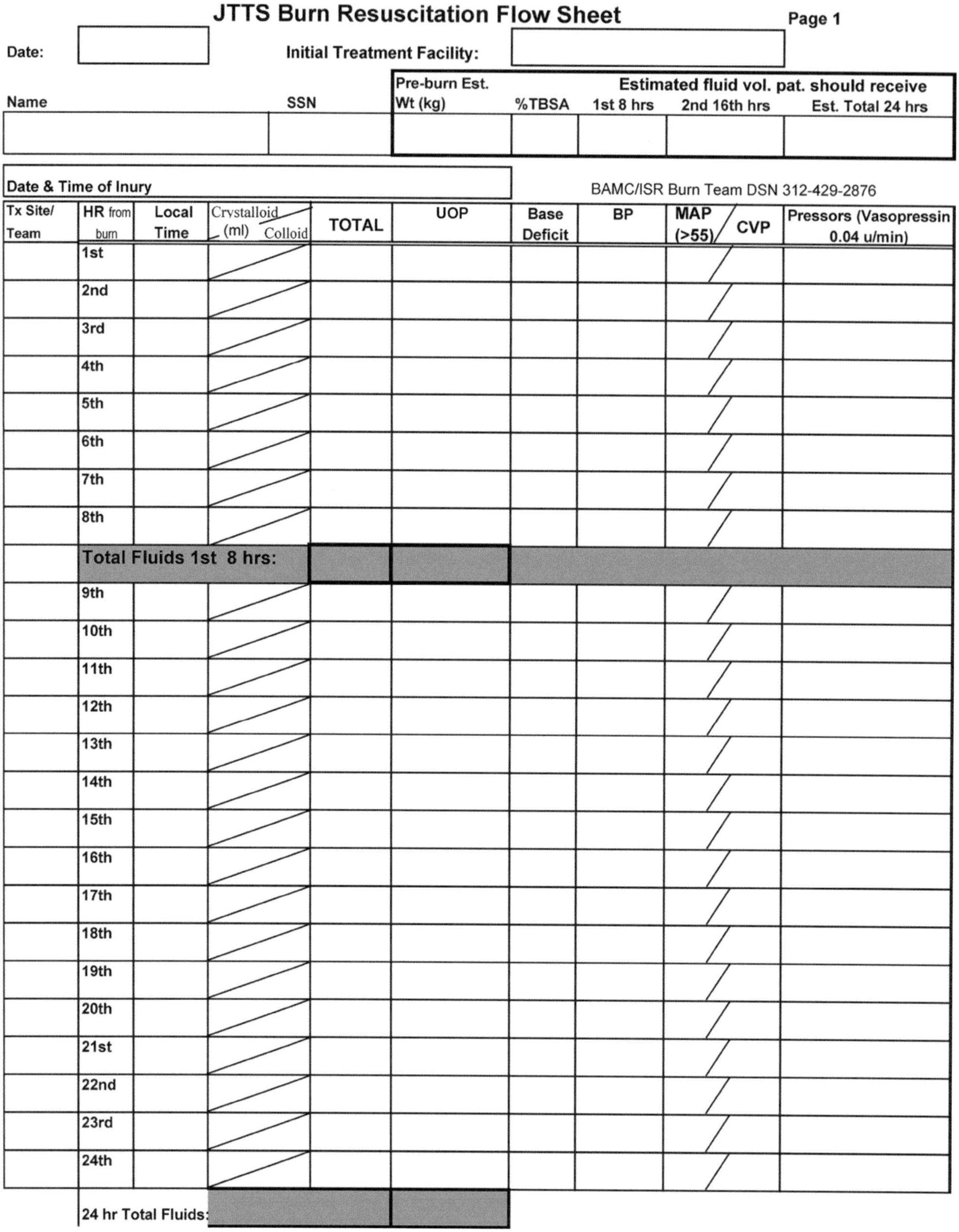

JTTS Burn Resuscitation Flow Sheet Page 1

Date: Initial Treatment Facility:

Name	SSN	Pre-burn Est. Wt (kg)	%TBSA	Estimated fluid vol. pat. should receive: 1st 8 hrs	2nd 16th hrs	Est. Total 24 hrs

Date & Time of Inury

BAMC/ISR Burn Team DSN 312-429-2876

Tx Site/ Team	HR from burn	Local Time	Crystalloid / Colloid (ml)	TOTAL	UOP	Base Deficit	BP	MAP (>55) / CVP	Pressors (Vasopressin 0.04 u/min)
	1st		/					/	
	2nd		/					/	
	3rd		/					/	
	4th		/					/	
	5th		/					/	
	6th		/					/	
	7th		/					/	
	8th		/					/	
	Total Fluids 1st 8 hrs:								
	9th		/					/	
	10th		/					/	
	11th		/					/	
	12th		/					/	
	13th		/					/	
	14th		/					/	
	15th		/					/	
	16th		/					/	
	17th		/					/	
	18th		/					/	
	19th		/					/	
	20th		/					/	
	21st		/					/	
	22nd		/					/	
	23rd		/					/	
	24th		/					/	
	24 hr Total Fluids:								

Fig. 4.1 Flow sheet used in the combat zone and en route for documentation of burn resuscitation

were burned as a result of an explosion. During the flight from LRMC to the USAISR, 160 (29.6%) burned casualties required only AE crews; 174 (32.2%) required CCATT-augmented AE crews; and 206 (38.1%) required the Burn Flight Team. Mean transit time for stable patients evacuated by AE crews was 7 days, and transit time for casualties evacuated by CCATT or Burn Flight Teams was less than 4 days.

Such rapid evacuation of patients with severe thermal injury carries both risks and benefits. The most notable risk is the inevitable degradation in care that occurs aboard the aircraft, despite the presence of CCATTs or BFTs. This is particularly important during the first 24 h postburn, during which rapidly evolving burn shock may make fluid resuscitation difficult even in a US burn center. The most notable benefits are the ability to complete excision and grafting of the burn wound within days of injury and to place the patient in the burn center before complications such as pneumonia make transport more hazardous [20]. Consideration of these risks and benefits argues in favor of a rather small "window" between hours 24 and 48, during which burn-patient evacuation off the battlefield is ideally accomplished.

Table 4.2 USTRANSCOM guidelines for Burn Flight Team Transport of patients during conflict in Iraq and Afghanistan

Burns involving 20% or more of the total body surface area
Inhalation injury requiring intubation
Burn and/or inhalation injury with PaO_2-to-FiO_2 ratio less than 200
High-voltage electric injury
Burns with concomitant traumatic injuries
Burn patients with injury/illness severity warranting Burn Flight Team assistance as determined by the attending, validating, or receiving surgeon

USTRANSCOM U.S. Transportation Command

4.2.4 Definitive Management of Burned Casualties

The management of thermally injured combat casualties follows standard principles. When possible, early burn wound excision (within the first 5–7 days of injury) with application of autograft is performed to close wounds. Cadaver allograft is used for temporary closure of excised burn wounds when adequate autograft is not available. Frequently, a "sandwich" of 1:1 meshed allograft over 4:1 meshed autograft is used to address massive injuries. In Chapman's review of long-term outcomes after combat-related burns, out of 285 combat-related burn patients, 35% had an associated traumatic injury [21]. Fractures, large soft tissue defects, and traumatic amputations are some of the more common injuries. These associated injuries make definitive wound closure challenging, increase the open surface area at risk for infection, and complicate long-term rehabilitation.

Military burn casualties remain inpatients at the USAISR Burn Center until all wounds are closed, inpatient rehabilitation needs are met, and nonmedical attendants (typically family members) have been educated in wound care and activities of daily living. Military personnel are then assigned to the Fort Sam Houston Warrior Transition Unit and discharged to local housing. Many blast-injured casual-

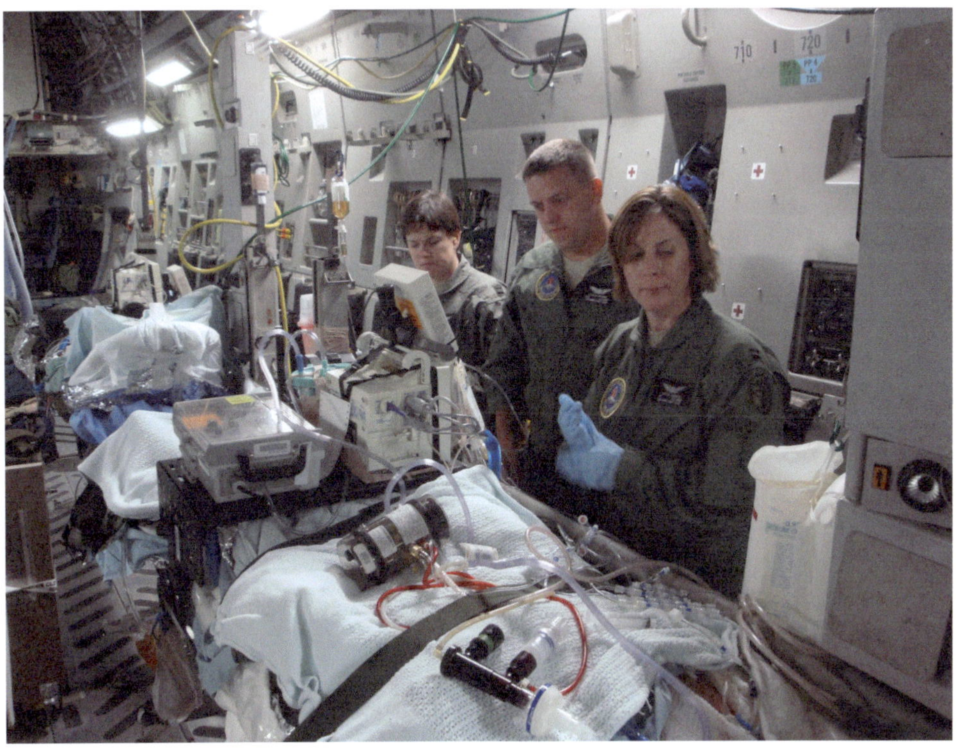

Fig. 4.2 U.S. Army Burn Flight Team members providing en route critical care to several thermally injured combat casualties

ties suffer traumatic amputations and require fitting and rehabilitation with extremity prostheses. The nearby Center for the Intrepid provides state-of-the-art amputee rehabilitation for these personnel.

Wolf and colleagues reviewed the outcomes of burned US combatants (evacuated from the combat zone) and civilians (from the local area in Texas) treated at the USAISR between April 2003 and May 2005 [22]. The authors hypothesized that due to the delays in evacuation and associated traumatic injuries, outcomes would be worse for the military burned casualties. Of 751 total patients cared for at the USAISR during the period studied, 273 were military personnel. Overall, the mortality of the US military personnel sustaining burns in the combat theaters was no different from locally evacuated civilians.

Of the 285 patients in Chapman's return-to-duty study mentioned above, 190 patients were categorized as having returned to duty. A total of 95 burned military casualties were medically discharged. Patients who were medically discharged had larger TBSA and full-thickness burn size, more frequently sustained inhalation injury and associated traumatic injuries, and had a higher injury severity score [21].

Full-thickness burns of the hands figure disproportionately into causing long-term disability. A study of the American Medical Association impairment guide (AMA) and the Disabilities of the Army, Shoulder, and Hand instrument (DASH) revealed that they both predicted the return-to-duty rate of combat casualties with hand burns. Other predictors of not returning to duty included larger TBSA, larger full thickness burn size, and a requirement for skin grafting of the hands [23]. These data indicate the importance of attention to hand burns throughout the burn care process as a major determinant of future functional outcomes.

4.2.5 Care of Host-Nation Burn Patients

One challenging aspect of military medical care in the deployed setting is the care of host-nation casualties (civilians and military personnel). The impetus for caring for these patients at US facilities stems from several sources. Article 56 of the 4th Geneva Convention of 1949 states that "the Occupying Power has the duty of ensuring and maintaining, with the cooperation of national and local authorities, the medical and hospital establishments and services, public health and hygiene in the occupied territory" [24]. Similarly, U.S. Army FM 8-10-14, *Employment of the Combat Support Hospital,* states that "Only urgent medical reasons will determine priority in the order of treatment to be administered. This means that wounded enemy soldiers may be treated before wounded Americans or allies (…) Civilians who are wounded or become sick as a result of military operations will be collected and provided initial medical treatment in accordance with theater policies and transferred to appropriate civilian authorities as soon as possible" [25]. In practice, this means that host-nation patients presenting to US forces with life-, limb-, or eyesight-threatening injuries have received initial care at US medical treatment facilities. Of these, burns figure prominently.

Whereas resuscitation and lifesaving surgery might conceivably be completed within roughly 2 days of injury for patients with non-thermal injuries, in the case of burn patients the threat to life continues until the wounds are fully closed. Evacuation out of the combat zone (i.e., evacuation to echelons higher than Role III hospitals) has not been available to host-nation patients. Furthermore, host-nation facilities on the current battlefield, whether in Iraq or in Afghanistan, have not been equipped to provide burn care comparable to that available in US Role III hospitals. Finally, disruption by war of critical infrastructure, to include (but not limited to) hospitals, degrades the host nation's ability to care for its citizens [26].

This constellation of factors—the Geneva Convention moral imperative, the duration of the threat to life caused by thermal injury, and the discrepancy between US and local capabilities—has made the disposition of host-nation burn patients problematic, and motivated US Role III hospitals to provide definitive care. But it would be incorrect to conclude that Role III hospitals were capable of providing the same level of care as a burn center in the USA. Lack of experience on the part of many providers, absence of multidisciplinary burn team members, limitations with respect to supplies, equipment, and physical plant, and patient-related factors such as delays in presentation heightened the challenge.

Because burn patient care is very costly with respect to supplies, manpower, and length of stay, and because bed space is limited at Role III facilities, it was necessary to expedite such treatment. Several techniques evolved over time to accomplish this. Patients with burns of up to 50–60% TBSA received definitive care at Role III hospitals. It became apparent that surgical care of patients with larger burns was futile; these patients were therefore triaged to comfort care. Excision and grafting of burns was performed at Role III hospitals within a day or two of admission (Fig. 4.3). Negative-pressure wound therapy (Vacuum-Assisted Closure, Acelity Inc., San Antonio, TX) was frequently used to speed up engraftment or to help prepare wound beds for grafting. Topical wound therapies, such as artificial skin (Biobrane, Smith & Nephew Inc., Andover, MA), silver-impregnated dressings (Silverlon, Argentum Medical LLC, Geneva, IL; others), and gamma-irradiated homograft (GammaGraft, Promethean LifeSciences Inc., Pittsburgh, PA) were used as appropriate. A small number of burned

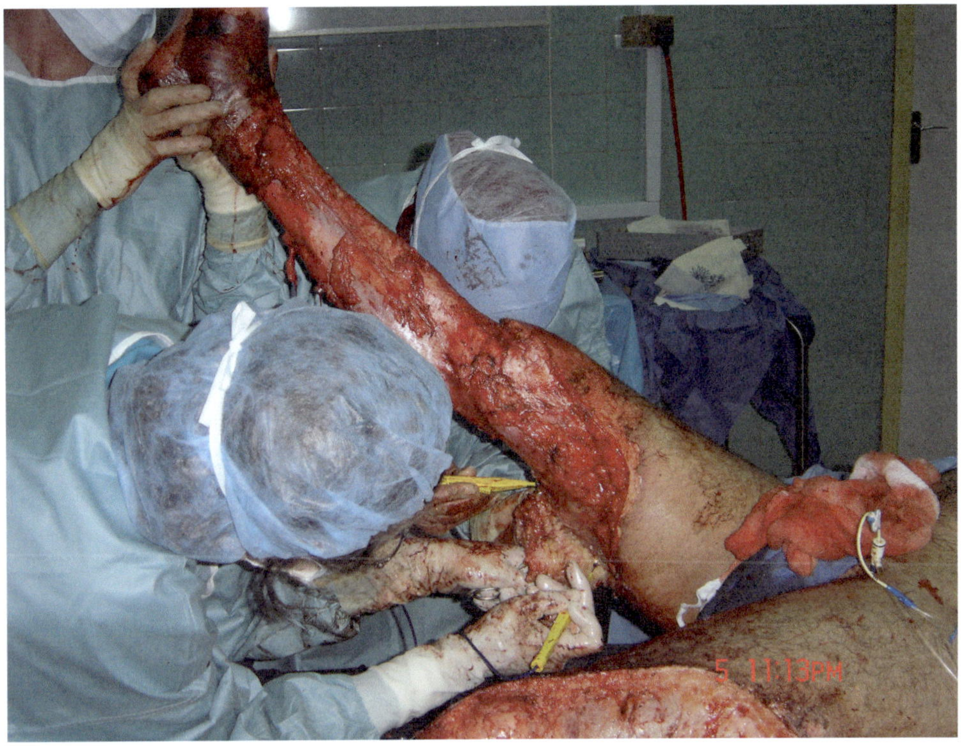

Fig. 4.3 Excision to fascia of infected lower extremity burns in an Iraqi male at the Combat Support Hospital (CSH) in Baghdad. Patient was transferred from a local facility 10 days after injury by an improvised explosive device (IED), and was successfully excised and grafted on day of admission to CSH

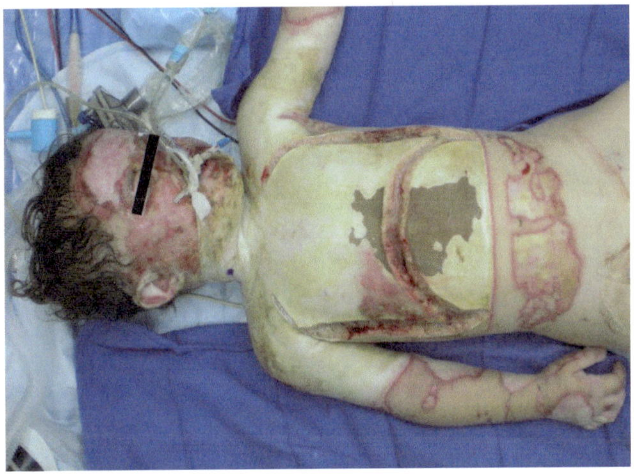

Fig. 4.4 Iraqi child selected for transfer to Shriners Institute in Boston, MA. Despite extensive full-thickness burns, patient was extubated and transitioned to oral medications before commercial flight

children were flown out of theater on commercial airlines by civilian charities for care at Shriners Institutes for Burned Children in the USA (Fig. 4.4) [27]. From these events, we can conclude that burn care, to include *definitive care of civilians of all ages* with major thermal injuries, is part of the usual workload of Role III hospitals on the modern battlefield; that these hospitals should have the supplies and equipment needed to provide definitive care to these patients; and that personnel should obtain experience with definitive burn care before deploying.

4.3 Disaster-Related Burns

Mass casualties as a result of fire have occurred with some regularity in the USA since the country was founded. The first large-scale fire occurred at Jamestown, Virginia in May 1607, decimating the colony [28, 29]. Worldwide, catastrophic fires have punctuated history due to their social and political implications. A recent development in the last two decades is the emergence of terrorism as a cause of mass casualty burns. Burn disasters are challenging because (1) burn victims are extremely resource- and time-intensive in their care needs and (2) burn expertise is normally concentrated in specialized centers, but local hospitals with no experience in the care of burns may be required to provide care of casualties for hours or days following a disaster.

Burn mass casualty incidents have provided unique opportunities for health care providers to review the treatment of these patients and to develop improvements in care. An excellent example of this is the Cocoanut Grove nightclub fire that occurred in Boston, MA in 1942. As a result of the attack on Pearl Harbor in 1941 (where half of the casualties were burned), by the time of the nightclub fire the Massachusetts General Hospital and Boston City Hospital were conducting research in burn care and had already developed guidelines for disaster preparedness. This work included the development of a blood bank, publication of a disaster manual, and accumulation of sterile supplies for multiple simultaneous operations [30]. Those who cared for victims of the Cocoanut Grove fire paved the way for future advances in burn care, in part by care-

Table 4.3 Recurring lessons learned from mass casualty fire disasters

1.	Value of disaster planning and rehearsal
2.	Command, control, communication
3.	Triage procedures
4.	Transport procedures
5.	Treatment strategies
6.	Personnel management
7.	Supplies and equipment
8.	Transfer to other facilities
9.	International response
10.	Rehabilitation and long-term follow-up

fully documenting their experiences. More recently, since the terrorist attacks in New York and Washington on 11 September 2001 and the bombing in Bali on 12 October 2002, awareness has increased regarding the importance of disaster preparedness specific to burns. The purpose of this section is to outline the epidemiology of burns suffered during mass casualty events, and to review techniques for triage, prehospital care, and resuscitation. The basic message is that although mass casualty events are chaotic, they unfold in a predictable manner; the "lessons learned" from these disasters are consistently observed, and can be used in the form of a checklist to help planners (see Table 4.3) [31].

4.3.1 Epidemiology

Barillo and Wolf performed a review of historic US fire catastrophes during the twentieth century. The largest number of significant fires was classified as "residential" and included fires in hotels, nursing homes, jails, and hospitals. Most fire disasters produce fewer than 25–50 survivors requiring inpatient care (with the total number decreasing over the twentieth century) [5]. This information should be used to guide planning efforts and disaster drills.

Fatally injured casualties from burn disasters typically die at the scene, during transport to a local hospital, or shortly after arrival to the hospital [32–41]. For example, the Iroquois Theater fire of 1903 in Chicago resulted in 602 deaths with a list of 571 fatalities published in the Chicago Tribune by the morning after the fire [32]. The Cocoanut Grove fire death toll was 492. Three hours after the fire occurred, the city mortuary had accounted for over 400 bodies in morgues around the city [33]. More recently, the 1990 Happy Land Social Club fire in Bronx, New York resulted in 87 deaths, all identified at the scene [42]; and the 1991 Imperial Foods plant disaster in Hamlet, North Carolina resulted in 25 deaths with 24 pronounced at the scene [35]. The Station Nightclub fire in Warwick, Rhode Island in 2003 occurred in a 1950s-era building that was not equipped with sprinklers when it ignited as a result of pyrotechnics during a concert [40]. Of the 439 people inside at the time of the fire, 96 people died at the scene and only an additional 4 died in surrounding area hospitals in the weeks following the incident. The predominance of early deaths in indoor fire disasters points to the importance of asphyxia (hypoxia and inhalation of toxic gases) and upper airway injury.

By contrast, the Ringling Brothers Circus in 1944 at Hartford, Connecticut led to a predominance of fatalities due to severe burns from the heavy canvas that was engulfed by flames and fell onto the crowd [38]. The canvas had been coated with paraffin dissolved in gasoline to make it waterproof. The open air tent resulted in only a few patients suffering inhalation injury [39]. In general, indoor fire disasters tend to cause smaller TBSA burns (in the survivors) than do outdoor fire disasters [43].

Medical response at the scene of the attack on the World Trade Center towers on 11 September 2001 was complicated by the fact that both towers collapsed, making evacuation and survival the primary mission of first responders [44–46]. A total of 39 survivors sustained significant burns, but had the towers not collapsed, many more thermally injured casualties might have required treatment [46–48]. The New York-Presbyterian Weill Cornell Center, with a total burn bed capacity of 40, received 18 patients by the 27th hour after the attack [49]. Nine were transferred directly from the scene and an additional nine were transferred from surrounding hospitals. Eight of the patients sustained burns involving more than 60% of the TBSA. Inhalation injury complicated the injuries of 14 patients admitted to the burn center.

4.3.2 Management

4.3.2.1 Prehospital

The scene of a burn catastrophe is best described as chaotic in the moments after the incident. In Arturson's review of the San Juanico, Mexico liquid petroleum gas (LPG) explosion in 1984, the author notes that no evacuation plan was in place to remove casualties from the scene. Evacuation routes away from the scene became clogged with private vehicles. Activation of the Army enabled resolution of the crisis [50].

Poor evacuation management affects outcomes, evidenced by the LPG tanker truck explosion in Los Alfaques, Spain in 1978 [51]. The incident caused a highway blockage, presenting two evacuation routes for patients needing further care. The group of 82 patients that was transported south had no en route medical care, traveled 150 km, and had an initial (first 4 days) survival rate of 45%. The 58 patients taken via the north evacuation route were provided care en route and experienced a 93% initial survival rate. A lack of field triage after the 1970 Osaka, Japan gas line explosion resulted in misutilization of hospital-based physicians [52].

The value of field triage was demonstrated after the MGM Grand Hotel fire in Las Vegas, Nevada in 1980. Over 3000 patients were triaged on the scene, allowing for evacuation of only 726 patients to hospitals and movement of 1700 minimally injured casualties to an off-site treatment center [53]. In order not to overwhelm the regional burn center, care should be provided on or close to the scene to both the minimal and expectant categories of patients [54]. Some have suggested that the on-site presence of a burn surgeon may facilitate triage of victims [41].

The importance of triage is highlighted by the fact that in disaster-related fires, approximately 80% of survivors will sustain burns of 20% or less of the TBSA [55]. The goal of triage in a fire disaster is to identify the other patients: that minority with critical but survivable injuries. In his analysis of terrorist bombings, Frykberg developed the concept of "critical mortality," that is, mortality in those survivors with Injury Severity Score (ISS) >15. He found that critical mortality varied widely in terrorist events, and that it was a linear function of the over-triage rate. That is, overwhelming the health care system with minimally injured patients distracts and degrades the care given to those in immediate need of lifesaving interventions [56]. The same principle applies to fire disasters.

Initial triage of burn victims should be performed based on the likelihood of death, which is primarily a function of age and burn size. The *lethal area fifty percent* (L_A50) defines the burn size which is lethal for 50% of a given population. At this time in modern burn centers, the L_A50 for a 20-year-old is a TBSA of 80% [57, 58]. Generalizing this relationship to other age groups means that when the (age + TBSA) = 100, mortality = 50%. This sum, age + TBSA, was originally described by Baux and is commonly referred to as the "Baux Score" [59]. Independent of age and burn size, inhalation injury also increases mortality risk. When inhalation injury is present, its effect on mortality can be taken into account by adding 17 to the Baux Score [57]. In a disaster in which inadequate resources exist to care for all patients, it may be appropriate to triage patients whose Baux Score >100 to the expectant category. Further, it may be necessary to further decrease the "cut point" for the expectant category, until the available resources match the number of patients who can be treated [60].

The ABA has published an age/TBSA survival grid that incorporates these concepts and that can be used to guide providers triaging burn victims (Fig. 4.5) [61]. It is not clear,

Appendix

Age/TBSA Survival Grid

Provided by Jeffrey R. Saffle, MD
Director, Intermountain Burn Center
Salt Lake City, UT

CAVEAT: This grid is intended only for mass burn casualty disasters where responders are overwhelmed and transfer possibilities are insufficient to meet needs.

This table is based on national data on survival and length of stay.

Triage Decision Table of Benefit-to-Resource Ratio based on Patient Age and Total Burn Size

Burn Size (%TBSA)

Age/ years	0 – 10%	11-20%	21-30%	31-40%	41-50%	51-60%	61-70%	71-80%	81-90%	91+%
0-1.99	High	High	Medium	Medium	Medium	Medium	Low	Low	Low	Expectant
2-4.99	Outpatient	High	High	Medium	Medium	Medium	Medium	Low	Low	Low
5-19.9	Outpatient	High	High	High	Medium	Medium	Medium	Medium	Medium	Low
20-29.9	Outpatient	High	High	High	Medium	Medium	Medium	Medium	Low	Low
30-39.9	Outpatient	High	High	Medium	Medium	Medium	Medium	Medium	Low	Low
40-49.9	Outpatient	High	High	Medium	Medium	Medium	Medium	Low	Low	Low
50-59.9	Outpatient	High	High	Medium	Medium	Medium	Low	Low	Expectant	Expectant
60-69.9	High	High	Medium	Medium	Medium	Low	Low	Low	Expectant	Expectant
70+	High	Medium	Medium	Low	Low	Expectant	Expectant	Expectant	Expectant	Expectant

Fig. 4.5 American Burn Association age/survival grid for triage during burn disasters resulting in multiple casualties

though, that such guidelines are easily utilized in an emergency by inexperienced personnel. We are concerned that non-burn providers may commit errors in burn size estimation to include overestimation of burn size by 100% or more [62]. Thus, burn triage should be performed by experienced burn providers whenever possible.

A three-level method can be used for on-scene triage in catastrophic fires [63]. Level 1 includes sorting patients as acute or non-acute. Level 2 triage categorizes patients into immediate, delayed, minimal, and expectant ("DIME"). Level 3 triage sorts based on priority of evacuation.

4.3.2.2 At the Hospital

If a burn provider is not available at the scene of a fire, burn triage should occur before casualties enter the emergency department as to not overwhelm the facility with patients, most of whom will be candidates for outpatient treatment.

Expansion of both hospital personnel and bed space is necessary. After the Station nightclub fire, physicians from the Rhode Island Hospital fortunately began receiving casualties during a shift change when two sets of staff were in house and available [40]. The trauma ward was cleared of inpatients, and burn bed capacity was increased by utilizing extra suction and oxygen mounts already present in the trauma ward rooms. This allowed rapid expansion and enabled admission of a large number of burn casualties.

Just as importantly, existing staff should be enabled to work more efficiently. Bedside paper charting may be more efficient than computer-based charting, especially if outside providers are brought in to assist [49]. Delegation of care can be performed, such that a burn surgeon and senior burn nurse provide oversight and managerial support and non-burn providers carry out daily care to include resuscitation, wound care, pain management, and rehabilitation [31, 64]. The stress on the hospital staff must be alleviated by implementation of a rotation schedule, a meal service, and a counseling program [65]. Following the Station nightclub fire, established protocols for burn care (e.g., resuscitation, wound care, ventilator management, donor site care, rehabilitation) streamlined the management of multiple burn patients and allowed for inexperienced providers to work effectively [40]. Yurt and colleagues noted that early and frequent coordination is required to maintain a smooth flow of patients into and out of the operating room [49].

Following catastrophic fires, movement of patients from one hospital to another may be required: from a non-burn hospital to a burn center, or from one burn center to another. The American Burn Association (ABA), recognizing the burn care should take place in burn centers, recommends the transfer of patients from non-burn hospitals to a burn center within 24 h. Furthermore, when a burn center's surge capacity is reached, "secondary triage" may be necessary, whereby patients are selected for transfer to other burn centers [66]. The ABA recommends that such transfers occur within the first 48 h postburn. Surge capacity is defined as 50% more patients than the normal maximum number of patients which the center can accommodate [61]. The policy is based on the recognition that exceeding surge capacity could result in degrading the quality of care which the center can realistically provide.

Transfer to other burn centers may require transport across state/province or even international borders. After the café fire in Volendam, Netherlands in 2001, 182 patients required hospital admission, some of whom were transferred to burn centers in Belgium and Germany [67]. Clearly, advance planning and resolution of administrative, legal, and financial hurdles facilitates such transfers.

Alternatively, personnel and other resources may be brought in to augment the capabilities of burn centers within the disaster zone. Days after the Bashkirian gas pipeline explosion in 1989, several international teams (including 17 personnel from the USAISR) arrived in Ufa, Russia and assisted in acute care, such as excision and autografting of burn wounds and rehabilitation [68–70]. Enthusiasm for international disaster relief should be balanced by realism. This was highlighted by an after-action review of the response to the Bam, Iran earthquake in 2003: to be effective, international medical teams should (1) arrive rapidly; (2) be self-sufficient; and (3) meet the actual, validated needs of the host nation [71].

4.3.2.3 Command, Control, and Communication

The city, region, state, and nation should have established plans for disaster management. These plans should be enacted early after a catastrophe and should cover (1) roles and responsibilities; (2) triage procedures; (3) operation of the incident command center; (4) evacuation routes and methods; and (5) the roles of hospitals in the area. Redundant methods of communication should link all of the above [31]. Communication should be established between the local burn center and neighboring and national burn centers to coordinate for evacuation and discuss bed availability [72]. Methods of communication that may be helpful include satellite telephones, international cellular phones, two-way radios, and the Internet. In any given disaster, some of these resources may not be functional.

4.3.3 National Burn Disaster Management in the USA

Burn beds are a scarce national resource. Currently, the USA has about 127 self-designated burn centers [73], of which 70 have been verified by the American Burn Association (Alice Zemelko, personal communication, 19 March 2018). Most of the approximately 1800 burn beds are occupied at any one point in time [73]. During the initial phase of combat operations in Iraq, the USAISR's daily census of national burn bed availability polled 70 burn centers selected based on proximity to aeromedical evacuation hubs as well as ABA verification status. The average number of burn beds identified during this process was 407 (range 196–584), from an average number of reporting centers of 43 (range 21–56). As a rule of thumb, then, an average of about 10 beds per reporting center were open on any given day, about half of which were ICU beds. The total number of open beds in the country is quite limited, and national burn disaster plans must be worked out in advance.

The US disaster response system is tiered, reflecting the principal of subsidiarity and a desire to place limits on federal involvement in local affairs. The tiers include (1) local, state, and regional responses; (2) a civilian Federal response; and finally (3) a national military response (Defense Support of Civil Authorities, DSCA).

4.3.3.1 Regional Response

The American Burn Association (ABA) participates actively in burn disaster planning. This role reflects several recent events which demonstrated the value of the ABA and in particular its regional organizations. Following the explosion at the West Pharmaceutical chemical plant in Kinston, NC, in 2003, initial reports indicated that 200–300 patients were inbound to the North Carolina Jaycee Burn Center. Pre-existing relationships fostered by the ABA facilitated communication between the burn center director and both the ABA central office, and the other burn centers throughout the Southern Region [74]. This and other experiences informed the development of the Southern Region Burn Disaster Plan, which calls for a central Communication Center [75].

Regional efforts in New York City after 9/11 led to a plan that would address up to 50/million (400) burn patients for the first 3–5 days postburn. This plan defined four tiers of hospitals: (1) burn centers; (2) trauma centers; (3) participating non-burn, non-trauma hospitals; and (4) other hospitals. The flow of patients is to be overseen by a Burn Logistics Coordinating Center. Patients are triaged to either Tier 1 hospitals (those with critical but survivable injuries) or to Tier 2 or 3 hospitals (those with either moderate or non-survivable injuries) [76].

The US government's current Mass Burn Event plan anticipates such participation by the ABA Regions in disaster response. The receiving burn center in the disaster zone is encouraged to contact its ABA Regional Burn Coordinating Center which, in turn, is responsible for coordinating the transfer of patients to available burn beds within the region [77].

4.3.3.2 Federal Response

Whereas overall responsibility for disaster management at the national level lies with the Department of Homeland Security's Federal Emergency Management Agency (FEMA), responsibility for medical care coordination lies with the Department of Health and Human Services's Office of the Assistant Secretary for Preparedness and Response (ASPR). The legal basis for federal assistance in a disaster is the Robert T. Stafford Disaster Relief and Emergency Assistance Act (Stafford Act). Following a presidential disaster declaration, the Federal government coordinates the provision of assistance via FEMA. Such support is categorized into various Emergency Support Functions (ESF). ESF-8 consists of Public Health and Medical Services, which is led by ASPR [78].

One key component of the medical response is the National Disaster Medical System (NDMS). NDMS functions are threefold: (1) medical response to the site, (2) movement of victims from the site to unaffected areas, and (3) assistance with definitive medical care in unaffected areas. NDMS's medical response to the disaster site may include Disaster Medical Assistance Teams (DMATs). DMATs are sponsored by a local major medical center, are comprised of physicians, nurses, and administrative staff, and are tasked with providing care during a disaster. A relatively new addition to the NDMS inventory is the Trauma and Critical Care Teams (TCCTs), which include a surgical capability [79]. Previously, 4 NDMS Burn Specialty Teams (BSTs) were formed to augment local burn capabilities in the event of a disaster. No specific NDMS burn teams exist at this time.

4.3.3.3 Military Response

The final tier in the national disaster plan incorporates the use of U.S. Department of Defense (DoD) forces under DSCA [80]. DoD medical support may include aeromedical transportation of patients out of the disaster area, in support of NDMS's evacuation mission. This is provided by the U.S. Air Force and is regulated by the Global Patient Movement Requirements Center (GPMRC) at Scott Air Force Base. During Hurricane Katrina, approximately 2600 patients were evacuated by this process [81].

DoD may also augment capabilities within the disaster zone. A U.S. Navy hospital ship, the USNS Comfort, arrived in New York City harbor 3 days after the attacks on 11 September 2001. It served primarily to provide on-board medical and psychological support to first responders [82]. Also, a U.S. Air Force Expeditionary Medical Support (EMEDS) unit deployed to Fort Dix, NJ, soon after 9/11 [83]. A U.S. Army Combat Support Hospital deployed to the New Orleans International Airport 8 days after Hurricane Katrina, later moving to the Convention Center, where it provided both primary and emergency care, to include surgery [84]. These experiences suggest that the DoD can deploy Role III care rapidly, but not immediately, to the scene of a disaster.

Following a domestic disaster, burn-specific expertise can be provided by the U.S. Army Burn Flight Team.

Although this team's primary mission is aeromedical evacuation of critically ill patients, it is also tasked with assessing, advising, and augmenting, a role which it repeatedly played following fire disasters in South America [31]. This team recently demonstrated its ability to establish a mobile burn ICU in a non-burn hospital ward following a multiple-casualty incident in Guam [85]. Small teams like this are not self-sufficient, however, and require additional logistical support for an expanded mission in the disaster zone.

4.4 Summary

Military operations and civilian mass casualty disasters confront providers with both tragedy and with the potential for strengthening the scientific and organizational foundation of burn care. Table 4.4 provides a list of advances that occurred following some of the major wars and fire disasters of the last 100 years. These advances were possible not only because of the galvanizing effect of the events, but also because committed multidisciplinary team members worked together to care for patients, to learn from their experiences, and to document those experiences in a disciplined fashion.

Table 4.4 Relationship between wars or disasters and advances in burn care

Event	Date	Examples of advances made	References
Rialto Theater Fire	1921	Concept of burn shock as plasma loss	Underhill [86]
Battle of Britain	1940	Burn reconstruction techniques	Mayhew [87]
Pearl Harbor	1941	US government burn research program	Lockwood [88]
Cocoanut Grove Nightclub fire	1942	Fluid resuscitation formulas; comprehensive description of care; fire code changes	Cope and Moore [89]; Saffle [90]
Cold War	1949	U.S. Army Burn Center	Artz [91]
Vietnam War	1966–72	Topical antimicrobial therapies; metabolic support	Moreau [92]; Pruitt [93]; Wilmore [94]
Gulf War	1990–1	National collaboration for burn bed reporting in the USA	Shirani [95]
World Trade Center and Pentagon attacks	2001	Improved regional disaster response plans	Leahy [76]
Iraq and Afghanistan Wars	2001–present	Rapid aeromedical evacuation; ABA-DoD multicenter research collaboration; burn resuscitation decision support; deployable extracorporeal life support	Renz [19]; Salinas [96]; Chung [97]; Cannon [98]

ABA American Burn Association; *DoD* U.S. Department of Defense

Summary Box

- Life-threatening burns (20% TBSA or greater) occur in about 20% of thermally injured combat casualties or civilian mass-casualty patients.
- The ISR Rule of 10s enables rapid calculation of the initial fluid rate for adult patients (weight 40–80 kg): rate = TBSA × 10.
- Definitive care of civilians of all ages with major thermal injuries is part of the usual workload of Role III military hospitals on the modern battlefield.
- Most recent fire disasters produced 25–50 burn patients requiring hospitalization.
- Burn size and age should be used to triage patients in a disaster.
- Burn-bed surge capacity is finite; secondary triage to other hospitals should be considered when capacity is exceeded.

References

1. Cancio LC, Horvath EE, Barillo DJ, Kopchinski BJ, Charter KR, Montalvo AE, et al. Burn support for Operation Iraqi Freedom and related operations, 2003 to 2004. J Burn Care Rehabil. 2005;26(2):151–61.
2. Champion HR, Bellamy RF, Roberts CP, Leppaniemi A. A profile of combat injury. J Trauma. 2003;54(5 Suppl):S13–9.
3. Kauvar DS, Wolf SE, Wade CE, Cancio LC, Renz EM, Holcomb JB. Burns sustained in combat explosions in Operations Iraqi and Enduring Freedom (OIF/OEF explosion burns). Burns. 2006;32(7):853–7.
4. Kauvar DS, Cancio LC, Wolf SE, Wade CE, Holcomb JB. Comparison of combat and non-combat burns from ongoing U.S. military operations. J Surg Res. 2006;132(2):195–200.
5. Barillo DJ, Wolf S. Planning for burn disasters: lessons learned from one hundred years of history. J Burn Care Res. 2006;27(5):622–34.
6. Allen BD, Whitson TC, Henjyoji EY. Treatment of 1,963 burned patients at 106th general hospital, Yokohama, Japan. J Trauma. 1970;10(5):386–92.
7. Eldad A, Torem M. Burns in the Lebanon War 1982: "the blow and the cure". Mil Med. 1990;155(3):130–2.
8. Voisine JJ, Albano JP. Reduction and mitigation of thermal injuries; what can be done (Report No. USAARL-96-03.). Fort Rucker, AL: U.S. Army Aeromedical Research Laboratory; 1996.
9. Chung KK, Blackbourne LH, Wolf SE, White CE, Renz EM, Cancio LC, et al. Evolution of burn resuscitation in Operation Iraqi freedom. J Burn Care Res. 2006;27(5):606–11.
10. Ennis JL, Chung KK, Renz EM, Barillo DJ, Albrecht MC, Jones JA, et al. Joint Theater Trauma System implementation of burn resuscitation guidelines improves outcomes in severely burned military casualties. J Trauma. 2008;64(2 Suppl):S146–51.

11. Markell KW, Renz EM, White CE, Albrecht ME, Blackbourne LH, Park MS, et al. Abdominal complications after severe burns. J Am Coll Surg. 2009;208(5):940–7.
12. Alvarado R, Chung KK, Cancio LC, Wolf SE. Burn resuscitation. Burns. 2009;35(1):4–14.
13. Barillo DJ, Cancio LC, Hutton BG, Mittelsteadt PJ, Gueller GE, Holcomb JB. Combat burn life support: a military burn-education program. J Burn Care Rehabil. 2005;26(2):162–5.
14. Anonymous. Joint Trauma System Clinical Practice Guideline (CPG). Burn Care (CPG ID: 12). 11 May 2016. https://jts.amedd.army.mil/assets/docs/cpgs/JTS_Clinical_Practice_Guidelines_(CPGs)/Burn_Care_11_May_2016_ID12.pdf. Accessed 30 Mar 2018.
15. Chung KK, Salinas J, Renz EM, Alvarado RA, King BT, Barillo DJ, et al. Simple derivation of the initial fluid rate for the resuscitation of severely burned adult combat casualties: in silico validation of the rule of 10. J Trauma. 2010;69(Suppl 1):S49–54.
16. D'Avignon LC, Chung KK, Saffle JR, Renz EM, Cancio LC, et al. Prevention of infections associated with combat-related burn injuries. J Trauma. 2011;71(2 Suppl 2):S282–9.
17. Anonymous. Annual research progress reports. Fort Sam Houston, TX: U.S. Army Institute of Surgical Research. p. 1967–72.
18. Grissom TE, Farmer JC. The provision of sophisticated critical care beyond the hospital: lessons from physiology and military experiences that apply to civil disaster medical response. Crit Care Med. 2005;33(1):S13–21.
19. Renz EM, Cancio LC, Barillo DJ, White CE, Albrecht MC, Thompson CK, et al. Long range transport of war-related burn casualties. J Trauma. 2008;64(2 Suppl):S136–44.
20. Kirksey TD, Dowling JA, Pruitt BA Jr, Moncrief JA. Safe, expeditious transport of the seriously burned patient. Arch Surg. 1968;96(5):790–4.
21. Chapman TT, Richard RL, Hedman TL, Chisholm GB, Quick CD, Baer DG, et al. Military return to duty and civilian return to work factors following burns with focus on the hand and literature review. J Burn Care Res. 2008;29(5):756–62.
22. Wolf SE, Kauvar DS, Wade CE, Cancio LC, Renz EP, Horvath EE, et al. Comparison between civilian burns and combat burns from Operation Iraqi Freedom and Operation Enduring Freedom. Ann Surg. 2006;243(6):786–92.
23. Chapman TT, Richard RL, Hedman TL, Renz EM, Wolf SE, Holcomb JB. Combat casualty hand burns: evaluating impairment and disability during recovery. J Hand Ther. 2008;21(2):150–8.
24. Anonymous. IV Geneva convention relative to the protection of civilian persons in time of war of 12 August 1949. http://www.un.org/en/genocideprevention/documents/atrocity-crimes/Doc.33_GC-IV-EN.pdf. Accessed 11 Mar 2018.
25. Anonymous. Employment of the Combat Support Hospital: tactics, techniques, and procedures (Field Manual 8-10-14). Washinton, DC: Headquarters, Department of the Army; 1994.
26. Levy BS, Sidel VW. Adverse health consequences of the Iraq War. Lancet. 2013;381(9870):949–58.
27. Schmidt PM, Sheridan RL, Moore CL, Scuba SC, King BT, Morrissey PM, et al. From Baghdad to Boston: international transfer of burned children in time of war. J Burn Care Res. 2014;35(5):369–73.
28. Smith D. Dennis Smith's history of firefighting in America: 300 years of courage. New York: Dial Press; 1978.
29. Goodman EC. Fire! The 100 most devastating fires through the ages and the heroes who fought them. New York: Black Dog & Leventhal; 2001.
30. Follett GP. The Boston fire: a challenge to our disaster service. Am J Nurs. 1943;43:4–8.
31. Cancio LC, Pruitt BA Jr. Management of mass casualty burn disasters. Int J Disaster Med. 2004;2:114–29.
32. Cowan D. Great Chicago fires: historic blazes that shaped a city. Chicago: Lake Claremont Press; 2001.
33. Moulton RS. Cocoanut grove night club fire. Boston: National Fire Protection Association. Accessed 11 Jan 1943.
34. Anonymous. Fire investigations: nursing home fire, Norfolk, VA, October 5, 1989. Quincy, MA: National Fire Protection Association; 1990.
35. Klem TJ. 25 die in food plant fire. NFPA J. 1992;86:29–35.
36. Finland M, Davidson CS, Levenson SM. Clinical and therapeutic aspects of the conflagration injuries in the respiratory tract sustained by victims of the Cocoanut Grove disaster. Med Health. 1946;25:215–83.
37. Schorow S. The Cocoanut Grove fire. Beverly, MA: Commonwealth Editions; 2005.
38. Kimball WY. Hartford city holocaust. NFPA Q; 1944. p. 9–21.
39. O'Nan S. The circus fire: a true story of an American tragedy. New York: Anchor; 2008.
40. Harrington DT, Biffl WL, Cioffi WG. The station nightclub fire. J Burn Care Rehabil. 2005;26(2):141–3.
41. Mackie DP, Koning HM. Fate of mass burn casualties: implications for disaster planning. Burns. 1990;16:203–6.
42. Gill JR, Goldfeder LB, Stajic M. The Happy Land homicides: 87 deaths due to smoke inhalation. J Forens Sci. 2003;48(1):1–3.
43. Arturson G. Analysis of severe fire disasters. In: Masselis M, Gunn SWA, editors. The management of mass burn casualties and fire disasters: proceedings of the first international conference on burns and fire disasters. Dordrecht: Kluwer Academic; 1992. p. 24–33.
44. Simon R, Teperman S. The World Trade Center attack: lessons for disaster management. Crit Care. 2001;5:318–20.
45. Asaeda F. The day that the START triage system came to a stop: observations from the World Trade Center disaster. Acad Emerg Med. 2002;9:255–6.
46. Bradt DA. Site management of health issues in the 2001 World Trade Center disaster. Acad Emerg Med. 2003;10:650–60.
47. Anonymous. Rapid assessment of injuries among survivors of the terrorist attack on the World Trade Center—New York City, September 2001. Morb Mortal Wkly Rep. 2002;51(1):1–5.
48. Anonymous. Centers for Disease Control and Prevention. Deaths in World Trade Center terrorist attacks—New York City, 2001. Morb Mortal Wkly Rep. 2002;51:16–8.
49. Yurt RW, Bessey PQ, Bauer GJ, Dembicki R, Laznick H, Alden N, et al. A regional burn center's response to a disaster: September 11, 2001, and the days beyond. J Burn Care Rehabil. 2005;26(2):117–24.
50. Arturson G. The tragedy of San Juanico—the most severe LPG disaster in history. Burns. 1987;13:87–102.
51. Arturson G. The Los Alfaques disaster: a boiling-liquid, expanding-vapour explosion. Burns. 1981;7(4):233–51.
52. Ishida T, Ohta M, Sugimoto T. The breakdown of an emergency system following a gas explosion in Osaka and the subsequent resolution of problems. J Emerg Med. 1985;2(3):183–9.
53. Buerk CA, Batdorf JW, Cammack KV, Ravenholt O. The MGM Grand Hotel fire: lessons learned from a major disaster. Arch Surg. 1982;117(5):641–4.
54. Sharpe DT. Management of burns in major disasters. NATNEWS. 1989;26(12):9–10.
55. Pruitt BAJ. Aeromedical transport and field care of burn patients in disaster situations. In: Haberal MA, Bilgin N, editors. Burn and fire disaster in the middle east. Ankara: Haberal Education and Research Foundation; 2001. p. 221–43.
56. Frykberg ER. Medical management of disasters and mass casualties from terrorist bombings: how can we cope? J Trauma. 2002;53(2):201–12.
57. Osler T, Glance LG, Hosmer DW. Simplified estimates of the probability of death after burn injuries: extending and updating the Baux score. J Trauma Acute Care Surg. 2010;68(3):690–7.

58. Pruitt BA Jr, Wolf SE, Mason AD Jr. Epidemiological, demographic, and outcome characteristics of burn injury. In: Herndon DN, editor. Total burn care. Philadelphia: Elsevier; 2007. p. 14–32.
59. Baux S. Contribution à l'étude du traitement local des brûlures thermiques étendues. Paris: AGEMP (Université de Paris [1896-1968]. Faculté de Médecine); 1961.
60. Bowen TE, Bellamy RF. Emergency war surgery: Second United States revision of the emergency war surgery NATO handbook. Washington, DC: U.S. Government Printing Office; 1988.
61. Anonymous. ABA Board of Trustees; Committee on Organization and Delivery of Burn Care. Disaster management and the ABA Plan. J Burn Care Rehabil. 2005;26(2):102–6.
62. Hammond JS, Ward CG. Transfers from emergency room to burn center: errors in burn size estimate. J Trauma. 1987;27:1161–5.
63. Briggs SM, Brinsfield KH. Advanced disaster medical response: manual for providers. Woodbury, CT: Cine-Med; 2014.
64. Mozingo DW, Barillo DJ, Holcomb JB. The Pope Air Force Base aircraft crash and burn disaster. J Burn Care Rehabil. 2005;26(2):132–40.
65. Cushman JG, Pachter HL, Beaton HL. Two New York City hospitals' surgical response to the September 11, 2001, terrorist attack in New York City. J Trauma. 2003;54(1):147–54.
66. Sheridan R, Barillo D, Herndon D, Solem L, Mohr W, Kadilack P, et al. Burn specialty teams. J Burn Care Rehabil. 2005;26(2):170–3.
67. Kuijper EC. The 2003 Everett Idris Evans memorial lecture: every cloud has a silver lining. J Burn Care Rehabil. 2004;25(1):45–53.
68. Becker WK, Waymack JP, McManus AT, Shaikhutdinov M, Pruitt BA Jr. Bashkirian train-gas pipeline disaster: the American military response. Burns. 1990;16(5):325–8.
69. Benmeir P, Levine I, Shostak A, Oz V, Shemer J, Sokolova T. The Ural train-gas pipeline catastrophe: the report of the IDF medical corps assistance. Burns. 1991;17(4):320–2.
70. Remensnyder JP, Ackroyd FP, Astrozjnikova S, Budkevitch LG, Buletova AA, Creedon CM, et al. Burned children from the Bashkir train-gas pipeline disaster. I. Acute management at Children's Hospital 9, Moscow. Burns. 1990;16(5):329–32.
71. Abolghasemi H, Radfar MH, Khatami M, Nia MS, Amid A, Briggs SM. International medical response to a natural disaster: lessons learned from the Bam earthquake experience. Prehosp Disaster Med. 2006;21(3):141–7.
72. Barillo DJ, Jordan MH, Jocz RJ, Nye D, Cancio LC, Holcomb JB. Tracking the daily availability of burn beds for national emergencies. J Burn Care Rehabil. 2005;26(2):174–82.
73. Iyer N, Barrera-Oro J, Turley D, Simon D, Selivanova O, Larsen J, et al. Next-generation burn care products and strategies draw on innovative ideas. Washington, DC: Office of the Assistant Secretary for Preparedness and Response, U.S. Department of Health and Human Services; 2017. https://www.phe.gov/ASPRBlog/pages/BlogArticlePage.aspx?PostID=237. Accessed 18 Mar 2018.
74. Cairns BA, Stiffler A, Price F, Peck MD, Meyer AA. Managing a combined burn trauma disaster in the post-9/11 world: lessons learned from the 2003 West Pharmaceutical plant explosion. J Burn Care Rehabil. 2005;26(2):144–50.
75. Barillo DJ, Dimick AR, Cairns BA, Hardin WD, Acker JE III, Peck MD. The Southern Region burn disaster plan. J Burn Care Res. 2006;27(5):589–95.
76. Leahy NE, Yurt RW, Lazar EJ, Villacara AA, Rabbitts AC, Berger L, et al. Burn disaster response planning in New York City: updated recommendations for best practices. J Burn Care Res. 2012;33(5):587–94.
77. Anonymous. Mass burn event overview. Office of the Assistant Secretary for Preparedness and Response (ASPR); Technical Resources, Assistance Center, and Information Exchange (TRACIE), US Department of Health and Human Services. 21 Feb 2016. https://asprtracie.s3.amazonaws.com/documents/aspr-aba-oem-mass-burn-event-overview.pdf. Accessed 19 Mar 2018.
78. Anonymous. Emergency Support Function #8—Public Health and Medical Services Annex. Jan 2008. https://www.fema.gov/media-library-data/20130726-1825-250458027/emergency_support_function_8_public_health___medical_services_annex_2008.pdf. Accessed 19 Mar 2018.
79. Anonymous. Trauma and Critical Care Teams. Office of the Assistant Secretary of Preparedness and Response, U.S. Department of Health and Human Services. 9 Sept 2017. https://www.phe.gov/Preparedness/responders/ndms/ndms-teams/Pages/tcct.aspx. Accessed 19 Mar 2018.
80. Anonymous. Department of Defense Directive 3025.18. Defense Support of Civil Authorities (DSCA). 29 Dec 2010. http://www.dco.uscg.mil/Portals/9/CG-5R/nsarc/DoDD%203025.18%20Defense%20Support%20of%20Civil%20Authorities.pdf. Accessed 19 Mar 2018.
81. Davis LE. Hurricane Katrina: lessons for army planning and operations. Santa Monica, CA: Rand Corporation; 2007.
82. Marvin DS. Bringing Comfort to New York City. 10 Sept 2016. https://health.mil/News/Articles/2016/09/10/Bringing-Comfort-to-New-York-City. Accessed 20 Mar 2018.
83. Sturkol ST. History shows strong response on 9-11 by AMC people. Air Mobility Command Public Affairs. 11 Sept 2009. http://www.af.mil/News/Article-Display/Article/119183/history-shows-strong-response-on-9-11-by-amc-people/. Accessed 21 Mar 2018.
84. Moore CJ. Army Nurses and Healthcare after Hurricane Katrina. Army Nurse Corps Association. https://e-anca.org/History/Topics-in-ANC-History/ANs_and_Katrina. Accessed 20 Mar 2018.
85. Barillo DJ, Cancio LC, Stack RS, Carr SR, Broger KP, Crews DM, et al. Deployment and operation of a transportable burn intensive care unit in response to a burn multiple casualty incident. Am J Disaster Med. 2010;5(1):5–13.
86. Underhill FP. The significance of anhydremia in extensive superficial burns. JAMA. 1930;95:852–7.
87. Mayhew ER. The reconstruction of warriors: Archibald McIndoe, the Royal Air Force and the Guinea Pig Club. London: Greenhill Books; 2004.
88. Lockwood JS. War-time activities of the National Research Council and the Committee on Medical Research; with particular reference to team-work on studies of wounds and burns. Ann Surg. 1946;124:314–27.
89. Cope O, Moore FD. The redistribution of body water and the fluid therapy of the burned patient. Ann Surg. 1947;126:1010–45.
90. Saffle JR. The 1942 fire at Boston's Cocoanut Grove nightclub. Am J Surg. 1993;166(6):581–91.
91. Artz CP. Burns in my lifetime. J Trauma. 1969;9(10):827–33.
92. Moreau AR, Westfall PH, Cancio LC, Mason AD Jr. Development and validation of an age-risk score for mortality predication after thermal injury. J Trauma. 2005;58(5):967–72.
93. Pruitt BA Jr, O'Neill JA Jr, Moncrief JA, Lindberg RB. Successful control of burn-wound sepsis. JAMA. 1968;203(12):1054–6.
94. Wilmore DW, Curreri PW, Spitzer KW, Spitzer ME, Pruitt BA Jr. Supranormal dietary intake in thermally injured hypermetabolic patients. Surg Gynecol Obstet. 1971;132(5):881–6.
95. Shirani KZ, Becker WK, Rue LW, Mason AD Jr, Pruitt BA Jr. Burn care during Operation Desert Storm. J US Army Med Dept. 1992;PB 8-92-1/2:37–9.
96. Salinas J, Chung KK, Mann EA, Cancio LC, Kramer GC, Serio-Melvin ML, et al. Computerized decision support system improves fluid resuscitation following severe burns: an original study. Crit Care Med. 2011;39(9):2031–8.
97. Chung KK, Lundy JB, Matson JR, Renz EM, White CE, King BT, et al. Continuous venovenous hemofiltration in severely burned patients with acute kidney injury: a cohort study. Crit Care. 2009;13(3):R62.
98. Allan PF, Osborn EC, Bloom BB, Wanek S, Cannon JW. The introduction of extracorporeal membrane oxygenation to aeromedical evacuation. Mil Med. 2011;176(8):932–7.

5 Population-Based Research Using Administrative Data to Evaluate Long-Term Outcomes in Burn Injury

Stephanie Mason, Rae Spiwak, and Sarvesh Logsetty

5.1 Introduction

The goal of population-based research is to answer research questions or hypotheses for a defined population [1]. Population-based research using administrative data can address some of the challenges in longitudinal studies, such as poor follow-up, and recollection bias [2]. Additionally, study findings can be generalizable to the entire population studied, not just a specific cohort. The population is usually defined by geographical boundaries, such as a province, state, and country [3]. However, populations may also be defined by membership in particular health maintenance organizations, such as Kaiser-Permanente Insurance program enrollees in the United States [2]. Such research can involve longitudinal assessment of individuals to assess exposure–outcome relationships and answer questions about individuals from a particular population [2].

Population-based research can be used to generate estimates of the incidence and prevalence of a particular disease or exposure in the defined population and to determine how these rates change over time at the population level. The variables associated with a given exposure in the population can also be estimated, and changes in the distribution of these factors over time can be characterized. By comparing the at-risk population with a not-at-risk population, the level of association of the risk factor with the outcome can be estimated. While population-based research can clarify associations of various factors and outcomes, caution should be used in assigning cause and effect based on these factors. Finally, given the ability to study a population, estimates of the association between particular exposures and outcomes can be generated that are relatively unbiased. This information can then be used in a number of ways, including informing the development of public health campaigns, healthcare service delivery and planning, and evaluating the results of policy or care changes. For example, the impact of burn prevention campaigns with defined implementation dates can be evaluated by comparing the pre- and post-intervention burn incidence rates in a given population. As well, the findings of population-based studies can help guide the creation of more specific clinical trials to better evaluate cause and effect.

S. Mason
Division of General Surgery, Department of Surgery, University of Toronto, Toronto, ON, Canada

R. Spiwak
Department of Psychiatry, University of Manitoba, Winnipeg, MB, Canada

S. Logsetty (✉)
Manitoba Firefighters Burn Unit, Departments of Surgery and Psychiatry, Rady Faculty of Health Sciences, University of Manitoba, Winnipeg, MB, Canada
e-mail: Sarvesh.Logsetty@umanitoba.ca

5.2 Population-Based Datasets

Conduct of population-based research depends on the availability of datasets that capture requisite data on the population of interest. Therefore, population-based studies generally utilize data sourced from administrative databases. These are massive repositories of data usually collected for non-research purposes, such as billing, pharmacy, education, and social supports. In healthcare, these are commonly maintained by hospitals, health maintenance organizations, and health insurance programs [4]. In countries with publicly funded and administered healthcare systems such as Canada, databases capture all eligible individuals and represent a near-complete sampling of the population. These datasets can capture information every time an individual interacts with the healthcare system, and record and store such information in an objective, standardized manner [2]. Separate datasets may exist for outpatient, emergency, hospital, and pharmacy claims. These can be linked via a unique, anonymous patient identifier to create a comprehensive record of healthcare utilization [4]. Further linkage to other data sources can enrich the dataset further; for example, claims data can be linked to socioeconomic information from census data, clinical information from clinical registries, or to survey data to gain information on patient lifestyle variables.

M. G. Jeschke et al. (eds.), *Handbook of Burns Volume 1*, https://doi.org/10.1007/978-3-030-18940-2_5

As an example, in Ontario, several health administrative databases can be linked and leveraged for research purposes. These are made available through the Institute for Clinical Evaluative Sciences (ICES). ICES is a section 45 prescribed entity under the Province of *Ontario's Personal Health Information Privacy Act*; as such, ICES collects and holds a large proportion of the administrative health data collected in Ontario for the purposes of health system planning and management [5]. Under this law, patients do not have to consent to the collection of their health data. In the absence of patient consent, ICES must uphold strict procedures to maintain patient privacy and confidentiality. These procedures include data encryption, physical security measures, anonymization of data, strict policies regarding access to data and dissemination of results, and regular audits [5]. These policies and procedures are implemented internally and enforced by the ICES privacy officer.

Similar to other Canadian provinces, the Ontario government administers a single-payer system that universally funds all hospital, laboratory, and necessary physician services for eligible residents; therefore, these data sources include records for virtually all residents in the province. Non-residents of Ontario, and individuals with lapsed healthcare coverage are not captured. These databases can be deterministically linked using an encrypted unique identifier based on each patient's Ontario Health Card Number. An example of the types of data contained in these datasets is presented in Table 5.1 [6].

Research-specific indices can also be generated using these datasets and applied to future projects. For example, the Ontario Marginalization Index (ONMARG) was created by researchers at the Centre for Research on Inner City Health (now the Centre for Urban Health Solutions) in Toronto to facilitate exploration of how multiple dimensions of social marginalization are concentrated at the local level, and how these factors are associated with health outcomes [7]. ONMARG is derived from 2006 census data and includes four dimensions of marginalization: residential instability, material deprivation, ethnic concentration, and dependency. The ONMARG for individuals is derived based on their census subdivision (smallest geographical unit), dissemination area, or local health integration authority (largest geographical unit). As such, the ONMARG does not represent individual-level data.

Health administrative databases are maintained in various other forms worldwide. Similar datasets are maintained in Manitoba, Canada, by the Manitoba Centre for Health Policy. These data can be used to evaluate functioning of the healthcare system and interactions with other publicly funded systems: education, justice. Other countries with large health administrative databases include Australia, Israel, and Taiwan. In the United States, the Veteran Affairs Clinical Database contains medical claims-based data for all Veterans, and Medicaid contains medical claims-based data for all recipients of social welfare. In the United Kingdom, the Hospital Episode Statistics database contains information on all hospital visits that are funded by the National Health Service.

Health administrative databases differ from registries that are maintained for research purposes. The National Burn Repository is perhaps the largest and most well-known database of burn-injured patients. It is maintained by the American Burn Association and represents an amalgamation of data voluntarily submitted by burn centers. Most of these burn centers are located in the United States; the 2016 report of data contained information from 96 US burn centers, in addition to 4 Canadian, 2 Swedish, and 1 Swiss burn center, representing more than 205,000 entries [8]. Although the NBR represents a rich source of burn-specific data, studies using this data are not considered population-based. The voluntary nature of burn centers reporting data to the NBR means that the data are a convenience sample of the burn-injured population, and not necessarily a representative sample. Furthermore, the NBR does not allow researchers to examine trends in the incidence of burn injury at the population level over time, or to relate outcomes to population-level variables. For example, data in the NBR might suggest a

Table 5.1 Ontario's population-based databases

Database	Data elements
Discharge Abstract Database (DAD)	• All acute care hospitalizations in Ontario after 1991 • Information regarding the admitting hospital, admission diagnosis, in-hospital interventions and length of stay, diagnoses contributing to the hospital stay, and discharge disposition
National Ambulatory Care Reporting System (NACRS)	• All ambulatory visits, including emergency department and outpatient visits information regarding presenting complaint, interventions, triage category, and discharge disposition
Ontario Mental Health Reporting System (OMHRS)	• All admissions to a mental health facility in Ontario, starting in 2005 DSM-IV axis I and axis II diagnoses at admission and discharge marital and employment status • Presence of specific psychiatric symptoms, information regarding self-harm attempts and their intent, and information regarding substance use
Registered Persons Database (RPDB)	• Demographic and vital statistics information date of last contact with healthcare system
Ontario Register General, Death (ORGD)	• Data on all deaths in Ontario date, location, and immediate, antecedent, and underlying cause of death

decrease in burn-related hospitalizations over time; however, the denominator (i.e., number of population at risk) is unknown. Nonetheless, the NBR is able to provide robust estimates of changes in burn patient demographics, incidence of complications during hospitalization, length of stay, and burn injury characteristics.

5.3 Advantages of Population-Based Research

There are several advantages to conducting population-based research using large health administrative databases. By the nature of such datasets, information about the healthcare utilization for all individuals in a given population is collected and stored objectively and consistently over time [2]. This facilitates the capture of information about a large number of individuals over indefinite periods of time, both prior to and following a given date, thereby permitting use of longitudinal study designs, with minimal loss to follow-up. The ability to "look back" in time before a given event overcomes the recall bias that can be associated with asking study participants to recall prior healthcare use, and allows adjustment or exclusion based on prior healthcare utilization. In the case of relatively rare events such as burn injury, population-based databases allow identification and follow-up of a large sample of burn-injured individuals, spanning an entire geographic region. As a result, with a relatively short and inexpensive study design, researchers can generate data about incidence, trends, and outcomes related to a given exposure in an entire population, over defined study periods. To gather such information using traditional research methods would be costly, time-consuming, and would be subject to losses to follow-up.

Population-based study designs also facilitate the relatively simple identification of a number of control members from the general population, matched on any number of patient characteristics, including but not limited to age, sex, geographic residence, socioeconomic status, and medical comorbidities. Identifying such controls in a retrospective or prospective cohort study would be incredibly onerous. The use of a controlled study design allows the description of relative, rather than just absolute risks.

5.4 Limitations of Population-Based Data

5.4.1 Ascertainment of Disorders and Burn Injury Characteristics

While administrative data has tremendous strengths, it is also limited in a variety of ways. Specifically, data are limited by ascertainment bias, and are ultimately representations of individuals who sought or received care from a care provider or were hospitalized [9]. As such, these health indicators report treatment use. While due to their severity, burn treatment rates are likely to reflect accurate rates of injury, sequalae such as mental disorders or suicidal behavior associated with the injury may be limited to individuals that sought care [10, 11]. Failure to seek help for mental disorders is a problem worldwide; certain populations, including males and older individuals, are less likely to seek care [12]. As a result, mental disorder measures that rely on administrative data are likely underestimated. While many diagnoses are available through the use of administrative data, some measures such as post-traumatic stress disorder (PTSD) are not always captured due to ICD coding challenges. For example, it is not possible to differentiate PTSD from other anxiety conditions using data housed at the Manitoba Centre for Health Policy unless the patient is hospitalized. Similarly, other measures related to burn injury might not be recorded accurately using administrative data such as burn depth and location. As a result, it is not always possible to examine injury characteristics and associated outcomes. While this limitation is present, administrative data can be augmented by specialized clinical databases which contain more detailed information specific burn injury, as is being done in Manitoba [13].

5.4.2 Social Factors

Social factors play an important role in an individual's health and response to injury [14, 15]. Factors such as social supports are an important component of recovery from injury, with increased perception of social support associated with improved quality of life post-burn injury [16]. Unfortunately, social measures including family supports following burn injury are not typically available in administrative data. Similarly, measures that may predict outcomes and quality of life among burn survivors including stigmatization, survivor guilt [17], and participation in burn survivor support groups [18] are also unavailable resulting in an incomplete picture of an individuals' adjustment to injury.

5.4.3 Immeasurable Time Bias and Loss to Follow-up

Immeasurable time bias and loss to follow-up are two potential limitations associated with the use of administrative data in the study of burn injury. Specifically, immeasurable time bias is when a health outcome or exposure is not measurable in a given period (such as cardiac events following pediatric burn injury) [19]. In Manitoba, medication used during hospitalizations is not captured, and as such medication use is available for outpatient visits only. Similarly, individuals who move out of province or who die over the study period would not contribute equal follow-up time in longitudinal studies. As such, different methodological and statistical approaches such as Cox Proportional Hazards Regression or offsets using log of person years may be used to account for censoring of incomplete observations or to ensure that follow-up periods reflect an individual's time at risk [20].

5.4.4 Lack of Randomization

While population-based data typically utilizes information from all individuals in a population, there is a lack of randomization. As such, the advantages of randomization including the assumption that known and unknown confounding factors are equal in both study and control groups and reduction of bias are not possible. While these limitations are present, both weighting and matching methods exist that may correct for selection biases in studies where random selection is not used. Specifically, propensity score matching (PSM) and inverse probability treatment weighting (IPTW) can be used to either create a composite score of selected covariates or assign more or less weight to individuals that have lower odds of being in a case or control group [21]. As such, case and control groups are equalized in the measures included in either the propensity score or weight. While these methods account for measurable confounders, it is important to recognize that unmeasured confounding factors are not accounted for, therefore residual confounding may impact estimates.

5.4.5 Health Indicator Coding

Health indicators available in administrative databases are vast. Databases may include vital statistics, hospital and medical claims, social services and education data and other registries [9]. While access to this data provides researchers and policymakers with tremendous opportunities, it is essential that defined, valid, and reliable health indicators are used. When using administrative data-derived indicators, it is essential to understand that data are collected for non-research purposes, including health system management and healthcare provider payments [22]. Therefore, investigators must carefully consider whether or not such indicators are appropriate measures of the variable of interest. Although some sources have cited the lack of data validation as a potential limitation of using administrative data in research [23], the reliability and validity of registries at the Manitoba Centre for Health Policy (MCHP) have been examined [24–26]. These studies provide support for the validation and utilization of measures related to the study of burn injury-related mental disorder outcomes, including measures of mood and anxiety disorder diagnoses [9]. A related limitation of using administrative data is how, or at what level, data are coded. In many cases, an individual may be coded as having either the presence or absence of disease (yes/no). When dichotomous outcomes or coding is present, it along with the research hypotheses will direct choice of statistical analyses.

5.4.6 Repeated Measures

As many administrative data studies use information that is collected over time, individuals will often contribute more than one data point over a study period. As a result, repeated measures are present. Such repeated data often violate the statistical assumption of independent observations [27]. Many methods exist to help account for these correlated (i.e., same individual) data. While analyses using administrative data are often complex and utilize multiple time points, it is essential to employ analyses that can accommodate the correlated nature of the data [28–31]. Paired *t*-tests and multivariate analysis of variance which are typically used for analyzing repeated measures may be limited in the analyses of such data [28, 31]. In this case, generalized estimating equations (GEE) facilitate regression analyses that take into consideration the correlated nature of complex data. GEE is an extension of generalized linear models and will ensure that correct inferences and estimates are produced [32].

5.5 Overcoming the Limitations Associated with Population-Based Data

5.5.1 Know Your Data

There are a number of ways that investigators can mitigate the limitations of using administrative datasets. Firstly, it is essential to have a thorough understanding of the methods by which their data is collected and coded, and the inherent limitations. This knowledge will facilitate an understanding of the limitations specific to a given project. For example, if using datasets that employ ICD-10 coding, investigators will be limited to this characterization of healthcare visits, which may not provide the granularity desired. Secondly, investigators should seek an understanding of the validity of the databases being used, including accuracy of coding. Many large administrative datasets will undergo validation studies on an ongoing basis in order to ensure data quality. For example, the Canadian Institute for Health Information (CIHI) utilizes a variety of measures to ensure accuracy and consistency in its databases [33]. In 2010, CIHI conducted a re-abstraction study which demonstrated 86% accuracy in reporting of the most responsible diagnosis for admission in the DAD [34]. Several other validation studies have demonstrated the accuracy of diagnoses codes in the DAD for the identification of inflammatory bowel disease, stroke, chronic obstructive pulmonary disease, and spinal cord injury [35–38].

5.5.2 Validation

Investigators planning to use health administrative databases in their research should consider conducting a validation study specific to their patient population of interest. To perform a validation study, a gold-standard dataset is required, against which the administrative data are compared [39]. This gold-standard may be derived from chart review, or from a pre-existing clinical dataset (such as the NBR). If a pre-existing clinical dataset is used, then its validity may have already been assured. This gold-standard dataset can then be compared against the administrative data to determine its validity. One such study was used to validate burn diagnosis codes in Ontario, Canada [40]. The authors utilized a prospectively maintained database from Canada's largest burn center as their gold-standard. This database was linked to a cohort of burn-injured individuals identified in the administrative dataset using patient-specific identifiers. Briefly, that study found that TBSA codes were highly sensitive and specific in identifying patients with ≥10 and ≥20% TBSA injuries (89/93% sensitive and 95/97% specific), with excellent agreement (κ, 0.85/κ, 0.88). Codes were weakly sensitive (68%) in identifying ≥10% TBSA full-thickness burn though highly specific (86%) with moderate agreement (κ, 0.46). The diagnoses codes had limited sensitivity (43%) to identify inhalation injury, but high specificity (99%) with moderate agreement (κ, 0.54). Burn mechanism had excellent coding agreement (κ, 0.84).

The above-mentioned validation study provides some important insights into the limitations of using administrative data to study burn outcomes. For example, burn depth was not reliably reported, owing to limitations of the ICD-10 coding system, and inhalation injury was underreported in the administrative datasets. Burn size and mechanism were accurately coded in the administrative data, while codes pertaining to the location of the burn were infrequently used. Therefore, this particular dataset is limited in its ability to provide details of burn depth or location and the potential association of these injury characteristics with any outcomes of interest. The ability to risk-adjust outcomes for these particular variables is also limited. Whether the limitations of Ontario's administrative databases are generalizable to other administrative databases is unknown; however, the limitations specific to ICD-10 coding are expected to be limitations of any database employing this coding structure.

5.5.3 Linkage with Other Datasets

To provide greater clinical granularity to administrative data, it may be possible to link a clinical database to an administrative dataset. Such an approach has been used to study burn injury in Manitoba. In this case, a specialized provincial burn database has been linked with administrative data, and enables detailed study and follow-up [13].

Such linkage can also overcome any challenges associated with identifying a specific cohort of burn-injured individuals in an administrative database because the cohort can be identified in the clinical database and then followed over time in the administrative dataset after linkage occurs. Records can be linked either deterministically through the use of patient identifiers, or probabilistically using various algorithms. A combination of deterministic and probabilistic linkage is also possible. The exact nature by which records can be linked, and how the data are stored, will depend on the specific privacy and data sharing regulations of the administrative database.

Successful linkage of a clinical database to an administrative dataset will allow investigators to answer a number of research questions, as both burn-specific clinical data as well as long-term healthcare utilization data will be available. In a sense, such a dataset combines the best of prospective cohort studies and large population-based studies, without the time, expense, and loss to follow-up that might be associated with prospective studies. However, the logistics and cost of generating such a linked dataset should not be underestimated and will vary from region to region. Linkage also offers an opportunity to validate the administrative data, using the clinical database as a gold-standard, as discussed above.

5.6 Population-Based Studies of Burn Injury

Population-based studies have not yet been widely used in burn care research. However, much of the long-term outcome data available in the burn literature has been derived from population-based studies, mainly in Canada, Australia, and Taiwan. These countries have in common a publicly funded healthcare system; therefore large, healthcare administrative databases are maintained for the purposes of tracking healthcare utilization of all individuals eligible for coverage.

Some of the first population-based burn research was conducted in Australia, using the Western Australia Data Linkage System [41]. Using this dataset, Fiona Wood and colleagues derived a cohort of all individuals admitted to hospital for burn injury in Western Australia, between 1983 and 2008. These data facilitated the description of the epidemiology of burn injury in Australia and demonstrated a decrease in burn-related hospitalizations and mortality over time [41]. This group went on to match burn survivors by age and sex to non-injured members of the general population to determine whether rates of late mortality and specific types of hospital admissions are higher among burn survivors. These studies demonstrated increased late mortality among childhood, adolescent, adult, and elderly burn survivors [42–44]; increased hospitalizations for cardiovascular diseases, infectious diseases, diabetes, gastrointestinal disease, and nervous system disease [45–49]. Their work clearly illustrates the advantages of population-based research for burn injury: long-term follow-up, the ability to match to members of the uninjured population, and the ability to characterize temporal trends in burn incidence and mortality, while identifying groups that remain at high risk, to whom prevention efforts should perhaps be targeted.

In Taiwan, investigators have leveraged the availability of population-based datasets to conduct both descriptive and matched cohort studies. They have used these datasets to describe the epidemiology and associated healthcare utilization of burn injury in Taiwan, including the outpatient burden of burn injury; they found that only 3.6% of all burn-injured patients were hospitalized for treatment [50]. Three matched cohort studies have demonstrated that burn survivors are at increased risk of ischemic stroke after burn although the absolute risk is quite low [51–53].

In Canada, investigators have similarly used population-based datasets to describe the epidemiology of burn injury and to characterize changes in regionalization of burn care over time [54]. An advantage of population-based datasets is the ability to study patients treated at both burn and non-burn centers and to compare their outcomes. In one Canadian study, the investigators found that burn-related mortality had improved significantly over time at burn centers, with significantly more variation in mortality rates at non-burn centers. Furthermore, in 2013, more than 25% of patients with major burn injury received their care at non-burn centers. This highlights some of the insights that can be gained using a population-based approach. These datasets have also been used similarly to those in Taiwan and Australia to infer long-term outcomes from healthcare utilization data. In one such study, readmissions and emergency department visits were common after burn injury, most often related to mental illness and unintentional injuries, while burn recidivism was rare [55]. Interestingly, this study demonstrated that burn center care was associated with significantly fewer emergency department visits and readmissions.

Finally, two Canadian population-based datasets to characterize the association between burn injury and mental illness. In one longitudinal matched cohort study, Logsetty et al. found high rates of psychopathology among burn patients both before and after their injury, compared to a control cohort [13]. Their study highlighted the importance of mental healthcare for burn-injured patients, and the potential role that pre-existing mental illness might have on burn outcomes. Mason et al. utilized an exposure-crossover design to conduct their longitudinal cohort study, therefore allowing each burn patient to act as their own control before and after injury. This study demonstrated high rates of mental illness both before and after burn injury, similar to the results of Logsetty et al. While the overall rate of mental illness did not increase after burn injury, patients with minimal pre-burn mental illness experienced significant increases in their rate of mental health emergencies after burn [56]. This study also demonstrated that self-harm risk doubles after burn injury, underscoring the potential role for screening for mental health disorders during burn follow-up.

The use of administrative data also allows creation of unique study design that would be very difficult in clinical studies. An example of this is evaluation of parents of pediatric burn survivors [57]. Using administrative data, it is possible to create a cohort of injured children, a cohort of controls (uninjured children), identify the parents from each cohort, and evaluate the mental health not only post child's injury, but also prior, thereby establishing if the rate of change in mental health caused by the injury is different from the control population. The obstacles in conducting this study, from identification of participants, consenting, dropout, and recollection bias would be insurmountable.

5.7 Conclusion

The studies discussed above offer only a small glimpse into the burn research possibilities afforded by the use of population-based datasets. As the focus of burn research shifts towards the measurement, evaluation, and improvement of long-term outcomes, both physical and psychological, population-based research will become an invaluable source of long-term outcome data for the burn investigator. The linkage of clinical databases, such as the NBR or other local registries, to population-based databases represents a powerful opportunity to study burn outcomes over both the short and long term, with the ability to generate comprehensive risk adjustment models, large sample sizes, long-term follow-up, and the ability to track and evaluate care provided both within and outside of burn centers. This knowledge will ultimately allow the creation of targeted interventions and care for individuals with burn injuries based on best evidence.

Summary Box

- Population-based research offers an opportunity to follow a large cohort of individuals over time and measure rates of healthcare utilization at the population level.
- This approach can be limited by a lack of clinical granularity in the data.
- Validation and linkage to other datasets can overcome these limitations.
- Many studies have successfully used a population-based approach to describe various outcomes after burn injury.

References

1. Lieb W, Vasan RS. Scientific contributions of population-based studies to cardiovascular epidemiology in the GWAS era. Front Cardiovasc Med. 2018;5:57. https://doi.org/10.3389/fcvm.2018.00057.
2. Gavrielov-Yusim N, Friger M. Use of administrative medical databases in population-based research. J Epidemiol Community Health. 2014;68:283–7. https://doi.org/10.1136/jech-2013-202744.
3. Szklo M. Population-based cohort studies. Epidemiol Rev. 1998;20:81–90.
4. Cadarette SM, Wong L. An introduction to health care administrative data. Can J Hosp Pharm. 2015;68:232–7.
5. ICES Report—2017. Prescribed Entity Review. 2017. https://www.ices.on.ca/~/media/Files/DataandPrivacy/ICES-Privacy-Report.ashx?la=en-CA.
6. ICES Data Dictionary. https://datadictionary.ices.on.ca/Applications/DataDictionary/Default.aspx. Accessed 24 Jul 2018.
7. Matheson FI, Dunn JR, Smith KLW, Moineddin R, Glazier RH. Canadian Marginalization Index (CAN-Marg) user guide version 1.0. Centre for Research on Inner City Health, St. Michael's Hospital; 2011.
8. American Burn Association. 2016 National Burn Repository: report of data from 2006-2015; 2016.
9. Martens P, Fransoo R, McKeen N, Burland E, Jebamani L, Burchill C, et al. Patterns of regional mental illness disorder diagnoses and service use in Manitoba: a population-based study. Winnipeg, MB: Manitoba Health; 2004.
10. Jutte DP, Brownell M, Roos NP, Schippers C, Boyce WT, Syme SL. Rethinking what is important: biologic versus social predictors of childhood health and educational outcomes. Epidemiology. 2010;21:314–23. https://doi.org/10.1097/EDE.0b013e3181d61e61.
11. Lix LM, Yogendran MS, Shaw SY, Burchill C, Metge C, Bond R. Population-based data sources for chronic disease surveillance. Chronic Dis Can. 2008;29:31–8.
12. Mojtabai R, Olfson M, Mechanic D. Perceived need and help-seeking in adults with mood, anxiety, or substance use disorders. Arch Gen Psychiatry. 2002;59:77–84.
13. Logsetty S, Shamlou A, Gawaziuk JP, March J, Doupe M, Chateau D, et al. Mental health outcomes of burn: a longitudinal population-based study of adults hospitalized for burns. Burns. 2016;42:738–44. https://doi.org/10.1016/j.burns.2016.03.006.
14. Patterson DR, Ptacek JT, Cromes F, Fauerbach JA, Engrav L. The 2000 Clinical Research Award. Describing and predicting distress and satisfaction with life for burn survivors. J Burn Care Rehabil. 2000;21:490–8.
15. Pavoni V, Gianesello L, Paparella L, Buoninsegni LT, Barboni E. Outcome predictors and quality of life of severe burn patients admitted to intensive care unit. Scand J Trauma Resusc Emerg Med. 2010;18:24. https://doi.org/10.1186/1757-7241-18-24.
16. Anzarut A, Chen M, Shankowsky H, Tredget EE. Quality-of-life and outcome predictors following massive burn injury. Plast Reconstr Surg. 2005;116:791–7.
17. Tarnowski KJ. Behavioral aspects of pediatric burns. Berlin: Springer Science and Business Media, LLC; 1994.
18. Badger K, Royse D. Helping others heal: burn survivors and peer support. Soc Work Health Care. 2010;49:1–18. https://doi.org/10.1080/00981380903157963.
19. Suissa S. Immeasurable time bias in observational studies of drug effects on mortality. Am J Epidemiol. 2008;168:329–35. https://doi.org/10.1093/aje/kwn135.
20. Bewick V, Cheek L, Ball J. Statistics review 12: survival analysis. Crit Care. 2004;8:389. https://doi.org/10.1186/cc2955.
21. Rosenbaum P. Observational studies. 2nd ed. New York: Springer; 2010.
22. Lix LM, Yogendren M, Burchill C, Metge C, McKeen N, Moore D, et al. Defining and validating chronic diseases: an administrative data approach. Winnipeg, MB: Manitoba Centre for Health Policy; 2006.
23. Tricco AC, Pham B, Rawson NSB. Manitoba and Saskatchewan administrative health care utilization databases are used differently to answer epidemiologic research questions. J Clin Epidemiol. 2008;61:192–7. https://doi.org/10.1016/j.jclinepi.2007.03.009.
24. Roos LL, Gupta S, Soodeen R-A, Jebamani L. Data quality in an information-rich environment: Canada as an example. Can J Aging. 2005;24(Suppl 1):153–70. https://doi.org/10.1353/cja.2005.0055.
25. Roos LL, Brownell M, Lix L, Roos NP, Walld R, MacWilliam L. From health research to social research: privacy, methods, approaches. Soc Sci Med. 2008;66:117–29. https://doi.org/10.1016/j.socscimed.2007.08.017.
26. Roos LL, Mustard CA, Nicol JP, McLerran DF, Malenka DJ, Young TK, et al. Registries and administrative data: organization and accuracy. Med Care. 1993;31:201–12.
27. Vittinghoff E, Glidden D, Shiboski S, McCulloch C. Regression methods in biostatistics: linear, logistic, survival and repeated measures models. New York: Springer US; 2005.
28. Twisk JWR. Longitudinal data analysis. A comparison between generalized estimating equations and random coefficient analysis. Eur J Epidemiol. 2004;19:769–76.
29. Zeger SL, Liang KY, Albert PS. Models for longitudinal data: a generalized estimating equation approach. Biometrics. 1988;44:1049–60.
30. Zeger SL, Liang KY. Longitudinal data analysis for discrete and continuous outcomes. Biometrics. 1986;42:121–30.
31. Hanley JA, Negassa A, Edwardes MD dB, Forrester JE. Statistical analysis of correlated data using generalized estimating equations: an orientation. Am J Epidemiol. 2003;157:364–75.
32. Liu J, Pei Y, Papasian CJ, Deng H-W. Bivariate association analyses for the mixture of continuous and binary traits with the use of extended generalized estimating equations. Genet Epidemiol. 2009;33:217–27. https://doi.org/10.1002/gepi.20372.
33. The CIHI Data Quality Framework. https://www.cihi.ca/en/data_quality_framework_2009_en.pdf.
34. CIHI Data Quality Study of the 2009-2010 Discharge Abstract Database. 2012. https://secure.cihi.ca/estore/productFamily.htm?pf=PFC1578&lang=fr&media=0.
35. Benchimol EI, Guttmann A, Mack DR, Nguyen GC, Marshall JK, Gregor JC, et al. Validation of international algorithms to identify adults with inflammatory bowel disease in health administrative data from Ontario, Canada. J Clin Epidemiol. 2014;67:887–96.

36. Gershon AS, Wang C, Guan J, Vasilevska-Ristovska J, Cicutto L, To T. Identifying individuals with physcian diagnosed COPD in health administrative databases. COPD. 2009;6:388–94.
37. Kothari R, Barsan W, Brott T, Broderick J, Ashbrock S. Frequency and accuracy of prehospital diagnosis of acute stroke. Stroke. 1995;26:937–41.
38. Welk B, Loh E, Shariff SZ, Liu K, Siddiqi F. An administrative data algorithm to identify traumatic spinal cord injured patients: a validation study. Spinal Cord. 2014;52:34–8.
39. Benchimol EI, Manuel DG, To T, Griffiths AM, Rabeneck L, Guttmann A. Development and use of reporting guidelines for assessing the quality of validation studies of health administrative data. J Clin Epidemiol. 2011;64:821–9. https://doi.org/10.1016/j.jclinepi.2010.10.006.
40. Mason SA, Nathens AB, Byrne JP, Fowler R, Gonzalez A, Karanicolas PJ, et al. The accuracy of burn diagnosis codes in health administrative data: a validation study. Burns. 2017;43:258–64. https://doi.org/10.1016/j.burns.2016.11.008.
41. Duke J, Wood F, Semmens J, Spilsbury K, Edgar DW, Hendrie D, et al. A 26-year population-based study of burn injury hospital admissions in Western Australia. J Burn Care Res. 2011;32:379–86. https://doi.org/10.1097/BCR.0b013e318219d16c.
42. Duke JM, Rea S, Boyd JH, Randall SM, Wood FM. Mortality after burn injury in children: a 33-year population-based study. Pediatrics. 2015;135:e903.
43. Duke JM, Boyd JH, Rea S, Randall SM, Wood FM. Long-term mortality among older adults with burn injury: a population-based study in Australia. Bull World Health Organ. 2015;93:400–6. https://doi.org/10.2471/BLT.14.149146.
44. Duke JM, Boyd JH, Randall SM, Wood FM. Long term mortality in a population-based cohort of adolescents, and young and middle-aged adults with burn injury in Western Australia: a 33-year study. Accid Anal Prev. 2015;85:118–24. https://doi.org/10.1016/j.aap.2015.09.011.
45. Duke JM, Randall SM, Fear MW, Boyd JH, Rea S, Wood FM. Understanding the long-term impacts of burn on the cardiovascular system. Burns. 2016;42:366–74. https://doi.org/10.1016/j.burns.2015.08.020.
46. Stevenson AW, Randall SM, Boyd JH, Wood FM, Fear MW, Duke JM. Burn leads to long-term elevated admissions to hospital for gastrointestinal disease in a west Australian population based study. Burns. 2016;43:665. https://doi.org/10.1016/j.burns.2016.09.009.
47. Vetrichevvel TP, Randall SM, Fear MW, Wood FM, Boyd JH, Duke JM. Burn injury and long-term nervous system morbidity: a population-based cohort study. BMJ Open. 2016;6:e012668. https://doi.org/10.1136/bmjopen-2016-012668.
48. Duke JM, Randall SM, Fear MW, Boyd JH, O'Halloran E, Rea S, et al. Increased admissions for diabetes mellitus after burn. Burns. 2016;42:1734–9. https://doi.org/10.1016/j.burns.2016.06.005.
49. Duke JM, Randall SM, Wood FM, Boyd JH, Fear MW. Burns and long-term infectious disease morbidity: a population-based study. Burns. 2017;43:273–81. https://doi.org/10.1016/j.burns.2016.10.020.
50. Chen S-H, Chen Y-C, Chen T-J, Ma H. Epidemiology of burns in Taiwan: a nationwide report including inpatients and outpatients. Burns. 2014;40:1397–405. https://doi.org/10.1016/j.burns.2014.01.014.
51. Chung S-D, Chen C-S, Lin H-C, Kang J-H. Increased risk for stroke in burn patients: a population-based one-year follow-up study. Burns. 2014;40:54–60. https://doi.org/10.1016/j.burns.2013.05.018.
52. Hung T-Y, Lee Y-K, Huang M-Y, Hsu C-Y, Su Y-C. Increased risk of ischemic stroke in patients with burn injury: a nationwide cohort study in Taiwan. Scand J Trauma Resusc Emerg Med. 2016;24:44. https://doi.org/10.1186/s13049-016-0236-1.
53. Chen C, Huang C-Y, Wang H-J, Chen C-I, Lin H-W. Stroke after burn: population data analysis. Burns. 2014;40:230–4. https://doi.org/10.1016/j.burns.2013.10.002.
54. Mason S, Nathens A, Byrne J, Gonzalez A, Fowler R, Karanicolas P, et al. Trends in the epidemiology of major burn injury among hospitalized patients: a population-based analysis. J Trauma Acute Care Surg. 2017;43:258–64.
55. Mason SA, Nathens AB, Byrne JP, Fowler RA, Karanicolas PJ, Moineddin R, et al. Burn center care reduces acute health care utilization after discharge: a population-based analysis of 1,895 survivors of major burn injury. Surgery. 2017;162:891. https://doi.org/10.1016/j.surg.2017.05.018.
56. Mason SA, Nathens AB, Byrne JP, Ellis J, Fowler RA, Gonzalez A, et al. Association between burn injury and mental illness among burn survivors: a population-based, self-matched, longitudinal cohort study. J Am Coll Surg. 2017;225:516. https://doi.org/10.1016/j.jamcollsurg.2017.06.004.
57. Enns J, Gawaziuk JP, Khan S, Chateau D, Bolton JM, Sareen J, et al. Mental and physical health outcomes in parents of children with burn injuries as compared with matched controls. J Burn Care Res. 2016;37:e18–26. https://doi.org/10.1097/BCR.0000000000000309.

6 Education in Burns

Sebastian Q. Vrouwe and Shahriar Shahrokhi

6.1 Introduction

Education and team building in burn care can be broken down into three main components: surgical education, mentorship, and interprofessional education. This brief chapter will highlight these in order to provide a framework for current trends and the future of education in this field. These ideas are not novel and they have been successfully implemented in other fields. Our goal is to harness this knowledge for implementation in burn care, thus not only improving education, but also enabling recruitment and retention of health care providers in this field.

6.2 Surgical Education

6.2.1 Background

Historically, the traditional method of educating a resident in the practice of surgery has been centered on the hospital-based, apprenticeship model, initially described by William Halsted over 100 years ago [1]. Skill acquisition has been reliant on observation, assisting and subsequently performing the task [2]. This is what many trainees have come to understand as the classic "see one, do one, teach one" mentality. Within this template, residents learn principles and gain experience while caring for real patients, and are given increasing amounts of responsibility to prepare them to practice independently. The skills and knowledge acquired during their training is contingent on exposure to the disease conditions and procedures encountered by their faculty, rather than curricular needs [3]. Given the varied patient population and practice patterns of each program, experience-based training in surgery does not ensure standardization of skills [4].

Scrutiny of the conventional framework has caused a significant "paradigm shift" towards a more objective standardized approach to education. The progression of technology in surgery, demand for improving patient safety and decreasing medical errors has created a need for innovation in surgical education [5]. Attendance by way of case logs insufficiently comments on surgical competence [6]. A long-term study by Drake et al. demonstrated that while operative volumes have rebounded following the introduction of work hour restrictions, the diversity of operative experience has narrowed with changing disease processes, technological advancement, subspecialization, and reductions in trainee autonomy [7]. The shifting dynamics of surgical education are both challenging and exciting for trainees and educators alike, as it provides the foundation to alter the future of this craft.

6.2.2 Competency-Based Medical Education

Over the past decade, there has been a paradigm shift towards the model of competency-based medical education (CBME), defined by the International CBME Collaborators as "an outcomes-based approach to the design, implementation, assessment, and evaluation of medical education programs, using an organizing framework of competencies" [8]. Their rationale for CBME has been summarized into four themes: (1) focusing on outcomes, (2) emphasizing abilities, (3) de-emphasizing time-based training, and (4) promoting greater learner-centeredness.

The Accreditation Council for Graduate Medical Education (ACGME) and Royal College of Physicians and Surgeons of Canada (RCPSC) are currently in the process of

S. Q. Vrouwe
Division of Plastic and Reconstructive Surgery, University of Toronto, Toronto, ON, Canada
e-mail: sebastian.vrouwe@med.usc.edu

S. Shahrokhi (✉)
Division of Plastic and Reconstructive Surgery, University of Toronto, Toronto, ON, Canada

Ross Tilley Burn Centre, Sunnybrook Health Sciences Centre, Toronto, ON, Canada
e-mail: shar.shahrokhi@sunnybrook.ca

M. G. Jeschke et al. (eds.), *Handbook of Burns Volume 1*, https://doi.org/10.1007/978-3-030-18940-2_6

implementing CBME in residency programs. The ACGME began phased implementation of the *Next Accreditation System* in 2013, in which milestones are developed within each specialty that will provide data on performance that graduates must achieve before entering unsupervised practice [9]. Similarly, the RCPSC officially initiated *Competence by Design* in 2017, which will be introduced in seven cohorts, extended to all specialties by 2022 [10].

Moving forward there are tremendous opportunities for innovation in surgical education, and specialists in burn care must collaborate to develop and clarify the competencies relevant to our field. The initial process of defining core competencies related to burn care began with the ACGME Milestone Projects for plastic surgery and general surgery [11, 12]. For establishing a CBME curriculum in plastic surgery, Knox et al. describes the following: identifying important principles and procedures, modeling new teaching strategies, and developing assessment models [13]. This framework gives a structured and systematic approach to curriculum development and is currently being implemented for burn unit rotations.

6.2.3 Simulation

The learning curve associated with new procedures carries inherent patient morbidity, as they require a level of technical skill and confidence normally gained through practice [14]. For example, the donor site morbidity of an improperly harvested split thickness skin graft is significant, especially if a second site is eventually required. Simulators are an objective and reproducible medium that can allow technology to facilitate the transition from beginner to expert, while standardizing education, decreasing costs, reducing patient risk, and improving outcomes [4]. The efficacy of simulators has been reported in the literature [14, 15], and their widespread application is seen in general surgery [16], plastic surgery [17], urology [18], neurosurgery [19], gynecology [20], and endoscopy [21]. Increasing prevalence of simulation in medical training has prompted the Accreditation Council for Graduate Medical Education (ACGME) and the American College of Surgeons (ACS), to implement a phased approach to formally require their use in surgical education.

The advent of simulators has forged a new era of excellence in surgery. The low-stress environment alleviates the anxiety of the operating room and enhances trainee learning, while allowing for mistakes and improvement without compromising patient care. The skills gained in this practical learning atmosphere have been proven to enrich performance in live operative models and therefore can be transferable to the operating room [22]. The concept, "physical and mental skills are learned through a long process of persistent and dedicated efforts with repetition to reinforce the activity" [2], is fundamental to the development of a successful surgeon. Fitts and Posner described the three stages of skill acquisition in 1967. The student must first intellectualize the process, second develop the proper motor behavior, and third subsequently repeat the skill, resulting in smooth performance through muscle memory [23]. The notion of "practice before the game" holds true for musicians and athletes, and similarly, simulation has been shown to be effective in surgical motor skill acquisition [24].

Several simulation tools relevant to burn training have been recently described in the literature. Sadideen et al. devised "The Burns Suite," a self-contained immersive simulation environment which guides trainees through a pediatric burn resuscitation [25]. Advantages of this learning tool include its low-cost and portability, as well as high face and content validity as judged by participants. Ur et al. developed and tested a biomimetic escharotomy trainer with discreet points of failure built in; their pilot study found that the model was considered realistic by participants and increased comfort levels in junior trainees [26]. Lastly, Gallagher et al. described and tested a simulator for tangential excision using a foam suture pad in novice, intermediate and expert subjects, who were prospectively assessed by blinded observers using an objective rating scale; all experts agreed that this tool would be useful prior to clinical performance of tangential excision [27].

Time is the key challenge faced by most programs establishing a skills lab. Trainee workload and responsibility is demanding and often prohibits dedication to practice. Similarly, the commitments of academic faculty limit their time to supervise and provide necessary feedback. For a skills curriculum to achieve optimal results, sufficient time allocation is imperative. Simulation training is a pivotal tool in surgical education, which should be adopted into the armamentarium of any residency program.

6.2.4 Education in the Internet Era

The widespread availability of online materials has permitted the shift of education away from the operating room. The issues of time constraints, patient safety, and geographical limitations have been greatly attenuated with the initiation of web-based learning. The Internet has also facilitated the development of global collaboration of medical education [5].

Currently, e-learning has been successfully integrated into surgical programs for instruction in areas including anatomy [28], course curriculum [29], procedural skills [30], and problem-based learning [31]. There are endless implementation strategies to supplement training. Individual programs can dictate the published content they wish to provide, ranging from links to journal articles and seminars, to modules and videos [5]. Online simulators are also becoming ubiquitous, creating a reusable, accurate, and self-directed model for the accession of knowledge and skills.

6.3 Mentorship

Mentoring relationships have been well established as an essential element for achieving growth and success in business, politics, and academia [32]. Within the health care system, although mentorship has clearly had a positive impact in nursing [33, 34], the literature in surgical training is limited. It is designed to provide support, encouragement, and professional vision [35], and has been described as crucial in surgical training [36] and influential in career path selection [37]. Faculty members who were mentored have more confidence, more productive research endeavors and greater career satisfaction [38–40], while a lack of mentoring is considered an important factor hindering career progress in academic medicine [41].

6.3.1 Peer Mentorship

Peer mentoring is defined as a relationship in which mentors and mentees are similar in professional status and they help each other and themselves through teaching and collaborative learning [42]. This model provides support in a non-evaluative environment [43], while promoting collegiality and a nurturing climate for personal and vocational growth [34]. It has been successfully applied in nursing, resulting in a less stressful and more comfortable environment [44, 45]. Students report increased self-confidence and social integration, mitigating much of the initial anxiety associated with a new rotation [34]. Mentors enjoy the satisfaction of service while honing their interpersonal and communication skills [46].

6.3.2 Hierarchical Mentorship

The classical model of mentorship involves a pupil learning skills and knowledge from a preceptor or established expert in the field. This allows for the transference of experience from one generation to the next. In addition to the obvious advantages to the trainee, hierarchical mentoring encompasses many benefits for the staff. Mentors develop a sense of pride and privilege in fulfilling their role of shaping the successors of their field. Medicine involves the pursuit of lifelong learning, and mentorship programs give the "lions" a chance to learn from the "cubs" in order to retool themselves in this progressively changing environment. This mutually beneficial relationship has also been shown to increase faculty retention [47].

6.3.3 What Is a Mentor?

A mentor is a trusted educator whose role extends far beyond the teaching of technical skills and clinical judgment in the clinics, operating room, and on the wards. They are role models who provide direction and instill values, while demonstrating effective communication, time management, and successful prioritization of multiple personal and professional commitments [48]. The relationship is dynamic and adapts over time to meet the needs of the mentee [49]. Although support is the primary principle, mentees need to be challenged and given both positive and negative feedback to enable professional development [50]. Successful execution of this role requires many important qualities that a mentor must possess. Competence, confidence, and commitment are three essential attributes vital to knowledgeable mentors who are respected in their field [51].

The ingredients that produce an outstanding mentor are rarely innate. "Mentorship has been a casually acquired trait with varying levels of success, but it is clear that the face of medicine and surgical training in the twenty-first century requires deliberate cultivation of mentors" [48]. It would be beneficial to implement staff development programs, highlighting effective mentoring skills and mentor responsibilities [47].

6.3.4 Implementation

Although informal mentoring occurs in the daily interactions with more senior surgeons, formal mentorship programs increase satisfaction and efficacy [36]. The success of the mentor relationship is significantly higher when mentees select their own mentors [36, 52]. Role preparation of both sides ensures a smooth introduction, as mentors need training, and mentees need objectives and reasonable expectations [33]. As with any new relationship, adequate meeting time is compulsory for the development of a trusting and fruitful alliance.

Mentorship primarily occurs because mentors consider it a rewarding feature of their profession. Increasing demands on faculty time and the current criteria for academic advancement have seriously threatened the future of mentorship. Scholarship over citizenship is currently the gauge for promotion in surgery; thus, mentoring descends to a lower priority being largely uncompensated and undervalued [38]. There is a need for novel ideas to enhance faculty participation in this cornerstone of surgical training. Institutional recognition and appreciation of mentors and publicly rewarding mentorship excellence will increase the prestige of the activity and faculty enrollment. Mentorship can also be adapted into the faculty evaluation process for promotion [38].

"Mentoring is a vital cog in the machinery of medical education" [50] and should be strongly considered in burn unit curricula.

6.4 Interprofessional Education

In medicine, physicians are largely educated in isolation of other health professionals, resulting in limited collaboration, communication, and coordination of care [53]. Many surgeons have been educated in a culture that places value on individual accomplishments; however, the importance of teamwork in medicine is becoming increasingly evident in the delivery of quality care and reduction of medical errors [54–59]. In complex care settings like burn units, a single health care professional is not equipped to handle the diversity of their patients' needs [60]. A strong, coherent team approach in a burn unit reduces mortality, shortens length of stay, and improves rehabilitation [61]. The relationship with other health care professionals has become an emphasis of modern surgical professionalism [62].

6.4.1 What Is Interprofessional Education?

Health Canada defines interprofessional education (IPE) as "socializing health care providers in working together, in shared problem solving and decision making, towards enhancing the benefits for patients; developing mutual understanding of, and respect for, the contributions of various disciplines; and instilling the requisite competencies for collaborative practice." The Centre for the Advancement of Interprofessional Education (CAIPE) similarly refers to IPE as instances when "two or more professions learn from and about each other to improve collaboration and the quality of care" [63]. IPE is a unique approach to learning, where knowledge is attained through social collaboration with other professions, and the learning process is equally as important as the content itself [53]. It improves the understanding of team member complementary skills and increases mutual accountability. The contact between professions is insufficient to build the communication, respect, and trust necessary for effective team performance [64]. Learning "as" a team, rather than simply "in" a team, enhances the collective capability [65].

6.4.2 Approaches to Interprofessional Education

There are numerous models to engage the members of the burn unit in interactive learning. These health professionals include students, surgical trainees at various levels of experience, occupational therapists, physiotherapists, social workers, nurses, respiratory therapists, dieticians, intensivists, surgeons, and any other specialists that are involved in the complex care of these patients. Exchange-based learning can be achieved through seminars, workshop discussions, and case study sessions, where members of the team can explore the realms of each other's roles in the setting of collaborative care [66]. Problem-based learning is an effective example of the action-based educational approach, as the team is actively involved in working together to determine the most suitable course of action. Simulation not only has educational merit in technical skill acquisition, it is also useful in the teaching of IPE when feedback is given in small instructor led groups simulating a real situation [67]. The growth of online resources has allowed asynchronous communication to overcome collaborative time scheduling and geographic constraints, while permitting practicing health care workers to learn together [68–72]. This model has been shown to be effective in teaching IPE [73].

Student feedback reveals that interprofessional education, through learning outside one's disciplinary boundaries, forges mutual respect [74, 75]. Interprofessional education provides the tools necessary to reduce the gaps in current practices by forming a profound comprehension of the patient care team.

6.5 Conclusions

This chapter has highlighted some of the current concepts in medical education relevant to burn care. While the foundations of surgical education were developed over a century ago by Halstead, novel ideas such as simulation, CBME, and e-learning continue to revolutionize the process of training the next generation of surgeons. Mentorship is an important component of surgical education, and strong mentors will pave the way for the next generation of burn care providers. Lastly, the multidisciplinary nature of burn care provides the ideal setting to promote and develop interprofessional education and can serve as a model for other complex patient populations.

Summary Box

- The training of surgeons is rapidly changing with the advent of simulation, competency-based medical education, and e-learning.
- Effective mentorship is required to train the next generation of burn care providers.
- The nature of the burn care team provides a model of quality interprofessional education.

References

1. Halstead W. The training of the surgeon. Bull Johns Hopkins Hosp. 1904;15:267–75.
2. Buscarini M, Stein JP. Training the urologic oncologist of the future: where are the challenges? Urol Oncol. 2009;27:193–8.
3. Sachdeva AK, Bell RH, Britt LD, Tarpley JL, Blair PG, Tarpley MJ. National efforts to reform residency education in surgery. Acad Med. 2007;82:1200–10.
4. Rosen JM, Long SA, McGrath DM, Greer SE. Simulation in plastic surgery training and education: the path forward. Plast Reconstr Surg. 2009;123:729–38.
5. Pugh CM, Watson A, Bell RH, Brasel KJ, Jackson GP, Weber SM, Kao LS. Surgical education in the internet era. J Surg Res. 2009;156:177–82.
6. Bell RH, Biester TW, Tabuenca A, Rhodes RS, Cofer JB, Britt LD, Lewis FR. Operative experience of residents in US general surgery programs: a gap between expectation and experience. Ann Surg. 2009;249:719–24.
7. Drake FT, Aarabi S, Garland BT, Huntington CR, McAteer JP, Richards MK, Zern NK, Gow KW. Accreditation Council for Graduate Medical Education (ACGME) Surgery Resident Operative Logs: the last quarter century. Ann Surg. 2017;265:923–9.
8. Frank JR, Snell LS, Ten CO, Holmboe ES, Carraccio C, Swing SR, Harris P, Glasgow NJ, Campbell C, Dath D, Harden RM, Iobst W, Long DM, Mungroo R, Richardson DL, Sherbino J, Silver I, Taber S, Talbot M, Harris KA. Competency-based medical education: theory to practice. Med Teach. 2010;32:638–45.
9. Nasca TJ, Philibert I, Brigham T, Flynn TC. The next GME accreditation system—rationale and benefits. N Engl J Med. 2012;366:1051–6.
10. Royal College of Physicians and Surgeons of Canada. Competence by design. 2017. http://www.royalcollege.ca/rcsite/cbd/competence-by-design-cbd-e.
11. Accreditation Council for Graduate Medical Education. The Plastic Surgery Milestone Project. 2015. http://www.acgme.org/Portals/0/PDFs/Milestones/PlasticSurgeryMilestones.pdf.
12. Accreditation Council for Graduate Medical Education. The Surgical Critical Care Milestone Project. 2015. http://www.acgme.org/Portals/0/PDFs/Milestones/SurgicalCriticalCareMilestones.pdf.
13. Knox ADC, Gilardino MS, Kasten SJ, Warren RJ, Anastakis DJ. Competency-based medical education for plastic surgery: where do we begin? Plast Reconstr Surg. 2014;133:702e–10e.
14. Fernandez GL, Page DW, Coe NP, Lee PC, Patterson LA, Skylizard L, St Louis M, Amaral MH, Wait RB, Seymour NE. Boot cAMP: educational outcomes after 4 successive years of preparatory simulation-based training at onset of internship. J Surg Educ. 2012;69:242–8.
15. Chipman JG, Schmitz CC. Using objective structured assessment of technical skills to evaluate a basic skills simulation curriculum for first-year surgical residents. J Am Coll Surg. 2009;209:364–370.e2.
16. Davies J, Khatib M, Bello F. Open surgical simulation—a review. J Surg Educ. 2013;70:618–27.
17. Podolsky DJ, Fisher DM, Wong KW, Looi T, Drake JM, Forrest CR. Evaluation and implementation of a high-fidelity cleft palate simulator. Plast Reconstr Surg. 2017;139:85e–96e.
18. Aydin A, Shafi AMA, Shamim Khan M, Dasgupta P, Ahmed K. Current status of simulation and training models in urological surgery: a systematic review. J Urol. 2016;196:312–20.
19. Kirkman MA, Ahmed M, Albert AF, Wilson MH, Nandi D, Sevdalis N. The use of simulation in neurosurgical education and training. A systematic review. J Neurosurg. 2014;121:228–46.
20. Kim-Fine S, Brennand EA. Surgical simulation and competency. Obstet Gynecol Clin North Am. 2016;43:575–90.
21. King N, Kunac A, Merchant AM. A review of endoscopic simulation: current evidence on simulators and curricula. J Surg Educ. 2016;73:12–23.
22. Gardner AK, Nepomnayshy D, Reickert C, Gee DW, Brydges R, Korndorffer JR, Scott DJ, Sachdeva AK. The value proposition of simulation. Surgery. 2016;160:546–51.
23. Fitts P, Posner M. Human performance. Belmont, CA: Cole; 1967.
24. Boehler ML, Schwind CJ, Rogers DA, Ketchum J, O'Sullivan E, Mayforth R, Quin J, Wohltman C, Johnson C, Williams RG, Dunnington G. A theory-based curriculum for enhancing surgical skillfulness. J Am Coll Surg. 2007;205:492–7.
25. Sadideen H, Wilson D, Moiemen N, Kneebone R. Proposing "the burns suite" as a novel simulation tool for advancing the delivery of burns education. J Burn Care Res. 2014;35:62–71.
26. Ur R, Holmes JH, Johnson JE, Molnar JA, Carter JE. Development of a burn escharotomy assessment tool: a pilot study. J Burn Care Res. 2016;37:e140–4.
27. Gallagher JJ, Goldin IM, O'Sullivan GM, Silverman EL, Mitchell KB, Yurt RW. Simulation of tangential excision: a test for construct validity. J Burn Care Res. 2015;36:558–64.
28. Choi A-RA, Tamblyn R, Stringer MD. Electronic resources for surgical anatomy. ANZ J Surg. 2008;78:1082–91.
29. Kalet AL, Coady SH, Hopkins MA, Hochberg MS, Riles TS. Preliminary evaluation of the Web Initiative for Surgical Education (WISE-MD). Am J Surg. 2007;194:89–93.
30. Chenkin J, Lee S, Huynh T, Bandiera G. Procedures can be learned on the web: a randomized study of ultrasound-guided vascular access training. Acad Emerg Med. 2008;15:949–54.
31. Corrigan M, Reardon M, Shields C, Redmond H. "SURGENT"—student e-learning for reality: the application of interactive visual images to problem-based learning in undergraduate surgery. J Surg Educ. 2008;65:120–5.
32. Roch GR. Much ado about mentors. Harv Bus Rev. 1979;57:14–20.
33. Sprengel AD, Job L. Reducing student anxiety by using clinical peer mentoring with beginning nursing students. Nurse Educ. 2004;29:246–50.
34. Sweet S, Fusner S. Social integration of the advanced placement LPN: a peer mentoring program. Nurse Educ. 2008;33:202–5.
35. Gilmour JA, Kopeikin A, Douché J. Student nurses as peer-mentors: collegiality in practice. Nurse Educ Pract. 2007;7:36–43.
36. Flint JH, Jahangir AA, Browner BD, Mehta S. The value of mentorship in orthopaedic surgery resident education: the residents' perspective. J Bone Joint Surg Am. 2009;91:1017–22.
37. McCord JH, McDonald R, Leverson G, Mahvi DM, Rikkers LF, Chen HC, Weber SM. Motivation to pursue surgical subspecialty training: is there a gender difference? J Am Coll Surg. 2007;205:698–703.
38. Levy BD, Katz JT, Wolf MA, Sillman JS, Handin RI, Dzau VJ. An initiative in mentoring to promote residents' and faculty members' careers. Acad Med. 2004;79:845–50.
39. Palepu A, Friedman RH, Barnett RC, Carr PL, Ash AS, Szalacha L, Moskowitz MA. Junior faculty members' mentoring relationships and their professional development in U.S. medical schools. Acad Med. 1998;73:318–23.
40. Ramanan RA, Phillips RS, Davis RB, Silen W, Reede JY. Mentoring in medicine: keys to satisfaction. Am J Med. 2002;112:336–41.
41. Jackson VA, Palepu A, Szalacha L, Caswell C, Carr PL, Inui T. "Having the right chemistry": a qualitative study of mentoring in academic medicine. Acad Med. 2003;78:328–34.
42. Topping KJ. The effectiveness of peer tutoring in further and higher education: a typology and review of the literature. High Educ. 1996;32:321–45.
43. Heinrich KT, Scherr MW. Peer mentoring for reflective teaching: a model for nurses who teach. Nurse Educ. 1994;19:36–41.

44. Becker MK, Neuwirth JM. Teaching strategy to maximize clinical experience with beginning nursing students. J Nurs Educ. 2002;41:89–91.
45. Sommer S. Active learning: cooperative, collaborative and peer learning. In: McKeachie W, Svinicki M, editors. Teaching tips: strategies, research, and theory for college and university teachers. Boston, MA: Houghton Mifflin Co.; 2006. p. 213–20.
46. Miller A. Mentoring students & young people: a handbook of effective practice. Sterling, VA: Stylus; 2002.
47. Benson CA, Morahan PS, Sachdeva AK, Richman RC. Effective faculty preceptoring and mentoring during reorganization of an academic medical center. Med Teach. 2002;24:550–7.
48. Möller MG, Karamichalis J, Chokshi N, Kaafarani H, Santry HP. Mentoring the modern surgeon. Bull Am Coll Surg. 2008;93:19–25.
49. Wensel TM. Mentor or preceptor: what is the difference? Am J Health Syst Pharm. 2006;63:1597.
50. Ramani S, Gruppen L, Kachur EK. Twelve tips for developing effective mentors. Med Teach. 2006;28:404–8.
51. Morton-Cooper A, Palmer A. Mentoring in practice. In: Morton-Cooper A, Palmer A, editors. Mentoring, preceptorship and clinical supervision. Malden, MA: Blackwell Science; 2000. p. 59–62.
52. Ford HR. Mentoring, diversity, and academic surgery. J Surg Res. 2004;118:1–8.
53. Sargeant J. Theories to aid understanding and implementation of interprofessional education. J Contin Educ Health Prof. 2009;29:178–84.
54. Campbell SM, Hann M, Hacker J, Burns C, Oliver D, Thapar A, Mead N, Safran DG, Roland MO. Identifying predictors of high quality care in English general practice: observational study. BMJ. 2001;323:784–7.
55. Morey JC, Simon R, Jay GD, Wears RL, Salisbury M, Dukes KA, Berns SD. Error reduction and performance improvement in the emergency department through formal teamwork training: evaluation results of the MedTeams project. Health Serv Res. 2002;37:1553–81.
56. Reeves S, Zwarenstein M, Goldman J, Barr H, Freeth D, Hammick M, Koppel I. Interprofessional education: effects on professional practice and health care outcomes. Cochrane Database Syst Rev. 2008;CD002213.
57. Risser DT, Rice MM, Salisbury ML, Simon R, Jay GD, Berns SD. The potential for improved teamwork to reduce medical errors in the emergency department. The MedTeams Research Consortium. Ann Emerg Med. 1999;34:373–83.
58. Stevenson K, Baker R, Farooqi A, Sorrie R, Khunti K. Features of primary health care teams associated with successful quality improvement of diabetes care: a qualitative study. Fam Pract. 2001;18:21–6.
59. Unützer J, Katon W, Callahan CM, Williams JW, Hunkeler E, Harpole L, Hoffing M, Della Penna RD, Noël PH, Lin EHB, Areán PA, Hegel MT, Tang L, Belin TR, Oishi S, Langston C, IMPACT Investigators, Improving Mood-Promoting Access to Collaborative Treatment. Collaborative care management of late-life depression in the primary care setting: a randomized controlled trial. JAMA. 2002;288:2836–45.
60. Al-Mousawi AM, Mecott-Rivera GA, Jeschke MG, Herndon DN. Burn teams and burn centers: the importance of a comprehensive team approach to burn care. Clin Plast Surg. 2009;36:547–54.
61. Gibran NS, Klein MB, Engrav LH, Heimbach DM. UW Burn Center. A model for regional delivery of burn care. Burns. 2005;31(Suppl 1):S36–9.
62. Kitto SC, Gruen RL, Smith JA. Imagining a continuing interprofessional education program (CIPE) within surgical training. J Contin Educ Health Prof. 2009;29:185–9.
63. Centre for the Advancement of Interprofessional Education (CAIPE). What is CAIPE? 2016. https://www.caipe.org/.
64. Sargeant J, Loney E, Murphy G. Effective interprofessional teams: "contact is not enough" to build a team. J Contin Educ Health Prof. 2008;28:228–34.
65. Barr H. An anatomy of continuing interprofessional education. J Contin Educ Health Prof. 2009;29:147–50.
66. Hammick M, Olckers L, Campion-Smith C. Learning in interprofessional teams: AMEE Guide no 38. Med Teach. 2009;31:1–12.
67. Issenberg SB, McGaghie WC, Petrusa ER, Lee Gordon D, Scalese RJ. Features and uses of high-fidelity medical simulations that lead to effective learning: a BEME systematic review. Med Teach. 2005;27:10–28.
68. Arias A, Bellman B. Networked collaborative research and teaching. In: Boschmann E, editor. The electronic classroom: a handbook for education in the electronic environment. Medford, NJ: Learned Information; 1995. p. 180–5.
69. Chen L, Gaines B. Modelling and supporting virtual cooperative interaction through the World Wide Web. In: Sudweeks F, McLaughlin M, Rafaeli S, editors. Networks and netplay: virtual groups on the Internet. Menlo Park, CA: AAAI; 1998. p. 221–42.
70. Harasim L, Hiltz S, Teles L, Turoff M. Learning networks: a field guide to teaching and learning online. Cambridge, MA: MIT; 1995.
71. Scardamalia M, Bereiter C. Computer support for knowledge-building communities. In: Koschmann T, editor. CSCL theory and practice of an emerging paradigm. Mahwah, NJ: L. Erlbaum Associates; 1996. p. 268–305.
72. Walsh K. Interprofessional education online: the BMJ Learning experience. J Interprof Care. 2007;21:691–3.
73. Luke R, Solomon P, Baptiste S, Hall P, Orchard C, Rukholm E, Carter L. Online interprofessional health sciences education: from theory to practice. J Contin Educ Health Prof. 2009;29:161–7.
74. Cooper H, Spencer-Dawe E, McLean E. Beginning the process of teamwork: design, implementation and evaluation of an inter-professional education intervention for first year undergraduate students. J Interprof Care. 2005;19:492–508.
75. Wilcock PM, Janes G, Chambers A. Health care improvement and continuing interprofessional education: continuing interprofessional development to improve patient outcomes. J Contin Educ Health Prof. 2009;29:84–90.

7 Burn Care Teams

Sarah Rehou and Marc G. Jeschke

7.1 Background

Teamwork is paramount in the delivery of healthcare. The burn care team, in particular, has always been an excellent model for a truly multidisciplinary and interdisciplinary team, as burn care providers must collaborate to maximize the success of patient care. The team is multidisciplinary because it utilizes the expertise of individuals from different disciplines but transcends to interdisciplinary by integrating the various approaches towards a shared goal. In a burn center, the set of goals is specific to the survival and quality of life of a burn patient.

7.1.1 Characteristics of an Effective Team

An effective burn team requires adequate team size, individuals with complementary backgrounds and skills, a balance of autonomy and authority, cohesion, open and inclusive, communication, and clearly defined measurable goals. This is essential for having the team being successful and working towards a common goal.

S. Rehou
Ross Tilley Burn Centre, Sunnybrook Health Sciences Centre, Sunnybrook Hospital, Toronto, ON, Canada

Sunnybrook Research Institute, Toronto, ON, Canada

M. G. Jeschke (✉)
Ross Tilley Burn Centre, Sunnybrook Health Sciences Centre, Sunnybrook Hospital, Toronto, ON, Canada

Faculty of Medicine, Institute of Medical Science, University of Toronto, Toronto, ON, Canada

Biological Sciences, Sunnybrook Research Institute, Toronto, ON, Canada

Division of Plastic and Reconstructive Surgery, Department of Surgery, Faculty of Medicine, University of Toronto, Toronto, ON, Canada

Department of Immunology, Faculty of Medicine, University of Toronto, Toronto, ON, Canada
e-mail: Marc.Jeschke@sunnybrook.ca

7.1.2 Burn Team Members

The special needs of burn patients are many and therefore the team has to be made out of multiple team players. There are numerous questions and issues that need to be addressed not only at hospital admission but also during hospitalization. These questions are contributors to burn patient outcomes and can only be addressed by a group of highly skilled healthcare professionals including burn surgeons, nurses, respiratory therapists, dietitians, physiotherapists, occupational therapists, social workers, pharmacists, speech-language pathologists, other support staff, and physicians such as physiatrists (rehabilitation physicians), psychiatrists, critical care physicians, anesthesiologists, and geriatric physicians.

7.1.3 Burn Surgeons

Historically, the attending surgeon was viewed as the "captain of the ship.". However, this rigid hierarchy in healthcare and, particularly in burns, has undergone a redesign to support team-based care. The burn surgeon is a general or plastic surgeon with expertise in critical care, operative, and reconstructive management of burn patients, complex wound patients, as well as Stevens-Johnson syndrome (SJS) and toxic epidermal necrolysis (TEN) or other complex dermatologic patients.

7.1.4 Nurses

Nurses make up the largest portion of the burn care team and are responsible for providing continuous care of the patient. Burn nurses possess unique skills to provide for not only the critical care requirements of each patient but also the important wound care needs. Due to the complex nature of burn injuries where patients can also be mechanically ventilated and receive renal support, nurses provide intensive physical care, administer medications, conduct dressing changes, maintain patient comfort, and communicate with patients

M. G. Jeschke et al. (eds.), *Handbook of Burns Volume 1*, https://doi.org/10.1007/978-3-030-18940-2_7

and families. Nursing acts as a liaison among the various multidisciplinary team members required to care for those with burn injuries ensuring a comprehensive holistic and supportive approach to care. Importantly, nurses are typically the first to observe any clinical changes in the patient and start any required intervention [1]. Therefore, nurses are central to the clinical course and assessment in clinical changes imperative for optimal patient outcomes. Care is provided using various assessments and critical thinking to identify slight changes in clinical condition.

7.1.5 Respiratory Therapists

Respiratory therapists are responsible for the management of the patient's airway including intubation and assisting in insertion, management, and weaning of the tracheostomy. They perform the institution, management, and discontinuing of ventilation with the use of arterial blood gas values. If required, they take patients on scans for the optimization of their care. Respiratory therapists give medication to help treat inhalation injuries and pulmonary disease. They participate during dressings with the team to ensure that the patients are breathing adequately and comfortably while being given sedation. We also perform indirect calorimetry to help optimize the patient nutritional status.

7.1.6 Dietitians

The registered dietitian's role in the burn unit is to monitor the dietary needs of the patients and provide nutritional recommendations and feeding regimens. Nutritional recommendations are adjusted to meet changing metabolic demands. The dietitian assesses multiple parameters including results of metabolic cart studies, laboratory markers in blood work, feeding tolerance, weight changes, and progression of wound healing and adjusts enteral feeds accordingly [2]. The dietitian is indispensable, especially for patients with pre-existing medical conditions, a complex social history associated with malnutrition, or a history of drug or alcohol misuse.

7.1.7 Occupational Therapists and Physiotherapists

Rehabilitation of the burn-injured patient is a continuum that commences from when the patient is admitted to hospital. The area and size of the burn and the patient's pre-existing comorbidities heavily influence the stages of rehabilitation. Therapists regularly assess the injury and progress of wound healing to implement treatment modalities in order to meet goals such as function, strength, and range of movement. Rehabilitation is essential to minimize the development of contractures and reduce scarring and can continue on an outpatient basis [3].

7.1.8 Physiatrists

The physiatrist has an important role in guidance and education around a patient's recovery, and short- and long-term functional goals. They work to increase both the patient's and family's understanding of the injury, medical management of burn-specific complications, and its impact on daily life. A vital part of the impact of burn injury includes quality of life, adjustment or coping skills, and managing changes in societal roles. Physiatrists also have a role in helping manage transitions of care from the acute care setting to discharge to rehabilitation, ambulatory, community, and return to work settings. As aforementioned, others and we suggest that it is important to have rehab team members attend to the patient even during acute hospitalization and not only when the patient left for rehab. Early integration of rehabilitation will improve outcomes and shorten length of stay.

7.1.9 Social Workers

The social worker is a crucial member of the burn center team who provides support and education for patients and families. The social worker conducts a comprehensive psycho-social assessment. Many aspects are included in the psycho-social assessment such as past medical history, including mental health, domestic violence and past trauma history, financial, employment, and housing considerations. Counseling is provided throughout hospitalization, discharge, and community reintegration phases to address practical needs and provide support to patients as they cope with the psychological and emotional issues that arise after injury including the risk of depression and PTSD. Social workers coordinate and advance an individualized discharge plan. The social worker also plays an important role in advance care planning and in end-of-life discussions.

7.1.10 Pharmacists

Pharmacists review and monitor all medications ordered for burn patients in hospital. They check to identify any allergies, drug interactions, and other potential safety concerns.

7.1.11 Physicians

Physicians from different specialties that are essential to the burn care team include anesthesiologists, critical care physicians, geriatric physicians, and psychiatrists. In addition to team members that are of different specialties, it is essential to have collaborations with other specialties, such as trauma, infectious disease, tissue bank, general surgery, internal medicine, and so on. When an issue occurs, these subspecialties are crucial to involve to help the patient to survive.

7.1.12 Students and Trainees

At teaching hospitals team members also include, students and trainees who are at burn centres for training and co-op palcements. Students come from a variety of professions and are integral to interprofessional teams.

7.1.13 Research Coordinator

The research coordinator's works under the direction of the principal investigator. The research coordinator facilitates, supports, and coordinates daily clinical trial activities. They work with the rest of the burn care team and the institutional review board or research ethics board to help ensure research activities are performed in accordance with any regulations.

7.2 Burn Centers and the Team

An aspect that has allowed burn care teams to flourish is of course burn centers or the dedication of units to burn patients. A joint program of the American Burn Association (ABA) and the American College of Surgeons (ACS) is Burn Center Verification. Achieving verification means that a burn center meets rigorous standards and indicates that the center provides high-quality patient care to burn patients [4].

Burn centers have led to the increased use of protocolized care and improved outcomes. The implementation of standardized protocols and guidelines for management during the resuscitation period and for complications like sepsis and pneumonia that can occur after burn injury are beneficial. Evidenced-based care is imperative for good patient outcomes and for a team to function because there is little margin for error in these critically ill patients.

Despite efforts to increase the quality of care through evidence-based medicine, medical errors still occur. A recent study estimated that deaths due to medical error surpassed respiratory disease as the third leading cause of death in the United States [5]. The Canadian Adverse Events Study found that of the approximately 2.5 million annual hospital admissions 7.5% of all patients suffered an adverse event because of healthcare management that resulted in death, disability, or a longer hospital stay [6]. While the cause of medical errors can be multifactorial, a common denominator relates to communication. Successful teams require effective communication, which is challenging. Part of the solution comes from quality improvement, engaging patient safety teams, documentation of performance, and setting goals for performance indicators. Quality improvement is most successful when executed by a multidisciplinary team.

7.3 Education

While each burn care provider completes their respective education and training, a vital aspect for a successful burn care team is education as a team. There are many different approaches to interprofessional learning like exchange-based learning (seminars, workshop discussions, and case studies), problem-based learning, and simulations [7]. Feedback from students showed that interprofessional education forged a mutual respect and a better understanding of the healthcare team [7]. Weekly education rounds should be attended by all members of the team and, importantly, taught by all members of the team.

7.4 Summary

In summary, a successful burn care team depends on various components; it needs to be open and inviting, dynamic, have a strong communication, trusting, and truly multidisciplinary. Only then the burn team can provide high-quality care for patients.

Summary Box

In summary, teamwork is paramount for the effective delivery of burn care. The team has to be multidisciplinary with every team member having an important impact and insight on patients care. It is in our opinion extremely crucial to build a safe and open environment for rounds and patients-related meetings, in fact to invite all team care providers to actively participate and contribute. As recently indicated by several studies, a certain aspect of continuity, as well as open invitations for contribution, are a key to achieve a better outcome.

References

1. Al-Mousawi AM, Mecott-Rivera GA, Jeschke MG, Herndon DN. Burn teams and burn centers: the importance of a comprehensive team approach to burn care. Clin Plast Surg. 2009;36(4):547–54.
2. Hall KL, Shahrokhi S, Jeschke MG. Enteral nutrition support in burn care: a review of current recommendations as instituted in the ross tilley burn centre. Nutrients. 2012;4(11):1554–65.
3. Procter F. Rehabilitation of the burn patient. Indian J Plastic Surg. 2010;43(Suppl):S101.
4. American Burn Association. Verification. http://ameriburn.org/quality-care/verification/. Published 2017. Updated 2018. Accessed 18 November.
5. Makary MA, Daniel M. Medical error-the third leading cause of death in the US. BMJ. 2016;353:i2139. https://doi.org/10.1136/bmj.i2139.
6. Baker GR, Norton PG, Flintoft V, et al. The Canadian adverse events study: the incidence of adverse events among hospital patients in Canada. CMAJ. 2004;170(11):1678–86.
7. Shahrokhi S, Jindal K, Jeschke MG. Three components of education in burn care: surgical education, inter-professional education, and mentorship. Burns. 2012;38(6):783–9.

Quality Improvement in Burn Care

8

Alan D. Rogers and Heinz Rode

8.1 Introduction

Few clinical sub-specialties require the kind of dedicated interdisciplinary involvement as burn surgery. There are countless opportunities for quality improvement (QI) interventions to optimize the care that is delivered for these patients at each stage. This chapter defines quality improvement and outlines its scope, introduces some of the various instruments and methods used for QI interventions, and highlights selected QI strategies as they pertain to burn care at the macro- and microsystem level. Principles and opportunities for benchmarking, verification and reporting are also included. The great challenge in relatively well-developed burn centres is to maintain a quality improvement focus in the execution of all activities, and to constantly evaluate how local practices can adapt to generalizable knowledge, while also advocating for prevention of burn injury and improvements in burn care in less developed settings.

8.2 The Scope of Quality Improvement and Patient Safety

Quality improvement is a proven, interdisciplinary approach to optimize the delivery of patient care, by continuously evaluating and testing how services are provided, and should be integral to the activities of all healthcare workers. The science of quality improvement has developed over the last two decades [1–4] and there is a growing appreciation for its role in evaluating the success or failures of complex interacting healthcare systems, the people who work within it, the variation in terms of outcomes resulting from the system, and how we make use of knowledge to affect these outcomes (Fig. 8.1).

Bailey described quality improvement as 'a broad range of activities of varying degrees of complexity and methodological and statistical rigour, through which healthcare providers develop, implement and assess small-scale interventions, identify those that work well, and implement them more broadly, in order to improve clinical practice' [5]. All stakeholders, including healthcare professionals, patients, their families, researchers, payers, planners, administrators and educators, may affect the changes that will lead to improved patient outcomes, better system performance and improved professional development [6].

Quality improvement may be applied in a macro-, meso- or microsystem, and can therefore be undertaken settings such as a small clinic, a unit, an operating room, an entire hospital, a group of hospitals, a university division or department, a provincial or national system, or even via an International organization.

The Institute of Medicine proposed a framework of six domains of healthcare quality. These have subsequently been expanded by Health Quality Ontario to incorporate nine attributes to describe a high-quality health system [7]. These include:

1. *Access*: Patients should have timely care at the appropriate setting by the appropriate healthcare provider.
2. *Efficacy*: Patients should receive healthcare that is evidence-based.
3. *Safety*: Patients should receive care that does not harm them.
4. *Patient-centric*: Care delivery should consider the preferences and values of individuals.

A. D. Rogers (✉)
Ross Tilley Burn Centre, Sunnybrook Health Sciences Centre, Toronto, ON, Canada

Division of Plastic and Reconstructive Surgery, Department of Surgery, University of Toronto, Toronto, ON, Canada
e-mail: alandavid.rogers@sunnybrook.ca

H. Rode
Red Cross War Memorial Children's Hospital, Rondebosch, Cape Town, South Africa

Division of Paediatric Surgery, University of Cape Town, Cape Town, South Africa
e-mail: Heinz.rode@uct.ac.za

M. G. Jeschke et al. (eds.), *Handbook of Burns Volume 1*, https://doi.org/10.1007/978-3-030-18940-2_8

Fig. 8.1 Resources, and how they are utilized within a system or process of care, influence outcomes

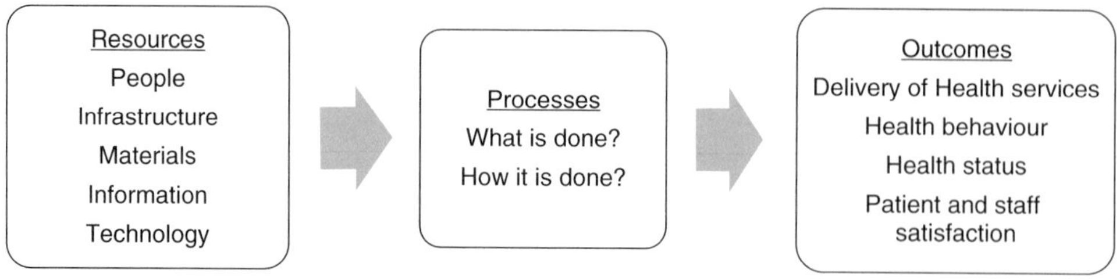

5. *Equity*: Care should be of a consistent standard irrespective of patient demographics, ethnicity, socioeconomic status, geographic origin, etc.
6. *Efficiency*: Healthcare should continuously evaluate its processes to reduce waste of resources, time and investment.
7. *Appropriately resourced*: The system should continuously evaluate its supply of providers, funding, information, equipment and facilities to meet its needs.
8. *Integrated*: Each component of the healthcare system should complement the others to optimize healthcare delivery.
9. *Promoting population health*: Healthcare systems should effectively treat and prevent illness and promote healthy lifestyles of all the people it serves.

Traditionally, most systems have placed the emphasis on safety and efficacy, while efficiency and equity are less frequently prioritized. Streamlined and reliable processes are less expensive to maintain than less efficient ones that might involve errors and rework. Quality improvement might aid an organization to avoid costs associated with failing processes, errors and sub-optimal outcomes. Quality improvement incorporates proactive processes that recognize problems before they occur, and is engaged in effective methods of reporting errors, addressing them if they do occur. Quality improvement involves the engagement of relevant stakeholders and as such, stimulates improvements in communication and might increase effective partnerships and funding opportunities [7].

To achieve a different level of performance, an organization's current system needs to change, but change per se does not necessarily result in improvement. A successful programme of quality improvement incorporates the following four key principles [7]:

1. Obtain a thorough understanding of the system or process.
2. Maintain the focus on patient care.
3. Encourage teamwork. Processes are frequently complex, involve more than one discipline or work area, and solutions often require creativity and sustainable staff engagement. Quality improvement will thus be facilitated because it is frequently multiple, iterative experiments of change. Although these teams may have often worked together in the past, QI initiatives often bring different teams together or encourage new approaches within stagnating teams.
4. Acquire and continuously evaluate reliable data. We must be able to distinguish between what is believed to be happening and what is actually happening, have reliable baseline and ongoing data, be able to monitor fidelity of the intervention, intervene if there are unintended consequences, and be able to demonstrate when change leads to an improvement. This will also ensure the sustainability of the intervention and allow translation to and comparison across sites.

Table 8.1 Prominent differences between Quality Improvement (QI) and traditional research

	Quality improvement	Traditional research
Primary goal	Improvement in local process or outcome	Generalizable knowledge
Cycle time	Rapid iterative tests of change	Longer data collection, definitive results
Context	Embraces context to allow for sustainability	Attempts to eliminate the impact of context; does not consider sustainability
Data analysis	Statistical control (Shewhart) and run charts; implicit; accept consistent bias	*T*-tests, *p*-values, chi-square and deviations; explicit; adjust for bias
Risk	Minimal risk. Ethics board review often not required; refer to ARECCI tool	May be some risk. Formal ethics board review required
Sample size	'Just enough' data	'Just in case' data
Examples of methods	Model for improvement, LEAN, Six Sigma	Randomized controlled trials, retrospective chart reviews
Hypothesis	Flexible	Fixed
Protocol	Adaptable; new tests of change	Strict adherence

Quality improvement interventions are quite distinct from traditional research (Table 8.1). Quality improvement involves the implementation of changes that are embraced by the members of the team who effect a change in a system or a practice. Not all changes are an improvement, but all improvements involve change. This change is usually based upon generalizable scientific knowledge. But translating this knowledge into action requires us to characterize the envi-

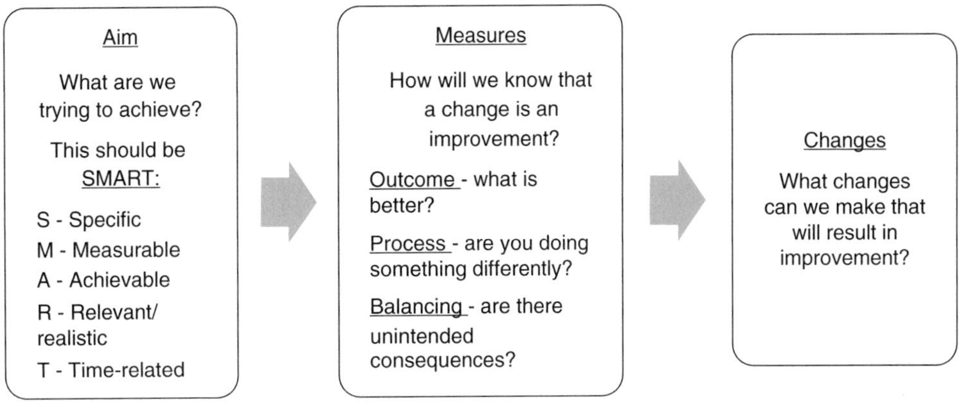

Fig. 8.2 The 'Model for Improvement' approach

ronments in which the care that we are delivering actually occurs. We require measurements of what is happening in the system prior to the intervention and once the intervention has been instituted. Quality improvement also gives us the ability to make iterative changes to the intervention, in real time, rather than waiting until the end of the intervention, as would be appropriate with a prospective trial, where a protocol would need to be followed, and research ethics board approval obtained.

In order for scientific knowledge to take hold, one needs to thoroughly understand the context in which it is being applied. If this context is variable, its effect may be difficult to understand. As a result, one needs to understand the traditions, culture, habits and processes of those who are likely to implement the intervention. Special forms of measurement are required to determine whether the intervention has been successful or that the change is in fact an improvement. For example, evidence-based interventions may be applied more or less effectively depending on the manner in which they are implemented. For example, standardization, education or forcing functions may be more appropriate in different contexts. The five knowledge systems involved in improvement, as proposed by Betaldien and Davidoff [6], include the available scientific evidence, context awareness, performance measurement, plans for change and execution of planned changes. QI is best implemented in an environment where its initiatives are supported by institutional leadership, is realistic given environmental and resource-related factors, and is well aligned with the organization's strategic objective. Quality improvement specialists have produced guidelines, referred to as the Squire guidelines, to assist in reporting initiatives in a scientific manner that is suitable for publication [4, 8].

In addition to reinforcing a change in culture, the science of QI provides tools to more effectively facilitate your efforts. Some of the structured improvement methods include the 'Model for Improvement', 'Six Sigma' and 'Lean'. Each of these methods offers evidence-based methods to achieve success in quality improvement. Each model reflects a common thread of analysis, implementation, and review, but focuses on different types of change concepts. There are two major quality improvement methodologies that specifically aim to evaluate processes. *Lean* methodology emphasizes the elimination of waste, and therefore the improvement of flow, by removing process steps that add little value, and improves the connections between these steps. *Six Sigma*, on the other hand, aims to improve quality by reducing variation. *Lean* is usually best applied to high-volume or frequent processes, while any process may be amenable to evaluation by *Six Sigma*. Both interventions are usually concluded within a few months. Lean is usually more ad hoc in nature, with minimal formal training required, while Six Sigma usually involves dedicated resources and broad-based training.

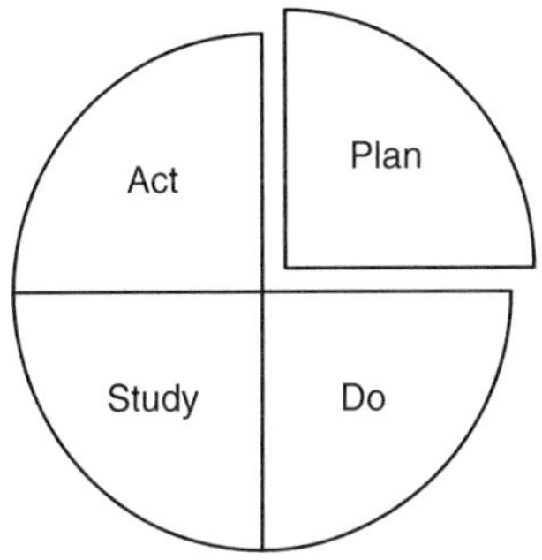

Fig. 8.3 PDSA Cycles. *Plan* a change; *Do* the test of change; *Study* the results; *Act* on the results

The *Model for Improvement* (Fig. 8.2) emphasizes distinct phases of identifying, defining and diagnosing a problem, before developing solutions and implementing interventions. This well-known testing model visually demonstrates incremental change through 'plan-do-study-act (PDSA)' cycles (Fig. 8.3). A family of measures, namely outcome, process and balancing measures, are required to comprehensively assess the intervention (Fig. 8.2) [7]. Examples of tools available to assist in the analysis of the identified problem/problems are tabulated (Table 8.2.).

Run charts and statistical process control charts are two methods of demonstrating results graphically. Run charts are

Table 8.2 Selected quality improvement tools to evaluate a system or process

Tool	Applications	Example
1. Fishbone/ Ishikawa diagram	Brainstorming strategy which assists to laying out all the possible causes	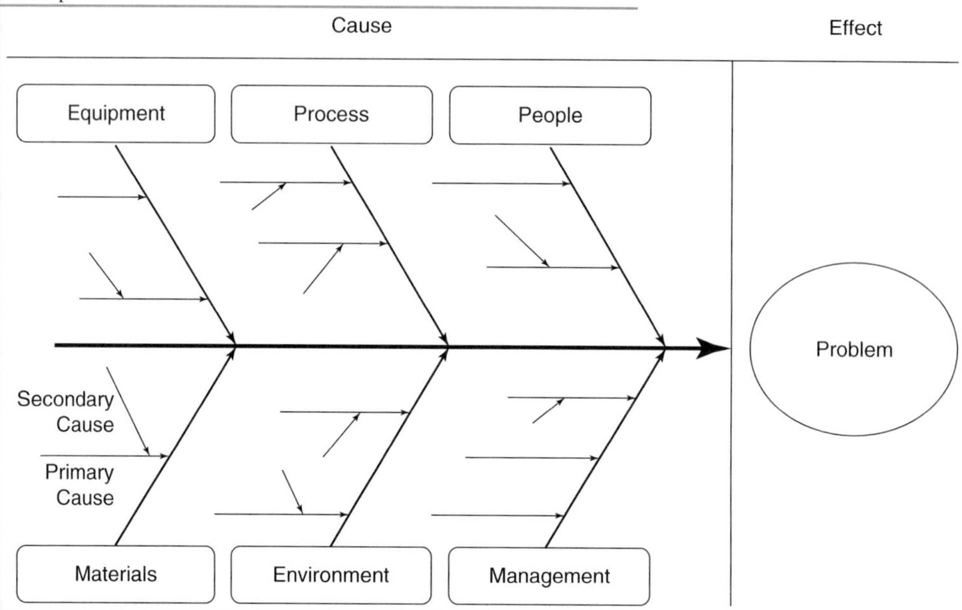
2. Five Why's	Assist in performing a root cause analysis	• Why do you think the CAUTI occurred? – The catheter was left in longer than needed • Why? – An order to remove it was not written • Why? – The nurse and doctor forgot to discuss the need for the catheter during rounds • Why? – Their rounding tool does not address urinary catheters • Why? – The tool was just revised and the urinary catheter daily assessment section was inadvertently deleted
3. Process mapping	Visually represents the steps undertaken during a process	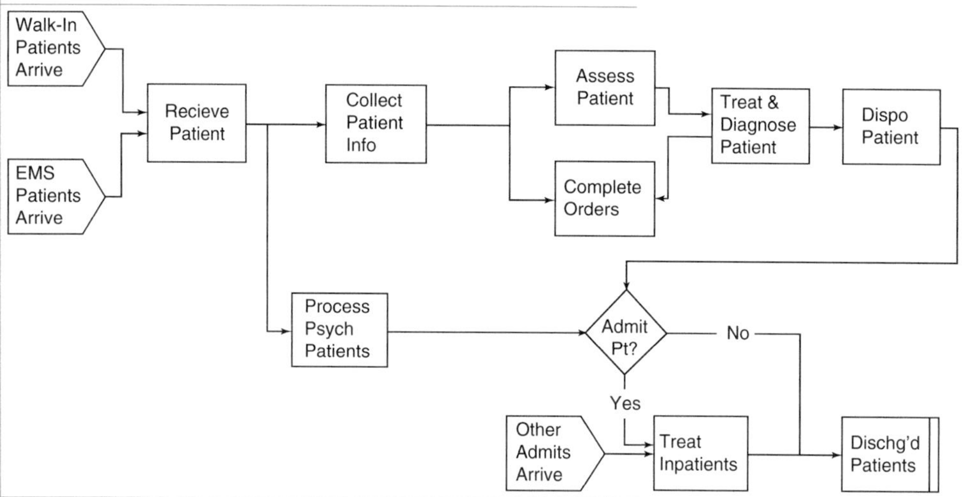

Table 8.2 (continued)

Tool	Applications	Example
4. Pareto charts	Causes are charted to identify the prominent reasons	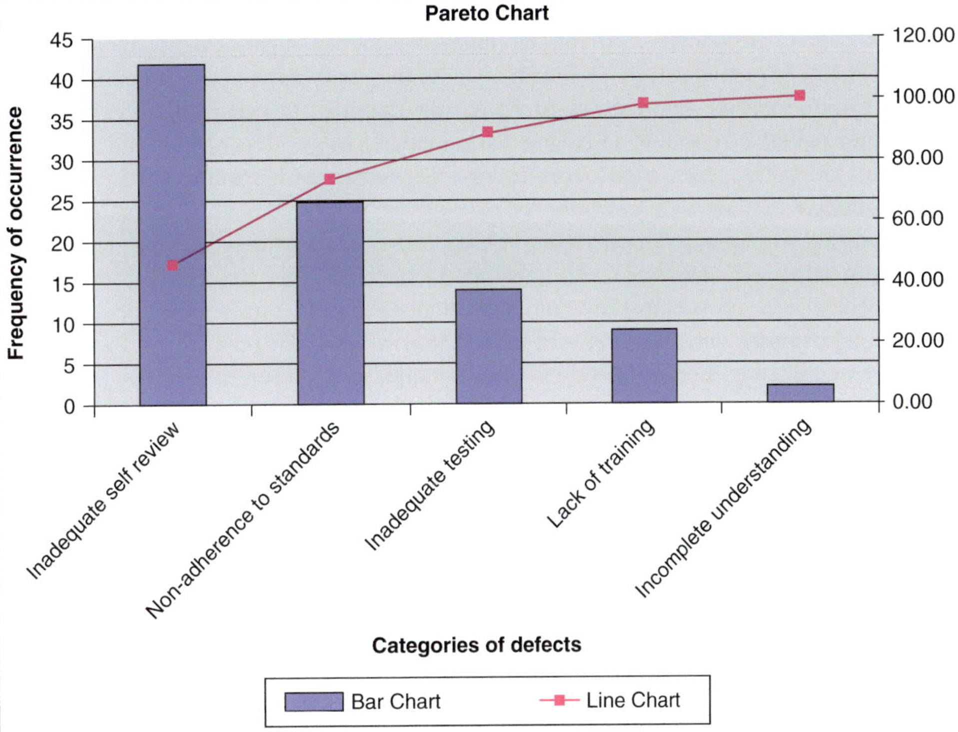

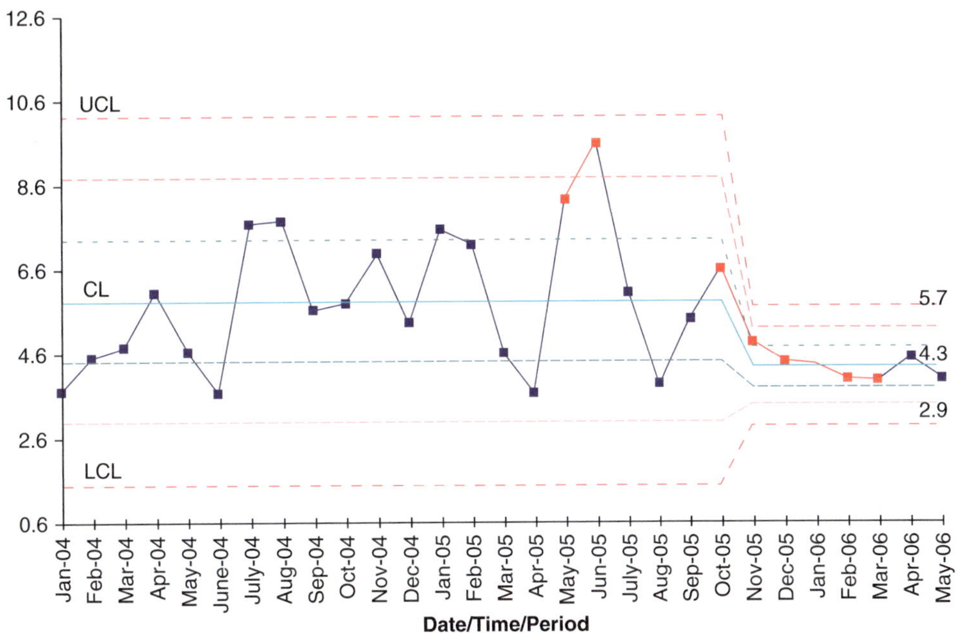

Fig. 8.4 A statistical process control chart demonstrating falls per 1000 patient days in a burn centre. The special cause variation is demonstrated in red: firstly, where two consecutive points fell beyond two standard deviations; and secondly, where six consecutive points were seen to decrease

simple to produce and interpret, and are guided by simple rules. Control charts are a more complex method, requiring a greater number of data points. They also have considerably more statistical power to detect improvements. Control charts have the ability to demonstrate whether a process shows common cause variation (i.e. normal variation) or special cause variation, which suggests that something has occurred, either positive or negative, to influence the results. Control limits are calculated to show standard deviations for the plotted data, and rules exist to demonstrate when special cause variation has indeed occurred. Different types of charts exist depending on the nature of the data. An example of special cause variation with respect to fall prevention in a burn centre is demonstrated on a control chart in Fig. 8.4.

In addition to courses offered by organizations such as the Institute of Healthcare Improvement (IHI), there are an increasing number of university certificate, diploma and master's degree programmes offering training in quality improvement and patient safety. This is in line with increasing recognition of its contribution to delivering quality healthcare, and QI is becoming a fundamental component of strategic priorities for high performing healthcare organizations.

Individuals with quality improvement training and experience add value in a variety of contexts within the hospital and specifically in burn units. In addition to undertaking quality improvement initiatives, some of the tools for which have been outlined earlier in this chapter, these individuals are frequently engaged in risk management and other patient safety related hospital functions. Examples of these include the assessment, prevention and management of medical errors, adverse events, and complications as diverse as infections, communication issues, medication errors, as well as surgical and diagnostic considerations. Quality improvement experts, either internal or external to the organization, may recommend a diverse range of solutions for safety-related issues incorporating, amongst other strategies, information technology, reporting, culturally sensitive programmes, training and educational initiatives, accreditation, workforce assessment and engagement solutions [9–11]. They are also well placed to implement processes for incident reporting, and are frequently called upon to facilitate and modernize clinical meetings such as those dedicated to discussing mortality and morbidities, and to obtain consensus for best practices [12–14].

Increasingly, governmental agencies and medical insurance services internationally are insisting that health services maintain outcome and process measures so that performance can be linked with payment and resource allocation. As in other surgical specialties, burn centres have begun to focus on a series of quality improvement indicators in their field. The involvement of burn surgeons (and professions allied to medicine) in activities of their various affiliations has undoubtedly been of value, as for example has been the impact of the American College of Surgeons' National Surgical Quality Improvement Program (NSQIP) on the process of QI applied to the practice of burn surgery [15].

8.3 Quality Improvement in Burn Care

Most of this textbook describes systems and processes relating to the quality care of patients with thermal injuries, incorporating prevention, acute management and rehabilitation. The authors have recommended, based on their expertise and the available evidence-base, how best to approach specific clinical scenarios. Quality improvement strategies are widely applicable to the care of patients with burn injuries, and a comprehensive review of the range of quality improvement interventions applied to the practice of the care of the burn injured patient would be impossible to limit to this chapter.

That being said, there remains a relative dearth of quality improvement interventions in the burn literature, using QI methods. As mentioned previously, quality improvement initiatives described for publication are distinct from traditional research publications and have different objectives. Unfortunately, quality improvement manuscripts submitted for publication are usually evaluated through a traditional research lens. In line with burn organizations' increasing requirement for quality improvement to form part of verification processes of burn centres, and the limited number of reviewers able to assess quality improvement submissions, there is considerable need to roll out quality improvement training amongst burn care practitioners. There are, however, a few prominent individuals, including Bessy and Gibran [16, 17] and other members of the American Burn Association (ABA) especially, who have made significant strides in advancing quality improvement as it applies to the delivery of burn care [18–24], and this culture has spread to other national and international burn organizations. Guidelines for the optimal care of patients with burn injuries have been published by several organizations, including the International Society for Burn Injuries (ISBI).

Quality improvement is nothing without reliable acquisition and evaluation of data. The nature of burn care is such that the best conclusions about clinical practices can often only be made by collecting data across regions, nationally and sometimes even internationally. In order to be able to compare outcomes, and then to derive broadly acceptable 'benchmarks', common definitions are required. Although organizations such as the American burn Association have published consensus documents about definitions for conditions such as sepsis, ventilator-associated pneumonia, wound infection, etc., considerable challenges still exist in their interpretation and application. As a result, reporting is variable and inconsistent between sites. This highlights the fact that valuable traditional research in burn care is becoming increasingly difficult to undertake without enormous resources, time and funding, while QI is increasingly being seen as a way to introduce tangible change within specific environments.

Although still a common cause of traumatic mortality globally, rates have declined significantly over the last three decades in modern burn centres [18, 25, 26]. Traditionally, mortality rates and hospital lengths of stay have been the key reported outcomes and have informed measures of excellence. But there are number of weaknesses inherent in utilizing these as prominent outcome measures: mortality rates will depend on factors beyond the control of the clinicians, including patient age, comorbidities and other factors [23, 25, 26]. Length of stay, and length of stay per percentage burn, are also flawed as measures depending on the nature of rehabilitation services available, the socio-economic factors in the community served, as well as geographical considerations, the need for follow-up, and patient comorbidities. But other broadly applicable outcome measures have been elusive. Without consensus on viable measures, we will have difficulty evaluating standards of care, comparing our services, interpreting research, and undertaking meaningful audit and quality improvement. Outcomes are very challenging to measure in patients with burn injuries owing to the heterogenous nature of the population in terms of the injury and the demographics of the patients, as well as a range of interrelating psychosocial factors [27–30].

As a result, there is a greater focus on long-term outcomes such as measures of disability, distress, social reintegration and quality of life: how best to measure these outcomes are at the forefront of debate within the burn fraternity. Patient-reported outcomes are currently very much in vogue in several areas in healthcare, not least plastic and reconstructive surgery. In the context of burn care, Klassen et al., for example, have recently validated a patient-reported outcome scale with respect to scar assessment, recognizing that healthcare workers' opinions about satisfactory outcomes are not necessarily shared by their patients [31, 32].

The National Burn Registry (NBR) collects a series of data submitted by participating burn centres for the purposes of research, and aims to promote improvements in the delivery of burncare by comparing different units, a concept referred to as benchmarking. Klein et al. [33], using data from the NBR, were able to compare outcomes with fixed accepted benchmarks in burn care at six academic burn centres. The authors evaluated the outcomes in 541 patients with major burn injuries between 2003 and 2009. The study demonstrated a 29% survival rate benefit for patients managed in these six academic burn centres compared to those patients in the NBR. Ten standard operating procedures were assessed including resuscitation strategies, blood glucose control, burn wound management, and antibiotic prophylaxis. The multi-organ failure rate in these units was as high as 27%; the authors proposed a benchmark of time to recovery of organ dysfunction as an excellent marker for good clinical care in the management of major burns.

Falder et al. reviewed seven core domains of assessment [Table 8.3], including skin, neuromuscular function, sensation and pain, psychological function, physical role function, community participation and perceived quality of life [18].

Table 8.3 Falder et al.'s seven core domains of assessment after burn injury

Core domains	Outcomes
Skin	Wound infection Sepsis Wound healing Scarring Need for reconstructive surgery
Neuromuscular function	Joint mobility Muscle strength Lower limb function Upper limb function Cardiovascular fitness
Sensory and pain	Pain intensity Itch
Psychological function	Posttraumatic stress disorder Depression
Community participation	Social reintegration
Perceived quality of life	
Physical role function	Functional independence Return to work

Similarly, Ryan et al. sought to evaluate the young adults burn outcome questionnaires (YABOQ) as a means of monitoring and predicting recovery and evaluating treatment [34, 35]. The study was undertaken over a 5-year period and was prospective, controlled and multicentre in nature, involving adults between the ages of 19 and 30 years who were interviewed at initial contact and then regularly up until 12 months after injury. The questionnaire evaluated 15 sectors, with recovery curves in itch, perceived appearance, social function limited by appearance, family concern and satisfaction with symptom relief, remaining below the reference control group at 2 years. The authors concluded that this tool was reliable at assessing multidimensional functional outcomes.

One way of improving the services offered by burn care facilities is to apply a process of objective peer-review, referred to as accreditation or verification. The American Burn Association (ABA) has published a number of criteria which are utilized to verify burn centres, and successful verification has become a mark of distinction for North American burn centres. To achieve burn centre verification, a centre must meet rigorous standards for organizational structure, personnel qualifications, resources, and medical care services from the time of injury to rehabilitation. These criteria are summarized in Table 8.4. The ABA Verification Programme strives for an objective, consistent, evidence-based process to assist burn centres to maintain quality by promoting patient safety, cost containment, regional education and outreach, injury prevention, innovation and research, and advocacy. A few burn centres in developed countries have recently also been verified by the ABA, and these criteria and principles have also been used and adapted in other countries [36, 37].

Table 8.4 Summarized criteria for verification of a burn centre by the American Burn Association

Category	Criterion
1. Facilities	Hospital and institutional support of the burn programme
	Located at a designated trauma centre
	Dedicated burn ICU beds with adequate census
	Timely access to an operating room appropriately set up for acute and reconstructive burn surgery
	Accredited source of allograft skin
	Access to a range of wound care materials, skin substitutes and antimicrobial dressings
	Dialysis, radiology and the laboratory support at all times
	Dedicated outpatient facilities, appropriate supply of wound dressings, splints and ability to perform minor procedures
	Affiliation to local university, with accredited, formalized resident/registrar and/or fellow training programmes
2. Burn surgeons	A burn director oversees all clinical aspects of administration
	Appropriate certification and experience which may include fellowship training in burn care
	EMSB/ABLS or equivalent training
	Commitment to research, audit, continuing education and quality improvement
	A director or delegate is available at all times
	24 h coverage and a call schedule
	Participation in regional, national and international meetings
	Able to perform or have access to timely reconstructive surgery
	Local, regional, national and international outreach, advocacy and teaching
3. Nursing	Nurse manager to oversee all nursing administration
	Continuous coverage of appropriately trained nurses in burn wound and ICU care
	Education programme
	Participation in regional, national and international meetings
	Involvement in Quality improvement
4. Physical and occupational therapists	Appropriate experience and credentials
	Oversee rehabilitation plan for all patients
	Continuous education programme involvement
	Quality improvement involvement
5. Multidisciplinary coverage	Operating room nurses with burn surgery experience and knowledge of protocols
	Physiatry consultant
	Psychology and psychiatry consultant referral system
	Anaesthesia, preferably dedicated, with allocated liaison/representative
	Respiratory therapists
	Paediatric (child life) and geriatric specific services as indicated
	Consulting services from all medical and surgical specialties
	Dedicated social worker
	Dedicated pharmacist with oversight over drug policies including antibiotic therapies and DVT prophylaxis
	Dedicated dietitian
6. Quality improvement	Weekly patient care conferences
	Monthly morbidity and mortality rounds to discuss adverse events, complications and to classify deaths as preventable or not preventable
	Oversight by non-involved external surgical critical care peer
	Multidisciplinary involvement
	Formal quality improvement training
	Ongoing quality improvement initiatives as part of the centre and hospital strategic plan, with an emphasis on safety
	Documentation, data collection, benchmark auditing and reporting systems
	Ability to identify weaknesses, intervene to correct, and undertake loop closure
	Formal incident reporting strategy
	Infection control policies and procedures compliance, with an emphasis on multidrug resistance and hospital-acquired infection
7. Other policies	Regularly reviewed and practical mass casualty plan
	Memorandum of understanding with other burn units and trauma centres
	Documented guidelines on patient care
	Guidelines on patient transport and transfers
	Peer support programmes
	Policies for polytrauma patients with burn injuries
	Close communication with rehabilitation facilities and community dressing and support nurses

Table 8.5 Selected benchmark criteria that may be utilized for organizational reporting of burn care

Selected outcome/benchmark criteria
Total fluid volume received (mL/kg)
Time to consultation for ambulatory patients and time to arrival from referral in patients requiring admission
Mortality rate [Burns less than 20% total body surface area (TBSA), 20–40% TBSA, more than 40% TBSA, over 60 years old]
Burn wound and surgical site infection rates
Time from acute burn injury to first surgery (or proportion within 72 h)
Time to recovery after organ dysfunction (e.g. length of dialysis, ventilation, etc.)
Time from acute burn injury to complete excision (or proportion within one week)
Time from acute burn injury 95% wound healing (or one week after last surgery)
Time to initiation of enteral feeding (e.g. proportion within 24 h)
Incidence of ventilator-associated pneumonia
Incidence of acute renal failure requiring dialysis
Incidence of catheter-associated urinary tract infections
Surgery for graft or flap loss
Proportion of cases of perioperative hypothermia
Mean length of stay per percentage burn
Proportion of patients managed on an ambulatory basis
Proportion of patients undergoing day case surgery
Mean length of stay per percentage burn
Readmission rate
Waiting time for reconstructive surgery after booking
Time to return to work
Incidence of pressure sores
Incidence of DVT
Proportion of patients followed up by own service (on-site or via telemedicine)
Proportion screened for PTSD and depression
Proportion seen by a social worker within 1 week

Some of the benchmarks that burn centres might use are tabulated (Table 8.5). Verification gives burn centres the opportunity to hone in on those areas of relative weakness and reinforce areas of strength. In line with evidence from numerous specialties, burn care literature has suggested that centres providing high-volume, focused and specialized care tend to offer improved outcomes with fewer complications and a lower overall cost compared to lower volume burn centres. Palmieri et al., for example [38], showed that verified burn centres in California admitted more patients per centre and treated more severely injured patients than non-verified centres, and offered improved outcomes.

The proposed benefits of being managed in a burn centre may have far greater impact than has previously been assessed, especially when one considers the healthcare needs of burn survivors well after discharge from hospital or even the rehabilitation process. Mason et al. reviewed data, from several population-based administrative databases, of 1895 patients who had sustained a burn injury. Patients who received their index acute burn care in a burn centre experienced significantly less need for subsequent unplanned acute care, fewer emergency department visits and acute hospital readmissions. Her work also highlighted that a considerable proportion of patients continue to receive their burn care outside the setting of burn centres. While the odds of death reduced significantly over the last 20 years, it is evident that this improvement has occurred as a result of regionalization, with greater numbers of patients managed in burn centres than previous years [39]. Mason also identified the relationship between mental health illness and burn injury, recognizing it as both a risk factor and sequelae of acute burn injury, and motivated for increased screening and targeted interventions after burn injury [40].

Burn centres are, at their best, regionalized self-contained facilities striving to offer excellence in burn care delivery. As such, burn centres are well placed to introduce QI initiatives, either independently, or as pilot studies for hospital-wide strategies [41–49]. Selected examples of published quality improvement projects are tabulated (Table 8.6).

Table 8.6 Selected quality improvement initiatives published in the burn literature

Reference	Summary
1. Fahlstrom et al. [41]	The authors demonstrated that a nurse-driven fluid resuscitation protocol improved endpoints, including lactate at 24 h after burn injury, and empowered nurses to titrate fluid themselves rather than consulting physicians
2. Maguiña et al. [42]	The authors undertook pressure mapping on bedding surfaces in the hospital and identified and introduced strategies to prevent pressure ulcer development
3. Edkins et al. [43]	The authors applied QI initiatives to optimize pain management using guidelines for multimodal anaesthesia, and also improved patient movement and efficiency through the perioperative phases
4. Popp et al. [44]	The authors were able to demonstrate a significant reduction in hospital-acquired infections in patients with major burn injury by regularly bathing patients in 0.9% chlorhexidine solution in sterile water
5. Mathews et al. [45]	Through a series of practice changes, the authors were able to demonstrate cost reductions without impairing quality of care
6. Philp et al. [46]	The authors prospectively evaluated their surgical approaches and techniques, as well as post-surgical practices to optimize aesthetic and functional results. They then implemented strategies to address areas for improvement
7. Rehou et al. [47]	The authors were able to demonstrate reductions in markers of inflammation and hospital stays by introducing a protocol of antioxidants for patients with major burn injury
8. Madni et al. [48]	The authors evaluated the allocation of intraoperative activities over an 18 month period, concluding that only 40% of available operating time was actually utilized for the procedure itself. They then considered and implemented strategies for quality improvement
9. Rogers et al. [49]	The authors applied 1 hour of preoperative warming for patients with major burn injury and demonstrated that the incidence of perioperative hypothermia, previously shown (by the same authors) to be deleterious to outcomes, can be successfully reduced

Summary Box

- Quality Improvement (QI) is a proven approach to optimize the delivery of patient care, by iteratively evaluating and testing service provision. Burn centres are ideally placed to introduce such initiatives, as they are, at their best, regionalized academic facilities with goal-directed pathways of care and protocols, with specially trained multidisciplinary staff and appropriate resources.
- Quality improvement is best introduced in an environment where there is a sound understanding of the system and the processes there, where the focus is always on exceptional patient care, where leaders recognise and reward teamwork, and where reliable data is available.
- In addition to introducing initiatives, QI specialists are empowered to aid the functioning of burn units by leading processes like mortality and morbidity meetings, overseeing data abstraction and reporting, assessing and responding to issues of safety, evaluating patient, family and staff feedback, and leading verification applications (as undertaken with the American Burn Association).
- What is distinct about QI when compared to traditional research, is the adaptability of interventions according to the results obtained, and the potential to significantly improve outcomes over a relatively short period of time.

References

1. Jain M, Miller L, Belt D, King D, Berwick DM. Decline in ICU adverse events, nosocomial infections and cost through a quality improvement initiative focusing on teamwork and culture change. Qual Saf Health Care. 2006;15(4):235–9. PMID:16885246.
2. Berwick DM. The science of improvement. JAMA. 2008;299(10):1182–4. https://doi.org/10.1001/jama.299.10.1182. PMID: 18334694.
3. Berwick DM. A user's manual for the IOM's 'Quality Chasm' report. Health Aff (Millwood). 2002;21(3):80–90. PMID: 12026006.
4. Berwick DM. A primer on leading the improvement of systems. BMJ. 1996;312(7031):619–22. PMID:8595340.
5. Bailey MA. The ethics of improving health care and safety: a Hastings center/AHRQ project. Garrison, NY: The Hastings Center; 2004.
6. Batalden PB, Davidoff F. What is "quality improvement" and how can it transform healthcare? Qual Saf Health Care. 2007;16(1):2–3. PMID: 17301192.
7. www.hqontario.ca/portals/0/Documents/qi/qi-quality-improve-guide-2012-en.pdf. Accessed 5 Jan 2018.
8. Ogrinc G, Davies L, Goodman D, Batalden P, Davidoff F, Stevens D. SQUIRE 2.0 (Standards for QUality improvement reporting excellence): revised publication guidelines from a detailed consensus process. Can J Diabetes. 2015;39(5):434–9. https://doi.org/10.1016/j.jcjd.2015.08.001.
9. Howell AM, Burns EM, Hull L, Mayer E, Sevdalis N, Darzi A. International recommendations for national patient safety incident reporting systems: an expert Delphi consensus-building process. BMJ Qual Saf. 2017;26(2):150–63. https://doi.org/10.1136/bmjqs-2015-004456. Epub 2016 Feb 22. PMID: 26902254.
10. Howell AM, Burns EM, Bouras G, Donaldson LJ, Athanasiou T, Darzi A. Can patient safety incident reports be used to compare hospital safety? Results from a quantitative analysis of the english national reporting and learning system data. PLoS One. 2015;10(12):e0144107. https://doi.org/10.1371/journal.pone.0144107. eCollection 2015. PMID:26650823.
11. Rabøl LI, Gaardboe O, Hellebek A. Incident reporting must result in local action. BMJ Qual Saf. 2017;26(6):515–6. https://doi.org/10.1136/bmjqs-2016-005971. Epub 2016 Aug 24. PMID: 27558307.
12. Calder LA, Kwok ES, Adam Cwinn A, Worthington J, Yelle JD, Waggott M, Frank JR. Enhancing the quality of morbidity and mortality rounds: the Ottawa M&M model. Acad Emerg Med. 2014;21(3):314–21. PMID:24628757. https://doi.org/10.1111/acem.12330.
13. Calder LA, Kwok ES, Adam Cwinn A, Worthington J, Yelle JD, Waggott M, Frank JR. Enhancing the quality of morbidity and mortality rounds: the Ottawa M&M model. Acad Emerg Med. 2014;21(3):314–21. https://doi.org/10.1111/acem.12330.
14. Kwok ESH, Calder LA, Barlow-Krelina E, Mackie C, Seely AJE, Cwinn AA, Worthington JR, Frank JR. Implementation of a structured hospital-wide morbidity and mortality rounds model. BMJ Qual Saf. 2017;26(6):439–48. https://doi.org/10.1136/bmjqs-2016-005459. Epub 2016 Jun 29.
15. Steinberg SM, Popa MR, Michalek JA, Bethel MJ, Ellison EC. Comparison of risk adjustment methodologies in surgical quality improvement. Surgery. 2008;144(4):662–7. ; discussion 662-7. PMID: 18847652. https://doi.org/10.1016/j.surg.2008.06.010.
16. Gibran NS. Importance of measuring outcomes after burns: why they matter. J Burn Care Res. 2017;38(3):e589–90. https://doi.org/10.1097/BCR.0000000000000543.
17. Mandell SP, Robinson EF, Cooper CL, Klein MB, Gibran NS. Patient safety measures in burn care: do National reporting systems accurately reflect quality of burn care? J Burn Care Res. 2010;31(1):125–9. https://doi.org/10.1097/BCR.0b013e3181cb8d00. PMID: 20061847.
18. Falder S, Browne A, Edgar D, Staples E, Fong J, Rea S, Wood F. Core outcomes for adult burn survivors: a clinical overview. Burns. 2009;35(5):618–41. https://doi.org/10.1016/j.burns.2008.09.002.. Epub 2008 Dec 25
19. Cioffi WG, Harrington DT. A multi-institutional benchmark of burn outcomes as a spur to further improvements in burn care. Ann Surg. 2014;259(5):842–3. https://doi.org/10.1097/SLA.0000000000000664. No abstract available. PMID: 24717373.
20. Dale EL, Hultman CS. Patient safety in burn care: application of evidence-based medicine to improve outcomes. Clin Plast Surg. 2017;44(3):611–8. https://doi.org/10.1016/j.cps.2017.02.015. Epub 2017 Apr 7.
21. Burd A. Burns: treatment and outcomes. Semin Plast Surg. 2010;24(3):262–80. https://doi.org/10.1055/s-0030-1263068. PMID: 22550448.
22. Abdelrahman I, Elmasry M, Steinvall I, Fredrikson M, Sjoberg F. Improvement in mortality at a National Burn Centre since 2000: was it the result of increased resources? Medicine (Baltimore). 2017;96(25):e6727. PMID: 28640072. https://doi.org/10.1097/MD.0000000000006727.
23. Hultman CS, van Duin D, Sickbert-Bennett E, DiBiase LM, Jones SW, Cairns BA, Weber DJ. Systems-based practice in burn care: prevention, management, and economic impact of health care-

associated infections. Clin Plast Surg. 2017;44(4):935–42. https://doi.org/10.1016/j.cps.2017.06.002. Epub 2017 Jul 29. PMID: 28888319.

24. Finnerty CC, Jeschke MG, Branski LK, Barret JP, Dziewulski P, Herndon DN. Hypertrophic scarring: the greatest unmet challenge after burn injury. Lancet. 2016;388(10052):1427–36. https://doi.org/10.1016/S0140-6736(16)31406-4. Review. PMID: 27707499.
25. Pereira C, Murphy K, Herndon D. Outcome measures in burn care. Is mortality dead? Burns. 2004;30(8):761–71. Review. PMID: 15555787.
26. Tompkins RG. Survival from burns in the new millennium: 70 years' experience from a single institution. Ann Surg. 2015;261(2):263–8. https://doi.org/10.1097/SLA.0000000000000623. Review. PMID: 24670865.
27. Hussain A, Dunn KW. Predicting length of stay in thermal burns: a systematic review of prognostic factors. Burns. 2013;39(7):1331–40. https://doi.org/10.1016/j.burns.2013.04.026. Epub 2013 Jun 13. Review. PMID: 23768707.
28. Moi AL, Haugsmyr E, Heisterkamp H. Long-term study of health and quality of life after burn injury. Ann Burns Fire Disasters. 2016;29(4).295–9. PMID: 28289366.
29. Öster C, Willebrand M, Ekselius L. Burn-specific health 2 years to 7 years after burn injury. J Trauma Acute Care Surg. 2013;74(4):1119–24; discussion 1124. PMID: 23511154. https://doi.org/10.1097/TA.0b013e318283cca0.
30. Schneider JC, Gerrard P, Goldstein R, DiVita MA, Niewczyk P, Ryan CM, Kowalske K, Zafonte R. The impact of comorbidities and complications on burn injury inpatient rehabilitation outcomes. PM R. 2013;5(2):114–21. https://doi.org/10.1016/j.pmrj.2012.07.014. Epub 2012 Sep 12. PMID:22981003.
31. Jones LL, Calvert M, Moiemen N, Deeks JJ, Bishop J, Kinghorn P, Mathers J, team PEGASUS. Outcomes important to burns patients during scar management and how they compare to the concepts captured in burn-specific patient reported outcome measures. Burns. 2017;43(8):1682–92. https://doi.org/10.1016/j.burns.2017.09.004. Epub 2017 Oct 12. PMID: 29031889.
32. Klassen AF, Ziolkowski N, Mundy LR, Miller CR, McIlvride A, DiLaura A, Fish J, Pusic AL. Development of a new patient-reported outcome instrument to evaluate treatments for scars: the SCAR-Q. Plast Reconstr Surg Glob Open. 2018;6:e1672. https://doi.org/10.1097/GOX.0000000000001672; Published online 24 April 2018.
33. Klein MB, Goverman J, Hayden DL, Fagan SP, McDonald-Smith GP, Alexander AK, Gamelli RL, Gibran NS, Finnerty CC, Jeschke MG, Arnoldo B, Wispelwey B, Mindrinos MN, Xiao W, Honari SE, Mason PH, Schoenfeld DA, Herndon DN, Tompkins RG. inflammation and host response to injury, and large-scale collaborative research program. Benchmarking outcomes in the critically injured burn patient. Ann Surg. 2014;259(5):833–41. https://doi.org/10.1097/SLA.0000000000000438.
34. Ryan CM, Schneider JC, Kazis LE, Lee A, Li NC, Hinson M, Bauk H, Peck M, Meyer WJ 3rd, Palmieri T, Pidcock FS, Reilly D, Tompkins RG, Multi-Center Benchmarking Study Group. Benchmarks for multidimensional recovery after burn injury in young adults: the development, validation, and testing of the American Burn Association/Shriners Hospitals for Children young adult burn outcome questionnaire. J Burn Care Res. 2013;34(3):e121–42. https://doi.org/10.1097/BCR.0b013e31827e7ecf.
35. Ryan CM, Parry I, Richard R. Functional outcomes following burn injury. J Burn Care Res. 2017;38(3):e614–7. https://doi.org/10.1097/BCR.0000000000000537. Review. PMID: 28328664.
36. ameriburn.org/quality-care/verification. Accessed 4 Mar 2018.
37. Holmes JH 4th, Carter JE, Neff LP, Cairns BA, d'Agostino RB Jr, Griffin LP, Meredith JW. The effectiveness of regionalized burn care: an analysis of 6,873 burn admissions in North Carolina from 2000 to 2007. J Am Coll Surg. 2011;212(4):487–93, 493.e1–6; discussion 493–5. PMID: 21463775. https://doi.org/10.1016/j.jamcollsurg.2010.12.044.
38. Palmieri TL, London JA, O'Mara MS, Greenhalgh DG. Analysis of admissions and outcomes in verified and nonverified burn centers. J Burn Care Res. 2008;29(1):208–12. https://doi.org/10.1097/BCR.0b013e31815f31b4. PMID: 18182924.
39. Mason SA, Nathens AB, Byrne JP, Fowler RA, Karanicolas PJ, Moineddin R, Jeschke MG. Burn center care reduces acute health care utilization after discharge: a population-based analysis of 1,895 survivors of major burn injury. Surgery. 2017;162(4):891–900. https://doi.org/10.1016/j.surg.2017.05.018. Epub 2017 Jul 13. PMID: 28712732.
40. Mason SA, Nathens AB, Byrne JP, Ellis J, Fowler RA, Gonzalez A, Karanicolas PJ, Moineddin R, Jeschke MG. Association between burn injury and mental illness among burn survivors: a population-based, self-matched, longitudinal cohort study. J Am Coll Surg. 2017;225(4):516–24. https://doi.org/10.1016/j.jamcollsurg.2017.06.004. Epub 2017 Jul 31. PMID: 28774550.
41. Fahlstrom K, Boyle C, Makic MB. Implementation of a nurse-driven burn resuscitation protocol: a quality improvement project. Crit Care Nurse. 2013;33(1):25–35. https://doi.org/10.4037/ccn2013385.
42. Maguiña P, Kirkland-Walsh H. Hospital-acquired pressure ulcer prevention: a burn surgeon's team approach. J Burn Care Res. 2014;35(5):e287–93. https://doi.org/10.1097/BCR.0000000000000057.
43. Edkins RE, Hultman CS, Collins P, Cairns B, Hanson M, Carman M. Improving comfort and throughput for patients undergoing fractionated laser ablation of symptomatic burn scars. Ann Plast Surg. 2015;74(3):293–9. https://doi.org/10.1097/SAP.0000000000000367. PMID: 25664406.
44. Popp JA, Layon AJ, Nappo R, Richards WT, Mozingo DW. Hospital-acquired infections and thermally injured patients: chlorhexidine gluconate baths work. Am J Infect Control. 2014;42(2):129–32. https://doi.org/10.1016/j.ajic.2013.08.015. PMID: 24485370.
45. Mathews JJ, Supple K, Calistro A, Gamelli RL. A burn center cost-reduction program. J Burn Care Rehabil. 1997;18(4):358–63; discussion 357. PMID: 9261705.
46. Philp L, Umraw N, Cartotto R. Late outcomes after grafting of the severely burned face: a quality improvement initiative. J Burn Care Res. 2012;33(1):46–56. https://doi.org/10.1097/BCR.0b013e318234d89f. PMID: 22002207.
47. Rehou S, Shahrokhi S, Natanson R, Stanojcic M, Jeschke MG. Antioxidant and trace element supplementation reduce the inflammatory response in critically ill burn patients. J Burn Care Res. 2018;39:1–9. https://doi.org/10.1097/BCR.0000000000000607.
48. Madni TD, Imran JB, Clark A, Arnoldo BA, Phelan HA 3rd, Wolf SE. Analysis of operating room efficiency in a burn center. J Burn Care Res. 2018;39:89–93. https://doi.org/10.1097/BCR.0000000000000572.
49. Rogers AD, Saggaf M, Ziolkowski N. Preoperative warming as part of a quality improvement initiative to prevent inadvertent intraoperative hypothermia in major burns. Burns. 2018. pii: S0305-4179(18)30097-4. https://doi.org/10.1016/j.burns.2018.02.012.

Burn Centers and the Multidisciplinary Team, Centralized Burn Care, and Burn Care Quality Control Work

9

Folke Sjöberg, Ingrid Steinvall, and Moustafa Elmasry

9.1 Change of Burn Care Volume

The incidence and prevalence of burn injuries is decreasing worldwide and in parallel there is an increase in outpatient type of care and a shortening in length of stay [1] that has been significant during the last 20 years [2, 3]. This is particularly so for the high income countries [4]. For the low income countries, data is still lacking [4]. This has led to a decreasing demand on health care volume for the care of burns. This has during the last 10 years been a contributing factor for a decrease in the availability of burn care facilities and has boasted the process for centralized care [5–7].

9.2 Burn Center

Historically, burn care was an entity that was early organized at separate locations within hospitals due to many factors, not least, at first due to the smell and the screaming of pain, that this patient group was constantly facing and which was disturbing other medical care, and later also due to the risk of bacterial contamination of the wounds posing a threat both to the patient himself and to other patients being treated for other diseases at the same hospital [8]. This fact has led to that the burn care process often has been unified in that the whole care process is undertaken at one location, by a separate staff, i.e., that both ICU/high dependence care, regular ward duties, and the outpatient clinics have been closely connected and not seldom placed at one combined location [9].

The fact that all facets of burn care has been provided at the same location has further stimulated different specialities to co-operate in daily care, and this is one cornerstone to what has been the successful co-operation within the multidisciplinary team, a success factor for medical care in general and burn care in particular [10, 11]. It is evident in the EBA guidelines the focus that has been placed on the multidisciplinary team is considered a significant player in the prosperous development of burn care [12].

The general opinion has been that the multidisciplinary and centralized way of administering burns has produced a favorable outcome for the patients. However in this process, there was early no scientific support for supplying such care in comparison to delivering burn care within other medical specialities. Now recently, more solid data for this approach has been documented [6, 13, 14] beside the work and evaluations made by the burn care organizations themselves, such as the International Society for Burn Injuries (ISBI) [15], American Burn Association [16], European Burns Association (EBA), or the Australian-New Zealand counterparts [17].

9.3 Burn Care Quality, Assessing, and Delivery of Burn Care Quality

Looking now at the care guidelines for burn care at the global level [15] or regionally such as in the USA (ABA; American Burn Association); Europe (EBA, European Burns Association) or Australia (ANZBA, the Australian and New Zealand Burns Association), there is a priority that burn care preferably should be undertaken at dedicated burn care facilities (Burn Centers or Burn Units). In these documents, especially for this book the EBA Guidelines provide recommendations as how to structure, manage the burn care process, and how to ascertain good burn

F. Sjöberg (✉)
Department of Clinical and Experimental Medicine, Linköping University, Linköping, Sweden
e-mail: folke.sjoberg@liu.se

I. Steinvall · M. Elmasry
Department of Clinical and Experimental Medicine, Linköping University, Linköping, Sweden

Department of Hand and Plastic Surgery, Linköping University Hospital, Linköping, Sweden
e-mail: ingrid.steinvall@regionostergotland.se; moustafa.elmasry@liu.se

M. G. Jeschke et al. (eds.), *Handbook of Burns Volume 1*, https://doi.org/10.1007/978-3-030-18940-2_9

care outcomes. In other words, this has been an attempt to accomplish high quality burn care. These ideas are founded scientifically already in the 70s by the care quality paradigm that was first published by Donabedian [18], in which quality of care was based and evaluated on three major parts: structure, process, and outcome [19].

In the burn care process, the structure and process have been described in the burn care Guidelines presented by the organizations just mentioned (ISBI/ABA/EBA/ANZBA) and the outcome part is most often claimed to be evaluated in quality registers [20] such as the TRACs database (American College of Surgeons national burn registry) or in separate scientific publications presenting burn care outcomes [21]. In the aim to assess quality of care, a lot of emphasis has been put on quality indicators [16, 22–24]. In this aspect, significant work has been undertaken within different medical specialities and especially the critical care sector can be refereed to [20]. In this area, a large number of quality of care indicators have been launched and vividly discussed. One problem is however, yet the lack of consensus when it comes to the choice of the most relevant ones. This is still debated and probably constitutes a significant part of the ongoing quality of care improving process. Within burn care, mortality (standardized mortality ratio (SMR)) has most often been the first quality of care marker addressed. In this aspect, the standard mortality ratio based on the Baux score constitutes a very good measure as it has very good predictability (High ROC AUC value) and the risk-adjusted mortality can be very well assessed and different levels of quality of care (from a mortality perspective) can be ascertained in cohorts that are of relevant size such as at, i.e., each burn center [25]. Risk-adjusted mortality thus may be yet the first and most important quality of burn care indicator and the LA50 measure may serve as one. This measure describes the burn size that in individuals lead to a 50% mortality risk/survival chance [26]. This value has improved from a burn size of 43% TBSA among young adults in 1947 compared to 66% TBSA in 2010 [26]. It is very interesting that when examining this outcome measure, especially in adults, it is evident that the largest improvement lately in mortality is not for the largest burn injuries TBSA% wise but for the injuries of a more intermediate size where the reduction in mortality is more pronounced [25]. Looking at this measure, it is evident that there is a large quality improvement that has occurred since first measures which was presented by Bull and Colleagues in Birmingham in 1949 [27]. Another that has been discussed, which at least from the theoretical perspective is important, and interesting is length of stay (LOS) [28]. It may be claimed a good measure of the time it takes to heal the burn wound and also the process of replacing and closing full thickness burn injuries. Its shortcomings depend on administrative routines and issues as well as, outpatient care procedures. In general, it has for long been claimed that a LOS of 1 day/TBSA% is a good measure of adequate care [29]; however, further knowledge gained of this indicator has added more substance to its value. Engrave and colleagues have been debating that LOS needs to be divided into two categories, i.e., full or partial thickness wounds. They argue that by doing so a better estimate of the burn care process may be obtained [21]. Others have presented data that supports this and more ideas on how to improve the LOS estimate and concomitantly its value as a quality of care indicator [1]. Most certainly, more indicators will be found valuable and effective in improving the burn care process.

9.4 Burn Center Verification

With the aim to improve burn care other initiatives for quality improvements have been launched and one very important is Burn Center verification. Such a program was started in the USA offering burn centers with a volume of more than 100 cases treated per year to apply. The evaluation process was based on the ABA Guidelines [30], but very important is also the quality of criteria list developed specifically in this process by ABA (Added under Appendix, below). The format of these describes the issues addressed in the verification process for adult and pediatric burn care.

Presently, also the EBA has launched a verification program, based on somewhat different criteria and work schedule, but still with a very similar fundament for burn care quality assessment is still aimed for. More information about this and the ongoing verifications are depicted on the EBA website.

In conclusion, burn care has evolved significantly over time and the framework to further improve burn care has been set both at the world (ISBI) and continent levels (e.g., ABA EBA and ANZBA). This process can be claimed to be more unified over time as all active parties seem to take impressions from each other and only retain such procedures that seem to adequately enhance the burn care quality process. It will be interesting to follow this process further into the future as it holds high promises for further progress.

Appendix: Verification Criteria

#	Criterion	Criterion level
1	The burn center hospital is currently accredited by the Joint Commission or equivalent	1
2	The burn center has an identifiable medical and administrative commitment to the care of the patient with burns	1
3	The burn center maintains an organizational chart of personnel within the burn center and the hospital	2
4	The burn center hospital maintains a specialized unit dedicated to acute burn care	1
5	The burn center has designated ICU capable beds	1
6	The burn center maintains an appropriate policy and procedure manual that is reviewed regularly with appropriate documentation by the burn center director and the nurse manager	1
7	Multidisciplinary patient care conferences are held and documented at least weekly	1
8	Renal dialysis, radiological services, including computed tomography scanning, and clinical laboratory services are available 24 h per day	2
9	The burn center has timely access to operating rooms available 24 h a day	1
10	A dedicated OR team with burn experience is available for the burn operating theatre	2
11	The burn center hospital's policies and procedures regarding the use of allograft tissues are in compliance with all federal, state, and the Joint Commission (or equivalent) requirements, and, when feasible and appropriate, with standards of the American Association of Tissue Banks (or equivalent)	1
12	The burn center has liaisons with a designated trauma center to coordinate care of patients with multi-trauma	1
13	The burn center must have a sufficient volume of acute burn admissions on an ongoing basis to demonstrate to the site reviewers and to the Verification Review Committee that the burn center has a quality burn care program; centers with less than 100 admissions per year should anticipate that site reviewers will audit patient charts for demonstration of quality of care	1
14	80% of admissions to the center must constitute acute burn injuries; for centers with numbers less than 100 admissions per year (including observation status patients) the center can consider that 5 new patient outpatients equates to 1 inpatient	1
15	Burn centers caring for pediatric patients and geriatric patients must demonstrate facilities, protocols, and personnel specific to the care of critically ill patients; centers with less than 100 admissions per year should anticipate that site reviewers will audit charts for demonstration of quality of care	1
16	The burn center maintains an average daily census of three or more patients with acute burns	1
17	No more than 5% of all patients with a primary diagnosis of a burn injury are admitted to another service per year (e.g., geriatrics, pediatrics, medicine)	1
18	The burn center has written guidelines for the triage, treatment, and transfer of burned patients from other facilities	1
19	The burn center maintains access to an EMS system for the transport of patients with burns from referral sources within the service area	1
20	The burn center offers input into the performance improvement of pre-hospital care of burn patients	2
21	The emergency department has written protocols mutually developed with the burn service for the care of acutely burned patients	2
22	The burn center interfaces with regional trauma centers to coordinate care of patients with multiple injuries and to develop regional educational programs, disaster planning, and advocacy efforts	2
23	The burn center has a written mass casualty disaster plan for the triage and treatment of those patients burned in a mass casualty incident occurring within its service area	1
24	The mass casualty disaster plan is reviewed and updated as needed and on an annual basis by EMS representatives and the burn center director	2
25	There are current (within the past 3 years) written memoranda of understanding with other burn centers regarding secondary triage	1
26	The burn center must maintain accurate and up-to-date contact information for burn surgeons and managers on the ABA website	2
27	The burn center director is a licensed surgeon (MD or DO) with board certification by American Board of Surgery or American Board of Plastic Surgery (or equivalent for international burn centers in which case a surgeon must co-manage the center)	1
28	The burn center director has completed a 1-year fellowship in burn treatment and/or has experience in the care of patients with acute burn injuries for 2 or more years during the previous 5 years	1
29	The burn center director has current ABLS (or equivalent) training	2
30	The burn center director is responsible for the direction of burn center administrative functions	1
31	The burn center director is responsible for the creation of policies and procedures within the burn center specifying all aspects of care for burned patients	1
32	The burn center director is responsible for ensuring that all burn center providers conform to the burn center's locally established policies and procedures	1
33	The burn center director is responsible for the coordination with regional EMS authorities regarding triage and transport of burn patients	1

#	Criterion	Criterion level
34	The burn center director is responsible for the approval of privileges for physicians participating in the burn service based on medical staff credentialing process	1
35	The burn center director is responsible for the development and active participation in internal and external continuing medical education programs in the care and prevention of burn injuries	1
36	Burn center director is responsible for direction and active participation in the burn center Quality and Process Improvement Programs	1
37	The burn center director is responsible for the communications on a regular basis with referring physicians regarding patients who have been transferred	1
38	In the event that the Burn Center Director is not available an accessible burn center staff surgeon is designated for administrative or clinical decisions	1
39	The Burn Center Director regularly participates in regional, national, or international burn meetings	1
40	The Burn Center Director has directed the total burn care of 50 or more acutely burned patients annually over a 3-year period	1
41	The Burn Center Director demonstrates ongoing involvement in burn-related research, community education, continuing medical education, prevention efforts, and local regional or national burn advocacy	1
42	Attending staff burn surgeons are licensed surgeons with board certification by American Board of Surgery, American Board of Plastic Surgery or equivalent based on review by Verification Committee	1
43	Attending staff burn surgeons have demonstrated expertise in burn treatment as evidenced by completion of a 1-year fellowship in burn treatment or by 2 or more years of mentored experience in the management of patients with acute burn injuries	1
44	Each attending staff surgeon must participate in continuing medical education in burn treatment	1
45	Attending staff surgeons have current ABLS (or equivalent) training	2
46	Each attending staff surgeon has participated, including primary decision-making, in the care of 35 or more acutely burned patients annually	1
47	The burn center maintains an on-call schedule for residents, qualified health care professionals, and attending staff surgeons for continuous responsibility of burn patients	1
48	All physicians (and physician extenders) who are routinely responsible for the care of burn patients conform to burn center criteria documenting appropriate training, patient care experience, continuing medical education, and commitment to the care of the burned patient	1
49	All physicians (and physician extenders) participating in the burn service are credentialed by the hospital medical staff credentialing process and are approved by the burn center director	1
50	Assigned burn center medical staff are promptly available on a 24-h basis	1
51	Specialty consultants (e.g., nephrology, cardiology, neurosurgery) are available in a timely manner determined by the acuity of the diagnosis	2
52	A dedicated anesthesia team with burn experience is available for the burn operating theater	2
53	The nurse manager is a licensed registered nurse (RN) in the state the burn center resides with a minimum of a baccalaureate degree in nursing	1
54	There is at least one nurse manager who is administratively responsible for the nursing care provided within the burn center for the unit he/she is assigned	1
55	In the eyes of the site reviewers, a nurse manager must have sufficient experience in burns and nursing leadership to lead the staff and manage the nursing program of the burn center	1
56	An organizational chart outlines the relationship between the nurse manager and other members of the burn team	2
57	An acuity-based or alternative equivalent staffing system is in place to determine nurse-staffing needs for patients in the burn center	2
58	There is a burn-specific competency-based training and continuing educational program for all nurses assigned to the burn center	1
59	The burn nurse manager routinely participates in multidisciplinary patient care rounds and there is adequate dissemination to the nursing staff	1
60	The nurse manager attends burn-specific continuing educational opportunities at least once every 2 years. These requirements can be addressed by attending regional, national, or international burn meetings; being an ABLS instructor; and being involved in the ABA	1
61	There is nurse representation within burn center quality improvement/performance improvement processes	1
62	A comprehensive rehabilitation program is designed for burned patients within 24 h of admission	1
63	Physical and occupational therapists in the burn center are appropriately licensed in their respective disciplines and demonstrate ongoing continuing education in burn rehabilitation	1
64	Therapy staffing is based upon burn center inpatient and therapy-specific outpatient activity with at least one designated full-time equivalent burn physical therapist and one occupational therapist but more depending on center volume	1
65	In-patients with an active rehabilitation plan must have care delivered as prescribed in the evaluation which should determine duration and frequency based on acuity, include goals, outcome, and plan for follow-up	1
66	Burn therapy services are provided 7 days per week for care of burn inpatients	1

#	Criterion	Criterion level
67	Burn therapists participate in multidisciplinary rounds and quality improvement	1
68	There is a competency-based burn therapy training program for all therapists assigned to the burn center	2
69	Therapists assigned to the burn unit must demonstrate burn therapy competence after initial training and at a minimum of once every 2 years	2
70	Burn team members are provided with a minimum of one regional, national, or international burn-related continuing education opportunity annually or demonstrate annual participation in internal educational process specific to burn care	2
71	Social service consultation is available to the burn service 7 days per week and on an as-needed basis in off-hours	1
72	A dietitian with adequate critical care and burn experience is available on a daily basis for consultation	1
73	A pharmacist with adequate critical care and burn experience is available on a 24-h basis	1
74	Respiratory therapists are available for the assessment and management of patients on the burn service on a continuous basis	1
75	A child life/recreational therapist is available for children cared for in the unit (for Pediatric Burn Centers)	1
76	A psychologist or psychiatrist is available to the burn service on an as-needed basis	1
77	The burn center has appropriate outpatient facilities to care for new outpatients and discharged patients	1
78	The outpatient facility ideally should be an integral and physical part of the burn center and should ideally be contiguous with/adjacent to the in-patient unit	2
79	If the outpatient services are at a site remote to the burn center, there must be adequate facilities for wound care	2
80	Outpatient examination room must be of adequate size to allow for dressing changes, wound cleansing, splinting, casting, and reapplication of wound dressings	1
81	The outpatient facility must be able to provide for appropriate pain management during wound care	2
82	For continuity of care, staffing of the outpatient area should be by multidisciplinary experienced burn team members approved by the burn center director and nurse manager	2
83	The outpatient staff participates in weekly multidisciplinary burn conferences and the burn center PI program	1
84	The burn center follows >75% of all patients who transition to the outpatient setting	1
85	The burn center provides coordinated transition of care to the outpatient status	1
86	The burn center provides appropriate follow-up after hospital discharge	1
87	The burn center provides brief psychological screening/intervention	1
88	The burn center provides evaluation of patient developmental status	2
89	The burn center provides access to burn-specific OT/PT evaluation and treatment	2
90	The burn center provides access to reconstructive surgery	2
91	The burn center provides access to peer support groups (such as but not exclusively a Phoenix Society SOAR program)	2
92	The burn center provides access to social service, pharmacist, and dietary consultations as needed	2
93	The burn center provides access to vocational counseling	2
94	No more than 5% of hospital admissions are transferred to another acute care facility	1
95	Physiatrist consultation is available	2
96	The burn center coordinates with local and/or regional rehabilitation centers for inpatient rehabilitation	1
97	The burn center coordinates with local and/or regional outpatient facilities for ongoing outpatient therapy needs of patients needing rehabilitation after discharge	1
98	The burn center director is responsible for the risk-adjusted performance improvement program	1
99	A multidisciplinary burn center committee oversees the performance improvement program, meets at least quarterly, and is integrated into the hospital QI structure	1
100	Sufficient QI documentation is available to verify problems, identify opportunities for improvement, resolve the problem, and provide loop-closure	1
101	The morbidity and mortality conferences are held at least monthly	1
102	The morbidity and mortality conferences include specialist peer staff members other than those practicing in the burn center	1
103	The morbidity and mortality conferences include discussion of all life-threatening complications and deaths with classification according to level of concern and preventability	1
104	The morbidity and mortality conferences include documentation of loop closure	1
105	The morbidity and mortality conferences are attended by clinical team members involved in the direct care of the burn patients who participate in at least 50% of the morbidity and mortality conferences	1
106	Sentinel events are discussed in a timely manner at multidisciplinary intensive reviews during which time a non-involved peer leads a discussion with all involved parties and areas for improvement and loop closure are identified	1
107	The burn service conducts audits of their benchmarked outcomes data (using available resources such as NBR, UHC, NHSN, or CMS) at least quarterly	1
108	The burn center develops ongoing PI projects to create a culture of safety and promote value-based programs	1
109	The burn center has policies for infection control with regular monitoring for hospital-acquired infections, multi-drug-resistant organisms, and compliance	1

#	Criterion	Criterion level
110	The burn center participates in the ABA's National Burn Repository and submits data every year	1
111	The burn center database includes all patients who are admitted to the burn center hospital for burn care	1
112	Burn team members are provided with a minimum of one regional, national, or international burn-related continuing education opportunity annually OR demonstrate annual participation in internal educational process specific to burn care	1
113	A burn center orientation and ongoing continuing education program documents staff competencies specific to age-appropriate care and treatment of burn patients, including critical care, wound care, and rehabilitation	1
114	The burn center offers regional education related to emergency and inpatient burn care such as that included the ABA Advanced Burn Life Support course	2
115	For centers that have residents involved in care of the burn patients an orientation program is provided for new residents	2
116	The burn center staff participates regularly in public burn outreach programs	2
117	Burn center staff is involved in local, regional, national, or international prevention outreach efforts	1
118	Burn center multidisciplinary staff under the leadership of the burn center director, work locally, regionally, or nationally to advocate for burn-related two health care issues	1
119	The burn center multidisciplinary staff is involved in research (including basic science, clinical, industry-sponsored, QI, multi-center) and presents posters or oral presentations at hospital based, regional, national, or international meetings	2

Summary Box

This chapter addresses issues mainly related to the construction and administration of the burn center paradigm, where centralized burn care is advocated due to decreasing incidence of burns in the western world, in conjunction with the outcome data that supports the specialized and improved care provided at such centers. A leading theme in the staffing process of burn centers has over the years been with a focus on care based on the multidisciplinary team, which has the ability to provide all the aspects specific for the advanced needs of the patients with burns. Furthermore, the chapter also examines ideas and factors important for the improvement and quality of burn care. Particularly quality indicators, guidelines, and the burn center verification process are addressed.

References

1. Abdelrahman I, Elmasry M, Olofsson P, et al. Division of overall duration of stay into operative stay and postoperative stay improves the overall estimate as a measure of quality of outcome in burn care. PLoS One. 2017;12(3):e0174579. https://doi.org/10.1371/journal.pone.0174579.
2. Brusselaers N, Monstrey S, Vogelaers D, et al. Severe burn injury in Europe: a systematic review of the incidence, etiology, morbidity, and mortality. Crit Care. 2010;14(5):R188. https://doi.org/10.1186/cc9300. cc9300 [pii]. [Published Online First: 2010/10/21].
3. Smolle C, Cambiaso-Daniel J, Forbes AA, et al. Recent trends in burn epidemiology worldwide: a systematic review. Burns. 2017;43(2):249–57. https://doi.org/10.1016/j.burns.2016.08.013.
4. Peck MD. Epidemiology of burns throughout the world. Part I: distribution and risk factors. Burns. 2011;37(7):1087–100. https://doi.org/10.1016/j.burns.2011.06.005.
5. Dokter J, Vloemans AF, Beerthuizen GI, et al. Epidemiology and trends in severe burns in the Netherlands. Burns. 2014;40(7):1406–14. https://doi.org/10.1016/j.burns.2014.03.003.
6. Mason SA, Nathens AB, Byrne JP, et al. Trends in the epidemiology of major burn injury among hospitalized patients: a population-based analysis. J Trauma Acute Care Surg. 2017;83(5):867–74. https://doi.org/10.1097/TA.0000000000001586.
7. Light TD, Latenser BA, Kealey GP, et al. The effect of burn center and burn center volume on the mortality of burned adults—an analysis of the data in the National Burn Repository. J Burn Care Res. 2009;30(5):776–82. https://doi.org/10.1097/BCR.0b013e3181b47ed2.
8. Monafo WW. Then and now: 50 years of burn treatment. Burns. 1992;18(Suppl 2):S7–S10.
9. Hardwicke J, Kohlhardt A, Moiemen N. The Birmingham Burn Centre archive: a photographic history of post-war burn care in the United Kingdom. Burns. 2015;41(4):680–8. https://doi.org/10.1016/j.burns.2015.01.008.
10. Elmasry M, Steinvall I, Abdelrahman I, et al. Changes in patterns of treatment of burned children at the Linkoping Burn Centre, Sweden, 2009-2014. Burns. 2017;43(5):1111–9. https://doi.org/10.1016/j.burns.2017.02.009.
11. Win TS, Nizamoglu M, Maharaj R, et al. Relationship between multidisciplinary critical care and burn patients survival: a propensity-matched national cohort analysis. Burns. 2018;44(1):57–64. https://doi.org/10.1016/j.burns.2017.11.003.
12. http://euroburn.org/documents-2/. Assessed http://euroburn.org/wp-content/uploads/2014/09/EBA-Guidelines-Version-4-2017-1.pdf.
13. Vrouwe SQ, Jeschke MG, Fish JS. Are we headed for a shortage of burn care providers in Canada? Burns. 2018;44(4):1000–4. https://doi.org/10.1016/j.burns.2017.11.009.
14. Mason SA, Nathens AB, Byrne JP, et al. Burn center care reduces acute health care utilization after discharge: a population-based analysis of 1,895 survivors of major burn injury. Surgery. 2017;162(4):891–900. https://doi.org/10.1016/j.surg.2017.05.018. [Published Online First: 2017/07/18].
15. Ahuja RB. ISBI PRACTICE GUIDELINES FOR BURN CARE: editorial. Burns. 2016;42(5):951–2. https://doi.org/10.1016/j.burns.2016.06.020.
16. Allwood J, Desmond L. Keeping on track with NATIONAL TRACS/ABA Burn Registry. J Burn Care Rehabil. 1998;19(1 Pt 1):66–72. [Published Online First: 1998/03/21].
17. Cassidy TJ, Edgar DW, Phillips M, et al. Transfer time to a specialist burn service and influence on burn mortality in Australia and New Zealand: a multi-centre, hospital based retrospective cohort study. Burns. 2015;41(4):735–41. https://doi.org/10.1016/j.burns.2015.01.016.
18. Donabedian A. The quality of medical care. Science. 1978;200(4344):856–64. [Published Online First: 1978/05/26].

19. Donabedian A. Evaluating the quality of medical care. 1966. Milbank Q. 2005;83(4):691–729. https://doi.org/10.1111/j.1468-0009.2005.00397.x. [Published Online First: 2005/11/11].
20. Sjoberg F, Walther S. Intensive care registries and the evolution of the concept of 'quality of care'—reflections from the 10-year anniversary symposium of the Swedish Intensive Care Registry. Acta Anaesthesiol Scand. 2012;56(9):1073–7. https://doi.org/10.1111/j.1399-6576.2012.02757.x. [Published Online First: 2012/09/13].
21. Engrav LH, Heimbach DM, Rivara FP, et al. Harborview burns—1974 to 2009. PLoS One. 2012;7(7):e40086. https://doi.org/10.1371/journal.pone.0040086.
22. Cleland H, Greenwood JE, Wood FM, et al. The Burns Registry of Australia and New Zealand: progressing the evidence base for burn care. Med J Aust. 2016;204(5):1951e–7. [Published Online First: 2016/03/18].
23. Cornell RG, Feller I, Roi LD, et al. Evaluation of burn care utilizing a national burn registry. Emerg Med Serv. 1978;7(6):107–14, 116–7. [Published Online First: 1978/10/09].
24. Watterson D, Cleland H, Darton A, et al. Developing clinical quality indicators for a Bi-National Burn Registry. Burns. 2011;37(8):1296–308. https://doi.org/10.1016/j.burns.2011.08.007. [Published Online First: 2011/10/04].
25. Steinvall I, Elmasry M, Fredrikson M, et al. Standardised mortality ratio based on the sum of age and percentage total body surface area burned is an adequate quality indicator in burn care: an exploratory review. Burns. 2016;42(1):28–40. https://doi.org/10.1016/j.burns.2015.10.032.
26. Jackson PC, Hardwicke J, Bamford A, et al. Revised estimates of mortality from the Birmingham Burn Centre, 2001-2010: a continuing analysis over 65 years. Ann Surg. 2014;259(5):979–84. https://doi.org/10.1097/SLA.0b013e31829160ca.
27. Bull JP, Squire JR. A study of mortality in a burns unit: standards for the evaluation of alternative methods of treatment. Ann Surg. 1949;130(2):160–73. [Published Online First: 1949/08/01].
28. Hussain A, Dunn KW. Predicting length of stay in thermal burns: a systematic review of prognostic factors. Burns. 2013;39(7):1331–40. https://doi.org/10.1016/j.burns.2013.04.026.
29. Johnson LS, Shupp JW, Pavlovich AR, et al. Hospital length of stay—does 1% TBSA really equal 1 day? J Burn Care Res. 2011;32(1):13–9. https://doi.org/10.1097/BCR.0b013e318204b3ab.
30. American Burn Association and American College of Surgeons Committee of Trauma. Guidelines for the operation of burn centers. J Burn Care Res. 2007;28(1):134–41.

Part II

Pre-hospital and Initial Management of Burns

10 The First Responders' Role in Managing Burn Care

Ken Webb

10.1 Introduction[1]

In the prehospital setting, there are a variety of first responders whose actions can have an impact on patient outcomes.

Prior to a patient finding their way to a facility where definitive care can be provided, first responders (often from different agencies), having a variety of skill sets and expertise, will perform a host of interventions to help the burn patient have the opportunity to have an optimal outcome. While rescuing, initiating and managing the care, and transporting the patient, there are a host of considerations and actions that require attention.

There needs to be a coordinated and collaborative approach to incident management between agencies. Police is the agency responsible for managing pedestrian (civilian) and vehicle traffic as well as securing a perimeter beyond the cold zone while supporting the movements and activities of the primary and secondary response agencies. The Emergency Medical Services (EMS) agency is the authority having jurisdiction for patient care. They will work with police and fire services to manage patient care through hazard mitigation to transport to definitive care. Fire services are usually the only all hazards response agency in the jurisdiction. Fire services will typically be responsible for the mechanics associated with life safety, hazard mitigation, initial patient care, and extrication of the affected parties.

A chapter in a textbook can never fully capture the scope and the nuisances of what can be required of the different agencies that respond to an emergency scene. This chapter is written from a fire service response perspective as it supports the overall response to any given incident. In many parts of Canada, fire services are trained to the emergency medical responder level and provide basic life support (BLS) care. This chapter is written from that perspective. All due respect should be afforded those agencies who are trained to deliver a higher level of care, including several fire services, that have advanced life support (ALS) capacity and response partners from EMS.

Fire and EMS service provider responses (BLS and ALS) and assessment and treatment protocols will be governed by local protocols and subject to medical oversight, direction, and quality assurance.

10.2 Responder/Patient Safety Considerations

As with all emergency scenes, the responders typically have a limited amount of control over what they will encounter in their inherited workspace. First responders do not have the luxury of working in relatively sanitary and controlled emergency rooms, treatment rooms, or operating rooms. There are a multitude of response considerations prior to the tones going off, the wheels moving, and the firefighters arrival on scene.

The mnemonic EMCA-P (Environment, Mechanism of Injury, Casualty Count, Assistance Required and Personal Protective Equipment) is a useful tool to help the first responder prepare to process the emergency they will inherit.

[1] From fall 2006 through spring 2015, Ken Webb was the Toronto Fire Services, Firefighter Prehospital Care, Program Manager at the Sunnybrook Centre for Prehospital Medicine. In this position, Ken oversaw program development, program deployment, and quality assurance for the Resuscitation Outcomes Consortium (ROC) participation in research to improve outcomes of patient suffering sudden cardiac arrests and a first responder symptom relief program for patients suffering anaphylactic reactions. Much of the material for this chapter was gleaned from the work performed during this period of time. Please consider this body of work as reference for this chapter: "TFS Education." Sunnybrook Centre for Prehospital Medicine. http://www.prehospitalmedicine.ca/tfs-education/.

K. Webb (✉)
Toronto Professional Firefighters Association,
Toronto, ON, Canada
e-mail: webb@torontofirefighters.org

M. G. Jeschke et al. (eds.), *Handbook of Burns Volume 1*, https://doi.org/10.1007/978-3-030-18940-2_10

10.2.1 Environment (E)

There are potential hazards associated with the uncontrolled environments that responders encounter. Responders are expected to quickly gain an appreciation of the potential hazards associated with the environment and to find ways to mitigate/manage the hazards so as to limit potential harm to them and to make the environment safer for the patient.

Is it winter? Is it summer? Is night or day? Is this a nuclear facility? Is the high-rise or house fire? Is this a chemical or biology laboratory at an educational facility or a laboratory at an industrial facility? Is this an electrical installation? Is it a biological waste handling facility? Is this an incident that is the result of a motor vehicle collision on a major highway or a busy intersection?

10.2.2 Mechanism of Injury (M)

How did the patient receive their burns?

There are many ways that patients can receive burns. Here are some of the ways and some hazard mitigation considerations:

- Thermal/flame burns—remove from the heat source, put out the fire
- Chemical—dilute, wash off, brush away if dry chemical
- Electrical—turn off the power, consider entry and exit wounds
- Nuclear—shielding and distance from the radioactive source are typically the appropriate measures

10.2.3 Casualty Count (C)

Triage should occur as survivors/patients are encountered to help establish the types of responders and transport capabilities that will be required.

Informing the closest emergency departments and specialized burn centers about the number of patients and estimated burn severity can help these facilities prepare for patient surges and make preliminary decisions about where different patients should be sent to.

10.2.4 Assistance Required (A)

Should command contact any public utilities or municipal services to support the operation? Are specialty fire apparatus required—hazmat, technical rescue? Would the patient benefit by having advanced life support (ALS) paramedic care, if available?

10.2.5 Personal Protective Equipment: PPE (P)

The rescuer should not become part of the problem. It is the individual's and the incident management team's responsibility to ensure the appropriate level of PPE is worn for the different types of hazards.

10.3 Arrival on Scene

In 2013, the International Association of Fire Fighters (IAFF) Charitable Foundation in collaboration with the American Burn Association published a guide for first responders, *First Responder Guide to Burn Injury Assessment & Treatment. Section 1: First Responder Initial Assessment and Management Procedures* that provides a five-step process to assist responders:

1. Stop the Burning Process
2. Initial Patient Assessment
3. Management of the Burn and Burn-Related Problems
4. Further Patient Management
5. Transport and Transfer
6. Management of Multiple-Burn Casualties

10.3.1 Stop the Burning Process

The basic "rule of thumb" is to cool, cool, cool, while taking into account considerations to what has caused the burn.

10.3.1.1 Thermal/Flame Burns

For thermal/flame burns, removing the patient from the burning environment, extinguishing and removing the burning clothing is a good start. Synthetic material/fabric will retain heat and will require active cooling. When removing burnt items of clothing be aware that deeper tissue involvement combined with synthetic material adhering to the wound requires responder attention and care. If material is adhering to a wound, carefully cut away clothing not adhering to the skin and leave the material remaining in the wound and actively cool (flush with water). Material/fabric adhering to the wound should not be removed on-scene as it can cause further tissue damage.

The cooling process requires a clean and reliable water source. Once removed from a reliable water source, during transport as an example, saline is typically what is used to continue cooling.

10.3.1.2 Chemical Burns

HAZMAT (hazardous material)/CBRNE (Chemical, Biological, Radiological, Nuclear, and Explosive) expertise may be required early in the incident so as to limit responder exposures. Emergency response guides are typically available to first responding fire-fighting crews. These are very helpful during the early stages of scene size-up and help the incident commander make decisions about responder safety, shielding, evacuation zones, etc. consult Material Safety Data Sheets (MSDS) and to utilize on-site specialists when they are available to provide information about the product and how best to protect the first responder from potential exposures and to remove the chemical from the patient's body tissue. Continuous flushing of the body area with running water is quite often what is prescribed to cool the burning, dilute/neutralize the substance. Acids and bases are common chemical properties. Acids should not be used to neutralize bases and vice versa; water is the best neutralizer.

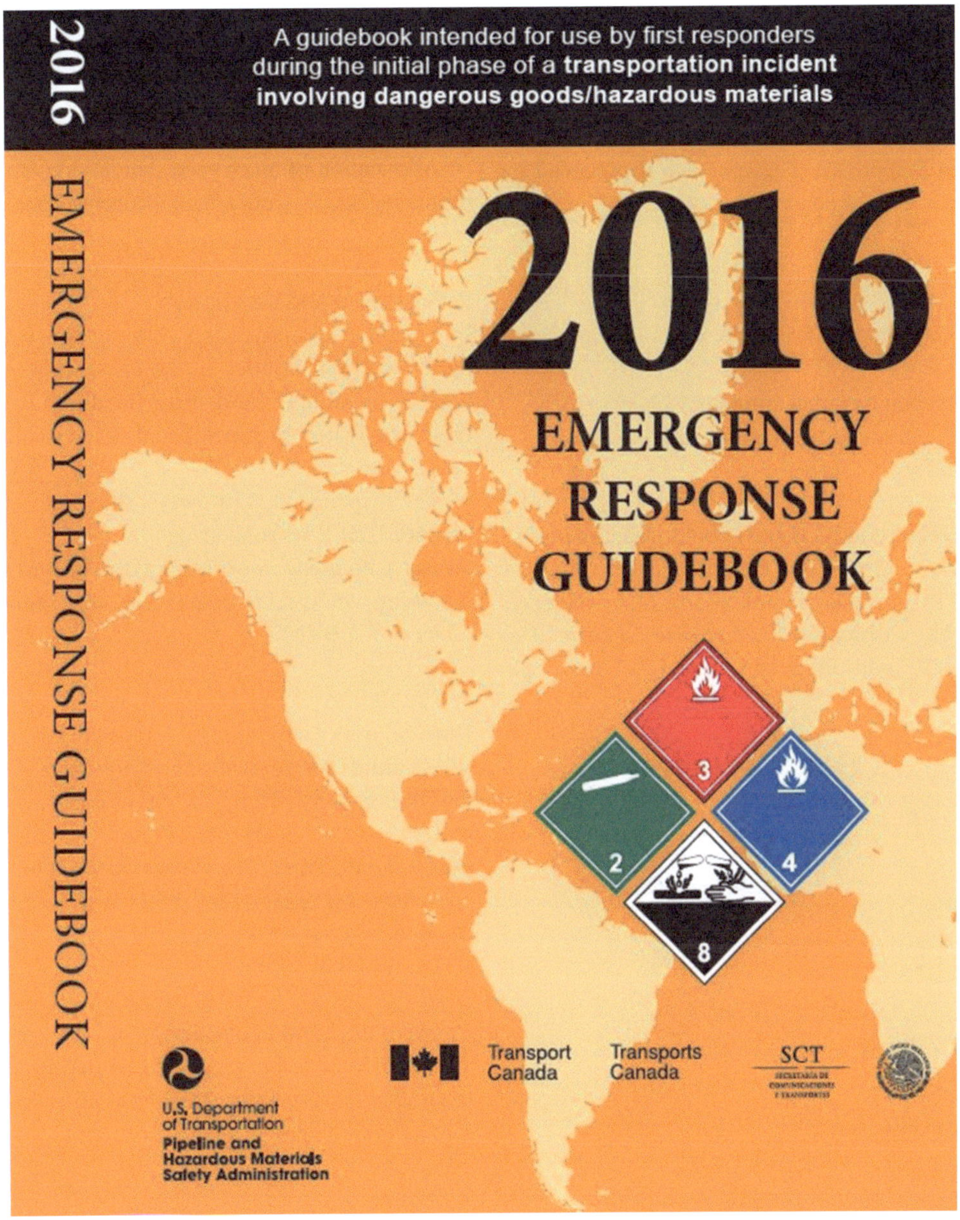

(© *2016 Emergency Response Guidebook*; source Transport Canada website; https://www.tc.gc.ca/eng/canutec/guide-menu-227.htm)

When a chemical comes in contact with body tissue and it causes a burn, it will continue burning while it remains in contact with the tissue. It is important for the first responder to

10.3.1.3 Electrical Burns

Responder safety is the priority. Turning off/eliminating the energy source may be as simple as unplugging an appliance and as complicated as having your local power authority turn off/isolate energy to the area in which you will be performing a rescue or providing initial patient assessment and care.

10.3.2 Initial Patient Assessment

Section 1: First Responder Initial Assessment and Management Procedures went onto suggest the utilization of the A-B-C-D-E-H 2 approach. The approach is preceded by assess the patient's level of consciousness (LOC). The mnemonic AVPU is useful for assessing LOC.

AVPU

- A—Alert; acknowledge rescuers presence and engage in interaction
- V—Verbal; respond to verbal stimulus
- P—Pain; have a response to a painful stimulus
- U—Unresponsive

An altered level of consciousness could indicate potential acute carbon monoxide poisoning, neurological impairment due to a trauma, or potentially other underlying conditions that will require further investigation. The mnemonics AEIOU and TIPS can be helpful with this investigation.

AEIOU TIPS

- A—Alcohol
- E—Epilepsy
- I—Insulin
- O—Overdose
- U—Uremia
- T—Trauma
- I—Infection
- P—Psychiatric
- S—Syncope

10.3.2.1 A-B-C-D-E-H

A: Airway Management with C-Spine Protection

Assess the airway for patency. Consider the mechanism of injury when assessing the airway. Is their soot around the nose? Is there swelling and soft tissue injuries in and around the airway that could result in the airway becoming blocked by edema? Superheated gases associated with fires can severely compromise a patient's airway. Airway compromise associated with the products of combustion can happen very quickly; constant monitoring of the status of the airway is critical.

Can the airway be opened easily with a head tilt chin lift? Is there possible c-spine injuries that would necessitate a jaw thrust to open and maintain the airway? The responder airway should be prepared to aggressively manage the airway. BLS skills and adjuncts (oropharyngeal OPA and supraglottic airways) may not be enough to secure a patent airway. Advanced airways (endotracheal intubation) that can secure the lower airway may be necessary. If these resources are available in your jurisdiction, they should be activated as soon as possible. Airway compromise in burn victims is a highly probable life-threatening concern.

Application of an oxygen delivery devise such as a non-rebreather mask would be appropriate therapy for all burn patients.

B: Breathing and Ventilation

Is breathing effective and sufficient to support life? Are there structural injuries to the chest limiting the effectiveness of breathing? Ineffective breathing or the absence of breathing is life threatening and needs to be resolved or the patient can die.

The responder's skill level will dictate how breathing is managed. BLS responders can use an OPA or a superglottic airway with a bag valve mask (BVM) to assist the patient's breathing while ALS responders will utilize endotracheal tubes with a BVM.

C: Circulation

Burn injuries often result in a rapid reassignment of fluids. These fluids cause swelling at the burn sights and divert the fluids away from the circulatory system. The burn patient's blood pressure should be monitored. Rapid assessment of the effectiveness can include pulse checks and electronic assessment (Electrocardiogram ECG) needs to be monitored.

Follow local protocols related to fluid replacement.

D: Disability (Brain Function)

This should have been considered during the LOC assessment, but the responder should use this opportunity to reassess and investigate further at this point.

E: Expose

If the affected areas had not been exposed during the "Stop the Burning" step, now would be a good time to perform this action. The responder's goal should continue to be to find ways to minimize the effects of the burning process so as to minimize further injury. The goal should be to find ways to minimize the opportunities for the patient to get worse. Here are some considerations during this step:

1. Jewelry can store heat energy and should be removed if it is likely to continue to transfer heat to the body.
2. Edema is associated with burns; rings on fingers should be removed from fingers and toes should there be the potential for swelling in these digits.
3. A rapid trauma assessment should be considered to see if there might be other injuries to the body; electrocution injuries can result in fractures and neurological deficits while blunt force trauma associated with falling debris in structure fires are easily missed if the rescuer is focused on the burn injury.
4. Debriding of imbedded melted material should not occur in the field so as to minimize the potential of causing further injury during the removal.
5. Initial assessment of the severity of the burn will also occur at this step.

The mnemonics CLAPS-D and TICS-D would be appropriate to use as part of a rapid trauma/body assessment (neck to knees) where undiscovered injuries could be life threatening if they are not discovered and managed.

The responder should look for:

- C—Contusions
- L—Lacerations
- A—Abrasions
- P—Penetrations
- S—Swelling/Symmetry
- D—Deformities/Distention

After looking for these injuries, the responder should palpate the body and assess for:

- T—Tenderness
- I—Instability
- C—Crepitus
- S—Subcutaneous Emphysema
- D—Deformity/Distention

Life-threatening injuries should be treated when found.

H: History

SAMPLE is a mnemonic that will be a helpful tool for gathering and managing information that can be passed onto the next level of care while the mnemonic OPQRST can be useful to gather information about pain.

S: Signs/Symptoms

An assessment of "Signs" requires the responder to use all their senses.

Can you see the patient has partial thickness burns to most of their chest and they are having difficulty moving air? Can you see soot around the patient's nose and mouth? Can you here "noisy" breathing? Can you smell the unforgettable sent of burning flesh? Can you see tissue involvement beyond the surrounding unbroken skin? Can you see entry and exit wounds associated with electrical burn injuries?

What can the patient tell you about their "symptoms"; pain they are feeling as a result of the incident? The mnemonic OPQRST can be helpful.

O: Onset

What were you doing when you started to feel the burning? When did you get burnt? Was the onset of pain gradual or rapid?

P: Provocation

What where you doing when you got burnt? Is there anything that makes you feel better or worse?

Q: Quality

Describe the pain to me? What does the pain feel like? (Avoid providing a "menu" as the patient is likely to pick from the menu just to shut you up.)

R: Radiation

Point to where it hurts the most and let me know if you feel pain anywhere else.

S: Severity

On a scale from 1 to 10, ten being the worst pain you have ever felt, rate your pain? (Don't be surprised if you get an answer like "20".)

T: Time

How long has the pain been going on? Has there been any change in the pain since the onset?

A: Allergies

Do you have any allergies? This may become important if the patient is allergic to antibiotics.

M: Medications

Are you taking any medications? What do you take the medications for? Where are your medications?

If readily available, the responder should gather medications for transport with the patient to a health care facility. The patient's heath card (medical insurance) would also be good to obtain should it be available.

P: Past Medical History

Are there any medical conditions you have that we should be aware of?

E: Event Leading

You may have already captured this information during the OPQRST component of your interview. If this information has yet to be gathered, this should be a reminder to find out or reconfirm what the patient was doing when they sustained their burns.

10.3.3 Management of the Burn and Burn-Related Problems

While managing the care for any type burn patient, attention needs to be paid to airway, breathing, and circulation. Airways can become narrowed due to edema caused by exposure to superheated gases and chemical exposures. Breathing could be compromised by superheated gases/chemicals damaging the lungs or by a decreased ability to effectively expand the thoracic cavity as a result of burns to the chest. Circulation could be compromised as a result of the adverse affects of a chemical exposure or electrocution.

A careful balance is required between cooling and helping the patient maintain body temperature as a result of a decreased ability to self-regulate temperature. Once the flame is out and active cooling has been provided, open wounds require the placement of dry, sterile, burn sheets so as to decrease potential for infection. Wet dressings can cause issues with the body's thermo-regulating system and possibly promote infection.

Chemical burns to the eye are common and require copious and continuous flow of water/saline to remove/dilute the chemical and stop the burning process. Avoid flushing chemicals from the affected eye to the non-affected eye. Consider removing contact lenses if possible as chemicals can become trapped under the lens, prolonging the exposure to the chemical.

Similar to synthetic clothing/fabric adhering to body tissue, hot tar creates a similar issue. The same rules apply in these types of burns; cool, cool, cool, do not remove the hardened tar that has adhered to underlying burnt tissue and transport to a burn center.

There are a variety of underlying/internal issues related to electrical burns, beyond the outward presenting burns, which should be considered when managing the initial care for patients who have suffered an electrical injury. These include but are not limited to:

- Cardiac issues; ventricular fibrillation, cardiac arrest
- Burns below the surface; muscle, tissue damage, and fractures
- Neurological damage; seizures
- Entry and exit wounds

Pain management is a challenge. First responders will encounter patients suffering with pain associated with their burns. The active cooling by using volumes of water poured over the burn area may not provide sufficint relief. BLS providers may be allowed to assist the patient to take their own oral pain relief medication (ibuprophin). An ALS provider is likely able to administer IV analgesics like morphine.

10.3.4 Further Patient Management

Ongoing monitoring of LOC and vital signs should occur while the patient is awaiting transport through to transport to a higher level of care.

Ongoing assessment of burn injuries and changes in status should be monitored and documented.

Splinting and bandaging should be considered so as to limit the potential of further injury during transport. In general, dressings and bandages should be applied loosely so as to allow for swelling and to avoid cutting off distal circulation. When practical, pre- and post-packaging assessment of distal circulation, sensation, and mobility should occur so as to limit the likelihood that the treatment does not make the patient's condition worse.

Loose/partial packaging will provide appropriate protection while allowing for assessment by the higher level of care during any transfer of care.

10.3.5 Transport and Transfer

Burn patients require attention by a higher level of care than is available outside a health care facility. Rapid transport to definitive care is ideal. Access to the closest emergency room may be necessary to provide appropriate care prior to transport to a burn center.

Consider the utilizing the American Burn Association's *Burn Center Referral Criteria'* document:

Courtesy of the
American Burn Association
Advanced Burn Life Support (ABLS)
Learn more about the ABA and ABLS at **www.ameriburn.org**

Burn Center Referral Criteria

A burn center may treat adults, children, or both.

Burn injuries that should be referred to a burn center include:

1. Partial thickness burns greater than 10% total body surface area (TBSA).
2. Burns that involve the face, hands, feet, genitalia, perineum, or major joints.
3. Third degree burns in any age group.
4. Electrical burns, including lightning injury.
5. Chemical burns.
6. Inhalation injury.
7. Burn injury in patients with preexisting medical disorders that could complicate management, prolong recovery, or affect mortality.
8. Any patient with burns and concomitant trauma (such as fractures) in which the burn injury poses the greatest risk of morbidity or mortality. In such cases, if the trauma poses the greater immediate risk, the patient may be initially stabilized in a trauma center before being transferred to a burn unit. Physician judgment will be necessary in such situations and should be in concert with the regional medical control plan and triage protocols.
9. Burned children in hospitals without qualified personnel or equipment for the care of children.
10. Burn injury in patients who will require special social, emotional, or rehabilitative intervention.

Excerpted from Guidelines for the Operation of Burn Centers (pp. 79-86), Resources for Optimal Care of the Injured Patient 2006, Committee on Trauma, American College of Surgeons

Severity Determination

First Degree (*Partial Thickness*)
Superficial, red, sometimes painful.

Second Degree (*Partial Thickness*)
Skin may be red, blistered, swollen. Very painful.

Third Degree (*Full Thickness*)
Whitish, charred or translucent, no pin prick sensation in burned area.

Percentage Total Body Surface Area (TBSA)

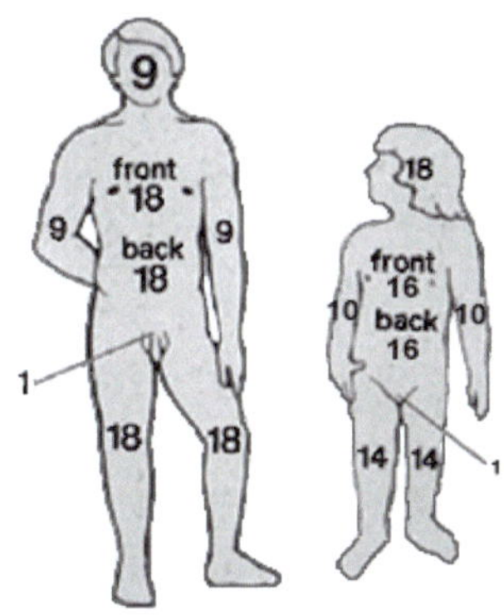

(Guidelines for the Operation of Burn Centers (pp. 79–86), Resources for Optimal Care of the Injured Patient 2006, Committee on Trauma, American College of Surgeons)

10.3.6 Management of Multiple-Burn Casualties

The *First Responder Guide to Burn Injury Assessment and Treatment* has made the following recommendations for triaging burn injury patients during multiple casualty incidents:

- *Triage Sorting Guidelines*
  - *The most critical patients, with a good likelihood of survival, are in the top priority.*
  - *Patients requiring emergency care soon, but not urgently, and having a good chance of recovery are in the next group.*

  - *Minor burn patients who can wait for care and the most critical patients with the least likelihood of survival are placed in the delayed categories.*
- *Triage Colored Tag Guidelines*
- *As patients are triaged, they are tagged with color tags to identify their category of care. Subsequent transport and definitive care are based on the category noted on the tag. The following criteria are common to triage tagging systems:*
  - *Immediate Care (Red)*
    - *Inhalation injury*
    - *Burns to more than 20% total body surface area (TBSA) in patients between ages 10 and 50 years (burns exceeding 20% can and will need fluid resuscitation)*
    - *Burns of more than 10% TBSA in patients age less than 10 or greater than 50 years*
    - *Chemical injury*
    - *Electrical injury*
    - *Associated, life-threatening injuries*
  - *Delayed Care (Yellow)*
    - *Burns of less than 20% TBSA in patients between the ages of 10 and 50 years*
    - *Full thickness burns of less than 5%*
- *Delayed Care (Green)*
  - *Minor injuries—not in need of emergency care (e.g., partial thickness burn to arms)*
- *Delayed Care (Black)*
  - *Survival unlikely (e.g., massive burns in elderly people)*

10.4 Special Populations

10.4.1 Geriatrics

These patients have gone through physiological changes that have a significant impact on how they can become burned, the severity of the burns, and how they recover. Neuropathways change in these patients making them less able to sense (feel) when they are being exposed to something that can cause a burn and slower to react making the time they are exposed to what is causing their burn last a little bit longer. A decreased brain mass can lead to a decreased ability to process stimuli from distal pain receptors, thus lengthening the time to send messages to withdraw from what is causing them pain.

Their skin has become thinner. This results in a decrease in pain receptors, reducing the number of signals being sent to the brain. The thin skin tissue can result in relatively minor exposures to causing catastrophic burn injuries. The decreased tissue available to begin with can result in much longer the healing processes.

Acute exposures to high temperatures can cause significant injuries in these patients due to their dulled sense of feeling and their slower reaction time. An example of this would be, while cooking, a patient reaches for an item in a cupboard above a stove. As they reach for the item they lose their balance and place their hand on the hot element of the stove.

The thermo-regulating system in these patients is often compromised and initial and ongoing management of their care becomes a challenge. Removing these individuals from what is causing their burns is a priority. Active cooling of the affected area is something that requires careful consideration.

Longer duration exposures to lower heat levels can cause significant burns due to the patient's dulled senses not providing enough stimuli to even realize they have sustained a burn. An example of this would be an elderly patient who uses a heat blanket or heating pad. A combination of a compromised thermo-regulating system and dulled senses could lead to the "cooking" of an area of the body where a prolonged exposure has occurred.

10.4.2 Pediatrics

These patients are susceptible to burn injuries. Their reduced body surface area make exposures potentially significantly worse; a 10 cm by 10 cm partial thickness thermal burn on the thorax of a 13-month-old baby would likely be worse that the same burn occurring to a 21-year-old patient. Pediatrics have proportionately smaller airways, increasing the negative impact of inhalation burn injuries; airways are smaller and tissue edema will narrow or block the airway more quickly.

Pediatric would benefit from the specialized ALS skill set as it relates to airway management. Early recognition that these recourses are required can mean the difference between life and death.

Pediatric patients have oral fixations; they learn about the world by putting items in their mouth. Electrical burns as a result of biting on energized electrical cords are not uncommon. These exposures can cause electrical dysfunction that can lead to cardiac arrest. The responder should prepare for that possibility. The energy delivered to the small body can also result in the other complications described earlier. Should the pediatric patient survive the impact of the initial exposure, a scab removed prematurely from the healing wound at the corner of the mouth can result in airway compromise complication and a circulation issue should there be significant blood loss.

10.5 Managing the Firefighter Removed from a Superheated Environment[2]

Providing a level of protection to firefighters as they enter superheated environments to save life and property has been a challenge taken on by industry through the centuries. Much work has been done over the last three decades to improve the quality of firefighter personal protective equipment (PPE). We are long removed from the minimal protection provided by hip waders and rain coats that were used by some of Canada's largest fire departments up to the early 1990s.

The 2018 PPE ensemble, combined with the latest in respiratory-protection devices, affords firefighters the best available opportunity to survive the hazards in a modern-construction dwelling containing materials that burn much more quickly and hotter than they did in 1990. The PPE industry and fire service professionals have worked diligently to use science and technological advancements to make significant improvements to PPE. Even with the advancements, situations still occur in which firefighters are seriously injured or killed as a result of acute exposure to the intense heat associated with hotter and faster-developing structure fires.

While attending the 2015 Canadian Burn Symposium in Toronto, listened to the harrowing story of Winnipeg firefighter Lionel Crowther. Lionel was working an overtime shift on the evening of Feb. 4, 2007, when he was dispatched as part of a response to a house fire. The circumstances of this event produced results that have changed Crowther's life. While attempting to conduct a primary search and initial interior fire attach Lionel and his crew encountered a change in fire conditions as a result of flow-path dynamics. Lionel suffered burns to 70% of his body, 30% of which were full-thickness burns. Captains Harold Lessard and Thomas Nichols died on scene and firefighter Ed Wiebe suffered injuries that put him in critical, but survivable, condition. Firefighters Darcy Funk and Scott Atchison sustained minor injuries.

Lionel was exposed to extreme heat levels for an extended period of time as he was unable to make an exit when fire conditions changed; he sustained burns that were likely caused by the compression of superheated gases trapped in his bunker gear. (For more about Crowther, go to https://afterthecocoon.com/burn-survivors/lionel-crowther/).

NFPA 1971 sets the minimum performance requirements for personal protective equipment (PPE) and also specifies the test methods by which the PPE is measured. The newest test is the stored energy test, which was added in 2013. Industry experts recognized the thermal protection offered by bunker gear also results in heat being stored in bunker gear. The trapped, superheated gas, when compressed at pinch points in the suit at the knees and the elbows, causes burns. Another common place where superheated gases are trapped is behind the backplate of the SCBA.

Lionel's story closely resembles that of Winnipeg firefighter Barry Borkowski, who suffered significant injuries on Oct. 9, 1994. Since retiring as a captain in 2005, Borkowski has worked to implement design changes to bunker gear.

The evolution of engineering of bunker gear has resulted in significant improvements in protection of firefighters; NFPA 1971 has evolved as a result of different types of firefighter injuries, and now measures more factors. But with the improvements have come some challenges: the retention of superheated gases inside the PPE envelope has resulted in burns during the handling of firefighters who have been removed from fires.

10.5.1 Common Burn Location in Firefighters

- Ears

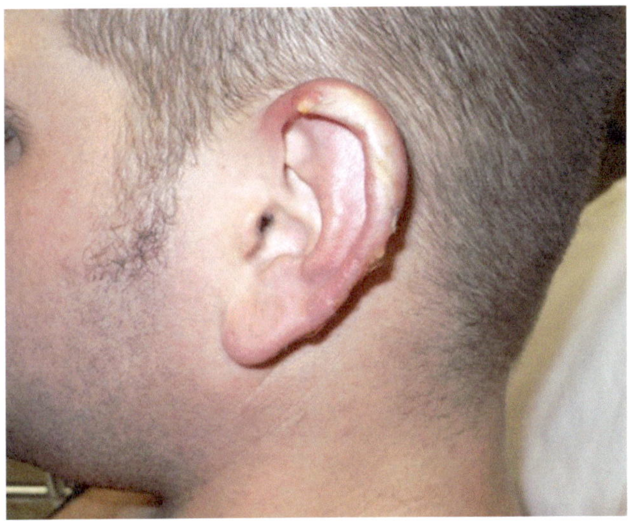

- Hands

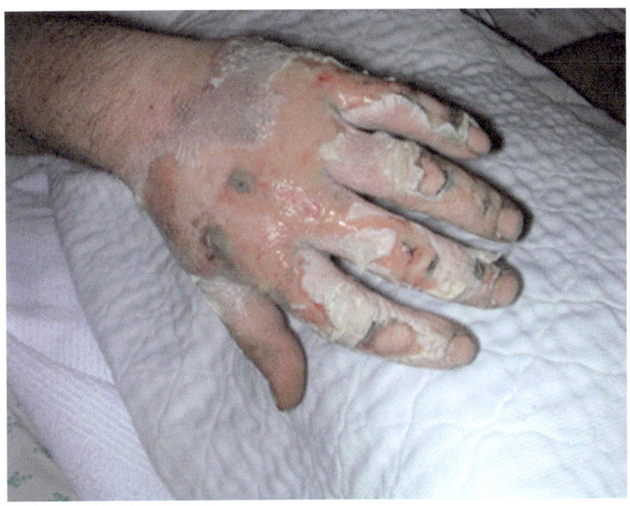

[2]Amended text first published in [...] with kind permission of © Fire Fighting in Canada | Canadian Firefighter...... All Rights Reserved.

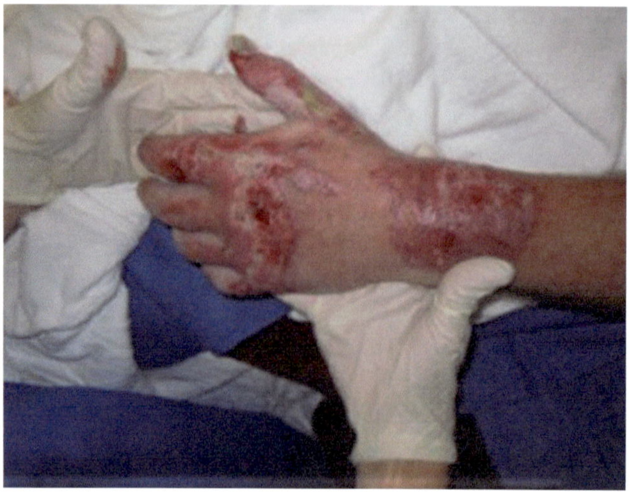

- Shoulders/Back

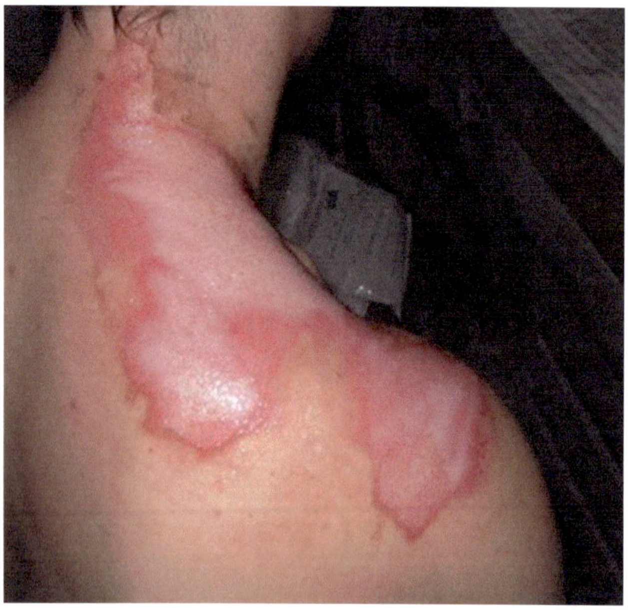

- Knees

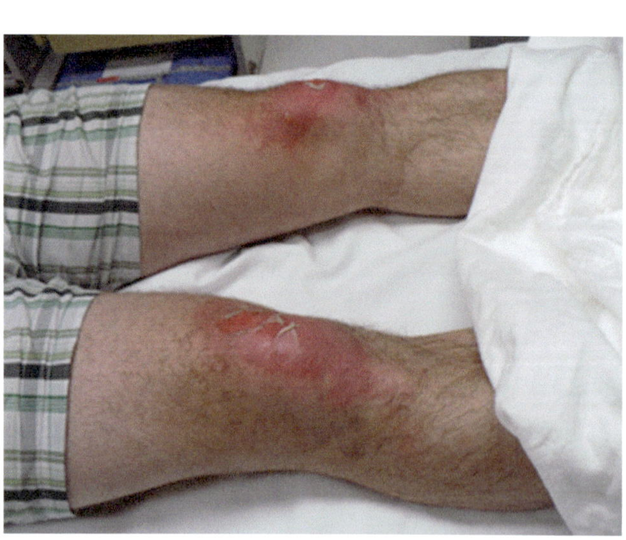

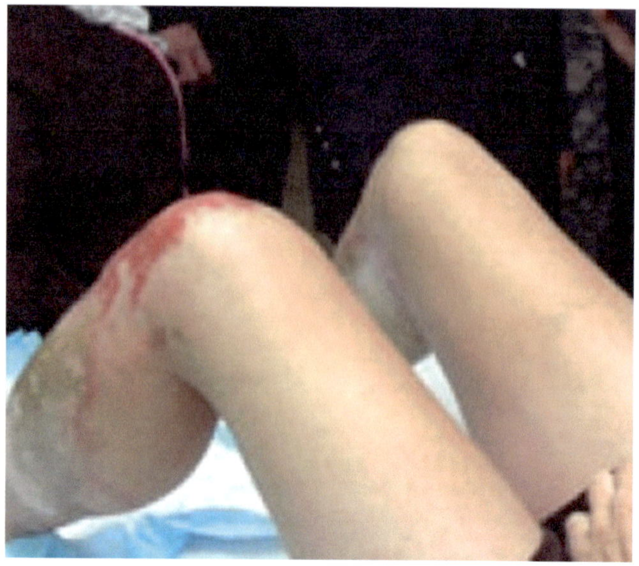

- Bends Behind Knees/Bends of Arms

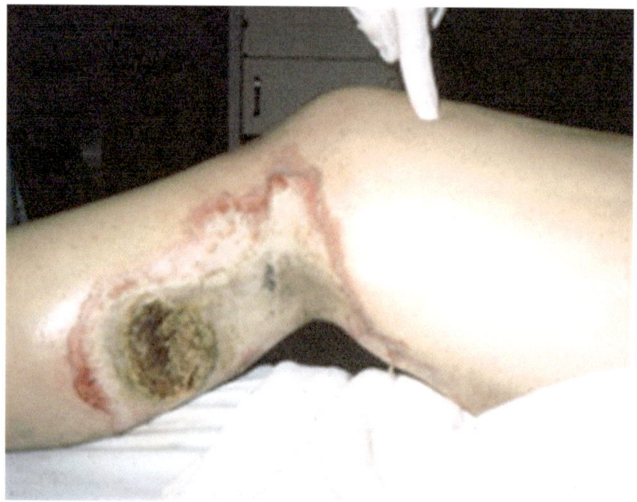

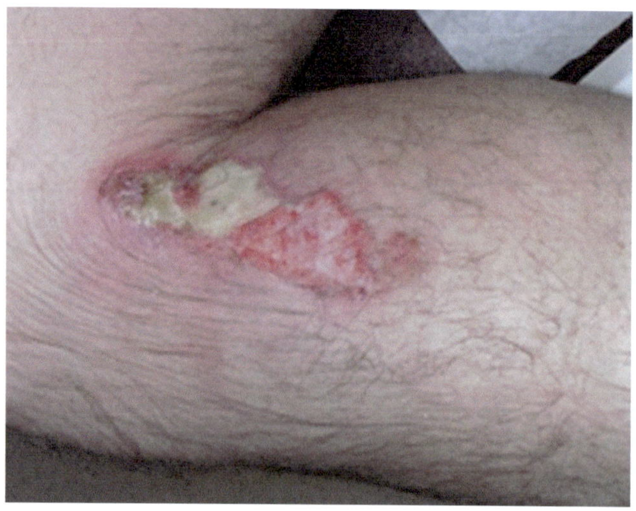

These figures are used with the kind permission of Lionel Crowther.

Fire services are recognizing the need to continually reflect on their practice. Similar to other industries, they are adopting the approach of continuous quality improvement through quality assurance. Firefighter injuries can be minimized via this process. The examples of the two firefighters who sustained injuries were the impetuous for reflection and need to revisit best practices.

In 2014, representatives from the International Association of Fire Fighters (IAFF) participated in the inaugural Canadian Burn Symposium. The IAFF was focused on addressing how first responders address the concerns of patients and responders at the scene of significant, life changing events, resulting from fire and other situations that can result in burns. At the 2014 symposium, much of the information presented contained American-specific details. IAFF Local 3888 was invited to attend the 2015 symposium hosted in Toronto. I was asked to participate as a presenter from a Canadian perspective. I co-presented with Judy Knighton, a registered nurse and burn specialist at the Ross Tilley Burn Centre at Sunnybrook Health Sciences Centre in Toronto. Knighton and I were tasked to identify best practices in handling and managing the care of responders who sustained burns. Knighton handled to the transport and treatment priorities in her presentation titled Emergency Management and Outpatient Care of the Person with Burns. I addressed management of the patient immediately following removal from the hazardous environment in my presentation, Managing the Handling of the Rescued Firefighter.

The process outlined below is the evolution of best practices.

Emotions among fellow firefighters run high when a firefighter is rescued from a fire. As with all hazardous situations in which patients are involved, the primary concern should be rescuer safety. It is important that the rescuers wear full PPE when managing care for a rescued firefighter, and be purposeful and careful when handling the superheated firefighter. The rescuers need to:

- Avoid off-gasing from firefighter
- Avoid skin contact with hot bunker gear

Considerations and steps to safely remove the PPE ensemble:

1. Have the firefighter remain standing
   - Allow some time for the PPE envelope to passively cool and off-gas or use a positive-pressure ventilation fan to speed up the process.
   - Do not use a hose line to cool the firefighter while he or she is in the PPE ensemble.
   - Use two rescuers to facilitate the removal of the PPE ensemble.
   - Protect the rescued firefighter from the stored heat in the bunker gear.
   - Avoid sitting, laying down, bending limbs prior to dissipating stored heat.

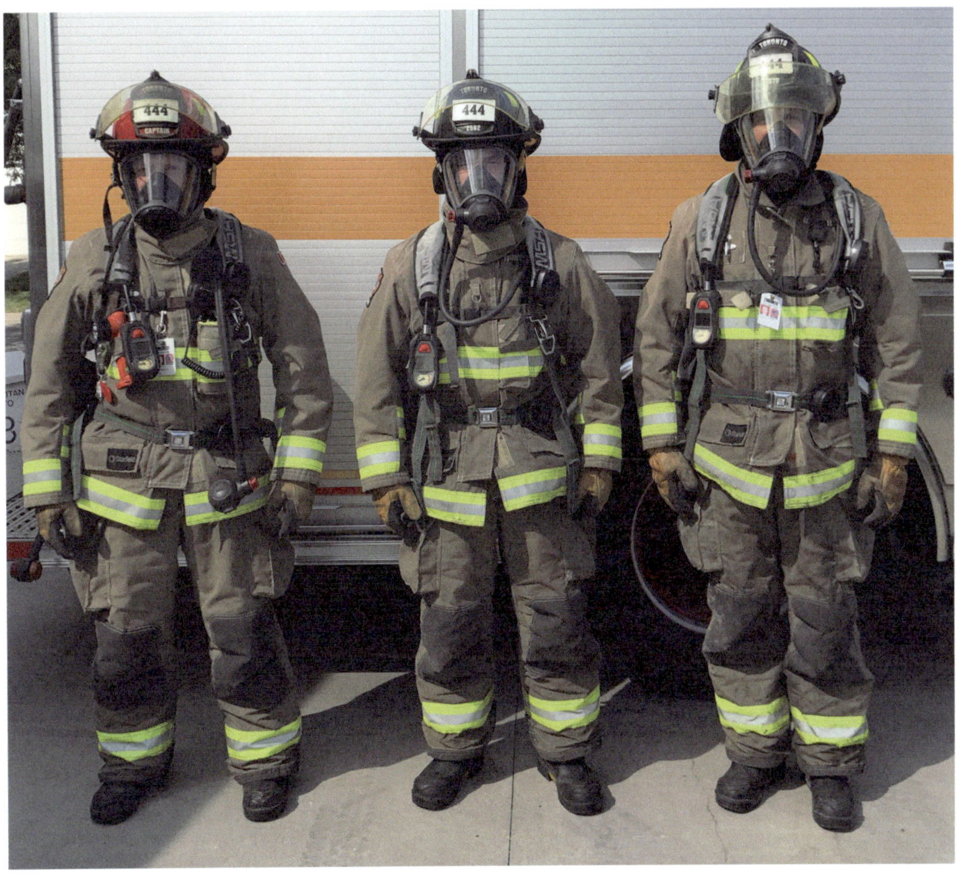

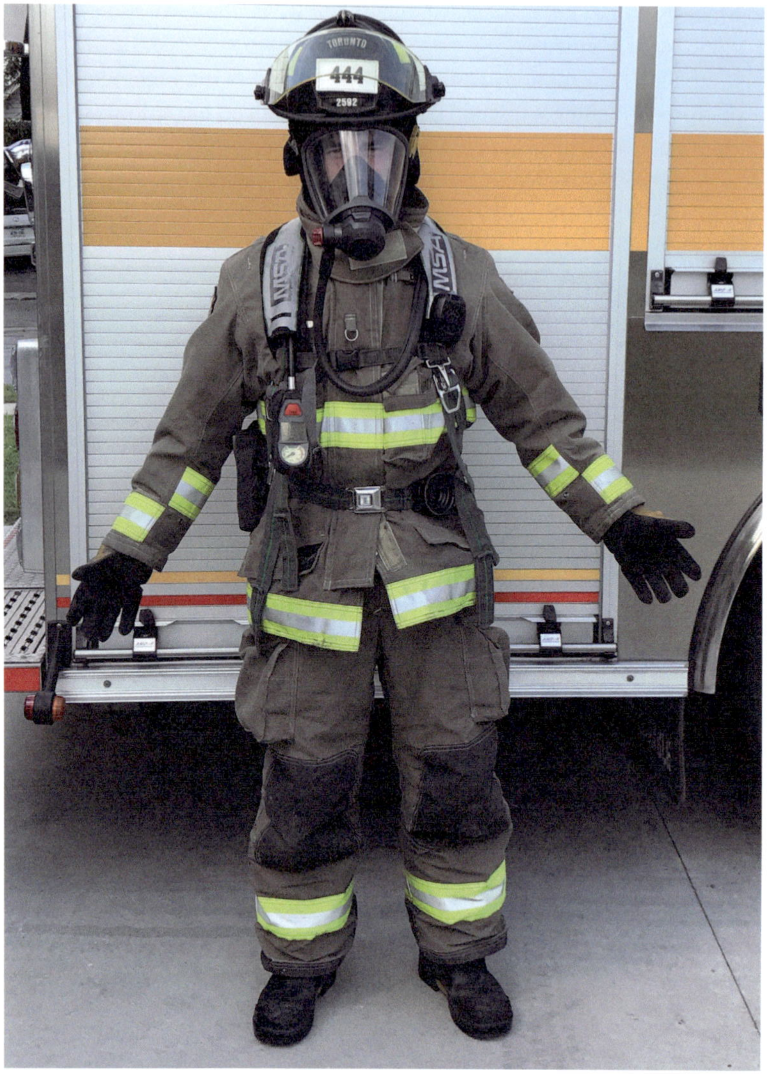

2. Loosen the SCBA shoulder straps; communicate your planned actions and co-ordinate the loosening

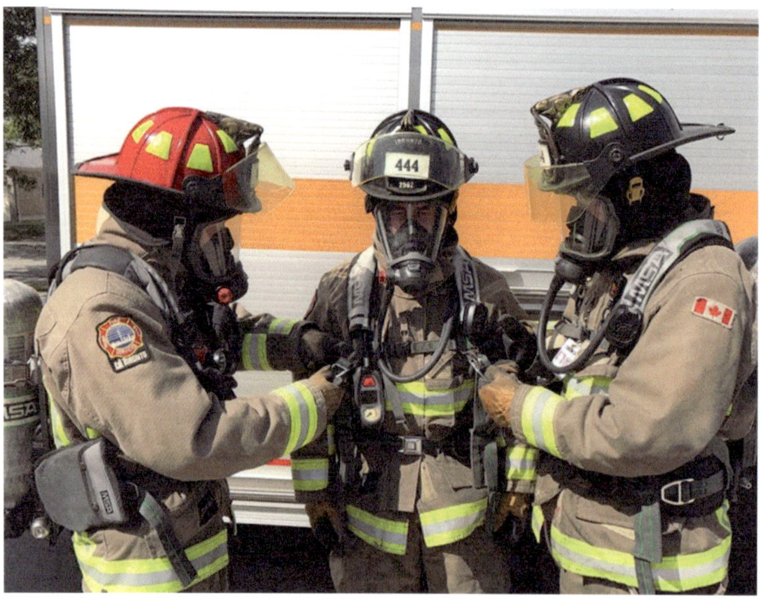

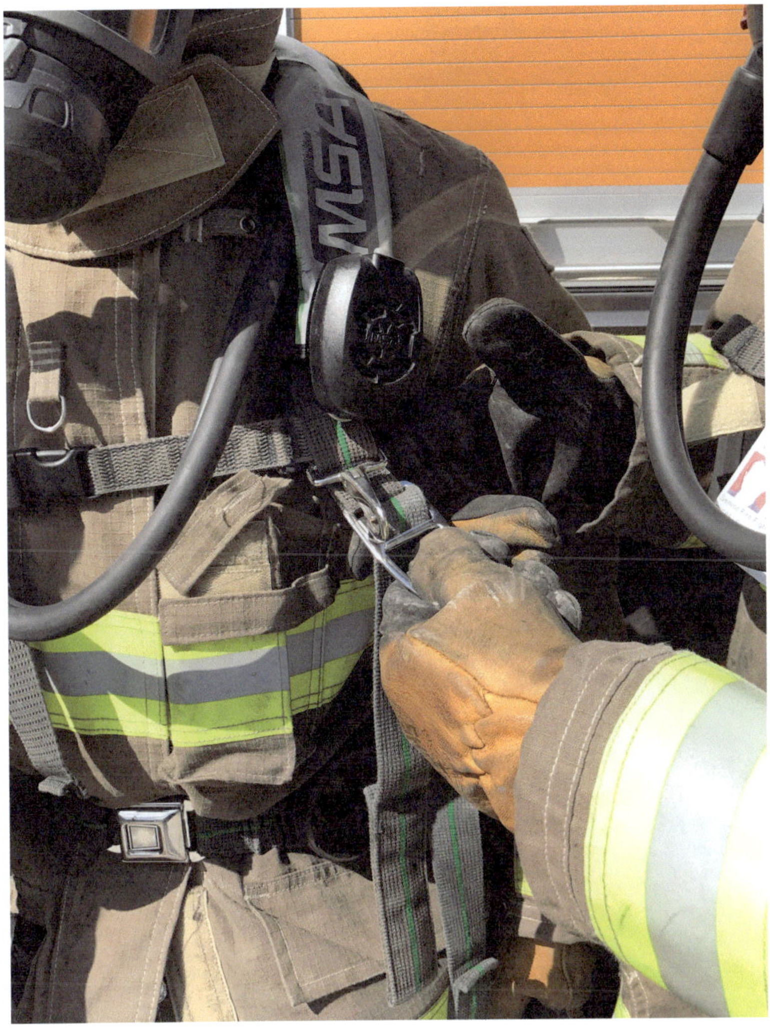

3. Disconnect the chest strap

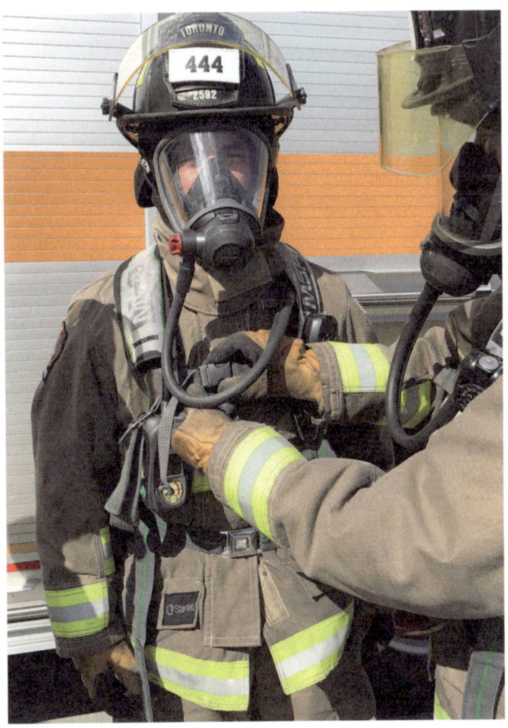

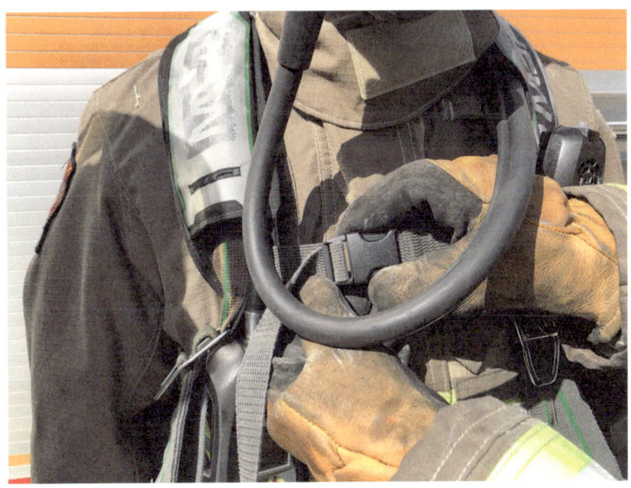

4. Loosen and unbuckle the waist belt

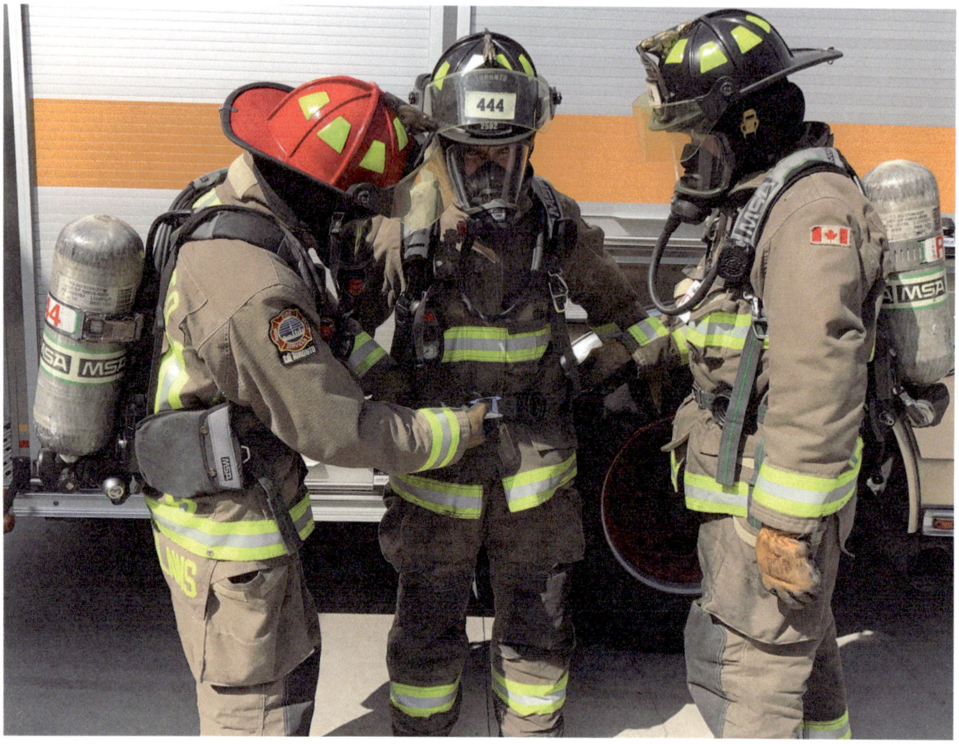

5. Remove and replace the neck flap

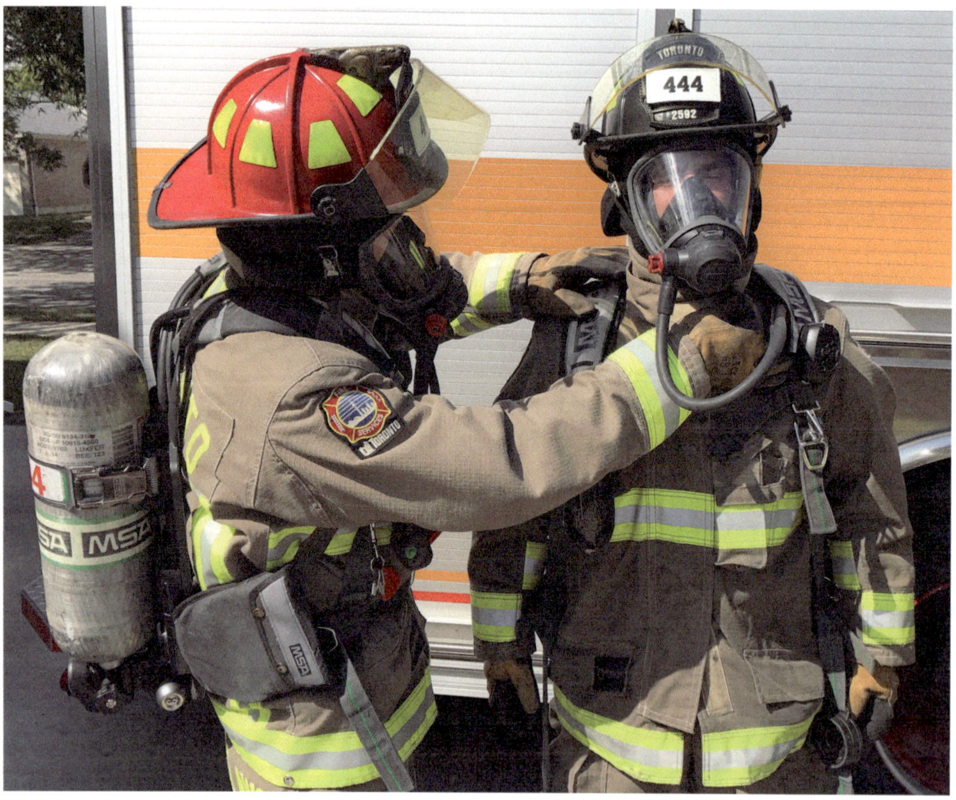

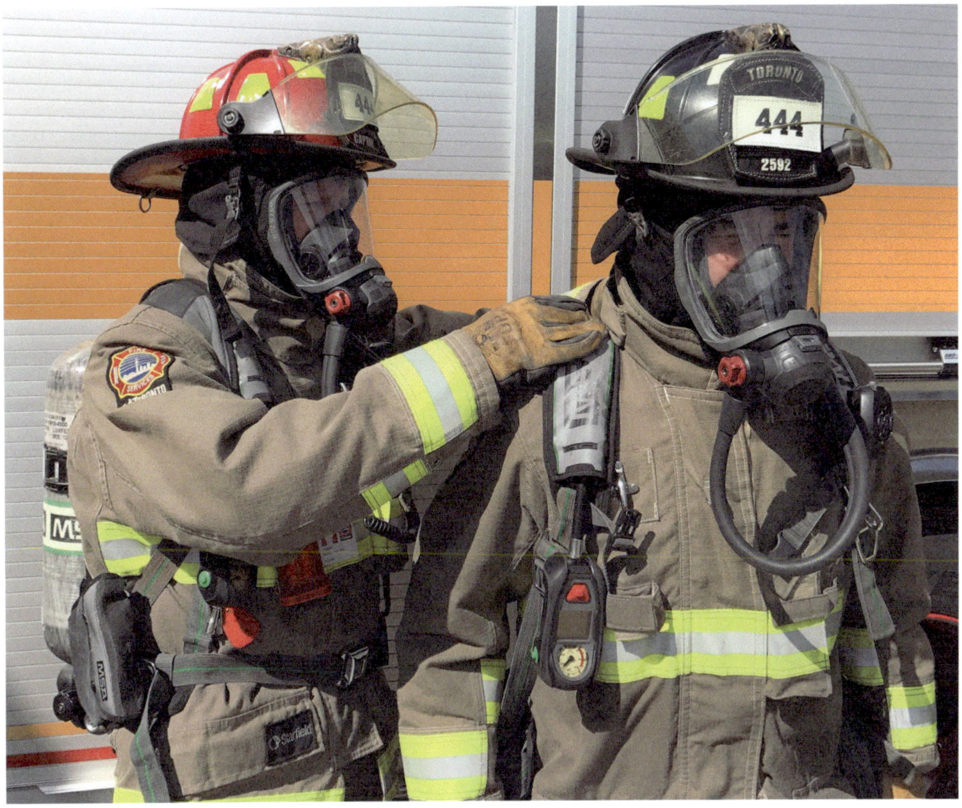

6. Open the front jacket flap while unclasping/unzipping the coat

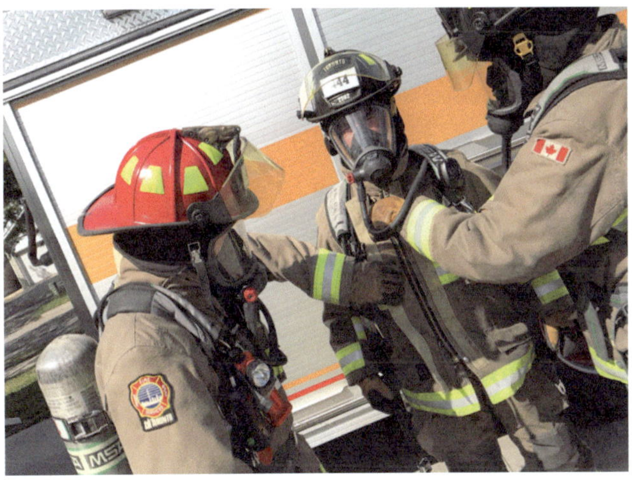

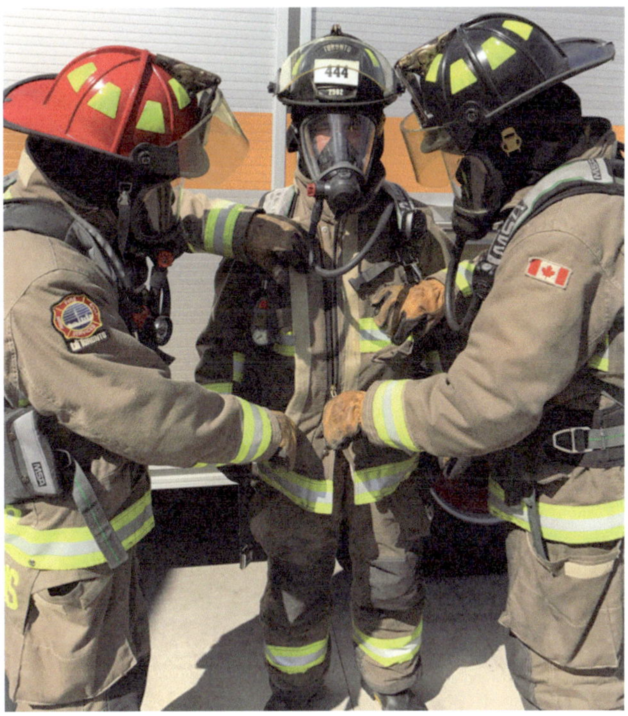

7. Open the jacket

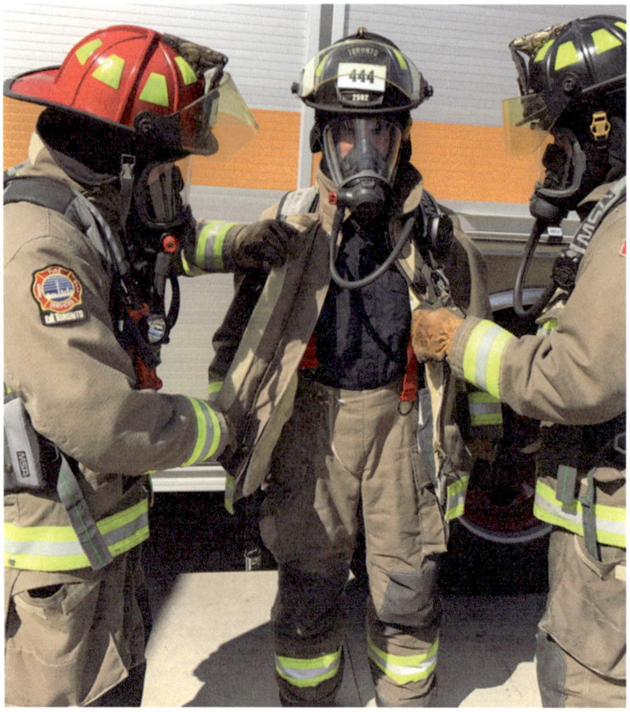

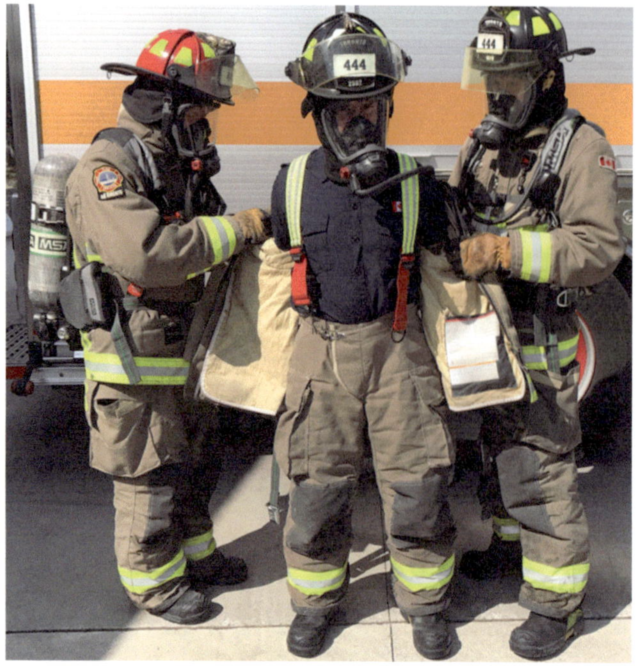

8. Roll the coat and the SCBA over the shoulders

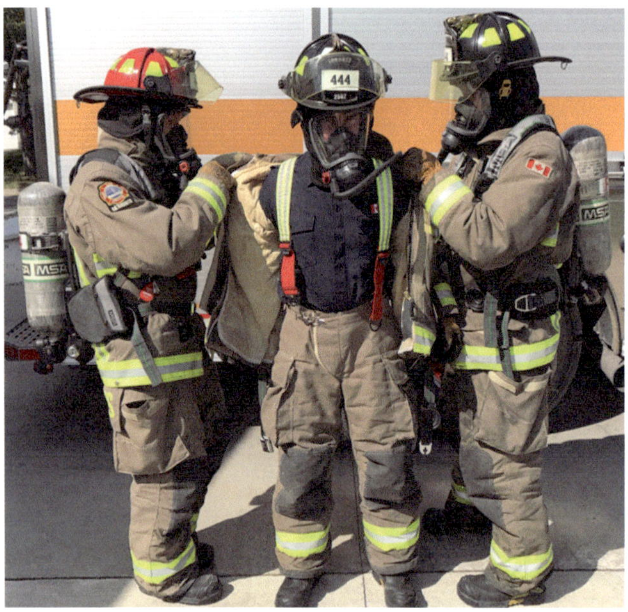

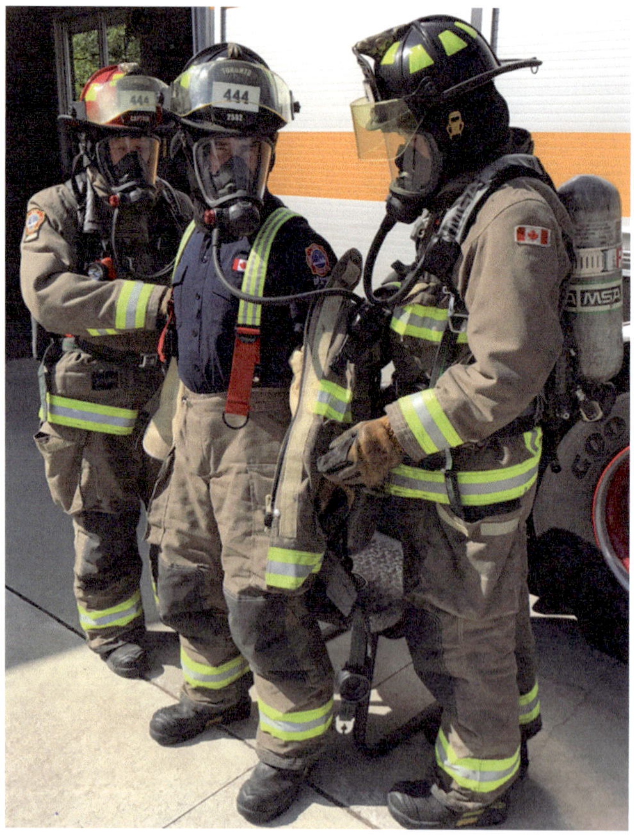

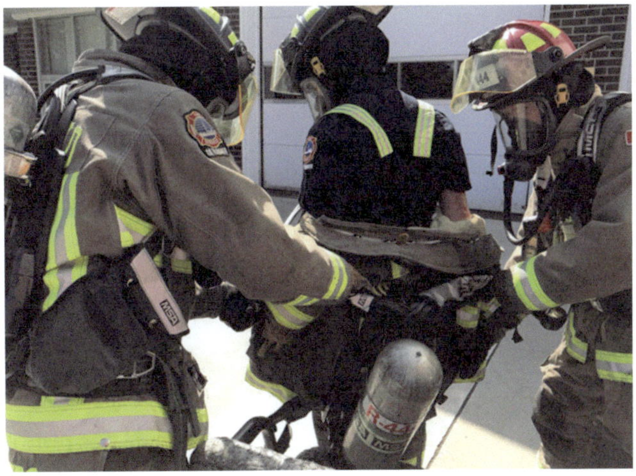

9. Remove gloves and the remainder of the coat

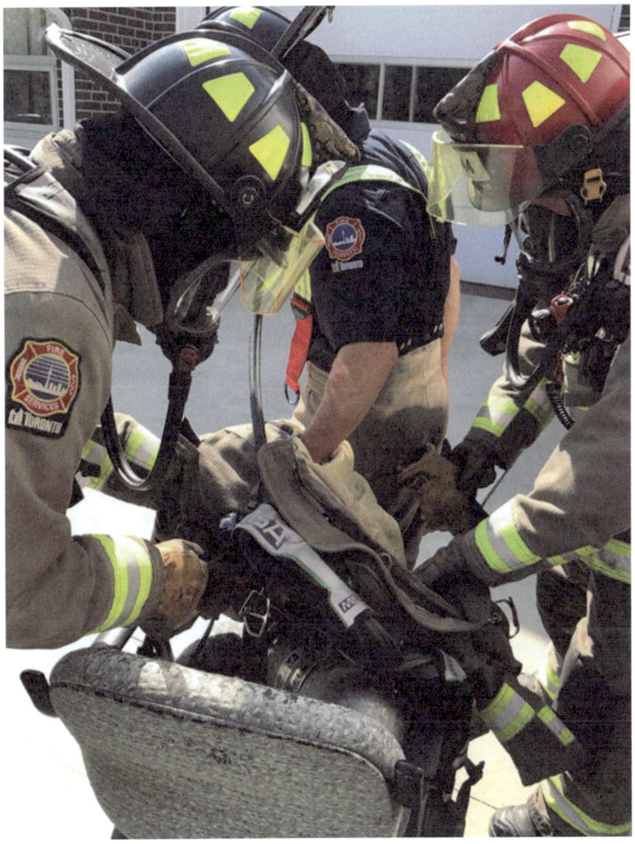

10. Unclasp the pants and remove the suspenders, letting the pants fall

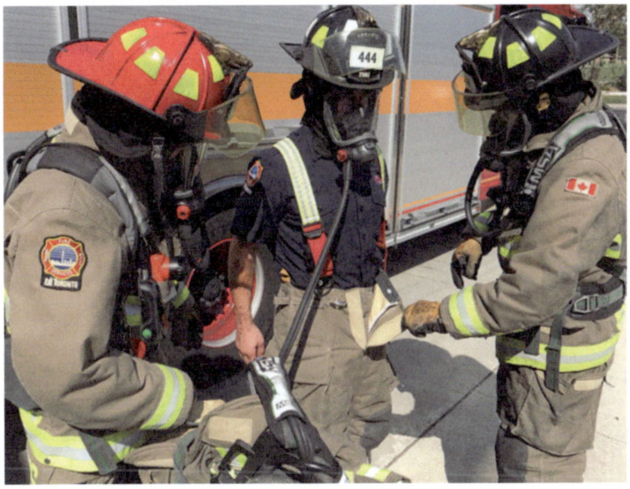

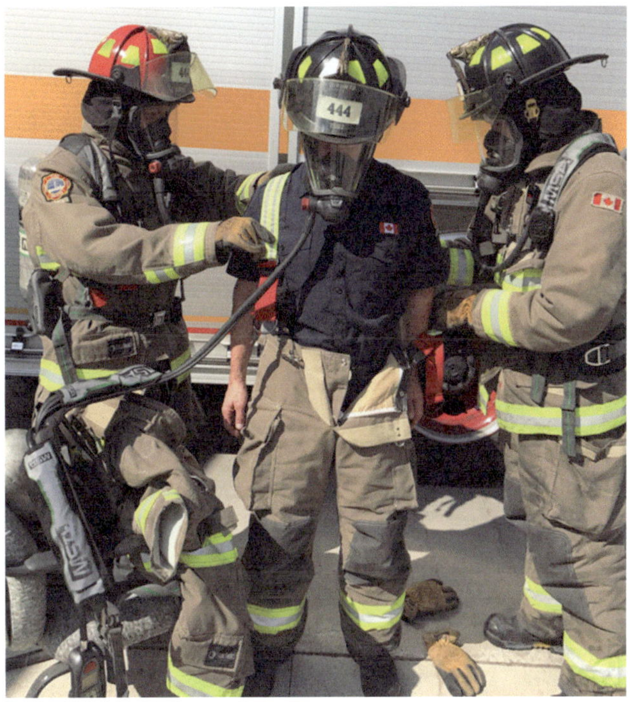

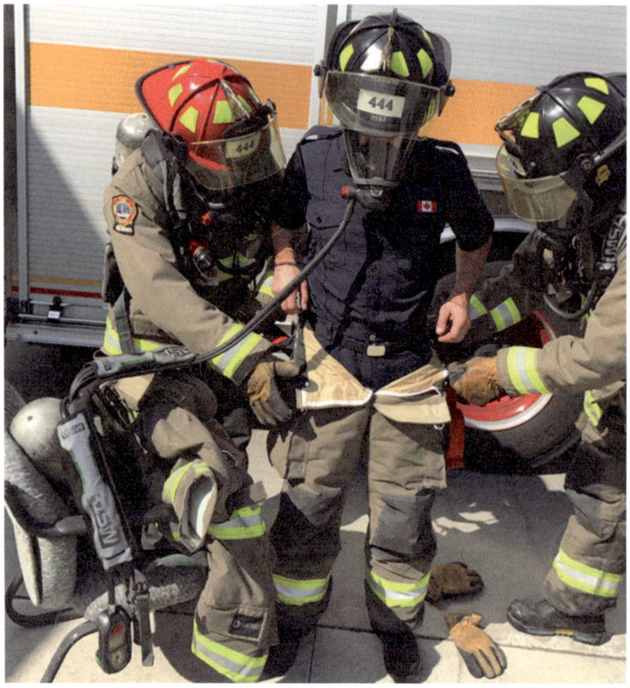

11. Roll the pants over the boots and assist in removal of boots

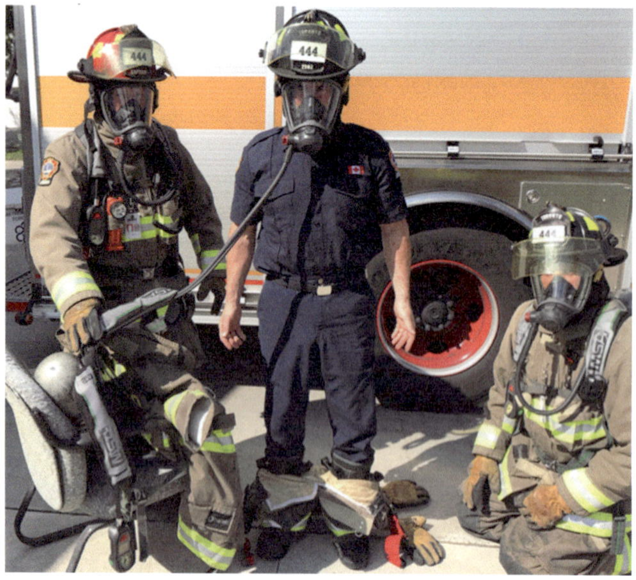

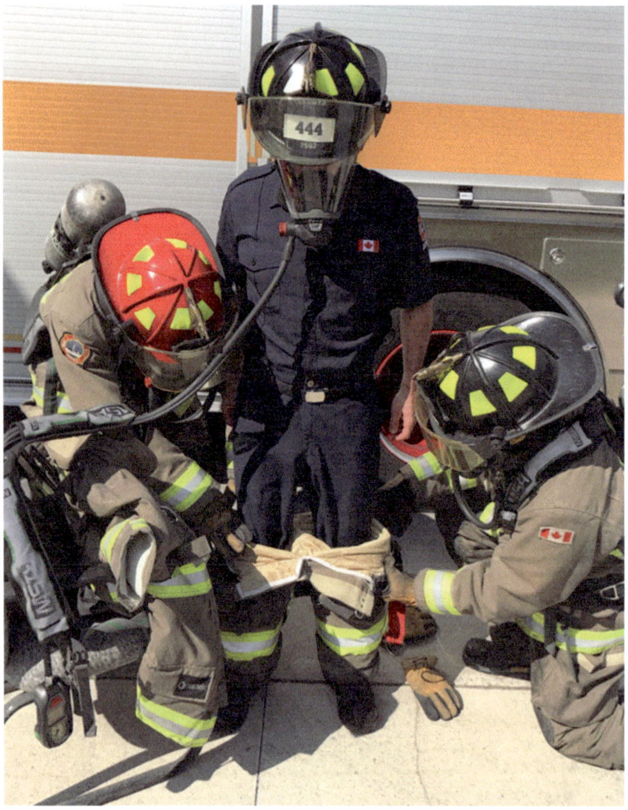

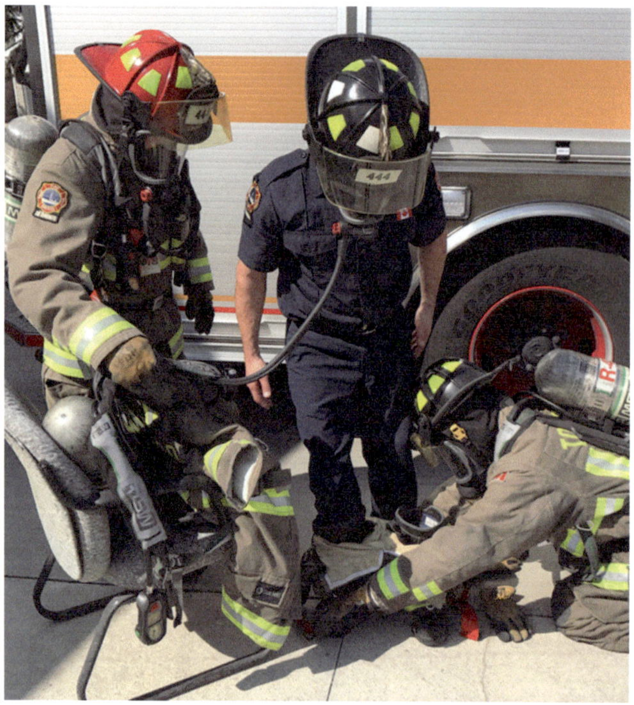

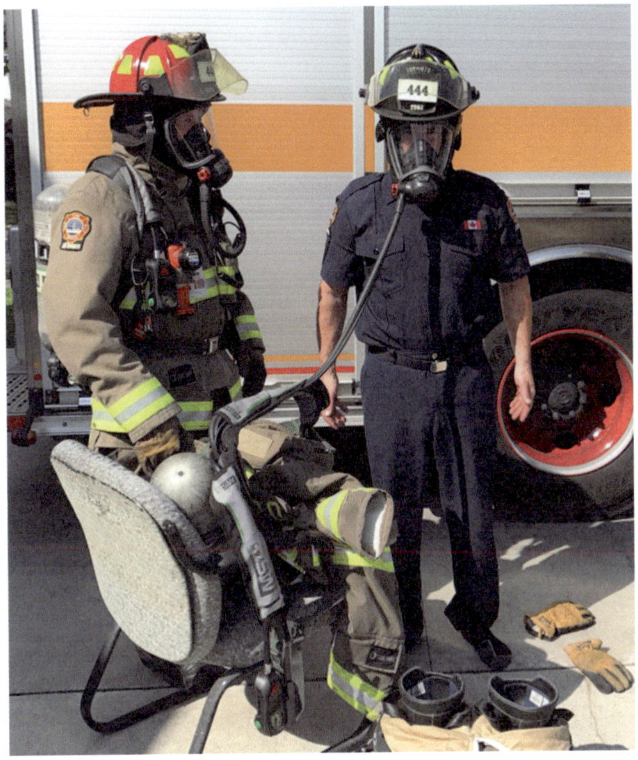

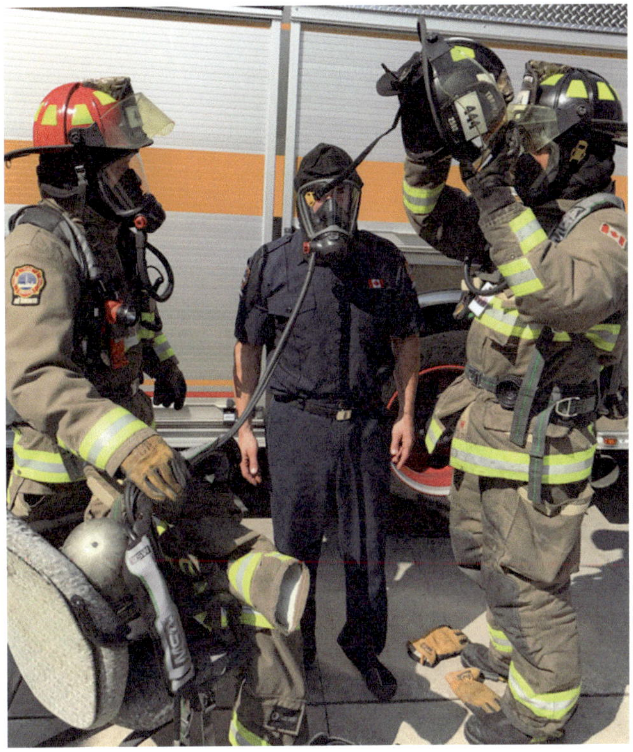

12. Remove helmet, balaclava, and mask

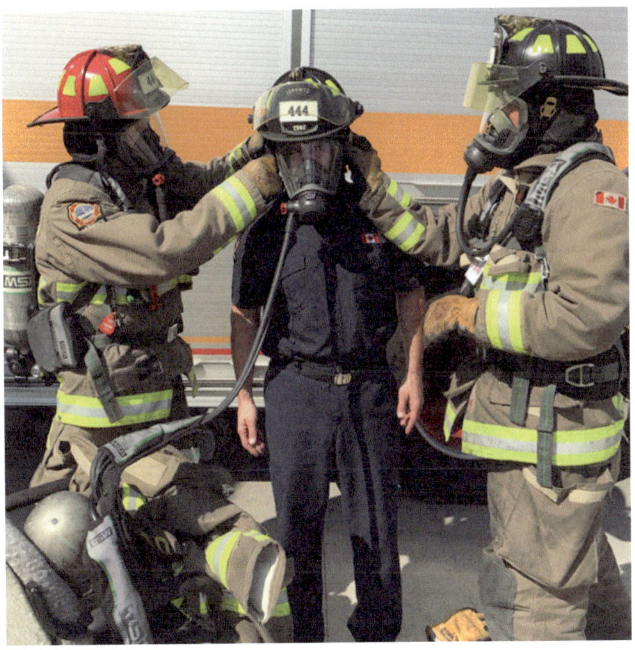

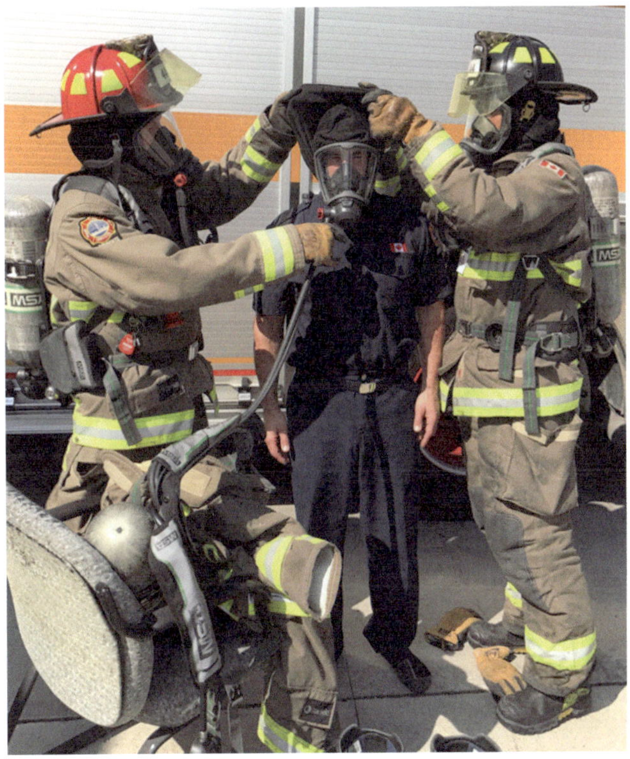

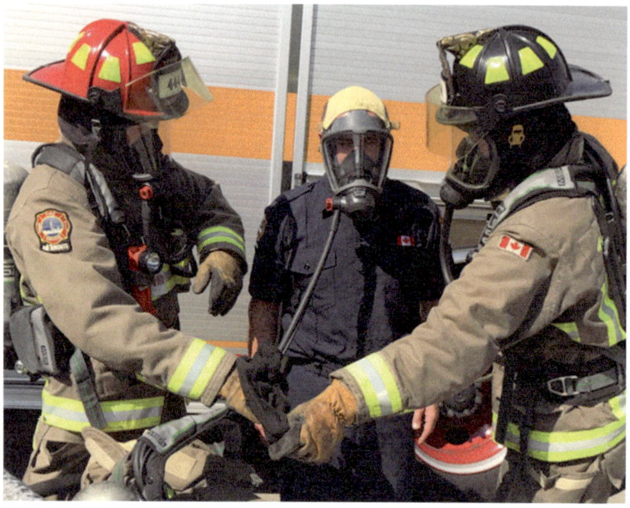

13. Remove the stage 2 regulator and face piece

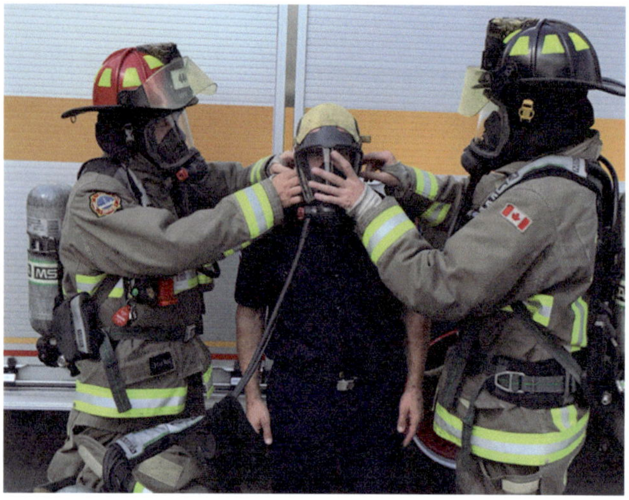

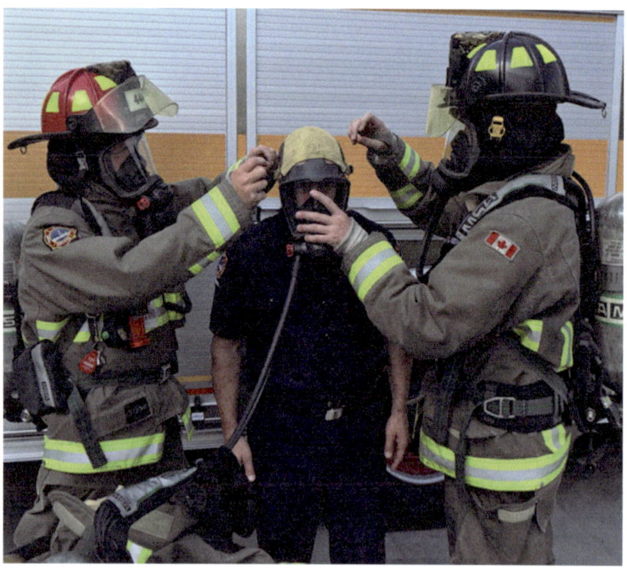

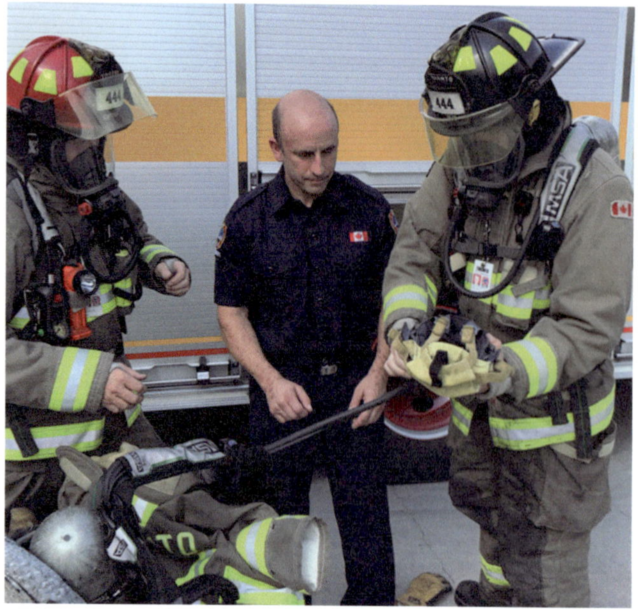

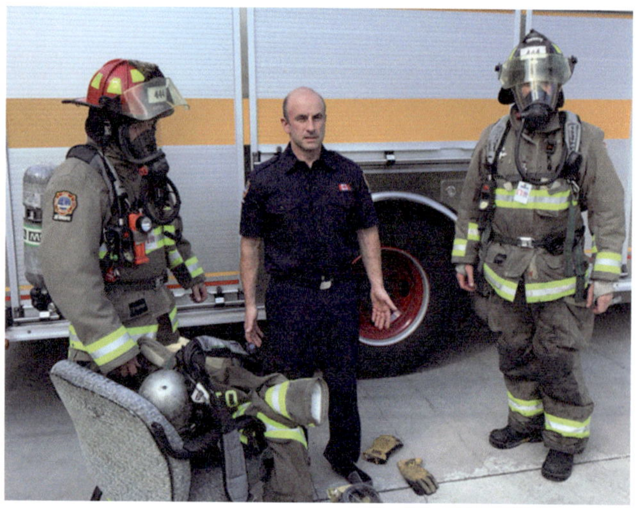

These figures are used with the permission of Ken Webb.

Initial burn treatment:

- Rapid access to definitive care ASAP
- Use water to cool small minor local burns
- Cut away clothing if necessary to avoid debriding when fabric remains in the burned tissue
- Protect open burn wound with dry sterile burn dressings
- Facilitate rapid transport to definitive care

Initial assessment of burns on scene are quite often not overly reliable; some burns that appear to be minor end up being severe while some burns that seem to be significant end up being less severe.

All regions in the country have burn centers associated with leading-edge hospitals that are best suited to manage the care of burn patients. It is worthwhile to ascertain where your firefighter will go when they sustain significant burn injuries. Our partners in emergency medical services will facilitate movement of firefighters to these facilities.

Fire services are very good at preplanning occupancies so they are aware of the different hazards. Situational awareness training is also helping firefighters recognize and react when fire conditions are about to change. These are initiatives designed to limit the risk to firefighters when emergencies occur. Through articles like this and presentations at conferences such as the Canadian Burn Symposium, we hope to spread the word about how to manage the superheated firefighter to limit injuries to the rescuer and the firefighter requiring rescue. These are low-incidence, high-risk situations that need to be planned for before they happen.

Summary Box

- First responders play an important role in managing the initial care of burn patients.
- Responder safety is the first priority when assessing the emergency scene.
- Utilizing a systematic approach to incident and patient care management will help maximize the potential of arriving at a successful outcome.
- Early identification and mitigation of the hazard and mechanism of injury associated with the burn will better position the first responders as they begin their initial treatment of the burn patient.
- Removing the patient from the source of the injury will help stop the burning.
- Early recognition and management of Airway, Breathing, and Circulation compromise is the first priority.
- Strategies to stop the burning based on the mechanism of injury are important to have in the top of mind.
- Identification of the severity of the burn will help the responder make the appropriate transport destination decision.
- Emotions run high following the removal of a firefighter from a superheated environment.
- Deliberate and planned removal of the firefighter's PPE will minimize unnecessary harm to the rescuer and the rescued firefighter.
- Initial care of burns and rapid transport to definitive care will improve outcomes.

Acknowledgements Geoff Boisseau (Captain, Toronto Fire Services)
Lionel Crowther (Firefighter, Winnipeg Fire Paramedic Services)
Ihor Iwanusiw (Firefighter, Toronto Fire Services)
Greg Byers (Acting Captain—Toronto Fire Services)
Mike Blacklaws (Captain, Toronto Fire Services)

Photo Credits

Fire Fighter Burn Injuries; Lionel Crowther (Firefighter, Winnipeg Fire Paramedic Services)

PPE Removal Sequence; Ken Webb

The base material regarding the management of the handling and care of the superheated firefighter was produced in the spring of 2015 and edited annually to reflect best practices for a presentation.

https://www.cdnfirefighter.com/specialized/burn-protocol-40822

This material was presented at the 2018 Canadian Burn Symposium: https://www.cpd.utoronto.ca/cdnburnsymposium/

References

1. Pollak AN, Barnes L, Ciotola JA, Gulli B. Emergency care and transportation of the sick and injured. 10th ed. Burlington: Jones & Bartlett Learning; 2013.
2. International Association of Fire Fighters. First responder guide to burn injury assessment & treatment. Washington, DC: International Association of Fire Fighters; 2013.
3. TFS Education. Sunnybrook Centre for Prehospital Medicine. http://www.prehospitalmedicine.ca/tfs-education/.
4. It happens in seconds: fire fighter burn injury awareness. http://ithappenedinseconds.org/when-a-firefighter-gets-burned/.
5. Fire Engineering.com. Firefighter burn injuries by Karen Owens. 1 Apr 2011. http://www.fireengineering.com/articles/print/volume-164/issue-4/departments/fire-service_ems/firefighter-burn-injuries.html.
6. Brown PL. Doffing superheated turnout gear. 16 June 2008. http://www.fireengineering.com/articles/2008/06/doffing-superheated-turnout-gear.html.

Prehospital Management of Burn Injuries

11

Folke Sjöberg

11.1 Introduction

11.1.1 Modern Care

In the last 20 years, large changes in burn care and in the background and logistics around the care for the burn injured have occurred which has implications for how burn care now should be administered and practically performed. Firstly, the incidence of burn injuries has decreased in the Western world and a decrease of about 30% is evident from e.g., since the eighties [1, 2]. In parallel, length of stay in the burn care facilities for the injured has been reduced to about 40% of what it was at that time [3, 4]. Thirdly, the outcome of burns has been significantly improved over the same time period. This may be exemplified by the 50% survival chance that was present for a 45% total burn surface area (TBSA%) burn in a 21-year-old in the late 1970s, which is to be compared to the corresponding 50% survival chance for 80–90% TBSA% burn in a patient of the same age today [5, 6]. Fourth, patients, with smaller burns, today are to a significant extent treated as outpatients and smaller injuries may have their surgery done as outpatients as well [7–9]. At the same time, an increasing proportion of the patients are in the elderly age groups where the same injury poses a larger threat as compared to in younger patients [10, 11]. In this age group, care is to a large extent influenced also by co-morbidities and the possibility to obtain good end results seen especially from the patient perspective [12].

Based on these changes, the approach to burn care has been to centralize this type of care to larger burn units and centers. This process is ongoing in most high income countries, however, with a variable intensity. The multidisciplinary approach to the care and the need to keep the care process unified for this patient group has led to that the centralization process has been pursued and the achieved improvement in outcome has been its driving force. The latter is exemplified by lower mortality rates a and shorter lengths of stay [6, 13, 14]. At the same time, such organizational changes bring about important care implications for the general medical practitioners and medical organizations [13, 14]. The decreased incidence and the centralized care reduce the magnitude of medical staff that have experience of these cases and that treats them on a regular basis. This then urgently calls for good teaching programs and a good organized care involving a well-designed communication between the referring doctor and the specialist. Especially the early management and stabilization of the patients needs to be optimized and well-functioning at any level of care as this care is often provided at a non-burn center by personnel with limited experience of burns. Importantly, as the outcome has been improved significantly in later times, the care to be provided needs to be optimized and the tolerance for any less successful results is low. It is relevant to note that there is an inherent risk in "over"-centralizing care even of small injuries that can be adequately treated at the local hospital [15]. Therefore, continuous teaching programs are important. This early part of the treatment has therefore been the target of specially organized teaching programs initially started through the advanced trauma life support (ATLS) concept [16, 17] followed by more specifically burn oriented programs such as: the American "Advanced Burn Life Support" course (ABLS; www.Ameriburn.org) provided by the American Burn Association and which is also taught outside the USA as, e.g., in Japan [18] or Sweden. This course is also available on line on the web [19]; or the Australian and New Zeeland "Emergency Management of Severe Burns (EMSB; www.anzba.org.au)" course which is also provided in other countries such as Britain, South Africa, Norway, and Finland [20, 21]. This chapter will therefore rely strongly on these principles as the strategies for the initial care are presented. These are important as they have implications for the success of the whole treatment process and the final outcome. As pointed out, the final care of the burn patients is in cases of significant burns

F. Sjöberg (✉)
Department of Clinical and Experimental Medicine, Linköping University, Linköping, Sweden
e-mail: folke.sjoberg@liu.se

M. G. Jeschke et al. (eds.), *Handbook of Burns Volume 1*, https://doi.org/10.1007/978-3-030-18940-2_11

undertaken at burn centers and the improved early stabilization and transport care that today can be offered is one of the reasons why modern burn care provides successful results and increased survival. From a teaching perspective, modern burn care in western countries may thus be described as most often provided at three locations: firstly, at the scene of the accident or very close by; secondly at a local hospital where also initial stabilization and the start of fluid therapy usually is undertaken; and finally the transport to the final care level, a tertiary referral burn unit or center. In densely populated areas, direct transport to the burn center is also an often employed alternative. Transport times are then usually in the range of less than 1 h. This chapter will review current principles for the care at these first two locations.

Another and today especially important treatment quality augmenting process is the increased use of the internet where updated information and referral strategies may be found as is exemplified by information provided by a burn center in England where plenty of information for patients, relatives, and importantly professionals may be found (http://www.bch.nhs.uk/Professional). In these settings, checklists etc. may facilitate the referral process and aid in promoting a good outcome for the patients. In parallel, the use of telemedicine may further improve the dialogue between the referring unit and the recipient. In this context, apps for mobile phones are being developed and by which detailed communication (burn size, depth assessment, etc.) can be made between caregivers without exposing the integrity of the patient. This is further elaborated upon in this chapter.

11.2 Early Management

Despite the improvements of burn care in general there is a significant improvement potential as treatment complications have been encountered in the early patient management and stressing the co-operation between the referral and receiving units is therefore undertaken prior to addressing early care. With modern technology (different modes of telemedicine) a close dialogue can be made between the referring and receiving hospitals and thus patient care can be optimized. A more detailed discussion regarding specific early treatment challenges encountered is therefore presented after the detailed description of early management principles presented below.

11.2.1 At the Site of Accident

The early and immediate care provided to a burn patient may vary depending on many factors, most of all related to: the type of injury (thermal, chemical, or electric); where the accident has occurred and its relation to different care levels and the available resources. The latter case, i.e., resource availability, being relevant in situations with large number of injuries, such as in disaster settings or similar circumstances and where other approaches and strategies also will come into play to ascertain good outcome [22]. In far, distant places the care may be started and undertaken by a companion or a bystander, which may also be the case in other settings immediately after the injury. The more organized assessment and care in the very early stage is otherwise most often done, in the western world, by paramedics from an ambulance rescue team or at times from rescue squads comprising personnel with higher medical education such as nurses and/or doctors or personnel from rescue groups arriving by, e.g., helicopter. At all levels, a similar approach is undertaken based on early trauma rescue principles (ATLS/ABLS). It may at this point be stressed that irrespectively at what level of care the treatment algorithms are undertaken a recommendation is that contact, whenever needed, is made with the next level of care and this can today be better undertaken.

This standard evaluation/care principles may mainly be divided into:

- primary assessment
- secondary assessment

which is followed by transportation to the next level of care.

The knowledge gained and the treatments undertaken under way need to be adequately registered and communicated properly to the next level, so that any important findings and interventions made are properly extended and especially in cases if problems or other difficulties are encountered they may be properly discussed.

Most urgently at the site of the fire or accident is to stop the fire process, electricity, or chemical exposure, and move the patient into a safe area. This may include getting the person out from a trapped situation in, e.g., a vehicle. Stopping the fire in, e.g., clothing is best done by suffocation of the fire (rolling and adding garments on the burning clothing), if not water or other type of fire extinguishers are within reach. Flushing with properly tempered fluid is very good as it not only extinguishes the fire but also cools the wound and thereby reduces the convection of heat and it reduces pain. Be aware of the risk for hypothermia. At this point, clothing and jewelry should be removed as they retain heat and may affect blood flow, as the extremities swell (e.g., jewelry/fingers). Early management also includes, if the exposure is based on chemicals, flushing with significant amounts of water and being aware of the contamination risk for others such as the rescue team, which shall take adequate precautions using gloves and gowns. If the eyes are involved, flushing becomes even more important prior to having the eyes examined by an ophthalmologist. It is also important to stress that neutralizing agents are contraindicated as they induce heat. In cases of accidents involving electricity, there is also a need to stop the current/voltage or using an insulator prior to getting into contact with the patient.

At the site of the accident, in the immediate period after the injury, the patient is cared for by regular ATLS/ABLS/EMSB or other well-organized trauma algorithms (ABC) and in their relevant order, i.e., A. Airway, B. Breathing, C. Circulation, D. Disability, E. Exposure—each specified in more detail below under primary/secondary assessment. Very important at this site is also to confirm or exclude other injuries that may be more important than the burn itself (see below the details for this under secondary survey). Pain treatment may be important in this setting especially if there is a somewhat longer initial transport. Pain relief is accomplished preferably by i.v. morphine in incremental doses in the larger burns if drugs are at this point available. It is also important to stress that there is an overrepresentation of abuse, psychiatric disorders, and criminality among burn injured patients. This may in certain circumstances have implications for the further care procedures. Most importantly at the site of the accident is to be aware of the risk of being infected/contaminated by Hepatitis B and C or HIV, which makes it important for the rescue personnel to take appropriate precautions (glasses/glows/gowns).

Wound care at the site of the accident is rather uncomplicated. Burnt textiles may be removed and the patient covered by clean sheets, to reduce the risk of contamination of the wound and also to maintain body temperature. There is no need for ointments or other local treatments at this stage. At times commercially available burn wound coverings may be presented at the site of injury but the potential positive effects of these are yet undocumented why clean sheets may always be preferred. Evaluating the wound may be difficult if the examiner has limited experience. In this setting, pictures sent by telecommunication, as previously mentioned, can be of significant value if such technology has been properly implemented.

In the case of isolated burn injuries, there is little need to force an uncontrolled early transport unless there is other life-threatening illnesses present. It has been suggested in guidelines of the ABA that if transport times are less than an hour, start of fluid treatment is not mandatory. Transport principles for the burn injured to the local hospital vary according to the local geographic situations, but often airborne transport (helicopter or fixed wing) in Europe is recommended when the transport time exceeds 2 h or is more than 100 km.

11.2.2 At a Local Hospital: Stabilization Prior to Transport to the Burn Center

11.2.2.1 Primary Assessment

The primary assessment scheme follows a strict order scheduled according to how urgent the intervention is. It should be done as early as possible and repeatedly controlled during the care of the patient. Some parts may be performed in less detail at e.g., the site of the accident as more is gained by rapid transport to the next care level or there is a risk of hypothermia, e.g., a detailed burn extent determination outside in the cold.

A. Airway

The airway is immediately assessed, evaluated, and dealt with. A compromised airway may be cared for by small means such as bending the neck backwards or pulling the yaw forward. Facial burns or upper airway edema may compromise the airway as time passes from the time of the accident—making intubation necessary. Oxygen transport difficulties within the lung are most often not present at the very early stage, but within hours, depending on inhalation injury and/or the development of ARDS a compromised gas exchange in the lung may be present, needing intubation and advanced respiratory treatment [23]. Unconsciousness, very uncommon in the uncomplicated burn setting unless there is a significant carbon monoxide or cyanide exposure, or another injury, may be a reason for a compromised airway and will call for an early intubation. Provide, then if possible, oxygen at 100% by a non-rebreathing mask to optimize oxygenation and treat possible carbon monoxide/cyanide effects. At this point also evaluate the spine for any concomitant injuries and the need for fixation—not to cause spinal cord injuries.

B. Breathing

In conjunction to the evaluation of the upper airway, the breathing pattern should be assessed and the lungs examined for proper functions (gas exchange and lung compliance) and especially in the case of circular thoracic burns, as these may compromise breathing mechanics as edema develops in the thoracic wall, which calls for escharotomies (See Fig. 11.1). This may be particularly important in small children as they rely more on auxiliary breathing muscles in their breathing.

C. Circulation

The circulatory status of the patient should be examined. It includes assessing the skin color, sensitivity, peripheral pulses, and capillary refill. Heart rate and blood pressure should also be included to confirm adequate organ perfusion. Be aware that heart rate effects need to be judged cautiously as it may also be affected by other reasons than hypovolemia, such as anxiety and/or pain. Blood pressure monitoring when done may be difficult, be aware of the risk for faulty or compromised measurements by, e.g., deep circumferential burns. In cases the peripheral circulation in the extremities is compromised, consider early escharotomies and invasive blood pressure measurements (See Fig. 11.1).

D. Disability

The burn injured patient during "normal" conditions in the acute phase should not have an altered level of consciousness

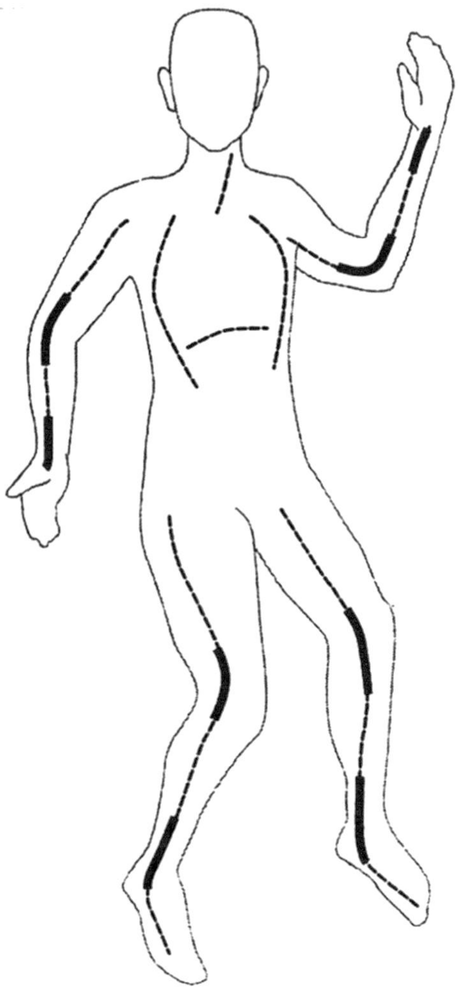

Fig. 11.1 Escharotomies. The lines indicate the location for escharotomies. Note that it is important that the cut is deep enough to accomplish a tissue release. This needs to be specifically addressed at the areas marked, as it is more difficult to assess the right tissue depth at these locations, i.e., close to the major joints

(LOC) even in cases of very severe burns. The LOC should be assessed, e.g., by the Glasgow Coma Scale (GCS). If the level of consciousness (LOC) is altered, suspect other underlying processes such as other trauma, carbon monoxide and/or cyanide intoxication, hypoxia, e.g., especially in a closed space and where fire is fierce, or other medical conditions such as stroke or diabetes.

E. Expose and Examine

The patient should be thoroughly examined and in order to do this removal of the clothing is necessary. Be aware of the risk for hypothermia. Jewelry, especially such as rings, should be removed due to the risk of compromising extremity (finger) blood flow as tissue edema develops. At this occasion, the important assessment of the burn injuries may be performed and evaluated. Important for the outcome is to initiate the fluid therapy early, which may be done at this point and when the extent of the burn injury becomes evident. A simplified fluid starting strategy has been suggested by the ABA for the very early burn care where a significant burn (>30%) is encountered. See Table 11.1 below.

11.2.2.2 Secondary Assessment

The complementary second assessment is undertaken rapidly after the first assessment and it is aimed at examining the patient thoroughly from head to toe, mainly in order to rule out other more important injuries that may pose a danger to the patient. One important point is that this examination needs to be undertaken in detail as the burn injury often is the most prominent injury and it may lead to that other injuries may be overlooked. If the assessment is done at larger facilities and there is a suspicion of other concomitant trauma, a regular trauma assessment algorithm may be undertaken and involving, e.g., ultrasound scan abdomen and/or (complementary) whole body CT scan.

Other issues to address at this point are to get a good medical history. This is important from mainly two aspects, firstly, the circumstances around the burn injury as it may help in determining the prognosis and may indicate the future burn treatment needs. Secondly, to assess the patients' present co-morbidities and ongoing medical treatments.

1. *Circumstances of the burn.* Where and when did it happen—what were the injury mechanisms (scald, flame, chemical, or electrical). Especially the factors, heat level (degrees) and exposure time (seconds) may signal the risk for deep injuries. Indoor accident and risk for inhalation injuries. Are other injury mechanisms present and relevant?
2. *Medical history.* Previous or associated illnesses (diabetes; hypertension; other heart, lung, or kidney disease)—Ongoing medical treatment, alcohol use or other (abuse), allergies. Time for last oral fluid or food intake. The tetanus immunization status—need for complementary injections?

11.2.2.3 Fluid Treatment

A cornerstone in the treatment of the burn injury is the fluid treatment. Usually i.v. fluid is provided to injuries larger than 15% total burn surface area % (TBSA%) [24, 25]. In order to provide fluid treatment intravenously, i.v. lines are needed. These are most commonly applied in the extremities in non-injured tissue, but in cases of massive burns also burned areas may be used. In larger burns, getting vascular access

Table 11.1 Patients with >30% TBSA obtain two large bore, indwelling venous catheters and a suggested simplified prehospital fluid management plan may be as is presented in this Table (11.1)

A simplified fluid management plan	
≤5 years	125 mL LR/h
6–13 years	250 mL LR/h
≥14 years	500 mL LR/h

may prove difficult and central i.v. lines may be mandatory as may an intraosseous cannula, or vein cutdown strategies in children. The fluid treatment may be initiated early at the scene of the accident, but should not significantly delay transportation. If transport is planned for more than 1 h, starting the i.v. fluid is most often recommended (see also Table 11.1). The background for the fluid needs for the burn patients is the rapid fluid loss to the injured tissue that is caused by the negative imbibition pressure, developing in the injured tissues secondary to the thermal injury and that "pulls" the fluid from the vascular space into the surrounding tissues. This effect is at its maximum after approximately 2 h, therefore the urgent time frame. Also a generalized permeability increase in the vascular tree is developing in parallel and that is due to the generalized inflammatory reaction that develops in the body after the burn injury. This effect is added to the effect by the imbibition pressure and they constitute the reason for the fluid needs of the burn injured [26]. The permeability change is claimed to subside at 8 h and most of it is undertaken within 24 h if the care is not complicated by sepsis and it is therefore most often recommended that the fluid provided is based on crystalloids until this time point [23, 27, 28]. In the USA fluids are based on lactated Ringer solutions, whereas many countries elsewhere do use acetated Ringer. In cases of refractory situations despite extensive fluid volume provided, the addition of colloids and/or vasoactive drugs may be relevant and needed [29, 30]. For most injuries, this is however uncommon. There are several fluid protocols in use worldwide today (Table 11.2) and the most commonly used is the one first presented by Dr. Baxter in the 1960s, called the Parkland formula as it was used initially at the Parkland Memorial Hospital in Dallas (Table 11.3) [32]. This scheme recommends in adults 2–4 mL/kg/TBSA% of crystalloids (Ringer's solution—lactate/acetate) for the first 24 h, 50% provided during the first 8 h, and 50% during the following 16 h. In children the corresponding fluid volume need is larger, that is 3–4 mL/kg/TBSA% and to this the normal 24 h fluid needs are added (Table 11.3). It is important to stress that the fluid volume suggested is to be closely adjusted according to endpoints—that is mainly urine output. In order to maintain perfusion of internal organs, the endpoint goal is for a urine output of 30 mL/h (or 0.5 mL/kg/h) in adults and 1 mL/kg/h in children. If insufficient urine output, a 30% increase in the fluid volume per hour provided is recommended. Alternatively, if urine output is too large a corresponding decrease is suggested.

It is important to stress that neither too little fluid nor too large fluid volumes in relation to the needs should be provided as it will lead to less successful results [33]. The needs vary largely between injuries and patients underlining the need for close surveillance and follow-up. In general and presently, in cases of less successful fluid resuscitations most often too large fluid volumes have been provided [30]. Too large fluid volumes will lead to deepening of the burn wound and secondary complications from other body compartments such as generalized large edema including cerebral, pulmonary edema and compartment situations, most importantly abdominal compartment syndrome [33]. Especially if using central circulatory endpoints rather than urine output during the first 12–18 h, such risk is higher [34]. Using the parkland formula, the patients appear "hypovolemic" as examined by central circulation techniques, e.g., echocardiography in the very early part of the resuscitation period [35, 36].

There are situations where larger fluid needs may be present. In general it has been claimed especially for inhalation or electrical injuries and in cases of a delayed start of fluid treatment. In the case of inhalation injuries the data supporting larger fluid needs are older and in newer investigations smaller effects of inhalation injury on the fluid needs have been seen [30]. In electrical injuries, the total tissue damage may be larger despite that the skin burn is less extensive. Other instances where larger fluid volumes are called for are in cases of high voltage electrical injuries or crush injures or

Table 11.2 Alternative fluid protocols (Modified from [31])

Crystalloid-based protocols	
Parkland	Ringer's lactate/acetate 2–4 mL/kg/TBSA%; half of the fluid during first 8 h
	Children: Ringer's lactate/acetate 3–4 mL/kg/TBSA%
Modified Brooke	Ringer's lactate/acetate 2 mL/kg/TBSA%
Colloid-based protocols	
Evans	NACl 1 mL/kg/TBSA%+ colloid 1 mL/kg/TBSA%+ 2000 mL glucose solution (5%)
Brooke	Ringer's lactate/acetate 1.5 mL/kg/TBSA%+ colloid 0.5 mL/kg %+ 2000 mL glucose solution (5%)
Slater	Ringer's lactate/acetate 2000 mL/24 + fresh frozen plasma 75 mL/kg/24 h
Dextran-based protocols	
Demling	Dextran 40 in NaCl (2 mL/kg/h in 8 h) + Ringer's lactate/acetate in sufficient amounts to induce a urine volume of 30 mL/h + fresh frozen plasma (0.5 mL/kg/h from 8 to 26 h post burn)
Hypertonic protocols	
Monafo	250 mEq Na/L. Amounts provided to induce a urine output of 30 mL/h
Warden	Ringer's lactate + 50 mEq sodium bicarbonate (total 180 mEq) during the first 8 h to induce a urine output of 30–50 mL/h. Thereafter Ringer's lactate with the same urinary output goal

Table 11.3 The Parkland protocol

Adults
Ringer's lactate/acetate 2–4 mL/kg/TBSA%. 50% provided during the first 8 h. The remaining fluid during the following 16 h
Children
Ringer's lactate/acetate 3–4 mL/kg/TBSA%. 50% provided during the first 8 h. The remaining fluid during the following 16 h. Normal 24 h fluid needs are added to this as glucose solution

when myo- och hemoglobinemia is present. Under these circumstances, an increased diuresis and alkalinization of the urine is recommended. The diuresis should reach 1–2 mL/kg/h (adults) and the pH of the urine should be kept alkaline preferably around or above 7. This is accomplished by adding sodium bicarbonate solution to the resuscitation fluids. This strategy should be continued as long as the pigments are present in the urine.

11.2.2.4 Burn Wound Evaluation

Most often the first burn wound evaluation is made under the heading "exposure" in the primary survey, at, e.g., the accident. A more thorough examination is then be made after the second survey. In evaluating the wound, it is important to have it adequately exposed and cleaned from debris and blisters, the latter situation calls for good analgesia or is done during general anesthesia. The risk of hypothermia should always be addressed. The wound evaluation is done mainly in two aspects, to determine, the depth and total percent body surface area injured (TBSA%). The depth is mainly important as it affects the treatment (surgical excision or not) and the TBSA% is important for the prognosis. TBSA% (including depth) is together with the age of the patient and the prevalence of inhalation injury, the most important prognostic factors for the injury. This will govern prognosis and also the fluid treatment.

Burn Wound Depth

How deep into the skin the injury progresses is dependent on several factors. Firstly, it depends on the thermal energy transferred to the tissue. This depends on the temperature and the exposure time; high temperature and longer exposure times increase the risk for significant injuries. The energy transfer process is further affected by the type of transfer, e.g., convection transfers more energy, and this is counteracted by the ability of the tissue to withstand the temperature (thicker skin—better resistance) or dissipate the heat (higher blood flow reduces the injury). In practice, this is exemplified by the lower risk for injuries on the back, in palms and soles with their thicker nature and the higher risk in elderly and children with their generally thinner skin.

Burn wound depth (see Fig. 11.2) has traditionally been divided into three levels according to anatomy, first degree—epidermal injury, second degree—dermal and third degree—subdermal burns. Today a two-level nomenclature is used which focuses more on treatment strategies: partial thickness burns (including epidermal and superficial dermal injuries first and superficial second degree burn; old nomenclature) and full thickness burns (including deep second degree and subdermal burns; old nomenclature). Modern care for partial thickness is conservative treatment, whereas full thickness burns are surgically excised and transplanted.

A burn involving the epidermis is usually erythematous and very painful but does not contain blisters. It is exemplified by a sunburn. The dead epidermis sloughs off and is replaced by regenerating keratinocytes within 2–3 days. A partial thickness burn wound is a superficial dermal burn and extends down to the papillary dermis and usually forms blisters. When the blisters are removed, the wound is pink, wet, and highly sensitive. Blanching is present. These wounds

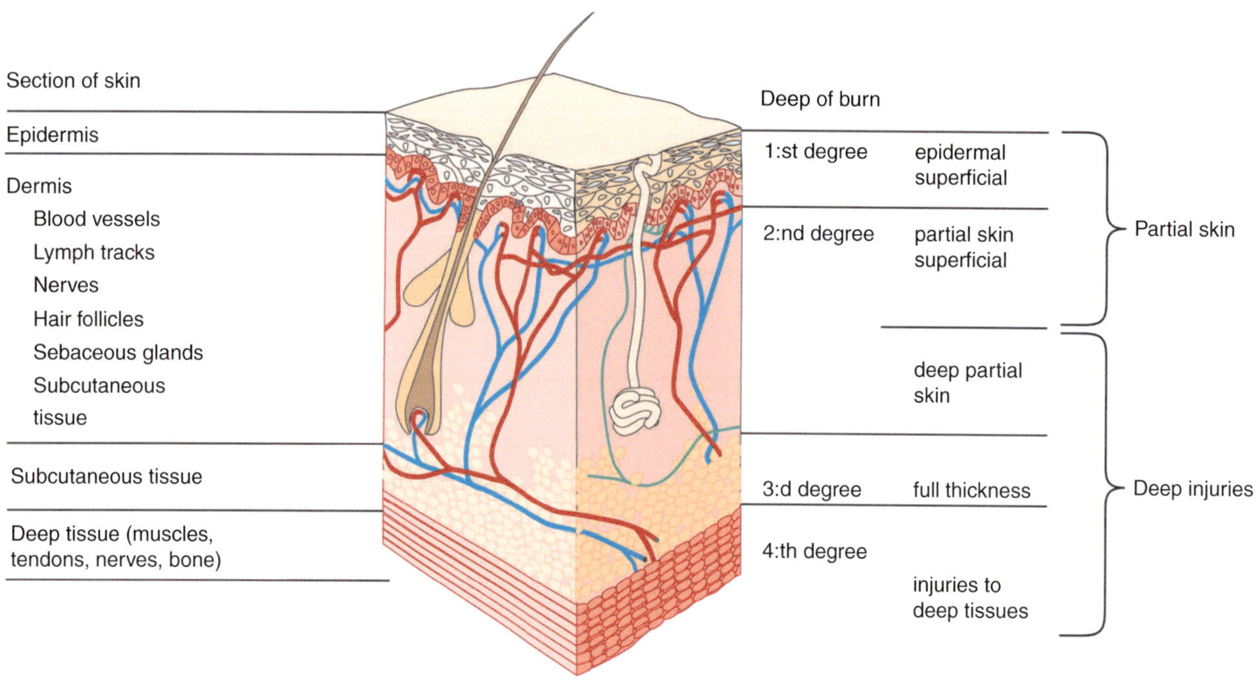

Fig. 11.2 Burn wound. Skin anatomy in relation to burn wound depth terminology

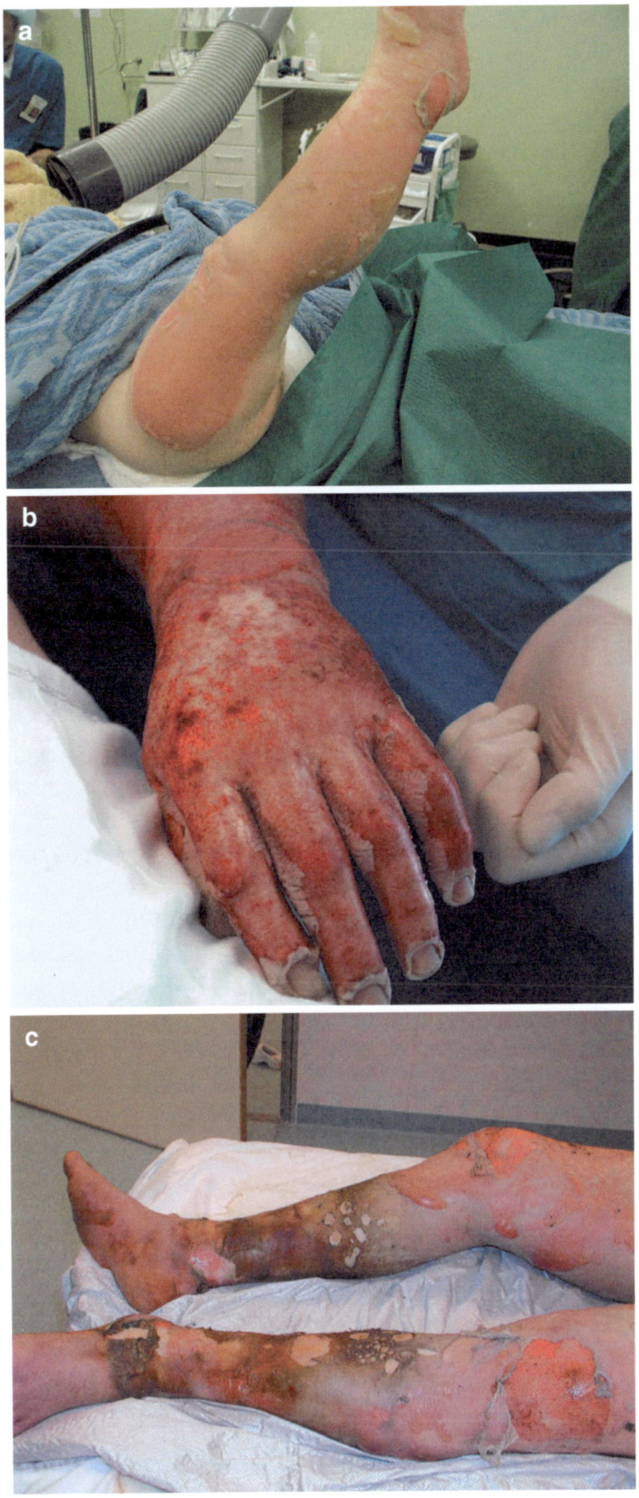

Fig. 11.3 Different burn depths (**a**–**c**) (Photos). (**a**) Superficial dermal burn wound—Partial thickness wound. (**b**) Deep dermal burn wound—Full thickness wound. (**c**) Full thickness wound extending down subdermally

heal within 2 weeks (Fig. 11.3a; Photo). Deep dermal wounds extend down to the reticular dermis and usually take more than 3 weeks to heal. These wounds also show blistering but the wound underneath has a mottled and white appearance. Blanching if at all present is slow. Sensitivity to pinprick is reduced and pain is described as discomfort rather than pain. See Fig. 11.3b (Photo). Full thickness wounds involve the entire dermis and extend to the underlying tissue. Appearance is described as charred, leathery, and firm. The wound is insensitive to touch and pinprick. See Fig. 11.3c (Photo). Deep dermal and full thickness wounds are surgically excised and autologous transplanted.

Burn Surface Area

The burned body surface area will as mentioned affect overall prognosis, the resources needed and not least from the practical perspective the immediate fluid treatment. It is therefore mandatory that it is done properly. From a practical perspective, the most commonly used technique is based on the rule of nines (See Fig. 11.4). In this setting, the body is divided into parts of 9% (arms and head) or multiples of nine (18%; each leg and each side of the torso/stomach and back); the corresponding chart for children (Fig. 11.4, lower) takes into account the larger size of the head and smaller legs in the smaller children (Fig. 11.4). If the ambition is to be more detailed, the chart of Lund and Browder is generally used [37]. In cases of dispersed injuries, it is common to apply the area of the palm and fingers (patient) as an estimate of 1% TBSA% of the injured [37].

11.2.2.5 Other Interventions at a Referring Hospital

When the patient is stabilized at a referring hospital, there are other interventions that may be done to progress the care and improve the situation for the patient prior to arrival at the burn center.

Pain Treatment

Pain early after the injury is very variable with patients at times experiencing severe pain, whereas others have more limited problems [38]. The extent of the pain is in each case difficult to predict in advance. Today most units base their pain treatment strategies on a multimodal pain strategy, which are based on several different principles. For the acute setting most often acetoaminophene (15 mg/kg × 4) is used in conjunction, when more significant pain is present, with i.v. administered opioids (e.g., morphine). The latter are provided in small incremental i.v. doses (1–2.5 mg), where the needs of the patients are monitored closely and the doses administered accordingly and thereby reducing the risk for a respiratory depression. The i.v. route is important in order to titrate the effect but also not least as it may be a poor uptake in hypoperfused tissue areas (s.c. or intramuscularly). Other more advanced pain strategies will be needed and employed during the further care of the patient, at the burn center.

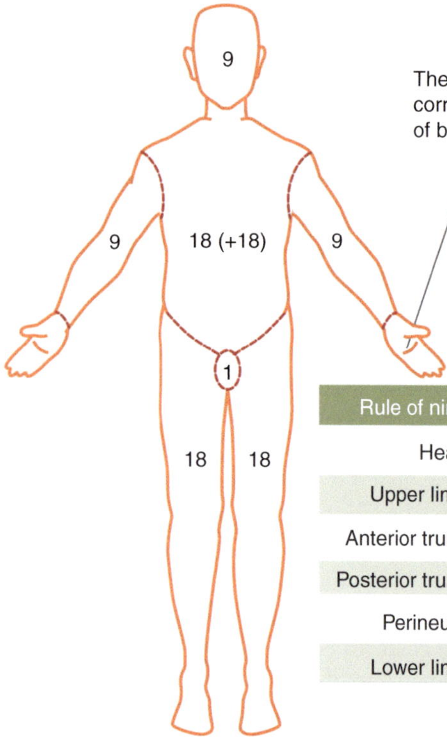

Rule of nine	Adult
Head	9 %
Upper limb	9 %
Anterior trunk	18 %
Posterior trunk	18 %
Perineum	1 %
Lower limb	18 %
	100 %

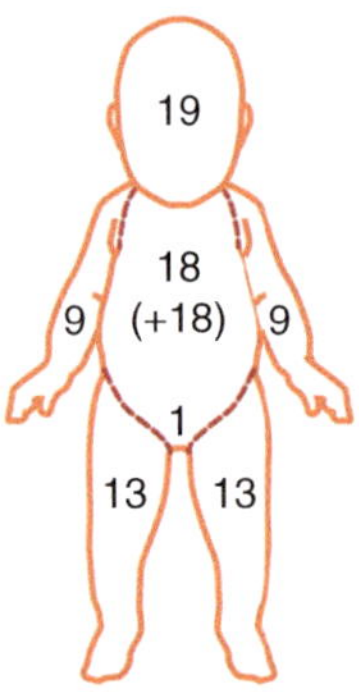

Rule of nine	Children < age of 10
Head	19 %
Upper limb	9 %
Anterior trunk	18 %
Posterior trunk	18 %
Perineum	1 %
Lower limb	13 % Plus half of age (years)
	100 %

For small children: Subtract 1 % from the head and add half percent to each leg for every year up to 10

Fig. 11.4 Total burn surface area (%). Rule of nine charts for an adult and a child

Urinary Catheter
Urine output is the main fluid treatment outcome measure. Therefore in order to monitor it, especially in larger burns a urinary catheter needs to be inserted. Modern catheters also have temperature sensors included in the intra-bladder portion of the catheter, which at the same time facilitates temperature surveillance. After insertion, urinary content of hemoglobin and myoglobin may be observable in such cases.

Decompression of the Stomach
Especially in the larger burns the stress response induces gastric, intestinal ileus and this is also further aggravated by the opioids provided for pain treatment. Therefore gastric decompression is often suggested by a nasogastric tube. Through this, also early enteral nutrition may be started and reducing the need for treatment with antacids for gastric ulcer prophylaxis [39]. The start of the enteral nutrition is made after the airway has been secured in cases of an impeding airway problem.

Temperature Control and Regulation
In the larger burns, maintaining body temperature is mandatory as one of the most important functions of the skin—temperature regulation—is affected by the burn. Also evaporative losses from the wounds generate further heat loss, which may further aggravate the situation. Therefore most often, active warming is needed. Temperature assessment needs to be properly done and one very good technique is to have thermistors in the intra-bladder part of the urinary catheter which senses the central body temperature. Good heating equipment includes heating ceilings; warm air mattresses (e.g., Bair Hugger®) or fluid heated mattresses (e.g., **Allon**®).

Invasive Blood Pressure Measurements: Central Circulation Surveillance and Central Venous Lines
Especially in larger burns (TBSA > 30%) the risk of circumferential extremity burns and major circulation effects increases. In these cases already at the referring hospital there might be a need to use invasive blood pressure monitoring and central circulatory surveillance, by, e.g., arterial thermodilution technique—e.g., the PICCO© system. This is not only important in adults [35] but has been shown also for children in which especially detection of burn sepsis [40] with circulatory effects is a well-known challenge within general pediatric ICU care [41] and where the invasive central circulatory surveillance has been strongly recommended [42–44]. It may thus be advantageous to, if properly skilled to do so, insert such catheters for use and measurements. It needs then, especially in the early phase after burn (0–12–24 h) to be stressed, that if the Parkland protocol is followed focus should remain on urinary output if arterial pressure, lactate and base excess are within relevant limits. Otherwise there is an imminent risk for fluid over resuscitation [34, 36, 38]. However, proper use of invasive monitoring in conjunction to adequate knowledge of the central circulatory parameters in burn shock resuscitation, a reduction in the use of inotropes may be accomplished, which at least from the theoretical perspective is advantageous. Already having such equipment in place is also valuable for the further resuscitation of the patient beyond the fluid resuscitation phase where sepsis is becoming more frequent and the major challenge [40, 45].

11.2.2.6 Referral to Burn Center
When the decision to refer the patient to a burn center is made, a physician to physician contact should be taken and the background of the patient and the details of the accident

should be properly communicated. Most often many interventions have been made since the accident and thereafter during transport or at the referral hospital. It is therefore important that all these are properly documented and that this documentation is properly communicated and transferred to the burn care physician. Especially the vital parameters, treatment interventions including fluid treatment and urine output should be documented and reported.

Referral criteria for burn center care may vary, but an often used table is that provided by the ABA, which also is applicable for most parts of Europe (e.g., Sweden), and which is close to that recommended by the European Burns Association (http://euroburn.org/wp-content/uploads/2014/09/EBA-Guidelines-Version-4-2017-1.pdf).

Burn Center Referral Criteria (EBA 2017)

- Patients with superficial dermal burns on more than:
  - 5% of TBSA in children under 2 years of age.
  - 10% of TBSA in children 3–10 years of age.
  - 15% of TBSA in children 10–15 years of age.
  - 20% of TBSA in adults of age.
  - 10% of TBSA in seniors over 65 years of age.

11.3 Transportation

Transportation of the burn victim may involve several steps—but most often two. The first is from the site of the accident to a local hospital, or to a similar point for stabilization. The second transport is from the referring hospital to the burn center, where the final treatment is provided. The first transport distance is often short and need for planning is less. Most often in Europe this is done by ambulance and the care during this transport is provided by paramedics or nurses which are stationed in the ambulance. The activities that have been undertaken at the scene of the accidents and during transport are then reported by the paramedics/nurse and/or documented in their report, which may be of complementary value when receiving the patient at the local hospital. In the report data regarding the patient, the circumstances at the scene as well as surveillance data may be found. At this point it is also important to identify the patient and obtain relevant data regarding relatives, so that information can be passed on or complementary questions regarding the background of the patient can be obtained.

The second transport is most often done from a local hospital, where the patient has been stabilized and some important burn-related treatments have been commenced, such as intubation/ventilatory treatment in cases of compromised airway, and fluid treatment for burn shock. In cases of circulatory compromise, escharotomies should have been performed. Also important is that in the early care other trauma-induced injuries should have been diagnosed and attended to—especially if urgent and/or life-threatening.

The choice of transport means depends on several factors of which local geography may be important, e.g., in an island or in an archipelago where airborne transport is almost obligatory. In general, transport exceeding 100 km often calls for airborne transport, such as helicopters or aircraft. Smaller hospitals may not have a helicopter landing facility and the first transport then involves an ambulance transport to the airfield. Tertiary referral hospitals (burn centers) in Europe most often have helicopter landing facilities. Specifically, if the patient needs ventilator or other specific intensive care treatments or interventions during transport a specially designed intensive care type ambulance is needed (Figs. 11.5 and 11.6).

It is important to stress the need for monitoring during transport, especially in major burns and in ventilated patients. For these patients, active heating devices, ventilators, and invasive blood pressure monitoring is relevant. It is important for the referring physician to be aware of the monitoring facilities provided by each type of transport system as this may pose a risk if the patient is not properly monitored and/or if interventions if needed are difficult or impossible to undertake during the transport. In some smaller helicopter types, critical care interventions may at times be difficult to perform and for such situations ground transport may be preferred. Also the referring physician needs to be updated on the skills and training of the transport surveillance personnel, who should be properly trained and have the relevant equipment for the transport that is planned.

11.4 Special Challenges in the Prehospital Setting, Referral Procedure, and Receiving Unit

11.4.1 Assessment of Burn Depth and Burn Surface Area Burned

As the incidence of burns is declining in most western countries and that changes in health care staffing may occur, there is a risk that the initial contact for the burn injured is with someone with limited experience of burn care and therefore there is an inherent need for a good communication between the referral unit and the receiving personnel. Today such communication can easily be undertaken by means of telemedicine, i.e., where detailed photographs even by modern apps in mobile telephones easily can be transferred. Modern technology can provide such information transfer without losing the integrity of the patient. An example may be found at (https://play.google.com/store/apps/details?id=com.wast.prehospitalcommunication), but proper versions are needed in order to ascertain patient integrity and compatibility with the computer systems of the involved hospitals. Information which is especially valuable in the prehospital setting is determining the depth and extent of the burn injury something known to be difficult not least for those less trained. It

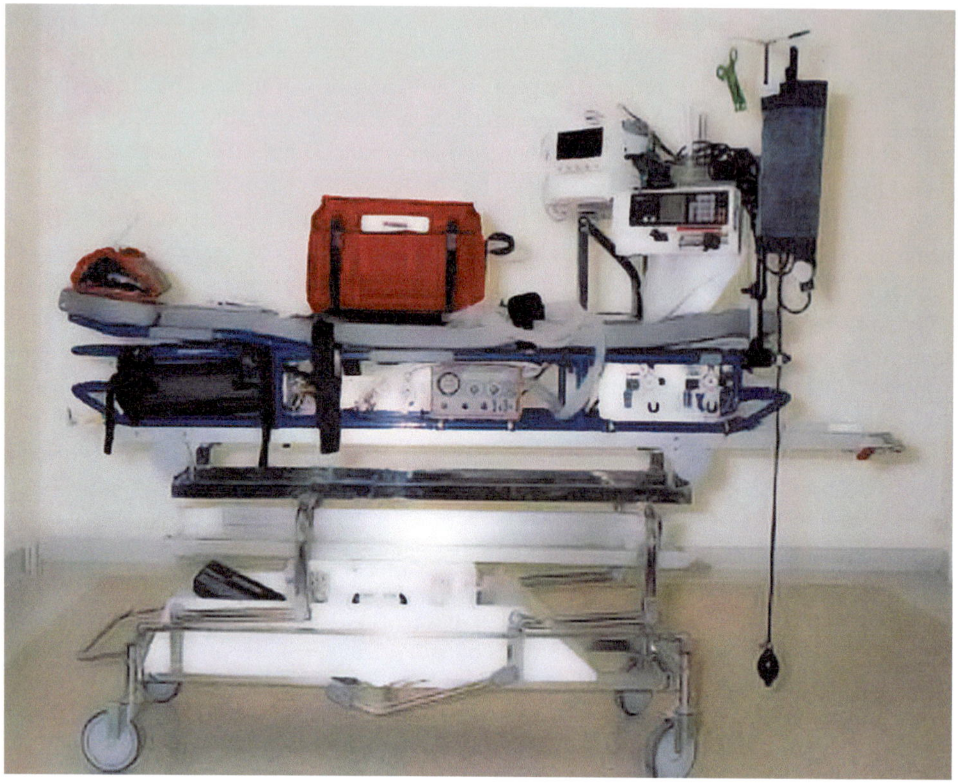

Fig. 11.5 Transportable critical care bed including equipment (text to be expanded)

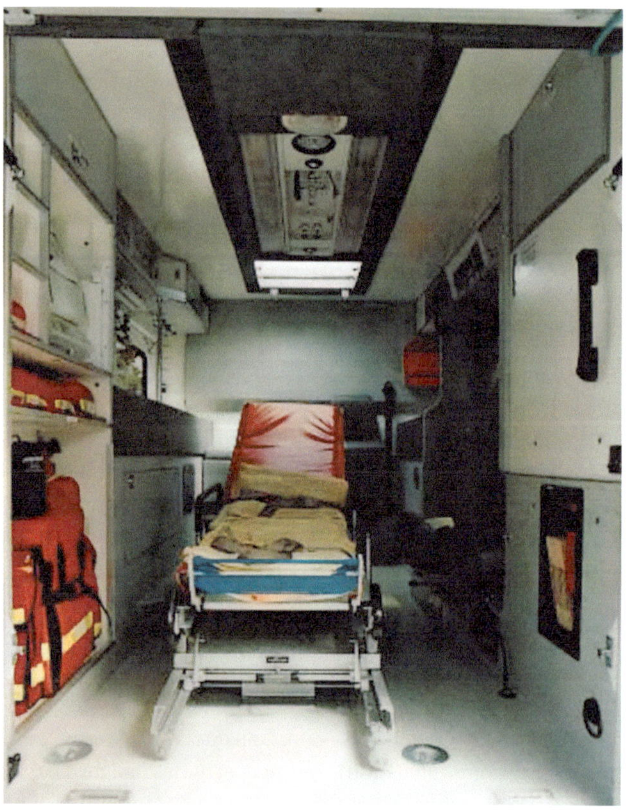

Fig. 11.6 Large interior of ambulance prepared for transporting critically ill patients (text to be expanded)

is therefore recommended that good communication between the referring and the receiving units is facilitated. Such procedures should be initiated and validated by preferably the tertiary burn center and its use properly communicated in the uptake area of the burn center.

11.4.2 Proper Indication for Intubation

In cases of gas exchange problems, the indication for intubation is less problematic [23]. However, confronted by facial burns the need for intubation to secure the airway may be more difficult to establish. In such cases, the use of telemedicine techniques may prove valuable as the referring physician/health worker may properly communicate with expertise at the burn center. This routine may reduce the need for unneeded intubations. It also makes the receiving unit aware of the present status of the patient in cases where changes occur during transport.

11.4.3 Fluid Resuscitation

In the time period years 2000–2010, an increase in the fluid treatment was noted in many publications and also fluid volumes were enhanced to the level that it was considered detrimental to the patient. This was referred to as the "fluid creep" and concomitantly significant discussions and teaching attempts have been focusing on reducing fluids to reach those levels considered more appropriate [29, 30]. In this context, increased reports of compartment syndrome complication have occurred. The risk of which increases significantly when the total volume exceeds 300 mL/kg/24 h [33]. However, there are recent indications that the pendulum has returned to a situation of too little fluid being provided [46]. Also when relatively very large volumes are provided within the Parkland strategy, the use of colloid rescue may be properly advised by the receiving hospital to reduce the risk for compartment syndrome [33]. Therefore the increased use of telemedicine or communication between referring and receiving unit may show further advantages.

Appendix: Referral and Transport Checklist

Organization, Logistics, and Communication

Sending hospitals contact recipient hospitals. Responsible physician at dispatch unit decides on transport method in consultation with the doctor on the receiving unit, and always has the medical responsibility for the transportation until this can be handed over to the receiving unit's medical doctor/specialist.

Those who transport patients should have the right skills for the task and should be used to transport/treat intensive care patients. For intubated or unstable patients, there should be two therapists in the care room and one of them must be specialist anesthetist.

All patient interventions before, during and after the transport should follow the patient, such as referral, list lists, surveillance lists, drug lists, hospital notes.

Other patient actions that are crucial for patient care after reception but not affecting treatment during transportation such as X-ray examination or hospital notes can be faxed to receiving in order not to delay transport. These documents shall, however, always be delivered at the receiving device by the time the patient arrives. X-rays should, if possible, be sent electronically.

Prior to transport, the transport team shall contact a dispatching hospital and receiving hospital and have relevant contact information (phone number/name) available under the entire transportation.

The mobile phone's benefit is superior to the potential risk of interference electronic equipment. With a plastic surgeon on the receiving unit, the chosen transport method is confirmed and preliminary arrival time communicated. Convey with receiving ICU doctors and discuss possible measures in case of deterioration of the patient's condition. The transport team shall inform the patient of the condition and assess the patient's general status before transport.

Examinations that should be carried out before transport:

- Trauma assessment
- Blood gas
- Relevant X-ray examinations
- Blood samples (Hemoglobin/Hct and coagulation)
- B-glucose
- Other relevant studies (possibly including blood grouping and base test)
  - ENT tubes and i.v. lines properly sutured

Monitoring

The basic principle of monitoring is that it must be at least the same monitoring level as at the sending hospital and should include:

- ECG with arrhythmia monitoring
- Invasive blood pressure measurement (invasive central circulation surveillance)
- Pulse oximetry
- Capnography (if the patient is intubated; controlled against arterial blood gas)
- Temperature measurement (if transport time exceeds 2–4 h, and with larger burns—continuous). For all larger burns, active heating should be secured by thermoregulated fluidized beds
- Diuresis (mL/h)

Treatment targets for all shipments are as follows (unless other target orders are given):

- SpO2 > 92%
- PCO2 4.5–5.5 kPa
- Temperature 37.5 °C
- Diuresis 0.5–1 mL/kg/h
- Blood gas and electrolytes within the normal reference range

Summary Box

The chapter describes the first evaluation and triage of the burn-injured patient and provides algorithms (ABLS/ATLS) for the early examination and stabilization (first 24 h) prior to transport. Based on present guidelines, details are provided in the ABCDE format for patient evaluation and finally especially challenging issues are addressed, together with referral and transport recommendations.

References

1. Akerlund E, Huss FR, Sjoberg F. Burns in Sweden: an analysis of 24,538 cases during the period 1987-2004. Burns. 2007;33(1):31–6.
2. Brigham PA, McLoughlin E. Burn incidence and medical care use in the United States: estimates, trends, and data sources. J Burn Care Rehabil. 1996;17(2):95–107.
3. Andel D, Kamolz LP, Niedermayr M, Hoerauf K, Schramm W, Andel H. Which of the abbreviated burn severity index variables are having impact on the hospital length of stay? J Burn Care Res. 2007;28(1):163–6.
4. Still JM Jr, Law EJ, Belcher K, Thiruvaiyarv D. Decreasing length of hospital stay by early excision and grafting of burns. South Med J. 1996;89(6):578–82.
5. Gomez M, Cartotto R, Knighton J, Smith K, Fish JS. Improved survival following thermal injury in adult patients treated at a regional burn center. J Burn Care Res. 2008;29(1):130–7.
6. Miller SF, Bessey PQ, Schurr MJ, Browning SM, Jeng JC, Caruso DM, et al. National Burn Repository 2005: a ten-year review. J Burn Care Res. 2006;27(4):411–36.
7. Mertens DM, Jenkins ME, Warden GD. Outpatient burn management. Nurs Clin North Am. 1997;32(2):343–64.
8. Moss LS. Outpatient management of the burn patient. Crit Care Nurs Clin North Am. 2004;16(1):109–17.
9. Tompkins D, Rossi LA. Care of out patient burns. Burns. 2004;30(8):A7–9.
10. Bessey PQ, Arons RR, Dimaggio CJ, Yurt RW. The vulnerabilities of age: burns in children and older adults. Surgery. 2006;140(4):705–15; discussion 15–7.
11. Sheridan R. Burns at the extremes of age. J Burn Care Res. 2007;28(4):580–5.
12. Thombs BD, Singh VA, Halonen J, Diallo A, Milner SM. The effects of preexisting medical comorbidities on mortality and length of hospital stay in acute burn injury: evidence from a national sample of 31,338 adult patients. Ann Surg. 2007;245(4):629–34.
13. Praiss IL, Feller I, James MH. The planning and organization of a regionalized burn care system. Med Care. 1980;18(2):202–10.
14. Yurt RW, Bessey PQ. The development of a regional system for care of the burn-injured patients. Surg Infect (Larchmt). 2009;10(5):441–5.
15. Vercruysse GA, Ingram WL, Feliciano DV. The demographics of modern burn care: should most burns be cared for by non-burn surgeons? Am J Surg. 2011;201(1):91–6.
16. Munzberg M, Mahlke L, Bouillon B, Paffrath T, Matthes G, Wolfl CG. [Six years of Advanced Trauma Life Support (ATLS) in Germany: the 100th provider course in Hamburg]. Unfallchirurg. 2010;113:561.
17. Soreide K. Three decades (1978-2008) of Advanced Trauma Life Support (ATLS) practice revised and evidence revisited. Scand J Trauma Resusc Emerg Med. 2008;16(1):19.
18. Sasaki J, Takuma K, Oda J, Saitoh D, Takeda T, Tanaka H, et al. Experiences in organizing Advanced Burn Life Support (ABLS) provider courses in Japan. Burns. 2010;36(1):65–9.
19. Cochran A, Edelman LS, Morris SE, Saffle JR. Learner satisfaction with Web-based learning as an adjunct to clinical experience in burn surgery. J Burn Care Res. 2008;29(1):222–6.
20. Lindford AJ, Lamyman MJ, Lim P. Review of the emergency management of severe burns (EMSB) course. Burns. 2006;32(3):391.
21. Stone CA, Pape SA. Evolution of the Emergency Management of Severe Burns (EMSB) course in the UK. Burns. 1999;25(3):262–4.
22. Haberal M. Guidelines for dealing with disasters involving large numbers of extensive burns. Burns. 2006;32(8):933–9.
23. Steinvall I, Bak Z, Sjoberg F. Acute respiratory distress syndrome is as important as inhalation injury for the development of respiratory dysfunction in major burns. Burns. 2008;34(4):441–51.
24. Cartotto R. Fluid resuscitation of the thermally injured patient. Clin Plast Surg. 2009;36(4):569–81.
25. Tricklebank S. Modern trends in fluid therapy for burns. Burns. 2009;35(6):757–67.
26. Lund T, Onarheim H, Reed RK. Pathogenesis of edema formation in burn injuries. World J Surg. 1992;16(1):2–9.
27. Vlachou E, Gosling P, Moiemen NS. Microalbuminuria: a marker of endothelial dysfunction in thermal injury. Burns. 2006;32(8):1009–16.
28. Vlachou E, Gosling P, Moiemen NS. Microalbuminuria: a marker of systemic endothelial dysfunction during burn excision. Burns. 2008;34(2):241–6.
29. Lawrence A, Faraklas I, Watkins H, Allen A, Cochran A, Morris S, et al. Colloid administration normalizes resuscitation ratio and ameliorates "fluid creep". J Burn Care Res. 2010;31(1):40–7.
30. Saffle JI. The phenomenon of "fluid creep" in acute burn resuscitation. J Burn Care Res. 2007;28(3):382–95.
31. Warden GD. Burn shock resuscitation. World J Surg. 1992;16(1):16–23.
32. Baxter CR, Shires T. Physiological response to crystalloid resuscitation of severe burns. Ann N Y Acad Sci. 1968;150(3):874–94.
33. Oda J, Yamashita K, Inoue T, Harunari N, Ode Y, Mega K, et al. Resuscitation fluid volume and abdominal compartment syndrome in patients with major burns. Burns. 2006;32(2):151–4.
34. Holm C, Mayr M, Tegeler J, Horbrand F, Henckel von Donnersmarck G, Muhlbauer W, et al. A clinical randomized study on the effects of invasive monitoring on burn shock resuscitation. Burns. 2004;30(8):798–807.
35. Bak Z, Sjoberg F, Eriksson O, Steinvall I, Janerot-Sjoberg B. Hemodynamic changes during resuscitation after burns using the Parkland formula. J Trauma. 2009;66(2):329–36.
36. Sjoberg F. The 'Parkland protocol' for early fluid resuscitation of burns: too little, too much, or ... even ... too late ...? Acta Anaesthesiol Scand. 2008;52(6):725–6.
37. The ABLS Manual. https://www.scribd.com/document/83859073/ABLS-Advanced-Burn-Life-Support-Provider-Manual. Assessed 8 Aug 2019.
38. Choiniere M, Melzack R, Rondeau J, Girard N, Paquin MJ. The pain of burns: characteristics and correlates. J Trauma. 1989;29(11):1531–9.
39. Raff T, Germann G, Hartmann B. The value of early enteral nutrition in the prophylaxis of stress ulceration in the severely burned patient. Burns. 1997;23(4):313–8.
40. Greenhalgh DG. Sepsis in the burn patient: a different problem than sepsis in the general population. Burns Trauma. 2017;5:23.
41. Potes C, Conroy B, Xu-Wilson M, Newth C, Inwald D, Frassica J. A clinical prediction model to identify patients at high risk of hemodynamic instability in the pediatric intensive care unit. Crit Care. 2017;21(1):282.
42. Branski LK, Herndon DN, Byrd JF, Kinsky MP, Lee JO, Fagan SP, et al. Transpulmonary thermodilution for hemodynamic measurements in severely burned children. Crit Care. 2011;15(2):R118.
43. Kraft R, Herndon DN, Branski LK, Finnerty CC, Leonard KR, Jeschke MG. Optimized fluid management improves outcomes of pediatric burn patients. J Surg Res. 2013;181(1):121–8.
44. Wurzer P, Branski LK, Jeschke MG, Ali A, Kinsky MP, Bohanon FJ, et al. Transpulmonary thermodilution versus transthoracic echocardiography for cardiac output measurements in severely burned children. Shock. 2016;46(3):249–53.
45. Greenhalgh DG. Defining sepsis in burn patients: still a long way to go. J Burn Care Res. 2017;38(6):e990–e1.
46. Soussi S, Deniau B, Ferry A, Leve C, Benyamina M, Maurel V, et al. Low cardiac index and stroke volume on admission are associated with poor outcome in critically ill burn patients: a retrospective cohort study. Ann Intensive Care. 2016;6(1):87.

12 Transfer, Telemedicine and Transportation in Pre-hospital Burn Management

Ryan E. Austin

12.1 Introduction

Burn centres serve as the gold standard in the treatment of patients with thermal injuries. However, a significant proportion of burn injuries occur in rural or remote locations without immediate access to a burn centre [1–3]. The declining incidence of thermal injuries has resulted in a decrease in the number of burn centres; as a result, the remaining facilities often provide service to large geographic regions with catchment areas of hundreds or even thousands of square kilometres [4]. Consequently, most thermally injured patients are initially assessed and triaged at a pre-hospital healthcare facility (i.e. a healthcare facility without specific burn care expertise) before considering transfer to a burn centre.

As a burn care provider, it is important to have an understanding of the transfer process for thermally injured patients. This chapter reviews the transfer and transportation of burn-injured patients from pre-hospital facilities to burn centres and reviews the role of telemedicine and technology in the pre-hospital management of burn injuries.

12.2 Transfer of Thermally Injured Patients

Once a thermally injured patient has been initially stabilized in the pre-hospital setting, one of the first questions that should be asked is 'Does this patient require transfer to a dedicated burn centre?' While this may seem like a straightforward question, multiple factors must be considered prior to making the decision to transfer (Table 12.1). In the ideal setting, all thermally injured patients would have access to the specialized care that a burn centre provides. However, the number of burn centres has declined in recent years, thereby limiting this resource availability [4, 5]. As a burn care provider, it is imperative to ensure that these limited resources are used as efficiently and effectively as possible to treat those thermally injured patients who most require burn centre care.

12.2.1 Pre-hospital Referral Guidelines

To assist pre-hospital healthcare providers in determining which patients may require transfer to a burn centre, several national burn associations have developed referral guidelines [6, 7] (Fig. 12.1). However, not all patients who meet referral guidelines require urgent transfer to a burn centre. Most burn injuries can be treated either on an outpatient basis or by local specialists with training in the management of burn injuries. There is a common misconception that these referral guidelines are actually transfer guidelines. While the difference between 'referral' and 'transfer' may seem semantic, this misconception may lead to potentially unnecessary acute burn transfers [8].

Despite the lack of well-defined transfer criteria, certain injury-specific factors are more likely to necessitate acute transfer to a burn centre [7]:

- Inhalation injury/airway compromise
- Burn size sufficient to require formal fluid resuscitation or intensive care monitoring
  - >10% total body surface area (TBSA) in children
  - >20% TBSA in adults
- Complex burn mechanism (e.g. chemical burn, electrical burn)
- Need for urgent surgical intervention (e.g. escharotomy)

Nevertheless, each thermal injury presents a unique set of patient-specific and injury-specific factors which must be taken into consideration as part of the transfer decision-making process.

R. E. Austin (✉)
The Plastic Surgery Clinic,
Mississauga, ON, Canada
e-mail: drraustin@theplasticsurgeryclinic.com

M. G. Jeschke et al. (eds.), *Handbook of Burns Volume 1*, https://doi.org/10.1007/978-3-030-18940-2_12

12.2.2 The Transfer Decision

Once the pre-hospital healthcare provider decides that a thermally injured patient may benefit from transfer to a burn centre, the next step is to establish direct communication with a burn care provider at a burn centre. The burn care provider will be able to review the circumstances of the thermal injury, as well as guide the pre-hospital provider regarding the management and ongoing resuscitation of the patient. Given the complex nature of burn injuries, direct communication between the most responsible healthcare providers is of the utmost importance to ensure that information is relayed clearly and accurately. Based on this information, the burn care provider will then be able to make a final determination regarding patient disposition and the need for acute transfer. The decision to transfer a thermally injured patient is not one that should be made by a pre-hospital healthcare provider unaided.

Table 12.1 Factors to be considered when determing the need for transfer of thermally injured patients

Factors influencing the need for transfer of thermally injured patients	
Pre-hospital factors	Experience treating burn injuries
	Knowledge of the treatment of burn injuries
	Resources for treating burn injuries
	Specialized intensive care/resuscitation requirements
Injury factors	Burn size, depth and location
	Airway involvement/inhalation injury
	Type of burn injury (e.g. flame, chemical and electrical)
	Concomitant injuries
	Need for urgent surgical intervention (e.g. escharotomy, fasciotomy, laparotomy)
	Need for eventual surgical intervention (e.g. burn excision and grafting)
Patient factors	Age
	Medical/psychiatric co-morbidities

Thermal injuries are complex by nature and may be overwhelming to healthcare providers unaccustomed to managing these injuries. In fact, the literature has documented that most pre-hospital healthcare providers have limited training and experience in treating thermally injured patients due to a lack of formal burn education during both medical school and residency training [9–12]. A study by Vrouwe et al. (2017) of Family Medicine and Emergency Medicine resident physicians, at a university training program associated with a regional burn centre, found that these primary care trainees encountered on average only 1–5 thermally injured patients during training and had limited to no burn-specific didactic or clinical teaching during their training. As a result, these primary care trainees self-reported being uncomfortable in the diagnosis and management of thermally injured patients [12].

Therefore, if primary healthcare providers are not being adequately trained or exposed to thermal injuries during training, it is not surprising that these providers have been well-documented to be significantly less accurate than burn care providers in the assessment of burn injuries (i.e. burn size and depth) [13–19]. Pre-hospital healthcare providers have a tendency to overestimate the size of small burns (<20% TBSA) and underestimate the size of large burns (>20% TBSA) [13, 14, 19, 20]. These errors in burn size estimates can be significant, with discrepancies as large as 560% of actual burn size reported in the literature [21]. Unfortunately, these inaccuracies regarding burn size estimation are further propagated by their direct impact on fluid resuscitation, as most resuscitation formulae are based on weight and %TBSA involvement [14, 20, 22–24].

Furthermore, the assessment and management of the airway by pre-hospital healthcare providers in burn-injured patients has come under increasing scrutiny. Multiple studies have demonstrated a tendency towards premature intubation of thermally injured patients in the pre-hospital setting. Though prophylactic intubation may seem benign, erring on the side of precaution, this intervention is not without its own

Fig. 12.1 American Burn Association (ABA) Burn Center Referral Criteria [6]

Burn injuries that should be referred to a burn center include:

- Partial thickness burns >10% TBSA
- Full thickness burns in any age group
- Burns involving the face, hands, feet, genitalia, perineum, or major joints
- Electrical burns, including lightning injury
- Chemical burns
- Inhalation injury
- Burn injury in patients with medical co-morbidities that could complicate management, prolong recovery, or affect mortality
- Burn injury with concomitant trauma (in which the burn injury poses the greatest risk of morbidity or mortality)
- Burned children in hospitals without qualified personnel or equipment for the care of children
- Burn injury in patients who will require special social, emotional, or rehabilitative intervention

inherent risks [25]. Studies have shown that among patients transferred to a burn centre having been intubated at a pre-hospital site, 30–60% are extubated within 24 h of arrival [21, 26–28].

In addition to %TBSA estimation and airway management, significant deficiencies have been reported in regard to pre-hospital documentation of treatment for thermally injured patients. Reviews of pre-hospital transfer records have found that documentation of burn size assessment, burn depth assessment, analgesia, tetanus status, and information for referral and follow-up are commonly inadequate or missing [29, 30].

These aforementioned errors in the initial assessment of burn injuries present a unique issue for the care of thermally injured patients. As a burn care provider, this highlights not only the importance of communication with pre-hospital healthcare providers to ensure accurate assessments prior to transfer but also the potential role for outreach and education on the management of thermally injured patients for pre-hospital healthcare providers.

12.2.3 Overtriage in Burn Transfers

As previously mentioned, not all thermally injured patients require acute transfer to a burn centre. An important aspect of ensuring appropriate utilization of burn centre resources involves minimizing the number of acute transfers for burns that could otherwise be managed on an outpatient basis. These patients, when transferred acutely with injuries that do not require burn centre admission, have been labelled in the literature as 'unnecessary', 'avoidable' or 'overtriaged' transfers.

Overtriage in the management of thermally injured patients is a complex issue and one that all burn care providers must be aware of. One of the main issues with overtriage is that it occupies burn centre beds that otherwise could be used by patients more in need of these intensive care services. One of the difficult issues with overtriage is that once these patients arrive at the burn centre, they may not be amenable for immediate discharge. Thermally injured patients often have multiple social issues affecting their disposition and repatriation, including

- Lack of immediate transportation back to home community
- Lack of housing in home community
- Need for ongoing hospitalization for non-burn medical/psychiatric co-morbidities

By transferring these patients away from their home community, they are distanced from family and social supports. It also becomes much more difficult to arrange the supports required for repatriation. A study by Austin et al. (2017) found that among overtriaged transfers, average burn centre length of stay was 2.8 days despite average burn size of only 5% TBSA [8].

Another issue with overtriage is the costs associated with transfer, both to the healthcare system and directly to the patient. Acute transfers for thermally injured patients can be quite expensive (see 12.4.4 *Cost of Burn Transportation*). In many cases, if hospitalization is not required, then the patient and their family are responsible for repatriation to the home community, which can be quite inconvenient [30]. In some cases, the patient may even be responsible for the costs of the transfer, which can be more expensive than the cost of the avoidable hospitalization [21, 31, 32].

Overtriage is an accepted risk in the management of acute thermal injuries, largely due to the potential risks of undertriage (i.e. not transferring burn-injured patients that require burn centre care). However, the issue becomes the rate at which overtriaged transfers occur for thermally injured patients. Studies have demonstrated that 17–30% of patients acutely transferred to a burn centre for thermal injuries were later deemed unnecessary [8, 31–33]. Latifi et al. (2017) investigated the reasons for burn centre transfer at a single institution and found that 45% of referrals to a single burn centre were made at the request of a patient or their family, while only 43% were referred due to a need for treatment at a burn centre [34].

While there are many possible explanations as to why overtriage occurs in thermally injured patients, four key factors have been identified [8].

- Inadequate knowledge of burn care
- Insufficient experience providing burn care
- Inadequate resources to provide burn care
- Incorrect initial assessment of burn injury

As a burn care provider, it is important to recognize these factors and identify their potential influence on transfers, so as to minimize the effects of overtriage. It is also important to make efforts to overcome these barriers whenever possible. During the transfer discussion, it is important to provide the pre-hospital healthcare provider with support and guidance and to appreciate that the pre-hospital healthcare provider managing a burn patients may be overwhelmed or limited by inadequate resources. Furthermore, the value of local and regional education and outreach initiatives cannot be overstated, to ensure that pre-hospital healthcare providers have the knowledge required to treat these complex patients.

12.3 Telemedicine in Pre-hospital Burn Care

The interaction between pre-hospital healthcare provider and burn care specialist is an integral part of the transfer process. Perhaps the most important aspect of this interaction is ensuring the accuracy of information conveyed about the burn injury itself, as this can directly impact patient care. Traditionally, this interaction would occur via telephone. While this real-time form of communication provides a direct connection between providers, it is limited by its reliance solely on the assessment and verbal description of the burn by the pre-hospital healthcare provider. Given the highly visual nature of burn injuries, providing a burn specialist the opportunity to visualize the burn injury would allow for a more reliable initial assessment. In recent years, advances in technology have made this possible with the integration of telemedicine into acute burn care.

12.3.1 Definition of Telemedicine

Any technology that allows healthcare providers to connect across a distance can be classified as 'telemedicine'. According to the World Health Organization, the official definition of telemedicine is "the delivery of healthcare services, where distance is a critical factor, by all health care professionals using information and communication technologies for the exchange of valid information [...] in the interests of advancing the health of individuals and their communities" [35]. This definition, though seemingly vague and broad, allows for the constant technological advancements that have changed the way medicine is practiced in the twenty-first century.

For the purposes of this chapter, however, the discussion of telemedicine focuses solely on those technologies that allow for the transmission of visual media (i.e. photographs and video) in the care of thermally injured patients.

12.3.2 Image Transfer in Telemedicine

Image transfer in telemedicine can be can be divided into two major categories, depending on the timing of the interaction between healthcare providers. In *synchronous* or 'real-time' telemedicine, individuals are simultaneously present for the exchange of information (e.g. videoconference). In *asynchronous* or 'store-and-forward' telemedicine, pre-recorded information is exchanged between individuals at different times (e.g. images sent via e-mail). In both synchronous and asynchronous telemedicine, information may be shared by any form of media (i.e. text, audio, photograph, video) [35].

Both categories of telemedicine have their advantages and disadvantages. While synchronous telemedicine provides real-time interaction between providers, establishing this live connection requires all parties to be available at the same time, and there must be access to a fast and reliable telecommunication network. On the other hand, while asynchronous telemedicine may have a delay in the interaction between providers, these connections are easier to arrange with less reliance on advanced telecommunication networks, and the ability for providers to review information at their leisure. For these reasons, asynchronous technology is the more commonly used method of communication for telemedicine in acute burn care [4].

12.3.3 Evidence for Telemedicine in Acute Burn Care

In the acute setting, telemedicine has two important roles in the management of thermally injured patients. First, visual assessment of burn injuries by a burn care specialist provides pre-hospital healthcare providers with additional resources for the initial management of burn-injured patients, including [21, 36]

- Assessment of inhalation injury and the need for intubation
- Assessment of burn size and depth
- Assessment of need for fluid resuscitation
- Assessment of need for surgical intervention

As previously mentioned, errors in the initial assessment of burn injuries by pre-hospital healthcare providers can significantly impact patient care. Saffle et al. (2004) found that 35% of patients transferred to a single burn centre would have had a substantial alteration in their care had telemedicine been available prior to transfer [21]. Multiple studies have shown high rates of potentially avoidable intubation among burn-injured patients, with 30–60% of patients intubated prior to transfer able to be safely extubated within 24 h of transfer [21, 26–28]. Furthermore, a prospective study by Wibbenmeyer et al. (2016) found that burn-injured patients transferred from referring centres that provided video images of the injuries prior to transfer had a significantly lower incidence of over- or under-resuscitation compared to referring centres that only had telephone communication [18]. By confirming the accuracy of initial burn injury assessment, telemedicine can help to prevent potential complications arising from primary assessment errors.

Second, telemedicine can improve the triage accuracy for acute thermal injuries, allowing for more informed transfer decisions and minimizing the effects of overtriage. Allowing a burn care provider to see images of a burn injury prior to deciding on the need for transfer improves confidence in the triage decision-making process. In situations where visual documentation is unavailable, there is a natural tendency to err on the side of caution so as to reduce the risk of undertriage. Wallace et al. (2007) found that the implementation of a telemedicine program for burns reduced the rate of unplanned clinic admissions from 21% down to 0% [37]. Den Hollander et al. (2017) found that the use of telemedicine led to an alteration of the transfer plan in 66% of referrals, with 38% of transfer referrals being avoided completely during an 8 month study period [38]. Saffle et al. (2009) demonstrated that the implementation of a regional telemedicine program altered the transfer plan in 55% of patients, with 42% of transfer referrals that would have previously required air transport able to receive local treatment only and another 12% able to be transported by private vehicle instead of by air [39]. Russell et al. (2015) were able to decrease air transport rates from 100% to 44% with the implementation of a telemedicine program [40].

As technology has improved and the potential benefits of telemedicine have been recognized, use of telemedicine in acute burn care has increased significantly. A 2012 study found that 84% of burn centres in the United States were using telemedicine, with the majority of centres reporting telemedicine use on a regular basis for both acute burn consultation and to aid in the determination of need for acute burn transfer [4]. Successful telemedicine programs have been implemented in both developed and developing nations, as well as cross-border international programs [38, 40–44]. These telemedicine programs have repeatedly demonstrated a high satisfaction rating among referring providers and patients [18, 37, 39, 40]. In 2017, the American Telemedicine Association developed guidelines for the establishment of a Teleburn network, which can aid in the development and implementation of telemedicine programs [5].

12.3.4 Accuracy of Burn Assessment Using Telemedicine

One of the key features required for the adoption of telemedicine in burn care is that the technology must allow burn care providers to accurately assess burn injuries, both in terms of burn size and burn depth.

Telemedicine has repeatedly demonstrated both high reliability and validity compared to in-person assessment for the estimation of burn size [39, 40, 45, 46]. Saffle et al. (2009) compared burn size estimates performed by burn physicians via telemedicine to in-person estimates and found high correlations [39]. Shokrollahi et al. (2007) demonstrated high intra- and inter-rater reliability comparing telemedicine evaluation to in-person evaluation of burn size [46]. Hop et al. (2014) compared burn size estimates made via telemedicine to laser Doppler imaging of burn size and again demonstrated good inter rater reliability and validity for the determination of burn size [45]. Even in dark skin types, telemedicine is at least as accurate as in-person evaluation of burn size [15]. However, when it comes to the assessment of burn size via telemedicine, experience does appear to play a role, with senior burn care providers being more accurate at estimation compared to providers with fewer years of experience [45].

In regard to the estimation of burn depth, the results of telemedicine have been slightly more mixed. While telemedicine can be used to distinguish full-thickness from partial-thickness burn injuries with a high degree of accuracy, determining the depth of partial-thickness burns (i.e. deep partial-thickness versus superficial partial-thickness) can be more difficult [46]. Boccara et al. (2011) reported that photographic evaluation of burn depth was equivalent to in-person assessment in 76% of cases, with most errors occurring amongst burns of intermediate depth [47]. Jones et al. (2003) also found that agreement on the depth of partial-thickness burns amongst four independent observers was lower than for either full-thickness or superficial burn injuries [47]. Boissin et al. (2015) found that amongst dark skin types, burn depth could be accurately assessed via telemedicine in 66% of cases [15]. In general, there seems to be a tendency to overestimate the depth of partial-thickness injuries when assessed via telemedicine [45]. Conversely, a study by Jones et al. (2005) found that inter-rater correlation of burn depth assessment ranged widely, from poor to good [46]. Hop et al. (2014) suggested that burn depth assessments via telemedicine were unreliable when compared to laser Doppler imaging assessment, though this technology is much more sensitive than clinical assessment alone [45]. However, it is important to remember that even experienced burn care providers only have a 50–76% accuracy rate for in-person determination of burn depth [17, 45].

Overall, telemedicine can be used to accurately assess thermal injuries for the purposes of initial management and triage. However, caution should be exercised if planning to use telemedicine alone to determine a clinical treatment plan, particularly if this plan is based on the assessment of burn depth. Hop et al. (2014) found that telemedicine alone could not be used to accurately determine the need for surgical debridement in small burn injuries (<10% TBSA) [45]. In situations where there is question about the need for potential surgical intervention, close follow-up and re-evaluation should be considered to monitor burn wound evolution over time.

12.3.5 Image Quality in Telemedicine

For accurate image assessment to occur via telemedicine, the image files must be of sufficient quality. Resolution in digital imaging is commonly defined by the number of pixels present in an image, with higher pixel counts representing higher-quality images. Early studies in telemedicine for burn injuries found that a modest image resolution of 800 × 600 pixels was sufficient for accurate image interpretation and that higher resolution images and larger file sizes were not required [48].

However, as technology has advanced, the standards for image resolution have evolved. In fact, the quality of camera technology in smartphones today far exceeds even what was available in high-end camera technology a decade ago.

As image quality increases however, so too does the file size. Though larger files contain more data and detail, file size can quickly become too large to send using standard telecommunications networks. To work around this, file size is often compressed during the process of image transfer to allow for quick and reliable image transmission. While image compression reduces file size, it also lessens image quality, particularly when employing standard compression methods typically used in telemedicine (i.e. JPEG) [50]. Roa et al. (1999) demonstrated that images may be compressed up to 50:1 while maintaining 90% accuracy in image assessment, though further compression reduced the accuracy of image assessment [49].

Current guidelines from the American Telemedicine Association have outlined the minimum image quality for telemedicine in burn care, as follows: [5]

- Photograph: 3-megapixel (MP) resolution with image compression not exceeding 20:1
- Video: 640 × 360 resolution at 30 frames per second

Most modern smartphones have specifications for both photographs and video that meet or exceed these minimum requirements [50].

On the receiving end, these images must be viewed on a display of sufficient resolution to allow for image interpretation. Previous studies in telemedicine for burn injuries have demonstrated that image resolution greater than 1024 × 768 pixels does not appear to benefit the viewer [50]. This image resolution is available on most modern smartphones. In fact, a study by Boissin et al. (2017) demonstrated that emergency providers preferred interpreting clinical photographs on a smartphone or tablet compared to a standard laptop computer screen [51]. The American Telemedicine Association guidelines, however, are slightly more stringent and suggest a minimum screen resolution of 1280 × 1024 pixels for image interpretation to avoid loss of image quality [5].

Often overlooked when discussing image quality in telemedicine is the quality of the captured image itself. Clinical photography in the acute traumatic setting can be difficult, and standard guidelines for image capture do not exist [38]. However, inadequate image capture may present significant issues for telemedicine, as poor-quality images make image interpretation difficult and less reliable [39]. Furthermore, patient care may be delayed by having to retake and resend poor-quality images. A study by Jones et al. (2004) of clinical photographs for plastic surgery and burn injuries found that 13% of transmitted images were inadequate for telemedicine analysis [48, 50]. Suggestions to improve the quality of image capture are presented in Table 12.2.

Table 12.2 Factors affecting image quality in the clinical photography of thermal injuries

Good-quality clinical photograph	Poor-quality clinical photograph
Multiple images of the sites of interest from varying distance (i.e. afar for frame of reference, medium and close-up for detail)	Too few images; images too zoomed-in without frame of reference; images too zoomed-out to provide sufficient detail
Image focused; image centred in camera frame	Blurry image; area of interest off-centre in image
Well-lit photographs with appropriate use of flash to minimize shadowing	Over- or under-lit photographs
Standardized, clean background	Distracting objects in background (e.g. blood, clothing, floor, jewellery, mirrors)
Ruler for standardized measurement when appropriate	Lack of standardized measurement between images

12.3.6 Smartphones and Telemedicine

One of the most significant advances in telemedicine over the past two decades has been the ubiquitous integration of the smartphone into daily life. With the ability to send and receive text, audio, photographs and video in both a synchronous and a store-and-forward manner, anybody with a smartphone essentially has a mobile telemedicine studio in their pocket, obviating the need for expensive infrastructure [36].

The technology in smartphones has improved exponentially over the past decade, and so too has their applicability in telemedicine. Take the iPhone® (Apple, Cupertino, CA) as an example. When the original iPhone® was released in 2007, it had a screen resolution of 320 × 480 pixels, a 2.0 MP camera, and was unable to record video. Compare this, only 10 years later, to the newest generation of the iPhone®, which boasts a screen resolution of 2436 × 1125 pixels, a 12MP camera, and the ability to record 3840 × 2160 pixel video at up to 60 frames per second; specifications that far exceed the minimum requirements for telemedicine image transmission outlined by the American Telemedicine Association [5]. A study by Boissin et al. (2015) found that among three major smartphone brands tested, all produced images that were as good quality as those produced by a digital camera [52].

As a result of these improvements, the role of the smartphone in the pre-hospital management of burn care has significantly increased. A study by Shokrollahi et al. (2007) found high inter- and intra-rater correlations in the determination of burn size and depth comparing photographs from a 1.0 MP smartphone camera to clinical assessment [46]. Den Hollander et al. (2017) found that based on telemedicine consultations from smartphone images alone they were able to avoid 38% of all pre-hospital referrals [38].

Furthermore, several burn-related applications have been created for use specifically with smartphones, focused on all areas of burn care from burn size and fluid resuscitation calculators to educational apps and even games [15, 53–56]. Applications have even been developed that allow pre-hospital providers to upload images of a burn injury and calculate burn size, with the application then determining initial fluid requirements and automatically alerting a burn specialist of the injury to initiate the telemedicine interaction [57]. As smartphone technology continues to advance, there is no doubt that its applicability to burn care will continue to develop.

12.3.7 Limitations of Telemedicine

Telemedicine systems can be difficult to implement. Traditionally, the greatest barrier to the implementation of telemedicine systems has been cost. With an average cost for a single portable telemedicine studio of $15,000–$20,000 (USD) and the start-up cost for a telemedicine network ranging from $50,000 to $110,000 (USD), these costs have historically been prohibitive [36, 50]. However, these cost estimates are for synchronous telemedicine systems. The cost of implementing an asynchronous system is far less, and costs will likely continue to decrease as advances in technology make these systems more readily available [37]. Furthermore, smartphone technology has made it possible for nearly anybody to perform both synchronous and asynchronous telemedicine [36].

Currently, the most significant barrier to the implementation of telemedicine systems in burn care is network security and patient privacy [4, 18, 58]. Most national healthcare agencies have developed legislation requiring that any personal health information, including images or videos, be transmitted across secured networks to ensure patient safety. The Health Insurance Portability and Accountability Act (HIPAA) in the United States is one of the most commonly cited examples of this legislation. The high costs associated with early telemedicine systems were, in large part, due to ensuring compliance with these regulations. However, these secured systems are often cumbersome to use, which may dissuade pre-hospital healthcare providers from using telemedicine communication [18]. Furthermore, as smartphones become more commonly used tools for telemedicine, the risk of unsecured interactions and privacy breeches may increase [59, 60]. All healthcare providers must be aware of the legislation governing the use of telemedicine where they practice to ensure that all communications comply with local laws [60, 61].

Other issues commonly cited as limitations to the implementation of telemedicine systems include a lack of well-defined guidelines for billing and remuneration for telemedicine services, difficulties with licensure across borders for burn centres that cover large geographic catchment areas, 'technophobia' and a lack of willingness to incorporate technology into the practice of medicine, and the reliance of telemedicine on information technology systems which may be affected by disruptions of the telecommunication network, such as in power outages or in the disaster setting [4, 39, 40, 58].

12.4 Transportation of Thermally Injured Patients

Once the decision has been made to transfer a thermally injured patient to a burn centre, the next determination is how the patient should be transported. In most situations, this decision is made by either the pre-hospital healthcare provider or by the emergency medical service (EMS) transport provider. When selecting the most appropriate method of transportation, multiple factors must be considered, including

- Injury severity/acuity
- Distance of transportation
- Accessibility of referring site
- Availability of EMS resources

Though most of these factors cannot be altered, as a burn care specialist, providing an accurate assessment of injury severity and acuity of transportation may directly impact selection of the method of transportation. This not only helps to ensure that patients are transported appropriately but also that transport resources are utilized efficiently and effectively.

When it comes to the transfer of thermally injured patients, the main goals of transportation are to ensure that the patients arrive at the burn centre

1. Safely, in stable condition
2. Within an appropriate period of time

In the transfer of thermally injured patients, the four most commonly utilized methods of transportation are private vehicle, ground ambulance (GEMS), helicopter (HEMS) and fixed-wing aircraft. While each option has its own unique advantages and disadvantages, the major difference between transportation methods relates largely to the speed of transportation, the distance they are able to travel and the cost of transport.

12.4.1 Preparation for Transportation

To maximize patient safety during transfer, patient optimization prior to transportation is critical [40, 62]. Resources available during transportation are limited, and procedural interventions (e.g. intravenous insertion and intubation) are much more difficult within the limited confines of an ambulance or helicopter. Adequate pre-transport optimization can help avoid potential complications. Burn care providers play an important role in pre-transport patient optimization, despite not being present on-site. Through frequent communication with both the pre-hospital healthcare team and the transportation team, it is important to ensure that a patient is suitable for transportation and to guide these providers regarding the needs of the thermally injured patient [40].

To optimize a thermally injured patient for transfer, all elements of the primary burn survey should be re-evaluated prior to transportation.

- *Airway*: Securing the airway prior to transportation is of the utmost importance, as an airway is more difficult to establish during transport once lost. However, unnecessary prophylactic intubation should be avoided to prevent undue risk to the patient. If there is doubt as to the security of the airway and the potential need for intubation, this should be discussed with the burn care provider prior to transportation.
- *Breathing*: Adequate oxygenation is important due to the increased metabolic demands in burn-injured patients. Oxygen saturation should be monitored in all patients throughout transportation, particularly if fluid resuscitation is ongoing, as generalized soft tissue oedema can impact respiratory demands. If the patient is intubated prior to transportation, ventilation settings should be reviewed with the burn care provider prior to transport. Difficulties in oxygenation or ventilation should be addressed prior to departing the pre-hospital healthcare facility.
- *Circulation*: Intravenous (IV) access is critical in thermally injured patients. Any patient being transferred via EMS should be sent with two large-bore peripheral IVs (minimum 18 gauge). Central venous access and arterial lines are commonly required in patients with larger burns; however, these are rarely placed in the pre-hospital setting and should never delay transfer. Fluid resuscitation with lactated Ringer's solution should be continued during transportation at the pre-calculated rate, if appropriate. For patients being transferred whilst undergoing active fluid resuscitation, a urinary catheter should be placed prior to transportation to allow for resuscitation monitoring. The goal for adequate fluid resuscitation is 0.5–1.0 cm^3/kg/h of urine output.
- *Disability*: Prior to transportation, the neurological status of the patient should be re-evaluated to ensure no interval change in the level of consciousness (LOC). Intoxication with drugs or alcohol is common in burn injuries and may affect LOC. Glasgow coma score (GCS) should be documented prior to transportation for all patients. Furthermore, a complete head-to-toe secondary survey should be performed to rule-out traumatic injuries that may be masked by the thermal injury.
- *Exposure*: All burn wounds should be kept clean during transportation. Burn wounds should be dressed with a non-stick base layer dressing (e.g. petroleum-impregnated gauze) and covered with gauze and an absorbent layer to minimize dressing saturation. Due to the risk of developing hypothermia during transportation, efforts must be made to keep the patient warm during transport. This may include covering the patient with warm blankets, use of an active warming device and warmed intravenous fluid resuscitation.

Thermal injuries can result in significant systemic physiologic derangement, and burn-injured patients can quickly and unpredictably become unstable during transportation. For this reason, all patients (with the exception of Private Vehicle transports) should be placed on continuous vital sign monitoring during transportation. This includes body temperature monitoring, as hypothermia is common in burn injuries.

12.4.2 Timing of Burn Transportation

In the ideal setting, patients with thermal injuries would be transferred to a burn centre as quickly as possible. However, unlike mechanical trauma injuries, burn-injured patients do not have a defined 'golden hour' that clearly affects patient outcomes [28]. Though the impact that transportation time has on patient outcomes has been studied, this metric is difficult to standardize due to disparity in transportation distance and injury severity. For example, a non-life-threatening 15% TBSA burn does not require the same transport urgency as a 30% TBSA burn with inhalation injury.

Reports of average transport times in the literature range widely, from less than 2 h to greater than 10 h for acute transfers [8, 28, 38, 62, 63]. Despite this variability, however, time to transportation has been shown to not significantly impact the outcome of thermally injured patients. A study by Bell et al. (2012) found that indirect referral to a burn centre from a pre-hospital facility did not influence the risk of mortality or hospital length-of-stay [64]. Cassidy et al. (2015) found that the only factor that independently affected mortality for indirect transfers was a transfer time >16 h among patients with inhalation injury [63].

Provided that adequate fluid resuscitation is initiated at the pre-hospital healthcare facility, there is no need for urgent surgical intervention and no evidence of inhalation injury, transportation may safely be delayed during the acute resuscitation phase. This certainly does not mean that transportation should be unduly postponed; instead, it simply means that not all thermally injured patients require transfer via the fastest method of transportation possible (i.e. air transportation) if there are other feasible options available. As a burn care provider, it is important to discuss these factors to help guide EMS and pre-hospital healthcare providers as to the appropriate level of transport urgency for every burn transfer.

12.4.3 Safety of Burn Transportation

The transportation of thermally injured patients is a practice that can be safely performed at any time, even during the ongoing acute resuscitation phase, with low complication rates (4.0–6.2%) [28, 62]. The most commonly reported complications during transportation include airway-related issues (e.g. accidental extubation, respiratory distress and inability to secure airway), loss of intravenous access, cardiac dysrhythmia and hemodynamic-related issues [28]. Hypothermia is also common in the transportation of thermally injured patients. A study by Klein et al. (2007) found that approximately 10% of patients transported to a regional burn centre were hypothermic at the time of arrival [28]. While there was a correlation between hypothermia and increasing total burn size, the duration of transportation did not appear to play a significant role [28]. However, the method of transportation may have a direct effect on the physiology of thermally injured patients. Though a review of aeromedical medicine is beyond the scope of this chapter, thermally injured patients transferred via helicopter or fixed-wing aircraft are known to experience decreased core temperature, increased oxygen demands and blood pressure fluctuations due to the changes in barometric pressures and altitude during air transportation [40].

12.4.4 Cost of Burn Transportation

Transportation of thermally injured patients can be associated with significant costs. Depending on injury severity and transport distance, these patients may require critical care EMS transfer teams, ongoing fluid resuscitation or even ventilation during transportation. These costs are further amplified when air transport is required due to aircraft maintenance expenses, pilot fees and fuel. However, not all patients require these specialized EMS services. In recent years, there has been an increased focus on improving the cost-efficiency of transportation for thermally injured patients. In general, there are two ways that the cost-efficiency of acute burn transportation can be improved [8]

1. Minimize the cost of transportation
2. Avoid wasteful use of transportation resources

One method of maximizing the cost-efficiency of burn transportation is to minimize transportation-related costs. Ideally, thermally injured patients should be transferred by the least expensive method of transportation possible, provided that

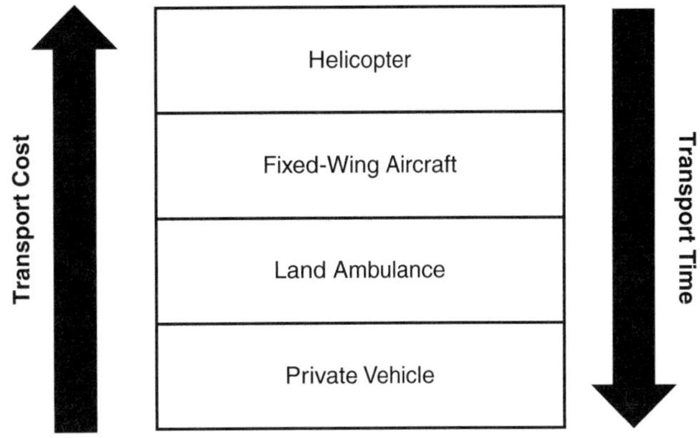

Fig. 12.2 The relationship between travel time and cost for commonly used methods of transportation in the transfer of thermally injured patients

this does not compromise patient outcome. Conceptually, a transportation hierarchy exists based on the inverse relationship between transportation cost and transport time [8] (Fig. 12.2). Private vehicle transportation, wherein the patient is transported to the burn centre by a relative or friend with no EMS personnel or equipment, has the lowest associated cost but is also the slowest method of transportation. This method of transportation is typically reserved for minor injuries requiring outpatient assessment or follow-up. Ground ambulance (GEMS) transfers are costlier, as they include EMS personnel and equipment. However, like private vehicle transports, GEMS transport times may be limited by distance as well as local traffic conditions. Helicopter (HEMS) transfers and fixed-wing aircraft are able to cover greater distances in significantly less time, though they are associated with the highest transportation costs. In cases where a combination of transportation methods is required (e.g. ambulance + helicopter), costs can further escalate. An understanding of the relationship between cost and transport time will allow both pre-hospital and burn care providers to select the most appropriate method of transportation while maximizing cost-efficiency.

A second method of maximizing the cost-efficiency of burn transportation is avoiding the wasteful use of transportation resources. As previously discussed, overtriage is a significant issue for burn centres. What often goes overlooked, however, are the costs associated with transporting these patients to a burn centre. This is particularly applicable for overtriaged patients that are transported by HEMS or fixed-wing aircraft. The cost for a one way HEMS trip can range from $4000 up to $30,000, which is approximately 10–15× higher than ground ambulance transfer costs [8, 32, 40]. These costs become even more significant with overtriage rates for HEMS burn transfers ranging from 12% to 65% [21, 31, 32, 65–68]. In fact, a single-centre study estimated that over a 2 year period, over $500,000 was wasted in the transportation of overtriaged patients by helicopter [69]. In some cases, the costs of HEMS transport for overtriaged patients can exceed the cost of hospitalization itself [21]. While some have argued that overtriage rates of 25–50% in the trauma setting should be considered acceptable given the risk of undertriage, there is no reason that these patients should be transported by the most expensive method of transportation, if at all avoidable [32]. By deescalating these transfers to a less expensive method of transportation, significant cost savings could be expected. Wibbenmeyer et al. (2016) demonstrated that they were able to deescalate the method of transportation from HEMS or GEMS to private vehicle in 6.3% of transfers [18]. Saffle et al. (2004) found that 18% of patients transferred by HEMS would have been appropriate for transfer by private vehicle instead [21]. The potential cost savings if these patients were transported by ambulance or private vehicle instead of helicopter could fund the development of telemedicine or outreach initiatives aimed at burn education for pre-hospital healthcare providers [8].

12.4.5 Development of Transportation Criteria

Transferring thermally injured patients via the most appropriate method of transportation maximizes the efficiency of transport resource utilization. The critical determination is whether or not air transport is required, as helicopter and fixed-wing aircraft costs far exceed land transfer costs [70]. In the trauma literature, pre-hospital triage scores have been developed to identify patients who would benefit from helicopter transport, however, similar guidelines do not exist for burn-injured patients [71–74]. To determine whether a thermally injured patient would benefit from air transportation, the following factors should be considered [67, 69]:

- *Distance*: Studies have demonstrated no benefit to helicopter transportation within a 180–200 miles (290–320 km) radius. Ground transportation within this radius typically adds no more than 2 h to the total travel time, which is well within the acceptable transfer window for thermal injuries. Beyond this distance helicopter use may be beneficial, depending on injury severity.
- *Inhalation Injury*: Patients with no evidence of inhalation injury can safely be transported by ground and do not typically require air transportation. Inhalation injury has been shown to independently impact patient mortality if transfer is delayed more than 16 h from time of injury, which must be considered [63]. However, not all patients with inhalation injury require air transportation.
- *Burn Size*: Patients with a burn size less than 20% TBSA can typically be safely transferred by ground transportation. Smaller burns typically have less physiologic derangement and are less likely to require intravenous fluid resuscitation, thereby reducing transfer urgency. Burns larger than 20% TBSA require fluid resuscitation and have greater physiologic derangement, making them more unstable by definition. Therefore, patients with larger burn size are more likely to benefit from faster transportation to a burn centre.
- *Surgical Emergency*: While early excision and grafting is common in burn surgery, this rarely occurs within the first 24–48 h following burn injury. Therefore, emergent surgical intervention for thermally injured patients is typically reserved for circumferential burns (i.e. escharotomy), compartment syndrome (i.e. fasciotomy or laparotomy) or for concomitant traumatic injuries. Patients not requiring urgent or emergent surgical intervention typically do not require air transportation and can be safely transported by ground.

While these are not intended to be strict criteria, these factors should be taken into consideration when determining the most appropriate method of transportation for thermally injured patients. If at all possible, efforts should be made to minimize the influence of non-injury-related factors on method of transportation (e.g. patient insurance status and competition between EMS service providers). Implementation of pre-transport telemedicine can help ensure safe, appropriate, and efficient utilization of transportation resources [75].

Summary Box

- Every thermal injury presents unique patient- and injury-specific factors that must be considered when determining the need for transfer to a regional burn centre.
- Burn referral guidelines are ***not*** transfer criteria.
- As a burn care provider, it is important to establish and maintain direct communication with the transferring centre. Many pre-hospital healthcare providers have limited experience treating burn injuries. Errors in the initial assessment of burn injuries can significantly impact acute resuscitation and the decision to transfer.
- Telemedicine is an important tool in burn care, allowing burn care providers to remotely assess thermal injuries for the purposes of initial management and triage. Though telemedicine (including smartphones) has demonstrated accuracy in the determination of burn size, assessment of burn depth may be less reliable.
- Burn care providers should provide the transferring centre with an accurate assessment of injury severity and acuity. This information can be combined with non-modifiable transportation factors (i.e. distance, accessibility of referring site, availability of EMS resources) to determine the most appropriate method of transportation.

- Thermally injured patients may be safely transported by land or air with low complication rates, even during the acute burn resuscitation period.
- Thermally injured patients can quickly and unpredictably become unstable; therefore, it is important that these patients are optimized prior to transfer. Informing EMS and the transfer centre regarding the requirements of thermally injured patients can help to ensure patient safety during transportation.
- The transfer of thermally injured patients can be associated with significant costs, particularly when air transportation is involved. To maximize cost-efficiency in burn transport, (1) patients should be transferred via the least costly method of transportation possible without compromising patient outcome and (2) overtriage to burn centres should be avoided.

Disclosures The authors declared no potential conflicts of interest with respect to the authorship and publication of this article. There are no sources of financial support to disclose regarding this article.

References

1. Duke J, Rea S, Semmens J, Wood F. Urban compared with rural and remote burn hospitalisations in Western Australia. Burns. 2012;38:591–8.
2. Han TH, Kim JH, Yang MS, Han KW, Han SH, Jung JA, et al. A retrospective analysis of 19,157 burns patients: 18-year experience from Hallym Burn Center in Seoul, Korea. Burns. 2005;31:465–70.
3. Kasana RA, Baba PU, Wani AH. Pattern of high voltage electrical injuries in the Kashmir valley: a 10-year single centre experience. Ann Burns Fire Disasters. 2016;29:259–63.
4. Holt B, Faraklas I, Theurer L, Cochran A, Saffle JR. Telemedicine use among burn centers in the United States. J Burn Care Res. 2012;33:157–62.
5. Theurer L, Bashshur R, Bernard J, Brewer T, Busch J, Caruso D, et al. American Telemedicine Association guidelines for teleburn. Telemed J E Health. 2017;23:365–75.
6. American Burn Association. Burn Center Referral Criteria. http://ameriburn.org/wp-content/uploads/2017/05/burncenterreferralcriteria.pdf. Accessed 11 Nov 2017.
7. NSW Agency for Clinical Innovation. NSW Burns Transfer Guidelines. https://www.aci.health.nsw.gov.au/__data/assets/pdf_file/0004/162634/Burns_Transfer_Guidelines_2013-14_-_web.pdf. Accessed 11 Nov 2017.
8. Austin RE, Schlagintweit S, Jeschke MG, MacDonald R, Ahghari M, Shahrokhi S. The cost of burn transfers: a retrospective review of 7 years of admissions to a regional burn center. J Burn Care Res. 2018;39(2):229–34.
9. Egro FM, Estela CM. The need for burns teaching: a cross-sectional study to assess burns teaching in the United Kingdom. Burns. 2014;40:173–4.
10. Lemon TI, Stapley S, Idisis A, Green B. Is the current UK undergraduate system providing junior doctors knowledge and confidence to manage burns? A questionnaire-based cohort study. Burns Trauma. 2016;3:1–5.
11. Zinchenko R, Perry FM, Dheansa BS. Burns teaching in UK medical schools: is it enough? Burns. 2016;42:178–83.
12. Vrouwe SQ, Shahrokhi S. Assessing primary care trainee comfort in the diagnosis and management of thermal injuries. J Burn Care Res. 2017;38:e739–44.
13. Hammond JS, Ward CG. Transfers from emergency room to burn center: errors in burn size estimate. J Trauma. 1987;27:1161–5.
14. Freiburg C, Igneri P, Sartorelli K, Rogers F. Effects of differences in percent total body surface area estimation on fluid resuscitation of transferred burn patients. J Burn Care Res. 2007;28:42–8.
15. Boissin C, Laflamme L, Wallis L, Fleming J, Hasselberg M. Photograph-based diagnosis of burns in patients with dark-skin types: the importance of case and assessor characteristics. Burns. 2015;41:1253–60.
16. Giretzlehner M, Dirnberger J, Owen R, Haller HL, Lumenta DB, Kamolz LP. The determination of total burn surface area: how much difference? Burns. 2013;39:1107–13.
17. Jaskille AD, Shupp JW, Jordan MH, Jeng JC. Critical review of burn depth assessment techniques: part I. Historical review. J Burn Care Res. 2009;30:937–47.
18. Wibbenmeyer L, Kluesner K, Wu H, Eid A, Heard J, Mann B, et al. Video-enhanced telemedicine improves the care of acutely injured burn patients in a rural state. J Burn Care Res. 2016;37:e531–8.
19. Harish V, Raymond AP, Issler AC, Lajevardi SS, Chang LY, Maitz PK, et al. Accuracy of burn size estimation in patients transferred to adult Burn Units in Sydney, Australia: an audit of 698 patients. Burns. 2015;41:91–9.
20. Collis N, Smith G, Fenton OM. Accuracy of burn size estimation and subsequent fluid resuscitation prior to arrival at the Yorkshire Regional Burns Unit. A three year retrospective study. Burns. 1999;25:345–51.
21. Saffle JR, Edelman L, Morris SE. Regional air transport of burn patients: a case for telemedicine? J Trauma. 2004;57:57–64.
22. Sadideen H, D'Asta F, Moiemen N, Wilson Y. Does overestimation of burn size in children requiring fluid resuscitation cause any harm? J Burn Care Res. 2017;38:e546–51.
23. Goverman J, Bittner EA, Friedstat JS, Moore M, Nozari A, Ibrahim AE, et al. Discrepancy in initial pediatric burn estimates and its impact on fluid resuscitation. J Burn Care Res. 2015;36:574–9.
24. Hagstrom M, Wirth GA, Evans GR, Ikeda CJ. A review of emergency department fluid resuscitation of burn patients transferred to a regional, verified burn center. Ann Plast Surg. 2003;51:173–6.
25. Costa Santos D, Barros F, Frazão M, Maia M. Pre-burn centre management of the airway in patients with face burns. Ann Burns Fire Disasters. 2015;28:259–63.
26. Cook TM, MacDougall-Davis SR. Complications and failure of airway management. Br J Anaesth. 2012;109(Suppl 1):i68–85.
27. Romanowski KS, Palmieri TL, Sen S, Greenhalgh DG. More than one third of intubations in patients transferred to burn centers are unnecessary. J Burn Care Res. 2016;37:e409–14.
28. Klein MB, Nathens AB, Emerson D, Heimbach DM, Gibran NS. An analysis of the long-distance transport of burn patients to a regional burn center. J Burn Care Res. 2007;28:49–55.
29. Smith S, Duncan M, Mobley J, Kagan R. Emergency room management of minor burn injuries: a quality management evaluation. J Burn Care Rehabil. 1997;18:76–80.
30. Bezuhly M, Gomez M, Fish JS. Emergency department management of minor burn injuries in Ontario, Canada. Burns. 2004;30:160–4.
31. Reiband HK, Lundin K, Alsbjorn B, Sorensen AM, Rasmussen LS. Optimization of burn referrals. Burns. 2014;40:397–401.
32. Kashefi N, Dissanaike S. Use of air transport for minor burns. J Burn Care Res. 2016;37:e453–60.
33. Face S, Dalton S. Consistency of total body surface area assessment in severe burns: implications for practice. Emerg Med Australas. 2017;29:429–32.
34. Latifi N-A, Karimi H. Why burn patients are referred? Burns. 2017;43:619–23.

35. World Health Organization. Telemedicine: opportunities and developments in Member States: report on the second global survey on eHealth. 2010. http://www.who.int/goe/publications/goe_telemedicine_2010.pdf. Accessed 11 Nov 2017.
36. Atiyeh B, Dibo SA, Janom HH. Telemedicine and burns: an overview. Ann Burns Fire Disasters. 2014;27:87–93.
37. Wallace DL, Smith RW, Pickford MA. A cohort study of acute plastic surgery trauma and burn referrals using telemedicine. J Telemed Telecare. 2007;13:282–7.
38. den Hollander D, Mars M. Smart phones make smart referrals: the use of mobile phone technology in burn care—a retrospective case series. Burns. 2017;43:190–4.
39. Saffle JR, Edelman L, Theurer L, Morris SE, Cochran A. Telemedicine evaluation of acute burns is accurate and cost-effective. J Trauma. 2009;67:358–65.
40. Russell KW, Saffle JR, Theurer L, Cochran AL. Transition from grant funding to a self-supporting burn telemedicine program in the western United States. Am J Surg. 2015;210:1037–42.
41. Mars M, Scott RE. Being spontaneous: the future of telehealth implementation? Telemed J E Health. 2017;23:766–72.
42. Fuzaylov G, Knittel J, Driscoll DN. Use of telemedicine to improve burn care in Ukraine. J Burn Care Res. 2013;34:e232–6.
43. Turk E, Karagulle E, Aydogan C, Oguz H, Tarim A, Karakayali H, et al. Use of telemedicine and telephone consultation in decision-making and follow-up of burn patients: initial experience from two burn units. Burns. 2011;37:415–9.
44. Syed-Abdul S, Scholl J, Chen CC, Santos MD, Jian WS, Liou DM, et al. Telemedicine utilization to support the management of the burns treatment involving patient pathways in both developed and developing countries: a case study. J Burn Care Res. 2012;33:e207–12.
45. Hop MJ, Moues CM, Bogomolova K, Nieuwenhuis MK, Oen IM, Middelkoop E, et al. Photographic assessment of burn size and depth: reliability and validity. J Wound Care. 2014;23:144–5.
46. Shokrollahi K, Sayed M, Dickson W, Potokar T. Mobile phones for the assessment of burns: we have the technology. Emerg Med J. 2007;24:753–5.
47. Jones OC, Wilson DI, Andrews S. The reliability of digital images when used to assess burn wounds. J Telemed Telecare. 2003;9(Suppl 1):S22–4.
48. Jones SM, Milroy C, Pickford MA. Telemedicine in acute plastic surgical trauma and burns. Ann R Coll Surg Engl. 2004;86:239–42.
49. Roa L, Gomez-Cia T, Acha B, Serrano C. Digital imaging in remote diagnosis of burns. Burns. 1999;25:617–23.
50. Wallace DL, Hussain A, Khan N, Wilson YT. A systematic review of the evidence for telemedicine in burn care: with a UK perspective. Burns. 2012;38:465–80.
51. Boissin C, Blom L, Wallis L, Laflamme L. Image-based teleconsultation using smartphones or tablets: qualitative assessment of medical experts. Emerg Med J. 2017;34:95–9.
52. Boissin C, Fleming J, Wallis L, Hasselberg M, Laflamme L. Can we trust the use of smartphone cameras in clinical practice? Laypeople assessment of their image quality. Telemed J E Health. 2015;21:887–92.
53. Wurzer P, Parvizi D, Lumenta DB, Giretzlehner M, Branski LK, Finnerty CC, et al. Smartphone applications in burns. Burns. 2015;41:977–89.
54. Kamolz LP, Lumenta DB, Parvizi D, Dirnberger J, Owen R, Holler J, et al. Smartphones and burn size estimation: "Rapid Burn Assessor". Ann Burns Fire Disasters. 2014;27:101–4.
55. Parvizi D, Giretzlehner M, Dirnberger J, Owen R, Haller HL, Schintler MV, et al. The use of telemedicine in burn care: development of a mobile system for TBSA documentation and remote assessment. Ann Burns Fire Disasters. 2014;27:94–100.
56. Morris R, Javed M, Bodger O, Gorse SH, Williams D. A comparison of two smartphone applications and the validation of smartphone applications as tools for fluid calculation for burns resuscitation. Burns. 2014;40:826–34.
57. Wallis LA, Fleming J, Hasselberg M, Laflamme L, Lundin J. A smartphone app and cloud-based consultation system for burn injury emergency care. PLoS One. 2016;11:e0147253.
58. Vyas KS, Hambrick HR, Shakir A, Morrison SD, Tran DC, Pearson K, et al. A systematic review of the use of telemedicine in plastic and reconstructive surgery and dermatology. Ann Plast Surg. 2017;78:736–68.
59. McKnight R, Franko O. HIPAA compliance with mobile devices among ACGME programs. J Med Syst. 2016;40:129.
60. Thomas VA, Rugeley PB, Lau FH. Digital photograph security: what plastic surgeons need to know. Plast Reconstr Surg. 2015;136:1120–6.
61. Greene AH. HIPAA compliance for clinician texting. J AHIMA. 2012;83:34–6.
62. Treat RC, Sirinek KR, Levine BA, Pruitt BA. Air evacuation of thermally injured patients: principles of treatment and results. J Trauma. 1980;20:275–9.
63. Cassidy TJ, Edgar DW, Phillips M, Cameron P, Cleland H, Wood FM, et al. Transfer time to a specialist burn service and influence on burn mortality in Australia and New Zealand: a multi-centre, hospital based retrospective cohort study. Burns. 2015;41:735–41.
64. Bell N, Simons R, Hameed SM, Schuurman N, Wheeler S. Does direct transport to provincial burn centres improve outcomes? A spatial epidemiology of severe burn injury in British Columbia, 2001-2006. Can J Surg. 2012;55:110–6.
65. Nicholson B, Dhindsa H. Helicopter transport in regionalized burn care: one program's perspective. Air Med J. 2016;35:355–9.
66. Chipp E, Warner RM, McGill DJ, Moiemen NS. Air ambulance transfer of adult patients to a UK regional burns centre: who needs to fly? Burns. 2010;36:1201–7.
67. Baack BR, Smoot EC, Kucan JO, Riseman L, Noak JF. Helicopter transport of the patient with acute burns. J Burn Care Rehabil. 1991;12:229–33.
68. Rhee KJ, Burney RE, Mackenzie JR, Conley J, LaGreca-Reibling K, Flora J. Therapeutic intervention scoring as a measure of performance in a helicopter emergency medical services program. Ann Emerg Med. 1986;15:40–3.
69. De Wing MD, Curry T, Stephenson E, Palmieri T, Greenhalgh DG. Cost-effective use of helicopters for the transportation of patients with burn injuries. J Burn Care Rehabil. 2000;21:535–40.
70. Taylor CB, Curtis K, Jan S, Newcombe M. Helicopter emergency medical services (HEMS) over-triage and the financial implications for major trauma centres in NSW, Australia. BMC Emerg Med. 2013;13:11.
71. Brown JB, Gestring ML, Guyette FX, Rosengart MR, Stassen NA, Forsythe RM, et al. Development and validation of the air medical prehospital triage score for helicopter transport of trauma patients. Ann Surg. 2016;264:378–85.
72. Thomas SH, Brown KM, Oliver ZJ, Spaite DW, Lawner BJ, Sahni R, et al. An evidence-based guideline for the air medical transportation of prehospital trauma patients. Prehosp Emerg Care. 2014;18(Suppl 1):35–44.
73. Wormer BA, Fleming GP, Christmas AB, Sing RF, Thomason MH, Huynh T. Improving overtriage of aeromedical transport in trauma: a regional process improvement initiative. J Trauma Acute Care Surg. 2013;75:92–6.
74. Delgado MK, Staudenmayer KL, Wang NE, Spain DA, Weir S, Owens DK, et al. Cost-effectiveness of helicopter versus ground emergency medical services for trauma scene transport in the United States. Ann Emerg Med. 2013;62:351–64.
75. Slater H, O'Mara MS, Goldfarb IW. Helicopter transportation of burn patients. Burns. 2002;28:70–2.

13 Admission of Burn Patients to the Burn Center Including Burn Wound Evaluation

Moustafa Elmasry, Ingrid Steinvall, Pia Olofsson, and Folke Sjöberg

13.1 Introduction

This chapter addresses the treatment algorithms and bundles to be undertaken at the second or last treatment level, the burn center [1, 2]. The burn center provides the last treatment level where also burn surgery is undertaken to cover full-thickness burn wounds. This chapter focuses on the early period of admission at the burn center usually encompassing the first 24–48 h after the burn, whereas the treatment strategies presented in the previous chapter focuses mainly on the triage and patient examination necessary for the acute care and proper prioritization for the next care level. One central aim has then been to do a proper trauma evaluation in line with a trauma triage guideline such as the ATLS and possibly also by a specific burn-based triage algorithm such as the ABLS [3–5] or the EMSB courses [6–8]. It is then important to strictly follow the algorithm so that no specific detail in the patient background or injury profile is overlooked—this strategy is then also continued at the receiving site as will be described below. Prior to referral contact is taken between the refereeing physician and the corresponding person at the receiving unit. As was stressed in the previous chapter, there are concerns that there may be details overlooked or the information may be hampered by at times the lack of experience at the referral site. This especially has been a topic of interest as burn care is constantly being further centralized as incidence numbers decline in most high-income western countries and the chance for different physician categories to be exposed to burns decline [9]. To facilitate the communication between referral and receiving units increasing focus has been directed at telemedicine tools that further enhances and facilitates communications [10–12]. Especially photos of injured tissues have been found valuable. Challenges that need special attentions in the early evaluation of the burn injured is related to the need for intubation, estimation of the burn size and depth and correspondingly the magnitude and titration of fluid treatment, and need of escharotomies. A significant portion of the early assessment that will also ensue at the burn center has already been described in detail in the previous chapter and therefore is only shortly mentioned now, and focus is instead directed to important issues to be examined and dealt with at the burn center.

M. Elmasry · I. Steinvall · P. Olofsson
Department of Hand and Plastic Surgery, Linköping University Hospital, Linköping, Sweden

Department of Clinical and Experimental Medicine, Linköping University, Linköping, Sweden
e-mail: moustafa.elmasry@liu.se; ingrid.steinvall@regionostergotland.se; Pia.Olofsson@regionostergotland.se

F. Sjöberg (✉)
Department of Clinical and Experimental Medicine, Linköping University, Linköping, Sweden
e-mail: folke.sjoberg@liu.se

13.2 Primary Admittance Protocol and Control

When the initial discussion has been undertaken with the burn center and the underlying information details of the patient has been transferred to the burn center, the first action is to prepare resources and equipment for the receiving process at the burn center. In a well-administered and trained burn center that means to activate the regular routines for new admittance. It may be advised that these procedures are well described in standard operating procedures (SOP) based on adequate guidelines [13, 14] as well as having checklist in place to control that each important procedure in the SOP is adequately followed. Such good examples for burn care may be found, e.g., in England [15]. It has been well documented that checklists within healthcare and not least intensive care may improve outcome [16–19]. Also good documentation principles are needed for follow-up purposes, quality assurance, and benchmarking. This includes entering data into quality registries [20–22] and for later follow-up reports used in burn center verification processes such as described for Europe [23], Australia [24], and the USA [25].

M. G. Jeschke et al. (eds.), *Handbook of Burns Volume 1*, https://doi.org/10.1007/978-3-030-18940-2_13

When the patient first arrives, control of previously obtained information is ascertained and it is ensured that the proper documentation is in place. In parallel, for the well-being of the patient, it is important that the different steps in the ABLS or the corresponding algorithm are regularly re-evaluated, so that the present medical status is ascertained and is in line with what has been reported earlier or if there are deviations, such as a deterioration in any of the vital parameters, the corresponding action is promptly undertaken.

13.3 Primary and Secondary Assessment

As stressed in the previous chapter, primary and secondary assessment is again made at the burn center. There are however a number of important issues that are relevant at this level where a more detailed and ambitious approach may be advocated.

13.4 ABCDE

Airway. Airway assessment can be more thoroughly evaluated, and the need or possibility to intubate can be more properly assessed using fiber-optic techniques examining the upper airway in detail for thermal injuries and the corresponding risk of immediate or later swelling, e.g., secondary to fluid resuscitation. If intubated acutely at the referring facility a decision on the management of the airway long term can now be made. This airway assessment is made and evaluated in relation to patient history and blood gas analysis (gas exchange/diffusion). In larger burns with bronchoscopy-verified inhalation injury with concomitant gas diffusion difficulties, an early tracheostomy should be considered [26]. It is important to thoroughly evaluate the airway by bronchoscopy and clear as much as possible of soot and debris at an early point. A thorough investigation at this point can also help predict the length of ventilator treatment [27]. Also the use of thoracic CT scans can help in delineating the extents of the inhalation injury [28–30]. Early ARDS development may occur but is not very common especially not in the very early phase after burn [31]. Early tracheostomy may facilitate treatment, based on completely without or with significantly reduced sedation and thus increasing the rehabilitative potential in early care [26]. Here it may be important to consider COPD in older patients with a smoking history, who might have fallen asleep while smoking and being injured, and who may have a pulmonary problem already prior to the accident. Increased fire accidents have also been noted in oxygen-treated COPD population [32].

Breathing. Again the restrictive effects of circular burns need to be re-assessed and the need for complementary escharotomies may be considered. In this situation, the restrictive effect of large fluid volumes may also be appreciated. At this point in time carbon monoxide and cyanide intoxication may be still relevant although oxygen may have been properly provided during transport in cases with suspect carbon monoxide poisoning. Blood levels need to be evaluated and especially in patients who have been extricated unconscious from the fire. It needs to be stressed that that may have been the primary reason for intubation. If carboxyhemoglobin levels in blood are not reduced, extended oxygen treatment is mandatory. There is no evidence for beneficial effects of hyperbaric oxygen treatment additional to an extended oxygen treatment administered through a ventilator or by nasal cannula in patients with smoke inhalation. If still considered it should be noted that treatment in hyperbaric oxygen chamber, including logistics and transport, may delay appropriate acute burn care including resuscitation, monitoring, and the need for additional escharotomies. Notes in the medical charts of cerebral effects, or the patient not having a normal level of consciousness (LOC), are indicators that need to be further examined. In unclear cases, the need of a cerebral CT scan may be mandatory to exclude other cerebral diseases.

Circulation. Is assessed as has been made at the referral site, including blood pressure and ECG, if needed as indicated by the medical history, cardiovascular risk factors, or due to the injury mechanism being an electrical one. Especially extremity perfusion needs to be assessed properly in cases of circular extremity burns with or without previous escharotomies. Here the use of Doppler techniques can improve accuracy although palpation of peripheral pulsation in the arms or audible pulsations using the hand Doppler is not a sure sign to escape escharotomy. The examination should be based on signs of capillary refill in the fingers/toes and on the swelling of the proximal tissues and if there is suspicion of compromised circulation even if suspected in the following few hours. In cases of electrical injuries, the risk of compartment issues needs to be considered and extremities at risk should be repeatedly examined.

Disability. Repeated examinations (e.g., Glascow coma scale) need to be made to ascertain that the LOC remains stable and uncompromised. In an elderly population, stroke, cardiovascular disease, or diabetes may have contributed to the circumstances for the accident and should be excluded in risk patients as it may need specific medical attention in parallel to the burn. Especially intracerebral hemorrhage may pose a challenge at this point [33].

Expose and Examine. This part is most particular for the early examination at the burn center as the organ of injury needs to be fully examined and scrutinized in conjunction with the planning process of wound care and importantly the ensuing surgery.

13.5 Burn Wound Evaluation and Treatment Planning Including Surgery

Evaluating the depth (partial/full thickness) and extent of burn injury (percentage of total body surface area burned, TBSA%) is crucial by many means not only because it is the most important factor for the overall outcome for the patient involving both short and long term [34, 35]; but also as it underlies the calculation for the fluid management. At this point however, from the burn center perspective, we will also focus on some specific details, such as early cleaning and debridement of the wound and also specifically address burn injury depth and the TBSA% estimate.

Cleaning and debridement. For this procedure, the circumstances for the burn wound assessment evaluation need to be optimized. Generally, it is undertaken in an operation like facility, with proper cleaning possibilities (tub) under clean conditions. In order to properly remove debris, blisters, and clean the skin, conscious sedation or general anesthesia is most often preferred. This procedure involves mechanical cleansing using cloth, brushes and scraping tools. It may be debated whether regular soap should be supported by antibacterial/cidal agents. Theoretically, the burn wound immediately after injury is sterile, but colonization may occur during any part of the transport process. Here also ointments with antibacterial properties are often used, but the science supporting either measures in this early phase is almost nonexistent.

Burn depth assessment. Over the years, this has been a hot topic, and not least, it has repeatedly been shown that the burn depth estimate varies between referral sites and burn centers, and importantly, it has also been shown to vary between different skilled surgeons. There are two important issues that need to be stressed today: first, depth estimate may be discussed and conveyed during the referral process between the referral site and the burn center by means of photography/telemedicine [10–12]. This will ensure a better primary estimate and more proper handling of the patient during the referral process. Second, it has been shown that technical instruments as the laser Doppler system can further improve even the skilled surgeons' estimate of the depth assessment [36–38]. This is today supported by the fact that several large burn centers in Europe use the Laser Doppler system to support decision-making as to the need for surgery. Scientifically it has been shown that by the use of two consecutive measurements in scald injures, 100% both sensitivity and specificity can be obtained [37]. This supports the further use and development of technical adjuncts in the burn depth assessment.

Burn extent estimate. As with the depth estimate, difficulties in getting uniform determinations of burn extent between referring and receiving parties are well acknowledged [39]. To simplify and optimize the process, the historical approach has been the use of the rule of nines and the Lund Browder chart as described in the previous chapter. In present times with an increasing computer capacity and support and Internet availability, other methods are emerging. These being either that the burn wound extent is being plotted on a three dimensional computer model i.e. in an app for fluid resuscitation estimates [40] or more importantly by photography/imaging systems generating three dimensional images of the injury extent on a three dimensional computer model [41]. In this setting, burn estimates in square centimeter can be provided. In the future it can be predicted that the registration of burn injuries using the two above-mentioned technologies may become the standard of care even in developing countries where such functions have already been launched on smartphone devices [41].

13.6 Secondary Assessment

As at the site of accident and the referral hospital, secondary assessment needs to be repeatedly undertaken to exclude a complication from other trauma than the burn. Often when refereed between hospitals and tertiary burn centers, the trauma responsible surgeon at the tertiary hospital is made aware of the burn injured being transported and transferred between institutions, and in case of a complication of the burn by regular trauma, the trauma organization is made aware and updated. Not seldom, the trauma team at the referral hospital has already arranged a trauma CT in unclear cases, and a detailed examination may have been done along the treatment path.

13.7 Early Burn Center Planning (at Admittance or Shortly After, <24–48 h) for Larger Injuries (>20/30%) Needing Surgery and Intensive Care

13.7.1 Very Early Intensive Care Planning at the Burn Center

Temperature. Temperature control is crucial in the burn ICU setting as it among many things may lead to infections; therefore, patients with larger burns need to be actively heated. This is best done by fluid-heated mattresses [42].

Vascular access. As discussed in the previous chapter, recommendations were made that invasive blood pressure measurements, central circulation surveillance, and central venous lines should be inserted and measurements started. If this has not been done previously, complementary instillations needs to be made at the center. Also in cases with early renal failure, a veno-venous line may be installed prior to the start of filtration or dialysis measures.

Early fluid therapy and continuous surveillance in the ICU period. From the fluid balance perspective, especially the risk of fluid over and under resuscitation needs to be acknowledged. In the time period 1995–2010, a significant concern was fluid over resuscitation, called the "fluid creep" also at the burn center level [43–46]. Presently there are indications that fluid under resuscitation is again beginning to be a problem [47, 48]. Urine output remains the main outcome parameter for the early fluid resuscitation.

To continuously have access to central circulation parameters has been increasingly important after the early fluid resuscitation period, and one system advocated and used by many in this respect in the burn setting [49–53] is the arterial thermodilution PiCCO system (Pulsion Medical Systems, Munich, Germany) [54]. It provides many useful surveillance parameters such as intrathoracic blood volume, which well depicts the patient fluid volume needs and can be used to titrate fluids in conjunction with pulse pressure variation (PPV), which also shows fluid volume needs but can be continuously assessed (in between every bolus for thermodilution), systemic vascular resistance (SVR), and extravascular lung water (EVLV). Another good argument for this system is also that it provides long-term intra-arterial assessment and is not usually as transient in function as are lines located in the radial or dorsal foot arteries. If difficult to apply in the femoral vessel due to, e.g., extensive burns, it has also been shown to function properly when either the central venous line is located in the femoral region [55–57] or the arterial catheter is placed in the proximal part of the brachial artery [58, 59]. Importantly, it needs to be stressed that the use of PiCCO system for fluid volume assessment in major pediatric burns have recently shown a positive outcome effect further supporting its general applicability in the burn ICU setting over even extended period of time [60]. It may then be advocated to use this mode of surveillance modality in the planning of the ICU period for larger burn injuries. Competing systems based on ultrasound technique may provide arguments based on ease to apply, but the parameters that may be assessed by this mode are significantly less. An important word of caution however needs be highlighted on invasive monitoring early after burn as the regular Parkland fluid resuscitation strategy provides a hypovolemic situation at 12 h post burn [49], and if not accepted in the resuscitation, a significant fluid over resuscitation will occur on a regular basis. This has been shown repeatedly in RCT trials [50, 51].

Further regarding the fluid balance, the risk of compartment problems, mainly abdominal compartment in very large burns when crystalloid fluid volumes exceed 300 mL/kg/24 h [61], needs to be remembered and the need for adjusted fluid strategies. The most popular approach is by adding colloids known as "colloid rescue" which significantly reduces the total fluid volumes provided [43, 62, 63]. Other and important alternatives include the use of hypertonic resuscitation fluids [64, 65], but caution is warranted as there has been shown risks of kidney affection in one study [66]. A common approach by many to reduce fluid needs in resuscitation of burns is by providing vitamin C. This has repeatedly been found successful and is therefore a strategy used by many, but the timing for the start of this treatment and the dosing is still debated [67].

It is important during the early care at the burn center to ascertain that the fluid resuscitation strategy is successful. This means that urine production is according to plan but also that the base excess and lactate are normalized early (another endpoint may be central venous saturation, SAT%). If not the patient is properly fluid resuscitated, i.e., these parameters normalize, organ failure will ensue and the risk of a mortality outcome increases [48].

If any doubts on the status of the abdominal compartment pressure, intra-abdominal compartment pressure measurements through the urinary catheter is recommended [61, 65].

There is limited risk of sepsis in this early phase after burn but surveillance for such signs of sepsis are important.

It may be underlined that the main use for arterial thermodilution surveillance starts at 24 h after burn in patients with large burns when the early burn shock period is coming to an end and the main focus is being directed to optimizing fluids for surgery and reducing risks of circulatory failure due to sepsis. At this point, 24 h after burn and if resuscitated by the Parkland strategy, the patient should be normovolemic, and the next 24 h should be directed toward reducing tissue edema. It is important to stress that definitions and treatment of sepsis have evolved in general [68], and it is well known that burn-related sepsis constitutes a particular and different challenge [69, 70]. When using the PiCCO system at 24 h after burn, the intrathoracic blood volume index (ITBVI) may serve as an excellent fluid volume estimate, and the fluids provided can properly be titrated against this value. Most often burn injured, even with large burns, should be without vasoactive support, and only when ITBVI is normal or slightly elevated and systemic vascular resistance index is low (together with a MAP <65–70 mmHg), there is a need for use of vasoconstrictors, as these are known to be injurious to both skin and intestine when used improperly.

Nutrition and mitigation of the hypermetabolic syndrome and its side effects. Important in the early burn center admittance period is to start enteral feeds as an early start increases the success rate [71–73]. Many advocate also putting the feeding tube beyond the pyloric region to increase the success rate however as of yet the scientific support for this is limited. In this perspective also, opioid receptor antagonists may be added to the gastrointestinal canal together with motility-stimulating agents to reduce the risk of opioid-induced obstipation and gut standstill—a not uncommon situation in burn care. Rectal catheters for fecal collection in patients with perineal injuries may be advocated, and some units even perform colostomies to reduce bacterial burden in the perineal burn wound. Nutrition may start at 25 kcal/kg/24 h and should be increased as data is emerging from indirect calorimetry readings on days 4–5 when most of the hypermetabolic effects are fully expressed, usually at a caloric level of +40% resting energy expenditure (REE) [74].

The hypermetabolic syndrome seen in larger burns carries a number of negative consequences for the burn injured [75, 76]. Importantly, a number of therapies have during the last 20 years been shown to mitigate the majority of the aspects of the hypermetabolic response [74, 77–83]. Interventions range from very early physical (early wound closure, thermoregulation, or exercise) to pharmacological; some strategies should be employed early during the acute hospitalization and can continue well into the rehabilitative stage. Early studies of β-blockade claim that although reduced adrenergic stress reduces hypermetabolic response after burns [77, 80, 81], modulation of additional mediators may lead to even greater reduction of the hypermetabolism. The combination of β-blockade with other therapies, including insulin, growth hormone, or oxandrolone, shows positive effects for the burn injured. The administration of growth hormone and propranolol reduces energy consumption, attenuates the systemic inflammatory response, reduces peripheral lipolysis, and alleviates side effects seen with rhGH alone [81]. When propranolol and insulin are given together, improvements in glucose turnover and growth are observed. More recently also positive long-term effects of propranolol and oxandrolone have been shown. The results of these studies show that mitigation of several aspects of the hypermetabolic response can further benefit patient recovery even more than when only based on a single treatment, and these interventions should start early. The expansion of these results, which mostly have been obtained in large pediatric burns, needs however to be further explored and confirmed in larger patient samples including burned adults and especially elderly as well.

Antibiotics. The use of prophylactic antibiotics early in care have been debated, and there are arguments supporting to wait for signs of infection prior to starting antibiotic treatment. This however makes close patient surveillance very important [84]. The use of antibiotic prophylaxis for newly burned patients upon admission to burn center has been studied extensively. In such a setting, two types of antibiotic prophylactic strategies were identified. First, local antibiotic prophylaxis in the form of creams and ointments, e.g., silver sulfadiazine. This however did not show any beneficial effects. Systemic prophylaxis has shown decreasing mortality in some studies but a review in 2010 concluded that the methods used in these studies were weak, and therefore, the role of systemic prophylactic antibiotics is still not validated. And in light of this, there is today no recommendation to use prophylactic antibiotics in burns [84]. The perioperative antibiotic prophylaxis has however shown a beneficial effect in the improvement in the survival of skin grafts.

Pain. From the pain perspective, there is a high variability of the pain perception among the patients early after burn, and pain remains a big concern for this patient group and a challenge throughout the care period [85, 86]. Most often background pain can be properly addressed but mobilization pain and pain during dressing changes constitute a major problem [85, 86]. A multimodal management approach is used to address nociceptive and neuropathic pain symptoms and contributing psychological factors. A combination of long-acting opioids for background pain and short-acting opioids for procedural and breakthrough pain is the standard of care. Dosing is titrated to account for altered pharmacokinetics due to impaired perfusion [87], metabolism, and plasma protein levels as well as opioid tolerance. Alternative treatments are increasingly used to avoid opioid misuse. Acetaminophen is efficacious in combination with opioids for minor burn. Adjuvant medications include NSAIDs, muscle relaxants, and anti-epileptics. However, also the use of gabapentin and other substances addressing specifically neuropathic pain components may be considered early, and these drugs are recommended as significant treatment effects are present [88] albeit pain remains a major issue in burn centers [89].

Ventilation. The need for continued invasive ventilations should be scrutinized early, and planning for longer such periods may be important on to which to base an early tracheotomy. If needed, a 6–8 mL/kg tidal volumes should be aimed for. Trying to avoid sedation is important to reduce the risk of PICS (post intensive care syndrome) [87] and the risk of developing delirium [90]. Unfortunately, as larger burn patients are often ventilator-dependent longer than general ICU patients, the risk for developing delirium and concomitantly cognitive dysfunction is larger; hence, adhering to a restrictive sedation strategy is important [90]. Presently there are arguments supporting sedation based on dexmedetomidine, which can possibly further reduce its incidence and consequences [91–93]. Early tracheostomy may thus be advantageous in this setting [26].

Laboratory investigations. Laboratory test has not seldom been issued already at the referring hospital, but still there is a need to follow the course of the burn, and therefore, a complete set of admittance laboratory test are usually issued at admittance to the burn center and should be specified in the SOPs. In this aspect, also a protocolized laboratory surveillance of the burn patients during the length of stay may be recommended and also for follow-up reasons [94]. Of specific importance is to assess if the patient is infected by hepatitis B/C, HIV as knowledge of these are important for safety reasons. Carboxyhemoglobin is another important test that needs to be controlled in the perspective both of oxygen treatment and prognostic as high levels of carboxyhemoglobin may herald the risk of later negative cognitive effects. Focus later in the care process should be directed to assessing signs of infection [68] (e.g., CRP/PCT and platelets) as well as markers for organ failure, i.e., if recording of SOFA (sequential organ failure score assessment) score is a standard at the unit, e.g., bilirubin and creatinine need to be taken on a regular basis (every third day). When taking laboratory samples from the patient, bacterial cultures are also very important. First, to assess any colonization of bacteria that has unfavorable resistance patterns, e.g., MRSA, which now can be transferred endemically and that may complicate the course of treatment. Such repeated cultures are also important as they can help in reducing the risk for obtaining opportunistic bacteria which may be difficult to isolate and eradicate from within the facility even after extensive cleaning procedures (e.g., Acinetobacter baumanii) [95].

13.8 Early Burn Wound Treatment and Surgery Planning

Early after admission and assessment of the burn extent and depth, proper planning for the ensuing dressing changes, burn excision, and grafting is a necessity. This constitutes the main stem and will most directly influence the effectiveness of the treatment plan. It involves both partial- and full-thickness wounds, which are treated by different protocols. According to recent ISBI guidelines, these procedures should be undertaken by an appropriately trained, prepared, and equipped burn team [14].

Different treatment approaches are available, and they vary between burn centers and at times between surgeons. One of the most important factors in this early planning is the depth of the injury.

Partial-thickness burns are treated conservatively with dressing changes, and spontaneous healing is expected to occur within 14 days unless invasive infection has complicated the healing course resulting in deepening of the burn and the need for excision. There is no universal consensus regarding dressing materials, and therefore, the materials that are used tends to vary between burn centers, national and internationally. However, a recent review has advocated the superiority of biological membranous dressings [96].

In case of *full-thickness burns*, planning for the excisional strategy is important. Simplifying this strategy it may be claimed to be based on two separate strategies, either early or late excision with the ensuing autografting. Also the timing of the auto grafting may vary, with some centers doing mostly early autografting after excision and others, who prefer to wait or at least have a observational period prior to grafting to ascertain a stable and proper wound bed to be present at grafting occasion [97].

13.8.1 Early Excision

Early excision and grafting is known to improve the outcome of burn care such as duration of hospital stay and scarring, and it is cost-effective. The early excision technique is widely known to have the best survival rates [98, 99]. Timing for early excision of burns varies, and it can start from the first day after injury, and even excisions up to day 10 after injury can be considered early excisions. Again there is a lack of consensus although most would consider early excision before day 3 after injury. The depth of excision may also vary, and generally tangential excision as first described by Janzekovic is most often used [100], and the less popular alternative excision method "fascial excision" is reserved for significantly deeper wounds in not seldom medically compromised patients, as the cosmetic outcome is less favorable [101].

The extent of burn injury often influences the strategy chosen for excision. Limited burns can most often and more easily be excised in one session with coverage with, e.g., temporary dressing until the wound bed is considered optimized, and then skin grafts are applied, or if the wound bed is considered optimal, direct skin grafting is made. With burns of larger extent, the strategy varies even more. In the early 90s, total excision of the burns was advocated in one or maximum two sessions with subsequent skin grafting [98, 99]. Nevertheless, another approach was proposed later by Still et al., where excisions were made in successions with temporary skin coverage followed by skin grafts after the wound bed was considered optimal [97]. This method proved a reduction of the duration of hospital stay in this specific study.

Temporary coverage of excised burns is otherwise a highly debated topic. Most authors would agree at times that optimization of the wound bed is needed. However, the timing and choice of covering materials are controversial. Most popular materials include donor skin (allografts), porcine xenografts, collagen-based scaffolds, and in the low cost range, Vaseline gauze. Research is limited in this area, and no study yet has convincingly shown superiority of any one procedural aspect or material. The choice of material today still depends mainly on the experience and training of the treating surgeon in conjunction with the availability and cost [102–105].

A later comparison by Elmasry and coworkers between delayed and an immediate total excision plan has not shown any superiority of either techniques in terms of duration of hospital stay [102, 103].

Present ISBI guidelines [14] states that "The first early excision should be aimed at excision and coverage of a large portion of the full thickness burn, and the largest areas that can be safely excised are to be chosen." Typically, these involve the front or back of the trunk or large areas on the limbs. The extent of the burn area excised in each operation is determined by the experience and approach of the surgical team in conjunction with the availability of autograft donor sites or skin substitutes. If the team is relatively inexperienced and/or there is little autograft available, less % TBSA burn is recommended to be excised during one surgical procedure to reduce operative risk and the risk of graft loss. After excision, all excised burn areas must be covered with autografts, skin allograft, or other skin substitutes [104, 105].

Technically early excision is not difficult; however, a well-trained surgical and anesthesia team should be available to carry out this task. In many areas where lack of training and resources exists, this task seems to be more difficult and do not provide the same outcomes [7, 106]. A specific recurring challenge is graft take and especially in previously grafted areas with graft loss [107].

Bleeding is also a considerable risk in excision burn surgery, and the whole team should have enough experience to control this situation rapidly and efficiently. This involves access to a blood bank with sufficient capacity. Usually, tangential excision is made using handheld dermatomes as Watson or Downy knives, and hemostasis is regularly achieved by the application of adrenaline-soaked dressings in conjunction with precise hemostasis of larger bleeding points by diathermy. The bipolar type is often the primary choice to limit the extent of tissue injury inflicted by the apparatus.

13.8.2 Late Excision

One rather uncommon technique, which needs to be mentioned in the area of late excision, is based on the chemical eschar binding properties by cerium. This approach is used by a smaller number of centers in Europe [108, 109].

Contrary to the previously described early excision plan, late excision is associated with lower costs and risk as long as the patient is not seriously infected or septic, the rates of which increases with burn size. Bleeding is less, and there is a possibility of doing direct skin grafting. In places with significantly reduced experience and resources, this technique may be recommended.

Summary Box

This chapter examines the treatment trajectory that the burn injured experience after having been triaged and stabilized at the scene of the accident or at the first receiving hospital. The early assessment and treatment at the tertiary treatment level, the burn center, is presented, which in many aspects is a further extrapolation and detailed approach extending and repeating the practices of the early ATLS/ABLS concepts that were used at the location of the accident or referring hospital. The start of the burn center-specific procedures are described, and it involves issues such as primary admittance protocol and control, extended primary and secondary assessment burn wound evaluation and treatment planning including surgery, early burn center planning (at admittance or shortly after, <24–48 h) for larger injuries (>20/30%) needing surgery and intensive care, and early burn wound treatment and surgery planning.

References

1. http://euroburn.org/documents-2/. Assessed http://euroburn.org/wp-content/uploads/2014/09/EBA-Guidelines-Version-4-2017-1.pdf.
2. American Burn Association and American College of Surgeons Committee of Trauma. Guidelines for the operation of burn centers. J Burn Care Res. 2007;28(1):134–41.
3. D'Asta F, et al. Introducing the advanced burn life support (ABLS) course in Italy. Burns. 2014;40(3):475–9.
4. Kearns RD, et al. Advanced burn life support for day-to-day burn injury management and disaster preparedness: stakeholder experiences and student perceptions following 56 advanced burn life support courses. J Burn Care Res. 2015;36(4):455–64.
5. Sasaki J, et al. Experiences in organizing Advanced Burn Life Support (ABLS) provider courses in Japan. Burns. 2010;36(1):65–9.
6. Lindford AJ, Lamyman MJ, Lim P. Review of the emergency management of severe burns (EMSB) course. Burns. 2006;32(3):391.
7. Rogers AD, et al. The Emergency Management of Severe Burns course in South Africa. S Afr J Surg. 2013;51(1):38.
8. Stone CA, Pape SA. Evolution of the Emergency Management of Severe Burns (EMSB) course in the UK. Burns. 1999;25(3):262–4.
9. Svee A, et al. Burns in Sweden: temporal trends from 1987 to 2010. Ann Burns Fire Disasters. 2016;29(2):85–9.
10. Atiyeh B, Dibo SA, Janom HH. Telemedicine and burns: an overview. Ann Burns Fire Disasters. 2014;27(2):87–93.
11. Saffle JR, et al. Telemedicine evaluation of acute burns is accurate and cost-effective. J Trauma. 2009;67(2):358–65.
12. Syed-Abdul S, et al. Telemedicine utilization to support the management of the burns treatment involving patient pathways in both developed and developing countries: a case study. J Burn Care Res. 2012;33(4):e207–12.
13. Ahuja RB. ISBI PRACTICE GUIDELINES FOR BURN CARE: Editorial. Burns. 2016;42(5):951–2.

14. Committee IPG, Steering S, Advisory S. ISBI practice guidelines for burn care. Burns. 2016;42(5):953–1021.
15. http://www.bch.nhs.uk/Professional.
16. Agarwala AV, et al. An electronic checklist improves transfer and retention of critical information at intraoperative handoff of care. Anesth Analg. 2015;120(1):96–104.
17. Brindley PG, et al. The "ABCs" of critical care teamwork: introduction of a practical checklist. J Crit Care. 2016;33:277–8.
18. Thongprayoon C, et al. The effect of an electronic checklist on critical care provider workload, errors, and performance. J Intensive Care Med. 2016;31(3):205–12.
19. Vukoja M, et al. Checklist for early recognition and treatment of acute illness: international collaboration to improve critical care practice. World J Crit Care Med. 2015;4(1):55–61.
20. Ajami S, Lamoochi P. Comparative study on National Burn Registry in America, England, Australia and Iran. J Educ Health Promot. 2014;3:106.
21. Cleland H. The Burns Registry of Australia and New Zealand: progressing the evidence base for burn care. Med J Aust. 2016;205(4):191.
22. McDonald-Smith GP. NATIONAL TRACS/ABA Burn Registry—the quest for quality burn data management. J Burn Care Rehabil. 1996;17(5):454–6.
23. http://euroburn.org/burn-centres-2/verification-burn-centre/.
24. https://anzba.org.au/quality/the-bi-nbr/bqip/.
25. http://ameriburn.org/quality-care/verification/.
26. Hosokawa K, et al. Timing of tracheotomy in ICU patients: a systematic review of randomized controlled trials. Crit Care. 2015;19:424.
27. Mosier MJ, et al. Predictive value of bronchoscopy in assessing the severity of inhalation injury. J Burn Care Res. 2012;33(1):65–73.
28. Koljonen V, et al. Multi-detector computed tomography demonstrates smoke inhalation injury at early stage. Emerg Radiol. 2007;14(2):113–6.
29. Reske A, et al. Computed tomography—a possible aid in the diagnosis of smoke inhalation injury? Acta Anaesthesiol Scand. 2005;49(2):257–60.
30. Yamamura H, et al. Chest computed tomography performed on admission helps predict the severity of smoke-inhalation injury. Crit Care. 2013;17(3):R95.
31. Steinvall I, Bak Z, Sjoberg F. Acute respiratory distress syndrome is as important as inhalation injury for the development of respiratory dysfunction in major burns. Burns. 2008;34(4):441–51.
32. Tanash HA, et al. Burn injury during long-term oxygen therapy in Denmark and Sweden: the potential role of smoking. Int J Chron Obstruct Pulmon Dis. 2017;12:193–7.
33. Pompermaier L, et al. Burned patients who die from causes other than the burn affect the model used to predict mortality: a national exploratory study. Burns. 2018;44(2):280–7.
34. Orwelius L, et al. Long term health-related quality of life after burns is strongly dependent on pre-existing disease and psychosocial issues and less due to the burn itself. Burns. 2013;39(2):229–35.
35. Steinvall I, et al. Standardised mortality ratio based on the sum of age and percentage total body surface area burned is an adequate quality indicator in burn care: an exploratory review. Burns. 2016;42(1):28–40.
36. Droog EJ, Steenbergen W, Sjoberg F. Measurement of depth of burns by laser Doppler perfusion imaging. Burns. 2001;27(6):561–8.
37. Mirdell R, et al. Accuracy of laser speckle contrast imaging in the assessment of pediatric scald wounds. Burns. 2018;44(1):90–8.
38. Mirdell R, et al. Microvascular blood flow in scalds in children and its relation to duration of wound healing: a study using laser speckle contrast imaging. Burns. 2016;42(3):648–54.
39. Goverman J, et al. Discrepancy in initial pediatric burn estimates and its impact on fluid resuscitation. J Burn Care Res. 2015;36(5):574–9.
40. https://play.google.com/store/apps/details?id=com.mulberrysoft.BRF_Android&hl=sv.
41. Parvizi D, et al. BurnCase 3D software validation study: burn size measurement accuracy and inter-rater reliability. Burns. 2016;42(2):329–35.
42. Kjellman BM, et al. Comparing ambient, air-convection, and fluid-convection heating techniques in treating hypothermic burn patients, a clinical RCT. Ann Surg Innov Res. 2011;5(1):4.
43. Atiyeh BS, et al. Acute burn resuscitation and fluid creep: it is time for colloid rehabilitation. Ann Burns Fire Disasters. 2012;25(2):59–65.
44. Cartotto R, Zhou A. Fluid creep: the pendulum hasn't swung back yet! J Burn Care Res. 2010;31(4):551–8.
45. Rogers AD, et al. Fluid creep in major pediatric burns. Eur J Pediatr Surg. 2010;20(2):133–8.
46. Saffle JR. Fluid creep and over-resuscitation. Crit Care Clin. 2016;32(4):587–98.
47. Mason SA, et al. Hold the pendulum: rates of acute kidney injury are increased in patients who receive resuscitation volumes less than predicted by the Parkland equation. Ann Surg. 2016;264(6):1142–7.
48. Soussi S, et al. Low cardiac index and stroke volume on admission are associated with poor outcome in critically ill burn patients: a retrospective cohort study. Ann Intensive Care. 2016;6(1):87.
49. Bak Z, et al. Hemodynamic changes during resuscitation after burns using the Parkland formula. J Trauma. 2009;66(2):329–36.
50. Csontos C, et al. Arterial thermodilution in burn patients suggests a more rapid fluid administration during early resuscitation. Acta Anaesthesiol Scand. 2008;52(6):742–9.
51. Holm C, et al. A clinical randomized study on the effects of invasive monitoring on burn shock resuscitation. Burns. 2004;30(8):798–807.
52. Holm C, et al. Haemodynamic and oxygen transport responses in survivors and non-survivors following thermal injury. Burns. 2000;26(1):25–33.
53. Holm C, et al. Effect of crystalloid resuscitation and inhalation injury on extravascular lung water: clinical implications. Chest. 2002;121(6):1956–62.
54. http://www.pulsion.com/.
55. Berbara H, et al. Pulmonary vascular permeability index and global end-diastolic volume: are the data consistent in patients with femoral venous access for transpulmonary thermodilution: a prospective observational study. BMC Anesthesiol. 2014;14:81.
56. Huber W, et al. Comparison of pulmonary vascular permeability index PVPI and global ejection fraction GEF derived from jugular and femoral indicator injection using the PiCCO-2 device: a prospective observational study. PLoS One. 2017;12(10):e0178372.
57. Schmidt S, et al. Effect of the venous catheter site on transpulmonary thermodilution measurement variables. Crit Care Med. 2007;35(3):783–6.
58. Antonini M, et al. [The PiCCO system with brachial-axillary artery access in hemodynamic monitoring during surgery of abdominal aortic aneurysm]. Minerva Anestesiol. 2001;67(6):447–56.
59. Clementi G. [Hemodynamic monitoring using a long radial catheter]. Minerva Anestesiol. 2002;68(4):231–5.
60. Kraft R, et al. Optimized fluid management improves outcomes of pediatric burn patients. J Surg Res. 2013;181(1):121–8.
61. Oda J, et al. Resuscitation fluid volume and abdominal compartment syndrome in patients with major burns. Burns. 2006;32(2):151–4.
62. Lawrence A, et al. Colloid administration normalizes resuscitation ratio and ameliorates "fluid creep". J Burn Care Res. 2010;31(1):40–7.
63. O'Mara MS, et al. A prospective, randomized evaluation of intra-abdominal pressures with crystalloid and colloid resuscitation in burn patients. J Trauma. 2005;58(5):1011–8.

64. Monafo WW, Chuntrasakul C, Ayvazian VH. Hypertonic sodium solutions in the treatment of burn shock. Am J Surg. 1973;126(6):778–83.
65. Oda J, et al. Hypertonic lactated saline resuscitation reduces the risk of abdominal compartment syndrome in severely burned patients. J Trauma. 2006;60(1):64–71.
66. Huang PP, et al. Hypertonic sodium resuscitation is associated with renal failure and death. Ann Surg. 1995;221(5):543–54; discussion 554–7.
67. Rizzo JA, et al. Vitamin C in burn resuscitation. Crit Care Clin. 2016;32(4):539–46.
68. Shankar-Hari M, et al. Developing a new definition and assessing new clinical criteria for septic shock: for the third international consensus definitions for sepsis and septic shock (Sepsis-3). JAMA. 2016;315(8):775–87.
69. Greenhalgh DG. Sepsis in the burn patient: a different problem than sepsis in the general population. Burns Trauma. 2017;5:23.
70. Greenhalgh DG. Defining sepsis in burn patients: still a long way to go. J Burn Care Res. 2017;38(6):e990–1.
71. Khorasani EN, Mansouri F. Effect of early enteral nutrition on morbidity and mortality in children with burns. Burns. 2010;36(7):1067–71.
72. Lu G, et al. Influence of early post-burn enteral nutrition on clinical outcomes of patients with extensive burns. J Clin Biochem Nutr. 2011;48(3):222–5.
73. Mosier MJ, et al. Early enteral nutrition in burns: compliance with guidelines and associated outcomes in a multicenter study. J Burn Care Res. 2011;32(1):104–9.
74. Hart DW, et al. Energy expenditure and caloric balance after burn: increased feeding leads to fat rather than lean mass accretion. Ann Surg. 2002;235(1):152–61.
75. Wilmore DW, et al. Catecholamines: mediator of the hypermetabolic response to thermal injury. Ann Surg. 1974;180(4):653–69.
76. Wilmore DW, et al. Effect of ambient temperature on heat production and heat loss in burn patients. J Appl Physiol. 1975;38(4):593–7.
77. Ali A, et al. Propranolol attenuates hemorrhage and accelerates wound healing in severely burned adults. Crit Care. 2015;19:217.
78. Finnerty CC, et al. Impact of stress-induced diabetes on outcomes in severely burned children. J Am Coll Surg. 2014;218(4):783–95.
79. Gore DC, et al. Association of hyperglycemia with increased mortality after severe burn injury. J Trauma. 2001;51(3):540–4.
80. Herndon DN, et al. Reversal of catabolism by beta-blockade after severe burns. N Engl J Med. 2001;345(17):1223–9.
81. Jeschke MG, et al. Combination of recombinant human growth hormone and propranolol decreases hypermetabolism and inflammation in severely burned children. Pediatr Crit Care Med. 2008;9(2):209–16.
82. Jeschke MG, et al. The effect of oxandrolone on the endocrinologic, inflammatory, and hypermetabolic responses during the acute phase postburn. Ann Surg. 2007;246(3):351–60; discussion 360–2.
83. Jeschke MG, et al. Intensive insulin therapy in severely burned pediatric patients: a prospective randomized trial. Am J Respir Crit Care Med. 2010;182(3):351–9.
84. Moiemen NS, ISBI Guideline Committee. Antibiotic stewardship in burns patients: ISBI guidelines. Burns. 2017;43(6):1366.
85. Choiniere M, Grenier R, Paquette C. Patient-controlled analgesia: a double-blind study in burn patients. Anaesthesia. 1992;47(6):467–72.
86. Choiniere M, et al. Comparisons between patients' and nurses' assessment of pain and medication efficacy in severe burn injuries. Pain. 1990;40(2):143–52.
87. Elliott D, et al. Exploring the scope of post-intensive care syndrome therapy and care: engagement of non-critical care providers and survivors in a second stakeholders meeting. Crit Care Med. 2014;42(12):2518–26.
88. Kaul I, et al. Use of gabapentin and pregabalin for pruritus and neuropathic pain associated with major burn injury: a retrospective chart review. Burns. 2018;44(2):414–22.
89. Morgan M, et al. Burn pain: a systematic and critical review of epidemiology, pathophysiology, and treatment. Pain Med. 2018;19(4):708–34.
90. Agarwal V, et al. Prevalence and risk factors for development of delirium in burn intensive care unit patients. J Burn Care Res. 2010;31(5):706–15.
91. Kawazoe Y, et al. Effect of dexmedetomidine on mortality and ventilator-free days in patients requiring mechanical ventilation with sepsis: a randomized clinical trial. JAMA. 2017;317(13):1321–8.
92. Rahme RJ, et al. Improving Neurosurgical Outcomes in the Intensive Care Unit: could dexmedetomidine make a difference in ventilator free days, neurological monitoring, and outcomes? World Neurosurg. 2016;94:556–8.
93. Reade MC, et al. Effect of dexmedetomidine added to standard care on ventilator-free time in patients with agitated delirium: a randomized clinical trial. JAMA. 2016;315(14):1460–8.
94. Sjoberg F, et al. Utility of an intervention scoring system in documenting effects of changes in burn treatment. Burns. 2000;26(6):553–9.
95. Herruzo R, et al. Two consecutive outbreaks of Acinetobacter baumanii 1-a in a burn Intensive Care Unit for adults. Burns. 2004;30(5):419–23.
96. Vloemans AF, et al. Optimal treatment of partial thickness burns in children: a systematic review. Burns. 2014;40(2):177–90.
97. Still JM Jr, et al. Decreasing length of hospital stay by early excision and grafting of burns. South Med J. 1996;89(6):578–82.
98. Herndon DN, et al. A comparison of conservative versus early excision. Therapies in severely burned patients. Ann Surg. 1989;209(5):547–52; discussion 552–3.
99. Munster AM, Smith-Meek M, Sharkey P. The effect of early surgical intervention on mortality and cost-effectiveness in burn care, 1978-91. Burns. 1994;20(1):61–4.
100. Janzekovic Z. A new concept in the early excision and immediate grafting of burns. J Trauma. 1970;10(12):1103–8.
101. Janzekovic Z. The burn wound from the surgical point of view. J Trauma. 1975;15(1):42–62.
102. Elmasry M, et al. Staged excisions of moderate-sized burns compared with total excision with immediate autograft: an evaluation of two strategies. Int J Burns Trauma. 2017;7(1):6–11.
103. Elmasry M, et al. Temporary coverage of burns with a xenograft and sequential excision, compared with total early excision and autograft. Ann Burns Fire Disasters. 2016;29(3):196–201.
104. Saffle JR. Closure of the excised burn wound: temporary skin substitutes. Clin Plast Surg. 2009;36(4):627–41.
105. Sheridan R. Closure of the excised burn wound: autografts, semipermanent skin substitutes, and permanent skin substitutes. Clin Plast Surg. 2009;36(4):643–51.
106. Allorto NL, Clarke DL, Thomson SR. A cost model case comparison of current versus modern management of burns at a regional hospital in South Africa. Burns. 2011;37(6):1033–7.
107. Abdelrahman I, et al. Division of overall duration of stay into operative stay and postoperative stay improves the overall estimate as a measure of quality of outcome in burn care. PLoS One. 2017;12(3):e0174579.
108. Garner JP, Heppell PS. Cerium nitrate in the management of burns. Burns. 2005;31(5):539–47.
109. Garner JP, Heppell PS. The use of Flammacerium in British Burns Units. Burns. 2005;31(3):379–82.

Burn Size Estimation, Challenges, and Novel Technology

14

Herbert L. Haller, M. Giretzlehner, and Stefan Thumfart

14.1 Introduction

Burn size, depth of burn, and age are the pillars of a scientific approach to burn treatment. So, the history of burn size estimation is a history of a developing scientific approach to burns. Progress based on a critical evaluation needs reliable data. Which advantage offer rules for burn center treatment based on the extent of burns when the reliability of primary evaluation must be questioned? How can we compare the quality of treatment, when the data on which the evaluation is based on depends on personal impression and are mixed with a subjective bias? How can we plan the costs of treatment without reliable data foundation!

The development of tools for accurate burn extent estimation is influenced by the contemporary technical standard and should lead to unique standards making studies comparable and less biased.

One Burn One Standard is an international intention, started at the ODBC (Committee on Organization and Delivery of Burn Care) of the American Burns Association on an initiative of James Jeng [1]. This was done as there was increasing evidence that the contemporary methods of registration and calculation of TBSA (Total Burned Surface Area) were highly prone to errors based on individual and technical reasons. The development of usable electronic burn surface area calculators showed the necessity to develop a generally accepted standard for TBSA registration and calculation. This problem was seen with high urgency as there was a tendency to develop into two different directions—two-dimensional and three-dimensional systems, showing different results. The existing rather erroneous methods of TBSA calculations with a mixture of non-electronically and electronically calculations in future will decrease the already poor level of comparability of burn injuries in studies, quality, workload, and cost controls.

H. L. Haller (✉) · M. Giretzlehner · S. Thumfart
Trauma Hospital Berlin, Trauma Hospital Linz, (ret), HLMedConsult, Leonding, Austria

Research Unit for Medical Informatics, RISC Software GmbH, Johannes Kepler University Linz, Upper Austrian Research GmbH, Hagenberg, Austria
e-mail: michael.giretzlehner@risc.uni-linz.ac.at; stefan.thumfart@risc-software.at

14.2 Extract of History of Burn Size Estimation

Documented knowledge of the correlation of burn severity and the probability of survival starts in Europe in the late eighteenth century with a report of Richter in 1788. It was only roughly described by Schjerning in 1884, and the coherence of size and mortality was doubted at this time, e.g., by Liman in 1882 [2]. Weidenfeld from University of Vienna established in 1879 a constant relationship of well-defined body areas to the whole-body surface area based on the calculations of Meeh [3]. He defined the relationship as proportions and not yet as a percentage. Riehl confirmed his findings in 1925 [4]. He together with von Zumbusch correlated the time of death with the extent of burns in a publication in 1905.

Berkow, not being aware of Weidenfeld's work, recalculated the surface area of parts of the body in five persons with very different physique using the formula of Dubois and Dubois [5]. While Berkow found an average error of 15% in the calculations of Meeh, he found an error rate of less than 5% in his calculations [2]. He found out that the body proportions of children were different and suggested to consider this fact. Berkow suggested the method to calculate the size of a burn as a percentage of total body surface area to be named after Weidenfeld and himself, which was not accepted.

In 1942, the treatment of burns on a scientific foundation got into the center of national interest not only because of the ongoing war. At this time a Burn Research Service had been established at the Boston City Hospital, and a National Burns and Trauma Research Committee had started. The determi-

M. G. Jeschke et al. (eds.), *Handbook of Burns Volume 1*, https://doi.org/10.1007/978-3-030-18940-2_14

nation of TBSA and the feasibility of a highly qualitative method got increasing importance as the treatment of shock based on the TBSA was started, suggested by the conference of the National Research Council in 1942.

CC. Lund and N.C. Browder, both members of Harvard Medical School, published their Lund Browder Chart in 1944 [6] with the aim to improve bodily proportions and to reduce errors. The chart was based on the surface calculations of Boyd [7]. They established clearly defined borders of the body regions and regarded different proportions during growth. The Lund Browder Chart was modified by many authors [8, 9] but remained in its original form in use until now.

Per Wallace (1979) he created together with Pulaski the "Rule of Nine" in 1949. Pulaski could demonstrate that he showed slides on this rule in 1950 at a symposium of the National Burns Research Council in Washington based on a cooperation with Tennison. This is the reason why this method is mostly credited to them by American authors [2]. The rule of nines was designed for a quick estimate of TBSA in a preclinical scenery.

The "Rule of Palms" according to Rossiter was based on the original Lund Browder Chart and is described in a "field surgery pocketbook" by Kirby and Blackburne in 1981 [10]. There are different understandings of this rule regarding what a "palm" is, whether it is with or without fingers [11]. This rule is a simple rule, and it is used alone or as an adjunct when using other methods like the Lund Browder to estimate the percentage of the burned area of a defined area of the body.

Following technical progress, IT-based systems started in the early 80s of the last century. In an intention to reduce calculation errors in estimating percentages, Wachtel published the use of computers to do so in 1983 followed by Nichter in 1984 (1985) [12, 13]. Both used Lund Browder Charts on screens which were calculated by computers and did pixel counts as a form of adapted two-dimensional planimetry. SAGE II (Surface Area Graphic Evaluation) is a system developed by Parshley in 1987 too using 2D charts which can be modified by age, weight, and height, and it uses the adapted planimetry of Lund Browder [14]. It is available online as free for single evaluations or as a registered form for multiple observations with costs.

Three-dimensional systems were developed and described first by Lee in 1994 [15, 16]. 3D Burn Vision was developed by a team of the University of Chicago and was sponsored by EPRI (Electric Power Research Institute). The release of the version 1.0 was in 1999 [17]. It was described in Comparison to Sage II in 2002 [14]. The project was stopped due to the end of funding.

Based on the increasing possibilities of IT technology, Burn Vision 3D had many forward-looking features like adaptation to sex, weight, height, and age. It was zoomable; you could rotate the model, it had a morph function, joints were movable, the results were storable in an electronic database and allowed multiple observations. Recording of degrees of burn, the area of allografts and autografts was possible. The available resolution of the model has not been described. Many ideas for further usability were developed in this project but could not be realized.

BurnCase 3D is a software project for three-dimensional registration and documentation of burn patients which was started as a student project in 2001. It is now run by RISC (Research Institute for Symbolic Computation) which is an 80% daughter of Johannes Kepler University in Linz, and 20% are owned by Upper Austrian Research. It runs as a research project where the members pay for an annual membership and can use the full features and influence the ongoing project and do have support. BurnCase 3D software and database runs on contemporary versions of Windows and can act as a standalone version or as a server with multiple clients serving for different departments or even hospital networks.

More recently, TBSA calculators as apps for smartphones and tablets were developed. Using graphic tablets for drawing burns had already been done by Nichter in 1984 [13]. Technical progress reduced the size of computers and screens to a cigarette box, having more power than the big computers in 1983. So a lot of apps was created to do TBSA calculation still based on the principles described after [18, 19].

A new approach is provided by Sheng and his system BurnCalc [20]. It consists of 3D scanning, 3D reconstruction, and interactive surface calculation. It is a technically high standard approach, which shows the possible high accuracy of 3D systems but the feasibility of this approach has not been demonstrated in clinical use.

These programs and apps could serve as treatment guides, but their use is limited due to laws for medical products and lacking certifications by the FDA or European Community.

14.3 Requirements for a Future Tool

To evaluate the requirements for a future tool, a weighting was performed. The results demonstrate a compromise between feasibility and accuracy to be the most promising way if technical means do not allow a 1:1 transfer of a photo or a scan to a model of the total body within a minimum of time under all conditions (preclinical as well as intubated and ventilated in the burns operating room or emergency room) (Table 14.1).

Table 14.1 Requirements for a documentation tool in burns

Requirements						
Environmental	Usability in IT-environment	0	0	100	25	100
	Equipment needed	50	100	50	0	50
	Usability in clinical settings	0	0	100	25	100
	Usability in preclinical settings	0	0	100	25	100
	Ease of use	100	75	75	0	50
Quality	Exactness	25	50	75	0	50
	Low inter-rater variability	0	50	75	100	100
Medical documentation	Enable timeline	0	0	75	100	100
	Enable automatic encoding	0	0	0	100	100
	Enable documentation of lateral	0	25	25	100	100
Physiology	Body shape	0	0	0	100	75
	Aging (of a surface point)	0	0	0	50	100
	Extreme body deformations	0	0	0	75	25
	Changing proportions	0	50	50	100	75
	Size	0	50	50	100	100
	Sex, age	0	0	0	100	100
		Planimetric	Lund Browder (adapted planimetric) manually	Lund Browder (adapted planimetric) electronically	3D scan	Adapted 3D model
		175	400	775	1100	1350

14.4 Challenges in TBSA Evaluation

14.4.1 Types of Errors in TBSA Calculations

14.4.1.1 Painting Error

Painting error is the error which occurs when a burn wound is transferred to a model. This means that more investigators see the same burn and paint it differently. This error can be determined by seeing a burn and drawing it on an evaluation sheet. The difference in extent and localization shows the transfer error.

14.4.1.2 Estimation Error

Estimation error is the error happening when the percentage of the area of the body burned already painted on the model is estimated by the investigator and declared as a certain percentage of the area. Estimation errors can be combined with transfer errors. The estimation error was investigated by Miller [21] who sent charts of hypothetical patients to burn units and found out that there were significant differences in the calculated burn size both by doctors and by nurses. This phenomenon was described by Berry as well [22], not using charts, but the calculations of TBSA.

He compared estimates of transferring facilities to the estimations of the centers to which patients were transferred. Out of 333 patients transferred, 105 documentation of an exact TBSA were found and could be used for this study. Only 12 patients showed the same estimations, 65 patients were rated higher by the transferring units, and 28 proved to be underestimated. The mean TBSA was 22,5%, so there were many burns not being extensive. The question remains whether the kind of error was simply misestimation or whether there was a specific intention to overestimation to find a good reason for the transfer. In average, the transferring hospitals estimated the TBSA 5% higher than the burn centers.

The error could even be bigger due to the general overestimation done by Lund Browder charts. This error has been described and investigated together with transfer error by Wachtel [23] although he used planimetry as "golden standard." The Lund Browder based charts showed a significant difference to the Rule of 9.

14.4.1.3 Inter-rater Error

The sum of the above-described errors is the inter-rater error caused by different estimates of one burned area by different estimators.

14.4.1.4 Calculation Error

Calculation error is the possible error, when calculations are done when summing up the total percentage of TBSA affected (miscalculations in additions, multiplications, percentage calculation) Usually this kind of error can be reduced when summing up the areas affected by the burn and do the control with the area not affected what should sum up to 100%.

14.4.1.5 Methodical Error

Methodical error is happening when a three-dimensional surface is transferred to the two-dimensional model, e.g., of Lund Browder or when a method attributes the wrong percentage to a certain area.

As an example: Lund Browder Error:

The chart is showing different percentages of the body surface, compared to objective methods like 3D body scan or measurement of real surfaces by spherical planimetry.

14.4.1.6 Model Error

Model error happens, when the model does not reflect the body shape of the patient. This error happens when obese patients or patients with an unusual body shape are reduced to average models which are not adapted.

14.4.2 BIAS Caused by Secondary Motivation

All methods are open for motivational error. In any system, you can draw bigger burns than they are. Photo comparison and overlay is a method to reduce this influence and make the evaluation more objective. Intended overestimation in 3D systems is more obvious than in 2D systems.

14.4.2.1 Motivation

An example of how to improve *motivation* was our investigation about burn size estimation by participants of international burn meetings. By the chance of winning a price (iPad), the standard deviation of estimates was reduced in comparison to other studies.

14.4.2.2 Funding

Another reason could be a *reimbursement strategy* of burns treatment. An example of this is a DRG Group dependent from TBSA.

14.4.2.3 Psychology and Vanity

A *psychological aspect* should not be missed: When a patient is successfully treated, it feels better to "diagnose" a big burn as this gives better self-esteem than the survival of a patient with a small burn and when a patient died despite our treatment it must have been a big burn as he would have survived otherwise. This happens, e.g., when benchmarking processes are done between centers.

14.5 Technical Aspects of TBSA Calculation Methods

14.5.1 Paperless and IT Less Documentation

14.5.1.1 A Simple Estimate by the First Guess

A simple estimate by the first guess is a time-saving method. Just by looking at a patient, TBSA is estimated. The method seems to be inexact, but Hintermüller could demonstrate that the results were nearly comparable to the "rule of palms" [24]. Both methods resulted in an overestimation of TBSA; the simple estimate was the most inexact method. This method often is hidden under the term "clinical assessment."

14.5.2 Paper-Based Charts

14.5.2.1 Simple Drawing

Long before the time when charts with relations existed , simple drawing in paper was done [2]. By mental arithmetic, the system is open to nearly all kinds of error combined with low inter-rater reliability.

14.5.2.2 Drawing on a Model on Paper

Example of this is the Lund Browder Chart. The burn extent and quality is drawn on a model on a piece of paper. Evaluation of the percentage of the areas affected and calculations must be done by estimate.

14.6 IT-Supported Drawings and Calculations

IT-based systems may still have a methodological error, but inter-rater reliability is much better than the hand and brain work, no matter whether they are two- or three-dimensional [24–27].

14.6.1 Two-Dimensional IT Systems

2D models are based on simple drawings of the human body on a plane screen of a computer. These models do not consider three dimensionalities of the human body, and in many applications, there is no space to register the lateral and other parts of the body.

Many 2D models do not reflect the difference in sex, body shape, size, and weight of the patients. On the other hand, they are easy to be handled but can only give a very crude overview about the type of burns and areas affected especially on the lateral body parts and miss the true extent of areas. Different types can be described:

14.6.1.1 Simple Planimetry

This refers to a simple pixel count in a two-dimensional picture. Some electronic devices use this approach.

14.6.1.2 Corrected Planimetry

Corrected planimetry is a pixel count in a two-dimensional picture corrected by a certain body percentage advised to a certain body area.

14.6.2 Examples for Corrected Planimetry Are

- Rule of nine [28].
- Rule of fives [29].
- Lund Browder and related charts [6].
- SAGE II.
- Some computerized charts partly accommodated to gender, height, weight, age, and body shape.
- Most smartphone apps are based on a two-dimensional calculation corrected by the Lund Browder percentages.

14.6.3 Three-Dimensional Systems

3D models can be adapted to the individual properties of the patients.

14.6.4 3D Models Can Be Better Adapted to the Reality

Three-dimensional systems avoid the methodological error of reduction to a 2D drawing. They can be adapted to body size, weight, sex, and body shape.

Existing methods show a high validity in grown-ups with BMI < 30 [27]. Limitations are in severe obesity or unusual body proportions. The accuracy of the model is dependent on the adaptation to the model to the individual patient's body shape and properties.

14.6.4.1 Individual Measurement Based Systems

Individual measurement based systems should show an accurate picture of the body of the patient to be evaluated such considering gender, height, weight, age, and body shape.

An exact 3D scan seems to be a total individual and exact 3D model. They have been mainly used in studies till now, having shortcomings themselves but also showing the weakness of other methods [30]. A complete 3D body scan consists of a series of sub-scans which must be adapted to one.

14.6.4.2 Model-Based Systems

Models are used and adapted to gender, height, weight, age, and body shape. A choice of a model out of a library is done by the system or the user. It is then adapted to the different qualities as far as the IT system provides. Adaptation can be based on measurements. The choice of a model out of a library can be partially or total IT supported based on these. Another way is just hoping that the model fits best to reality out of the offered choice by visual compliance.

Lund Browder offers one model with one standard type of body shape. The proportions of certain body parts can be adapted to different ages. Just one model to draw on it represents three different models, and by this, it is a library based system.

14.6.4.3 Examples for 3D Methods

- Rule of palms [31]
- Measurement by comparing to the known surface:
  - Rapid Burn Assessor [32]
  - EPRI 3D Vision [14]
  - BurnCase 3D [33–35]
  - 3D Scanners [36]

14.7 Error Types Dependent on Methods (Table 14.2)

14.7.1 Methodological Error

14.7.1.1 The Methodological Errors of Two-Dimensional Charts

The Projection Error

In a front and/or backside view, the true size of an area affected can only be shown as the projection of a three-dimensional area on a plane area, not showing the true size. When an additional lateral picture exists, the same happens as a projection on a sagittal plane with the same shortcomings [13, 23, 37]. This error can be calculated by mathematical rules.

Calculation of Projection Error

The human body can be interpreted as a series of cylinders and cubes (Fig. 14.1).

In a lateral burn and a chart cutting the body in a two-dimensional anterior and posterior half, the area or percentage covered by the burn can be calculated (Fig. 14.2):

Table 14.2 Susceptibility to error types of different methods

	Painting error	Estimation error	Calculation error	Methodological error	Open for motivational error
Paper based	*****	*****	*****	*****	***
IT-based 2D	***	****	–	***	***
IT-based 3D	*	–	–	*(dep. on body shape)	***

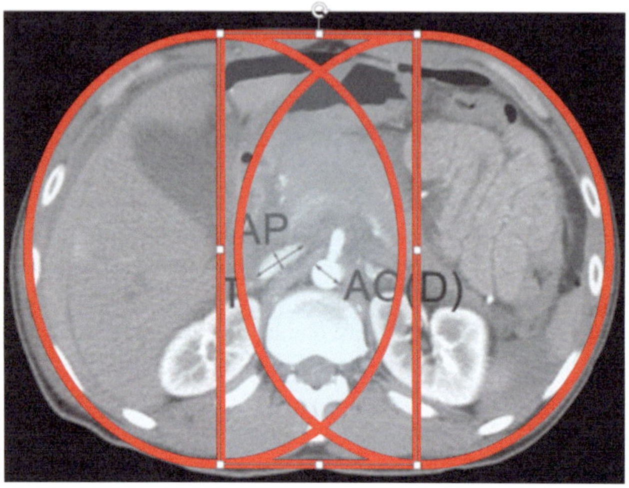

Fig. 14.1 Shows how a body can be abstracted to circles and rectangles

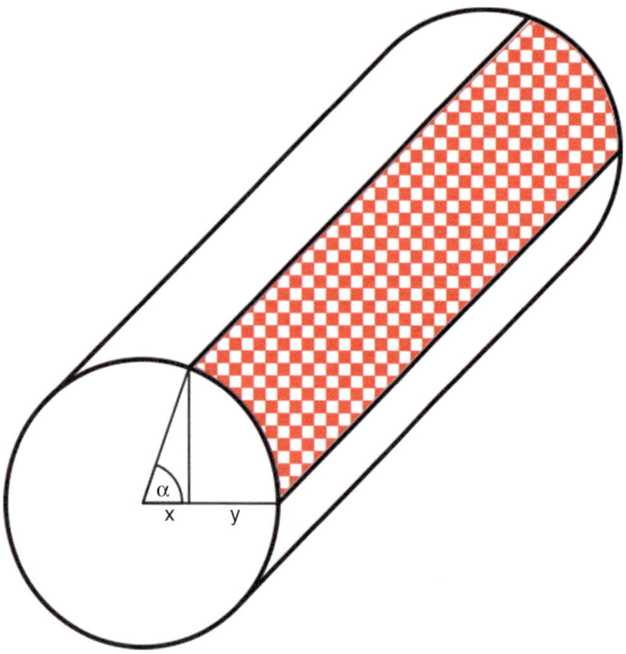

Fig. 14.2 Projection of a burnt area on a plane 2D system compared to 3D beginning from 0° to alpha: y is the projection of the circle segment to the plane

Presumed: radius = 1, height = 1, the area of the plane projection can be calculated by the formula $(1 - x) *1$ where $x = \cos$ (alpha).

$Y = 1 - \cos$(alpha); Projected area = (1 − cos(alpha) × 1). In a three-dimensional measurement, the red area can be calculated as follows: $(2r\pi \times \alpha) *h/360$ = 2pi × alpha)/360

The relation between the two-dimensional and three-dimensional area in the lateral body parts where the form of the body corresponds to a circle shape can be calculated depending on the angle α (Table 14.3).

The numbers in the table above are only calculated for one-quarter of the body and as total angles.

Result: In a lateral wound between 0° and 10° it can be demonstrated that the 3D registration calculates 11 times the area which is calculated by the 2D registration and 1.5 times for the whole area of a quarter of the body cylinder and the double amount when the anterior and the posterior quarters are affected.

Calculation of Projection of Segments of 10° Each (Fig. 14.3)

To calculate the area as a projection of segments which means not as true angles but as the segment between, e.g., 10 and 20°, a different calculation for the relation between 2D and 3D must be done.

The calculation for *the plane 2D area is*

Presumed $r = 1$, $h = 1$; Area 1 = $r (\cos(\beta) - \cos(\alpha)) *h$ where r and h are eliminated as 1

And for the 3D documentation: $2r\pi*(\alpha - \beta) \times h$ where r and h are eliminated as 1

This number stays the same for all 10-degree slices (Fig. 14.4 and Table 14.4).

Result: It can be shown that the projection of wounds lateral from 60° only shows between 90 and 8% of the true area. This effect is doubled when the anterior and the posterior quarters are affected!

14.7.1.2 The Standardization Error

The standardization error is the error happening when the measurement has an immanent system error due to the type of standardization of the measurement. This can be demonstrated by showing the different results of different methods of measurement.

This can be demonstrated by computer simulation:

Lund Browder chart was compared to the male and female 3D model (BurnCase 3D) and male and female scan models and to Make Human Taiwanese models based on the measurements of Yu. Typical areas of the body were selected, and

Table 14.3 Cumulated difference in true 3D areas to projected 2D areas from

α	Area 2D	Area 3D	Percentage 2D area of 3D area	Percentage 3D area of 2D area	Difference 3D-2D
0–10	0.01519225	0.17453278	0.08704524	11.4882794	0.15934053
0–20	0.06030738	0.34906556	0.17276806	5.78810686	0.28875818
0–30	0.1339746	0.52359833	0.25587285	3.90819117	0.38962374
0–40	0.23395556	0.69813111	0.33511693	2.98403304	0.46417555
0–50	0.35721239	0.87266389	0.40933559	2.44298326	0.5154515
0–60	0.5	1.04719667	0.47746523	2.09439333	0.54719667
0–70	0.65797986	1.22172944	0.53856429	1.85678852	0.56374959
0–80	0.82635182	1.39626222	0.5918314	1.68967041	0.5699104
0–90	1	1.570795	0.63662031	1.570795	0.570795

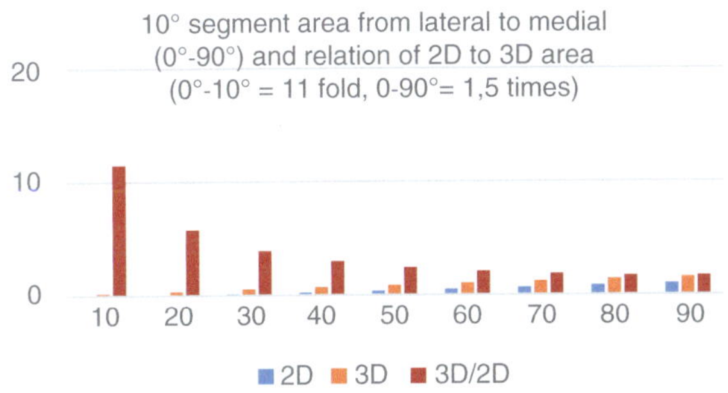

Fig. 14.3 How much of a 3D area (10° segment) do you really see in 2D projection?

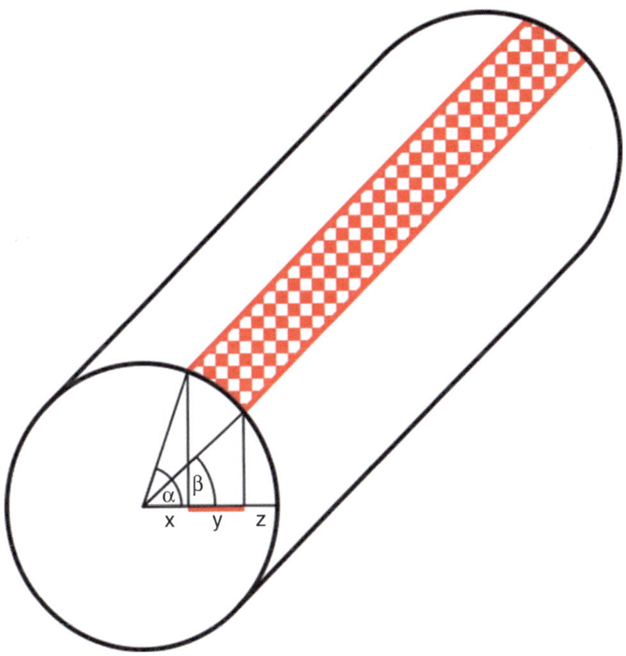

Fig. 14.4 Shows how a 10° cylinder segment is projected to a 2D plane

the total percentage of body surface area as indicated by the different systems were compared.

Models used: (Table 14.5)

The standardization error is a technical error and the individual errors by the investigators are not reflected.

14.8 Description, Critics, and Literature of Different Methods

14.8.1 Which Rules Are Used in Common Practice? (Table 14.6)

Although burn surgeons mostly declare to use a special procedure (per SOP) in determining TBSA, when demonstrating how they do, a combination of methods is used, where the rule of the palm is a basic tool (personal experience of the authors). The rule of nines seems to be the most used method.

14.8.2 Rule of Palm

14.8.2.1 Rule

The surface of the patient's palm is about 1% of the total body surface. There are different usages of this rule, whether palm is to be calculated with or without fingers [11].

14.8.2.2 Critics

The rule of palm leads to an overestimation of the real extent of the burn injury. In adults, the extent of a palm varies between 0.75% [11] and 0.94% of the total body surface [47]. There are principal gender-related differences as the palm of a man is 0.85% [11], and the palm of a woman is 0.79% [48] of the total body surface in normal BMI. The isolated palm is 0.5% in men and 0.4% in women [11]. In children, the palm is 0.92% and the palm 0.52% [47].

The rule of the palm is influenced by the BMI as the true area of the palm does not change in the same amount than body surface area in a BMI > 31 [49] both in men and women. Butz [50] describes the dependency of the real palmar surface from BMI and formula of BSA calculation and

Table 14.4 Shows the numeric differences between a 3D cylinder segment and its projection to a single plane

Angle	cos	cos > - Cos <	Segment 3D	2D/3D∗100 percentage projected on 2D	3D/2D
0–10	1	0.01519225	0.17453278	8.7045236	11.4882794
10–20	0.98480775	0.04511513	0.17453278	25.8490885	3.86860836
20–30	0.93969262	0.07366722	0.17453278	42.2082419	2.36920553
30–40	0.8660254	0.09998096	0.17453278	57.2849192	1.74566014
40–50	0.76604444	0.12325683	0.17453278	70.6210232	1.41600894
50–60	0.64278761	0.14278761	0.17453278	81.8113431	1.22232439
60–70	0.5	0.15797986	0.17453278	90.5158668	1.10477868
70–80	0.34202014	0.16837197	0.17453278	96.4701117	1.03659049
80–90	0.17364818	0.17364818	0.17453278	99.493161	1.00509421

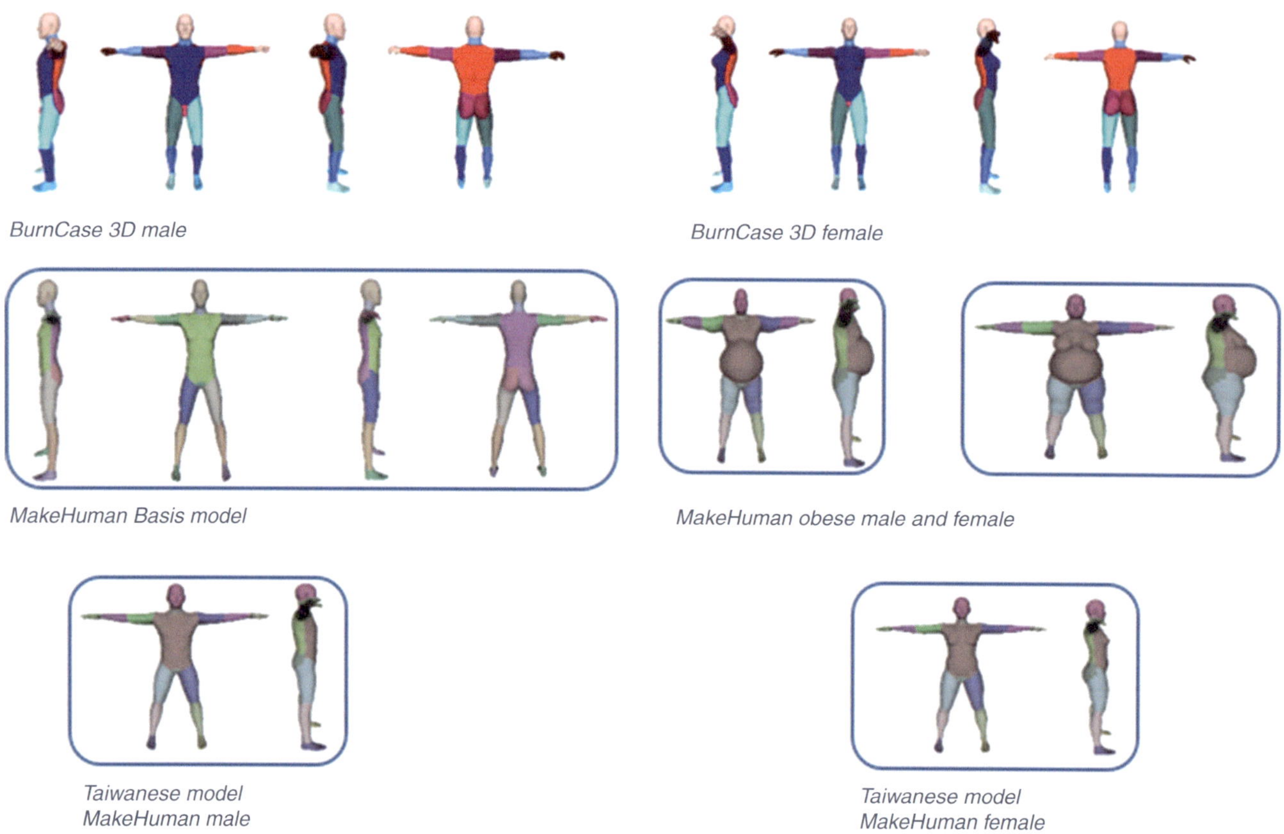

Fig. 14.5 Shows the different models tested for comparison

found values in a BMI of 18.5–24, between 0.95 (Mosteller and Dubois) and 0.99 (Yu et al.) [50]. In a BMI ≥ 40, the values differed between 0.61 (Livingston and Scott) and 0.73 (Du-Bois and Du-Bois).

The degree of overestimation in practical use varies. Hintermüller found a variance from +173% to +41.55% of the true area and a standard deviation of 19.91% and an average overestimation of 70.88% in the total area of 7 wounds evaluated. The error was bigger in small wounds than in large wounds.

The method could be the reason for severe overestimation up to 100% in A&E departments as described by Laing [51]. He describes a clear dependency from the specialty or grade of the assessor in the A&E department. Doctors varied between 117 and 7% of overestimation although using a Lund Browder chart. This could be caused by the rule of palms to assist in Lund Browder evaluation. Cone described an average overestimation of 75% by referring physicians [52]. Sheng et al. describe an overestimation by the combined use of Chinese rule of nines and the rule of palms between 12 and 30% in 17 wounds evaluated [20].

14.8.2.3 Validation

The rule of palm has been tested for validity by Rossiter [11]. He measured the size of the palms in 70 subjects (36 male, 34 female) and compared it to BSA calculations by a formula (which formula is not described). Evaluations were

Table 14.5 Results of comparison of body areas in different models

Method	Lund Browder	BurnCase 3D		Yu et al.	Make Human obese		Make Human model adapted to average of Taiwanese Body Bank	
		Male	Female		Male	Female	Male	Female
Region	% BSA	% BSA	% BSA	% BSA	% BSA	% BSA	% BSA	% BSA
Head	7	6.71	7.36	7.43	5.76	6.09	8.26	8.06
Neck	2	1.39	1.38	2.67	1.05	0.98	1.5	1.09
Anterior trunk	13	13.32	12.9	14.94	20.6	20.56	13.68	15.46
Posterior trunk	13	9.78	8.27	10.97	11.76	10.38	10.7	9.88
Right buttock	2.5	3.01	3.38	2.55	2.87	3.34	2.32	3.06
Left buttock	2.5	3	3.21	2.55	2.88	3.37	2.33	3.1
Genitals	1	1.17	0.26	0	0.44	0.5	0.41	0.5
Right upper arm	4	4.39	4.88	4.11	4.31	4.07	4.42	4.02
Left upper arm	4	4.36	4.82	4.11	4.41	4.16	4.51	4.13
Right lower arm	3	3.64	3.24	2.99	3.15	2.89	2.93	2.65
Left lower arm	3	3.63	3.21	2.99	3.15	2.88	2.93	2.65
Right hand	2.5	2.2	2.08	2.32	2.02	1.7	2.5	1.98
Left hand	2.5	2.2	2.07	2.32	2.02	1.7	2.5	1.98
Right thigh	9.5	11.25	12.24	9.93	9.03	10.25	10.38	11.14
Left thigh	9.5	11.07	12.11	9.93	8.94	10.1	10.29	11.01
Right shank	7	5.97	6.2	6.83	6.34	6.2	6.98	6.62
Left shank	7	6.14	6.14	6.83	6.34	6.2	6.98	6.62
Right foot	3.5	3.4	3.13	3.28	2.47	2.31	3.19	3.03
Left foot	3.5	3.39	3.13	3.28	2.47	2.31	3.19	3.03

Table 14.6 Usage of rules accordimg to literature

Publication	Rule of palms	Rule of Nines	Lund Browder	Electronic	Combination of LB and R. of 9 s	Not described or others
Miller percentage [21]		35	33		1.75	21
Giretzlehner [41]						
DAV percentage	37.3	38.8	10.4		29.4	9
EBA percentage	41.8	37.3	24.1		41.2	4.8
Ziegler percentage [43]		71	18	29		

done as well by Sheridan [53], Nagel and Schunk [47], Amirsheybani [54], Jose [55, 56], and others.

14.8.2.4 Result

A palm is not 1% of body surface area [57]. Severe overestimation of TBSA can be expected when using the rule of palms due to inaccuracy in definition and usage, varying between 10 and 70%. The inter-rater error is expected to be high.

14.8.3 Rule of Nines per Pulaski and Tennison (Wallace)

14.8.3.1 Description

In his publication in 1951 [58], following percentages are given arms 9% of total body surface each, legs 18% each, chest and back 18% each, head 7%, neck 2%, hands and feet, genitals 1% each. There is no adaption to sex, weight, height, and different body shapes.

14.8.3.2 Critics

The rule was intended for preclinical use in a disaster or mass casualty situation. The application of the rule of nines often leads to an overestimation of the real extent of the burn injury [22, 23], especially in patients with an increased body mass index [59]. In patients weighing more than 80 kg, it is more promising to apply a rule of fives, under 10 kg a rule of eights [59]. Not regarding different body shapes leads to an overestimation of extremity burns and underestimation of torso burns [29]. In normal weighted patients, the back and the torso are overrepresented by the rule of nines when compared to the results of 3D scans [36].

14.8.3.3 Validation

This rule was intended as fast orientation in the place of the accident. Its simplicity contributed to a wide use even in burn centers. The author found no validation study of the rule of nines. The inter-rater error is expected to be high.

14.8.3.4 Result

The rule of nines is very dependent on the BMI and usually leads to severe overestimations. It was one of the most common rules in the investigation of Giretzlehner [41]. He found an average overestimation (= estimate – true value) by use of the rule of nines and Lund Browder of 138%. The rule is considered inaccurate by many authors [13, 22, 23, 60].

14.8.4 Lund Browder Chart [6]

14.8.4.1 Description

The Lund Browder Chart assigns various age groups to various body proportions. One model is attributing different percentages of BSA to special areas, which are defined by their borders. It cannot be adapted to sex, weight, height and body shape and five different ages.

It uses adapted planimetry for the calculation procedure. It is regarded as "the most accurate procedure" by most authors [61].

14.8.4.2 Critics

Several authors have shown an overestimation of the extent of the burn injury when applying the Lund Browder Chart, maybe as it is based on only one type of physique. Various forms of corpulence and different weight categories cannot be considered as well as different body shapes and changes in proportions between the given ages.

14.8.4.3 Validation

When evaluating the Lund Browder Chart, the challenge is to compare it to objective measurements. Usually, the "*golden standard*" in comparisons is an experienced senior surgeon of the burn center. This is no objective method. Computerized planimetry only can improve the calculation of the percentage of burns of an identified area without calculating the real extent as this method has the projection error immanent. Computerized methods like 3D measurements or stereogrammetry seem to be adequate [61]. Another method is the evaluation with paper squares. Klippel described concerns about the validity of the chart which had not been validated by an expert panel and that the anthropometric data used were more than 60 (now 100) years old [62].

14.8.4.4 Results

The comparison to 3D methods sometimes shows severe overestimations by this method (see table).

Differences between investigators estimating the same patient can be found due to different surroundings (e.g., A&E department, preclinical evaluation, and burn center) where many types of error are possible. Such studies have mainly been performed when patients were transferred to a burn unit after primary evaluation. Big differences were found in many studies [63–66]. Most of the preclinical evaluations were compared to burn center evaluation what again was a Lund Browder Chart.

14.8.4.5 Overestimation

Table 14.7 shows estimation errors published in the literature:

14.8.4.6 Underestimation

Underestimation is only diagnosed when compared to an "expert Lund Browder Chart." It happens less frequently than overestimation and when mainly in extensive burns.

14.8.5 Inter-rater Error

Inter-rater error is the error when two investigators evaluate the same burn differently. A high inter-rater error makes data not sufficient for scientific use.

Table 14.7 Over- and underestimation when using own method chart

Author	Over-under estimation	Info	Golden standard
Alm 2003 [38]	Average plus 17.18%	Overestimation in 90%	Paper squares
Nichter 1985 [13] cited in Neuwalder 2002 [14]	Average plus 29–49%	Mean estimate 21.1 for a 10.8% burns	Acetate rip-off planimetry of affected area in computer
Nichter [13]	Mean rater plus 90% TBSA paper chart	Mean overestimation found was 12.48%	2D computer against true area
Berry [39]	Standard distribution of error 20.5 TBSA	Overestimation in 94 of 256 cases (37%)	Burn unit assessment (LB)
Martin Lundy [40] Military Operational Surgical Group	Underestimated avg—12%		2 Burn Center experts using Lund Browder
Martin Lundy [40] CPSS (Burns + plastic Surgeons)	Overestimate + 1%		2 Burn Center experts using Lund Browder
Giretzlehner [41]	Overestimation of plus 77–161%	Estimation from photos	3D computer model (BurnCase 3D)
Berry [42]	Overestimation 12% (39.4% versus 34.9%)		2D system manually versus 2D system computerized

Table 14.8 Inter-rater error as shown in literature

Author/year	Chart	True size TBSA	Average std. dev in % BSA	Add. info	Method of comparison	
Neuwalder [14]	2D computerized and 3D computerized	n.a.	n.a.	Can reduce overestimation and increase accuracy to 0.5% error	Technical comparison	
Wachtel et al. 2000 [23]	Univ. San Diego Cal.	50.50	±5.86%	No 3D comparison	Computer planimetry	
Wachtel et al. 2000 [23]	Univ. San Diego Cal. Rule of Nines	52.36	±6.32	No 3D comparison	Computer planimetry	
Martin 2013 [40] MOST cohort	Mod. Lund Browder Chart	64.5 Avg. eval.: 52.53	±10.03	No 3D comparison	Comparison to "expert Lund Browder"	
Martin 2013 [40] CSPSS cohort	Mod. Lund Browder Chart	64.5 Avg. eval.: 65.68	±10.29	No 3D comparison	Comparison to "expert Lund Browder"	
Retrouvey [44]	Lund Browder	Median 10%	±1.5% average (1.4–2.2)	Compared to BurnCase 3D	Est. error of +14% to +22% by use of LB	
Electronic systems:						
Berry [42]	Electronic Lund Browder Chart				Interobserver variability 0.995	
Parvizi [27]	3D electronic calculator model based	20.7; 27.2; 16.5	0.9 1.5 0.1	0.1863 0.01088 0.00495	Intra-class correlation 98% CI 95%	BurnCase 3D
Sheng 2016 [20]	3D electronic calculator based on 3D scans				Intra-class correlation 99.9%	BurnCalc

Table 14.8 shows the inter-rater error in literature.

14.8.5.1 Conclusion

The Lund Browder Chart mostly leads to an overestimation of the real burn and is prone to a high inter-rater error. These overestimations are bigger in small burns and smaller in larger burns [22, 39]. Big burns have the trend to be underestimated by Lund Browder Chart (only compared to Lund Browder performed by experts). As the total burn size is limited to 100%, it is obvious that bigger burns are less overestimated having this mathematical limit.

Results: 3D systems have less inter-rater errors and high intra-class correlations compared to the truth. As they are based on different calculation methods, different results are to be expected. Hintermüller compared 2D electronic system (Mersey Burns) to a 3D electronic system (BurnCase 3D). In her evaluation, Mersey Burns was linked to an overestimation of 32% to the ground truth with a range of 17.8%, while BurnCase 3D showed an overall difference to the ground truth of average −4.53% with a range of 7.6%. So, it was superior to the other methods. Similar findings were described by Goldberg [25, 46].

14.8.6 Electronic Systems

14.8.6.1 Two-Dimensional Systems

One example of a two-dimensional electronic system is Mersey Burns. It has been approved by Medicines and Healthcare Regulatory Affairs Agency in the UK [18]. The App showed in comparison to Auburn [18] nearly the same ease of use and frequency of errors. The real TBSA evaluated was not investigated, and the electronic calculations of both programs were based on a 2D Lund Browder Chart.

Examples for this are [19] (Tables 14.9 and 14.10).

14.8.6.2 3D Systems as Apps

Examples for 3D apps:

14.8.7 3D Systems as Desktop Programs

Desktop programs are mostly designed for usage in burn centers. They can act as standalone versions or as a network of computers.

14.8.7.1 BurnCase 3D

Description

It is a Windows-based desktop program and database for 3D registration and storage and electronic processing of burns information. Most challenges of modern burn care are considered by the developers. Its strength is the simple and

Table 14.9 Technical and other specifications of different systems

App	Method	Min res	Medical implications	Medical product	Literature on medline
BurnCare	Lund Browder	Minimum 1% square	Gives suggestion for resuscitation	No	None available
Mersey Burns	Lund Browder		Parkland	Medicines and Healthcare products Regulatory Agency (MHRA) authority as a class I medical device in the United Kingdom [18]	[18, 24, 45]
NurseCalc	Rule of Nines	1 Unit (extremity)	Just TBSA	No	None
BurnCalc	Lund Browder				
uBurn	Rule of Nines		Parkland	No	[18, 24]

Table 14.10 Apps and used methods

App	Method	Min res	Medical implications	Medical Product	Literature on medline
3D Burn	3D model adapted	?	Parkland formula	No	Not found
BurnMed Lite	3D model adapted	9704 triangles total	TBSA	No	[46]
BurnCase 3D	3D model adapted	90,000 triangles	TBSA, TBSA superficial, deep, partially deep, BMI, Parkland B.E.E. Caloric requirements	No	[24]

intuitive user interface, allowing quick data input without the need for sophisticated training [24].

The model is build up as a 3-dimensional mesh of over 90,000 connected triangles with each smaller than 1 cm^2. By specifying age, sex, height, and weight, and choosing an appropriate 3D standard model the system generates an automatically adapted virtual body surface which fits the patient's body shape. It incorporates the 12 most widely accepted TBSA estimation formulas in the scientific literature. Also, the adaptation algorithm considers the growth behavior of different body regions to reach realistic body expansion.

The burned surface area is marked on the 3D body surface by standard mouse or touchpad interaction. Consequently, the marked area appears in a significant color and pattern, thus visualizing different burn degrees or even surgical procedures, dressings, or medications. The covered surface area as well as affected percentage of the TBSA and several medical scores and indices (ASBI, Baux, Baxter-Parkland, etc.) are calculated in real time and presented on the user interface immediately after drawing.

14.8.7.2 Special Features

Can Be Used as a Network Server or Client

The system is designated for network use in a hospital or within hospitals as well as a standalone feature.

It can cooperate with BurnCase 3D app, to work as a central data collection tool in mass casualties where pictures and datasheets can be transferred as well.

Creation of a Timeline

Such an acquisition of a 3D state can be created and revisited at different points in time throughout the whole treatment. Thus, a comprehensive 3-dimensional track of the complete treatment history is created and stored in the database for every patient. So the history of burns treatment can be documented, percentage of graft loss can be documented as well as the time to heal [67].

Additional Database for Injury-Related Data

Additional burn-related information such as the course of the accident, first aid, complications, former illnesses, and condition on admission can also be acquired and stored to the database. To be able to supervise all changes to the stored data, *BurnCase 3D* keeps track of every data acquisition or deletion in a separate changelog. This data collection is compatible with the United States' National Trauma Registry (NTRACS).

Intelligent Picture Archieves

The system enables picture storage and retrieval by an intelligent link to patient, date, procedure, diagnosis, and much more in a simple and intuitive way.

Improvement of Accuracy by Picture Overlay

To further increase the level of accuracy, an integrated digital picture archive provides visual verification by superimposing pictures on the 3D model. An intuitive model-picture-registration algorithm has been implemented, which allows the physician to easily move the virtual body in the position of the patient on any digital picture. By doing so, the whole burn surface estimation procedure becomes as easy as sketching the border of burn wounds on a picture, however without subjective influences.

This can be done with true or false color pictures as produced by burn depth classification methods.

Addition of Burn Depth Diagnosis

CCD cameras with appropriate classification software as developed by Dr. Werner Eisenbeiß and Dr. Jörg Marotz in Lübeck, Germany at Delphi-Optics GmbH or other methods like Laser-Doppler-Measurement (Moore Instruments, UK) or Infrared Spectroscopy (NRCC, Canada) can also be used as classification input for *BurnCase 3D* and leads to an automatic and objective characterization and documentation of burn injuries.

Automated Encoding

The system encodes automatically all diagnostic procedures per ICD and operation procedures.

Workload Description Based on ICD and Surgical Procedure Codes

At the end of treatment, the total used ICD codes and OPS codes are generated to enable the comparison of workload and to generate DRGs.

14.8.8 Validation

14.8.8.1 Accuracy and Interobserver Error

BurnCase 3D was validated in a study comparing computer measurements of seven wounds in each of three models (male-female, child) to the real extent of wounds measured by detaching the wound areas from the models and planimetric measurements [27, 68]. It showed an average deviation of measurements to the ground truth of 0.2% and an intra-class correlation of 98. So, it proved to be "a valid and reliable tool for the determination of percentage burned TBSA in standard models."

14.8.8.2 The Dependency of Results from Training

Hintermüller demonstrated that after an introduction into the program of just 1-min paramedics achieved an intra-class correlation of 96% and an average standard deviation of estimates <1.2%.

It has been observed that the use of a 3D evaluation tool even reduced the overestimation when using Lund Browder Charts.

14.8.9 Limitations

14.8.9.1 Severe Obesity or Unusual Body Shape

Validation was done using standard models of manikins. Although an adaptation of the models can be done to an "obesity type," this adaptation is limited by a higher BMI (~30) or by unusual body shape. Further model development is in progress.

14.8.9.2 Children

TBSA evaluation in children was described as an unsolved problem [69]. Lund Browder only offers models of a newborn baby, a baby about 1 year and a juvenile model with about 12 years. In the MICA Study (Measurements for Infants, Children, and Adolescents) the team of Kinderklinik Linz measured the proportions of 2529 children [70] and created 12 proportionally correct models for different age groups, which can be adapted to weight sex and height. These models were integrated into BurnCase 3D. An evaluation has been started.

14.8.9.3 Results

BurnCase 3D is reliable and easy to use tool with many different features. It shows the highest accuracy and lowest inter-rater error of all tools in clinical practice [27].

14.8.9.4 3D Pictures

3D pictures together with an objectivation of size (e.g., by the ruler, a fixed distance of photos or a grid pattern [71]) can be a good method to determine burns extent especially in small burns with high accuracy.

Critique: Results are given in absolute square cm, the calculation of TBSA percentage demands BSA estimation by a formula. So this method is only perfect in small burns [72].

14.8.9.5 3D Scans

3D scans can be useful for accurate determination of the size of a burn wound, as these systems once calibrated give the absolute size of an area.

14.8.10 Partial Scans

Partial scans are used to produce compression devices, e.g., for the head. The usual method of a plaster cast is replaced by a 3D scan of the face and the scars. A compression mask can be produced by a 3D print. The degree of compression must be determined by a special algorithm.

14.8.11 Total Scans

14.8.11.1 Description

When there are bigger burns or unusual body shapes, 3D scan needs a total body scan from all aspects (e.g., planta pedis, palms of the hand). Only a scan can determine the surface of the body so scans of axilla, perineum and other are necessary. So about eight total scans are necessary to reconstruct a body exactly [56]. These scans must be assembled as a "total body scan picture" which demands an evaluation of the composition procedure. To evaluate changes on the surface, the 3D scan from a point cloud must be stored in a model where each surface point can be followed up over the timeline.

14.8.11.2 Critique

Till now no usable 3D scan for a total body scan in a burns environment has been published. BurnCalc [20] shows the accuracy of a 3D scan but does not tell how to use in an environment with a ventilated and sedated patient. The storage in a point cloud does not allow follow-up of a certain point of the surface over different scans.

14.9 Consequences of Wrong TBSA Evaluation

14.9.1 Over-Resuscitation

Shock treatment in burn injuries was one of the greatest progresses in burns treatment when it was implicated by a feasible rule like the one of Parkland created by Baxter and shires in 1968. The rules implicated were mainly based on the extent of burns as a percentage of TBSA [73]. In *1979*, an NIH-sponsored conference on burn care was summarized with a statement that burn patients should be resuscitated *with as little fluid as possible to maintain organ perfusion.* Initial fluid therapy should consist of isotonic crystalloid at a volume between 2 and 4 mL/kg/%TBSA for the first 24 h and titrated to maintain *urine output of 30–50 mL/h* [74].

In the years' complications in burns, treatment was found in increasing number which was not documented before [73]. Abdominal compartments led the attention to the fact that most centers used amounts of fluids for resuscitation which were sometimes severely more than the calculated 4 mL/kg/TBSA%.

Many reasons may be causal for this.

First, there was the trend to optimize resuscitation to "super-normal" values [75]. Small boluses of fluid were given to the point that cardiac output did not increase any more. By following this procedure, very high volumes were applied. "More" simply was accepted as better. First results seemed promising, but in a multicenter trial, supra-normal values did not provide a better outcome [76].

Sympathetic activation by vasoconstrictor substances as catecholamine or angiotensin 2 increases CVP and releases NAP. This happens in the primary situation of the injury where pain raises pressure and makes tachycardia.

NAP mediates the shredding of the glycocalyx which is responsible for the tightening or leakage of vessels [77, 78]. This effect can be aggravated by the application of additional fluid [79].

Early shredding of the glycocalyx may establish early capillary leakage, demanding higher amounts of fluid later [80]. The low-volume responders could be differentiated from the high-volume responders in the very early phase which was within the first 4 h [81]. "Difference developed after two hours and remained so" [81]. So the very early phase of resuscitation is determining the later run. Once initiated, "fluid begets more fluid" [80]! Control by urine output fails in the case of severe capillary leakage. This can be seen in Friedrich who investigated supra-Baxter resuscitation and found no difference in 24-h urine output between groups of high-volume resuscitation and low-volume resuscitation [82]. The same can be seen in the paper of Engrav where she showed that the average urine output did not increase although the fluid administrations did [83].

Initial overestimation of TBSA increases all the previous effects. Over-resuscitation caused by overestimation will happen during the primary transport where no urine output is measured. The consequences of burn edema cannot be reversed later. It is common in emergency departments.

14.9.2 Complications Due to Burn Edema

Complications of burn edema as pulmonary dysfunction and increased intra-abdominal and intercompartmental are well described [73]. Mortality has not been proven due to high-volume resuscitation. Local complications like reduced take rates of dermatomes too are not investigated and described till now. Low-volume resuscitation reduces the risk for MODS and makes a improved lung function in the early phase [84]. After all "suboptimal fluid resuscitation in burn, patients leads to greater burn depth and extension of the shock period [85]."

14.9.3 Missing Accuracy in Studies

A scientific approach to burns treatment is based on accurate TBSA calculation. This has been generally accepted, and different intentions are going on an international level. The OBOS (One Burn One Standard) initiative of the ABA [1], the one world one burn of ISBI, and the standardization initiatives of the German-Speaking Association for Burns Treatment [86, 87] try to set up standards for burns treatment. The necessity of standards was well recognized in, e.g., the "Inflammation and the Host Response to Injury study." The creation of SOPS was seen as necessary for this study to create high-quality clinical endpoints in burn care as a basis for further evaluation of genetic and proteomic changes and its influence on inflammation [88]. Unfortunately, this study like others is based on an evaluation of TBSA by Lund Browder Chart, ignoring the immanent errors like over- or underestimations and inter-rater error of these methods. Even if in a very expert surrounding doing TBSA evaluations, the validity of data based on methods and errors is basic to further conclusions. An inter-rater error of 10% as reported by Wachtel and others [13, 23] can change results and significances and can simply be changed by the use of electronic media.

14.9.4 Wrong Distribution of Patients

14.9.4.1 Distribution to Burn Centers

Burn size is the most important parameter whether to transfer patients to burn centers or not. TBSA evaluation happens either preclinically or in the emergency department. It is common knowledge that TBSA evaluated preclinically or in an emergency department, in an Emergency Department, where burns treatment is not common knowledge often differs severely from later TBSA evaluation in the burn center [63, 66]. In a recent study [89], it was demonstrated that 59% of the burn patients were administered more fluid, based on the primary evaluation than was necessary after evaluation in the burn center. The percentage of overestimation of TBSA found by Goverman was 339%. Burn size was overestimated in 94% of all children transferred. The degree of overestimation could even be higher as the "golden standard" for burn center evaluation was Lund Browder chart. As according to the ABA rules certain percentages of TBSA are an indication for transfer to a burn center, this could lead to an overuse of the resources of burn centers and avoidable costs for transports [90].

14.9.4.2 Distribution in Mass Casualties

In mass casualties, the utilization of burn center resources is critical. Dependent on TBSA and other parameters, the distribution of burn victims must be guided. Wrong estimates can contribute to wrong decisions about further treatment, causing complications or missing adequate treatment.

Summary Box

- TBSA is one of the essential parameters for the prognosis in burns. It influences not only outcome parameters but also workload, material needs, and need for staff, and most of burn-science is based on it.
- When inhomogeneous data of burned surface area are used, results from scientific studies can lose their pretended significances, and wrong conclusions can be drawn.
- Due to its importance, it must be based on exact data; accurate *burn size evaluation* should *replace estimation*. Technical solutions have progressed and enable burn surgeons to provide accurate data without significant interobserver variation. Different types of error can be avoided, and personal motives lose their relevance.
- This chapter shows methods and errors and demonstrates why three-dimensional IT solutions are to be preferred to hand paints. The perfect feature is a combination of usability under different environments which does not only evaluate TBSA in an individually adapted model but is combined with burn depth evaluation in a fast procedure for the whole body.
- Research and development are on its way to this goal.

References

1. Hickerson WL, Ryan CM, Conlon KM, Harrington DT, Foster K, Schwartz S, et al. What's in a name? Recent key projects of the committee on organization and delivery of burn care. J Burn Care Res. 2015;36(6):619–25.
2. Klasen HJ. Size. Hist. Burn. Rotterdam: Erasmus; 2004. p. 23ff.
3. Meet K. Oberflächenmessungen des menschlichen Körpers. Z Biol. 1879;15:125–47.
4. Riehl. Zur Therapie schwerer Verbrennungen. Wien Klin Wochenschriift. 1925;37:833–4.
5. Dubois D, Dubois E. A formula to estimate the approximate surface area if height and weight be known. Arch Intern Med. 1916;17:863–71.
6. Lund C, Browder N. The estimation of areas of burns. Surg Gynecol Obstet. n.d.;79:352–8.
7. Boyd E. The growth of the surface area of the human body. Minneapolis: Univ Minnesota Press; 1935.
8. Neaman KC, Andres LA, McClure AM, Burton ME, Kemmeter PR, et al. A new method for estimation of involved BSAs for obese and normal-weight patients with burn injury. J Burn Care Res. 2011;32:421–8.
9. Wilson GR, Fowler CA, Housden PL. A new burn area assessment chart. Burns. 1987;13:401–5.
10. Kirby NG, Blackburn G. Field surgery pocket book. London: The Stationery Office Books; 1981.. ISBN-10: 0117723606 ISBN-13: 978-0117723603
11. Rossiter ND, Chapman P, Haywood IA. How big is a hand? Burns. 1996;22:230–1.
12. Wachtel TL, Brimm JE, Knight MA, Heisterkamp S, Frank HA, Inancsi W, et al. Research: computer assisted estimation of the size of burns. J Burn Care Rehabil. 1983;4:255–9.
13. Nichter LS, Williams J, Bryant CA, Edlich RF. Improving the accuracy of burn-surface estimation. Plast Reconstr Surg. 1985;76:428–33.
14. Neuwalder JM, Sampson C, Breuing KH, Orgill DP. A review of computer-aided body surface area determination: SAGE II and EPRI's 3D Burn Vision. J Burn Care Rehabil. 2002;23:55–9; discussion 54.
15. Lee RC, Kieska G, Mankani MH. A three-dimensional computerized burn chart: stage I: development of three-dimensional renderings. J Burn Care Rehabil. 1994;15:80–3.
16. Mankani MH, Kicska G, Lee R. A three-dimensional computerized burn chart—stage II: assessment of accuracy. J Burn Care Rehabil. 1994;15:191–3.
17. Mult EPRI J. 1999. http://eprijournal.com/wp-content/uploads/2016/02/1999-Journal-No.-4.pdf.
18. Morris R, Javed M, Bodger O, Hemington Gorse S, Williams D, Gorse SH, et al. A comparison of two smartphone applications and the validation of smartphone applications as tools for fluid calculation for burns resuscitation. Burns. 2013;40:826–34.
19. Wurzer P, Parvizi D, Lumenta DB, Giretzlehner M, Branski LK, Finnerty CC, et al. Smartphone applications in burns. Burns. 2015;41:977–89.
20. Sheng W, Zeng D, Wan Y, Yao L, Tang H, Xia Z. BurnCalc assessment study of computeraided individual threedimensional burn area calculation. J Transl Med. 2014;12:1–6.
21. Miller SF, Finley RK, Waltman M, Lincks J, Sidney F. Burn size estimate reliability: a study. J Burn Care Rehabil. 1991;12:546–59.
22. Berry CC, Wachtel T, Frank HA. Differences in burn size estimates between community hospitals and a Burn Center. J Burn Care Rehabil. 1982;3:176–8.
23. Wachtel TL, Berry CC, Wachtel EE, Frank HA. The inter-rater reliability of estimating the size of burns from various burn area chart drawings. Burns. 2000;26:156–70.
24. Hintermüller C. Estimation of total burn surface area: a comparison of four different methods. Salzburg: Paracelsus Medical University; 2016.
25. Wachtel TL, Brimm JE, Knight MA, Heisterkamp S, Frank HA, Inancsi W, et al. Research: computer-assisted estimate of the area and depth of burn. J Burn Care Rehabil. 1983;4:255–9.
26. Siegel JB, Wachtel TL, Brimm JE. Automated documentation of burn injuries. J Trauma. 1986;26:44–6.

27. Parvizi D, Giretzlehner M, Wurzer P, Klein LD, Shoham Y, Bohanon FJ, et al. BurnCase 3D software validation study: burn size measurement accuracy and inter-rater reliability. Burns. 2016;42:329–35.
28. Knaysi GA, Crikelair GF, Cosman B. The role of nines: its history and accuracy. Plast Reconstr Surg. 1968;41:560–3.
29. Williams RY, Wohlgemuth SD. Does the "rule of nines" apply to morbidly obese burn victims? J Burn Care Res. 2013;34:447–52.
30. Yu C-Y, Lo Y-H, Chiou W-K. The 3D scanner for measuring body surface area: a simplified calculation in the Chinese adult. Appl Ergon. 2003;34:273–8.
31. Jose RM, Roy DK, Vidyadharan R, Erdmann M. Burns area estimation—an error perpetuated. Burns. 2004;30:481–2.
32. Giretzlehner M, Owen R, Dirnberger J, Haller LK. Rapid burn assessor. In: European Burns Association, editor. Abstr. B. 15th Eur. Burn. Assoc. Congr. Vienna; 2013, p. 24.
33. Giretzlehner M, Dirnberger J, Luckeneder T, Haller HL, Rodemund C. BurnCase 3D: a research product for effective and time-saving documentation of burn injuries. Ann Burns Fire Disasters. 2004;XVII(2):64–72.
34. Haller H. Data collection in burn injuries—rationale for BurnCase 3D. Osteosynth Trauma Care. 2007;15:34–41.
35. Haller HL, Dirnberger J, Giretzlehner M, Rodemund C, Kamolz L. "Understanding burns": research project BurnCase 3D—overcome the limits of existing methods in burns documentation. Burns. 2009;35:311–7.
36. Yu C-YY, Lin C-HH, Yang Y-HH. Human body surface area database and estimation formula. Burns. 2010;36:616–29.
37. Nichter LS, Bryant CA, Edlich RF. Efficacy of burned surface area estimates calculated from charts—the need for a computer-based model. J Trauma. 1985;25:477–81.
38. Alm J. Retrospective study of TBSA-B calculating; Manually estimated Burnchart versus computerized Burn Charts. In: Progr. Abstr. - 10 Congr. Eur. Burn. Assoc. Bergen, European Burns Association. 2003, p. 158.
39. Berry MG, Goodwin TI, Misra RR, Dunn KW, Collis N, Smith G, et al. Accuracy of burn size estimation and subsequent fluid resuscitation prior to arrival at the Yorkshire Regional Burns Unit. A three year retrospective study. Burns. 1999;25:0–6.
40. Martin NA, Lundy JB, Rickard RF. Lack of precision of burn surface area calculation by UK Armed Forces medical personnel. Burns. 2014;40(2):246–50.
41. Giretzlehner M, Dirnberger J, Owen R, Haller HL, Lumenta DB, Kamolz L-P. The determination of total burn surface area: how much difference? Burns. 2013;39:1–7.
42. Berry MG, Goodwin TI, Misra RR, Dunn KW. Digitisation of the total burn surface area. Burns. 2006;32:684–8.
43. Ziegler B, Hirche C, Horter J, Kiefer J, Alfred P, Kremer T, et al. In view of standardization part 2: management of challenges in the initial treatment of burn patients in Burn Centers in Germany, Austria, and Switzerland. Burns. 2016;43:4–11.
44. Retrouvey H, Chan J, Shahrokhi S. Comparison of two-dimensional methods versus three-dimensional scanning systems in the assessment of total body surface area estimation in burn patients. Burns. 2018;44(1):195–200.
45. Barnes J, Duffy A, Hamnett N, McPhail J, Seaton C, Shokrollahi K, et al. The Mersey Burns App: evolving a model of validation. Emerg Med J. 2015;32(8):637–41. https://doi.org/10.1136/emermed-2013-203416.
46. Goldberg H, Klaff J, Spjut A, Milner S. A mobile app for measuring the surface area of a burn in three dimensions: comparison to the Lund and Browder assessment. J Burn Care Res. 2014;35:480–3.
47. Nagel TR, Schunk JE. Using the hand to estimate the surface area of a burn in children. Pediatr Emerg Care. 1997;13:254–5.
48. Amirsheybani HR, Crecelius GM, Timothy NH, Pfeiffer M, Saggers GC, Manders EK. Natural history of the growth of the hand: part II—hand length as a treatment guide in the pediatric trauma patient. J Trauma. 2000;49:457–60.
49. Berry MG, Evison D, Roberts AH. The influence of body mass index on burn surface area estimated from the area of the hand. Burns. 2001;27:591–4.
50. Butz DR, Collier Z, O'Connor A, Magdziak M, Gottlieb LJ, Connor AO, et al. Is palmar surface area a reliable tool to estimate burn surface areas in obese patients? J Burn Care Res. 2015;36:87–91.
51. Laing JHE, Sanders R. Assessment of burn injury in the accident and emergency department: a review of 100 referrals to a regional burns unit. Ann R Coll Surg Engl. 1991;73:329–31.
52. Cone JB. What's new in general surgery: burns and metabolism. J Am Coll Surg. 2005;200:607–15.
53. Sheridan RL, Petras L, Basha G, Salvo P, Cifrino C, Hinson M, et al. Planimetry study of the percent of body surface represented by the hand and palm: sizing irregular burns is more accurately done with the palm. J Burn Care Rehabil. 1995;16:605–6.
54. Amirsheybani HR, Crecelius GM, Timothy NH, Pfeiffer M, Saggers GC, Manders EK. The natural history of the growth of the hand: I. Hand area as a percentage of body surface area. Plast Reconstr Surg. 2001;107:726–33.
55. Jose RM, Roy DK, Wright PK, Erdmann M. Hand surface area—do racial differences exist? Burns. 2006;32:216–7.
56. Yu C-Y, Hsu Y-W, Chen C-Y. Determination of hand surface area as a percentage of body surface area by 3D anthropometry. Burns. 2008;34:1183–9.
57. Thom D. Appraising current methods for preclinical calculation of burn size—a pre-hospital perspective. Burns. 2017;43(1):127–36.
58. Wallace A. The exposure treatment of burns. Lancet. 1951;1:501–3.
59. Livingston EH, Lee S. Percentage of burned body surface area determination in obese and nonobese patients. J Surg Res. 2000;91:106–10.
60. Nichter LS, Bryant CA, Edlich RF, Williams J, Bryant CA, Edlich RF, et al. Efficacy of burned surface area estimates calculated from charts—the need for a computer-based model. J Trauma. 1985;25:477–81.
61. Miminas DA. A critical evaluation of the Lund and Browder chart. Wounds UK. 2007;3:58–68.
62. Klippel CH. Surface area versus skin area. N Engl J Med. 1979;301:730.
63. Hammond JS, Ward CG. Transfers from emergency room to burn center: errors in burn size estimate. J Trauma. 1987;27:1161–5.
64. Freiburg C, Igneri P, Sartorelli K, Rogers F. Effects of differences in percent total body surface area estimation on fluid resuscitation of transferred burn patients. J Burn Care Res. 2007;28:42–8.
65. Irwin LR, Reid CA, McLean NR. Burns in children: do casualty officers get it right? Injury. 1993;24:187–8.
66. Berkebile BL, Goldfarb IW, Slater H. Comparison of burn size estimates between prehospital reports and burn center evaluations. J Burn Care Rehabil. n.d.;7:411–2.
67. Benjamin NC, Wurzer P, Voigt CD, Benjamin DA, Herndon DN. Using a 3D tool to document and determine graft loss: a mini-review and case report. Burns. 2016;42(4):e65–9.
68. Wurzer P, Giretzlehner M, Klein D, Shoham Y, Haller HL, Branski LK. BurnCase 3D software validation study: burn size measurement accuracy, test-retest reliability and inter-rater reliability (239). In: Ann. Burn. Fire Disasters - Vol. XXVIII – Suppl. EBA - Sept. 2015. p. 2015.
69. Chan QE, Barzi F, Cheney L, Harvey JG, Holland AJ. Burn size estimation in children: still a problem. Emerg Med Australas. 2012;24:181–6.
70. Thumfart S, Giretzlehner M, Höller J, Ehrenmüller M, Pfurtscheller K, Haller H, et al. Proportionally correct 3D models of Infants, children and Adolescents for precise burn size measurement (187). Ann Burns Fire Disasters. 2015;XXVIII:5–6.
71. Stockton KA, McMillan CM, Storey KJ, David MC, Kimble RM. 3D photography is as accurate as digital planimetry tracing in determining burn wound area. Burns. 2015;41:80–4.
72. Wurzer P, Giretzlehner M, Kamolz L-P. 3D photography is an accurate technique for measuring small wound areas. Burns. 2015;41:196–7.

73. Cartotto R, Zhou A. Fluid creep: the pendulum hasn't swung back yet! J Burn Care Res. 2008;31:551–8.
74. Schwartz SI. Supportive therapy in burn care. Consensus summary on fluid resuscitation. J Trauma. 1979;19:876–7.
75. Velmahos GC, Demetriades D, Shoemaker WC, Chan LS, Tatevossian R, Wo CC, et al. Endpoints of resuscitation of critically injured patients: normal or supranormal? Ann Surg. 2000;232:409–18.
76. Rhee P. Chapter 5: Shock, electrolytes, and fluid. Nineteenth. Elsevier Inc.; 2012.
77. Jacob M, Chappel D. Mythen und Fakten der perioperativen Infusionstherapie. Anästhesiol Intensivmed. 2009;50: 358–76.
78. Bruegger D, Schwartz L, Chappell D, Jacob M, Rehm M, Vogeser M, et al. Release of atrial natriuretic peptide precedes shedding of the endothelial glycocalyx equally in patients undergoing on- and off-pump coronary artery bypass surgery. Basic Res Cardiol. 2011;106:1111–21.
79. Lobo DN, Stanga Z, Aloysius MM, Wicks C, Nunes QM, Ingram KL, et al. Effect of volume loading with 1 liter intravenous infusions of 0.9% saline, 4% succinylated gelatine (Gelofusine) and 6% hydroxyethyl starch (Voluven) on blood volume and endocrine responses: a randomized, three-way crossover study in healthy volunteers. Crit Care Med. 2010;38:464–70.
80. Chung KK, Wolf SE, Cancio LC, Alvarado R, Jones JA, McCorcle J, King BT, Barillo DJ, Renz EM, Blackbourne LH. Resuscitation of severely burned military casualties: fluid begets more fluid. J Trauma. 2009;67:231–7; discussion 237.
81. Cancio LC, Chávez S, Alvarado-Ortega M, Barillo DJ, Walker SC, McManus AT, et al. Predicting increased fluid requirements during the resuscitation of thermally injured patients. J Trauma. 2004;56:404–13; discussion 413-4.
82. Friedrich JB, Sullivan SR, Engrav LH, Round KA, Blayney CB, Carrougher GJ, et al. Is supra-Baxter resuscitation in burn patients a new phenomenon? Burns. 2004;30:464–6.
83. Engrav LH, Heimbach DM, Rivara FP, Kerr KF, Osler T, Pham TN, et al. Harborview burns—1974 to 2009. PLoS One. 2012;7:e40086.
84. Zhang J, Xiang F, Tong D, Luo Q, Yuan Z, Yan H, et al. [Comparative study on the effect of restrictive fluid management strategy on the early pulmonary function of patients with severe burn]. Zhonghua Shao Shang Za Zhi. 2012;28:165–9.
85. Guilabert P, Usúa G, Martín N, Abarca L, Barret JP, Colomina MJ. Fluid resuscitation management in patients with burns: update. Br J Anaesth. 2016;117(3):284–96.
86. Ziegler B, Hirche C, Horter J, Kiefer J, Grützner PA, Kremer T, et al. In view of standardization part 2: management of challenges in the initial treatment of burn patients in Burn Centers in Germany, Austria and Switzerland. Burns. 2016;43:559–66.
87. Münzberg M, Ziegler B, Fischer S, Wölfl CG, Grützner PA, Kremer T, et al. In view of standardization: comparison and analysis of initial management of severely burned patients in Germany, Austria and Switzerland. Burns. 2015;41:6–11.
88. Silver GM, Klein MB, Herndon DN, Gamelli RL, Gibran NS, Altstein L, et al. Standard operating procedures for the clinical management of patients enrolled in a prospective study of Inflammation and the Host Response to Thermal Injury. J Burn Care Res. 2007;28:222–30.
89. Goverman J, Bittner EA, Friedstat JS, Moore M, Nozari A, Ibrahim AE, et al. Discrepancy in initial pediatric burn estimates and its impact on fluid resuscitation. J Burn Care Res. 2015;36(5):574–9.
90. Vercruysse GA, Ingram WL, Feliciano DV. Overutilization of regional burn centers for pediatric patients—a healthcare system problem that should be corrected. Am J Surg. 2011;202:802–9.

Early Management of Burn Patients and Fluid Resuscitation

15

David G. Greenhalgh

15.1 Introduction

The initial management of the burn patient has a significant impact on his/her ultimate outcome. Failure to adequately address airway or breathing problems can be devastating. Under- or over-resuscitation can be just as problematic. Insufficient resuscitation can lead to renal failure, burn depth progression, and even death. Even more prevalent has been over-resuscitation, a term that has been coined "fluid creep" [1]. Providing too much fluid may lead to pulmonary edema or acute respiratory distress syndrome (ARDS), heart failure, burn depth progression, and various forms of compartment syndrome (extremity, thoracic or abdominal). While the concept of fluid resuscitation is relatively simple, the performance of most burn teams is frequently quite poor [2]. The simple fact that there are multiple resuscitation formulas that are all relatively inaccurate suggests that there is a long way to go in optimizing initial burn shock resuscitation. The goal of this chapter is to briefly describe the "ABCs" of the initial management of burns. Since there are chapters on airway management and breathing problems, those topics will just be touched upon. The major focus will be to present issues related to "C"—Circulation in the first 24–48 h after a major burn.

15.2 Airway, Breathing, Circulation: The "ABCs"

All major burns should be treated by the "trauma strategy" of addressing the "ABCs"—airway, breathing, and circulation. "Airway" is first because loss of an airway can lead to death within minutes. The main concern for "airway" is swelling of the upper airway leading to total obstruction. The degree of swelling is proportional to the extent of burn, depth of injury, and involvement of the face. The major decision point is whether to intubate the patient or not. This topic is covered elsewhere. There are several issues related to "breathing" that are special to burns. The first issue is hypoxia since fire in an enclosed space competes with the patient for oxygen. The next issue is related to carbon monoxide poisoning which interferes with oxygen binding to the hemoglobin molecule and thus impairs oxygen delivery. Patients may also suffer from acute respiratory distress syndrome (ARDS) and constriction from circumferential chest burns or abdominal compartment syndrome. Finally, smoke inhalation injury leads mucosal sloughing and ultimately increases mortality related to the size burn. Again, these breathing issues will be covered in another chapter. The major focus of this chapter will be on burn resuscitation.

15.3 Pathophysiology of Initial Burn Shock

Any injury causes edema due to the release of local mediators. If one sprains an ankle, is punched in the eye or bangs his thumb, there is local swelling. The same local response occurs after a small burn. Local injury leads to the release of many mediators including histamine, serotonin, bradykinins, leukotrienes, α-thrombin, and platelet activating factor. The purpose of these mediators is to increase vasodilation and vascular permeability in order to allow delivery of factors that assist with fighting infection and initiating wound healing. The large number of mediators that participate in permeability changes suggests that there is significant redundancy in the system. Studies from the past support this redundant system since blocking any one mediator had little effect on the extent of capillary leak.

The molecular and cellular signaling that increase cellular permeability is quite well known and reviewed in a recent publication [3]. In response to mediator binding to a receptor, there is increased efflux of water and small molecules

D. G. Greenhalgh (✉)
Shriners Hospitals for Children Northern California, Sacramento, CA, USA

Burn Division, Firefighters Regional Burn Center at University of California, Davis, Sacramento, CA, USA

Department of Surgery, University of California, Davis, Davis, CA, USA
e-mail: dggreenhalgh@ucdavis.edu

M. G. Jeschke et al. (eds.), *Handbook of Burns Volume 1*, https://doi.org/10.1007/978-3-030-18940-2_15

that occurs both between and through the endothelial cells. The three adhesion molecules that hold the endothelial cells together are "tight junctions," "adherens junctions," and "gap junctions." Each type of junction is composed of many different known molecules, which will not be covered here. The *tight junction* is relatively constant and is not the main connection that changes in response to signaling. The *gap junction* has the primary function of being a conduit for cell to cell communication. The *adherens junction* is the main regulator of permeability. The extracellular component of the adherens junction consists of cadherin molecules that protrude into the gap between endothelial cells. The cadherin molecules on opposing cells actually "swap" parts of their molecules to create the junction. This swapping is reversed to allow increased permeability. In addition, molecules of the adherens junction extending within the cytoplasm are linked to f-actin within the cytoplasm. The f-actin binds to nonmuscular myosin to create a muscle-like motor that responds to signals to increase permeability. The link to actin/myosin is also utilized as a sensor to detect tension within the capillary lumen. When signaling molecules such as histamine bind the G-protein-coupled receptor (GPCR), the Rho signaling pathway up-regulates GTP (guanosine triphosphate) to pull the endothelial cell gap open. This is an over-simplification of a very complex process.

Classic teaching describes the "Starling Equation" as the main regulator of vascular permeability [4].

$$\textbf{Starling's Equation}: Q = K_f\left(P_{cap} - P_i\right) - \sigma\left(\pi_p - \pi_i\right)$$

Q—Fluid filtration rate
K_f—Capillary filtration coefficient (capillary surface area x hydraulic conductivity)
P_{cap}—Capillary hydrostatic pressure
P_i—Interstitial hydrostatic pressure
σ—Reflection coefficient (Permeability)
π_p—Plasma oncotic pressure
π_i—Interstitial oncotic pressure

After a deep burn, the fluid filtration rate (Q) increases drastically. All components of the Starling equation contribute to the increase in capillary fluid filtration rate [5]. The capillary filtration coefficient (K_f) increases 2–3 times normal after a burn. Capillary hydrostatic pressure (P_{cap}) increases as a result of increased vasodilation in response to the injury, especially in superficial burns. Interestingly, interstitial hydrostatic pressure (P_i) becomes more negative because of the breakdown of proteins to create smaller and more osmotically active molecules that draw water into the interstitial space. Another theory to explain this negative interstitial pressure suggests that structural changes in collagen and hyaluron contribute to the negative interstitial pressure. The reflection coefficient (σ) clearly decreases with increased permeability. A reflection coefficient of 1 means that no molecule passes through the capillary wall and at 0 there is free flow of macromolecules. Normal reflection coefficient is 0.9 but the value drops after a burn. The plasma oncotic pressure (π_p) drops as macromolecules, especially albumin leaks out of the capillary. The value drops by as much as 50% after a burn. The interstitial oncotic pressure (π_i) increases as albumin and other large molecules escape.

There are other factors that affect the amount of fluid leaking across the capillary wall. The destruction of collagen leads to increased "interstitial compliance," which in essence, means that there is more room for interstitial expansion. The most important factor that regulates the amount of edema is the rate of lymphatic resorption of fluids [6]. If lymphatic flow is decreased, such as with compartment syndromes, then less fluid is resorbed back into the intravascular space.

The Starling equation has been found to be more complex than previously considered. On the inner surface of the endothelial cells, there is a glycocalyx layer consisting of membrane-bound glycoproteins and proteoglycans that acts like a sponge [6–9]. The endothelial glycocalyx layer acts as the main oncotic space that determines transcapillary fluid flow. The Starling equation has been revised to be [8]:

$$Q = K_f\left(P_{cap} - P_i\right) - \sigma\left(\pi_p - \pi_g\right)$$

In this formula, π_i (interstitial oncotic pressure) has been replaced with π_g (subglycocalyx oncotic pressure). This endothelial glycocalyx layer is usually destroyed by local burn injury (and local sepsis) leading to greater fluid loss [10]. The capillaries of the uninjured tissue maintain this layer and thus do not have the same volume of fluid loss. This mechanism may partially explain why oncotic fluids have some efficacy in some part of burn resuscitation.

15.4 A Practical Guide to Burn Resuscitation

Burn shock resuscitation has not been perfected by any means. The fact that there are many different formulas and preferred fluids indicates that no method works very well. The debate on the appropriate volume and endpoints has been going on for over 50 years [11, 12]. The question of whether to use crystalloid versus colloid has also been debated for decades. It is clear that there have been more problems with providing too much fluid—a problem called "fluid creep" [1, 2, 13–15]. Much of the problem of over-resuscitation has been the result of failing to respond to indicators of over-resuscitation such as excessive urine output [2]. It is clear that providing too much fluid does lead to many complications such as respiratory failure and compartment syndromes. The initial resuscitation will influence the ultimate outcome of burn patients. Therefore, it is essential that caregiver optimize burn shock resuscitation.

It is intuitively obvious that fluid resuscitation should be dictated by the patient's response to fluids. Unfortunately, the endpoints of burn resuscitation are poorly defined [11, 12, 16]. Clearly, formulas provide an estimate of fluid volume based on an "average" patient. But not all burns are the same. It is clear that more fluids are required for any patient who has a deeper burn, delay in resuscitation, smoke inhalation injury, other injuries or receives escharotomies. Drugs and alcohol, commonly associated with burns, also increase the amount of fluid required for resuscitation. The age of the patient also influences the volume required for resuscitation. Young children have higher daily fluid requirements per weight than adults [17, 18], so it is not surprising that their fluid requirements are greater per kilogram than adults. The elderly need fewer fluids than younger adults. Since it is expected that there would be so much variability, it is essential to have guidelines to direct fluid resuscitation.

If one plots the amount of fluid required during burn shock resuscitation, a curve is created with large amounts of fluids required at the start. The fluid requirements rapidly decrease as distant capillary leaks close, and over time, the leak rate slows to a stable maintenance rate. Clearly, the concept that a patient requires "half" of the fluids at 8 h is erroneous and this part of the Parkland Formula needs to be eliminated from the burn literature. The fluid rate must be reduced based on the patient response. The current standard is to target urine output as an indicator for adequate resuscitation. **For adults the urine output target is 0.5 mL/kg/h and for children less than 30 kg the goal is 1.0 mL/kg/h.** It is clear that urine output is not perfect but if one really reduces fluids to avoid urine output rates greater than those targets, most patients do fairly well. There have been attempts to develop other more accurate endpoints but as of yet, no great endpoints exist [16].

Therefore, the purpose of any burn resuscitation formula is to provide an estimate as to the starting fluid rate. After determining the starting rate, all formulas should be ignored and fluids should be adjusted based on the patient's response. There are many burn resuscitation guidelines that have been described but the most commonly used formula is the "Parkland Formula" [19]. The Parkland Formula is probably most commonly used since it is very simple:

- **Parkland Formula: 4 mL/kg/%TBSA Burn**
  - **Start at a rate to give half during the first 8 h**
  - ***Do not worry about the second 16 h, just decrease fluids to target urine output of 0.5 mL/kg/h***

As an example, for a 100 kg patient with 80% TBSA burns:

- 4 × 100 × 80 = 32,000 mL
- Start rate to give half during the first 8 h = 16,000 mL or start at 2000 mL/h
- Target urine output = 50 mL/h

If urine output is too low, increase fluids, and if urine output is high, reduce fluids. Since there is a concern for providing too much fluid, some guidelines (American Burn Association's Advanced Burn Life Support) have suggested using the Parkland Formula at a lower rate (2 mL/kg/%TBSA burn) for superficial burns and raising the rate for patients with deeper burns [20]. The target of 2 mL/kg/%TBSA burn is what is recommended by the Brooke Formula. In actuality, the starting rate is of lesser concern as long as the fluid rate is adjusted based on the patient's urine output and other physiologic responses.

It has been documented that small children with burns tend to need more fluids per weight than adults [17, 18]. There is a tendency to need up to 6 mL/kg/%TBSA burn. The explanation for this greater need is that because of their small size, there is a relative increase in the proportion of daily basal fluid requirements. In other words, the daily basal requirements become a greater percentage of the resuscitation fluid requirements. To adjust for the increased fluid requirements in children, we simply add daily basal fluid requirements to the Parkland Formula.

- **Pediatric Burn Resuscitation:**
  - **Daily Basal Fluid Requirements + 4 mL/kg/%TBSA**
  - **Start rate to give half during the first 8 h**
  - ***Do not worry about the second 16 h, just decrease fluids to target urine output of 0.5 mL/kg/h if >30 kg or 1 mL/h if <30 kg***
- **Daily Basal Fluid Requirements**
  - **<30 kg = 2000 × Body Surface Area (BSA)**
  - **>30 kg = 1500 × Body Surface Area**
- **or**
  - **100 mL/kg for the first 10 kg**
  - **+ 50 mL/kg for 10–20 kg**
  - **+ 20 mL/kg for >20 kg**

As an example, for a 10 kg infant, (BSA 0.5 m^2), with 50% TBSA burn

- Daily Basal Fluid Requirements (using either formula)
  - 2000 × 0.5 (BSA) = 1000 mL/day or by the other formula
  - 100 m/kg × 10 kg = 1000 mL/day
- Parkland Formula = 4 × 10 × 50 = 2000 mL

- **Total** Resuscitation **Volume = 1000 mL + 2000 mL = 3 000 mL in 24 h**
- Give half in the first 8 h = 1500 mL/8 h = **187.5 mL/h**
- Target **urine output = 10 mL/h**

15.5 Endpoints of Burn Shock Resuscitation

Currently the most commonly used endpoint of resuscitation is urine output [19] but it is clear that that guideline is fairly inaccurate. It is common for uninjured people to have periods of low urine output during periods of exercise or mild dehydration—without any sequelae. The same can be said for burn patients who can tolerate short periods of urine output. The philosophy of "permissive hypovolemia" [21, 22] or "permissive hypooliguria" [23] is practiced in many places where fluids are not increased for urine outputs as low as 0.3 mL/kg/h for short periods. There are also periods during burn resuscitation when the patient has greater than the target urine output but they are hypotensive. It is not clear what to do in this situation—many just increase fluids anyway. Others may provide vasopressors to increase blood pressure but there is the risk that vasoconstriction to the injured skin might increase burn depth. In addition, it is not uncommon for the patient's hemoglobin and hematocrits to rise as an indicator of hemoconcentration. Using the hemoglobin or hematocrit to guide resuscitation tends to lead to the administration of excessive fluids since experience suggests that it takes time for hemodilution to occur. Another option is to measure lactate levels since higher levels are an indication of poor perfusion [24–27]. Again, it is not uncommon for the patient to have higher lactate levels while making adequate urine.

Because of these problems, many burn teams have used more advanced methods of detecting cardiac output and hemodynamics during burn shock. Using central venous pressures (CVP) is unreliable since they rarely rise above normal levels despite excessive urine output [28–31]. The use of pulmonary catheters has also been shown to over-resuscitate burn patients [30, 31]. More modern noninvasive devices have not been any better in guiding resuscitation [12, 16, 32]. In special cases, such as patients with renal or cardiac failure, these devices may be all that is available to guide resuscitation. Fortunately, most healthy patients can tolerate a wide range of inadequate or excessive volumes of fluid.

The major problem in the modern burn unit is from providing too much fluid, not under-resuscitating. There has been an increase in effort to understand why "fluid creep" has become a problem [1, 2, 13–15]. One problem is that the many endpoints do not align. If the patient is not making good urine output, the tendency is to increase volumes. It is clear, however, that many times over-resuscitation is the result of failing to respond to the patient's response. It is not uncommon to observe a failure to reduce fluids despite excessive urine output. One solution is to utilize nurse-based protocols that provide guidelines for adjusting resuscitation fluids [2, 24]. This problem has also prompted investigators to develop computer-based devices that automatically adjust fluids based on urine flow [33–35]. Another theory is that the increased use of opioids has led to increased vasodilation and thus the need for more fluids [36]. This "opioid creep" phenomenon might be reduced by avoiding automatic narcotic drips and providing pain medications on an as needed basis. The other theory is that when a patient is placed on a ventilator the positive chest pressure reduces venous return [37]. More fluids are required in order to overcome the increased thoracic pressure. Clearly, there is still a great deal of work required to understand how to optimize fluids during burn shock.

15.6 Maintenance Fluid Rate

The signals that create the capillary leak syndrome of burn shock gradually decrease and eventually disappear around 24 h after the injury. Initially, distant uninjured capillary beds close, and later the capillaries beneath the burn close. At this point, burn shock is completed. The problem is that there are no good indicators of when burn shock has resolved. One method of determining when burn shock has been completed is to calculate the **maintenance fluid rate** that is expected when there is no capillary leak. One can easily determine basal fluid rates (as described above) but the fluid losses are even greater than basal calculations since destruction of the epidermis eliminates the barrier to water loss. Fortunately, one can approximate evaporative rate based on the following formulas [38]:

- **Evaporative Water Loss**
  - **<30 kg = (35 + % TBSA burn) × BSA = mL/h**
  - **>30 kg = (25 + % TBSA burn) × BSA = mL/h**

We then consider burn shock to be completed when the resuscitative volume reaches the sum of basal requirements + evaporative water loss:

Maintenance Fluid Rate = Daily Basal Fluid Rate + Evaporative Water Losses

As an example, for a 10 kg infant, 10 kg, BSA 0.5 m^2, 50% TBSA burn

- Basal Fluid Requirements = 100 mL/kg × 10 = 1000 mL for 24 h or 40 mL/h
  - Evaporative Fluid Rate = (35 + 50) × 0.5 = 42.5 mL/h
  - Maintenance Fluid Rate = 82.5 mL/h (1020 mL/day)

Therefore, when the fluid rate for burn resuscitation drops to the calculated maintenance rate, 82.5 mL/h, we consider the patient to be resuscitated and we switch the fluid to D5½NS with 20 mEq KCl. After the initial resuscitation, urine output becomes unreliable due to the resorption of resuscitative fluids and fluids provided in the operating room. In addition, the hypermetabolic changes often lead to spilling glucose or proteins so urine output tends to be high despite normovolemia. We leave the daily fluid target at the maintenance rate until the wound starts to close. Fine tuning of the rate is based on the blood urea nitrogen and creatinine.

15.7 The Choice of Fluid for Resuscitation

The classic teaching has always been to provide an isotonic crystalloid fluid—usually lactated Ringer's (LR) solution during burn shock. The rationale for using an isotonic crystalloid was that during shock the gap created between the endothelial cells was so large that many proteins, including albumin, passed into the interstitial space. The leak of large proteins occurs not only at the burn site but also away from the burn [39–42]. There is no sense to provide colloid if it were to leak into the interstitial space. Even worse, the extravasated proteins would increase interstitial oncotic pressure and tend to drive more fluid into the interstitium. This protein leakage does occur but capillary leak away from the burn tends to be less severe and tends to close within 6–12 h. In addition, serum albumin levels drop precipitously due to leakage and dilution. There must be a point where the plasma oncotic pressure becomes so low that more fluid leaks than is necessary. Because of this fact, many burn teams are utilizing oncotic fluids more commonly than in the past [19].

There are pros and cons behind using crystalloids versus colloids. Crystalloids have been favored for many years because they are effective most of the time. There is little risk of transmitting infectious organisms compared to human-derived products. They are significantly less expensive than colloids and much easier to store. Therefore they are readily available for the field situation. The main downside for crystalloids is that they are freely permeable from the intravascular space to the interstitial space. Since the interstitial space has 3 times the volume of the intravascular space, one must replace 3–4 times the volume of lost intravascular fluid. In other words, if a patient loses 1 L of blood, then, in theory, one must give 3–4 L of isotonic crystalloid to replace that blood loss. In addition, proteins create the osmotic intravascular pressure that keeps fluid in the intravascular space. As more crystalloid is delivered, the intravascular osmotic pressure gradually decreases to a point that even greater leakage of fluids out of the intravascular space. In theory, this extra interstitial fluid would predispose a patient with large fluid requirements to higher risks of extremity, thoracic and intra-abdominal compartment syndromes. In addition, one may be at higher risk for pulmonary and cardiac compromise. Fortunately, most healthy patients can tolerate the extra volume and will later excrete the extra fluid.

Colloids, in theory, should reduce the volume of fluid needed to resuscitate a patient who is in shock. Colloids should replace blood loss in a 1:1 ratio, so that only 1 L of colloid would be required to replace 1 L of blood loss. In addition, colloids increase the intravascular osmotic pressure to reduce fluid loss through the capillaries. The downside of colloids is that they are more expensive than crystalloids; and there is a slight risk for infectious transmission, at least for human products such as albumin or fresh frozen plasma. The other problem that has been described in the past was that many proteins, including albumin, leak across the capillaries during burn shock. The argument against their use is that since they freely leak out they are wasted and even harmful [39–42]. It is possible that increasing the osmotic pressure in the interstitial space will "draw" more fluids from the intravascular space. In other words, colloids are fine if there is no capillary leak, but if there is an ongoing capillary leak then they are potentially harmful.

After a major burn injury, there is leakage of albumin and other proteins at the burn site and, in addition, distant from the burn site. The capillary leak at the uninjured capillary sites is less severe and lasts 6–12 h. In addition, the albumin levels frequently drop to very low levels (<1 mg/dL) [43–45] so that after several hours there is very little intravascular osmotic pressure to prevent further fluid loss. Therefore, after 6–12 h the addition of exogenous albumin to reduce fluid administration makes sense. When burn directors around the world were surveyed, it was discovered that while most initiated resuscitation with crystalloid, most "cheated" at some time during the first 24 h by adding albumin or another colloid to the resuscitation [19]. During the resuscitation discussion at the 2016 Burn State of the Science meeting [12], most participants admitted to using either albumin or fresh frozen plasma at some time during burn resuscitation. The remaining major dilemma is whether colloids should be started immediately or hours later when crystalloid resuscitation was failing. Everyone agreed that a multicenter prospective trial testing the validity of crystalloid versus colloid is needed.

Several studies have compared the use of albumin versus crystalloids for all types of resuscitation. The use of albumin was tempered by the Cochrane Collaborative, which in 1998 stated that the use of albumin increased the risk of death [46]. In 2012 and 2013, however, the same group reviewed 24 trials and found no difference in mortality [47, 48]. Very large trials have been performed, but not in burn patients. The "Saline versus Albumin Fluid Evaluation (SAFE) Trial" found no increase in mortality in a study with nearly 7000 patients [49]. The "Early Albumin Resuscitation During Septic Shock (EARSS) Study" [50] and "Albumin Italian Outcome Sepsis (ALBIOS) Study" [51] also found no difference in mortality. In 2014, a meta-analysis of all three of the above studies suggested a small reduction in mortality with the use of albumin [52].

There are fewer studies with the use of albumin in burns, and the number of patients is much smaller than the above studies. There are two approaches to studying the use of albumin for burn resuscitation—"immediate use" or delivering albumin as a "rescue" when crystalloid resuscitation volumes exceed predictive values. There were two studies from the 1970s that compared albumin versus crystalloid starting at the initiation of burn resuscitation [53, 54]. Both revealed that the immediate use of albumin reduced the fluids required for resuscitation. The study by Goodwin, et al. found that albumin could lower fluid requirements during burn resuscitation but they found that albumin increased lung water compared to the use of lactated Ringer's solution [55]. This study led to the philosophy that albumin usage during burn resuscitation had potential adverse consequences. In 2006, Cooper et al. performed a prospective trial comparing lactated Ringer's solution versus lactated Ringer's solution containing 5% albumin [56]. They found an insignificant reduction in fluids with the addition of albumin. The philosophy at the time was that there was no need to provide albumin at the start of burn resuscitation.

As stated earlier, albumin was being provided later during resuscitation as burn caregivers "cheated" by adding albumin to improve resuscitations that were providing excessive amounts of fluids [19]. At the same time, the concept of "fluid creep"—providing way too much fluid—was the topic of the burn community. The concept of providing albumin as a "rescue" to reduce fluid requirements in patients not meeting target resuscitation goals became popular. The concept is that around 6–12 h the capillary leak starts to close at the same time as the intravascular osmotic pressures drop to extremely low levels (albumin levels often <1 mg/dL). It makes sense that at 6–12 h, increasing the intravascular osmotic pressures with albumin would slow capillary leakage and reduce fluid requirements. The first study examining albumin for rescue, from Utah, utilized the protocol to add 5% albumin (1/3 rate) to 2/3 rate lactated Ringer's solution if the patient was receiving volumes twice the Parkland formula (>4 mL/kg/% burn) [57]. This study demonstrated that adding albumin could reduce the amount of fluids used later in the course and it suggested a reduction in mortality. The United States military reviewed their protocol of adding 5% albumin if fluid rates were >6 mL/kg/% burn, and they added vasopressin if the patient was hypotensive [58]. They demonstrated a reduction in abdominal compartment syndrome (36% versus 18%, $p = 0.0315$). Another study suggested that albumin might reduce extremity compartment syndromes and renal failure [59]. Two more recent studies from Utah clearly demonstrated that the initiation of albumin had a dramatic effect changing the trajectory of resuscitation from greater than target back to reasonable levels [60, 61]. Finally, a report from Michigan suggested that use of albumin for "rescue" reduced the incidence of abdominal compartment syndrome, ventilator days, oxygenation, vasopressor use, and mortality [62]. The volumes, however, were not different in this retrospective trial. Two meta-analyses on the use of albumin on burn resuscitation have been recently published which reveal no differences in mortality, renal failure, and respiratory failure with the use of albumin [63, 64]. In addition, there was a reduction in fluid volumes and compartment syndromes. While the controversy over the use of albumin seems to be lessened, there is still a need for a larger prospective study to evaluate the role of albumin.

There are other colloids that are available but their use has fallen into disfavor. Hydroxyethyl starch (HES) solutions have been used for burn resuscitation since the 1980s [65, 66]. A prospective trial from England compared Hartmann's solution (crystalloid) versus 1/3 of the predicted crystalloid was replaced with 6% HES. Those patients receiving HES required less fluid and had less interstitial edema [67]. In the same year, another study compared burn patients resuscitated with lactated Ringer's solution to hyperoncotic 10% HES in 30 patients [68]. The fluids required with HES were less but not statistically significant. The major concern was the finding that the patients treated with HES had a higher mortality and a 25% incidence of renal failure [68]. In 2013, the same group performed another trial with 6% HES 48 burn patients [69]. They found no differences in the amount of fluid delivered, but mortality and renal failure were not different in this study [69]. The use of HES for resuscitation in any patient was greatly discouraged after two very large randomized prospective trials demonstrated a higher risk for renal failure and mortality [70, 71]. The use of gelatins or dextran solutions has not gained favor for any major resuscitation. There are some centers that use fresh frozen plasma for burn shock resuscitation. O'Mara et al. demonstrated that using fresh frozen plasma for resuscitation reduced total resuscitative volumes, weight gain, intra-abdominal pressures, and base deficit compared to lactated Ringer's solution [72]. The main protein in fresh frozen plasma is albumin so one could argue that it is just another formulation of albumin.

15.8 High Dose Vitamin C and Other Methods to Reduce Inflammation

Ascorbic acid (vitamin C) has gained popularity in many burn centers as an inexpensive drug to reduce burn-related oxidative stress and thus reduce fluid requirements for burn resuscitation. The initial animal studies were performed by Matsuda and Tanaka who found that adding vitamin C to lactated Ringer's solution would reduce the fluids required for burn resuscitation compared to lactated Ringer's solution alone [73–75]. They next performed an unblinded prospective trial in 37 burn patients adding 66 mg/kg/h vitamin C to lactated Ringer's solution. They found that the high dose vitamin C significantly reduced fluid volumes and improved oxygenation compared to lactated Ringer's alone [76]. Kahn and Lentz found similar reductions in fluid requirements with no increase in complications [77, 78]. When discussing different vitamin C protocols at the Resuscitation Special Interest Group of the 2017 Annual Meeting of the American Burn Association, all centers admitted that vitamin C would induce paradoxical diuresis and that one must beware of hypovolemia [12]. Kahn and Lentz, for instance, stated they would provide fresh frozen plasma if there were signs of hypovolemia. There is a need to expand the studies of the use of high dose vitamin C to determine its efficacy and safety. There is the theoretic potential for renal failure and hypovolemic shock [79]. Hopefully, multicenter trials will lead to a definitive answer to the use of vitamin C.

Another method of reducing oxidative stress and other signals of inflammation is to remove the inciting agents from the blood. The burn team at Utah proposed the use of exchange transfusions for small children and plasmapheresis to "rescue" patients from excessively high volume resuscitations [80–82]. Their data suggest that both techniques reduce fluid requirements. More recently, the teams in Seattle [83] and Wake Forest [84] have supported these findings with 37 and 21 patients, respectively. More expansive studies are needed to corroborate the effectiveness of therapeutic plasma exchange in burn resuscitation.

15.9 Complications of Excessive Fluids

Providing inadequate volumes of resuscitation leads to the complications of hypovolemic shock such as renal failure, increased burn depth, and ultimately death. To compensate for hypovolemia, catecholamines are released which in turn lead to vasoconstriction to peripheral capillary beds, especially the skin and extremities. Typically, the burn is divided into three zones: zone of coagulation where the skin is destroyed, zone of stasis where capillary blood flow is decreased due to leukocyte crowding, and the zone of erythema due to vasodilation. With inadequate resuscitation capillary flow is further decreased in the zone of stasis, which increases the chance of burn depth progression. Therefore, providing adequate fluid resuscitation during burn shock is essential to optimizing an optimal outcome.

Clearly, not providing enough fluid leads to adverse outcomes but this knowledge has led to tendency to provide excessive amounts of fluid, described as "fluid creep" [1, 2, 13–15]. It is clear, however, that providing too much fluid has its own set of complications including extremity compartment syndromes, and intrathoracic and intra-abdominal compartment syndromes. There has also been a description of blindness from increased intraocular pressure [85]. In addition, excessive fluid can enter the lungs to exacerbate the risks for acute respiratory distress syndrome or worsen smoke inhalation injury. Too much fluid can overwhelm the heart and lead to congestive heart failure. Excessive edema leads to a greater distance for nutrients to travel from the capillaries to the wound, so it has been associated with impaired wound healing. While these complications may occur with appropriate burn resuscitation, they are clearly increased with excessive over-resuscitation.

Extremity compartment syndromes are caused by pressures within a closed muscle compartment that lead to impaired capillary flow to the enclosed muscle. There are two factors that lead to compartment syndromes in burned extremities: significant capillary leakage within an enclosed muscle compartment and a deep circumferential burn that will not expand. In other words, small superficial and circumferential burns that are relatively small do not lead to compartment syndromes. Deep, full-thickness and circumferential burns do not expand and are at risk for compartment syndromes. The classic symptom of compartment syndromes is pain that is caused by ischemia to the muscle. The pain is worsened with passive motion. Unfortunately, many patients have so much pain due to the burn itself that compartment syndromes are missed. Therefore, one should always be cognizant that compartment syndromes may occur in patients with deep circumferential burns.

The diagnosis of extremity compartment syndrome may not always be simple. The risks are greater for the problem if the patient has larger and deeper circumferential burns. Some caregivers feel there is no compartment syndrome if the extremity has a distal pulse. Unfortunately, compartment damage may occur in the presence of distal pulses. In order to lose the distal pulse, the compartment pressure must be higher than systolic blood pressure. It requires compartment pressures of around 30 mmHg to lose capillary flow to the muscle, so damage often occurs despite having distal pulses [86]. If there is a question of compartment tightness, one may easily measure pressures by placing an 18 gauge needle on monitor (such as central venous pressure monitor) and inserting it into the compartment. If the pressure is >30 mmHg, then escharotomies are usually indicated. If the patient has very large and deep burns, I will often perform escharotomies early in the course of the initial resuscitation. Failure to perform escharotomies when indicated may lead to muscle necrosis and potentially, amputations. As a worst case scenario, I had one patient with 80% TBSA burns sent to us 4 days after injury who required bilateral above knee amputations because most of the extremity muscle had died. He had never had escharotomies. There is very little downside to performing escharotomies since those same wounds will ultimately require grafting.

Escharotomies are usually performed at the bedside with conscious sedation. We use ketamine for children, and fentanyl and midazolam for adults. An escharotomy is a “cut through eschar” and eschar is the coagulated proteins replacing the skin as a result of the burn. To minimize bleeding, a cautery is used to create incisions into the fat on the medial and lateral sides of the extremity. The incision should extend continuously from the proximal to distal extents of the burn (Fig. 15.1). Bleeding should be controlled prior to completion. The extremity should then be checked to ensure that the muscle compartments are <30 mmHg and if not, then fasciotomies should be performed. For the lower leg, there are four compartments—anterior, lateral, superficial posterior, and deep posterior. Since the anterior compartment is the smallest, it is at highest risk for ischemic damage. I have seen several patients with foot drop because of anterior compartment damage [86]. Fasciotomies of the lower extremity are also bedside procedures that can be performed with escharotomies. Usually, only the lateral and anterior compartments require releases for thermal burns. The lateral escharotomy is performed over the lateral compartment so the dissection is carried down to the fascia and a small nick is made in the lateral fascia. Scissors then are pushed up and down to open up the entire fascia (Fig. 15.1). Dissection is then performed a little anteriorly until the anterior compartment is visualized and the same procedure is performed. If there is a need for posterior fasciotomies, the medial escharotomy incision is deepened to the fascia and both the superficial and deep posterior fascia can be opened approximately 1 cm medial to the tibia. The deep fascia is just a few millimeters below the superficial fascia. Forearm fasciotomies are a little more complicated since the carpal tunnel needs to be released with the flexor compartment. Forearm releases are usually performed in the operating room to facilitate exposing the median nerve. A curvilinear incision is made up the forearm for the flexor surface. A straight incision is used for the extensor fascia. There is a separate compartment called the “mobile wad” (brachioradialis, extensor carpi radialis brevis, extensor carpi radialis longus muscles) but that compartment is rarely released.

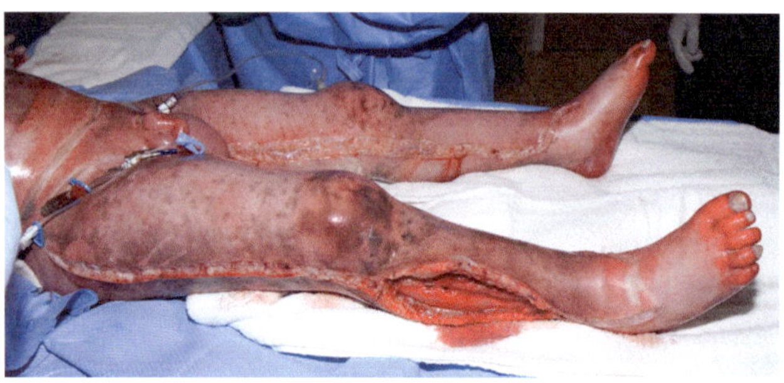

Fig. 15.1 Escharotomies were performed to both medial and lateral aspects of the legs in this child with deep circumferential burns. After the escharotomies were completed, the compartment pressures were still >30 mmHg so anterior and lateral fasciotomies were performed

Deep circumferential chest burns may also restrict chest excursion as indicated by the need for increased ventilator pressures. Escharotomies may need to be performed through the mid-axillary line from the shoulders to the pelvis to release the chest. Usually, another release is performed horizontally between the chest and abdomen. The other compartment that is at risk is the abdominal cavity. The first description of abdominal compartment syndrome in a burn patient was by Greenhalgh and Warden in 1994 [87]. During resuscitation, the peritoneal cavity may fill up with enough fluid to create pressures that increase peak inspiratory pressure, compress the renal veins and interfere with venous return. The three classic signs are elevated peak inspiratory pressures, minimal urine output (since renal flow is impaired), and hemodynamic instability. While the problem has been attributed to excessive fluid delivery, there are occasional patients who develop abdominal compartment pressures despite careful monitoring of resuscitative rates. One may measure intra-abdominal pressures through the bladder and intra-abdominal hypertension is considered to present at 20 mmHg and abdominal compartment syndrome is present at >30 mmHg. If the patient has the three cardinal signs and the abdominal pressure is >30 mmHg, there are several treatment options. First, chest and abdominal escharotomies may be performed. The patient should also have a nasogastric tube and Foley catheter to ensure that those organs are not distended. Percutaneous drainage of the abdominal cavity has been described and may be effective [88]. In our experience, however, the relief is often only temporary. The definitive treatment is to perform a laparotomy. Typically, a large amount of serous fluid is released with marked improvements within an hour. The abdominal contents are temporarily covered with a silicone sheet. It used to felt that a laparotomy for abdominal compartment syndrome in a burn patient was routinely fatal but we have had significant numbers of survivors [89]. We have also found that it is possible to close the abdomen within 1–2 days without any problem. If the abdomen is closed rapidly, there are few problems but after a couple of weeks there is loss of domain and it is not possible to close the abdomen. In this case, the abdominal contents can be covered with a biologic mesh and after formation of granulation tissue it can be grafted. The hernia is then repaired months after discharge.

There are other complications of over-resuscitation that should be mentioned. The burn team in Seattle has reported blindness after a major burn that was attributed to increased intraocular pressures [85]. They have advocated performing lateral canthotomies if there is an elevation of the intraocular pressure. I have never seen that complication but it is probably worthwhile to be concerned about higher pressures within the globe. Excessive volume overload can also stress the heart, especially in the elderly where relative failure might occur. In addition, one must also be concerned with over-resuscitation in any patient who has the combination of traumatic or ischemic brain injury combined with a large burn. With loss of the blood-brain barrier, there is leakage of fluid into the cranial vault. This combination is often fatal since there is a tendency to develop intracranial herniation.

15.10 Conclusion

Appropriate resuscitation of the burn patient will provide the patient with the massive burn the best opportunity for survival. Simply paying close attention to prevent over- or under-resuscitation will improve outcomes. Formulas should only be used as a starting point for resuscitation. After determining the starting volume, all subsequent adjustments should be guided by the patient's physiologic response. Hopefully, better endpoints will be developed in the future but for now urine output is the best guide. Classic teaching has always been to use isotonic crystalloids for burn shock resuscitation, but recently, there has been evidence to support the addition of colloids, especially albumin to the resuscitation strategy. Hopefully, multicenter, randomized, prospective trials will be performed to answer the optimal resuscitation strategy. Optimal resuscitation will minimize the complications of over-resuscitation but despite best practices, compartment syndromes may develop so the burn team needs to be prepared to treat them.

Summary Box

- A systemic capillary leak that is caused by mediators released at the burn site occurs in all burns >15–20% TBSA.
- Endothelial cells have receptors that detect these mediators. In response, endothelial cells relax junctions between the cells to allow leakage of water, electrolytes, and proteins.
- The glycocalyx on the surface of endothelial cells moderates the capillary leak.
- Formulas for burn resuscitation should only be used to determine the initial fluid resuscitation rates. All further adjustments should be based on the patient's response to fluids.
- Urine output is currently the standard used to dictate fluid resuscitation. The use of newer methods of determining fluid status and cardiovascular response is being evaluated.
- While isotonic crystalloids have been the standard resuscitation fluids, newer data suggests that the use of colloids may reduce fluid requirements.
- One should monitor the patient for compartment syndromes and early escharotomies or fasciotomies may save tissue or limbs.

References

1. Pruitt BA Jr. Protection from excessive resuscitation: "pushing the pendulum back". J Trauma. 2000;49:567–8.
2. Saffle JR. The phenomenon of fluid creep in acute burn resuscitation. J Burn Care Res. 2007;28:382–95.
3. Komarova YA, Kruse K, Mehta D, Mali AB. Protein interactions at endothelial junctions and signaling mechanisms regulating endothelial permeability. Circ Res. 2017;120:179–206.
4. Starling EH. On the absorption of fluids from connective tissue spaces. J Physiol. 1896;19:312–26.
5. Demling RH. The burn edema process: current concepts. J Burn Care Rehabil. 2005;26:207–27.
6. Woodcock TE, Woodcock TM. Revised Starling equation and the glycocalyx model of transvascular fluid exchange: an improved paradigm for prescribing intravenous fluid therapy. Br J Anaesth. 2012;108:384–94.
7. Myburgh JA, Mythen MG. Resuscitation fluids. N Engl J Med. 2013;369:1243–51.
8. Kottke MA, Walters TJ. Where's the leak in vascular barriers? A review. Shock. 2016;46:S20–36.
9. Ushiyama A, Kataoka H, Iijima T. Glycocalyx and its involvement in clinical pathophysiologies. J Intensive Care. 2016;4:59–70.
10. Johansson P, Stensballe J, Ostrowski S. Shock induced endotheliopathy (SHINE) in acute critical care illness—a unifying pathophysiologic mechanism. Crit Care. 2017;21:25–32.
11. Greenhalgh DG. Burn resuscitation. J Burn Care Res. 2007;28:555–65.
12. Cartotto R, Greenhalgh DG, Cancio C. Burn state of the science. Fluid resuscitation. J Burn Care Res. 2017;38:e596–604.
13. Cartotto RC, Innes M, Musgrave MA, Gomez M, Cooper AB. How well does the Parkland Formula estimate actual fluid resuscitation volumes? J Burn Care Rehabil. 2002;23:258–65.
14. Cartotto R, Zhou A. Fluid creep: the pendulum hasn't swung back yet! J Burn Care Res. 2010;31:551–9.
15. Engrav LH, Colescott PL, Kemalyan N, et al. A biopsy of the use of the Baxter Formula to resuscitate burns or do we do it like Charlie did? J Burn Care Rehabil. 2002;23:258–65.
16. Paratz JD, Stockton K, Paratz ED, et al. Burn resuscitation—hourly urine output versus alternative endpoints: a systemic review. Shock. 2014;42:295–306.
17. Merrell SW, Saffle JR, Sullivan JJ, et al. Fluid resuscitation in thermally injured children. Am J Surg. 1986;152:664–8.
18. Graves TA, Cioffi WG, McManus WF, et al. Fluid resuscitation of infants and children with massive thermal injury. J Trauma. 1988;28:1656–9.
19. Greenhalgh DG. Burn resuscitation: the results of the ISBI/ABA survey. Burns. 2010;36:176–82.
20. Advanced Burn Life Support. Emergency Care of the Burn Patient. American Burn Association, Chicago, Illinois, 2018
21. Arlati S, Storti E, Pradella V, et al. Decreased fluid volume to reduce organ damage: a new approach to burn shock resuscitation. Resuscitation. 2007;72:371–8.
22. Walker TLJ, Urriza Rodriguiz DU, Coy K, et al. Impact of reduced resuscitation fluid on outcomes of children with 10-20% body surface area scalds. Burns. 2014;40:1581–6.
23. Kulkarni S, Harrington DT, Heffernan D, et al. Tolerance of oliguria improves burn resuscitation. J Burn Care Res. 2013;34:S113.
24. Cancio L, Chavez S, Alvarado-Ortega M, et al. Predicting increased fluid requirements during the resuscitation of thermally injured patients. J Trauma. 2004;56:404–14.
25. Choi J, Cooper A, Gomez M, et al. The relevance of base deficits after burn injuries. J Burn Care Rehabil. 2000;21:499–504.
26. Cochran A, Edelman LS, Saffle JR, Morris SE. The relationship of serum lactate and base deficit in burn patients to mortality. J Burn Care Res. 2007;28:231–40.

27. Andel D, Kamolz LP, Roka J, et al. Base deficit and lactate: early predictors of morbidity and mortality in patients with burns. Burns. 2007;33:973–8.
28. Marik PE, Baran M, Vahid B. Does central venous pressure predict fluid responsiveness? A systematic review of the literature and the tale of the seven mares. Chest. 2008;134:172–8.
29. Shippey CR, Appel PL, Shoemaker WC. Reliability of clinical monitoring to assess blood volume in critically ill patients. Crit Care Med. 1984;12:107–12.
30. Osman D, Ridel C, Ray P, et al. Cardiac filling pressures are not appropriate to predict hemodynamic response to volume challenge. Crit Care Med. 2007;35:64–8.
31. Kumar A, Anel R, Bunnell E, et al. Pulmonary artery occlusion pressure and central venous pressure fail to predict ventricular filling volume, cardiac performance, or the response to volume infusion in normal subjects. Crit Care Med. 2004;32:691–9.
32. Tokarik M, Sjöberg F, Balik M, et al. Fluid therapy LiDCO controlled trial-optimization of volume resuscitation of extensively burned patients through noninvasive continuous real-time hemodynamic monitoring LiDCO. J Burn Care Res. 2013;34:537–42.
33. Hoskins SL, Elgjo GI, Lu J, et al. Closed loop resuscitation of burn shock. J Burn Care Res. 2006;27:377–85.
34. Salinas J, Drew G, Gallagher J, et al. Closed-loop and decision-assist resuscitation of burn patients. J Trauma. 2008;64:S321–32.
35. Salinas J, Chung KK, Mann EA, et al. Computerized decision support system improves fluid resuscitation following severe burns: an original study. Crit Care Med. 2011;39:2031–8.
36. Sullivan SR, Freidrich JB, Engrav LH. Opioid creep is real and may be the cause of fluid creep. Burns. 2004;30:583–90.
37. Mackie DP, Spoelder EJ, Paauw RJ, et al. Mechanical ventilation and fluid retention in burn patients. J Trauma. 2009;67:1233–8.
38. Warden GD. Burn shock resuscitation. World J Surg. 1992;16:16–23.
39. Baxter CR, Shires T. Physiological response to crystalloid resuscitation of severe burns. Ann N Y Acad Sci. 1968;150:874–94.
40. Baxter CR, Marvin J, Curreri PW. Fluid and electrolyte therapy of burn shock. Heart Lung. 1973;2:707–13.
41. Pruitt BA Jr. Fluid and electrolyte replacement in the burned patient. Surg Clin North Am. 1978;58:1291–312.
42. Pruitt BA Jr. The burn patient: II. Later care and complications of thermal injury. Curr Probl Surg. 1979;16:1–95.
43. Demling RH, Smith M, Bodai B, et al. Comparison of postburn capillary permeability in soft tissue and lung. J Burn Care Rehabil. 1981;15:86–92.
44. Harms BA, Bodai BI, Kramer GC, Demling RH. Microvascular fluid and protein flux in pulmonary and systemic circulations after thermal injury. Microvasc Res. 1982;23:77–86.
45. Vlachou E, Moieman NS. Microalbuminemia: a marker of endothelial dysfunction in thermal injury. Burns. 2006;32:1009–16.
46. Cochrane Injuries Group. Human albumin administration in critically ill patients: systematic review of randomized controlled trials. BMJ. 1998;317:235–40.
47. Perel P, Roberts I. Colloids versus crystalloids for fluid resuscitation in critically ill patients. Cochrane Database Syst Rev. 2012;(6):CD000567. https://doi.org/10.1002/14651858.CD000567.pub5.
48. Perel P, Roberts I, Ker K. Colloids versus crystalloids for fluid resuscitation in critically ill patients. Cochrane Database Syst Rev. 2013;(2):CD000567. https://doi.org/10.1002/14651858.CD000567.pub6.
49. The SAFE Study Investigators. A comparison of albumin and saline for fluid resuscitation in the intensive care unit. N Engl J Med. 2004;350:2247–56.
50. Charpentier J, Mira JP. EARSS study group. Efficacy and tolerance of hyperoncotic albumin administration in septic shock patients: the EARSS Study. Intensive Care Med. 2011;37(Suppl 1):S115.
51. Caironi P, Tognoni G, Masson S, et al. Albumin replacement in patients with severe sepsis or septic shock. N Engl J Med. 2014;370:1412–21.
52. Wieddermann CJ, Joannidid M. Albumin replacement in severe sepsis or septic shock. N Engl J Med. 2014;371:83–4.
53. Recinos PR, Hartford CA, Ziffren SE. Fluid resuscitation of burn patients comparing a crystalloid with a colloid containing solution: a prospective study. J Iowa Med Soc. 1975;65:426–32.
54. Jelenko C 3rd, Williams JB, Wheeler ML, et al. Studies in shock and resuscitation, I: use of a hypertonic, albumin-containing, fluid demand regimen (HALFD) in resuscitation. Crit Care Med. 1979;7:157–67.
55. Goodwin CW, Dorethy J, Lam V, Pruitt BA Jr. Randomized trial of efficacy of crystalloid and colloid resuscitation on hemodynamic response and lung water following thermal injury. Ann Surg. 1983;197:520–31.
56. Cooper AB, Cohn SM, Zhang HS, Hanna K, Stewart TE, Slutsky AS, ALBUR Investigators. Five percent albumin for adult burn shock resuscitation: lack of effect on daily multiple organ dysfunction score. Transfusion. 2006;46:80–9.
57. Cochran A, Morris SE, Edelman LS, Saffle JR. Burn patient characteristics and outcomes following resuscitation with albumin. Burns. 2007;33:25–30.
58. Ennis JL, Chung KK, Renz EM, et al. Joint Theater Trauma System implementation of burn resuscitation guidelines improves outcomes in severely burned military casualties. J Trauma. 2008;64(2 Suppl):S146–51; discussion S151–2.
59. Dulhunty JM, Boots RJ, Rudd MJ, et al. Increased fluid resuscitation can lead to adverse outcomes in major burn injured patients, but low mortality is achievable. Burns. 2008;34:1090–7.
60. Lawrence A, Faraklas I, Watkins H, et al. Colloid administration normalizes resuscitation ratio and ameliorates "fluid creep". J Burn Care Res. 2010;31:40–7.
61. Faraklas I, Lam V, Cochran A, et al. Colloid normalizes resuscitation ratio in pediatric burns. J Burn Care Res. 2011;32:91–7.
62. Park SH, Hemilla MR, Whal WL. Early albumin use improves mortality in difficult to resuscitate burn patients. J Trauma. 2012;73:1294–7.
63. Navickis RJ, Greenhalgh DG, Wilkes MM. Albumin in burn shock resuscitation: a meta-analysis of controlled clinical studies. J Burn Care Res. 2016;37:e268–78.
64. Eljaiek R, Heylbroeck C, Dubois M-J. Albumin administration for fluid resuscitation in burn patients: a systemic review and meta-analysis. Burns. 2017;43:17–24.
65. Waters LM, Christenson MA, Sato RM. Hetastarch: an alternative colloid in burn shock management. J Burn Care Rehabil. 1989;10:11–5.
66. Waxman K, Holness R, Tominaga G, et al. Hemodynamic and oxygen transport effects of pentastarch in burn resuscitation. Ann Surg. 1989;209:341–5.
67. Vlachou E, Gosling P, Moieman NS. Hydroxyethylstarch supplementation in burn resuscitation—a prospective randomized controlled trial. Burns. 2010;36:984–91.
68. Béchir M, Puhan MA, Neff SB, et al. Early fluid resuscitation with hyperoncotic hydroxyethyl starch 200/0.5 (10%) in severe burn injury. Crit Care. 2010;14:R123.
69. Béchir M, Puhan MA, Fasshauer M, Schuepbach RA, Stocker R, Neff TA. Early fluid resuscitation with hydroxyl ethyl starch 130/0.4 (6%) in severe burn injury: a randomized controlled double blind clinical trial. Crit Care. 2013;17:R299.
70. Myburgh JA, Finfer S, Bellomo R, et al. Hydroxyethyl starch or saline for fluid resuscitation in intensive care. N Engl J Med. 2012;367:1901–11.

71. Perner A, Haase N, Guttormsen AB, et al. Hydroxyethyl starch 130/0.42 versus Ringer's acetate in severe sepsis. N Engl J Med. 2012;367:124–34.
72. O'Mara MS, Slater H, Goldfarb IW, Caushaj PF. A prospective, randomized evaluation of intra-abdominal pressures with crystalloid and colloid resuscitation in burn patients. J Trauma. 2005;58:1011–8.
73. Matsuda T, Tanaka H, Williams S, et al. Reduced fluid volume requirements for resuscitation of third degree burns with high dose vitamin C. J Burn Care Rehabil. 1991;12:525–32.
74. Matsuda T, Tanaka H, Shimazaki S, et al. High-dose vitamin C therapy for extensive deep dermal burns. Burns. 1992;18:127–31.
75. Sakurai M, Tanaka H, Matsuda T, et al. Reduced resuscitation fluid volume for second degree experimental burns with delayed initiation of vitamin C therapy (beginning 6 h after injury). J Surg Res. 1997;73:24–7.
76. Tanaka H, Matsuda T, Miyagantani Y, et al. Reduced resuscitation volumes in severely burned patients using ascorbic acid administration. A randomized prospective study. Arch Surg. 2000;135:326–31.
77. Kahn SA, Beers RJ, Lentz CW. Resuscitation after severe burn injury using high-dose ascorbic acid: a retrospective review. J Burn Care Res. 2011;32:110–7.
78. Lentz CW, Huelskamp S, Reid D. Adjuvant high dose ascorbic acid reduces both the volume of burn resuscitation fluids and the time to complete resuscitation in burn shock. J Burn Care Res. 2014;46:S107.
79. Lin J, Falwell S, Greenhalgh DG, et al. High dose ascorbic acid for burn shock resuscitation may not improve outcomes. J Burn Care Res. 2018;39(5):708–12.
80. Warden GD, Strata RJ, Saffle JR, et al. Plasma exchange therapy in patients failing to resuscitate from burn shock. J Trauma. 1983;23:945–51.
81. Kravitz M, Warden GD, Sullivan JJ, Saffle JR. A randomized trial of plasma exchange in the treatment of burn shock. J Burn Care Rehabil. 1989;10:17–26.
82. Strata RJ, Saffle JR, Kravitz M, et al. Exchange transfusion therapy in pediatric burn shock. Circ Shock. 1984;12:203–12.
83. Klein MB, Edwards JA, Kramer CB, et al. The beneficial effects of plasma exchange after severe burn injury. J Burn Care Res. 2009;30:243–8.
84. Neff LP, Alman JM, Holmes JH. The use of therapeutic plasma exchange (TPE) in the setting of refractory burn shock. Burns. 2010;36:372–8.
85. Sullivan SR, Ahmadi AJ, Singh CN, et al. Elevated orbital pressure: another untoward effect of massive resuscitation after burn injury. J Trauma. 2006;60:72–6.
86. Brown RL, Greenhalgh DG, Kagan RJ, Warden GD. The adequacy of limb escharotomies/fasciotomies after referral to a major burn center. J Trauma. 1994;37:916–20.
87. Greenhalgh DG, Warden GD. The importance of intra-abdominal pressure measurements in burned children. J Trauma. 1994;36:685–90.
88. Latenser BA, Kowel-Vern A, Kimball D, et al. A pilot study comparing percutaneous decompression with decompressive laparotomy for acute abdominal compartment syndrome in thermal injury. J Burn Care Rehabil. 2002;23:190–5.
89. Hobson KG, Young KM, Ciraulo A, Palmieri TL, Greenhalgh DG. Release of abdominal compartment syndrome improves survival in patients with burn injury. J Trauma. 2002;53:1129–34.

16 Novel Resuscitation Strategies and Technology

Chris Meador and George Kramer

Challenges of Fluid Resuscitation of Burn Injury: Optimal trauma fluid resuscitation is controversial and a frequent topic at scientific proceedings and reviews [1–4]. The controversy may be greatest in burns, where a variety of different treatments are under discussion and clinical testing [4]. Classic formulas are taught, but their application varies. Education and training are challenging amidst declining per capita severe burn incidents and staff turnover. In addition, a sizeable portion of burn resuscitations are not "normal" and present unique challenges to bedside caregivers. Can technology improve care in this daunting environment?

Severe burns cause a variety of physiological changes and sequelae throughout the "golden day," the first 24 h post burn. After burn trauma, direct injury and inflammatory agents increase capillary porosity, allowing plasma and its protein molecules to enter the interstitial space. This permeation reduces the colloid osmotic gradient, which shifts fluids from the vascular space to the interstitial space. Untreated vascular fluid loss results in reduced cardiac output, reduced tissue perfusion and ultimately organ ischemia, failure, and death. Fluid therapy is the first choice for maintaining tissue perfusion. Lactated Ringer's is typically utilized as a basic volume supporting fluid to avoid these under-resuscitation outcomes. However, overuse of fluid therapy can be equally deleterious. Fluid overload in burns is widely recognized and has been termed fluid creep [5]. Fluid overload can result in poor outcomes, including pulmonary edema, abdominal or extremity compartment syndrome, retinal detachment, poor wound healing, and mortality [1, 6, 7]. Since fluid therapy can both support and hinder outcomes, it must be guided by the patient's changing physiological status. The goal of fluid resuscitation is to maintain global and end organ perfusion with the least amount of fluid.

Resuscitation Formulas: There are two commonly referenced guidelines which describe *both* the starting rate and an estimate of total volume to be given by 24 h post burn. For instance, a guideline may suggest a patient receive a total of 16 L in 24 h and start at 1000 mL/h. The Parkland formula (4 mL per kg per percent total body surface area (TBSA) burned volume in 24 h) is the most well-known "formula" internationally, published by Charles Baxter [8, 9]. Baxter's team at Parkland Hospital resuscitated 277 patients using primarily cardiac output based on dye dilution measurements. Baxter reported that those patients received an average of 3.5 mL per kg per TBSA and had an acceptable early survival rate [8]. In animals, Baxter's work found that giving a higher rate of fluids in the first 8 h provided a better cardiac output recovery response than giving a straight amount during the first 24 h [8]. In order to develop a simple guideline for fluid resuscitation without invasive cardiac output monitoring, the average volume number was rounded up to 4 (mL per kg per TBSA) and a starting rate was derived as the 24 h volume divided by 2 then divided by 8.

However, use of the Parkland formula's starting rate can be problematic. A review by Chung et al. found that fluid therapy initiated at the Parkland starting rate resulted in actual fluids given by 24 h to be nearly 50% above the Parkland 24 h volume; whereas, if fluid therapy was started at half Parkland, or the Modified Brooke formula rate (2 mL per kg per %TBSA in 24 h), actual fluids given averaged 3.8 mL per kg per TBSA, notably just below the Parkland formula volume at 24 h but above Baxter's published average volume [10]. These data suggest that either hourly reductions in infusion are not aggressive enough to match urinary output targets or that more fluids administered early drives more fluids to be given later in resuscitation. The American Burn Association recently changed its Advanced Burn Life Support (ABLS) guidelines to have pre-hospital caregivers

C. Meador (✉)
Arcos, Inc., Missouri City, TX, USA
e-mail: chris.meador@arcosmedical.com

G. Kramer
Arcos, Inc., Missouri City, TX, USA

University of Texas Medical Branch, Galveston, TX, USA
e-mail: gkramer@utmb.edu

M. G. Jeschke et al. (eds.), *Handbook of Burns Volume 1*, https://doi.org/10.1007/978-3-030-18940-2_16

start at the Brooke rather than Parkland rate for adults [11]. For pediatric patients, halfway between Brooke and Parkland is suggested as a starting rate.

Use of Urinary Output (UO) as a Target Endpoint: As Baxter suggested, the most often used goal or target of fluid therapy of burn shock is an adequate UO, based on the rationale that adequate UO equates with adequate renal blood flow, end organ perfusion, and cardiac output [8, 9]. The UO bioassay of effectiveness of fluid therapy or specific target levels has never been proven. However, ABLS guidelines recommend a target UO goal of 0.5 mL per kg per hour (30–50 mL per hour) for adults and 1.0 mL per kg per hour for pediatric patients weighing less than 40 kg [11].

Adjusting fluids hourly is important. The cumulative physiological cost of fluid requires clinical vigilance, titrating fluids down when higher rates are no longer needed. A 35-year meta-analysis evidences the practical difficulty of vigilance, with most studies documenting fluids given well in excess of Baxter's guideline and mean 24 h UO above target levels [4, 12]. These data validate the phenomenon of widespread fluid creep.

In addition to UO, caregivers seek to maintain normal or decreasing lactate levels and prevent hypotension and elevated heart rates, as these variables are further indicators of inadequate cardiovascular function. "Chasing" these variables with increased fluid infusion rates may also contribute to fluid overload, so early use of pressors and inotropes might be preferred.

Other Resuscitation Endpoints: As above, other endpoint variables are used for assessing hemodynamic support and resuscitation effectiveness in general. A technological approach can be provided by a variety of invasive and noninvasive cardiac output monitors based on thermal dilution (Pulsion PiCCO, Edwards EV-1000, LiDCO) or bioimpedance (Cheetah's NICOM and Cardiotronic's ICON). Cardiac output can also be estimated using pulse contour analysis of arterial waveforms (Edwards EV-1000 and Pulsion PiCCO). In particular, intrathoracic blood volume and cardiac output as measured by transpulmonary thermal dilution has been suggested for burns [13]. Generally, only descriptive studies have evaluated hemodynamic monitoring versus UO endpoint in burn resuscitation [14]. Advanced hemodynamic monitoring has largely failed to be effective in guiding fluid therapy of burns. Use of hemodynamic endpoints has most often been reported to lead to over-resuscitation [15]. Another approach has been the use of metabolic markers, such as lactate, to help guide fluid therapy [16]. Lactate and base excess are widely used as an indicator for when resuscitation is inadequate, but they have not been shown useful as a prospective endpoint to guide hourly care. Pending new research results, UO as an endpoint appears to be the best single variable to guide fluid therapy in burns.

Electronic Urinary Output Monitor (eUOM): UO is most often measured manually with graduated urimeters that allow the nurse to measure accumulated UO and then to dump the UO in a large collection bag. An advancement is the development of eUOMs that measure UO using weight (Adaptec SensicaUO), capacitive sensors (Navamedic Sippi), ultrasound of accumulated UO (Bard Criticore), or UO in a small collection chamber (Potrero Medical Accuryn). One advantage of all eUOMs is that they reduce volume assessment errors and time errors when measuring UO either before or after the hour. A 15-min error causes a 25% error in hourly flow rate. Most eUOMs do not necessarily correct for air locks that trap urine in the drainage tubing and bladder [17]; however, the Accuryn uses a double-lumen drainage tube and pump to clear the drainage tube every 5 min [18]. Finally, the greatest benefit of eUOMs may be the clinical value of continuous UO data. Algorithms may be able to process such data to provide more effective and timely recommendations to infusion rate to bring UO to target levels.

Resuscitation Solutions: Several resuscitation strategies have emerged based on fluid type. The antioxidant vitamin C in high doses (66 mg per kg per hour) is advocated by some groups who report lower fluid infused volumes and less complications [19, 20]. High dose vitamin C is a strong diuretic and thus precludes the use of UO as endpoint. There is no standard approach to guiding fluids when Vitamin C is used. Rizzo's analysis of vitamin C resuscitation protocols found wide disparity in practice [21]. Thus, to date, vitamin C does not lend itself to a single endpoint variable, nor has it been protocolized.

Over the last 15 years, practitioners have utilized albumin more frequently in ratio with Lactated Ringer's, as a rescue intervention when the in/out ratio reaches an indexed level [22, 23] or as an adjunct therapy when UO does not respond to Lactated Ringer's alone. Some burn centers use albumin as the primary resuscitation fluid for pediatric patients after 8 h post burn. Most groups use albumin on a case-by-case basis based on clinical expertise and experience, but typically advocate starting it after 8-h post injury, based on the rationale that the capillary leak may largely be repaired by that time point. Cartotto has written extensively on the use of albumin in burns [24, 25]. The value and best use of albumin in burn care may be determined by an ongoing prospective observational trial sponsored by the US Army and American Burn Association.

Clinical Decision Support (CDS): Until recently, computational tools for burn resuscitation were simply printed tools, calculators, or apps which provided a quicker way to calculate the Parkland formula based on body weight and burn size [26, 27]. Some burn centers utilize Excel spreadsheets to perform calculations for initial fluid rates and hourly titrations. One paper tool utilized for bedside resuscitation is a decision tree flow chart that suggests hourly changes in infusion rate. Adjustment to infusion rate of 10 or

20% is based on the last hour's UO being above or below target levels [22, 28]. Bedside "nurse-driven" resuscitation using decision tree flowcharts have been implemented as Quality Improvement projects [28–30].

Recently, a predictive model and infusion algorithm was developed for adult patients to guide hourly fluid rates. The Salinas model was based on data from 39 burn patients that related fluid infusions to burn size and resultant UO [31, 32]. Whereas paper protocols use only the last hour of data and a limited set of fixed 10–20% changes to infusion rates, the predictive algorithm uses 3 h of physiological trends and a mathematical model to predict the infusion rate most likely to achieve target UO in the next hour. However, predictive algorithms are limited in part by demographics of the patient population that contributed data to the algorithm's development. A predictive algorithm for "adults" will not be as specific as a predictive algorithm for "adults with gross myoglobinuria" or "adolescents above 40 kg."

One commercialized CDS tool (Arcos Burn Navigator) incorporates the Salinas model to provide hourly decision support along with novel resuscitation displays that provide situational awareness of the fluid status and UO levels during the resuscitation process [33]. One display is a volume graph showing total fluids infused since time of burn, with Baxter and Modified Brooke guidelines overlaid and total 24 h volume projection (Fig. 16.1). Such computer drawn graphs would be too tedious and time-consuming for clinicians to manually create, yet provide a useful visual representation of the fluid resuscitation.

A single-center cohort study showed that computerized decision support can increase how often patients meet UO goals, reduce total fluids given, reduce ventilator days, and may contribute to a reduction in mortality [32]. These results occurred even when 20% or more of the recommendations are rejected by clinicians. The rejection rate may reflect a limitation of the recommendation for the most complicated patients, general skepticism, or proof that the graphical aids and alerts are useful apart from the recommendations. For patient safety, an essential feature of any computerized resuscitation system is the ability for clinicians to override a recommended fluid rate at any time.

In practice, satisfaction with CDS seems to be based on a confidence level obtained with use and familiarity, which results in less need for late night consults between nurses and physicians. It should be noted that when urinary output is not responding to fluid rate increases, or a high 24 h fluid volume is projected, the computer alerts the bedside caregiver to contact the attending physician. CDS technology is a tool to aid, not replace, physician judgment.

Limitations of current CDS: The use of UO is both a strength and a weakness of computerized decision support. UO remains the primary target endpoint today, albeit with notable limitations when it cannot be used. End stage renal disease, hyperglycemia, and high blood alcohol (EtOH) lev-

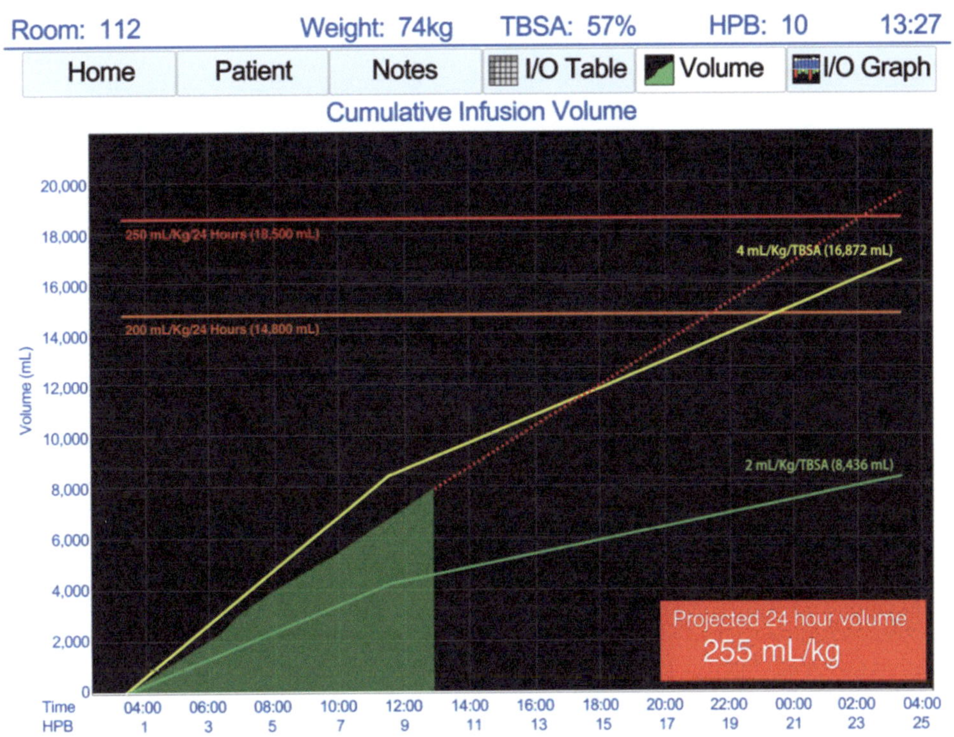

Fig. 16.1 Graph from Burn Navigator showing current volume (green), Parkland (yellow) and Modified Brooke (bright green) guidelines and projected 24-hour fluid volume

els make urine output a falsely low or falsely high surrogate of organ perfusion. Those scenarios require users to rely more on hemoglobin, lactate, and hemodynamic indicators for titrating fluids. Gross myoglobinuria and hematuria necessitate a kidney preservation strategy of higher target UO rates to clear high renal concentrations of toxins.

Current CDS approaches face two main limitations: manual data entry and fluid "non-responders," who are generally defined as patients whose urine output does not increase after increasing infusion rates, or patients whose UO is adequate but only with excessively high infusion rates and a large positive net fluid balance. Patients with a total infused volume over 250 mL/kg, regardless of burn size, are at risk for abdominal compartment syndrome, which is associated with high rates of morbidity and increased mortality [10, 34]. Some patients are non-responders only temporarily, so physicians may tolerate oliguria for 1–3 h during the first 10 h post burn [35]. However, many patients will continue to be non-responders after 10 h post burn. If clinicians continue to increase a crystalloid fluid, such as Lactated Ringer's, for chronic non-responders, then over-resuscitation and morbidities can result.

Medical providers need to remain vigilant toward intervening. Albumin is a common intervention for many burn centers facing non-responders. Although CDS tools can provide alerts and suggest considering albumin, use of albumin varies greatly by burn center and physician judgment. Albumin therapy typically requires a separate medical prescription order.

Future Technology and Automation: Clinical computerized decision support systems can be advanced in two broad ways. First, by improving approaches to UO confounding situations, as seen with electrical injuries, end stage renal disease or vitamin C use. Adjusting the UO targets higher or lower may be sufficient in some cases; however, incorporation of other endpoint variables and multivariable models may be needed. The second way is by automating UO data collection and fluid titration.

Open Loop Resuscitation: A potential improvement to manual data entry and computerized decision support would be "open loop" CDS, which involves communication and controls between an eUOM, a CDS computer, and IV infusion pumps (Fig. 16.2). Data entry would be automatic, hourly recommendations could be generated, and the caregiver could accept them or change the infusion rate per clinical judgment. When accepting recommendations, a single button push sets the pump each hour. By reducing manual data entry, technology can free clinicians for the more important tasks of clinical assessments and therapies. Automating data entry may reduce occasional data entry mistakes, which are not well tracked in daily care.

Fully Automated Resuscitation. Beyond open loop is "closed loop" resuscitation (Fig. 16.3). The concept of automated, or closed loop, burn resuscitation is not new. Bowman et al. obtained a US patent in 1981 [36]; however, their invention had limited research and was not commercialized [37]. In the last decade, the U.S. Department of Defense has been heavily funding internal and external resuscitation research, beginning a renaissance of autonomous critical care technology development [38–41]. Automated burn resuscitation seeks two main goals: reduce tedious manual data entry and mistakes and enable titration frequency to approach physiological response.

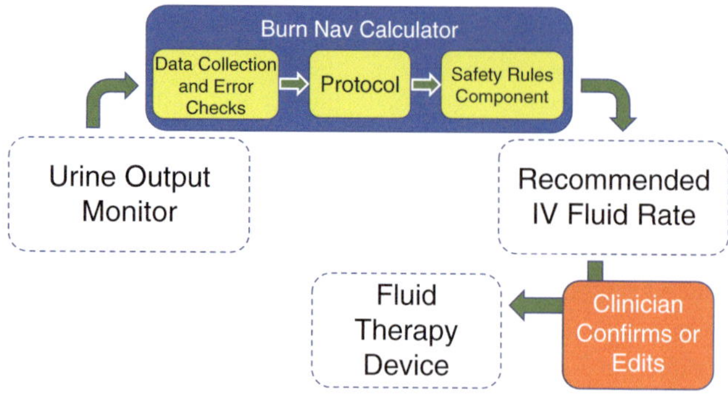

Fig. 16.2 Workflow for hourly fluid updates on open-loop Clinical Decision Support system

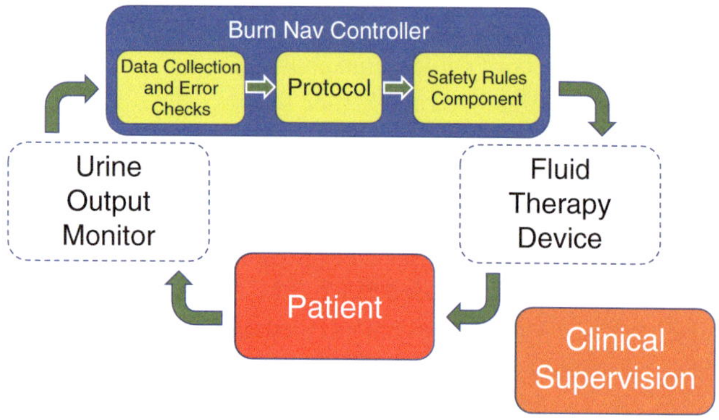

Fig. 16.3 Data and control workflow for closed-loop fluid resuscitation

The response time of UO to fluid and drugs can be on the order of minutes, not an hour. A bolus of fluid delivered over 5 min takes another roughly 5–10 min to result in an increase in UO in the bladder. Fenrich presented sheep data when an automated system adjusted fluids every 10 min based on UO and infusion rates [42]. This frequency of titration would be far too impractical for clinicians to conduct with competing clinical duties, yet promises optimal resuscitation.

In the distant future, a fully automated system may set the UO target based on the patient scenario, run the resuscitation, titrating and weaning fluids, and then announce that the resuscitation phase is over. The U.S. Food and Drug Administration is defining levels of automation and laying the path toward approving physiological closed loop controllers [43].

The connection between a physiologic-based controller and an infusion pump is not a technical challenge, but a regulatory and business challenge with patient safety overtones. Infusion pump companies are extremely reluctant to allow remote rate commands by a third-party device (even an FDA cleared device) since adding such a capability requires a significant cybersecurity defense for the pump's open port.

A clinician might wonder why the therapeutic device isn't also the controller; why have two devices instead of one? Infusion pump companies are typically very large companies due to the advanced engineering required to develop and market an infusion pump and the significant safety hurdles that must be maneuvered. On the other hand, companies pioneering closed loop controllers are typically small and heavily reliant on federal development funds. Large, established companies expect to see little improvement in revenues from adding a closed loop feature or controller, particularly for a market as small as burn resuscitation. Despite these business challenges, we suggest that with the pull of the U.S. Department of Defense and with a clear regulatory environment, manufacturers will come to an arrangement on increasing levels of device interaction and automation.

16.1 Conclusion

Burn resuscitation is a complex and ongoing area of research. Challenges include use of surrogate endpoints, the need for physiological vigilance, tedious infusion rate changes, and high variation in patient response to therapy. Emerging strategies, such as use of high dose vitamin C, and evolving strategies, such as use of albumin, offer more options for resuscitative interventions. Novel technologies allow additional visualization and monitoring capabilities and present a vision for automating therapy in the future.

Summary Box

Following severe burn trauma, vascular fluid loss can result in reduced cardiac output, reduced tissue perfusion, and ultimately organ ischemia, failure, and death. Fluid therapy can be effective for maintaining tissue perfusion, but shortcomings with classic methods of burn resuscitation have been linked to fluid overload. In response, alternative approaches to standard of care have been developed, such as use of albumin, high doses of vitamin C and nurse-driven care. A significant recent advancement has been development of electronic urinary output monitors (eUOMs). Another major advancement is Clinical Decision Support (CDS). The Salinas model is a predictive algorithm developed to guide hourly fluid therapy using physiological trends to predict optimal infusion rates. Arcos Burn Navigator, a CDS tool, incorporates the Salinas model to provide decision support and resuscitation displays. It is anticipated that the future of fluid resuscitation will be "open loop" CDS, which involves coordination between a decision support computer, eUOM and IV infusion pumps; and "closed loop" resuscitation, a fully automated system that will customize a urine output target, run the resuscitation, then alert when the resuscitation phase is complete.

References

1. Saffle JI. The phenomenon of "fluid creep" in acute burn resuscitation. J Burn Care Res. 2007;28(3):382–95.
2. Cartotto R, Greenhalgh D, Cancio C. Burn state of the science. J Burn Care Res. 2017;38(3):e596–604.
3. Gibran NS, Wiechman S, Meyer W, Edelman L, Fauerbach J, Gibbons L, et al. Summary of the 2012 ABA Burn Quality Consensus conference. J Burn Care Res. 2013;34(4):361–85.
4. Cancio LC, Bohanon FJ, Kramer G. Burn resuscitation. Total burn care. London: Elsevier; 2017.
5. Pruitt BA Jr. Protection from excessive resuscitation: "pushing the pendulum back". J Trauma. 2000;49(3):567–8.
6. Cartotto R, Zhou A. Fluid creep: the pendulum hasn't swung back yet! J Burn Care Res. 2010;31(4):551–8.
7. Cancio L, Burrows J, Khan M, Salinas J, Kramer G. Stemming the tide of fluid creep (225). Crit Care Med. 2013;41(12):A51.
8. Baxter CR. Fluid volume and electrolyte changes in the early post burn period. Clin Plast Surg. 1974;1:693–703.
9. Baxter CR, Shires GT. Physiological response to crystalloid resuscitation of severe burns. Ann N Y Acad Sci. 1968;150:874–94.
10. Chung KK, Wolf SE, Cancio LC, Alvarado R, Jones JA, McCorcle J, et al. Resuscitation of severely burned military casualties: fluid begets more fluid. J Trauma. 2009;67(2):231–7; discussion 7.
11. American Burn Association. Advanced Burn Life Support Course (ABLS), Instructor's manual. Chicago: American Burn Association; 2015.
12. Kramer G, Khan M, Serio-Melvin ML, Fenrich C, Chung K, Cancio LC, et al. Metrics for assessing the effectiveness of burn resuscitation. J Burn Care Rehabil. 2013;34(2):S114.
13. Holm C, Melcer B, Horbrand F, Worl H, von Donnersmarck GH, Muhlbauer W. Intrathoracic blood volume as an end point in resuscitation of the burn patient. J Trauma. 2000;48(4):728–34.
14. Paratz JD, Stockton K, Paratz ED, Blot S, Muller M, Lipman J, et al. Burn resuscitation—hourly urine output versus alternative endpoints: a systematic review. Shock. 2014;42(4):295–306.
15. Aboelatta Y, Abdelsalam A. Volume overload of fluid resuscitation in acutely burned patients using transpulmonary thermodilution technique. J Burn Care Res. 2013;34(3):349–54.
16. Jeng J, Lee K, Jablonski K, Silva C, Jordan MH. Serum lactate and base deficit suggest inadequate resuscitation of burn patients:

application of a point of care laboratory instrument. Proc Am Burn Assoc. 1995;27:142.
17. Garcia MM, Gulati S, Liepmann D, Stackhouse GB, Greene K, Stoller ML. Traditional Foley drainage systems—do they drain the bladder? J Urol. 2007;177(1):203–7; discussion 7.
18. Kramer GC, Luxon E, Wolf J, Burnett DR, Nanduri D, Friedman BC. Inaccuracy of urine output measurements due to urinary retention in catheterized patients in the burn ICU. J Burn Care Res. 2017;38(1):e409–e17.
19. Kahn SA, Beers RJ, Lentz CW. Resuscitation after severe burn injury using high-dose ascorbic acid: a retrospective review. J Burn Care Res. 2011;32(1):110–7.
20. Tanaka H, Matsuda T, Yukioka T, Matsuda H, Shimazaki S. High dose vitamin C reduces resuscitation fluid volume in severely burned patients. Proc Am Burn Assoc. 1996;28:77.
21. Rizzo JA, Rowan MP, Driscoll IR, Chung KK, Friedman BC. Vitamin C in burn resuscitation. Crit Care Clin. 2016;32(4):539–46.
22. Faraklas I, Lam U, Cochran A, Stoddard G, Saffle J. Colloid normalizes resuscitation ratio in pediatric burns. J Burn Care Res. 2011;32(1):91–7.
23. Salinas J, Fenrich C, Chung K, Kramer G, Serio-Melvin M, Zonies D, et al., editors. Albumin rescue: it just takes time. ABA Conf; 2012. Seattle, Supplement to J Burn Care Res. 2012;33(2):S108.
24. Cartotto R, Callum J. A review of the use of human albumin in burn patients. J Burn Care Res. 2012;33(6):702–17.
25. Cartotto R, Greenhalgh D. Colloids in acute burn resuscitation. Crit Care Clin. 2016;32(4):507–23.
26. Smith CE, Milner SM. The burn wheel: a guide to burn resuscitation. Emerg Med Serv. 2001;30(3):76–7, 90.
27. Wurzer P, Parvizi D, Lumenta DB, Giretzlehner M, Branski LK, Finnerty CC, et al. Smartphone applications in burns. Burns. 2015;41(5):977–89.
28. Faraklas I, Cochran A, Saffle J. Review of a fluid resuscitation protocol: "fluid creep" is not due to nursing error. J Burn Care Res. 2012;33(1):74–83.
29. Mann EA, Heffernan J, Serio-Melvin M, Mitchell C, Miller K, Haglund J, et al. Burn resuscitation 2010—current practices and the nurse's role. J Burn Care Res. 2011;32(2):S101.
30. Fahlstrom K, Boyle C, Makic MB. Implementation of a nurse-driven burn resuscitation protocol: a quality improvement project. Crit Care Nurse. 2013;33(1):25–35.
31. Salinas J, Kramer G, Mann EA, Chung KC, Gibson D, Serio-Melvin M, et al. Computer decision support system improves fluid management during resuscitation of burn patients. J Burn Care Res. 2009;30(20):S46.
32. Salinas J, Chung K, Mann E, Cancio LC, Kramer GC, Serio-Melvin ML, et al. Computerized decision support system improves fluid resuscitation following severe burns: an original study. Crit Care Med. 2011;39(9):2031–8.
33. Cancio LC, Salinas J, Kramer GC. Protocolized resuscitation of burn patients. Crit Care Clin. 2016;32(4):599–610.
34. Ivy ME, Atweh NA, Palmer J, Possenti PP, Pineau M, D'Aiuto M. Intra-abdominal hypertension and abdominal compartment syndrome in burn patients [comment]. J Trauma. 2000;49(3):387–91.
35. Serio-Melvin ML, Salinas J, Chung KK, Collins C, Graybill JC, Harrington DT, et al. Burn shock and resuscitation: proceedings of a Symposium Conducted at the Meeting of the American Burn Association, Chicago, IL, 21 April 2015. J Burn Care Res. 2017;38(1):e423–e31.
36. Bowman RJ, Westenskow DR, inventors; University of Utah (Salt Lake City, UT), assignee. Closed-loop infusion system, both method and apparatus, based on real time urine measurement. United States Patent 4,291,6921981 September 29.
37. Bowman RJ, Westenskow DR. A microcomputer-based fluid infusion system for the resuscitation of burn patients. Trans Biomed Eng. 1981;28(6):475–9.
38. Kramer GC, Kinsky MP, Prough DS, Salinas J, Sondeen JL, Hazel-Scerbo ML, et al. Closed-loop control of fluid therapy for treatment of hypovolemia. J Trauma. 2008;64(4 Suppl):S333–41.
39. Salinas J, Drew G, Gallagher J, Cancio LC, Wolf SE, Wade CE, et al. Closed-loop and decision-assist resuscitation of burn patients. J Trauma. 2008;64(4 Suppl):S321–32.
40. Marques N, Ford B, Khan M, Kinsky M, Deyo D, Mileski W, et al. Automated closed-loop resuscitation of multiple hemorrhages. Disaster Mil Med. 2017;3:1.
41. Marques N, Whitehead W, Upendar KR, Funston J, Kinsky M, Khan M, et al. Physician directed versus computerized closed loop control of blood pressure using phenylephrine in a swine model. Anesth Analg. 2017;125:110–6.
42. Fenrich C, Kramer G, Salinas J. An automated burn resuscitation decision support system (BRDSS-A). Symp; 2013. In: Proc Mil Res Sci.
43. Parvinian B, Scully C, Wiyor H, Kumar A, Weininger S. Regulatory considerations for physiological closed-loop controlled medical devices used for automated critical care: Food and Drug Administration Workshop Discussion Topics. Anesth Analg. 2018;126(6):1916–25.

Part III

Critical Care and Acute Phase After Burn

17 Respiratory Management in Burn Care

Kevin N. Foster

17.1 Introduction

Airway and respiratory management are necessary and important components of burn care because a significant minority of burn patients requires intubation and mechanical ventilation, often for weeks or even months. Burn patients require respiratory management for two major reasons: the presence of smoke inhalation injury (II) and/or a large percent total body surface area (% TBSA) burn. Inhalation of the products of combustion causes a cascade of injury and inflammatory response that typically leads to respiratory failure and the need for intubation and ventilation. Likewise, a large % TBSA thermal injury (typically ≥30% TBSA) imposes such a large systemic metabolic load on patients that intubation and ventilation are almost always necessary. This chapter reviews general concepts of airway and respiratory management in burn patients.

17.2 Airway Management

17.2.1 Endotracheal intubation

As noted previously, the two major indications for endotracheal intubation in burn patients are inhalation injury and a large % TBSA burn. Each of these indications has several individual components.

Inhalation injury (II) is classically caused by breathing in the hot products of combustion. The smoke produced by such combustion typically has hundreds of toxic chemicals. These chemicals react with airway and alveolar cells producing injury and initiating an intense inflammatory response. This injury and inflammatory response ultimately causes airway obstruction, impaired ciliary function and surfactant production, thickening of the alveolar-capillary membrane, ventilation-perfusion mismatch, hypoxemia, hypercarbia, acidosis, and respiratory failure [1–5]. II can be classified into injury above larynx which is caused primarily by heat, and injury below the larynx which is typically caused by chemical exposure. Patients with upper airway (heat) injury often require intubation because the local edema and tissue swelling from the burn injury may cause upper airway obstruction. Patients with lower airway and lung injury (chemical) often require intubation because of respiratory failure. Not infrequently patients will have both upper airways and lower airway and lung injury simultaneously [6].

The suspicion of an II (either upper or lower) often is enough of an indication for intubation. However, not all patients exposed to smoke will require intubation. It can be difficult to determine early in a patient's clinical course if that patient will develop significant upper airway edema to cause obstruction and/or enough lower airway and lung injury to cause respiratory failure. Close observation with preparation to intervene immediately is a prudent course. If the patient is to be transported to another facility and obtain a definitive airway during transport is likely to be difficult, then prophylactic intubation is warranted. Ultimately, if the course is uncertain, then intubation is the wisest choice. If the intubation proves unnecessary, then the endotracheal tube can be removed. Conversely, if the patient is not intubated and subsequently requires intubation, the procedure may be very difficult because of upper airway edema and obscuring of the airway and landmarks.

Thus, patients with evidence of upper airway injury upon presentation or developing during observation, such as obvious orinasal burns, swelling, erythema, stridor, or hoarseness should be promptly intubated. Likewise, patients with evidence of lower airway and lung injury such as a history of closed space injury, the presence of true carbonaceous sputum either coughed up or suctioned, an elevated carboxyhemoglobin level >10% (see below), stridor, or hoarseness should also be promptly intubated.

K. N. Foster (✉)
Department of Surgery, The Arizona Burn Center—Valleywise Health, Phoenix, AZ, USA
e-mail: kevin_foster@dmgaz.org

M. G. Jeschke et al. (eds.), *Handbook of Burns Volume 1*, https://doi.org/10.1007/978-3-030-18940-2_17

A third component of II is carbon monoxide (CO) poisoning. CO is produced by virtually every type of fire. CO preferentially binds to hemoglobin over oxygen and causes hypoxemia. The degree of CO poisoning is determined by the degree of binding to hemoglobin to produce carboxyhemoglobin (COHg). This is measured as a percent of hemoglobin bound to CO. Most patients have baseline levels of COHg close to 0%. Mild to moderate symptoms occur with levels of 20–30%, severe symptoms with levels of 30–50%, and death with levels >50%. Documentation or suspicion of CO poisoning (levels >10%) mandates prompt intubation and placing the patient on 100% FiO_2. The half-life of COHg can be reduced from 4 h on room air to less than 60 min with 100% oxygen [7].

Finally, there are rare instances where the lower airway and lung suffer direct thermal injury. Examples of this are inhalation of hot steam or inhalation of hot or flaming liquids such as flaming fuel. These situations almost always warrant immediate intubation.

The second major indication for early intubation in burn patients is the presence of a large %TBSA burn injury. The generalized inflammatory response to burn injury and the resulting soft tissue edema from that response plus the large fluid volume resuscitation often leads to airway edema even in the absence of an II or direct burns to the face and head. The metabolic load from the large thermal injury adds additional stress. Finally, the high levels of analgesia and sedation usually required to maintain adequate pain control and comfort in a burn patient often could not be administered safely in the absence of intubation and ventilation. There is no mandatory cut-off for % TBSA above which intubation is necessary. However, 30% TBSA seems a reasonable level at which to consider intubation and is the cut-off recommended by Acute Burn Life Support.

Another consideration in addition to the size of the burn is their anatomic location. Upper body burns (head and neck, torso above the nipples, upper extremities) may cause airway edema even if the airway and surrounding structures are not directly involved. This potentially dangerous situation should be recognized early and intubation performed before airway edema makes it difficult.

Finally, a last indication for intubation is a decreased level of consciousness (DLOC). This may occur with or without II and/or a large %TBSA burn. There are numerous reasons for this DLOC including hypoxia, hypercarbia, medications, substance abuse, associated traumatic injury, II, CO poisoning, etc. These patients should be immediately intubated and a thorough investigation into the cause of the decreased level of consciousness initiated.

Once the decision has been made to intubate, the entire team should be assembled and the most experienced person should intubate. Equipment should include a functioning bag and mask with 100% FiO_2, suctioning device, ventilator, laryngoscope, and appropriate medications. Adjuncts to facilitate visualization of the vocal cords and airway include a fiberoptic bronchoscope and glideslope. The team should be prepared to perform an emergency cricothyroidotomy or tracheostomy if standard endotracheal intubation fails.

17.2.2 Tracheostomy

There are several controversies surrounding the use of elective tracheostomy in burn patients requiring prolong ventilation. The first controversy is whether tracheostomy is indicated ("to trach or not to trach?"). If one believes that tracheostomy is in fact indicated, the next issue is the timing of the tracheostomy (1 week post-injury? 2 weeks? 3 weeks?). Once one has decided when to perform a tracheostomy, the next issue is how to perform. The general choices are traditional, operative, open tracheostomy versus bedside percutaneous dilational tracheostomy, or some combination of the two. A final question is whether a neck burn impacts any of the other three issues presented. Let's look at each of these in greater detail.

The advantages of tracheostomy include easier suctioning, better maintenance of oral hygiene, better ventilator mechanics, more secure, better tolerated requiring less sedation, and easier weaning from ventilation [8]. Disadvantages include necessity for an invasive procedure, easier colonization of respiratory tract, and possible development of a tracheoinnominate fistula. Studies on the effectiveness and safety of tracheostomy prior to the mid-1990s were mostly retrospective and did not provide good data. Early studies tended to report high complication rates and poorer outcomes with tracheostomy [9]. More recent studies report low complication rates and better outcomes [10].

Saffle et al. [11] randomized burn patients to early tracheostomy (4 days post-injury) or conventional treatment with ventilation via standard endotracheal tube until day 14 at which time the patients underwent tracheostomy. There were no differences in the two groups in length of stay, need for ventilator support, incidence of pneumonia, or survival. The early tracheostomy group demonstrated improvement in PAO_2/FiO_2 ratio within 24 h of the procedure. However, there was a significantly great number of patients in the conventional treatment group who were extubated compared to the early tracheostomy group. The authors concluded that early tracheostomy offered no particular advantage or disadvantage over conventional management.

Palmieri et al. [12] reported a retrospective review of 38 severely burn children who underwent tracheostomy at a mean time of 3.9 days after admission. Peak inspiratory pressure, PaO_2/FiO_2 ratio, pulmonary compliance, and ventilatory volumes all improved following tracheostomy. There were no tracheostomy-related deaths, no tracheostomy site infections, and no post-tracheostomy tracheal stenosis. The authors concluded that early tracheostomy in this population of burn patients was safe and effective, and that it resulted in a more secure airway and improvement in ventilator management.

Aggarwal et al. [13] reported a retrospective comparison of burn patients who received tracheostomy ($n = 48$) with burn patients who had ventilation with endotracheal intubation only ($n = 84$). The tracheostomy group had significantly larger % TBSA burns, a significantly greater incidence of inhalation injury, and a lower probability of survival based on the Abbreviated Burn Severity Index (ABSI). Duration of ventilation, length of hospital and ICU stay, and incidence of pulmonary infection were all greater in the tracheostomy group, but mortality was equivalent between the two groups.

The second controversy regarding tracheostomy is the timing of tracheostomy. Reports of tracheostomy performed as early as 3 [14] or 4 [11, 12] days after the initiation of mechanical ventilation have demonstrated safety and efficacy for the procedure and timing. A recent survey of ventilator practices showed that most (67%) of respondents considered tracheostomy after 2 weeks of mechanical ventilation. Reasons for earlier tracheostomy included large % TBSA burn, burns of the head and neck, failed extubation attempts and poor fluid resuscitation status. Additional considerations for early tracheostomy were severe traumatic brain injury and predicted prolonged need for mechanical ventilation [15].

The third controversy regarding tracheostomy is the choice of technique, either a traditional open tracheostomy or a bedside percutaneous dilational tracheostomy. The traditional method is performed in the operating room under general anesthesia. The neck is dissected through an anterior incision, the trachea is exposed, and the tracheostomy is place under direct vision. The percutaneous method is performed at the bedside usually under IV sedation with or without monitored anesthesia care. A needle is percutaneously placed into the trachea under bronchoscopic visualization. A guideline is placed through the needle, a dilator is used to dilate the track and the tracheostomy site, and a tracheostomy tube is placed. In the survey of ventilation practices, 78% of burn surgeons preferred to perform tracheostomy in the operating room [15]. Comparative trials of the two techniques have generally demonstrated either no difference in outcomes, or fewer complications and lower cost with the percutaneous technique [16–19].

The final issue is that of tracheostomy use in a patient with a neck burn. This remains controversial and the evidence for one clinical path over another is lacking [8]. As noted above, head and neck burns may be an indication for tracheostomy or even early tracheostomy. Smailes et al. studied this and found a higher incidence of stoma infections in grafted necks if the autograft was not fully adhered and healed to the neck. They recommended performing tracheostomy only after the neck autograft was completely healed, and suggested 10 days post-graft [19].

In conclusion, tracheostomy appears to be a useful tool in burn care, and the advantages largely outweigh its disadvantages. The most common timing for tracheostomy is approximately 2 weeks after the onset of ventilation although early tracheostomy (3–4 days) may be beneficial in some situations. Open tracheostomy is the preferred method of tracheostomy. However, percutaneous tracheostomy is safe and may offer some advantages over open. Patients with neck burns can safely undergo tracheostomy, but the procedure is best performed after excision and autografting.

17.3 Ventilator Management

Burn patients with injuries ≥30% TBSA or burn patients with inhalation injury typically require mechanical ventilation, often for weeks or even months. Burn patients are somewhat unique in the fact that they have normal lungs and normal lung function, at least at the time of initiation of mechanical ventilation. Obviously, patients with inhalation injury have lung pathology, and the inflammatory response of burn injury may induce some pathophysiologic changes in otherwise normal lungs. This makes evaluation of ventilator studies somewhat difficult because most of these studies have been done in patients with lung pathology such as acute lung injury (ALI), acute respiratory distress syndrome (ARDS), pneumonia, and others. Compounding this problem is the fact that burn patients have not infrequently been excluded from ventilator studies. Let's now examine the various ventilator management strategies used in burn patients. We will start with the two most common ventilation management strategies for patients with ARDS: lung protective ventilation and the open-lung approach. We will conclude with several less common ventilation strategies.

17.3.1 Lung Protective Mechanical Ventilation

The Acute Respiratory Distress Syndrome Network (ARDS Net) trial in 2000 has had a profound effect on ventilator management. The trial compared ventilation with lower tidal volumes (6 mL/kg) to ventilation with traditional higher volumes (12 mL/kg). The lower tidal volume group demonstrated significantly lower mortality and greater number of ventilator-free days. Mean plateau pressures were also significantly lower in the lower tidal volume group. Subsequent studies have confirmed the safety and efficacy of lower tidal volume ventilation. It has become known as lung protective ventilation [20].

Lung protective ventilation (LPV) is appropriate and indicated for burn patients with and without inhalation injury. Initial ventilator setting goals in these patients are a tidal volume of 6–8 mL/kg with respiratory rate and positive end-expiratory pressure (PEEP) to attain normal arterial blood gas values for PAO_2, $PACO_2$, and pH, and with peak inspiratory pressures (PIP) less than 35 cm H_2O. Numerous studies have validated the effectiveness of lung protective ventilation in patients with ARDS, ALI, and other pulmonary disorders requiring ventilation management [21–25].

Lung protective ventilation may present challenges in burn patients because of unique features of burn pathophysiology. Burn injury and fluid resuscitation results in soft tissue swelling and edema. Body wall and torso edema may be significant enough to decrease chest wall compliance. Under these circumstances, it may be necessary to increase tidal volume to compensate for decreased compliance. Likewise, a thermal burn extending over most or all of the torso may adversely decrease chest wall compliance. This is particularly true for circumferential and/or full-thickness burns.

17.3.2 The Open-Lung Approach to Mechanical Ventilation and Positive End-Expiratory Pressure (PEEP)

The protective lung strategy aims to reduce lung strain by decreasing lung volumes and pressures. The second strategy, the open-lung approach (OLA), aims to decrease dynamic strain on alveoli. The purported advantages of OLA include improved oxygenation and ventilation, decreased atelectasis, and decreased shear injury from opening and closing of alveoli [26]. The hallmarks interventions of the OLA are: (1) to open alveoli with recruitment maneuvers, and then (2) keep them open with PEEP [27].

Recruitment maneuvers (RMs) comprise a variety of techniques used to temporarily increase intrapulmonary pressures and expand airless and atelectatic alveoli. The overall goal of RMs is to increase the number of open alveoli, improve lung aeration, increase the surface for gas exchange, and ultimately improve oxygenation. One key to successful recruitment is to use RMs that effectively open collapsed alveoli but do not over-distend and injure the alveoli. Indeed, one objection to RMs is that if they are improperly implemented, adverse effects such as hypotension, barotrauma, or oxygen desaturation can occur. There are several RMs that have been demonstrated to be effective including sigh breaths, sustained inflation, assisted ventilation, prone positioning, and stepwise increase in airway pressure and/or PEEP. The ideal RM protocol (type, frequency, duration, peak pressure, etc.) is not known and patient response to an RM is impossible to predict. Thus, RMs must be individualized. There is ample clinical data to support the concept that stepwise RMs tend to better improve oxygenation with less adverse hemodynamic or respiratory consequences than traditional abrupt RMs. Once a successful PM has been performed, the second hallmark of OLA ventilation is to maintain alveolar patency with PEEP [28–30].

PEEP in the context of mechanical ventilation (also known as extrinsic or applied PEEP) is positive pressure applied by the ventilator at the end of expiration. PEEP helps to keep alveoli in the open position and prevent their collapse. There are numerous advantages to PEEP. It helps to recruit alveoli and prevent trauma to them by keeping them open. It improves oxygenation by increasing surface area for gas exchange. It increases functional residual capacity and diminishes ventilation-perfusion mismatches. It increases pulmonary compliance. Disadvantages to PEEP include the inability to fully expire leading to breath stacking or auto-PEEP, and possibly decreasing cardiac return and thus decreasing cardiac output [31]. The ideal level of PEEP to be utilized in OLA ventilation is not known. As with RMs, a balance must be attained between PEEP that is too low and fails to maintain open alveoli and PEEP that is too high and causes barotrauma leading to worsening of oxygenation and possibly hemodynamic instability. A number of appropriately powered, well-conducted prospective clinical trials have been performed to determine the optimal level of PEEP. None of these trials individually or in combination has provided a definitive answer to the optimal PEEP question [27, 32–37]. The following simple methods have been suggested (this list is not exhaustive) [38]:

- Use a relatively high PEEP: 15 to 20 cm H_2O
- Use ARDSNet PEEP-FiO_2 escalation tables (PEEP set based on oxygenation)
- Titrate PEEP to maximum static compliance
- Set PEEP to slightly above the lower inflection point of pressure-volume curve
- Use stepwise recruitment to find lowest PEEP with maximal oxygenation

17.3.3 Permissive Hypercapnia

Permissive hypercapnia (PH) is a ventilation strategy often used as an adjunct to LPV and/or OLA. The lower tidal volumes used in these ventilation approaches can result in CO2 retention. Attempts to normalize this hypercapnia may result in larger tidal volumes or higher pressures and may defeat the purpose of the employed ventilation strategies. PH allows abnormally high PCO_2 levels to permit ventilation with low tidal volumes. PH is not detrimental; indeed, it has been shown to have beneficial effects on lung and other tissues and organs. PH may attenuate lung injury and edema and decrease cytokine release. It increases cardiac output and oxygen carrying capacity and decreases peripheral vascular resistance. PH increases cerebral oxygenation [39]. Most studies have shown a benefit with the use of PH [40, 41] although one large database study demonstrated a higher mortality with PH use [42]. The ideal technique of PH and the optimal PCO_2 level remain to be defined.

17.3.4 High Frequency Percussive Ventilation

High frequency percussive ventilation (HFPV) is a unique mode of ventilation that imposes high frequency, subtidal percussive volume breaths onto conventional pressure ventilation breaths. This delivers intrapulmonary percussion (similar to chest physiotherapy) that helps to loosen debris, mobilize secretions, and facilitate removal from the lungs and airways while supporting recruitment and gas exchange. This function ultimately increases oxygenation and lowers airway pressures. HFPV is administered to patients using a special ventilator, the Volumetric Diffusive Respirator®-4 (VDR-4) which is time-cycled and pressure-driven. Early retrospective studies comparing HFPV with conventional ventilation generally found that HFPV improved oxygenation, lower airway pressures and barotrauma, reduced the incidence of ventilator-associated pneumonia, and improved survival [43–46]. Two subsequent comparative trials demonstrated improved oxygenation a lower airway pressures with HFPV compared to conventional ventilation. There was no difference in VAP rate or mortality between the two groups [47, 48]. A recent clinical trial comparing HFPV with LPV demonstrated no significant difference in primary or secondary outcomes in the two groups with the exception of need for rescue ventilation which significantly lowers in the HFPC group [49]. The mechanism of action of HFPV seems ideally suited for patients with inhalation injury, and existing evidence supports its use in this population. More evidence-based study is needed to draw definite conclusions [50–64].

17.3.5 High Frequency Oscillatory Ventilation

High frequency oscillatory ventilation (HFOV) works by delivering very small tidal volumes (1–4 mL/kg) at very high respiratory rates or frequencies (3–15 Hz) using an oscillatory pump combined with continuous application of high mean airway pressure. This functions to maintain alveolar recruitment and to prevent lung injury from over-distension or loss of alveolar recruitment. Oxygenation is controlled primarily by the mean airway pressure and ventilation is controlled primarily by the frequency, which affects both respiratory rate and tidal volume. The advantages of HFOV are that it decreases ventilator-induced lung injury, mobilizes secretions, and separates oxygenation and ventilation (CO_2 clearance) processes. The disadvantages of HFOV is that it requires deep sedation and usually chemical paralysis, the higher pressures cause a higher risk for hemodynamic instability, and there is de-recruitment once the HFOV is terminated [65, 66]. HFOV has been shown to be safe and effective as a salvage or rescue ventilator mode. Three clinical trials comparing HFOV with conventional ventilation failed to show any significant benefit with HFOV [67–69]. One trial demonstrated increased adverse effects [68] and one trial demonstrated an increased mortality [67]. A recent meta-analysis, which did not include two of the three clinical trials above, suggested that HFOV improved oxygenation (P/F ratios) and decreased mortality with no increase in adverse events [70]. There has been some experience with HFOV is several burn centers and the results have generally been satisfactory [71–83]. Currently, HFOV cannot be recommended as a primary therapy in burn patients. However, it should be considered in patients with complicated or severe lung injury, and as a salvage ventilator when conventional ventilation methods fail.

17.3.6 Airway Pressure Release Ventilation

Airway Pressure Release Ventilation (APRV) functions by applying a continuous airway pressure (P high) for a relatively long period of time (T high). Periodically, this pressure is released to a lower pressure (P low) for a short period of time (T low). Then the ventilator is cycled back to P high. This provides alveolar recruitment and prevents alveolar collapse, allowing for excellent gas exchange and oxygenation and ventilation. One of the unique aspects of APRV is that it is a very comfortable ventilator mode. Patients do not require additional sedation or analgesia. And patients can breathe spontaneously at both the P high and P low levels [84]. There is minimal information on the use of APRV in burn patients [85].

17.3.7 Extracorporeal Membranous Oxygenation

Extracorporeal membranous oxygenation (ECMO) utilizes cardiopulmonary bypass technology to temporarily provide oxygen and carbon dioxide gas exchange in patients with severe respiratory failure. ECMO is unique in that it does not rely on the lungs for gas exchange. ECMO is of proven benefit in neonates and there is a growing body of evidence that it may also be effective in older pediatric and adult patients [86]. There is a fairly substantial burn experience with ECMO although most reports are case reports or case histories [87–101]. A recent report from a survey of the American Burn Association National Burn Repository database identified 30 patients treated with ECMO. Overall outcomes were acceptable, and the authors concluded that ECMO is a viable option for supporting critically ill burn patients, especially those who have failed conventional ventilation management [102].

17.4 Adjuncts to Ventilation

17.4.1 Bronchodilators

Bronchodilators work by opposing cholinergic bronchoconstriction causing bronchodilation, decreased resistance to airflow, increased compliance, and increased gas exchange. Bronchodilators include ß2-adrenegic agonists such as albuterol and salbutamol, muscarinic antagonists such as ipratropium bromide and tiotropium bromide, and ß agonists such as epinephrine. Studies of bronchodilator use in burn patients generally show benefit in burn by improving P/F ratio, decreased airway pressures, and possibly by decreasing host immune response [88, 103–105].

17.4.2 Inhaled Anticoagulants

Inhaled heparin has been used as an adjunct in the ventilator management of burn and inhalation injury patients. Heparin helps to prevent formation and aids in dissolution of fibrin casts and clots which form in the airways of ventilated patients. This improves oxygenation and decreases barotrauma. Heparin use is usually combined with NAC to take advantage of its mucolytic and anti-inflammatory properties. Often a ß2-adrenegic agonist is given with the heparin-NAC combination to help open the airways for better drug delivery and to prevent bronchospasm that NAC may incite. Two studies have document benefit from a heparin-NAC regimen in burn patients with increases in compliance, oxygenation, and survival and decreases in pulmonary resistance and mortality [106, 107]. In contrast, another similar study found no benefit to heparin-NAC [108]. A recent retrospective, case-control study demonstrated that nebulized heparin (10,000 units) use resulted in a significant decrease in ventilator-free days compared to controls. There was no difference in length of stay, mortality, VAP, or bleeding complications [109]. A systematic review of inhaled anticoagulation regimens for the treatment of smoke inhalation-associated lung injury confirmed decreased morbidity and increased survival with the use of inhaled anticoagulants [110].

17.4.3 Mucolytic Agents

N-acetylcysteine (NAC) is a mucolytic that exerts its effects by reducing disulfide bonds on mucous protein and decreasing its viscosity. In addition to its properties as a reducing agent, NAC also provides cysteine for glutathione synthesis and may thus have an added anti-inflammatory effect. Animal studies and studies in patients with chronic obstructive pulmonary disease (COPD) have demonstrated efficacy [5, 111–113].

17.5 Ventilator-Associated Pneumonia

Ventilator-associated pneumonia is an expected complication of ventilator therapy in burn patients. The incidence of VAP is about 35% [114] or 22–26 cases per 1000 ventilator days [115, 116]. Burn patients are susceptible to VAP because of immunosuppression, inhalation injury, prolonged ventilation, wound colonization, and infectious processes elsewhere. VAP typically begins with colonization of the upper aerodigestive tract followed by aspiration of microbe into the airways and lung, followed by colonization of these areas followed by infection. Diagnosis of VAP in the burn setting is challenging because burn patients at baseline have finding consistent with systemic infection, including fever, leukocytosis, tachycardia, and tachypnea. Diagnosis of VAP usually rests on a clinical gestalt based on changes or new findings in vital signs coupled with increasing and/or new purulent respiratory secretions, increase in ventilator support, and new findings on chest radiograph. The diagnosis is confirmed with protected bronchoalveolar lavage specimen(s) sent for quantitative culture and sensitivity. If VAP is suspected, then the patient is started on broad-spectrum antibiotics based on the expected or likely pathogens, covering for both Gram-positive and Gram-negative microorganisms. Once culture and sensitivities are obtained, the antibiotic regimen is de-escalated appropriately.

Summary Box

This chapter outlines a brief review of irway and respiratory managment of the burn injured patient.

References

1. Cha S, Kim C, Lee J, et al. Isolated smoke inhalation injuries: acute respiratory dysfunction, clinical outcomes, and short term evolution of pulmonary function with the effects of steroids. Burns. 2007;33(2):200–9.
2. Ching JA, Ching YH, Shivers SC, et al. An analysis of inhalation injury diagnostic methods and patient outcomes. J Burn Care Res. 2016;37(1):e27–32.
3. Hassan Z, Wong JK, Bush J, et al. Assessing the severity of inhalation injuries in adults. Burns. 2010;36(2):212–6.
4. Ikonomidis C, Lang F, Radu A, et al. Standardizing the diagnosis of inhalation injury using a descriptive score based on mucosal injury criteria. Burns. 2012;38(4):513–9.
5. Mlcak R, Suman O, Herndon D. Respiratory management of inhalation injury. Burns. 2007;33(1):2–13.
6. Walker PF, Buehner MF, Wood LA, et al. Diagnosis and management of inhalation injury: an updated review. Crit Care. 2015;19:351.
7. Kealey GP. Carbon monoxide toxicity. J Burn Care Res. 2009;30(1):146–7.
8. Purdue G. To trach or not to trach. J Burn Care Res. 2009;30(1):192–3.

9. Eckhauser F, Billote J, Burke J, et al. Tracheostomy complicating massive burn injury. A plea for conservation. Am J Surg. 1974;127(4):418–23.
10. Clark W, Bonaventura M, Myers W, et al. Smoke inhalation and airway management at a regional burn unit: 1974 to 1983. II airway management. J Burn Care Rehabil. 1990;11(2):121–34.
11. Saffle JR, Morris SE, Edelman L. Early tracheostomy does not improve outcome in burn patients. J Burn Care Rehabil. 2002;23(6):431–8.
12. Palmieri T. Benefits of early tracheostomy in severely burned children. Crit Care Med. 2002;30(4):922–4.
13. Aggarwal S, Smailes S, Dziewulski P. Tracheostomy in burns patients revisited. Burns. 2009;35(7):962–6.
14. Lipovy B, Brychta P, Rihova H, et al. Effect of timing of tracheostomy on changes in bacterial colonisation of the lower respiratory tract in burned children. Burns. 2013;39(2):255–61.
15. Chung KK, Rhie RY, Lundy JB, et al. A survey of mechanical ventilator practices across burn centers in North America. J Burn Care Res. 2016;37(2):e131–9.
16. Caruso D. Percutaneous dilatational tracheostomy. J Burn Care Res. 2009;30(1):194–5.
17. Feldman M, Milner S, Dhanjani K, et al. Semi-open percutaneous tracheostomy inburn patients. Burns. 2011;37(6):1072–8.
18. Gravvanis A, Tsoutsos D, Iconomou T, et al. Percutaneous versus conventional tracheostomy in burned patients with inhalation injury. World J Surg. 2005;29(12):1571–5.
19. Smailes ST, Ives M, Richardson P, et al. Percutaneous dilational and surgical tracheostomy in burn patients: incidence of complications and dysphagia. Burns. 2014;40(3):436–42.
20. The ARDS Network. Ventilation with lower tidal volumes as compared with traditional tidal volumes for acute lung injury and the acute respiratory ditress syndrome. NEJM. 2000;342(18):1301–8.
21. Amato M, Barbas C, Medieros D, et al. Effect of a protective lung strategy on mortality in ARDS. N Engl J Med. 1998;338:347–454.
22. Brouchard L, Roudot-Toraval F, Roupie E. Tidal volume reduction for prevention of ventilator-induced lung injury in ARDS. Am J Respir Crit Care Med. 1998;158(6):1831–8.
23. Brower R, Stanholz C, Fessler H, et al. Prospective randomized controlled trial comparing traditional vs. reduced volumes for ALI or ARDS. Crit Care Med. 1999;27:1492–8.
24. Neto A, Cardoso S, Manetta J, et al. Association between use of lung-protective ventilation with lower tidal volumes and clinical outcomes among patients without acute respiratory distress syndrome. JAMA. 2012;308(16):1651–9.
25. Stewart T, Meade M, Cook D, et al. Evaluation of a strategy to prevent barotrauma in patients at high risk for ARDS: pressure and limited volume ventilation group. N Engl J Med. 2000;342:1301–8.
26. Spieth PM, Guldner A, Carvalho AR, et al. Open lung approach vs acute respiratory distress syndrome network ventilation in experimental acute lung injury. Br J Anaesth. 2011;107(3):388–97.
27. Meade M, Cook D, Guyatt G, et al. Ventilation strategy using low tidal volumes, recruitment maneuvers, and high positive end-expiratory pressure for acute lung injury and acute respiratory distress syndrome. JAMA. 2008;299(6):637–45.
28. Keenan J, Formenti P, Marini J. Lung recruitment in acute respiratory distress syndrome: what is the best strategy? Curr Opin Crit Care. 2014;20(1):63–8.
29. Santos RS, Silva PL, Pelosi P, et al. Recruitment maneuvers in acute respiratory distress syndrome: the safe way is the best way. World J Crit Care Med. 2015;4(4):278–86.
30. Suzumura E, Figeiro M, Normillo-Silva K, et al. Effects of alveolar recruitment maneuvers on clinical outcomes in patients with acute respiratory distress syndrome: a systematic review and meta-analysis. Intensive Care Med. 2014;40(9):122701240.
31. Rubenfeld G. How much PEEP in acute lung injury. JAMA. 2010;303(9):883–4.
32. ART Investigators Writing Group. Effect of lung recruitment and titrated positive end-expiratory pressure (PEEP) vs low PEEP on mortality in patients with acute respiratory distress syndrome: a randomized clinical trial. JAMA. 2017;318(14):1335–45.
33. Briel M, Meade M, Mercat A, et al. Higher vs lower positive end-expiratory pressure in patients with acute lung injury and acute respiratory distress syndrome: systematic review and meta-analysis. JAMA. 2010;303(9):865–73.
34. Brower R, Lanken P, Malntyre N, et al. Higher versus lower positive end-expiratory pressures in patients with the acute respiratory distress syndrome. N Engl J Med. 2004;351(4):327–36.
35. Guerin C. The preventive role of higher PEEP in treating severely hypoxemic ARDS. Minerva Anesthesiol. 2011;77(8):835–45.
36. Kacmarek R, Villar J, Sulemanji D. Open lung approach for the acute respiratory distress syndrome: a pilot, randomized controlled trial. Crit Care Med. 2016;44(1):32–42.
37. Mercat A, Richard J, Vielle B, et al. Positive end-expiratory pressure setting in adults with acute lung injury and acute respiratory distress syndrome: a randomized controlled trial. JAMA. 2008;299(6):646–55.
38. Deranged Physiology. Optimal PEEP for open lung ventilation in ARDS. http://www.derangedphysiology.com/main/required-reading/respiratory-medicine-and-ventilation/Chapter 5.1.2.1/optimal-peep-open-lung-ventilation-ards. Accessed 14 July 2016.
39. Bautista A, Akca O. Hypercapnia: is it protective in lung injury? Med Gas Res. 2013;3(23):1–6.
40. Amato M, Barbas C, Medeiros D, et al. Effect of a protective-ventilation strategy on mortality in the acute respiratory distress syndrome. N Engl J Med. 1998;338:347–54.
41. Fuchs H, Rossmann N, Schmid MB, et al. Permissive hypercapnia for severe acute respiratory distress syndrome in immunocompromised children: a single center experience. PLoS One. 2017;12(6):e0179974.
42. Nin N, Muriel A, Penuelas O, et al. Severe hypercapnia and out- come of mechanically ventilated patients with moderate or severe acute respiratory distress syndrome. Intensive Care Med. 2017;43:200–8.
43. Cioffi WG, Graves TA, McManus WF, et al. High-frequency percussive ventilation in patients with inhalation injury. J Trauma Injury Infec Crit Care. 1989;29(3):350–4.
44. Cioffi WG Jr, Rue LW 3rd, Graves TA, et al. Prophylactic use of high-frequency percussive ventilation in patients with inhalation injury. Ann Surg. 1991;213(6):575–80; discussion 580-2.
45. Cortiella J, Mlcak R, Herndon D. High frequency percussive ventilation in pediatric patients with inhalation injury. J Burn Care Rehabil. 1999;20(3):232–5.
46. Reper P, Dankaert R, van Hille F, et al. The usefulness of combined high-frequency percussive ventilation during acute respiratory failure after smoke inhalation. Burns. 1998;24(1):34–8.
47. Reper P, Wibaux O, Van Laeke P, et al. High frequency percussive ventilation and conventional ventilation after smoke inhalation: a randomised study. Burns. 2002;28(5):503–8.
48. Carmen B, Cahill T, Warden G. A prospective randomized comparison of the volume diffusive respirator vs conventional ventilation for ventilation of burned children. J Burn Care Rehabil. 2002;23(6):444–8.
49. Chung KK, Wolf SE, Renz EM, et al. High-frequency percussive ventilation and low tidal volume ventilation in burns: a randomized controlled trial. Crit Care Med. 2010;38(10):1970–7.
50. Al Ashry HS, Mansour G, Kalil AC, et al. Incidence of ventilator associated pneumonia in burn patients with inhalation injury treated with high frequency percussive ventilation versus volume control ventilation: a systematic review. Burns. 2016;42(6):1193–200.

51. Eastman A, Holland D, Higgins J, et al. High-frequency percussive ventilation improves oxygenation in trauma patients with acute respiratory distress syndrome: a retrospective review. Am J Surg. 2006;192(2):191–5.
52. Gallagher TJ, Boysen PG, Davidson DD, et al. High-frequency percussive ventilation compared with conventional mechanical ventilation. Crit Care Med. 1989;17(4):364–6.
53. Godet T, Jabaudon M, Blondonnet R, et al. High frequency percussive ventilation increases alveolar recruitment in early acute respiratory distress syndrome: an experimental, physiological and CT scan study. Crit Care. 2018;22(1):3.
54. Hall JJ, Hunt JL, Arnoldo BD, et al. Use of high-frequency percussive ventilation in inhalation injuries. J Burn Care Res. 2007;28(3):396–400.
55. Hiller KN, Morgan CK. High-frequency percussive ventilation for severe inhalation injury. Anesthesiology. 2014;120(4):998.
56. Kacmarek RM, Villar J. Clinical repercussions of high-frequency percussive ventilation: a burning issue. Crit Care Med. 2010;38(10):2069–70.
57. Kunugiyama SK, Schulman CS. High-frequency percussive ventilation using the VDR-4 ventilator: an effective strategy for patients with refractory hypoxemia. AACN Adv Crit Care. 2012;23(4):370–80.
58. Lucangelo U, Antonaglia V, Gullo A, et al. High-frequency percussive ventilation. Crit Care Med. 2005;33(9):2155; author reply 2155–6.
59. Lucangelo U, Fontanesi L, Antonaglia V, et al. High frequency percussive ventilation (HFPV). Principles and technique. Minerva Anestesiol. 2003;69(11):841–8, 848–51.
60. Reper P, Van Bos R, Van Loey K, et al. High frequency percussive ventilation in burn patients: hemodynamics and gas exchange. Burns. 2003;29(6):603–8.
61. Rizkalla NA, Dominick CL, Fitzgerald JC, et al. High-frequency percussive ventilation improves oxygenation and ventilation in pediatric patients with acute respiratory failure. J Crit Care. 2014;29(2):314.e1–7.
62. Salim A, Martin M. High-frequency percussive ventilation. Crit Care Med. 2005;33(3 Suppl):S241–5.
63. Salim A, Miller K, Dangleben D, et al. High-frequency percussive ventilation: an alternative mode of ventilation for head-injured patients with adult respiratory distress syndrome. J Trauma Injury Infect Crit Care. 2004;57(3):542–6.
64. Spapen H, Borremans M, Diltoer M, et al. High-frequency percussive ventilation in severe acute respiratory distress syndrome: a single center experience. J Anaesthesiol Clin Pharmacol. 2014;30(1):65–70.
65. Ferguson N, Slutsky A. Point: high-frequency ventilation is the optimal physiological approach to ventilate ARDS patients. J Appl Physiol. 2008;104(4):1230–1.
66. Bouchut J, Godard J, Claris O. High-frequency oscillatory ventilation. Anesthesiology. 2004;100(4):1007–12.
67. Ferguson ND, Cook D, Guyatt G, et al. High-frequency oscillation in early acute respiratory distress syndrome. N Engl J Med. 2013;368(9):795–805.
68. The HIFI Study Group. High-frequency oscillatory ventilation compared with conventional mechanical ventilation in the treatment of respiratory failure in preterm infants. N Engl J Med. 1989;320(2):88–93.
69. Young D, Lamb S, Shah S, et al. High-frequency oscillation for acute respiratory distress syndrome. N Engl J Med. 2013;368(9):806–13.
70. Sud S, Sud M, Friedrih J, et al. High-frequency ventilation versus conventional ventilation for treatment of acute lung injury and acute respiratory distress syndrome. Cochrane Database Systemic Review. 2013;28(2):CD004085.
71. Andersen FA, Guttormsen AB, Flaatten HK. High frequency oscillatory ventilation in adult patients with acute respiratory distress syndrome—a retrospective study. Acta Anaesthesiol Scand. 2002;46(9):1082–8.
72. Cartotto R. High frequency oscillatory ventilation in burn patients. Acta Anaesthesiol Scand. 2003;47(4):495; author reply 496.
73. Cartotto R. High-frequency oscillatory ventilation (HFOV) in trauma patients. J Trauma Injury Infect Crit Care. 2007;62(5):1315–6.
74. Cartotto R, Cooper AB, Esmond JR, et al. Early clinical experience with high-frequency oscillatory ventilation for ARDS in adult burn patients. J Burn Care Rehabil. 2001;22(5):325–33.
75. Cartotto R, Ellis S, Gomez M, et al. High frequency oscillatory ventilation in burn patients with the acute respiratory distress syndrome. Burns. 2004;30(5):453–63.
76. Cartotto R, Ellis S, Smith T. Use of high-frequency oscillatory ventilation in burn patients. Crit Care Med. 2005;33(3 Suppl):S175–81.
77. Cartotto R, Walia G, Ellis S, et al. Oscillation after inhalation: high frequency oscillatory ventilation in burn patients with the acute respiratory distress syndrome and co-existing smoke inhalation injury. J Burn Care Res. 2009;30(1):119–27.
78. Cooper AB, Islur A, Gomez M, et al. Hypercapnic respiratory failure and partial upper airway obstruction during high frequency oscillatory ventilation in an adult burn patient. Can J Anaesth. 2002;49(7):724–8.
79. Greathouse ST, Hadad I, Zieger M, et al. High-frequency oscillatory ventilators in burn patients: experience of Riley Hospital for Children. J Burn Care Res. 2012;33(3):425–35.
80. Mehta S, Lapinsky SE, Hallett DC, et al. Prospective trial of high-frequency oscillation in adults with acute respiratory distress syndrome. Crit Care Med. 2001;29(7):1360–9.
81. Rowan CM, Cristea O, Greathouse ST, et al. Preemptive use of high-frequency oscillatory ventilation in pediatric burn patients. J Burn Care Res. 2013;34(2):237–42.
82. Walia G, Jada G, Cartotto R. Anesthesia and intraoperative high-frequency oscillatory ventilation during burn surgery. J Burn Care Res. 2011;32(1):118–23.
83. Wang SG, Guo GH, Fu ZH, et al. Comparison of conventional mandatory ventilation and high frequency oscillatory ventilation for treatment of acute lung injury induced by steam inhalation injury. Burns. 2006;32(8):951–6.
84. Dries DJ, Marini JJ. Airway pressure release ventilation. J Burn Care Res. 2009;30(6):929–36.
85. Dries DJ. Key questions in ventilator management of the burn-injured patient (second of two parts). J Burn Care Res. 2009;30(2):211–20.
86. Peek GJ, Clemens F, Elbourne D, et al. CESAR: conventional ventilatory support vs extracorporeal membrane oxygenation for severe adult respiratory failure. BMC Health Serv Res. 2006;6:163.
87. Askegard-Giesmann JR, Besner GE, Fabia R, et al. Extracorporeal membrane oxygenation as a lifesaving modality in the treatment of pediatric patients with burns and respiratory failure. J Pediatr Surg. 2010;45(6):1330–5.
88. Asmussen S, Maybauer DM, Fraser JF, et al. Extracorporeal membrane oxygenation in burn and smoke inhalation injury. Burns. 2013;39(3):429–35.
89. Burke CR, Chan T, McMullan DM. Extracorporeal life support use in adult burn patients. J Burn Care Res. 2017;38(3):174–8.
90. Chou NK, Chen YS, Ko WJ, et al. Application of extracorporeal membrane oxygenation in adult burn patients. Artif Organs. 2001;25(8):622–6.
91. Goretsky MJ, Greenhalgh DG, Warden GD, et al. The use of extracorporeal life support in pediatric burn patients with respiratory failure. J Pediatr Surg. 1995;30(4):620–3.

92. Hilt T, Graves DF, Chernin JM, et al. Successful use of extracorporeal membrane oxygenation to treat severe respiratory failure in a pediatric patient with a scald injury. Crit Care Nurse. 1998;18(6):63–72.
93. Kane TD, Greenhalgh DG, Warden GD, et al. Pediatric burn patients with respiratory failure: predictors of outcome with the use of extracorporeal life support. J Burn Care Rehabil. 1999;20(2):145–50.
94. Lessin MS, el-Eid SE, Klein MD, et al. Extracorporeal membrane oxygenation in pediatric respiratory failure secondary to smoke inhalation injury. J Pediatr Surg. 1996;31(9):1285–7.
95. Nelson J, Cairns B, Charles A. Early extracorporeal life support as rescue therapy for severe acute respiratory distress syndrome after inhalation injury. J Burn Care Res. 2009;30(6):1035–8.
96. Nosanov LB, McLawhorn MM, Vigiola Cruz M, et al. A National Perspective on ECMO utilization use in patients with burn injury. J Burn Care Res. 2017;39(1):10–4.
97. O'Toole G, Peek G, Jaffe W, et al. Extracorporeal membrane oxygenation in the treatment of inhalation injuries. Burns. 1998;24(6):562–5.
98. Ombrellaro M, Goldthorn JF, Harnar TJ, et al. Extracorporeal life support for the treatment of adult respiratory distress syndrome after burn injury. Surgery. 1994;115(4):523–6.
99. Patton ML, Simone MR, Kraut JD, et al. Successful utilization of ECMO to treat an adult burn patient with ARDS. Burns. 1998;24(6):566–8.
100. Pierre EJ, Zwischenberger JB, Angel C, et al. Extracorporeal membrane oxygenation in the treatment of respiratory failure in pediatric patients with burns. J Burn Care Rehabil. 1998;19(2):131–4.
101. Soussi S, Gallais P, Kachatryan L, et al. Extracorporeal membrane oxygenation in burn patients with refractory acute respiratory distress syndrome leads to 28% 90-day survival. Intensive Care Med. 2016;42(11):1826–7.
102. Nayyar A, Charles AG, Hultman CS. Management of pulmonary failure after burn injury: from VDR to ECMO. Clin Plast Surg. 2017;44(3):513–20.
103. Jacob S, Zhu Y, Jonkam C, et al. Effect of bronchodilators on bronchial gland cell proliferation after inhalation and burn injury in sheep. J Burn Care Res. 2013;34(4):386–93.
104. Jonkam C, Zhu Y, Jacob S, et al. Assessment of combined muscarinic antagonist and fibrinolytic therapy for inhalation injury. J Burn Care Res. 2012;33(4):524–31.
105. Lopez E, Fujiwara O, Lima-Lopez F, et al. Nebulized epinephrine limits pulmonary vascular hyperpermeability to water and protein in ovine with burn and smoke inhalation injury. Crit Care Med. 2016;44(2):e89–96.
106. AC M, Rivero A, Ziad S, et al. Influence of nebulized unfractionated heparin and N-acetylcysteine in acute lung injury after smoke inhalation. J Burn Care Rehabil. 2009;30:249–56.
107. Desai M, Mlcak R, Richardson J, et al. Reduction on mortality in pediatric patients with inhalation injury with aerosolized heparin/acetylcysteine therapy. J Burn Care Rehabil. 1998;19:210–2.
108. Holt J, Saffle J, Morris S. Use of inhaled heparin/N-acetylcysteine in inhalation injury: does it help? J Burn Care Res. 2008;29:192–5.
109. McIntire AM, Harris SA, Whitten JA, et al. Outcomes following the use of nebulized heparin for inhalation injury (HIHI Study). J Burn Care Res. 2017;38(1):45–52.
110. Miller AC, Elamin EM, Suffredini AF. Inhaled anticoagulation regimens for the treatment of smoke inhalation-associated acute lung injury: a systematic review. Crit Care Med. 2014;42(2):413–9.
111. Konukoglu D, Cetinkale O, Bulan R. Effects of N-acetylcysteine on lung glutathione levels in rats after burn injury. Burns. 1997;23(7–8):541–4.
112. Brown M, SDesai M, Traber L, et al. Dimethylsulfoxide with heparin in the treatment of smoke inhalation injury. J Burn Care Rehabil. 1988;9:22–5.
113. Sadowska A, Verbraecken J, D'arquennes K, et al. Role of N-acetylcysteine in the management of COPD. Ther Clin Risk Manag. 2006;2(1):3–18.
114. Younan D, Griffin R, Swain T, et al. A comparison of clinical characteristics and outcomes of ventilator-associated pneumonias among burn patients by diagnostic criteria set. Shock. 2017;48(6):624–8.
115. Santucci S, Gobara S, Santos S, et al. Infections in a burn intensive care unit: experience of seven years. J Hosp Infections. 2003;53:6–13.
116. Wibbenmeyer L, Danks RR, Faucher LD, et al. Prospective analysis of resistance in a burn population. J Burn Care Res. 2006;27:152–60.

18 Pathophysiology of Burn Injuries

Marc G. Jeschke and Gerd G. Gauglitz

Burn injury represents a significant problem worldwide. More than one million burn injuries occur annually in the United States. Although most of these burn injuries are minor, approximately 40,000–60,000 burn patients require admission to a hospital or major burn center for appropriate treatment every year [1]. The devastating consequences of burns have been recognized by the medical community and significant amounts of resources and research have been dedicated, successfully improving these dismal statistics: Recent reports revealed a 50% decline in burn-related deaths and hospital admissions in the United States over the last 20 years; mainly due to effective prevention strategies, decreasing the number and severity of burns [2, 3]. Advances in therapy strategies, due to improved understanding of resuscitation, enhanced wound coverage, better support of hypermetabolic response to injury, more appropriate infection control and improved treatment of inhalation injury, based on better understanding of the pathophysiologic responses after burn injury have further improved the clinical outcome of this unique patient population over the past years. This chapter describes the present understanding of the pathophysiology of a burn injury including both the local and systemic responses, focusing on the many facets of organ and systemic effects directly resulting from hypovolemia and circulating mediators following burn trauma.

M. G. Jeschke (✉)
Faculty of Medicine, Institute of Medical Science, University of Toronto, Toronto, ON, Canada

Biological Sciences, Sunnybrook Research Institute, Toronto, ON, Canada

Ross Tilley Burn Centre, Sunnybrook Health Sciences Centre, Sunnybrook Hospital, Toronto, ON, Canada

Division of Plastic and Reconstructive Surgery, Department of Surgery, Faculty of Medicine, University of Toronto, Toronto, ON, Canada

Department of Immunology, Faculty of Medicine, University of Toronto, Toronto, ON, Canada
e-mail: Marc.Jeschke@sunnybrook.ca

G. G. Gauglitz
Department of Dermatology and Allergology, Ludwig Maximilians University, Munich, Germany
e-mail: Gerd.Gauglitz@med.uni-muenchen.de

18.1 Local Changes

Locally, thermal injury causes coagulative necrosis of the epidermis and underlying tissues, with the depth of injury dependent upon the temperature to which the skin is exposed, the specific heat of the causative agent, and the duration of exposure.

Burns are classified into five different causal categories/etiologies and depths of injury. The causes include injury from flame (fire), hot liquids (scald), contact with hot or cold objects, chemical exposure, and/or conduction of electricity. The first three induce cellular damage by the transfer of energy, which induces coagulative necrosis. Chemical burns and electrical burns cause direct injury to cellular membranes in addition to the transfer of heat.

The skin, which is the largest organ on the human body, provides a staunch barrier in the transfer of energy to deeper tissues, thus confining much of the injury to this layer. Once the inciting focus is removed, however, the response of local tissues can lead to injury in the deeper layers. The area of cutaneous or superficial injury has been divided into three zones: zone of coagulation, zone of stasis, and zone of hyperemia. The necrotic area of burn where cells have been disrupted is termed the *zone of coagulation*. This tissue is irreversibly damaged at the time of injury. The area immediately surrounding the necrotic zone has a moderate degree of insult with decreased tissue perfusion. This is termed the *zone of stasis* and, depending on the wound environment, can either survive or go on to coagulative necrosis. The zone of stasis is associated with vascular damage and vessel leakage [4]. Thromboxane A_2, a potent vasoconstrictor, is present in high

M. G. Jeschke et al. (eds.), *Handbook of Burns Volume 1*, https://doi.org/10.1007/978-3-030-18940-2_18

concentrations in burn wounds, and local application of inhibitors improves blood flow and decreases the zone of stasis. Antioxidants, bradykinin antagonists, and subatmospheric wound pressures also improve blood flow and affect the depth of injury [5–8]. Local endothelial interactions with neutrophils mediate some of the local inflammatory responses associated with the zone of stasis. Treatment directed at the control of local inflammation immediately after injury may spare the zone of stasis, indicated by studies demonstrating the blockage of leukocyte adherence with anti-CD18 or anti-intercellular adhesion molecules monoclonal antibodies improves tissue perfusion and tissue survival in animal models [9]. The last area is the *zone of hyperemia,* which is characterized by vasodilation from inflammation surrounding the burn wound. This region contains the clearly viable tissue from which the healing process begins and is generally not at risk for further necrosis.

18.1.1 Burn Depth

Local changes appear in the tissue when the amount of absorbed heat exceeds the body system's compensatory mechanisms. On a molecular level protein degradation begins at a temperature of 40 °C. This degradation leads to alterations in cell homeostasis. This is reversible if the temperature is lowered. Starting at 45 °C proteins are permanently denatured. This is reflected by local tissue necrosis. The speed with which permanent tissue damage can appear is dependent on time exposed and temperature:

45–51 °C	within minutes
51 and 70 °C	within seconds
Above 70 °C	less than a second

The depth and severity of the burn are also determined by the ability of the contact material to transfer heat, a factor referred to as the specific heat. This is especially important in scald and contact burns. The knowledge about the material type allows for a more accurate estimate of tissue damage.

Definition: Burn depth is determined by the time of exposure, the temperature at which the burn occurred, and the caloric equivalent of the burn media.

Another determinant of the severity of burn is the location of the burn wound and the age of the burn patient. The thickness of the skin layers increases from the age of 5 up to the age of 50. In elderly patients, the thickness starts to decrease at the age of 65. The epidermis can vary by location from 0.03 up to 0.4 mm. The depth of burn varies depending on the degree of tissue damage. Burn depth is classified into degree of injury in the epidermis, dermis, subcutaneous fat, and underlying structures.

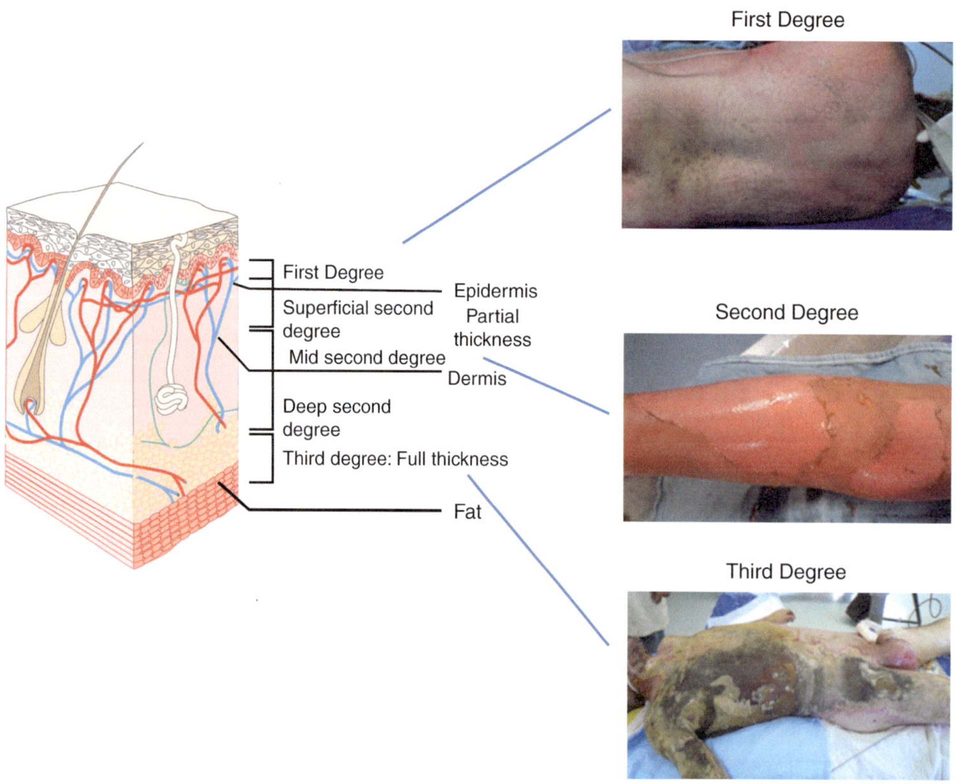

(a) *I degree: Superficial burn of the epidermis*

First-degree burns are painful, erythematous, and blanch to the touch with an intact epidermal barrier. Examples include sunburn or a minor scald from a kitchen accident. These burns do not result in scarring, and treatment is aimed at comfort with the use of topical soothing salves with or without aloe and oral nonsteroidal anti-inflammatory agents.

(b) *IIa degree: Burn including epidermis and superficial dermis*

(c) *IIb degree: Burn including epidermis and deep dermis*

Second-degree burns are divided into two types: superficial and deep. All second-degree burns have some degree of dermal damage, by definition, and the division is based on the depth of injury into the dermis. Superficial dermal burns are erythematous, painful, blanch to touch, and often blister. Examples include scald injuries from overheated bathtub water and flash flame burns. These wounds spontaneously re-epithelialize from retained epidermal structures in the rete ridges, hair follicles, and sweat glands in 1–2 weeks. After healing, these burns may have some slight skin discoloration over the long term. Deep dermal burns into the reticular dermis appear more pale and mottled, do not blanch to touch, but remain painful to pinprick. These burns heal in 2–5 weeks by re-epithelialization from hair follicles and sweat gland keratinocytes, often with severe scarring as a result of the loss of dermis.

(d) *III degree: Burn including epidermis and dermis and subcuticular layer*

Third-degree burns are full-thickness through the epidermis and dermis and are characterized by a hard, leathery eschar that is painless and black, white, or cherry red. No epidermal or dermal appendages remain; thus, these wounds must heal by re-epithelialization from the wound edges. Deep dermal and full-thickness burns require excision with skin grafting from the patient to heal the wounds in a timely fashion.

(e) *IV degree: All dermal layers including fascia, muscles, and/or bones*

Fourth-degree burns involve other organs beneath the skin, such as muscle, bone, and brain.

Currently, burn depth is most accurately assessed by judgment of experienced practitioners. Accurate depth determination is critical to wound healing as wounds that will heal with local treatment are treated differently than those requiring operative intervention. Examination of the entire wound by the physicians ultimately responsible for their management then is the gold standard used to guide further treatment decisions. New technologies, such as the multi-sensor laser Doppler flow-meter, hold promise for quantitatively determining burn depth [10].

18.1.2 Burn Size

Determination of burn size estimates the extent of injury. Burn size is generally assessed by the "rule of nines." In adults, each upper extremity and the head and neck are 9% of the TBSA, the lower extremities and the anterior and posterior trunk are 18% each, and the perineum and genitalia are assumed to be 1% of the TBSA. Another method of estimating smaller burns is to equate the area of the open hand (including the palm and the extended fingers) of the patient to be approximately 1% TBSA and then to transpose that measurement visually onto the wound for a determination of its size. This method is crucial when evaluating burns of mixed distribution.

Children have a relatively larger portion of the body surface area in the head and neck, which is compensated for by a relatively smaller surface area in the lower extremities. Infants have 21% of the TBSA in the head and neck and 13% in each leg, which incrementally approaches the adult proportions with increasing age. The Berkow formula is used to accurately determine burn size in children.

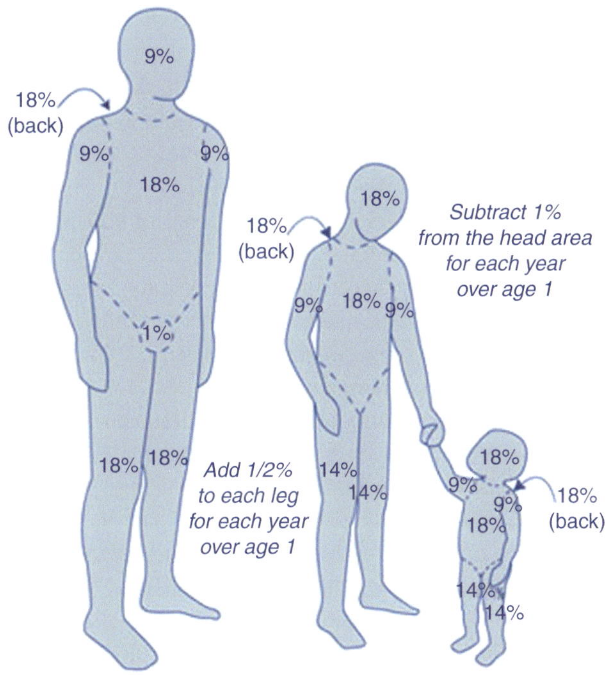

18.1.2.1 Etiology

The causes include injury from flame (fire), hot liquids (scald), contact with hot or cold objects, chemical exposure, and/or conduction of electricity. The first three induce cellular damage by the transfer of energy, which induces a coagulation necrosis. Chemical burns and electrical burns cause direct injury to cellular membranes in addition to the transfer of heat.

18.2 Systemic Changes

The release of cytokines and other inflammatory mediators at the site of injury has a systemic effect once the burn reaches 30% of total body surface area (TBSA). Cutaneous thermal injury greater than one-third of the total body surface area invariably results in the severe and unique derangements of cardiovascular function called burn shock. Shock is an abnormal physiologic state in which tissue perfusion is insufficient to maintain adequate delivery of oxygen and nutrients and removal of cellular waste products. Before the nineteenth century, investigators demonstrated that after a burn, fluid is lost from the blood and blood becomes thicker; and in 1897, saline infusions for severe burns were first advocated [11, 12]. However, a more complete understanding of burn pathophysiology was not reached until the work of Frank Underhill [13]. He found that unresuscitated burn shock correlates with increased hematocrit values in burned patients, which are secondary to fluid and electrolyte loss after burn injury. Increased hematocrit values occurring shortly after severe burn were interpreted as a plasma volume deficit. Cope and Moore showed that the hypovolemia of burn injury resulted from fluid and protein translocation into both burned and non-burned tissues [14].

Over the last 80 years an extensive record of both animal and clinical studies has established the importance of fluid resuscitation for burn shock. Investigations have focused on correcting the rapid and massive fluid sequestration in the burn wound and the resultant hypovolemia. The peer-reviewed literature contains a large experimental and clinical database on the circulatory and microcirculatory alterations associated with burn shock and edema generation in both the burn wound and non-burned tissues. During the last 40 years, research has focused on identifying and defining the release mechanisms and effects of the many inflammatory mediators produced and released after burn injury [15].

It is now well recognized that burn shock is a complex process of circulatory and microcirculatory dysfunction that is not easily or fully repaired by fluid resuscitation. Severe burn injury results in significant hypovolemic shock and substantial tissue trauma, both of which cause the formation and release of many local and systemic mediators [16–18]. Burn shock results from the interplay of hypovolemia and the release of multiple mediators of inflammation with effects on both the microcirculation as well as the function of the heart, large vessels, and lungs. Subsequently, burn shock continues as a significant pathophysiologic state, even if hypovolemia is corrected. Increases in pulmonary and systemic vascular resistance (SVR) and myocardial depression occur despite adequate preload and volume support [18–22]. Such cardiovascular dysfunctions can further exacerbate the whole body inflammatory response into a vicious cycle of accelerating organ dysfunction [17, 18, 23]. Hemorrhagic hypovolemia with severe mechanical trauma can provoke a similar form of shock.

18.2.1 Hypovolemia and Rapid Edema Formation

Burn injury causes extravasation of plasma into the burn wound and the surrounding tissues. Extensive burn injuries are hypovolemic in nature and characterized by the hemodynamic changes similar to those that occur after hemorrhage, including decreased plasma volume, cardiac output, urine output, and an increased systemic vascular resistance with resultant reduced peripheral blood flow [16, 18, 24–26]. However, as opposed to a fall in hematocrit with hemorrhagic hypovolemia due to transcapillary refill an increase in hematocrit and hemoglobin concentration will often appear even with adequate fluid resuscitation. As in the treatment of other forms of hypovolemic shock, the primary initial therapeutic goal is to quickly restore vascular volume and to preserve tissue perfusion in order to minimize tissue ischemia. In extensive burns (>25%TBSA), fluid resuscitation is complicated not only by the severe burn wound edema, but also by extravasated and sequestered fluid and protein in non-burned soft tissue. Large volumes of resuscitation solutions are required to maintain vascular volume during the first several hours after an extensive burn. Data suggests that despite fluid resuscitation normal blood volume is not restored until 24–36 h after large burns [27].

Edema develops when the rate by which fluid is filtered out of the microvessels exceeds the flow in the lymph vessels draining the same tissue mass. Edema formation often follows a biphasic pattern. An immediate and rapid increase in the water content of burn tissue is seen in the first hour after burn injury [25, 28]. A second and more gradual increase in fluid flux of both the burned skin and non-burned soft tissue occurs during the first 12–24 h following burn trauma [17, 28]. The amount of edema formation in burned skin depends on the type and extent of injury [25, 29] and whether fluid resuscitation is provided as well as the type and volume of fluid administered [30]. However, fluid resuscitation elevates blood flow and capillary pressure contributing to further fluid extravasation. Without sustained delivery of fluid into the circulation edema fluid is somewhat self-limited as plasma volume and capillary pressure decrease. The edema development in thermal-injured skin is characterized by the extreme rapid onset of tissue water content, which can double within the first hour after burn [25, 31]. Leape and colleagues found a 70–80% water content increase in a full-thickness burn wound 30 min after burn injury with 90% of this change occurring in the first 5 min [26, 32, 33]. There was little increase in burn wound water content after the first hour in the nonresuscitated animals. In resuscitated animals or animals with small wounds, adequate tissue perfusion continues to "feed" the edema for several hours. Demling and others used dichromatic absorptiometry to measure edema development during the first week after an experimental partial-thickness burn injury on one hind limb in sheep [28]. Even though edema was rapid with over 50% occurring in the first hour, maximum water content did not occur until 12–24 h after burn injury.

18.2.2 Altered Cellular Membranes and Cellular Edema

In addition to a loss of capillary endothelial integrity, thermal injury also causes change in the cellular membranes. Baxter found in burns of >30% a systemic decrease in cellular transmembrane potentials as measured in skeletal muscle away from the site of injury [20]. It would be expected that the directly injured cell would have a damaged cell membrane, increasing sodium and potassium fluxes, resulting in cell swelling. However, this process also appears in cells that are not directly heat-injured. Micropuncture techniques have demonstrated partial depolarization in the normal skeletal muscle membrane potential of −90 mV to levels of −70–−80 mV; cell death occurs at −60 mV. The decrease in membrane potentials is associated with an increase in intracellular water and sodium [34–36]. Similar alterations in skeletal membrane functions and cellular edema have been reported in hemorrhagic shock [34, 36] also in the cardiac, liver, and endothelial cells [37–39]. Early investigators of this phenomenon postulated that a decrease in ATP levels or ATPase activity was the mechanism for membrane depolarization, however, other research suggests that it may result from an increased sodium conductance in membranes or an increase in sodium-hydrogen antiport activity [35, 38]. Resuscitation of hemorrhage rapidly restores depolarized membrane potentials to normal, but resuscitation of burn injury only partially restores the membrane potential and intracellular sodium concentrations to normal levels, demonstrating that hypovolemia alone is not totally responsible for the cellular swelling seen in burn shock [40]. A circulating shock factor(s) is likely to be responsible for the membrane depolarization, [41–43] but surprisingly, the molecular characterization of such a circulating factor has not been elucidated; suggesting that it has a complex structure. Data suggests it has a large molecular weight, >80 kDalton [44]. Membrane depolarization may be caused by different factors in different states of shock. Very little is known about the time course of the changes in membrane potential in clinical burns. More importantly, we do not know the extent to which the altered membrane potentials affect total volume requirements and organ function in burn injury or even shock in general.

18.2.3 Mediators of Burn Injury

Many mediators have been proposed to account for the changes in permeability after burn, including histamine, b serotonin, bradykinin, prostaglandins, leukotrienes, platelet-activating factor, and catecholamines, among others [10, 45–49]. The exact mechanism(s) of mediator-induced injury are of considerable clinical importance, as this understanding would allow for the development of pharmacologic modulation of burn edema and shock by mediator inhibition.

Histamine: Histamine is most likely to be the mediator responsible for the early phase of increased microvascular permeability seen immediately after burn. Histamine causes large endothelial gaps to transiently form as a result of the contraction of venular endothelial cells [50]. Histamine is released from mast cells in thermal-injured skin; however, the increase in histamine levels and its actions are only transient. Histamine also can cause the rise in capillary pressure (Pc) by arteriolar dilation and venular contraction. Statistically significant reductions in burn edema have been achieved with histamine blockers and mast cell stabilizers when tested in acute animal models [50]. Friedl et al. demonstrated that the pathogenesis of burn edema in the skin of rats appears to be related to the interaction of histamine with xanthine oxidase and oxygen radicals [51]. Histamine and its metabolic derivatives increased the catalytic activity of xanthine oxidase (but not xanthine dehydrogenase) in rat plasma and in rat pulmonary artery endothelial cells. In thermally injured rats, levels of plasma histamine and xanthine oxidase rose in parallel, in association with the uric acid increase. Burn edema was greatly attenuated by treating rats with the mast cell stabilizer, cromolyn, complement depletion or the H_2 receptor antagonist, cimetidine; but was unaffected by neutrophil depletion [52–54]. Despite encouraging results in animals, beneficial antihistamine treatment of human burn injury has not been demonstrated although antihistamines are administered to reduce risk of gastric ulcers.

Prostaglandins: Prostaglandins are potent vasoactive autocoids synthesized from the arachidonic acid released from burned tissue and inflammatory cells and contribute to the inflammatory response of burn injury [55, 56]. Macrophages and neutrophils are activated through the body; infiltrate the wound and release prostaglandin as well as thromboxanes, leukotrienes, and interleukin-1. These wound mediators have both local and systemic effects. Prostaglandin E2 (PGE2) and leukotrienes LB_4 and LD_4 directly and indirectly increase microvascular permeability [57]. Prostacyclin (PGI2) is produced in burn injury and is also a vasodilator, but also may cause direct increases in capillary permeability. PGE2 appears to be one of the more potent inflammatory prostaglandins, causing the post-burn vasodilation in wounds, which, when coupled with the increased microvascular permeability amplifies edema formation [58, 59].

Thromboxane: Thromboxane A_2 (TXA_2) and its metabolite, thromboxane B_2 (TXB_2) are produced locally in the burn wound by platelets [50]. Vasoconstrictor thromboxanes may be less important in edema formation; however, by decreasing blood flow they can contribute to a growing zone of ischemia under the burn wound and can cause the conversion of a partial-thickness wound to a deeper full-thickness wound. The serum level of TXA and TXA_2/PGI_2 ratios are increased significantly in burn patients [60]. Heggers showed the release of TXB_2 at the burn wound was associated with local tissue ischemia, and that thromboxane inhibitors prevented the progressive dermal ischemia associated with thermal injury and thromboxane release [61, 62]. The TXA_2 synthesis inhibitor anisodamine also showed beneficial macrocirculatory effects by restoring the hemodynamic and rheological disturbances towards normal. Demling showed that topically applied ibuprofen (which inhibits the synthesis of prostaglandins and thromboxanes) decreases both local edema and prostanoid production in burned tissue without altering systemic production [63]. On the other hand, systemic administration of ibuprofen did not modify early edema, but did attenuate the post-burn vasoconstriction that impaired adequate oxygen delivery to tissue in burned sheep [64]. Although cyclooxgenase inhibitors have been used after burn injury, neither their convincing benefit, nor their routine clinical use has been reported.

Kinins: Bradykinin is a local mediator of inflammation that increases venular permeability. It is likely that bradykinin production is increased after burn injury, but its detection in blood or lymph can be difficult owing to the simultaneous increase in kininase activity and the rapid inactivation of free kinins. The generalized inflammatory response after burn injury favors the release of bradykinin [65]. Pretreatment of burn-injured animals with aprotinin, a general protease inhibitor, should have decreased the release of free kinin, but no effect on edema was noted [66]. On the other hand, pretreatment with a specific bradykinin receptor antagonist reduced edema in full-thickness burn wound in rabbits [8].

Serotonin: Serotonin is released early after burn injury [67]. This agent is a smooth-muscle constrictor of large blood vessels. Antiserotonin agents such as ketanserin have been found to decrease peripheral vascular resistance after burn injury, but have not been reported to decrease edema [67]. On the other hand, the pretreatment effect of methysergide, a serotonin antagonist, reduces hyperemic or increases blood flow response in the burn wounds of rabbits, along with reducing the burn edema [8]. Methysergide did not prevent increases in the capillary reflection coefficient or permeability [68]. Ferrara and colleagues found a dose-dependent reduction of burn edema when methysergide was given pre-burn to dogs, but claimed that this was not attributable to blunting of the regional vasodilator response [68]. Zhang et al. reported a reduction in nonnutritive skin blood flow after methysergide administration to burned rabbits [69].

Catecholamines: Circulating catecholamines epinephrine and norepinephrine are released in massive amounts after burn injury [17, 70, 71]. On the arteriolar side of the microvessels, these agents cause vasoconstriction via alpha 1 receptor activation, which tends to reduce capillary pressure, particularly when combined with the hypovolemia and the reduced venous pressure of burn shock [50]. Reduced capillary pressure may limit edema and induce interstitial fluid to reabsorb from non-burned skin, skeletal muscle, and visceral organs in nonresuscitated burn shock. Further, catecholamines, via β-agonist activity, may also partially inhibit increased capillary permeability induced by histamine and bradykinin [50]. These potentially beneficial effects of catecholamines may not be operative in directly injured tissue and may also be offset in non-burned tissue by the deleterious vasoconstrictor and ischemic effects. The hemodynamic effects of catecholamines will be discussed later in the chapter.

Oxygen Radicals: Oxygen radicals play an important inflammatory role in all types of shock, including burn. These short-lived elements are highly unstable reactive metabolites of oxygen; each one has an unpaired electron, creating them into strong oxidizing agents [72]. Superoxide anion (O_2^-), hydrogen peroxide (H_2O_2), and hydroxyl ion (OH^-) are produced and released by activated neutrophils after any inflammatory reaction or reperfusion of ischemic tissue. The hydroxyl ion is believed to be the most potent and damaging of the three. The formation of the hydroxyl radical requires free ferrous iron (Fe_2) and H_2O_2. Evidence that these agents are formed after burn injury is the increased lipid peroxidation found in circulating red blood cells and biopsied tissue [53, 72, 73]. Demling showed that large doses of deferoxamine (DFO), an iron chelator, when used for resuscitation of 40% TBSA in sheep, prevented systemic lipid peroxidation and decreased the vascular leak in non-burned tissue while also increasing oxygen utilization [74]. However, DFO may have accentuated burned tissue edema, possibly by increasing the perfusion of burned tissue.

Nitric oxide (NO) simultaneously generated with the superoxide anion can lead to the formation of peroxynitrite ($ONOO^-$). The presence of nitrotyrosine in burned skin found in the first few hours after injury suggests that peroxynitrite may play a deleterious role in burn edema [75]. On the other hand, the blockade of NO synthase did not reduce burn edema, while treatment with the NO precursor arginine reduces burn edema [76]. NO may be important for maintaining perfusion and limiting the zone of stasis in burned skin [77]. Although the pro- and anti-inflammatory roles of NO remain controversial, it would appear that the acute beneficial effects of NO generation out-weigh any deleterious effect in burn shock.

Antioxidants, namely agents that either directly bind to the oxygen radicals (scavengers) or cause their further metabolism, have been evaluated in several experimental studies [78, 79]. Catalase, which removes H_2O_2 and superoxide dismutase (SOD), which removes radical O_{2-}, have been reported to decrease the vascular loss of plasma after burn injury in dogs and rats [53, 78].

The plasma of thermally injured rats showed dramatic increases in levels of xanthine oxidase activity, with peak values appearing as early as 15 min after thermal injury. Excision of the burned skin immediately after the thermal injury significantly diminished the increase in plasma xanthine oxidase activity [51, 53]. The skin permeability changes were attenuated by treating the animals with antioxidants (catalase, SOD, dimethyl sulfoxide, dimethylthiourea) or an iron chelator (DFO), thus supporting the role of oxygen radicals in the development of vascular injury as defined by increased vascular permeability [53]. Allopurinol, a xanthine oxidase inhibitor, markedly reduced both burn lymph flow and levels of circulating lipid peroxides, and further prevented all pulmonary lipid peroxidation and inflammation. This suggests that the release of oxidants from burned tissue was in part responsible for local burn edema, as well as distant inflammation and oxidant release [73]. The failure of neutrophil depletion to protect against the vascular permeability changes and the protective effects of the xanthine oxidase inhibitors (allopurinol and lodoxamide tromethamine) suggests that plasma xanthine oxidase is the more likely source of the oxygen radicals involved in the formation of burn edema. These oxygen radicals can increase vascular permeability by damaging microvascular endothelial cells [51, 53]. The use of antioxidants has been extensively investigated in animals, and some clinical trials suggest benefit. Antioxidants (vitamin C and E) are routinely administered to patients at many burn centers. High doses of antioxidant ascorbic acid (vitamin C) have been found to be efficacious in reducing fluid needs in burn-injured experimental animals when administered post-burn [80–82]. The use of high doses (10–20 g per day) of vitamin C was shown to be effective in one clinical trial, but ineffective in another [83, 84]. High dose vitamin C has not received wide clinical usage.

Platelet Aggregation Factor: Platelet aggregation (or activating) factor (PAF) can increase capillary permeability and is released after burn injury [66, 85]. Ono and colleagues showed in scald-injured rabbits that TCV-309 (Takeda Pharmaceutical Co Ltd., Japan), a PAF antagonist, infused soon after burn injury blocked edema formation in the wound and significantly inhibited PAF increase in the damaged tissue in a dose-dependent manner. In contrast, the superoxide dismutase content in the group treated with TCV-309 was significantly higher than that of the control group [85]. These findings suggest that the administration of large doses of a PAF antagonist immediately after injury may reduce burn wound edema and the subsequent degree of burn shock by suppressing PAF and superoxide radical formation.

Angiotensin II and Vasopressin: Angiotensin II and vasopressin or antidiuretic hormone (ADH) are two hormones that participate in the normal regulation of extracellular fluid volume by controlling sodium balance and osmolality through renal function and thirst [50]. However, during burn shock where sympathetic tone is high and volume receptors are stimulated, both hormones can be found in supranormal levels in the blood. Both are potent vasoconstrictors of terminal arterioles with little effect on the venules. Angiotensin II may be responsible for the selective gut and mucosal ischemia, which can cause translocation of endotoxins and bacteria and the development of sepsis and even multi-organ failure [86, 87]. In severely burn-injured patients, angiotensin II levels were elevated two to eight times normal in the first 1–5 days after burn injury with peak levels occurring on day 3 [88]. Vasopressin had peak levels of 50 times normal upon admission and declined towards normal over the first 5 days after burn injury. Vasopressin, along with catecholamines may be largely responsible for increased system vascular resistance and left heart afterload, which can occur in resuscitated burn shock. Sun and others used vasopressin-receptor antagonist in rats with burn shock to improve hemodynamics and survival time, while vasopressin infusion exacerbated burn shock [89].

Corticotropin-releasing Factor: Corticotropin-releasing factor (CRF) has proven to be efficacious in reducing protein extravasation and edema in burned rat paw. CRF may be a powerful natural inhibitory mediator of the acute inflammatory response of the skin to thermal injury [90].

18.2.3.1 Hemodynamic Consequences of Acute Burns

The cause of reduced cardiac output (CO) during the resuscitative phase of burn injury has been the subject of considerable debate. There is an immediate depression of cardiac output before any detectable reduction in plasma volume. The rapidity of this response suggests a neurogenic response to receptors in the thermally injured skin or increased circulating vasoconstrictor mediators. Soon after injury a developing hypovolemia and reduced venous return undeniably contribute to the reduced cardiac output. The subsequent persistence of reduced CO after apparently adequate fluid therapy, as evidenced by a reduction in heart rate and restoration of both arterial blood pressure and urinary output, has been attributed to circulating myocardial depressant factor(s), which possibly originates from the burn wound [21, 22]. Demling and colleagues showed a 15% reduction in CO despite an aggressive volume replacement protocol after a 40% scald burn in sheep [28]. However, there are also sustained increases in catecholamine secretion and elevated systemic vascular resistance for up to 5 days after burn injury [70, 88]. Michie and others measured CO and SVR in anesthetized dogs resuscitated after burn injury [91]. They found that CO fell shortly after injury and then returned towards normal, however, reduced CO did not parallel the blood volume deficit. They concluded that the depression of CO resulted not only from decreased blood volume and venous return, but also from an increased SVR and from the presence of a circulating myocardial depressant substance. Thus, there are multiple factors that can significantly reduce CO after burn injury. However, resuscitated patients suffering major burn injury can also have supranormal CO from 2 to 6 days post-injury. This is secondary to the establishment of a hypermetabolic state.

18.2.3.2 Hypermetabolic Response to Burn Injury

Marked and sustained increases in catecholamine, glucocorticoid, glucagon, and dopamine secretion are thought to initiate the cascade of events leading to the acute hypermetabolic response with its ensuing catabolic state [92–100]. The cause of this complex response is not well understood. However, interleukins 1 and 6, platelet-activating factor, tumor necrosis factor (TNF), endotoxin, neutrophil-adherence complexes, reactive oxygen species, nitric oxide, and coagulation as well as complement cascades have also been implicated in regulating this response to burn injury [101]. Once these cascades are initiated, their mediators and by-products appear to stimulate the persistent and increased metabolic rate associated with altered glucose metabolism seen after severe burn injury [102].

Several studies have indicated that these metabolic phenomena post-burn occur in a timely manner, suggesting two distinct pattern of metabolic regulation following injury [103]. The first phase occurs within the first 48 h of injury and has classically been called the "ebb phase" [103, 104], characterized by decreases in cardiac output, oxygen consumption, and metabolic rate as well as impaired glucose tolerance associated with its hyperglycemic state. These metabolic variables gradually increase within the first 5 days post-injury to a plateau phase (called the "flow" phase), characteristically associated with hyperdynamic circulation and the above-mentioned hypermetabolic state. Insulin release during this time period was found to be twice that of controls in response to glucose load [105, 106] and plasma glucose levels are markedly elevated, indicating the development of an insulin resistance [106, 107]. Current understanding has been that these metabolic alterations resolve soon after complete wound closure. However, recent studies found that the hypermetabolic response to burn injury may last for more than 12 months after the initial event [92, 93, 100, 108]. We found in recent studies that sustained hypermetabolic alterations post-burn, indicated by persistent elevations of total urine cortisol levels, serum cytokines, catecholamines, and basal energy requirements, were accompanied by impaired glucose metabolism and insulin sensitivity that persisted for up to 3 years after the initial burn injury [109].

A 10–50-fold elevation of plasma catecholamines and corticosteroid levels occur in major burns which persist up to 3 years post-injury [49, 109–112]. Cytokine levels peak immediately after burn, approaching normal levels only after 1-month post-injury. Constitutive and acute phase proteins are altered beginning 5–7 days post-burn and remain abnormal throughout acute hospital stay. Serum IGF-I, IGFBP-3, parathyroid hormone, and Osteocalcin drop immediately after the injury tenfold, and remain significantly decreased up to 6 months post-burn compared to normal levels [111]. Sex hormones and endogenous growth hormone levels decrease around 3 weeks post-burn [111].

For severely burned patients, the resting metabolic rate at thermal neutral temperature (30 °C) exceeds 140% of normal at admission, reduces to 130% once the wounds are fully healed, then to 120% at 6 months after injury, and 110% at 12 months post-burn [92, 111]. Increases in catabolism result in loss of total body protein, decreased immune defenses, and decreased wound healing [92].

Immediately post-burn patients have low cardiac output characteristic of early shock [113] However, 3–4 days post-burn, cardiac outputs are greater than 1.5 times that of non-burned, healthy volunteers [111]. Heart rates of pediatric burn patients' approach 1.6 times that of non-burned, healthy volunteers [114]. Post-burn, patients have increased cardiac work [110, 115]. Myocardial oxygen consumption surpasses that of marathon runners and is sustained well into rehabilitative period [115, 116]. There is profound hepatomegaly after injury. The liver increases its size by 225% of normal by 2 weeks post-burn and remains enlarged at discharge by 200% of normal [111].

Post-burn, muscle protein is degraded much faster than it is synthesized [111, 114]. Net protein loss leads to loss of lean body mass and severe muscle wasting leading to decreased strength and failure to fully rehabilitate [117, 118]. Significant decreases in lean body mass related to chronic illness or hypermetabolism can have dire consequences.

- 10% loss of lean body mass is associated with immune dysfunction.
- 20% loss of lean body mass positively correlates with decreased wound healing.
- 30% loss of lean body mass leads to increased risk for pneumonia and pressure sores.
- 40% loss of lean body mass can lead to death [119 #365]

Uncomplicated severely burned patients can lose up to 25% of total body mass after acute burn injury [120]. Protein degradation persists up to nearly 1-year post severe burn injury resulting in significant negative whole body and cross-leg nitrogen balance [110, 118, 121]. Protein catabolism has a positive correlation with increases in metabolic rates [118]. Severely burned patients have a daily nitrogen loss of 20–25 g/ m^2 of burned skin [110, 122]. At this rate, a lethal cachexia can be reached in less than 1 month [122]. Burned pediatric patients' protein loss leads to significant growth retardation for up to 24 months post-injury [123].

Severe burn causes marked changes in body composition during acute hospitalization. Severely burned children lost about 2% of their body weight (−5% LBM, −3% BMC, and −2% BMD) from admission to discharge. Total fat and percent fat increased from admission to discharge by 3% and 7%, respectively.

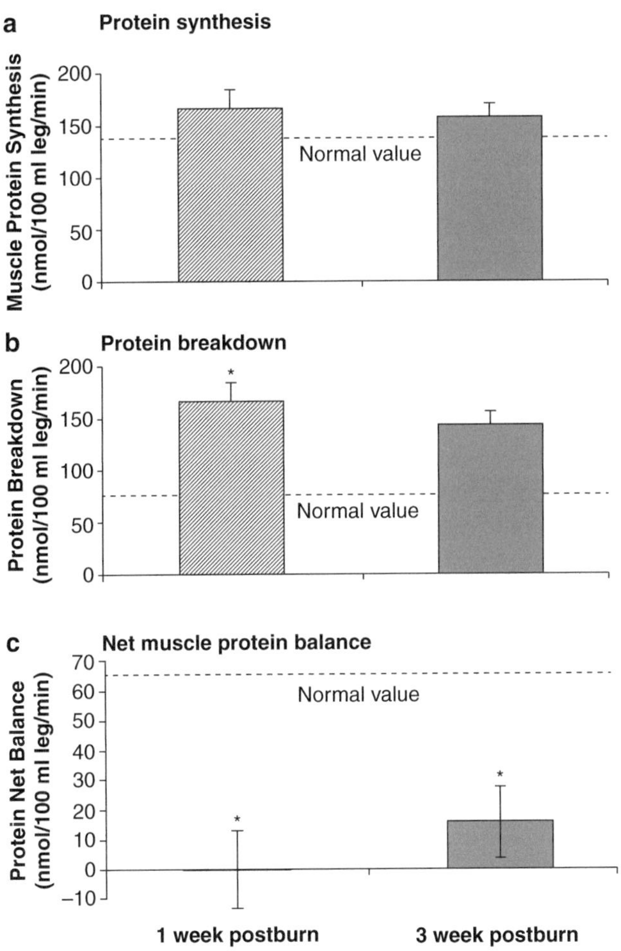

Septic patients have a particularly profound increase in metabolic rates and protein catabolism up to 40% more compared to those with like-size burns that do not develop sepsis [118]. A vicious cycle develops, as patients that are catabolic are more susceptible to sepsis due to changes in immune function and immune response. Modulation of the hypermetabolic, hypercatabolic response, thus preventing secondary injury is paramount in the restoration of structure and function of severely burned patients.

Elevated circulating levels of catecholamines, glucagon, and cortisol after severe thermal injury stimulate free fatty acids and glycerol from fat, glucose production by the liver, and amino acids from muscle [103, 124, 125]. Specifically, glycolytic-gluconeogenic cycling is increased 250% during the post-burn hypermetabolic response coupled with an increase of 450% in triglyceride-fatty acid cycling [126]. These changes lead to hyperglycemia and impaired insulin sensitivity related to post-receptor insulin resistance demonstrated by elevated levels of insulin, fasting glucose, and significant reductions in glucose clearance [127–130].

18.2.3.3 Glucose Metabolism

Glucose metabolism in healthy subjects is tightly regulated: under normal circumstances, a postprandial increase in blood glucose concentration stimulates release of insulin from pancreatic β-cells. Insulin mediates peripheral glucose uptake into skeletal muscle and adipose tissue and suppresses hepatic gluconeogenesis, thereby maintaining blood glucose homeostasis [131, 132]. In critical illness, however metabolic alterations can cause significant changes in energy substrate metabolism. In order to provide glucose, a major fuel source to vital organs, release of the above-mentioned stress mediators oppose the anabolic actions of insulin [133]. By enhancing adipose tissue lipolysis [125] and skeletal muscle proteolysis [134], they increase gluconeogenic substrates, including glycerol, alanine, and lactate, thus augmenting hepatic glucose production in burned patients [131, 132, 135]. Hyperglycemia fails to suppress hepatic glucose release during this time [136] and the suppressive effect of insulin on hepatic glucose release is attenuated, significantly contributing to post-trauma hyperglycemia [137]. Catecholamine-mediated enhancement of hepatic glycogenolysis, as well as direct sympathetic stimulation of glycogen breakdown, can further aggravate the hyperglycemia in response to stress [132]. Catecholamines have also been shown to impair glucose disposal via alterations of the insulin signaling pathway and GLUT-4 translocation muscle and adipose tissue, resulting in peripheral insulin resistance [131, 138]. Cree and colleagues [137] showed an impaired activation of Insulin Receptor Substrate-1 at its tyrosine binding site and an inhibition of AKT in muscle biopsies of children at 7 days post-burn. Work of Wolfe and colleagues indicates links between impaired liver and muscle mitochondrial oxidative function, altered rates of lipolysis, and impaired insulin signaling post-burn attenuating both the suppressive actions of insulin on hepatic glucose production and on the stimulation of muscle glucose uptake [106, 125, 136, 137]. Another counter-regulatory hormone of interest during stress of the critically ill is glucagon. Glucagon, like epinephrine, leads to increased glucose production through both gluconeogenesis and glycogenolysis [139]. The action of glucagons alone is not maintained over time; however, its action on gluconeogenesis is sustained in an additive manner with the presence of epinephrine, cortisol, and growth hormone [133, 139]. Likewise, epinephrine and glucagon have an additive effect on glycogenolysis [139]. Recent studies found that pro-inflammatory cytokines contribute indirectly to post-burn hyperglycemia via enhancing the release of the above-mentioned stress hormones [140–142]. Other groups showed that inflammatory cytokines, including tumor necrosis factor (TNF), interleukin (IL)-6, and monocyte chemotactic protein (MCP)-1 also act via direct effects on the insulin signal transduction pathway through modification of signaling properties of insulin receptor substrates, contributing to post-burn hyperglycemia via liver and skeletal muscle insulin resistance [143–145]. Alterations in metabolic pathways as well as pro-inflammatory cytokines, such as TNF, have also been implicated in significantly contributing to lean muscle protein breakdown, both during the acute and convalescent phases in response to burn injury [121, 146]. In contrast to starvation, in which lipolysis and ketosis provide energy and protect muscle reserves, burn injury considerably reduces the ability of the body to utilize fat as an energy source.

Skeletal muscle is thus the major source of fuel in the burned patient, which leads to marked wasting of lean body mass (LBM) within days after injury [110, 147]. This muscle breakdown has been demonstrated with whole body and cross-leg nitrogen balance studies in which pronounced negative nitrogen balances persisted for 6 and 9 months after injury [118]. Since skeletal muscle has been shown to be responsible for 70–80% of whole body insulin-stimulated glucose uptake, decreases in muscle mass may significantly contribute to this persistent insulin resistance post-burn [148]. The correlation between hyperglycemia and muscle protein catabolism has been also supported by Flakoll and others [149] in which an isotopic tracer of leucine was utilized to index whole body protein flux in normal volunteers. The group showed a significant increase in proteolysis rates occurring without any alteration in either leucine oxidation or non-oxidative disposal (an estimate of protein synthesis), suggesting an hyperglycemia-induced increase in protein breakdown. Flakoll and others [149] further demonstrated that elevations of plasma glucose levels resulted in a marked stimulation of whole body proteolysis during hyperinsulinemia. A 10–15% loss in lean body mass has been shown to be associated with significant increases in infection rate and marked delays in wound healing [150]. The resultant muscle weakness is further shown to prolong mechanical ventilatory requirements, inhibits sufficient cough reflexes, and delays mobilization in protein-malnourished patients, thus markedly contributing to the incidence of mortality in these patients [151]. Persistent protein catabolism may also account for delay in growth frequently observed in our pediatric patient population for up to 2 years post-burn [123].

Septic patients have a particularly profound increase in metabolic rates and protein catabolism up to 40% more compared to those with like-size burns that do not develop sepsis [92, 152, 153]. A vicious cycle develops, as patients that are catabolic are more susceptible to sepsis due to changes in immune function and immune response. The emergence of multidrug-resistant organisms has led to increases in sepsis, catabolism, and mortality [153–155]. Modulation of the hypermetabolic, hypercatabolic response, thus preventing secondary injury is paramount in the restoration of structure and function of severely burned patients.

Lipid metabolism has recently gained interest in the field of hypermetabolism with the discovery of changes in the structure and function of adipose tissue, called browning. Lipolysis with the change in lipidomic profiling and browning of the adipose could explain in part why hypermetabolism is persistently elevated and is associated with various detrimental outcomes on a clinical level but also on cellular levels.

18.2.3.4 Cardiovascular System: Myocardial Dysfunction

Myocardial function can be compromised after burn injury due to overload of the right heart and direct depression of contractility shown in isolated heart studies [156, 157]. Increases in the afterload of both the left and right heart result from SVR and PVR elevations. The left ventricle compensates and CO can be maintained with increased afterload by augmented adrenergic stimulation and increased myocardial oxygen extraction. The right ventricle has a minimal capacity to compensate for increased afterload. In severe cases, desynchronization of the right and left ventricles is deleteriously superimposed on a depressed myocardium [158]. Burn injury greater than 45% TBSA can produce intrinsic contractile defects. Several investigators reported that aggressive early and sustained fluid resuscitation failed to correct left ventricular contractile and compliance defects [157–159]. These data suggest that hypovolemia is not the only mechanism underlying the myocardial defects observed with burn shock. Serum from patients failing to sustain a normal CO after thermal injury have exhibited a markedly negative inotropic effect on in vitro heart preparations, which is likely due to the previously described shock factor [160]. In other patients with large burn injuries and normal cardiac indices, little or no depressant activity was detected.

Sugi and colleagues studied intact, chronically instrumented sheep after a 40% TBSA flame burn injury and smoke inhalation injury, and smoke inhalation injury alone. They found that maximal contractile effects were reduced after either burn injury or inhalation injury [161, 162]. Horton and others demonstrated decreased left ventricular contractility in isolated, coronary perfused, guinea pig hearts harvested 24 h after burn injury [163]. This dysfunction was more pronounced in hearts from aged animals and was not reversed by resuscitation with isotonic fluid. It was largely reversed by treatment with 4 mL/kg of hypertonic saline dextran (HSD), but only if administered during the initial 4–6 h of resuscitation [164, 165]. These authors also effectively ameliorated the cardiac dysfunction of thermal injury with infusions of antioxidants, arginine and calcium channel blockers [166–168]. Cioffi and colleagues in a similar model observed persistent myocardial depression after burn when the animals received no resuscitation after burn injury [169]. As opposed to most studies, Cioffi reported that immediate and full resuscitation totally reversed abnormalities of contraction and relaxation after burn injury. Murphy et al. showed elevations of a serum marker for cardiac injury, Troponin I, for patients with a TBSA >18%, despite good cardiac indices [170]. Resuscitation and cardiac function studies emphasize the importance of early and adequate fluid therapy and suggest that functional myocardial depression after burn injury may not occur in patients receiving prompt and adequate volume therapy.

The primary mechanisms by which burn shock alters myocardial cell membrane integrity and impairs mechanical function remain unclear. Oxygen-derived free radicals may play a key causative role in the cell membrane dysfunction that is characteristic of several low-flow states. Horton et al. showed that a combination therapy of free radical scavengers SOD and catalase significantly improved burn-mediated defects in left ventricular contractility and relaxation when administered along with adequate fluid resuscitation (4 mL/kg per percent of burn). Antioxidant therapy did not alter the volume of fluid resuscitation required after burn injury [166].

18.2.3.5 Effects on the Renal System

Diminished blood volume and cardiac output result in decreased renal blood flow and glomerular filtration rate. Other stress-induced hormones and mediators such as angiotensin, aldosterone, and vasopressin further reduce renal blood flow immediately after the injury. These effects result in oliguria, which, if left untreated will cause acute tubular necrosis and renal failure. Twenty years ago, acute renal failure in burn injuries was almost always fatal. Today newer techniques in dialysis became widely used to support the kidneys during recovery [171]. The latest reports indicate an 88% mortality rate for severely burned adults and a 56% mortality rate for severely burned children in whom renal failure develops in the post-burn period [172, 173]. Early resuscitation decreases risks of renal failure and improves the associated morbidity and mortality [174].

18.2.3.6 Effects on the Gastrointestinal System

The gastrointestinal response to burn is highlighted by mucosal atrophy, changes in digestive absorption, and increased intestinal permeability [175]. Atrophy of the small bowel mucosa occurs within 12 h of injury in proportion to the burn size and is related to increased epithelial cell death by apoptosis [176]. The cytoskeleton of the mucosal brush border undergoes atrophic changes associated with vesiculation of microvilli and disruption of the terminal web actin filaments. These findings were most pronounced 18 h after injury, which suggests that changes in the cytoskeleton, such as those associated with cell death by apoptosis, are processes involved in the changed gut mucosa [177]. Burn also causes reduced uptake of glucose and amino acids, decreased absorption of fatty acids, and reduction in brush border lipase activity [178]. These changes peak in the first several hours after burn and return to normal at 48–72 h after injury, a timing that parallels mucosal atrophy.

Intestinal permeability to macromolecules, which are normally repelled by an intact mucosal barrier, increases after burn [179]. Intestinal permeability to polyethylene glycol 3350, lactulose, and mannitol increases after injury, correlating to the extent of the burn [180]. Gut permeability increases even further when burn wounds become infected. A study using fluorescent dextrans showed that larger molecules appeared to cross the mucosa between the cells, whereas the smaller molecules traversed the mucosa through the epithelial cells, presumably by pinocytosis and vesiculation [181]. Mucosal permeability also paralleled increases in gut epithelial apoptosis.

Changes in gut blood flow are related to changes in permeability. Intestinal blood flow was shown to decrease in animals, a change that was associated with increased gut permeability at 5 h after burn [182]. This effect was abolished at 24 h. Systolic hypotension has been shown to occur in the hours immediately after burn in animals with a 40% TBSA full-thickness injury. These animals showed an inverse correlation between blood flow and permeability to intact *Candida* [183].

The best treatment to alleviate mucosal atrophy is early initiation of enteral nutrition, usually within 8–12 h post-burn. Glutamine and other antioxidants have been shown to improve enteral inflammatory driven pathways as well as gut function.

Despite the need for liver function and integrity the liver is profoundly affected post-burn and in our opinion a central contributor to post-burn morbidity and mortality [111, 184]. The liver has several myriad functions that are each essential for survival:

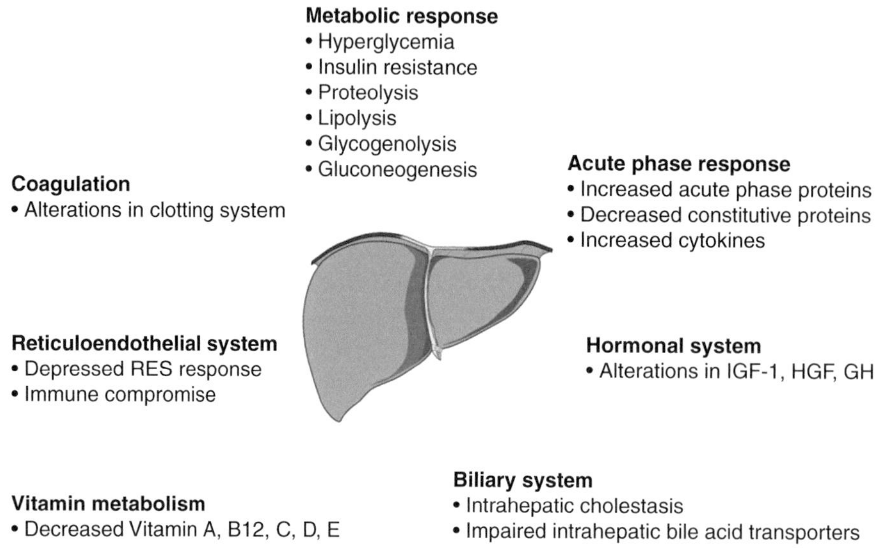

All of these hepatic functions are affected by a thermal injury, and we have strong evidence that hepatic biomarkers predict and determine morbidity and mortality in severely burned patients. We, therefore, believe that the liver is central for post-burn outcome and we propose that attenuation of liver damage and restoration of liver function will improve morbidity and mortality of severely burned patients [111].

There is currently no treatment for hepatic dysfunction or failure post-burn. Animal and in vitro studies suggested a beneficial effect on hepatic apoptosis and function with the use of insulin and Propranolol.

The pancreas may or may not be affected after burn. There is little evidence that looks at the endocrine and paracrine function of the pancreas after burn; it is only well documented that if pancreatitis occurs after burn this is associated with a high morbidity and mortality.

18.2.3.7 Effects on the Immune System

Burns cause a substantial hyperinflammation but also a global depression in immune function, which is shown by prolonged allograft skin survival on burn wounds. Burned patients are then at great risk for a number of infectious complications, including bacterial wound infection, pneumonia, and fungal and viral infections. These susceptibilities and conditions are based on depressed cellular function in all parts of the immune system, including activation and activity of neutrophils, macrophages, T lymphocytes, and B lymphocytes. With burns of more than 20% TBSA, impairment of these immune functions is proportional to burn size.

Macrophage production after burn is diminished, which is related to the spontaneous elaboration of negative regulators of myeloid growth. This effect is enhanced by the presence of endotoxin and can be partially reversed with granulocyte colony-stimulating factor (G-CSF) treatment or inhibition of prostaglandin E_2 [185]. Investigators have shown that G-CSF levels actually increase after severe burn. However, bone marrow G-CSF receptor expression is decreased, which may in part account for the immunodeficiency seen in burns [186]. Total neutrophil counts are initially increased after burn, a phenomenon that is related to a decrease in cell death by apoptosis [187]. However, neutrophils that are present are dysfunctional in terms of diapedesis, chemotaxis, and phagocytosis. These effects are explained, in part, by a deficiency in CD11b/CD18 expression after inflammatory stimuli, decreased respiratory burst activity associated with a deficiency in p47-phox activity, and impaired actin mechanics related to neutrophil motile responses [188, 189]. After 48–72 h, neutrophil counts decrease somewhat like macrophages with similar causes [186].

T-helper cell function is depressed after a severe burn that is associated with polarization from the interleukin-2 and interferon-γ cytokine-based T-helper 1 (TH1) response towards the TH2 response [190]. The TH2 response is characterized by the production of interleukin-4 and interleukin-10. The TH1 response is important in cell-mediated immune defense, whereas the TH2 response is important in antibody responses to infection. As this polarization increases, so does the mortality rate [191]. Administration of interleukin-10 antibodies and growth hormone has partially reversed this response and improved mortality rate after burn in animals [192, 193]. Burn also impairs cytotoxic T-lymphocyte activity as a function of burn size, thus increasing the risk of infection, particularly from fungi and viruses. Early burn wound excision improves cytotoxic T-cell activity [194].

18.2.3.8 Summary and Conclusion

Thermal injury results in massive fluid shifts from the circulating plasma into the interstitial fluid space causing hypovolemia and swelling of the burned skin. When burn injury exceeds 20–30% TBSA, there is minimal edema generation in non-injured tissues and organs. The Starling-forces change to favor fluid extravasation from blood to tissue. Rapid edema formation is predominating from the development of strongly negative interstitial fluid pressure (imbibition pressure) and to a lesser degree by an increase in microvascular pressure and permeability.

Secondary to the thermal insult, there is release of inflammatory mediators and stress hormones. Circulating mediators deleteriously increase microvascular permeability and alter cellular membrane function by which water and sodium enter cells. Circulating mediators also favor renal conservation of water and salt, impair cardiac contractility, and cause vasoconstrictors, which further aggravates ischemia from combined hypovolemia and cardiac dysfunction. The end result of this complex chain of events is decreased intravascular volume, increased systemic vascular resistance, decreased cardiac output, end-organ ischemia, and metabolic acidosis. Early excision of the devitalized tissue appears to reduce the local and systemic effects of mediators released from burned tissue, thus reducing the progressive pathophysiologic derangements. Without early and full resuscitation therapy, these derangements can result in acute renal failure, vascular ischemia, cardiovascular collapse, and death.

Edema in both the burn wound and particularly in the non-injured soft tissue is increased by resuscitation. Edema is a serious complication, which likely contributes to decreased tissue oxygen diffusion and further ischemic insult to already damaged cells with compromised blood flow increasing the risk of infection. Research should continue to focus on methods to ameliorate the severe edema and vasoconstriction that exacerbate tissue ischemia. The success of this research will require identification of key circulatory factors that alter capillary permeability, cause vasoconstriction, depolarize cellular membranes, and depress myocardial function. Hopefully, methods to prevent the release and to block the activity of specific mediators can be further developed in order to reduce the morbidity and mortality rates of burn shock. The profound and overall metabolic alterations post-burn associated with persistent changes in glucose metabolism and impaired insulin sensitivity also significantly contribute to adverse outcome of this patient population and constitute another challenge for future therapeutic approaches of this unique patient population.

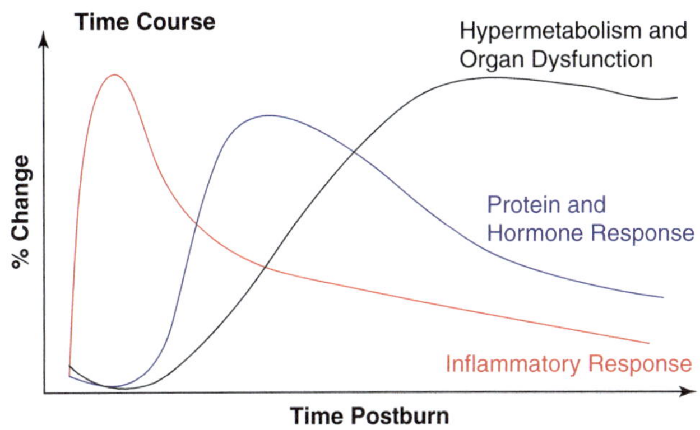

Summary Box

The pathophysiologic response after burn injury is one of the most formidable and complex ones after any injury. It is impossible to normalize this response. However due to recent advances in the inflammatory metabolic cellular and stress responses, various patterns have now been identified that potentially allow modification and perturbation. This now leads to the question, how to ideally and optimally alter these responses. Again, it is imperative to note that there are a time- and course-dependent differences and that alteration may have different effects at different times. Additionally, treatment of one single pathway seems over simplistic and will most likely not lead to improved outcomes. Therefore, diligent thoughts and careful consideration about intervention need to be conducted.

Conflicts of Interest and Source of Funding This study was supported by National Institutes of Health R01-GM087285-01. CFI Leader's Opportunity Fund: Project #25407 and Canadian Institutes of Health Research (CIHR) grant #123336. Authors have no conflicts of interest to declare.

References

1. Nguyen TT, Gilpin DA, Meyer NA, et al. Current treatment of severely burned patients. Ann Surg. 1996;223(1):14–25.
2. Brigham PA, McLoughlin E. Burn incidence and medical care use in the United States: estimates, trends, and data sources. J Burn Care Rehabil. 1996;17(2):95–107.
3. Wolf S. Critical care in the severely burned: organ support and management of complications. In: Herndon DN, editor. Total burn care. 3rd ed. London: Saunders Elsevier; 2007.
4. Vo LT, Papworth GD, Delaney PM, et al. A study of vascular response to thermal injury on hairless mice by fibre optic confocal imaging, laser Doppler flowmetry and conventional histology. Burns. 1998;24(4):319–24.
5. Heggers JP, Loy GL, Robson MC, et al. Histological demonstration of prostaglandins and thromboxanes in burned tissue. J Surg Res. 1980;28(2):110–7.
6. Herndon DN, Abston S, Stein MD. Increased thromboxane B2 levels in the plasma of burned and septic burned patients. Surg Gynecol Obstet. 1984;159(3):210–3.
7. Morykwas MJ, David LR, Schneider AM, et al. Use of subatmospheric pressure to prevent progression of partial-thickness burns in a swine model. J Burn Care Rehabil. 1999;20(1 Pt 1):15–21.
8. Nwariaku FE, Sikes PJ, Lightfoot E, et al. Effect of a bradykinin antagonist on the local inflammatory response following thermal injury. Burns. 1996;22(4):324–7.
9. Chappell VL, LaGrone L, Mileski WJ. Inhibition of leukocyte-mediated tissue destruction by synthetic fibronectin peptide (Trp-9-Tyr). J Burn Care Rehabil. 1999;20(6):505–10.
10. Holland AJ, Martin HC, Cass DT. Laser Doppler imaging prediction of burn wound outcome in children. Burns. 2002;28(1):11–7.
11. Cockshott WP. The history of the treatment of burns. Surg Gynecol Obstet. 1956;102:116–24.
12. Haynes BW. The history of burn care. In: Boswick JAJ, editor. The art and science of burn care. Rockville: Aspen Publishers; 1987. p. 3–9.
13. Underhill FP, Carrington GL, Kapsinov R, et al. Blood concentration changes in extensive superficial burns, and their significance for systemic treatment. Arch Intern Med. 1923;32:31–9.
14. Cope O, Moore FD. The redistribution of body water and fluid therapy of the burned patient. Ann Surg. 1947;126:1010–45.
15. Youn YK, LaLonde C, Demling R. The role of mediators in the response to thermal injury. World J Surg. 1992;16(1):30–6.
16. Aulick LH, Wilmore DW, Mason AD, et al. Influence of the burn wound on peripheral circulation in thermally injured patients. Am J Phys. 1977;233:H520–6.
17. Settle JAD. Fluid therapy in burns. J R Soc Med. 1982;1(75):7–11.
18. Demling RH. Fluid replacement in burned patients. Surg Clin North Am. 1987;67:15–30.
19. Demling RH, Will JA, Belzer FO. Effect of major thermal injury on the pulmonary microcirculation. Surgery. 1978;83(6):746–51.
20. Baxter CR. Fluid volume and electrolyte changes of the early postburn period. Clin Plast Surg. 1974;1(4):693–709.
21. Baxter CR, Cook WA, Shires GT. Serum myocardial depressant factor of burn shock. Surg Forum. 1966;17:1–3.
22. Hilton JG, Marullo DS. Effects of thermal trauma on cardiac force of contraction. Burns Incl Therm Inj. 1986;12:167–71.
23. Clark WR. Death due to thermal trauma. In: Dolecek R, Brizio-Molteni L, Molteni A, Traber D, editors. Endocrinology of thermal trauma. Philadelphia: Lea & Febiger; 1990. p. 6–27.
24. Lund T, Reed RK. Acute hemodynamic effects of thermal skin injury in the rat. Circ Shock. 1986;20:105–14.
25. Arturson G. Pathophysiological aspects of the burn syndrome. Acta Chir Scand. 1961;274(Supp 1):1–135.
26. Leape LL. Kinetics of burn edema formation in primates. Ann Surg. 1972;176:223–6.
27. Cioffi WG Jr, Vaughan GM, Heironimus JD, et al. Dissociation of blood volume and flow in regulation of salt and water balance in burn patients. Ann Surg. 1991;214(3):213–8; discussion 218–20.
28. Demling RH, Mazess RB, Witt RM, et al. The study of burn wound edema using dichromatic absorptiometry. J Trauma. 1978;18:124–8.
29. Lund T, Wiig H, Reed RK. Acute postburn edema: role of strongly negative interstitial fluid pressure. Am J Phys. 1988;255:H1069.
30. Onarheim H, Lund T, Reed R. Thermal skin injury: II. Effects on edema formation and albumin extravasation of fluid resuscitation with lactated Ringer's, plasma, and hypertonic saline (2,400 mosmol/l) in the rat. Circ Shock. 1989;27(1):25–37.
31. Arturson G, Jakobsson OR. Oedema measurements in a standard burn model. Burns. 1985;1:1–7.
32. Leape LL. Early burn wound changes. J Pediatr Surg. 1968;3:292–9.
33. Leape LL. Initial changes in burns: tissue changes in burned and unburned skin of rhesus monkeys. J Trauma. 1970;10:488–92.
34. Shires GT, Cunningham JN Jr, Baker CRF, et al. Alterations in cellular membrane dysfunction during hemorrhagic shock in primates. Ann Surg. 1972;176(3):288–95.
35. Nakayama S, Kramer GC, Carlsen RC, et al. Amiloride blocks membrane potential depolarization in rat skeletal muscle during hemorrhagic shock (abstract). Circ Shock. 1984;13:106–7.
36. Arango A, Illner H, Shires GT. Roles of ischemia in the induction of changes in cell membrane during hemorrhagic shock. J Surg Res. 1976;20(5):473–6.
37. Holliday RL, Illner HP, Shires GT. Liver cell membrane alterations during hemorrhagic shock in the rat. J Surg Res. 1981;31:506–15.
38. Mazzoni MC, Borgstrom P, Intaglietta M, et al. Lumenal narrowing and endothelial cell swelling in skeletal muscle capillaries during hemorrhagic shock. Circ Shock. 1989;29(1):27–39.
39. Garcia NM, Horton JW. L-arginine improves resting cardiac transmembrane potential after burn injury. Shock. 1994;1(5):354–8.
40. Button B, Baker RD, Vertrees RA, et al. Quantitative assessment of a circulating depolarizing factor in shock. Shock. 2001;15(3):239–44.
41. Evans JA, Darlington DN, Gann DS. A circulating factor(s) mediates cell depolarization in hemorrhagic shock. Ann Surg. 1991;213(6):549–57.
42. Trunkey DD, Illner H, Arango A, et al. Changes in cell membrane function following shock and cross-perfusion. Surg Forum. 1974;25:1–3.
43. Brown JM, Grosso MA, Moore EE. Hypertonic saline and dextran: impact on cardiac function in the isolated rat heart. J Trauma. 1990;30:646–51.
44. Evans JA, Massoglia G, Sutherland B, et al. Molecular properties of hemorrhagic shock factor (abstract). Biophys J. 1993;64:A384.
45. Anggard E, Jonsson CE. Efflux of prostaglandins in lymph from scalded tissue. Acta Physiol Scand. 1971;81(4):440–7.
46. Holliman CJ, Meuleman TR, Larsen KR, et al. The effect of ketanserin, a specific serotonin antagonist, on burn shock hemodynamic parameters in a porcine burn model. J Trauma. 1983;23(10):867–71.
47. Majno G, Palade GE. Studies on inflammation. 1. The effect of histamine and serotonin on vascular permeability: an electron microscopic study. J Biophys Biochem Cytol. 1961;11:571–605.
48. Majno G, Shea SM, Leventhal M. Endothelial contraction induced by histamine-type mediators: an electron microscopic study. J Cell Biol. 1969;42(3):647–72.
49. Wilmore DW, Long JM, Mason AD Jr, et al. Catecholamines: mediator of the hypermetabolic response to thermal injury. Ann Surg. 1974;180(4):653–69.
50. Goodman-Gilman A, Rall TW, Nies AS, et al. The pharmacological basis of therapeutics. New York: Pergamon Press; 1990.
51. Friedl HS, Till GO, Tentz O, et al. Roles of histamine, complement and xanthine oxidase in thermal injury of skin. Am J Pathol. 1989;135(1):203–17.
52. Boykin JV Jr, Manson NH. Mechanisms of cimetidine protection following thermal injury. Am J Med. 1987;83(6A):76–81.

53. Till GO, Guilds LS, Mahrougui M, et al. Role of xanthine oxidase in thermal injury of skin. Am J Pathol. 1989;135(1):195–202.
54. Tanaka H, Wada T, Simazaki S, et al. Effects of cimetidine on fluid requirement during resuscitation of third-degree burns. J Burn Care Rehabil. 1991;12(5):425–9.
55. Harms B, Bodai B, Demling R. Prostaglandin release and altered microvascular integrity after burn injury. J Surg Res. 1981;31:27–8.
56. Anggard E, Jonsson CE. Efflux of prostaglandins in lymph from scalded tissue. Acta Physiol Scand. 1971;81:440–3.
57. Arturson G. Anti-inflammatory drugs and burn edema formation. In: May R, Dogo G, editors. Care of the burn wound. Basel: Karger; 1981. p. 21–4.
58. Arturson G, Hamberg M, Jonsson CE. Prostaglandins in human burn blister fluid. Acta Physiol Scand. 1973;87:27–36.
59. LaLonde C, Knox J, Daryani R. Topical flurbiprofen decreases burn wound-induced hypermetabolism and systemic lipid peroxidation. Surgery. 1991;109:645–51.
60. Huang YS, Li A, Yang ZC. Roles of thromboxane and its inhibitor anisodamine in burn shock. Burns. 1990;4:249–53.
61. Heggers JP, Loy GL, Robson MC, et al. Histological demonstration of prostaglandins and thromboxanes in burned tissue. J Surg Res. 1980;28:11–5.
62. Heggers JP, Robson MC, Zachary LS. Thromboxane inhibitors for the prevention of progressive dermal ischemia due to thermal injury. J Burn Care Rehabil. 1985;6:46–8.
63. Demling RH, LaLonde C. Topical ibuprofen decreases early post-burn edema. Surgery. 1987;5:857–61.
64. LaLonde C, Demling RH. Inhibition of thromboxane synthetase accentuates hemodynamic instability and burn edema in the anesthetized sheep model. Surgery. 1989;5:638–44.
65. Jacobsen S, Waaler BG. The effect of scalding on the content of kininogen and kininase in limb lymph. Br J Pharmacol. 1966;27:222.
66. Hafner JA, Fritz H. Balance antiinflammation: the combined application of a PAF inhibitor and a cyclooxygenase inhibitor blocks the inflammatory take-off after burns. Int J Tissue React. 1990;12:203.
67. Carvajal H, Linares H, Brouhard B. Effect of antihistamine, antiserotonin, and ganglionic blocking agents upon increased capillary permeability following burn edema. J Trauma. 1975;15:969–75.
68. Ferrara JJ, Westervelt CL, Kukuy EL, et al. Burn edema reduction by methysergide is not due to control of regional vasodilation. J Surg Res. 1996;61(1):11–6.
69. Zhang XJ, Irtun O, Zheng Y, et al. Methysergide reduces nonnutritive blood flow in normal and scalded skin. Am J Phys. 2000;278(3):E452–61.
70. Wilmore DW, Long JM, Mason AD, et al. Catecholamines: mediator of the hypermetabolic response to thermal injury. Ann Surg. 1974;80:653–9.
71. Hilton JG. Effects of sodium nitroprusside on thermal trauma depressed cardiac output in the anesthesized dog. Burns Incl Therm Inj. 1984;10:318–22.
72. McCord J, Fridovieh I. The biology and pathology of oxygen radicals. Ann Intern Med. 1978;89:122–7.
73. Demling RH, LaLonde C. Early postburn lipid peroxidation: effect of ibuprofen and allopurinol. Surgery. 1990;107:85–93.
74. Demling R, Lalonde C, Knox J, et al. Fluid resuscitation with deferoxamine prevents systemic burn-induced oxidant injury. J Trauma. 1991;31(4):538–43.
75. Rawlingson A, Greenacre SA, Brain SD. Generation of peroxynitrite in localised, moderate temperature burns. Burns. 2000;26(3):223–7.
76. Lindblom L, Cassuto J, Yregard L, et al. Importance of nitric oxide in the regulation of burn oedema, proteinuria and urine output. Burns. 2000;26(1):13–7.
77. Lindblom L, Cassuto J, Yregard L, et al. Role of nitric oxide in the control of burn perfusion. Burns. 2000;26(1):19–23.
78. Slater TF, Benedetto C. Free radical reactions in relation to lipid peroxidation, inflamnation and prostaglandin metabolism. In: Berti F, Veto G, editors. The prostaglandin system. New York: Plenum Press; 1979. p. 109–26.
79. McCord JM. Oxygen-derived free radicals in post ischemic tissue injury. N Engl J Med. 1979;312:159–63.
80. Tanaka H, Matsuda H, Shimazaki S, et al. Reduced resuscitation fluid volume for second-degree burns with delayed initiation of ascorbic acid therapy. Arch Surg. 1997;132(2):158–61.
81. Tanaka H, Lund T, Wiig H, et al. High dose vitamin C counteracts the negative interstitial fluid hydrostatic pressure and early edema generation in thermally injured rats. Burns. 1999;25(7):569–74.
82. Dubick MA, Williams CA, Elgjo GI, et al. High dose vitamin C infusion reduces fluid requirements in the resuscitation of burn injured in sheep. Shock. 2005;24(2):139–44.
83. Tanaka H, Matsuda T, Yukioka T, et al. High dose vitamin C reduces resuscitation fluid volume in severely burned patients. Proc Am Burn Assoc. 1996;28:77.
84. Fischer SF, Bone HG, Powell WC, et al. Pyridoxalated hemoglobin polyoxyethylene conjugate does not restore hypoxic pulmonary vasoconstriction in ovine sepsis. Crit Care. 1997;25(9):1151–9.
85. Ono I, Gunji H, Hasegawa T, et al. Effects of a platelet activating factor antagonist on edema formation following burns. Burns. 1993;3:202–7.
86. Fink MP. Gastrointestinal mucosal injury in experimental models of shock, trauma, and sepsis. Crit Care Med. 1991;19(5):627–41.
87. Cui X, Sheng Z, Guo Z. Mechanisms of early gastro-intestinal ischemia after burn: hemodynamic and hemorrheologic features [Chinese]. Chin J Plast Surg Burns. 1998;14(4):262–5.
88. Crum RL, Dominie W, Hansbrough JF. Cardiovaseular and neuroburnoral responses following burn injury. Arch Surg. 1990;125:1065–70.
89. Sun K, Gong A, Wang CH, et al. Effect of peripheral injection of arginine vasopressin and its receptor antagonist on burn shock in the rat. Neuropeptides. 1990;1:17–20.
90. Kiang JG, Wei-E T. Corticotropin-releasing factor inhibits thermal injury. J Pharmacol Exp Ther. 1987;2:517–20.
91. Michie DD, Goldsmith RS, Mason AD Jr. Effects of hydralazine and high molecular weight dextran upon the circulatory responses to severe thermal burns. Circ Res. 1963;13:46–8.
92. Hart DW, Wolf SE, Mlcak R, et al. Persistence of muscle catabolism after severe burn. Surgery. 2000;128(2):312–9.
93. Mlcak RP, Jeschke MG, Barrow RE, et al. The influence of age and gender on resting energy expenditure in severely burned children. Ann Surg. 2006;244(1):121–30.
94. Przkora R, Barrow RE, Jeschke MG, et al. Body composition changes with time in pediatric burn patients. J Trauma. 2006;60(5):968–71.
95. Dolecek R. Endocrine changes after burn trauma–a review. Keio J Med. 1989;38(3):262–76.
96. Jeffries MK, Vance ML. Growth hormone and cortisol secretion in patients with burn injury. J Burn Care Rehabil. 1992;13(4):391–5.
97. Klein GL, Bi LX, Sherrard DJ, et al. Evidence supporting a role of glucocorticoids in short-term bone loss in burned children. Osteoporos Int. 2004;15(6):468–74.
98. Goodall M, Stone C, Haynes BW Jr. Urinary output of adrenaline and noradrenaline in severe thermal burns. Ann Surg. 1957;145(4):479–87.
99. Coombes EJ, Batstone GF. Urine cortisol levels after burn injury. Burns Incl Therm Inj. 1982;8(5):333–7.
100. Norbury WB, Herndon DN. Modulation of the hypermetabolic response after burn injury. In: Herndon DN, editor. Total burn care. 3rd ed. New York: Saunders & Elsevier; 2007. p. 420–33.
101. Sheridan RL. A great constitutional disturbance. N Engl J Med. 2001;345(17):1271–2.
102. Pereira C, Murphy K, Jeschke M, et al. Post burn muscle wasting and the effects of treatments. Int J Biochem Cell Biol. 2005;37(10):1948–61.

103. Wolfe RR. Review: acute versus chronic response to burn injury. Circ Shock. 1981;8(1):105–15.
104. Cuthbertson DP, Angeles Valero Zanuy MA, Leon Sanz ML. Post-shock metabolic response. 1942. Nutr Hosp. 2001;16(5):175–82.
105. Galster AD, Bier DM, Cryer PE, et al. Plasma palmitate turnover in subjects with thermal injury. J Trauma. 1984;24(11):938–45.
106. Cree MG, Aarsland A, Herndon DN, et al. Role of fat metabolism in burn trauma-induced skeletal muscle insulin resistance. Crit Care Med. 2007;35(9 Suppl):S476–83.
107. Childs C, Heath DF, Little RA, et al. Glucose metabolism in children during the first day after burn injury. Arch Emerg Med. 1990;7(3):135–47.
108. Jeschke MG, Mlcak RP, Finnerty CC, et al. Burn size determines the inflammatory and hypermetabolic response. Crit Care. 2007;11(4):R90.
109. Gauglitz GG, Herndon DN, Kulp GA, et al. Abnormal insulin sensitivity persists up to three years in pediatric patients post-burn. J Clin Endocrinol Metab. 2009;94(5):1656–64.
110. Herndon DN, Tompkins RG. Support of the metabolic response to burn injury. Lancet. 2004;363(9424):1895–902.
111. Jeschke MG, Chinkes DL, Finnerty CC, et al. Pathophysiologic response to severe burn injury. Ann Surg. 2008;248(3):387–401.
112. Wilmore DW, Aulick LH, Pruitt BA Jr. Metabolism during the hypermetabolic phase of thermal injury. Adv Surg. 1978;12:193–225.
113. Cuthbertson DP, Angeles Valero Zanuy MA, Leon Sanz ML. Post-shock metabolic response. 1942. Nutr Hosp. 2001;16(5):176–82; discussion 175–6.
114. Herndon DN, Hart DW, Wolf SE, et al. Reversal of catabolism by beta-blockade after severe burns. N Engl J Med. 2001;345(17):1223–9.
115. Baron PW, Barrow RE, Pierre EJ, et al. Prolonged use of propranolol safely decreases cardiac work in burned children. J Burn Care Rehabil. 1997;18(3):223–7.
116. Minifee PK, Barrow RE, Abston S, et al. Improved myocardial oxygen utilization following propranolol infusion in adolescents with postburn hypermetabolism. J Pediatr Surg. 1989;24(8):806–10; discussion 810–1.
117. Bessey PQ, Jiang ZM, Johnson DJ, et al. Posttraumatic skeletal muscle proteolysis: the role of the hormonal environment. World J Surg. 1989;13(4):465–70; discussion 471.
118. Hart DW, Wolf SE, Chinkes DL, et al. Determinants of skeletal muscle catabolism after severe burn. Ann Surg. 2000;232(4):455–65.
119. Chang DW, DeSanti L, Demling RH. Anticatabolic and anabolic strategies in critical illness: a review of current treatment modalities. Shock. 1998;10(3):155–60.
120. Newsome TW, Mason AD Jr, Pruitt BA Jr. Weight loss following thermal injury. Ann Surg. 1973;178(2):215–7.
121. Jahoor F, Desai M, Herndon DN, et al. Dynamics of the protein metabolic response to burn injury. Metabolism. 1988;37(4):330–7.
122. Kinney JM, Long CL, Gump FE, et al. Tissue composition of weight loss in surgical patients. I. Elective operation. Ann Surg. 1968;168(3):459–74.
123. Rutan RL, Herndon DN. Growth delay in postburn pediatric patients. Arch Surg. 1990;125(3):392–5.
124. Wolfe RR, Goodenough RD, Burke JF, et al. Response of protein and urea kinetics in burn patients to different levels of protein intake. Ann Surg. 1983;197(2):163–71.
125. Wolfe RR, Herndon DN, Jahoor F, et al. Effect of severe burn injury on substrate cycling by glucose and fatty acids. N Engl J Med. 1987;317(7):403–8.
126. Yu YM, Tompkins RG, Ryan CM, et al. The metabolic basis of the increase of the increase in energy expenditure in severely burned patients. JPEN J Parenter Enteral Nutr. 1999;23(3):160–8.
127. Gauglitz GG, Halder S, Boehning DF, et al. Post-burn hepatic insulin resistance is associated with Er stress. Shock. 2010;33(3):299–305.
128. Gauglitz GG, Finnerty CC, Herndon DN, et al. Are serum cytokines early predictors for the outcome of burn patients with inhalation injuries who do not survive? Crit Care. 2008;12(3):R81.
129. Gauglitz GG, Toliver-Kinsky TE, Williams FN, et al. Insulin increases resistance to burn wound infection-associated sepsis*. Crit Care Med. 2010;38(1):202–8.
130. Wilmore DW, Mason AD Jr, Pruitt BA Jr. Insulin response to glucose in hypermetabolic burn patients. Ann Surg. 1976;183(3):314–20.
131. Gearhart MM, Parbhoo SK. Hyperglycemia in the critically ill patient. AACN Clin Issues. 2006;17(1):50–5.
132. Robinson LE, van Soeren MH. Insulin resistance and hyperglycemia in critical illness: role of insulin in glycemic control. AACN Clin Issues. 2004;15(1):45–62.
133. Khani S, Tayek JA. Cortisol increases gluconeogenesis in humans: its role in the metabolic syndrome. Clin Sci (Lond). 2001;101(6):739–47.
134. Gore DC, Jahoor F, Wolfe RR, et al. Acute response of human muscle protein to catabolic hormones. Ann Surg. 1993;218(5):679–84.
135. Carlson GL. Insulin resistance and glucose-induced thermogenesis in critical illness. Proc Nutr Soc. 2001;60(3):381–8.
136. Wolfe RR, Durkot MJ, Allsop JR, et al. Glucose metabolism in severely burned patients. Metabolism. 1979;28(10):1031–9.
137. Cree MG, Zwetsloot JJ, Herndon DN, et al. Insulin sensitivity and mitochondrial function are improved in children with burn injury during a randomized controlled trial of fenofibrate. Ann Surg. 2007;245(2):214–21.
138. Hunt DG, Ivy JL. Epinephrine inhibits insulin-stimulated muscle glucose transport. J Appl Physiol. 2002;93(5):1638–43.
139. Gustavson SM, Chu CA, Nishizawa M, et al. Interaction of glucagon and epinephrine in the control of hepatic glucose production in the conscious dog. Am J Physiol Endocrinol Metab. 2003;284(4):E695–707.
140. Mastorakos G, Chrousos GP, Weber JS. Recombinant interleukin-6 activates the hypothalamic-pituitary-adrenal axis in humans. J Clin Endocrinol Metab. 1993;77(6):1690–4.
141. Lang CH, Dobrescu C, Bagby GJ. Tumor necrosis factor impairs insulin action on peripheral glucose disposal and hepatic glucose output. Endocrinology. 1992;130(1):43–52.
142. Akita S, Akino K, Ren SG, et al. Elevated circulating leukemia inhibitory factor in patients with extensive burns. J Burn Care Res. 2006;27(2):221–5.
143. Fan J, Li YH, Wojnar MM, et al. Endotoxin-induced alterations in insulin-stimulated phosphorylation of insulin receptor, IRS-1, and MAP kinase in skeletal muscle. Shock. 1996;6(3):164–70.
144. del Aguila LF, Claffey KP, Kirwan JP. TNF-alpha impairs insulin signaling and insulin stimulation of glucose uptake in C2C12 muscle cells. Am J Phys. 1999;276(5 Pt 1):E849–55.
145. Sell H, Dietze-Schroeder D, Kaiser U, et al. Monocyte chemotactic protein-1 is a potential player in the negative cross-talk between adipose tissue and skeletal muscle. Endocrinology. 2006;147(5):2458–67.
146. Baracos V, Rodemann HP, Dinarello CA, et al. Stimulation of muscle protein degradation and prostaglandin E2 release by leukocytic pyrogen (interleukin-1). A mechanism for the increased degradation of muscle proteins during fever. N Engl J Med. 1983;308(10):553–8.
147. Saffle JR, Graves C. Nutritional support of the burned patient. In: Herndon DN, editor. Total burn care. 3rd ed. London: Saunders Elsevier; 2007. p. 398–419.
148. DeFronzo RA, Jacot E, Jequier E, et al. The effect of insulin on the disposal of intravenous glucose. Results from indirect calorimetry and hepatic and femoral venous catheterization. Diabetes. 1981;30(12):1000–7.
149. Flakoll PJ, Hill JO, Abumrad NN. Acute hyperglycemia enhances proteolysis in normal man. Am J Phys. 1993;265(5 Pt 1):E715–21.

150. McClave SA, Snider HL. Use of indirect calorimetry in clinical nutrition. Nutr Clin Pract. 1992;7(5):207–21.
151. Arora NS, Rochester DF. Respiratory muscle strength and maximal voluntary ventilation in undernourished patients. Am Rev Respir Dis. 1982;126(1):5–8.
152. Greenhalgh DG, Saffle JR, Holmes JHT, et al. American burn association consensus conference to define sepsis and infection in burns. J Burn Care Res. 2007;28(6):776–90.
153. Williams FN, Herndon DN, Hawkins HK, et al. The leading causes of death after burn injury in a single pediatric burn center. Crit Care. 2009;13(6):R183.
154. Murray CK, Loo FL, Hospenthal DR, et al. Incidence of systemic fungal infection and related mortality following severe burns. Burns. 2008;34(8):1108–12.
155. Pruitt BA Jr, McManus AT, Kim SH, et al. Burn wound infections: current status. World J Surg. 1998;22(2):135–45.
156. Martyn JAJ, Wilson RS, Burke JF. Right ventricular function and pulmonary hemodynamics during dopamine infusion in burned patients. Chest. 1986;89:357–60.
157. Adams HR, Baxter CR, Izenberg SD. Decreased contractility and compliance of the left ventricle as complications of thermal trauma. Am Heart J. 1984;108(6):1477–87.
158. Merriman TW Jr, Jackson R. Myocardial function following thermal injury. Circ Res. 1962;11:66–9.
159. Horton JW, White J, Baxter CR. Aging alters myocardial response during resuscitation in burn shock. Surg Forum. 1987;38:249–51.
160. Baxter CR, Shires GT. Physiological response to crystalloid resuscitation of severe burns. Ann N Y Acad Sci. 1968;150:874–94.
161. Sugi K, Newald J, Traber LD. Smoke inhalation injury causes myocardial depression in sheep. Anesthesiology. 1988;69:A 111.
162. Sugi K, Theissen JL, Traber LD, et al. Impact of carbon monoxide on cardiopulmonary dysfunction after smoke inhalation injury. Circ Res. 1990;66:69–75.
163. Horton JW, Baxter CR, White J. Differences in cardiac responses to resuscitation from burn shock. Surg Gynecol Obstet. 1989;168(3):201–13.
164. Horton JW, White DJ, Baxter CR. Hypertonic saline dextran resuscitation of thermal injury. Ann Surg. 1990;211(3):301–11.
165. Horton JW, Shite J, Hunt JL. Delayed hypertonic saline dextran administration after burn injury. J Trauma. 1995;38(2):281–6.
166. Horton JW, White J, Baxter CR. The role of oxygen derived free radicles in burn-induced myocardial contractile depression. J Burn Care Rehabil. 1988;9(6):589–98.
167. Horton JW, Garcia NM, White J, et al. Postburn cardiac contractile function and biochemical markers of postburn cardiac injury. J Am Coll Surg. 1995;181:289–98.
168. Horton JW, White J, Maass D, et al. Arginine in burn injury improves cardiac performance and prevents bacterial translocation. J Appl Physiol. 1998;84(2):695–702.
169. Cioffi WG, DeMeules JE, Gameili RL. The effects of burn injury and fluid resuscitation on cardiac function in vitro. J Trauma. 1986;26:638–43.
170. Murphy JT, Horton JW, Purdue GF, et al. Evaluation of troponin-I as an indicator of cardiac dysfunction following thermal injury. J Trauma. 1998;45(4):700–4.
171. Leblanc M, Thibeault Y, Querin S. Continuous haemofiltration and haemodiafiltration for acute renal failure in severely burned patients. Burns. 1997;23(2):160–5.
172. Chrysopoulo MT, Jeschke MG, Dziewulski P, et al. Acute renal dysfunction in severely burned adults. J Trauma. 1999;46(1):141–4.
173. Jeschke MG, Barrow RE, Wolf SE, et al. Mortality in burned children with acute renal failure. Arch Surg. 1998;133(7):752–6.
174. Wolf SE, Rose JK, Desai MH, et al. Mortality determinants in massive pediatric burns. An analysis of 103 children with > or = 80% TBSA burns (> or = 70% full-thickness). Ann Surg. 1997;225(5):554–65; discussion 565–9.
175. LeVoyer T, Cioffi WG Jr, Pratt L, et al. Alterations in intestinal permeability after thermal injury. Arch Surg. 1992;127(1):26–9; discussion 29–30.
176. Wolf SE, Ikeda H, Matin S, et al. Cutaneous burn increases apoptosis in the gut epithelium of mice. J Am Coll Surg. 1999;188(1):10–6.
177. Ezzell RM, Carter EA, Yarmush ML, et al. Thermal injury-induced changes in the rat intestine brush border cytoskeleton. Surgery. 1993;114(3):591–7.
178. Carter EA, Udall JN, Kirkham SE, et al. Thermal injury and gastrointestinal function. I. Small intestinal nutrient absorption and DNA synthesis. J Burn Care Rehabil. 1986;7(6):469–74.
179. Deitch EA, Rutan R, Waymack JP. Trauma, shock, and gut translocation. New Horiz. 1996;4(2):289–99.
180. Deitch EA. Intestinal permeability is increased in burn patients shortly after injury. Surgery. 1990;107(4):411–6.
181. Berthiaume F, Ezzell RM, Toner M, et al. Transport of fluorescent dextrans across the rat ileum after cutaneous thermal injury. Crit Care Med. 1994;22(3):455–64.
182. Horton JW. Bacterial translocation after burn injury: the contribution of ischemia and permeability changes. Shock. 1994;1(4):286–90.
183. Gianotti L, Alexander JW, Fukushima R, et al. Translocation of Candida albicans is related to the blood flow of individual intestinal villi. Circ Shock. 1993;40(4):250–7.
184. Jeschke MG, Micak RP, Finnerty CC, Herndon DN. Changes in liver function and size after a severe thermal injury. Shock. 2007;28(2):172–7.
185. Gamelli RL, He LK, Liu H, et al. Burn wound infection-induced myeloid suppression: the role of prostaglandin E2, elevated adenylate cyclase, and cyclic adenosine monophosphate. J Trauma. 1998;44(3):469–74.
186. Shoup M, Weisenberger JM, Wang JL, et al. Mechanisms of neutropenia involving myeloid maturation arrest in burn sepsis. Ann Surg. 1998;228(1):112–22.
187. Chitnis D, Dickerson C, Munster AM, et al. Inhibition of apoptosis in polymorphonuclear neutrophils from burn patients. J Leukoc Biol. 1996;59(6):835–9.
188. Rosenthal J, Thurman GW, Cusack N, et al. Neutrophils from patients after burn injury express a deficiency of the oxidase components p47-phox and p67-phox. Blood. 1996;88(11):4321–9.
189. Vindenes HA, Bjerknes R. Impaired actin polymerization and depolymerization in neutrophils from patients with thermal injury. Burns. 1997;23(2):131–6.
190. Hunt JP, Hunter CT, Brownstein MR, et al. The effector component of the cytotoxic T-lymphocyte response has a biphasic pattern after burn injury. J Surg Res. 1998;80(2):243–51.
191. Zedler S, Bone RC, Baue AE, et al. T-cell reactivity and its predictive role in immunosuppression after burns. Crit Care Med. 1999;27(1):66–72.
192. Kelly JL, Lyons A, Soberg CC, et al. Anti-interleukin-10 antibody restores burn-induced defects in T-cell function. Surgery. 1997;122(2):146–52.
193. Takagi K, Suzuki F, Barrow RE, et al. Recombinant human growth hormone modulates Th1 and Th2 cytokine response in burned mice. Ann Surg. 1998;228(1):106–11.
194. Hultman CS, Yamamoto H, deSerres S, et al. Early but not late burn wound excision partially restores viral-specific T lymphocyte cytotoxicity. J Trauma. 1997;43(3):441–7.

Organ Responses and Organ Support

19

Craig R. Ainsworth, Julie A. Rizzo, and Kevin K. Chung

Abbreviations

AKI	Acute kidney injury
AKIN	Acute kidney injury network
ARDS	Acute respiratory distress syndrome
BD	Base deficit
CVP	Central venous pressure
CRRT	Continuous renal replacement therapy
ICU	Intensive care unit
IHD	Intermittent hemodialysis
JTTS	Joint Theater Trauma System
LTVV	Low tidal volume ventilation
RIFLE	Risk injury failure loss end-stage
RRT	Renal replacement therapy
$ScvO_2$	Central venous oxygen saturation
SV	Stroke volume
SVV	Stroke volume variation
TBSA	Total body surface area

19.1 Introduction

Severe burn injury is a massive physiologic insult to the human body. The trauma to tissue caused by large burns results in an intense immune-inflammatory and hypermetabolic response that can be greater than other forms of severe critical illness and trauma. To address the highly complex and morbid physiologic derangements caused by burn injury, multi-disciplinary teams in burn intensive care units have aggressively sought ways to support injured and failing organs while the patient undergoes initial resuscitation and subsequent surgeries for excision and grafting. High impact advances in the critical care of burn patients with organ failure in recent decades include: multi-modal pain management, prevention of resuscitation morbidity using resuscitation protocols and decision support devices, advances in assessing the adequacy of resuscitation, the use of medications and physical therapy to prevent the loss of lean muscle mass, the use of high frequency percussive ventilation and other rescue modes when treating burn patients with severe acute respiratory distress syndrome and inhalation injury, the early use of renal replacement therapy (RRT) in patients with acute kidney injury (AKI), the recognition and management of gut failure, and the use of multi-organ support technologies. This chapter seeks to detail the physiologic organ response to severe burn injury and the means of organ support being used in current practice.

C. R. Ainsworth · J. A. Rizzo
Burn Center, United States Army Institute of Surgical Research, Fort Sam Houston, TX, USA
e-mail: craig.r.ainsworth.mil@mail.mil; julie.a.rizzo.mil@mail.mil

K. K. Chung (✉)
Department of Medicine, Uniformed Services University, Bethesda, MD, USA
e-mail: kevin.k.chung.mil@mail.mil

19.2 Central Nervous System

Burn patients suffer severe pain that does not always correlate with burn thickness or the area affected [1]. If this pain is managed inappropriately, it can result in physiologic derangements, anxiety, and post-traumatic stress disorder [2]. Inappropriate management of pain medications and sedatives in patients who are intubated and receiving mechanical ventilation can result in an increased incidence of delirium. This can thwart weaning from mechanical ventilation and prolong the intensive care unit (ICU) length of stay. Burn patients are at an increased risk of developing delirium due to the high incidence of mental health disorders and substance abuse among patients with burn injury [3]. Clinicians who treat burn patients must address constantly present background pain, take steps to mitigate procedural pain, and make medication available on an as-needed basis to address breakthrough pain.

M. G. Jeschke et al. (eds.), *Handbook of Burns Volume 1*, https://doi.org/10.1007/978-3-030-18940-2_19

Tools for treating burn pain include opioid analgesics, acetaminophen, NSAIDS, gabapentin, and ketamine. The use of NSAIDs is often limited by their nephrotoxicity and the damage that they can cause gastrointestinal mucosa. Medications that can help reduce the perception of pain include clonidine, dexmedetomidine, and benzodiazepines. The management of pain, agitation, and delirium are discussed in other chapters of this textbook.

19.3 Pulmonary

Approximately one-third of patients with burn injury require mechanical ventilation with that number increasing in patients with inhalation injury [4]. The primary difference between mechanical ventilation and our normal spontaneous breathing is that mechanical ventilation utilizes positive pressure whereas our normal breathing is done using negative pressure. While positive pressure can recruit alveoli, increase functional residual capacity, and improve gas exchange, it can also cause barotrauma to the lungs, reduce venous return to the heart, and decrease cardiac output. Understanding basic modes of mechanical ventilation will help the clinician be able to appropriately support this organ system when respiratory failure is caused by a burn injury or inhalation injury.

Control and Assist Control Ventilation. These are volume-cycled modes that deliver a preset tidal volume at a programmed respiratory rate and inspiratory flow rate without respect to the patient's respiratory effort. The control mode cannot be triggered by the patient and as such causes patients significant discomfort and results in patient-ventilator dyssynchrony. As such, this mode is usually used on heavily sedated and paralyzed patients in the operating room. The assist control mode will deliver the preset settings at a minimum and will allow the patient to trigger breaths when the ventilator senses that the patient is generating at least 2 cmH_2O of negative pressure. Patients are more comfortable being able to trigger their own breaths, and this mode will allow them to take a larger tidal volume breath than the preprogrammed tidal volume if they desire. Both the peak inspiratory pressure and plateau pressure should be serially measured in patients on this mode to avoid barotrauma.

Time-Cycled Pressure Control Ventilation. In patients with ARDS, the functional lung that can be aerated is a small fraction of the diseased lung. This small portion of functional lung has been referred to as a baby lung in literature on ARDS [5]. Because volume-cycled modes will deliver the tidal volume programmed, regardless of the pressure needed to deliver that tidal volume, patients on volume-cycled modes are at increased risk of barotrauma. Time-cycled pressure control ventilation delivers the breath at a preset flow rate and maximal inspiratory pressure. The breath is terminated at a preset time so the tidal volume delivered will be variable and that volume will be based on the compliance of the patient's lung and the amount of air that can be delivered at the preset flow rate while staying under the maximum programmed pressure. Clinicians who use this form of ventilation need to serially assess the adequacy of ventilation as the patient's lung compliance changes over time.

Synchronized Intermittent Mandatory Ventilation. The mode was initially developed as a weaning mode of ventilation with the principle being that it would allow patients to take spontaneous breaths in between programmed time or volume-cycled breaths. Technological advances allowed for synchronization of the breaths so that the machine did not deliver a pre-programmed breath on top of a spontaneous breath. Additionally, clinicians can provide varying levels of pressure support according to patient needs for the spontaneously triggered breaths. Clinicians believed that overtime as the patient's lung compliance improved that the programmed respiratory rate would decrease and the spontaneous respiratory rate would increase to the point that eventually the patient would be triggering and pulling nearly all of their minute ventilation and could thus be extubated. This however has not proved to be the case; when SIMV weaning is compared to weaning using pressure support or a T-piece, it has been demonstrated to be the most ineffective method of weaning [6].

Pressure Support Ventilation. In this mode, the patient triggers the breath when they generate a minimal negative pressure, usually (−)2 cmH_2O. The breath is delivered with a preset flow and pressure limit. Since these breaths are flow cycled, they will terminate once the patients inspiratory demand falls below the pre-programmed level. Thus for an awake patient who wants to be able to control the size and frequency of their own breaths, this is an ideal mode that will help avoid patient-ventilator dyssynchrony. This is not a good mode for patients who are heavily sedated or receiving neuromuscular blockade as the patient will not be able to trigger the ventilator. Once patients are awake and calm and able to spontaneously breathe, pressure support ventilation can be a good weaning mode as the preset inspiratory pressure can be weaned over time until it is at a low enough level and the patient can be extubated.

Inverse Ratio Ventilation. Usually, breaths are delivered by a ventilator with a short inspiratory time and a prolonged expiratory time with ratios of 1:2 or 1:4 being common. When inverse ratio ventilation is used, these ratios are reversed and longer inspiratory times are utilized with ratios from 1:1 to 2:1 being common. The principle behind the reversal of ratios is that the rapid initial flow rate will increase mean airway pressure and result in alveolar recruitment and that this recruitment effect won't be lost during the decelerating flow period of the inspiratory phase. This mode is used to improve oxygenation in patients with reduced pulmonary compliance as the prolonged inspiratory time will allow for more gas exchange to occur in areas of lung with ventilation and perfusion mismatch. These patients are usually difficult to ventilate due to their decreased compliance so the inverse ratios are applied to pressure controlled modes so as to avoid barotrauma.

High Frequency Percussive Ventilation. High frequency percussive ventilation (HFPV) has been associated with improved outcomes in patients with inhalation injury [7]. It facilitates the clearance of respiratory secretions, carbonaceous deposits, and endobronchial casts composed of sloughed bronchial mucosa. It is the author's mode of choice in the initial management of patients with inhalation injury as gas exchange goals can be met using lower inspiratory pressures. The breaths delivered to the patient are time-cycled with preset inspiratory and expiratory pressure limits and sub-tidal breaths cycled at a frequency of 400–800 per minute are superimposed on top. Patients with inhalation injury initially managed with HFPV had better chances of meeting gas exchange goals and not requiring rescue modes of ventilation when compared to patients receiving low tidal volume ventilation [8].

Airway Pressure Release Ventilation. It delivers continuous positive airway pressure at a preset time under a pressure limit with brief, intermittent releases. This mode works best in patients who are able to spontaneously breathe during the time that they are at the preset high pressure. This mode is an open lung strategy as it recruits alveoli in the under ventilated juxta-diaphragmatic portions of the lung as opposed to conventional positive pressure ventilation that tends to deliver breaths only to the already functional lung units. While there are no multi-center, randomized controlled trials demonstrating this mode to be superior to conventional positive pressure ventilation, there are numerous small trials and many experienced clinicians that have noted improved oxygenation, alveolar recruitment, improved hemodynamic performance, and decreased sedative requirements in patients being ventilated in this mode [9].

Acute respiratory distress syndrome (ARDS) complicates the course of 40–54% of patients with burn injury who require mechanical ventilation [10, 11]. ARDS is diagnosed using the Berlin criteria when there are bilateral opacities on chest imaging that are not due to cardiogenic pulmonary edema, atelectasis, or pleural effusions within 1 week of a known clinical insult. Echocardiography should be performed to rule out hydrostatic causes of edema if no risk factor for ARDS is present. See Table 19.1 for a description of how the severity of ARDS is categorized. Strategies for managing ARDS in patients with burn injury include low tidal volume ventilation (LTV) and other open lung ventilation strategies, usage of neuromuscular blockade, prone positioning, inhaled pulmonary vasodilators, and usage of extra corporeal membrane oxygenation.

Table 19.1 Berlin criteria for assessing the severity of a patient's ARDS

Mild	PaO_2/FiO_2 ratio from 200 to 300 mmHg with PEEP or CPAP $\geq$ 5 cmH_2O
Moderate	PaO_2/FiO_2 ratio from 100 to 200 mmHg with PEEP $\geq$ 5 cmH_2O
Severe	PaO_2/FiO_2 ratio < 100 mmHg with PEEP $\geq$ 5 cmH_2O

The use of LTV in patients with burn injury has been extrapolated from the ARDSNet study, which is controversial due to the fact that this trial excluded patients with burn injury [12]. A single center, randomized controlled trial was performed on 62 patients with burn injury that randomized them to either LTV or mechanical ventilation with a high frequency percussive ventilator [8]. Baseline demographics, percentage of total body surface area (TBSA) burned, and rates of inhalation injury were similar in both groups. Nearly one-third of patients in the LTV group failed to meet predetermined goals for oxygenation and ventilation and had to be placed on a rescue mode of mechanical ventilation. Two thirds of patients with smoke inhalation failed LTV. Burn injury and the loss of chest wall compliance due to edema or burn eschar, the hyper-catabolic state associated with burns and other variables make LTV a less effective treatment strategy.

Therapies for Refractory Hypoxemia in Patients with ARDS. Severe hypoxia induces vasoconstriction of the pulmonary vasculature which in turn causes pulmonary hypertension [13]. It is hypothesized that vasodilation of blood vessels perfusing aerated lung tissue with inhaled pulmonary vasodilators would redistribute blood from less ventilated regions of lung, reducing shunt fraction and correcting pulmonary hypertension. This process should then improve oxygenation and decrease mortality; however, it has not proven to be the case in randomized clinical trials [14]. Meta-analysis of the data from randomized trials reveals that while inhaled nitric oxide will improve oxygenation it does not decrease mortality and may increase rates of AKI [15]. The role of inhaled nitric oxide as a therapy for refractory hypoxemia is unclear.

Prone positioning is a viable treatment for refractory hypoxemia in adult burn-injured patients with severe ARDS. In a trial involving 18 burn ICU patients, the average PaO_2 to FiO_2 ratio increased from an average value of 87 prior to prone positioning to 236 at 36 hours after initiating prone positioning [16]. While facial ulcers developed on 4 patients, there were no unintentional extubations.

Extracorporeal membrane oxygenation (ECMO) technology has improved in the last decade with respect to its use in burn-injured patients [17]. In our burn center, the survival to hospital discharge rate for patients with severe ARDS due to burn injury, inhalation injury, or toxic epidermal necrolysis treated with ECMO is 57% [18]. This is a viable treatment strategy to reduce mortality in properly selected patients.

19.4 Cardiovascular

Burn injury can disturb multiple physiologic variables that affect the function and performance of the circulatory system. Volume loss into burned and non-burned tissue results in intravascular volume depletion which reduces the venous return to the heart, resulting in decreased cardiac output. Large TBSA burns induce myocardial depression which can cause a global decrease in contractility and a reduced left ventricular ejection fraction. This myocardial depression is pronounced during the initial presentation and this is usually followed by a hyper-dynamic phase in which cardiac output is augmented by an increase in heart rate and a reduction in afterload caused by vasodilation which is mediated by inflammatory cytokines. When patients with burn injury develop hypotension, clinicians will usually attribute this to volume depletion and vasodilation, and it is often the case early in the patient's resuscitation. Clinicians should put forth effort to make an accurate determination of the patient's intravascular volume status as unnecessary fluids or fluid creep can cause edema to form in the brain, lungs, bowel wall, renal parenchyma, skin and soft tissue. Determining intravascular volume status using the physical exam, vital signs, intake and output flow sheets, urine output, and calculating insensible losses is difficult to do reliably and in a way that is easy to reproduce among members of a care team. Any one, or many, of these parameters can be confounded by factors other than intravascular volume and this assessment relies upon multiple points of data rather than any one gold standard measure.

Right sided or static measures of hemodynamics and cardiovascular performance, namely the central venous pressure and pulmonary artery occlusion pressure have been demonstrated to be inaccurate in healthy patients, let alone those that are critically ill [19]. For this reason, dynamic measures of cardiac performance such as using an arterial line to calculate arterial wave form pulse pressure variation or stroke volume variation, cardiac output and cardiac index or using beside transthoracic or transesophageal echocardiography in real time is preferred.

When an intravascular volume assessment reveals that the patient has been adequately resuscitated and the patient remains hypotensive with a mean arterial pressure less than 65 mmHg, vasopressor therapy should be initiated. While there are no large, multi-center randomized controlled trials on this subject, our practice is to initiate vasopressin first followed by norepinephrine, epinephrine, and phenylephrine. The use of vasopressin in burn patients already on norepinephrine had a norepinephrine sparing effect and resulted in graft loss in only one of 30 patients involved in the study [20]. In patients with echocardiographic evidence of myocardial depression and left ventricular systolic dysfunction, clinicians should consider the use of dobutamine. Additionally, if patients have high vasopressor requirements, especially in the setting of septic shock, clinicians should consider initiating stress dose corticosteroids (hydrocortisone 100 mg IV every 8 h) for relative adrenal insufficiency associated with sepsis. [21].

19.5 Renal

Over the last decade, various diagnostic criteria have been proposed and validated in multiple populations, including surgical patients. These include the Risk Injury Failure Loss End-stage (RIFLE) criteria, the Acute Kidney Injury Network (AKIN) criteria and most recently the Kidney Disease Improving Global Outcomes (KDIGO) criteria. See Table 19.2 regarding the clinical and laboratory criteria for diagnosing AKI using the KDIGO criteria. Fenoldopam is a selective dopamine-1 receptor agonist approved for the treatment of hypertensive emergencies that in low doses (0.03–0.09 μg/kg/min) has been used to treat burn-injured patients with AKI. The patients who received fenoldopam in a retrospective study had varying degrees of AKI and initiating fenoldopam resulted in increased urine production, increased systolic blood pressure, and decreased serum creatinine levels. These effects were seen in the first 24 h and continued to improve through 48 h [22]. The use of this medication can sometimes prevent the patient from having to receive renal replacement therapy.

Traditional complications of AKI that would warrant immediate initiation of renal replacement therapy are included in Table 19.3.

The literature demonstrates that early and intensive RRT may provide the best benefit for critically ill patients, particularly in those with AKI diagnosed early in their clinical course. Critically ill burn patients who develop AKI have mortality rates that are over 20% higher than the general critical care population [23, 24]. Historically, these patients were often not considered candidates for intermittent hemodialysis (IHD) due their hemodynamic instability by the time they developed a traditional indication for RRT. Continuous veno-venous hemofiltration (CVVH) is known to be well tol-

Table 19.2 KDIGO staging criteria for patients with AKI

	Creatinine criteria	Urine output criteria
Stage 1	↑ 0.3 mg/dL in 48 h or by >50% over 7 days	<0.5 mL/kg/h for >6 h
Stage 2	↑ Creatinine of >100%	<0.5 mL/kg/h for >12 h
Stage 3	↑ Creatinine of >200%	<0.3 mL/kg/h for ≥24 h or anuria for ≥12 h

Table 19.3 Traditional indications for initiating renal replacement therapy

Complication	Criteria for initiating renal replacement therapy
Metabolic acidosis	Refractory to sodium bicarbonate infusion
Electrolyte imbalance	Hyperkalemia refractory to medical management
Toxic ingestion	Small molecular size and low level protein binding so as to be cleared by dialysis
Uremia	Uremic encephalopathy, pericarditis, gastropathy, or bleeding due to uremic platelets
Intravascular volume overload	Pulmonary edema refractory to diuretic therapy

erated in the setting of shock. In a recent study, patients with greater than 40% total body surface area burn and AKIN stage 3 AKI or AKIN stage 2 AKI with shock were started on CVVH, even if they did not meet traditional criteria for initiating RRT. When these patients were compared to historical controls, they had a 24% lower in-hospital mortality rate, a 33% lower 28-day mortality rate, a dramatic reduction in vasopressor requirement and an average PaO_2/FiO_2 ratio increase of 153 within 24 h [25]. What mode of renal replacement therapy will provide maximal benefit to the patient, at what dose and when therapy should be initiated are questions that investigators have sought to answer with the best data available. We review these controversies below.

Mode. In a review of nine randomized trials comparing outcomes in patients placed on intermittent compared to continuous therapy, there was no standardization of the timing, criteria for initiation or dose of renal replacement therapy [26]. This review concluded that there was no statistically significant evidence that the initial RRT modality influenced mortality or recovery of renal function. There was a trend observed that CRRT was associated with less hemodynamic instability and better control of the patient's fluid balance. Another meta-analysis reviewed 23 randomized controlled trials and 16 observational studies to investigate if there was any difference in rates of renal recovery among severe AKI survivors [27]. Pooled analysis of the RCT's did not reveal a statistically significant difference in renal recovery based on RRT modality used. A pooled analysis of the observational studies did demonstrate a higher rate of renal recovery among patients receiving continuous therapy.

The main factor to be considered in deciding to use intermittent or continuous RRT is the patient's hemodynamic stability. Advanced age, female gender, diabetes, low blood pressure prior to dialysis, hypoalbuminemia, and higher BMI are all associated with increased risk for intradialytic hypotension [28]. If removal of intravascular volume exceeds the patient's ability to refill their plasma volume, then hypotension will occur. The level of sodium in the dialysate, plasma albumin levels and hydrostatic capillary force all influence plasma refill [29]. The patient's osmolality declines during dialysis due to the rapid removal of urea and shifts in plasma sodium concentrations which will lead to slower plasma refill and eventually hypotension [29]. For patients who are hemodynamically unstable or who cannot tolerate large volume shifts and rapid changes in plasma osmolality, continuous modalities offer the benefit of renal replacement therapy with less risk of hypotension. Patients with neuro-trauma or other conditions that elevate intra-cranial pressure cannot tolerate the osmotic shifts that occur during IHD and it is contraindicated in this patient population [30].

Dose of Renal Replacement Therapy. The currently recommended dose for renal replacement therapy is 20–25 mL/kg/h [30]. Most patients do not have day after day of uninterrupted CRRT. Therapy can be interrupted by trips to radiology for imaging studies or dysfunction with the circuit caused by clotting or malfunction of the dialysis access line. In one study, interruptions in RRT ranged from 8 to 28% of the total treatment time [31]. Clinicians should target a prescription of 25–30 mL/kg/h and above so as to account for interruptions in therapy and insure that the patient is receiving the minimal delivered dose of 20–25 mL/kg/h. The current recommended dose is based on several clinical trials that compared different doses of renal replacement therapy and their impact on clinical outcomes. The VA/NIH Acute Renal Failure Trial Network randomized 1124 patients with acute kidney injury and failure of at least one non-renal organ or sepsis to intensive therapy (CRRT dose of 35 mL/kg/h) or less intensive therapy (CRRT dose of 20 mL/kg/h). The primary end point was all-cause mortality by day 60. There was no difference in the rate of all-cause mortality, or in duration of renal replacement therapy, or the rate of renal recovery [32]. The RENAL Replacement Therapy Study Investigators conducted a multi-center, randomized controlled trial to compare the effect of different doses of renal replacement therapy on 90-day mortality. They randomized patients with AKI and critical illness to post-dilution CVVH with a dose of 40 or 25 mL/kg/h. There was no statistically significant difference in all-cause 90-day mortality or renal recovery or duration of renal replacement therapy [33].

Given the seeming absence of any benefit to higher doses, the KDIGO guideline recommends a dose of 20–25 mL/kg/h for CRRT in AKI [30]. However, this may not be the case for patients with post-surgical AKI. In a recent Cochrane review, post-surgical patients who developed AKI had a statistically significant reduction in mortality if they received a dose greater than 35 mL/kg/h [34]. This was based on two studies that enrolled 531 patients and was deemed by reviewers to be high quality evidence. We therefore recommend the consideration of an initial higher delivered dose of 35 mL/kg/h of RRT for patients with post-surgical AKI, especially when dealing with severe metabolic disturbance.

Timing. The literature demonstrates that early and intensive RRT may provide the best benefit for critically ill patients.

Two recently published trials attempted to answer the question of when to initiate renal replacement therapy in AKI. The Artificial Kidney Initiation in Kidney Injury (AKIKI) study group performed a multi-center randomized controlled trial on patients with KDIGO stage 3 AKI who required mechanical ventilation and catecholamine infusion. These patients did not have a life-threatening complication directly related to renal failure and were designated to an early or delayed strategy for RRT initiation [35]. Early initiation consisted of starting RRT at the time of randomization. Delayed initiation consisted of starting RRT when the patient developed a potentially life-threatening complication of AKI to include severe hyperkalemia, metabolic acidosis, pulmonary edema, BUN higher than 112 mg/dL, or oliguria for more than 72 h after randomization. The primary outcome was survival at 60 days. The results of the trial demonstrated no difference in mortality but did demonstrate an increased incidence of catheter-related blood stream infection in the early initiation group and half of the patients in the delayed initiation arm never needed renal replacement therapy. While the trial did not demonstrate a mortality reduction attributable to early initiation, it may be that waiting to initiate RRT once the patient has KDIGO stage 3 AKI is already too late to see a benefit in "early" initiation.

The Early Versus Late Initiation of Renal Replacement Therapy in Critically Ill Patients with Acute Kidney Injury (ELAIN) randomized clinical trial was a single center study that randomized 231 patients with KDIGO stage 2 AKI and plasma neutrophil gelatinase-associated lipocalin levels higher than 150 ng/mL to early initiation of RRT (within 8 h of diagnosis of KDIGO stage 2 AKI) or delayed initiation (within 12 h of diagnosis of KDIGO stage 3 AKI) or no initiation [36]. Ninety-day mortality in the early RRT group was 39% and 54% in the delayed group. In the early group, 53% experienced renal recovery whereas in the delayed group 38% experienced renal recovery. Duration of renal replacement therapy and hospital length of stay were also shorter in the early initiation group. These results led the authors to call for larger, multi-center trials to be performed using a similar protocol so as to demonstrate whether these results can be generalized to all critical care patients with KDIGO stage 2 AKI.

19.6 Gastrointestinal

The pathophysiology of burn shock includes end-organ hypoperfusion and the gastrointestinal (GI) tract is at high risk during the acute phase of burn resuscitation and also during episodes of sepsis. The risk of intestinal ischemia is further increased with increasing burn size, high resuscitation volumes, and the use of vasoactive agents [37]. Intestinal ischemia results in a disruption of the barrier function of the mucosa, resulting in the movement of bacteria and/or endotoxin into the mesenteric lymph nodes and systemic tissues, termed translocation. Life-threatening bacteremia with associated abdominal sepsis can quickly ensue. Treatment is primarily focused on prevention with controlled resuscitation, judicious use of vasoactive agents, early enteral nutrition, and close monitoring.

Gastrointestinal dysfunction, not related to burn shock or the resulting hypoperfusion, occurs commonly after burn injury. The liberal use of opioid-based analgesia, electrolyte imbalances, prolonged immobility, endocrine abnormalities, and septic episodes are factors that contribute to the increased prevalence of GI dysfunction in critically ill burn patients. Common manifestations of GI dysfunction include increased gastric secretions, tube feeding intolerance, reduced intestinal motility resulting in paralytic ileus, mucosal ulceration, and constipation. Constipation and late defecation is common in burn patients and treatment should be aimed at prevention by understanding the multi-factorial etiology and implementing appropriate therapy early. Osmotic laxatives, such as lactulose and polyethylene glycol, and stool softeners, such as docusate, are first-line agents. These are often all that is needed to prevent or treat constipation. Opioid-based analgesia is a mainstay of pain control in burned patients. Acting on the μ-receptor centrally produces analgesia but stimulation of this receptor in the mucosal layer of the GI tract causes reduced peristalsis and inhibition of intestinal ion and fluid secretion, resulting in opioid-induced bowel dysfunction, most commonly manifested by constipation. μ-receptor antagonists, such as naloxone and methynaltrexone, are agents that can reverse the peripheral effects of opioids while preserving the central analgesic effects. Naloxone dosing is often 2 mg orally every 4 hours, methynaltrexone is dosed at 12–24 mg subcutaneously daily [38]. The side effect profile of these agents is minimal; they are recommended for patients on opioids who fail laxative therapy. Acute colonic pseudo-obstruction is a well-recognized cause of lower GI tract dysfunction in burn patients, presenting with abdominal distention and pain and obstipation [39]. Abdominal imaging demonstrates a massive dilation of the colon, most often the cecum and right colon. Conservative management, including correction of electrolyte abnormalities as well as nasogastric and rectal decompression, is often successful. If unsuccessful, neostigmine is recommended as the next line of therapy as it stimulates muscarinic receptors in the colon to promote motility. Continuous monitoring is required during administration of this medication with common adverse effects being bradycardia that is responsive to atropine, abdominal cramping, and excessive salivation [40].

19.7 Conclusion

Improvements in organ support of the severely burned have reduced mortality in recent decades. This is due to improvements in resuscitation and the prevention of resuscitation morbidities, improvements, and widespread implementation of advanced forms of mechanical ventilation, renal replacement therapy, and strategies to mitigate the hypercatabolic state associated with burns. These treatment modalities are delivered by highly trained specialists who compose a multidisciplinary team dedicated to the care of critically injured burn patients until their organs can resume their normal physiologic function.

Summary Box

- Severe burn injury is a massive physiologic insult to the human body, greater than other forms of severe critical illness and trauma.
- Critical care is a process of frequent physiologic monitoring coupled with procedural or pharmacologic interventions.
- Organ failure is common after severe burns.
- Adequate organ support is paramount to improving outcomes.

References

1. Richardson P, Mustard L. The management of pain in the burns unit. Burns. 2009;35:921–36.
2. Summer GJ, Puntillo KA, Miakowski C, et al. Burn injury pain: the continuing challenge. J Pain. 2007;8:533–48.
3. Palmu R, Suominen K, Vuola J, et al. Mental disorders among acute burn patients. Burns. 2010;36:1072–9.
4. Belenkiy SM, Buel AR, Cannon JW, et al. Acute respiratory distress syndrome in wartime military burns: application of the Berlin criteria. J Trauma Acute Care Surg. 2014;76:821–7.
5. Gattinoni L, Marini JJ, Psenti A, et al. The "baby lung" became an adult. Intensive Care Med. 2016;42:663–73.
6. Alia I, Esteban A. Weaning from mechanical ventilation. Crit Care. 2000;4:72–80.
7. Allan PF, Osborn EC, Chung KK, et al. High-frequency percussive ventilation revisited. J Burn Care Res. 2010;31:510–20.
8. Chung KK, Wolf SE, Renz EM, et al. High-frequency percussive ventilation and low tidal volume ventilation in burns: a randomized controlled trial. Crit Care Med. 2010;38:1970–7.
9. Jain SV, Kollisch-Singule M, Sadowitz B, et al. The 30-year evolution of airway pressure release ventilation (APRV). Intensive Care Med Exp. 2016;4:11–29.
10. Dancey DR, Hayes J, Gomez M, et al. ARDS in patients with thermal injury. Intensive Care Med. 1999;25:1231–6.
11. Liffner G, Bak Z, Reske A, et al. Inhalation injury assessed by score does not contribute to the development of acute respiratory distress syndrome in burn victims. Burns. 2005;31:263–8.
12. The Acute Respiratory Distress Syndrome Network. Ventilation with lower tidal volumes as compared with traditional tidal volumes for acute lung injury and the acute respiratory distress syndrome. N Engl J Med. 2000;342:1301–8.
13. Zapol WM, Snider MT. Pulmonary hypertension in severe acute respiratory failure. N Engl J Med. 1977;296:476–80.
14. Afshari A, Brok J, Moller AM, et al. Inhaled nitric oxide for acute respiratory distress syndrome (ARDS) and acute lung injury in children and adults. Cochrane Database Syst Rev. 2010;(7) https://doi.org/10.1002/14651858.CD002787.Epub2010/07/09.pub2.
15. Adhikari NK, Burns KE, Friedrich JO, et al. Effect of nitric oxide on oxygenation and mortality in acute lung injury: systematic review and meta-analysis. BMJ. 2007;334:779.
16. Hale DF, Cannon JW, Batchinsky AI, et al. Prone positioning improves oxygenation in adult burn patients with severe acute respiratory distress syndrome. J Trauma Acute Care Surg. 2012;72:1634–9.
17. Asmusen S, Maybauer DM, Fraser JF, et al. Extracorporeal membrane oxygenation in burn and smoke inhalation injury. Burns. 2013;39:429–35.
18. Ainsworth CR, Dellavolpe J, Chung KK, et al. Outcomes in the use of extracorporeal membrane oxygenation on adult US Army Burn Center patients with severe ARDS. Unpublished case series.
19. Kumar A, Anel R, Bunnell E, et al. Pulmonary artery occlusion pressure and central venous pressure fail to predict ventricular filling volume, cardiac performance, or the response to volume infusion in normal subjects. Crit Care Med. 2004;32:691–9.
20. Cartotto R, McGibney K, Smith T, et al. Vasopressin for the septic burn patient. Burns. 2007;33:441–51.
21. Rhodes A, Evans LE, Alhazzani W, et al. Surviving sepsis campaign: international guidelines for management of sepsis and septic shock: 2016. Crit Care Med. 2017;45:486–552.
22. Simmons JW, Chung KK, Renz EM, et al. Fenoldapam use in a burn intensive care unit: a retrospective study. BMC Anesthesiol. 2010;10:9.
23. Chung KK, Stewart IJ, Gisler C, et al. The Acute Kidney Injury (AKIN) criteria applied in burns. J Burn Care Res. 2012;33(4):483–90.
24. Stewart IJ, Tilley MA, Cotant CL, et al. Association of AKI with adverse outcomes in burned military casualties. Clin J Am Soc Nephrol. 2012;7(2):199–206.
25. Chung KK, Lundy JB, Matson JR, et al. Continuous venovenous hemofiltration in severely burned patients with acute kidney injury: a cohort study. Crit Care. 2009;13:R62.
26. Bagshaw SM, Berthiaume LR, Delaney A, Bellomo R. Continuous versus intermittent renal replacement therapy for critically ill patients with acute kidney injury: a meta-analysis. Crit Care Med. 2008;36:610.
27. Schneider AG, Bellomo R, Bagshaw SM, et al. Choice of renal replacement therapy modality and dialysis dependence after acute kidney injury: a systematic review and meta-analysis. Intensive Care Med. 2013;39:987.
28. Flythe JE, Xue H, Lynch KE, et al. Association of mortality risk with various definitions of intradialytic hypotension. J Am Soc Nephrol. 2015;26:724–34.
29. Assimon MM, Flythe JE. Intradialytic blood pressure abnormalities: the highs, the lows and all that lies between. Am J Nephrol. 2015;42:337–50.
30. Kidney Disease Improving Global Outcomes (KDIGO) Acute Kidney Injury Work Group. KDIGO clinical practice guideline for acute kidney injury. Kidney Int. 2012;2(Suppl):1–138.
31. Monti G, Herrera M, Kindgen-Milles D, et al. The dose responsive multicenter international collaborative initiative (DO-RE-MI). Contrib Nephrol. 2007;156:434–43.
32. Palevsky PM, Zhang JH, O'Conner TZ, et al. Intensity of renal support in critically ill patients with acute kidney injury. N Engl J Med. 2008;359:1–14.
33. Bellomo R, Cass A, Cole L, et al. Intensity of continuous renal-replacement therapy in critically ill patients. N Engl J Med. 2009;361:1627–38.
34. Fayad AI, Buamscha DG, Ciapponi A, et al. Intensity of continuous renal replacement therapy for acute kidney injury. Cochrane Database Syst Rev. 2016;(10):CD010613.

35. Gaudry S, Hajage D, Schortgen F, et al. Initiation strategies for renal-replacement therapy in the intensive care unit. N Engl J Med. 2016;375(2):122–33.
36. Zarbock A, Kellum JA, Schmidt C, et al. Effect of early vs delayed initiation of renal replacement therapy on mortality in critically ill patients with acute kidney injury: the ELAIN randomized clinical trial. JAMA. 2016;315(20):2190–9.
37. Markell KW, Renz EM, White CE, et al. Abdominal complications after severe burns. J Am Coll Surg. 2009;208:940–7.
38. Lundy JB, Chung KK, Ainsworth CR, et al. Update on severe burn management for the intensivist. J Intensive Care Med. 2016;31:499–510.
39. Ives A, Muller M, Pegg S. Colonic pseudo-obstruction in burns patients. Burns. 1996;22:598–601.
40. Law NM, Bharucha AE, Undale AS, et al. Cholinergic stimulation enhances colonic motor activity, transit and sensation in humans. Am J Physiol Grastrointest Liver Physiol. 2001;281:1228–37.

Critical Care in Burns

20

Luis R. Taveras, Marc G. Jeschke, and Steven E. Wolf

20.1 Introduction

Severe burns represent around 436,000 ambulatory care visits to hospital emergency departments in the United States [1]. A significant portion of these burns are minor; nevertheless between 40,000 and 60,000 burn patients undergo admission to a hospital [2]. Of all cases, nearly 4000 people die of complications related to the burn [3]. During the 1940s and 1950s, the burn size lethal to 50% of the population was 42% of total body surface area (TBSA). More recently, this number has increased to more than 90% TBSA in selected groups of patients. The devastating consequences of burns have been recognized by the medical community, and significant amounts of resources and research have been dedicated to improve our understanding and enhancing the way we manage patients, successfully improving these dismal statistics [3–5]. This significant improvement is secondary to the establishment of specialized burn centers, refinements in resuscitation strategies, advances in critical care, sepsis management and infection control, early excision of burn wounds, enhanced wound coverage, better support on the metabolic response to burns, and improved treatment of inhalation injury [5, 6].

A major burn involves more than 20% TBSA, and one that involves 40% TBSA or more is termed "massive." Increased morbidity and mortality are directly proportional to burn size. There is a distinction noted at around 60% TBSA for pediatric patients and around 40% TBSA for adult burn patients [7]. This subset of patients benefits the greatest from specialized burn centers and intensive care. Severe burns are devastating injuries affecting nearly every organ system and leading to significant morbidity and mortality [3–6, 8]. The presence of inhalation injury further increases mortality, up to 20% added mortality for patients in the 50% lethality region [9–11].

Patients with severe burns share several characteristics with other critically ill patients; nonetheless, there are noteworthy differences:

- Patients suffer a cutaneous exudative losses of fluids, proportional to the TBSA. These fluids contain large amounts of proteins, minerals, and micronutrients.
- The injured body surface area poses an enormous catabolic challenge.
- The loss of the skin barrier increases risk of infection; moreover, significant immunosuppression results following major burn.
- The duration of inflammatory and hypermetabolic response is immediate and long-lasting.
- Venous access is compromised secondary to the destruction of the skin at puncture sites.
- Long stays in the ICU and prolonged nutritional support are indicated.

Total length of hospital stay and the proportion of intensive care unit days is variable and highly dependent on TBSA. Overall, the mean length of stay is approximately 2 days per percent burn, based on the National Burn Repository

L. R. Taveras
Division of Burn, Trauma, and Critical Care, Department of Surgery, University of Texas—Southwestern Medical Center, Dallas, TX, USA
e-mail: steven.wolf@utsouthwestern.edu

M. G. Jeschke
Faculty of Medicine, Institute of Medical Science, University of Toronto, Toronto, ON, Canada

Biological Sciences, Sunnybrook Research Institute, Toronto, ON, Canada

Ross Tilley Burn Centre, Sunnybrook Health Sciences Centre, Sunnybrook Hospital, Toronto, ON, Canada

Division of Plastic and Reconstructive Surgery, Department of Surgery, Faculty of Medicine, University of Toronto, Toronto, ON, Canada

Department of Immunology, Faculty of Medicine, University of Toronto, Toronto, ON, Canada
e-mail: Marc.Jeschke@sunnybrook.ca

S. E. Wolf (✉)
Department of Surgery, University of Texas Medical Branch, Galveston, TX, USA
e-mail: swolf@utmb.edu

M. G. Jeschke et al. (eds.), *Handbook of Burns Volume 1*, https://doi.org/10.1007/978-3-030-18940-2_20

report. It ranges from 1.5 to 3 days per % TBSA in patients with less than 20% TBSA to patients with burns greater than 60% TBSA, respectively [12]. ICU stay can represent 20% of the total hospital stay in both adult and pediatric patients. In a cohort by Maan et al., the mean length of stay in the ICU was 0.32 ± 0.02 days per % burn while the length of stay in the general burn ward was 0.68 ± 0.06 days per % burn [13].

Deaths secondary to burns generally occur either immediately after the injury or weeks later as a result of infection/sepsis, multisystem organ failure, or hypermetabolic responses [6, 14]. Therefore, this chapter is divided into critical care during early phases and late phases. The quality of the complex care of burn patients is directly related to the outcome and survival of burn patients. The key aspects for the care are:

1. *Prehospital and initial management of burns*: an adequate and timely response, evaluation of the burns, treatment of the burn patient, resuscitation, initial pain management, and transport
2. *Early hospital phase*: admission to a burn center,escharatomies/fasciotomies, resuscitation, treatment of inhalation injury, critical care to maintain organ perfusion and function
3. *Later hospital phase*: wound care including burn wound closure operations, infection control, attenuation of hypermetabolism, maintaining organ function, and rehabilitation efforts

In this chapter, we focus on critical care components that have been shown to contribute to improved outcomes after burn. Prehospital and early management as well as fluid management will be discussed at length.

20.2 Early Hospital Phase

In the initial management, the therapeutic goal for burn patients is the prevention of organ failure, an effort that begins with adequate resuscitation [15–19]. Resuscitation and all current formulas are discussed in detail in another chapter in this book. However, resuscitation is also one of the key aspects of the early phase in critical care.

Once the burn patient is received by the accepting burn center, the patient usually is evaluated and treated in a room for wound cleaning and treatment (tubroom). This visit includes cleansing, an evaluation of burn wounds, possible escharotomies/fasciotomies, intubation including bronchoscopy and a diagnosis of inhalation injury, the placement of arterial and venous access, the placement of a Foley catheter, early analgesia, and adequate dressing care. When these interventions are finished, the central element of critical care is the monitoring of vital signs and subsequent regulation of homeostasis. Monitoring can include:

- Invasive arterial blood pressure
- Noninvasive blood pressure (not recommended for large burns >40% TBSA)
- Urine output
- Central venous pressure
- Oxygen saturation and respiratory rate
- Blood gas with lactate
- Ventilation settings
- Invasive and noninvasive hemodynamic monitoring (i.e., cardiac output, cardiac index, stroke volume, stroke volume variation)
- Serum organ markers
- Central and peripheral tissue perfusion markers

20.2.1 Cardiovascular Management and Resuscitation

Immediately following injury, inflammatory shock mediators are released from the burned skin. These include histamine, serotonin, bradykinin, nitric oxide, lipid peroxides, prostaglandins, derived oxygen and nitric oxide-free radicals, thromboxane, cytokines (interleukins and TNF), and platelet aggregating factor with the subsequent coagulation cascade. Additionally, numerous mechanisms affect the endothelial cells, by these mechanisms the connections between these cells could become compromised and the proteins that make up those connections might be altered [20]. The response is proportional to the injury, and systemic effects of these mediators will become obvious with burns exceeding 20–25% TBSA [21] though as little as 10% TBSA can induce edema in nonburned tissues. This phase lasts for 24–72 h and is characterized by increased vascular permeability, fluid shifts resulting in intravascular hypovolemia, and the formation of edema. The massive histamine release will cause an early increase in the permeability of local and systemic capillaries, initiating a massive capillary leak enabling large molecules such as albumin to escape into the interstitial space. Serotonin and bradykinin will cause the persistence of this phenomenon during the first 18–24 h. Due to the loss of plasma, a steep increase in hematocrit is observed.

The generalized edema after burns starts developing as soon as 2–4 h after injury and follows a biphasic pattern: an early rapid phase and a slower increase during the next 12–36 h [22, 23]. A slow resolution of the increased permeability will start between 8 and 12 h depending on the burn size. During this resolution phase, extravasated plasma proteins and resuscitation fluids will remain sequestered in extravascular spaces of nonburned and burned soft tissue. Edema formation will exceed the capacity of the lymph vessels to evacuate fluid. The rate of resorption from lymphatics is faster in partial-thickness rather than full-thickness burns.

The difference in rates of resorption is thought to be due to the destruction of lymphatics in full-thickness burns [24]. The speed of the edema progression will depend on the quality of the resuscitation: a rapid early delivery of large amounts of resuscitation fluids increases the edema formation and worsens the compromised local microcirculation, worsening ischemia in the injured tissues. In addition to the capillary leak, fluid losses can directly be attributed to the wound exudates (1–2 L/10% TBSA during the first 24 h, decreasing thereafter until closure of the wound) and evaporation, and these losses include plasma proteins (30 g of protein/10% TBSA/day), minerals, and trace elements.

Burn shock is the result of the significant loss of fluids described as a combination of hypovolemic and distributive shock. A component of cardiogenic shock has also been recognized. Myocardial dysfunction after burns has been repeatedly demonstrated both in humans and animals. Neuroendocrine responses will contribute to the worsening of the hemodynamic condition by increasing cardiac afterload due to the massive release of endogenous norepinephrine and epinephrine. This is further complicated by the decrease in preload due to the hypovolemic stage. Cardiac function is affected by mitochondrial burn-induced oxidative stress. Oxygen-free radicals and lipid peroxides play an important role. In burns over 40% TBSA cardiac intrinsic contractile defects are observed, which are only partially reversed by fluid resuscitation and antioxidants [25]. Troponin I increases in a large proportion of the patients with major burns, reflecting intrinsic tissue damage.

Resuscitation should aim to maintain organ perfusion through: urinary output of 0.5 mL/h, stabilization of the heart rate, maintenance of a mean arterial pressure (MAP) of ≥60 mmHg; normal lactate and base excess levels. These parameters will generally reflect the patient's resuscitation status [3, 26, 27]. The majority of burn surgeons use the Parkland formula for the initial resuscitation [17]. A computer decision support system (Burn Resuscitation Decision Support System) was developed in an effort to guide resuscitation based on hourly urine output. Its use has been associated with a reduction in crystalloid volume used, ventilator days, and mortality, and with an increase in the frequency of urine output within the target range [28, 29].

Inadequate resuscitation, either under- or over-resuscitation (Table 20.1), can have deleterious effects on the patient. Over-resuscitation is associated with significant generalized edema resulting in respiratory failure, abdominal compartment syndrome, and ocular and extremity compartment syndromes.

The continuous monitoring of the arterial blood pressure ensures adequate organ perfusion and is a key aspect in the initial post-burn phase. In burns over 40% TBSA, invasive monitoring may be required. Chronic hypertensive patients may benefit from a greater MAP, which can vary. The most common problem during the first 24–48 h after burn is hypotension with very few patients having hypertension. Adequate MAP and organ perfusion can be achieved by:

- Adequate fluid resuscitation (e.g., Parkland 4 cc/kg/m^2 burn of Ringer's lactate)
- Albumin substitution after 8–12 h after burn if initial fluid resuscitation fails (5% albumin 75–125 cc/h)
- Transfusion of packed red blood cells
- Dobutamine if low cardiac index (0.5–1 μg/kg/min)
- Norepinephrine or epinephrine in cases of fluid-resistant hypotension
- Vasopressin in refractory distributive shock (up to 0.03 units/min)

If a patient is hypertensive (systolic > 200 mmHg or diastolic > 120 mmHg) and has signs of over-resuscitation, the recommendation is to decrease the vasopressors, decrease fluids, and decrease albumin in stages until target MAP is achieved. If the patient is not on vasopressors, inotropes, and hypertensives, recommendations are:

- Nitroprusside (up to 10 μg/kg/min)
- Labetalol (10–20 mg)
- Nicardipine (5 mg/h)

In patients with associated trauma and altered mental status that exhibit unexplained early arterial hypertension, the presence of traumatic brain injury should be considered.

Rates of infusion during resuscitation tend to be attenuated following hour 13 after injury. Even when comparing different resuscitation strategies, Salinas et al. showed a sustained increase in urine output after the 12 h mark [28]. This effect, might be secondary to a relative and progressive myocardial recovery. After 24–48 h, the patients generally become spontaneously hyperdynamic and the fluid delivery

Table 20.1 Assessment of resuscitation

Under-resuscitation	Over-resuscitation
Oliguria < 0.3 mL/kg/h	Polyuria > 1.0 mL/kg/h
Hemoglobin > 18 g/dL (Hct > 55%)	Decreasing PaO_2/FiO_2, →pulmonary edema
Sodium > 145 mEq/L	Increasing pulmonary artery wedge pressure, central venous pressure (CVP)
Cardiac index < 2 L/min/m^2	Rapidly increasing cutaneous edema
Mixed venous oxygen saturation (SvO_2) < 55%	Fluid delivery > Ivy index (fluid delivery > 250 mL/Kg body weight) [30]
Plasma lactate > 2 mmol/L or increasing	Intra-abdominal hypertension
Base deficit < −5 mmol/L or decreasing	Compartment syndrome

should be drastically reduced to about 30–40% of that infused during the first 24 h. As the microvasculature starts to seal and peripheral blood flow is increased to the burned areas, the physiology shifts to a decreased vascular permeability, increased heart rate, and decreased peripheral vascular resistance resulting in an increase in cardiac output. The patients' metabolic rate is increased to nearly three times that of their basal metabolic rate [31].

20.2.1.1 Crystalloids

Adequate resuscitation is a key element of early burn critical care [15–19]. Maintenance of organ perfusion during burn shock depends upon the restoration of intravascular volume. The principles of burn fluid resuscitation were developed in the early 1950s. The most common algorithm, the Parkland formula, calculates a total volume of crystalloid to be given over the first 24 h according to 4 mL × weight (kg) × TBSA (%) [15, 17, 27, 32, 33]. Drs. Baxter and Shires published their seminal article in 1968 after experiments on animal models followed by their early experience with burn patients. They used animal models to determine direct extracellular fluid volume changes in the early post-burn period. Subsequently, 11 patients were treated experimentally with the volumes estimated by the experimental burns. They proposed that in the first 24 h post-burn, hemodynamics appear to be closely in correlation with functional extracellular fluid volume maintenance but unrelated to volume thereafter. Even in this early work, significant changes in cardiac output were noticed in burn subjects [34].

In accordance with the American Burn Association, the resuscitation formula is only to be used as a guideline for resuscitation in burn shock [16–18, 26, 33]. The endpoints (urine output of 0.5 cc/kg/h, MAP > 60) which traditionally had been used for fluid resuscitation are not always adequate. With the advent of goal-directed therapy (base deficit, lactate, cardiac index and/or output, and stroke volume variation) [15, 27, 32, 33, 35, 36], it has become apparent that traditional formulas may inadequately estimate fluid requirements. The Parkland formula is deficient in calculating the fluid requirements for resuscitation in patients with: a large burn size, deeper burns, an inhalation injury, delays in resuscitation, current alcohol or drug use, and an electrical injury, leading to inadequate/inappropriate resuscitation.

Patients with severe burns and electrical injuries receive far greater crystalloid volumes than predicted, resulting in "fluid creep" [16, 17, 27, 36, 37] with its inherent complications such as: pulmonary edema, pleural effusions, pericardial effusions, abdominal compartment syndrome, extremity compartment syndrome, and the conversion of burns to deeper wounds. In addition, increasing the fluid administration in burned patients significantly increases the risk of developing acute respiratory distress syndrome (ARDS), pneumonia, bloodstream infections, multiorgan failure, and death [26]. Given the risk of abdominal compartment syndrome with large burns and its dire consequences, intra-abdominal pressure monitoring is therefore recommended in burns involving more than 30% TBSA [30].

The selection of crystalloid for resuscitation has been debated extensively. Exudates and edema fluid are known to be isotonic, containing the same amounts of electrolytes and protein as plasma. Whatever the formula, the fluid used must contain sodium in sufficient concentration to deliver about 0.5 mmol/kg/%TBSA by 48 h to prevent water intoxication associated with hypotonic fluids. Ringer's lactate solution is a common option. However, the use of other alternatives is acceptable. The use of normal saline can induce acidemia due to the disassociation of ions of sodium and chloride in the solution, further exacerbating the acidosis associated with burn injury. Hypertonic saline has been associated with hypernatremia, renal failure, and mortality when used in burn resuscitation.

By day 3, the interstitial fluids that have accumulated during the first 24–48 h start to mobilize and be excreted. This might be augmented by active stimulation of diuresis using loop diuretics, sometimes in combination with an aldosterone antagonist.

As the resuscitation phase approaches an end, it becomes important to determine the total daily maintenance fluid requirement, which can be calculated by:

$$\text{Basal Fluid } (1500\ \text{mL} \times \text{BSA}\left[\text{m}^2\right]) + \text{Evaporative Water Loss } (\left[\left(25 + \text{TBSA}(\%)\right] \times \text{BSA}\left[\text{m}^2\right] \times 24\ \text{h}\right)$$

However, calculated fluid balances are difficult to calculate, as they do not account the exact amount of exudative losses through the burn wounds (about 0.5–1.0 L/10% TBSA/day). The condition may be complicated by the use of fluidized or air beds, which cause an even greater loss of free water.

20.2.1.2 Colloids

The use of albumin in burn patients is not well defined and to date no prospective randomized trial in burn patients shows an advantage or disadvantage of albumin administration for burn resuscitation, maintenance, or burn infection/sepsis [17, 38]. The use of albumin and its timing is controversial.

Many burn care providers believe that albumin has a positive effect in the case of burn resuscitation as a rescue modality. The use of colloids reduces the amounts of total fluids administered, decreasing the risks of over-resuscitation and consequently decreasing the risk of intra-abdominal compartment syndrome. The use of albumin has been related to decreased mortality and a decreased incidence of extremity compartment syndrome and renal failure [39–41]. Huzar et al. has proposed the use of thrombelastography (TEG) to predict patients who will require supranormal resuscitation. The risks of over-resuscitation have been described elsewhere in this chapter but the early identification of these patients might prompt an earlier use of colloids [42].

To the contrary, Cochrane systematic reviews show no benefit in mortality with colloids over crystalloids alone. No difference in outcomes was seen among the many colloid solutions; moreover, the use of hydroxyethyl starch might increase mortality [43, 44]. The use of TEG and thromboelastometry (ROTEM) can aid in the decision of which colloid to use, and fresh frozen plasma (FFP) could be favored in patients with a concurrent hypocoagulable state [42]. The use of FFP is associated with transfusion-associated lung injury and anaphylaxis. Since colloids are substantially more expensive than crystalloids and might have potentially fatal complications, their use should be individualized. In patients with comorbidities sensitive to fluid changes, such as renal or cardiac insufficiency, the use of colloids is justified. Some have proposed the protocolized use of albumin in patients with hypoalbuminemia (<2.0 g/dL) or in those for whom resuscitation is failing [45].

20.2.1.3 Transfusion

Transfusion guidelines are currently under investigation. Transfusion requirements should be aligned with a patient's operative plan and rehabilitation efforts. If significant burn excision is planned, the patient ought to be optimized and a low starting hemoglobin concentration is not recommended. During the rehabilitation phase, anemia can compromise activity levels. The results of delayed or impaired rehabilitation are not inconsequential in this patient group [46].

A target level of at least 7 g/dL is reasonable, but if a patient is premorbid with impaired cardiac function or poor oxygen delivery, we consider reaching hemoglobin levels of 8 mg/dL. A recent prospective randomized multicenter trial contrasted a liberal transfusion strategy with a restrictive modality and found that with a restrictive approach, the blood product utilization halved. Major outcomes evaluated, such as bloodstream infection, mortality, and organ dysfunction, were not worse than the liberal strategy [47].

20.2.1.4 Vasopressors/Inotropes

Vasopressors or inotropes can be used when indicated in difficult to resuscitate patients. Usually during the first 8–12 h, vasopressors should be avoided as vasoconstriction can have adverse effects. The evidence in favor of using one vasopressor or a combination over others is scarce in the literature and continues to be debated. Titration is usually dependent on mean arterial pressure with a goal of greater than 60 mmHg, though even this can be debated. Normal filling pressures should not be an objective, as this strategy causes over-resuscitation and its multitude of subsequent complications. A study by Evans et al., based on an animal model, showed that the potency of α-adrenergic receptor agonists to increase mean arterial pressure within 24 h after burn is reduced, and the potency and efficacy of a vasopressin receptor agonists are increased. Severe burn sensitizes intrinsic vasopressin receptor reactivity in resistance arteries. While this data might assist in selecting a vasopressor drug, it is unknown if early use of vasopressors will positively impact outcomes [48].

Dobutamine as an inotrope can improve cardiac function if cardiac output or cardiac index is low (<3). The classic vasopressors, epinephrine and norepinephrine, should be used with caution. Vasopressin is currently being studied in various trials, and we await the results. In the critical care population, vasopressin did not improve outcomes compared to catecholamines. In addition, there are case reports that show no benefit with vasopressin but an increased incidence of adverse effects, which is usually associated with high doses of vasopressin (>2.4 IU). However, it appears that doses between 1.2 IU and 2.4 IU are relatively safe and can improve blood pressure to meet goals. The use of vasopressin as a second-line agent has also been suggested. Dopamine, another inotropic agent, is used by some but generally is not widely used in burns.

20.2.2 Invasive and Noninvasive Monitoring

Monitoring of vital signs and other measures in large burns is crucial. Resuscitation endpoints, including clinical, hemodynamic, and biochemical parameters, might improve outcomes of resuscitation. The exclusive use of formulas can be misleading as fluid requirements can be impacted by other factors such as burn depth, inhalation injury, associated injuries, age, a delay in resuscitation, escharotomies/fasciotomies, and the use of alcohol or drugs [16].

Another study evaluating base deficit and lactate levels during burn resuscitation confirmed increased mortality with increased base deficit and lactate derangement. The study authors noted that the normalization of base deficit within 24 h after burn correlated with improved outcomes compared to patients with prolonged elevated base deficit [49]. These findings have been corroborated in other studies in burned patients [50, 51]. Therefore, increased tissue hypoxia may represent under-resuscitation and result in increased organ dysfunction and higher mortality.

Pulse contour analysis is based on the shape of the arterial waveform from either a femoral or radial arterial catheter. Prospective data regarding pulse contour analysis in burn patients are currently lacking. Transesophageal echocardiography, partial carbon dioxide rebreathing, and impedance electrocardiography are some of the other methods used to determine cardiac output. Tissue perfusion monitors, such as gastric tonometers and subcutaneous devices, have been tested without substantial clinical application.

Cardiovascular monitoring requirements will depend on the extent of injury and the presence of inhalation injury. Volume status and cardiac performance are especially difficult to evaluate in the burned victim. In particular, burned extremities may impede the ability to obtain a blood pressure reading by a sphygmomanometer (blood pressure cuff). Generally, in cases with burns over 20% TBSA an arterial catheter will be used for blood pressure monitoring, in those patients who are intubated due to inhalation injury or airway protection. Blood gas determinations will, in addition, enable the monitoring of arterial lactate and the evolution of acid-base status. With increasing severity of burns and in patients over 60 years, information about cardiac output becomes more valuable.

Hemodynamic findings in early invasive cardiovascular monitoring will be variable. Massive burns are generally associated with cardiogenic shock even in the youngest patients and will invariably be present in the elderly during the early phase. The etiology includes increased afterload caused by high levels of stress hormones, direct depression of the myocardium by cytokines, lipoperoxides, intravascular hypovolemia with low preload, and vasoplegia [25, 52].

Pulmonary catheters may be used in patients with massive burns and major cardiopulmonary comorbidities. Invasive hemodynamic monitoring via a pulmonary artery catheter allows the direct and continuous measurement of central venous pressure (CVP), pulmonary capillary wedge pressure, cardiac output, systemic vascular resistance, oxygen delivery, and oxygen consumption. Pulmonary artery catheter-guided therapy has been studied most extensively in trauma and critically ill surgical patients. Hemodynamic data derived from the pulmonary artery catheters appears to be beneficial to ascertain cardiovascular performance in certain situations (inadequate noninvasive monitoring, difficulty in defining endpoints of resuscitation). The cardiac output and cardiac index are useful in determining cardiac sufficiency. Pulmonary capillary wedge pressure and systemic vascular resistance are markers of volume status and shock. Potential complications of pulmonary artery catheter placement include arrhythmias, blood clots, and blood vessel damage. However, the general practicability, risk-benefit ratio, and lack of mortality reduction when using a pulmonary artery catheter have been widely criticized. At the moment, there are no studies in burned patients to provide evidence-based recommendations. In order to overcome the disadvantages of the pulmonary artery catheters, less invasive techniques have been developed.

A novel approach for burn patients has been the use of thermodilution catheters to determine cardiac function, resistance, and lung water [18, 53, 54]. The use of these catheters may enable focused and algorithm-driven therapy that may improve the resuscitation phase, but currently, only a few small studies have been published, which does not allow major conclusions to be drawn; these catheters however do show promise for optimizing resuscitation [18].

Transpulmonary thermodilution can provide similar information to a pulmonary artery catheter, with the use of a central line and an arterial line. With transpulmonary thermodilution (TPTD), a cold saline bolus is injected into the central venous circulation, and the subsequent change in blood temperature is measured by a thermistor-tipped arterial catheter. This is connected to a commercially available device (PiCCO) that calculates flows and volumes from the dilution curves. In addition to cardiac output and systemic vascular resistance measurement, TPTD allows an estimation of global end-diastolic volume and intrathoracic blood volume, both of which are indicators of cardiac preload, and extravascular lung water, a marker of pulmonary edema. The use of TPTD goal-directed therapy based on intrathoracic blood volume and extravascular lung water measurements in critically ill patients has been studied in various prospective trials and shows promising results. The evidence for the use of TPTD is contradictory but the obtained data are reproducible and have a reasonable correlation with data obtained from pulmonary artery catheters [54].

The following algorithm (Fig. 20.1) has been used to optimize fluid resuscitation and cardiac performance in the acute setting as well as during the ICU stay [18]:

Other methods, such as pulse contour analysis and transesophageal echocardiography (TEE), are alternatives for determining hemodynamic parameters [55], while subcutaneous gas tension and gastric tonometry have been used as markers of resuscitation.

20.2.2.1 Urine Output

Hourly urine output (UOP) continues to be the most commonly used endpoint for resuscitation. We have limited evidence that other methods, more invasive or more expensive, can result in better outcomes [56].

Urinary output in the acute phase of a burn is indicative of adequate organ perfusion and its suggested target is 0.5–1.0 mL/kg/h. In children, urine output is targeted to 1 mL/kg/h. Certain situations, including electrical or crush injury with associated rhabdomyolysis, merit additional monitoring and fluid loading [46]. However, urine output is not always an adequate indicator and can be affected by the burn itself,

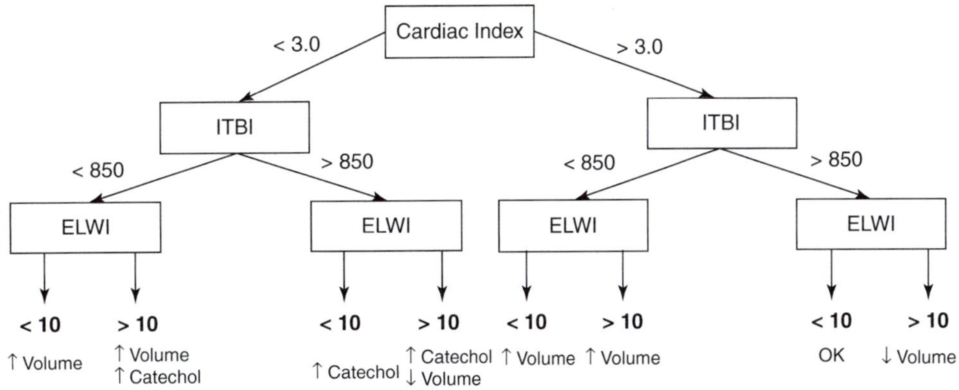

Fig. 20.1 Algorithm for fluid resuscitation based on transpulmonary thermodilution parameters. *ITBI* intrathoracic blood volume index, *ELWI* extravascular lung water index

infusion of antioxidants during resuscitation, cardiac or renal comorbidities, and central or peripheral renal insufficiency.

20.2.2.2 Central Venous Pressure

CVP is a rough marker for preload and hence filling of the patient. CVP should be measured correctly at the level of the heart with a subclavian or jugular line in place. The range of an adequate CVP in burned adults is 4–8 mmHg, and 2–6 mmHg in burned children. The use of CVP as an endpoint for resuscitation has been challenged as it can be highly influenced by external or abdominal pressures, limiting its reliability to monitor intravascular volume [57].

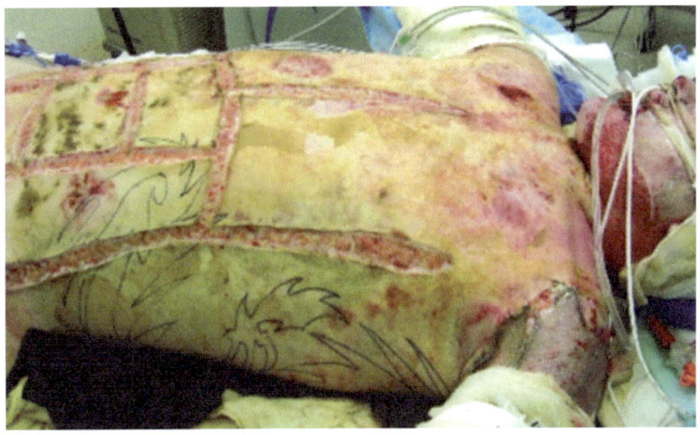

Fig. 20.2 Escharotomies [61]

20.2.3 Intra-abdominal Hypertension and Abdominal Compartment Syndrome

With overenthusiastic fluid delivery, increasing intra-abdominal pressures (IAP) and consequently abdominal compartment syndrome (ACS) becomes a matter of concern in both adult and pediatric burn patients [30, 58]. The Ivy index (250 mL/kg fluid resuscitation) is a cut-off value beyond which trouble is nearly certain [30].

Large volume resuscitation, restricted wall compliance due to burn eschar, and a systemic inflammatory response syndrome resulting in intestinal edema can increase IAP. An intra-abdominal pressure greater than 12 mmHg is called intra-abdominal hypertension, as long as it is not associated with organ failure. Abdominal compartment syndrome is characterized by new organ failure secondary to intra-abdominal pressure with a pressure over 20 mmHg. Intra-abdominal pressure monitoring is useful for a TBSA of >30%. Burned patients with a TBSA over 40% are at higher risk of developing abdominal compartment syndrome, as the systemic inflammatory effect is proportional to the burn size, as well as to the fluid resuscitation to ensure end-organ perfusion. In high-risk patients, the intra-abdominal pressure should be measured every 6 h, or hourly in patients with an Ivy index over 200 mL/kg [59]. Significant morbidity/mortality is associated with the presence of intra-abdominal hypertension and abdominal compartment syndrome; reported mortality can be as high as 75%. An increase in pressure can have consequences in extra-abdominal organs such as decreased cardiac preload resulting in reduced cardiac output. Further, decreased intrathoracic volume limits physiologic lung function (resulting in hypoventilation and hypoxia), and a decrease in renal and splanchnic blood flow results in further ischemia and edema [60]. Abdominal pressure should be controlled by judicious diuresis, inotropic support, positive pressure ventilation, gastric and rectal decompression, sedation, analgesia, and neuromuscular blockade. Continuous renal replacement therapy (CRRT) is a more aggressive option. If the abdomen is burned, checkerboard escharatomies need to be performed (Fig. 20.2). When other measures have failed, a decompressive laparotomy is indicated.

20.2.4 Respiration

Respiratory rate, respiratory effort, breath sounds, and skin color reflect oxygenation and provide objective measure-

Table 20.2 Indications for intubation

$PaO_2 < 60$ mmHg
$PaCO_2 > 50$ mmHg (acutely)
P/*F* ratio < 200
Impending respiratory/ventilatory failure
Severe upper airway edema
Severe facial burn
Burns over 40% TBSA
Clinical signs of severe inhalation injury: edema, blisters, or ulceration during laryngoscopy

ments of breathing. A respiratory rate of less than 10 or greater than 30 is a sign of impending respiratory failure. The use of accessory muscles, manifested by supraclavicular, intercostal, subcostal, or sternal retractions, as well as the presence of grunting or nasal flaring, are signs of increased work of breathing. Auscultation of breath sounds provides a clinical determination of tidal volume. Skin color deteriorates from pink, to pale, to mottled, to blue as hypoxemia progresses. These signs must be followed from the primary survey to avoid respiratory failure. Patients with probable respiratory failure should receive rapid, aggressive, and definitive airway management. There are a number of indications for intubation (Table 20.2) [3, 5]: Oral intubation with the largest appropriate endotracheal tube is the preferred method for obtaining airway access and should be accomplished early if impending respiratory failure or ventilatory obstruction is anticipated. In children, the signs of impending airway obstruction might be obscure. A high level of suspicion is indicated to prevent negative outcomes. In this population, if cuffed endotracheal tubes are going to be used, data have suggested that a small air leak should be maintained to prevent the development of tracheo-esophageal fistula [62].

Effective gas exchange should be determined in an arterial blood gas analysis. Oxygen saturation should be over 85%. The respiratory rate should be 8–20 in adults and 14–38 in children.

20.2.4.1 Ventilation Settings

Detailed descriptions of the different ventilation modes are beyond the scope of this text. In short, positive end-expiratory pressure (PEEP) is useful in supporting oxygenation. The level of PEEP required should be established by empirical trials and reevaluated on a regular basis. PEEP levels should start at 5 cm H_2O and be increased in 2–3 cm increments. PEEP trials should be done to optimize oxygenation and cardiac output. The effectiveness of continuous positive airway pressure or PEEP is related to the surface tension abnormalities and the marked tendency for atelectasis in these patients.

Pressure control ventilation with permissive hypercapnia is the current preferred method of treatment for ventilated patients. In general, plateau pressures above 35 cm H_2O are concerning but in conditions where there is a decreased chest wall compliance as in patients with extensive burns, greater ranges might be acceptable. To accomplish the goal of limiting plateau pressures, pCO_2 can be permitted to rise (permissive hypercapnia) unless other contraindications exist that demand a more normal pCO_2 or pH.

If pulmonary edema continues, the amount of PEEP and of oxygen should be elevated to maintain adequate gas exchange. Low-tidal volumes (5–8 mL/kg) with PEEP may be needed to improve oxygenation. In general, peak flow rates should be adjusted as needed to satisfy patient inspiratory demands. As for the inspiratory/expiratory (I:E) ratio, the inspiratory time should be long enough to deliver the tidal volume at flow rates that will not result in airway turbulence and high peak airway pressures. The normal *I*:*E* ratio is 1:2. This may be adjusted to increase the ratio if oxygenation becomes difficult. With inspired oxygen concentration as a starting point and until the level of hypoxemia is determined, a patient placed on a ventilator should receive an oxygen concentration of 100%. Decrease the FiO_2 as ABG improves. Keep in mind that chest and abdominal wall burns can result in poor compliance and high inspiratory pressures.

In efforts to choose a ventilation mode that is lung protective but at the same time appropriately oxygenates and ventilates, nonconventional modes are often used. A low-tidal volume strategy in burn patients with inhalation injury can be challenging as there is a restrictive and obstructive pathophysiology. Chest wall eschar, edema, and bulky dressings as well as bronchospasm and debris-related bronchial obstruction contribute to this effect.

High-frequency percussive ventilation (HFPV) is a time-cycled, pressure-limited mode of ventilation that delivers sub-tidal volumes at high rates. Tidal volumes are determined by peak inspiratory pressure settings and volume provided by oscillatory function. The use of HFPV is typically restricted to a rescue modality for oxygenation failure although some have reported that use of this strategy as a primary mode for those with inhalation injury results in decreased use of rescue modes. It has been used in adult ARDS but its application in the burn/inhalation injury population is limited. HFPV has demonstrated improved oxygenation at lower peak airway pressures when compared to a low-stretch strategy. The percussive effect in HFPV is thought to facilitate the evacuation of airway debris and mucous plugs. In a randomized controlled trial, Chung et al. concluded that no significant difference between HFPV and low-tidal volume modes with respect to the lung protection provided with a decreased use of rescue modalities [63].

The experience with extracorporeal membrane oxygenation (ECMO) for burn patients is scarce but it can be useful in selected cases that have failed other modes with refractory hypoxemia [64].

Table 20.3 Extubation criteria

PaO_2/FiO_2 ratio > 250
Maximum inspiratory pressure > 60 cm H_2O
Spontaneous tidal volume > 5–7 mL/kg
Spontaneous vital capacity > 15–20 mL/kg
Maximum voluntary ventilation > twice the minute volume
Cough peak flow > 60 L/min
None to moderate amount of secretions (suction frequency)
Audible leak around the endotracheal tube with deflated cuff
Adequate secretions management (cough/gag reflexes)

An increased duration of mechanical ventilation is associated with worse outcomes, including a higher incidence of ventilation-associated pneumonia and mortality. Efforts should be made to discontinue mechanical ventilation as soon as it is safe (Table 20.3). However, premature extubation and subsequent reintubation have severe detrimental effects. In burns, extubation failure is associated with an extended duration of ventilation, ICU stay, and hospital length of stay. Mortality as well is affected by the outcomes of extubation [65].

20.2.4.2 Tracheostomy

Tracheostomy is safe in burn patients. The decision to perform one should be weighed with the timing of the grafting of the neck. There is no consensus on timing. Patients with major burns and significant inhalation injury will likely benefit the most as they will undergo multiple surgical interventions and lengthy mechanical ventilation. In patients with damage to the vocal cords secondary to the inhalation injury, tracheostomy should be considered to prevent further damage to the vocal cords and airway.

20.2.5 Inhalation Injury

Inhalation injury is a significant confounder in burn injury, increasing morbidity and mortality. Of all major burns, approximately 20–30% are associated with a concomitant inhalation injury, with a mortality of 25–50% when patients undergo ventilatory support for more than 1 week after injury [3, 5, 66]. However, the incidence of inhalation injury is typically co-linear with burn size and severity, decreasing its use as a predictor of outcomes.

Inhalation injury can be classified into three types: thermal injury (mostly limited to the upper airway), chemical injury of the respiratory tract and systemic toxicity due to metabolic asphyxiants, or a combination of these insults [67]. The severity of inhalation injury is directly proportional to early oxygenation challenges, complex hospitalization, increased fluid resuscitation requirements, ventilation demands, and mortality [68].

A significant portion of fire-related deaths result not from cutaneous burns, but from inhalation of the toxic products of combustion [33, 66, 69, 70]. Many of these compounds may act together, increasing mortality. This is especially true of carbon monoxide (CO) and hydrogen cyanide, where a synergism has been found that increases tissue hypoxia and acidosis in addition to decreasing cerebral oxygen consumption and metabolism. Carbon monoxide levels higher than 15–20% should be treated with 100% endotracheal oxygen. The use of hyperbaric oxygen is controversial and its availability is restricted [71].

Cyanide can be the result of the burning of many household products, especially those that contain cotton, wool, and nylon. Cyanide toxicity associated with inhalation injury remains a diagnostic dilemma, as markers for cyanide toxicity (elevated blood lactate, elevated BD, or metabolic acidosis) can also represent under-resuscitation, associated trauma, CO poisoning, or hypoxia. Regardless, aggressive resuscitation and administration of 100% oxygen remains a mainstay of treatment. Controversy remains as to the need for specific antidotes in cyanide poisoning [72]. The use of hydroxocobalamin (a standard in prehospital care in some European centers) has not been as widely accepted in North America. A retrospective review conducted in a center in the United States determined that its use was associated with a lower rate of pneumonia, faster effective extubation, and a decrease in intensive care unit stay when compared with controls [73]. There is minimal evidence for the role of cyanide antidotes in smoke inhalation injury; therefore, aggressive supportive therapy aimed at allowing for the hepatic clearance of cyanide without specific antidotes should be the first line of treatment.

Other possible contributing toxic substances are hydrogen chloride (produced by polyvinyl chloride degradation), nitrogen oxide, and aldehydes, which can result in pulmonary edema, chemical pneumonitis, or respiratory irritability. Direct thermal damage to the lung is seldom seen except as a result of high-pressure steam, which has 4000 times the heat-carrying capacity of dry air. Laryngeal reflexes and the efficiency of heat dissipation in the upper airway prevent heat damage to the lung parenchyma.

The clinical course of patients with inhalation injury is divided into three stages:

- *First stage*: *Acute pulmonary insufficiency*. Patients with severe lung injuries show acute pulmonary insufficiency from 0 to 36 h after injury with asphyxia, carbon monoxide poisoning, bronchospasm, upper airway obstruction, and parenchymal damage.
- *Second stage*: *Pulmonary edema*. This second stage occurs in 5–30% of patients, usually from 6 to 72 h post burn and is associated with a high mortality rate.

- *Third stage*: *Bronchopneumonia*. This appears in 15–60% of these patients and has a reported mortality of 50–86%. Bronchopneumonia occurs typically 3–10 days after burn injury and is often associated with the expectoration of large mucus casts formed in the tracheobronchial tree. Early pneumonias are usually due to penicillin-resistant *Staphylococcus* species, whereas after 3–4 days, the change of flora on the burn wound is reflected in the appearance in the lung of Gram-negative species, especially *Pseudomonas* species.

The early detection of bronchopulmonary injury is critical in improving survival after a suspected inhalation injury. Clinical indicators and adjuncts include [33, 66, 74]:

- A history of exposure to smoke in a closed space
- Altered mental status (stuporous or unconscious patients)
- Facial burns, singed nasal vibrissae, bronchorrhea, sooty sputum, wheezing or rales on auscultation
- Laboratory findings of hypoxemia, elevated levels of carbon monoxide
- Chest X-ray findings. Can be an insensitive method because they may remain normal as long as 7 days post burn.
- Bronchoscopy. Should be the standard diagnostic method on every burn patient.

The most specific method to define parenchymal injury is ^{133}Xe lung scanning, which involves intravenous injection of radioactive xenon gas followed by serial chest scintiphotograms. This technique identifies areas of air trapped due to partial or total obstruction of small airways by demonstrating areas of decreased alveolar gas washout. Fiberoptic bronchoscopy remains the gold standard to establish the diagnosis of inhalation injury and to determine severity (Fig. 20.3). Inhalation injury can be graded using the scale by Endorf and Gamelli (Table 20.4) [70].

The treatment of the inhalation injury should be started immediately, with the administration of 100% oxygen via a face mask or nasal cannula. This serves to reverse the effects of carbon monoxide poisoning and aids in its clearance, as 100% oxygen lowers its half-life time from 250 to less than 50 min. The role of hyperbaric oxygen remains controversial although both physiological data and some randomized trial data suggest a potential benefit in terms of a reduction in cognitive sequelae; hence, it has been included in the guidelines of the Undersea and Hyperbaric Medical Society [71, 76].

Several clinical studies have shown that pulmonary edema was not prevented by fluid restriction, as the interstitial fluid after thermal and inhalation injury is caused mainly by the inflammatory process [77]. Although overhydration could increase pulmonary edema, inadequate hydration increases the severity of pulmonary injury by the sequestration of polymorphonuclear cells and leads to increased mortality.

Prophylactic antibiotics for inhalation injury are not used, but are clearly indicated for documented lung infections. Empiric choices for treatment of pneumonias prior to culture results should include coverage of methicillin-resistant

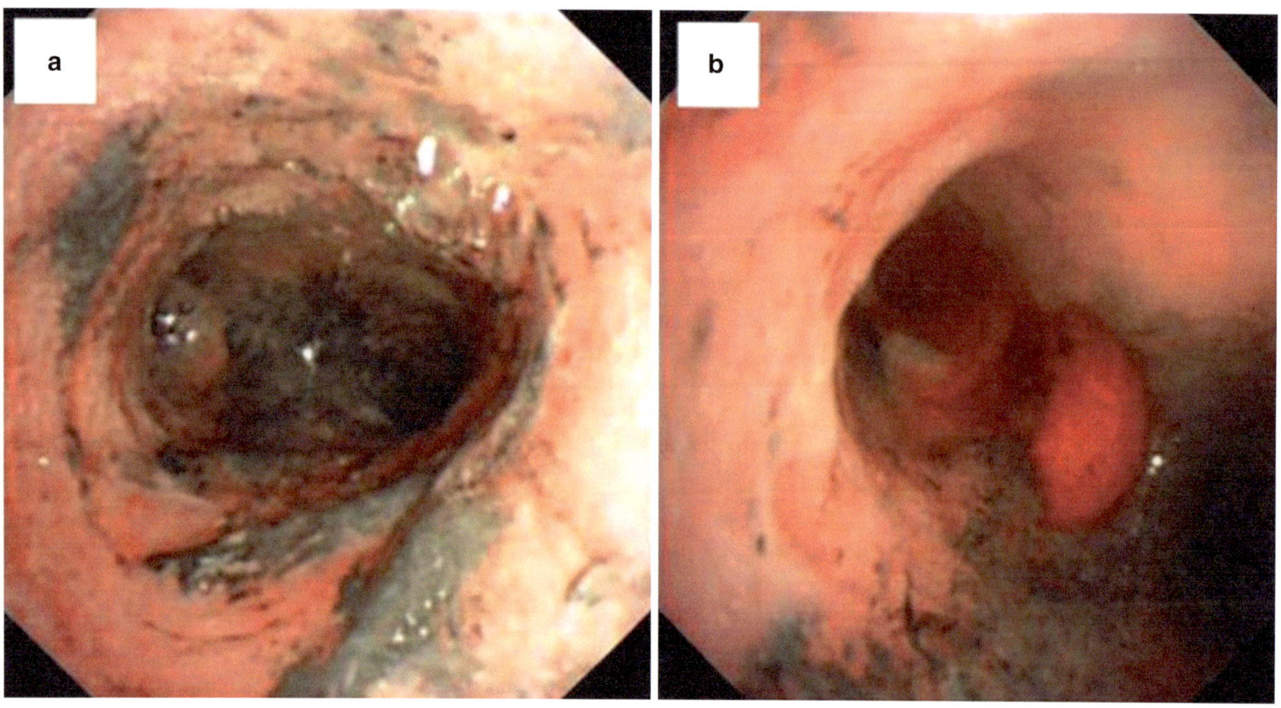

Fig. 20.3 (**a**) Trachea with severe edema, erythema, and carbon soot deposition. (**b**) Formation of pseudomembrane [75]

Table 20.4 Inhalation injury scale

Grade 0 (no injury)
Absence of carbonaceous deposits, erythema, edema, bronchorrhea, and obstruction
Grade I (mild injury)
Minor or patchy areas of erythema, carbonaceous deposits in proximal or distal bronchi (any one of these or a combination)
Grade II (moderate injury)
Moderate degree of erythema, carbonaceous deposits, bronchorrhea with or without compromise of the bronchi (any one of these or a combination)
Grade III (severe injury)
Severe inflammation with friability, copious carbonaceous deposits, bronchorrhea, bronchial obstruction (any one of these or a combination)
Grade IV (massive injury)
Evidence of mucosal sloughing, necrosis, endoluminal obliteration (any one of these or a combination)

Staphylococcus aureus in the first few days after burn (these infections develop within the first week after burn) and of Gram-negative organisms (especially *Pseudomonas* or *Klebsiella*), which mostly occur after 1 week after burn. Systemic antibiotic regimes are based on serially monitored sputum cultures, bronchial washings, or transtracheal aspirates.

Inhalation injury results in airway obstructive casts, which are composed of mucus secretions, denuded airway epithelial cells, inflammatory cells, and fibrin [11]. The presence of fibrin solidifies the airway content forming the firm cast that is hard to remove by a single cough or even by aggressive airway toilet. Therefore, prevention and dissolution of airway fibrin deposition is crucial in effective airway management.

Inhalation injury is one of the most important predictors of morbidity and mortality in burn patients. When present, inhalation injury increases mortality up to 15 times [33, 66, 72, 78]. Inhalation injury prompts endotracheal intubation, which in turn increases the incidence of pneumonia. Pneumonia can increase mortality in up to 60% in these patients. Patients usually recover full pulmonary function and late complications are not the rule. In patients who have been recently extubated, cough after swallowing might represent an early sign of a tracheo-esophageal fistula. Scarring of the airway can cause stenosis, rupture, and dysphonia, requiring voice therapy and occasionally surgery.

20.2.5.1 Pharmacological Management

The following are used to manage inhalation injuries:

- Bronchodilators (albuterol/salbutamol) for smooth muscle relaxation and bronchospasm inhibition
- Muscarinic antagonists (tiotropium) to decrease airway pressures and mucus secretions
- Nebulized heparin to inhibit cast formation controlling fibrin creation
  - A systematic review in 2014 highlighted proof of the potential benefits of inhaled heparin and similar alternatives. Inhaled anticoagulation regimens in both preclinical and clinical studies improve survival and decrease morbidity without altering systemic markers of clotting and anticoagulation. In some preclinical and clinical studies, inhaled anticoagulants were associated with a favorable effect on survival [79]. A multicenter randomized controlled trial by Glas et al. [80] is currently underway to assess nebulized heparin versus placebo in inhalation injury, and it is expected to be completed by the end of 2017.
- Nebulized acetylcysteine, a mucolytic with anti-inflammatory properties that attenuates reactive oxygen species damage
- Nitric oxide to improve oxygenation
  - Nitric oxide has been used to improve oxygenation in treating hypoxic pulmonary vasoconstriction and to improve ventilation/perfusion mismatches and therefore tissue oxygenation. However, Enkhbaatar and colleagues have reported increased levels of nitric oxide in lung tissue secondary to inhalation injury and that the resultant loss of hypoxic vasoconstriction worsens ventilation-perfusion mismatch [81].
- Hypertonic saline to induce effective coughing
- Nebulized racemic epinephrine, which has been shown to be safe to use with no significant resultant hemodynamic changes. It reduces mucosal edema and produces bronchodilation [82].
- Inhaled epoprosprostenol, which is used mainly in ARDS and decreases pulmonary artery pressure, produces vasodilation, and inhibits platelet aggregation. It results in decreased ventilation-perfusion mismatch [83].
- Corticosteroids are contraindicated. The theoretical benefits of corticosteroid therapy include a reduction in mucosal edema, reduced bronchospasm, and the maintenance of surfactant function. However, in several animal and clinical studies, mortality increased with the administration of corticosteroids, and bronchopneumonia showed more extensive abscess formation.

20.2.6 Immune Response and Inflammation

The inflammatory response constitutes an organized defense mechanism aimed at protecting the body from further damage, restoring homeostasis, and promoting wound repair. This includes a local reaction to injury, a systemic response, massive cytokine production, immune and endocrine changes, increased protein catabolism, and the rearrangement of hepatic synthesis priorities. Cytokine production is strongly enhanced after major burns, and the balance between pro-inflammatory and anti-inflammatory mediators in acute injury is lost [84]; the phenomenon further increases infectious complications. The intensity of this reaction is correlated with mortality [85, 86]. Although inflammation is perceived as beneficial, its persistence for long periods of time can cause various derangements in the normal physiology. These metabolic and inflammatory changes can persist for up to 3 years. The changes can result in insulin resistance, increased fracture risk, growth and development retardation, increased cardiac work and cardiac dysfunction development, impaired strength and muscle function, hormonal abnormalities, and an increased risk for infections and sepsis. All the aforementioned can lead to organ dysfunction and failure, possibly resulting in mortality for the patient [87].

In healthy subjects, the endogenous antioxidant defense mechanisms are sufficient to cope with moderate free radical overproduction. In major burns, these defenses are overwhelmed, leaving space for the deleterious effects of reactive oxygen species, with proximity oxidation of nucleotides, proteins, and lipids. The endogenous antioxidant defenses become acutely depleted by the massive production of reactive oxygen species derived from both oxygen and nitric oxide.

The pro-inflammatory cytokines (particularly IL-6) are responsible for the redistribution of micronutrients (including those with antioxidant properties) from the circulating compartment to tissues and organs with high synthetic and cell replication activity.

20.2.7 Serum Organ Markers

Baseline measures of organ function from the initial phase after injury throughout ICU and hospital stay are highly useful. The most feasible measures are serum markers of organ function or dysfunction/damage [5].

- Cardiac markers: troponin, A- and B-natriuretic peptide, CK
- Liver: AST, ALT, bili, ALKP
- Pancreas: amylase, lipase
- Kidney: BUN, creatinine
- Hematology: CBC including coagulation, differential including bands
- Hormonal: cortisol including ACTH challenge, thyroid axis, GnRH

For longitudinal observation, it is recommended to obtain admission values and measures values once or twice per week.

20.3 Late Hospital Phase

The later phase includes performing critical practices to maintain organ function, control infection and sepsis, and alleviate hypermetabolism. This section will focus on maintaining organ function and on the complications of long-term ICU sequelae, as infection and sepsis and hypermetabolism are discussed in detail in later chapters.

20.3.1 Central Nervous System

Anoxic brain injury was a leading cause of death in burn patients, which has been replaced by sepsis and multiple organ failure [14]. Adequate resuscitation and early intubation have improved mortality in burn patients [19, 33]. However, neurological disturbances are commonly observed in such patients. The possibility of cerebral edema and raised intracranial pressure must be considered during the early fluid resuscitation phase, especially in the case of associated brain injury or high voltage electrical injury. The inhalation of neurotoxic chemicals, of carbon monoxide, or hypoxic encephalopathy may adversely affect the central nervous system [33, 66, 69, 72]. Other factors include hypo-/hypernatremia, hypovolemic shock, sepsis, antibiotic overdosage (e.g., penicillin), and possible oversedation or withdrawal effects from sedative drugs. If increased intracranial pressure is suspected, neurosurgery consultation needs to be considered and intracranial pressure monitoring and therapy initiated.

In general, severe burn injury is associated with nonspecific atrophy of the brain that normally resolves over time, and no intervention is needed. Hung et al. suggested that burned patients have a higher risk of ischemic stroke that persists for more than 1 year after injury [88].

20.3.1.1 Pain, Sedation, and Delirium

Pain and anxiety will generally require rather large doses of opioids and sedatives (benzodiazepines mainly). Continuous infusion regimens will generally be successful in maintaining pain within acceptable ranges. Sedation and analgesia should be assessed frequently. In the case of analgesia, for patients with intact communication skills, self-reporting scales are preferred. If the patient has a limited ability to use a self-reporting numeric rating scale (NRS), scales like the Behavioral Pain Scale (BPS) and Critical Care Pain Assessment Tool (CPOT) are available. Sedatives can be targeted using appropriate scores on the Richmond Agitation Sedation Scale (RASS) or Riker Sedation Agitation Scale scores (SAS). Thus, the sequelae associated with oversedation and opioid creep are prevented, namely fluid creep and effects on the central and peripheral cardiovascular system

[37]. Consideration should be given to the use of NMDA receptor antagonists, such as ketamine or gabapentin, which have important opioid-sparing effects in order to decrease the need for opioids and benzodiazepines [3, 5]. Multimodal pain management combining a long-acting opioid for background pain, a short-acting opioid for procedures, an anxiolytic, an NSAID, acetaminophen, and gabapentin for neuropathic pain control [3, 5] targeted to the Riker Sedation Agitation Scale and SAS scores and Behavioral Pain Scale scores should provide adequate analgesia and sedation.

Delirium is commonplace in mechanically ventilated patients and patients with prolonged hospital stays. Its presence results in longer hospitalization and increased mortality and costs. Patients can experience long-term cognitive impairment. Patients should be monitored for delirium frequently using the Confusion Assessment Method for ICU (CAM-ICU) or the Intensive Care Delirium Screening Checklist. Methods to prevent and treat delirium include early mobility and rehabilitation, sleep hygiene, adequate oxygenation, and the limited use of benzodiazepines.

20.3.1.2 Intensive Care Unit-Acquired Weakness

Survival and organ function have been the main outcome measures for burn patients; however, recently long-term outcomes have been the focus of burn care providers. Long-term outcomes include those of the peripheral nervous system and muscular system, derangements of which can manifest as neuromyopathy. In the burn population, the incidence of neuromyopathy is approximately 2–29%. Frequently, the first sign can be difficulty weaning the patient off mechanical ventilation [89]. The importance of positioning and the prevention of peripheral nerve compression is well known and ingrained in the daily practices of most critical care units. The main risk factors for neuropathy include multiple organ failure, muscular inactivity, prolonged periods of ventilation, hyperglycemia, and the use of corticosteroids and neuromuscular blockers. In a recent publication by de Jonghe et al. [90], early identification and treatment of conditions leading to multiple organ failure (especially sepsis and septic shock), avoiding unnecessary deep sedation and excessive hyperglycemia, promoting early mobilization, and weighing the risk and benefits of corticosteroids might reduce the incidence and severity of ICU-acquired weakness.

20.3.1.3 Thermal Regulation

Temperature regulation is altered with a "resetting" of the hypothalamic temperature above normal values [91–93]. The teleological advantage of maintaining an elevated core temperature following burn injury is not fully understood, but major burns destroy the insulating properties of the skin, while the patients strive for a temperature of 38.0–38.5 °C. Moreover, grafted skin has an impaired sweat response and cutaneous vasodilation, which persists to up to 8 years [94]. Sometimes, it is difficult to differentiate between elevated temperatures due to a central reset or due to other causes such as infection or fever. Cultures become useful if temperatures are persistently over 39 °C.

Catecholamine production contributes to changes associated with several cytokines, including interleukin-1 and interleukin-6. Any attempt to lower the basal temperature by external means will result in augmented heat loss, thus increasing the metabolic rate. The ambient temperature should be maintained between 28 and 33 °C to limit heat loss and the subsequent hypermetabolic response [4]. The metabolic rate is increased as a consequence of several factors such as the catecholamine burst, the thermal effects of pro-inflammatory cytokines, and evaporative losses from the wounds, which consumes energy, causing further heat loss. Evaporation causes extensive fluid loss from wounds, approximating 3750 mL/m^2/%TBSA burns [3, 5]. Every liter of evaporated fluid corresponds to a caloric expenditure of about 600 kcal.

Besides hyperthermia, another very important contributor to poor outcomes is hypothermia. Burn patients frequently experience hypothermia (defined as a core temperature below 35 °C) on admission, in the ICU, during operations, and during sepsis [3, 5]. Time to recover from hypothermia has been shown to be predictive of outcomes in adults, with time to revert to normothermia being longer in non-survivors. Considering that hypothermia favors infections and delays wound healing, the maintenance of perioperative normothermia is of utmost importance. Tools for doing so include warming the ambient room temperature, intravenous fluid warming systems, and warming blankets. The temperature of the bed should be set at 38 ± 0.5 °C. However, this is contraindicated in the febrile patient, as it complicates fluid therapy due to largely unpredictable free water losses, and respiratory management due to the supine position. The patient may benefit from an additional 1–4 L of free water per day (as D5W IV or enteral free water) to prevent dehydration. These additional requirements are difficult to assess in the absence of bed-integrated weight scales.

20.3.2 Heart

Critically ill patients, including burn patients, are at a higher risk of developing in-hospital cardiac events, explained by the increased cardiac demand due to the injury burden and a hypermetabolic state. The adrenergic surge can trigger cardiac disturbances [95]. The burn population is unique as a consequence of the in-volume and electrolyte shifts. Arrhythmias are among the most common complications [96]. The resultant cardiomyopathy can require the use of inotrope therapy for maintaining end-organ perfusion.

Another complication that can occur is cardiac ischemia. Ischemic events can lead to a manifest heart or to temporary cardiac ischemia. If a myocardial infarction occurs, Cardiology consultation is especially beneficial if procedural intervention is required.

20.3.3 Lung

Pulmonary complications in the early phase are pulmonary edema and inhalation injury that were discussed previously. Pulmonary complications that occur during an ICU or hospital stay include ventilation-associated pneumonia (VAP)/pneumonia and acute respiratory distress syndrome (ARDS).

20.3.3.1 Ventilator-Associated Pneumonia (VAP)

Mechanically ventilated burn patients have a high incidence of VAP, which results in significant morbidity and mortality. VAP prevention should be a paramount feature of critical care of these patients. Preventative measures are usually grouped in bundles that include recumbent position and elevating the head, oral care, ulcer and deep venous thrombosis prophylaxis, subglottic suctioning, hand hygiene, daily spontaneous breathing trials, and daily sedation interruption [97]. The implementation of such bundles has produced a decreased risk of developing VAP in burn patients [98]. VAP early in admission is mostly caused by *S. aureus*, whereas those that occur late in the hospital course are caused by opportunistic bacteria such as methicillin-resistant *S. aureus*, *P. aeruginosa*, and *A. baumannii* [99].

The American Burn Association guidelines for the prevention, diagnosis, and treatment of VAP in burn patients were published in 2009 [27, 100]. The guidelines are as follows:

- Mechanically ventilated burn patients are at a high risk for developing VAP, with the presence of inhalation injury as a unique risk factor in this patient group.
- VAP prevention strategies should be used in mechanically ventilated burn patients.
- A clinical diagnosis of VAP can be challenging in mechanically ventilated burn patients where systemic inflammation and acute lung injury are prevalent. Therefore, a quantitative strategy, when available, is the preferable method to confirm the diagnosis of VAP.
- An 8-day course of targeted antibiotic therapy is generally sufficient to treat VAP; however, resistant *S. aureus* and Gram-negative bacilli may require a longer treatment duration.
- An effort should be made to reduce the ventilator days.

A suggested protocol (shown below) considers the length of stay for empiric antibiotic selection:

Early phase (less than 5 days)

- Ceftriaxone 1 g IV q24 h ± cloxacillin 1–2 g IV q4–6 h
- Levofloxacin 750 mg IV/po q24 h if penicillin allergy

Late phase (admitted for >5 days)

- Piperacillin/tazobactam 4.5 g IV q6 h (renal dosing required)
- ±vancomycin 1 g IV q12 h (with pre- and post-levels around the third dose)
- If penicillin allergy
  - Tobramycin 2 mb/kg q8h (in non-obese patients) with creatinine clearance > 70 ml/min + vancomycin 1 gram IV q 12 h with monitoring by pre- and post- levels with the 3rd dose

    or
  - Meropenem 500 mg IV q6 h (renal dosing required)

20.3.4 Gastrointestinal System

The effect of thermal injury on the gastrointestinal system was identified in 1970 with the description of Curling's ulcer. During the initial hours, splanchnic blood flow is reduced, except for flow to the adrenals and to the liver. Poorly perfused organs shift towards anaerobic metabolism, leading to acidosis. Adequate fluid resuscitation restores perfusion to a great extent.

The gut is extremely vulnerable to changes in perfusion and nutrition. Even short ischemia can lead to gut atrophy associated with several complications. Early enteral feeding should be initiated no later than 12 h after injury. The benefits of this strategy are numerous: increasing blood flow to the splanchnic compartment before edema makes it impossible, maintaining pyloric function, maintaining intestinal motility, and reducing significantly infectious complications [101, 102]. Current recommendations are to place a nasogastric feeding tube as well as post-pyloric feeding tube.

During the initial phase after burn as well as after each ischemia reperfusion, gastrointestinal function, including pyloric function, is vastly depressed. A true paralytic ileus will ensue for many days if the gastrointestinal tract is not used. Opiates and sedatives further depress the gastrointestinal function and constipation is frequent and may become critical with the development of ileus and fecal impaction. Prevention should be initiated from admission using fiber-containing enteral diets, lactulose (osmotic cathartic), and enemas when the other measures have failed. Regular bowel movements need to be diligently monitored.

Gut complications may be life-threatening; in addition to the already mentioned abdominal compartment syndrome and opioid-induced bowel dysfunction and constipation, patients may develop acute colonic pseudoobstruction (Ogilvie syndrome), ischemic and non-ischemic bowel necrosis, and intestinal hemorrhage. A careful tight supervision of bowel function with daily examinations is therefore mandatory, particularly in perioperative periods with intraoperative hemorrhage leading to hypovolemia, which exposes the patient to gut hypoperfusion and their threatened complications. Wolf et al. examined over 1800 patients admitted to their unit and recorded development of abdominal complications. Primary abdominal complications occurred in approximately 1 in 20 patients. Abdominal compartment syndrome and/or ischemic bowel presented in 2.8% of their cohort and was associated with a 78% mortality. Incidence of these complications were directly proportional to burn size. Associated conditions were high acute resuscitation volumes, use of vasopressor agents, and enteral tube feedings, although causation could not be determined [103]. Abdominal complications in severe burns are common, and the best treatment is prevention.

Stress ulcer prophylaxis is mandatory, and its common use has virtually eliminated diffuse gastric bleeding as a common source of morbidity and mortality in the severely burned. Early enteral nutrition and H2 blockers (ranitidine) or proton pump inhibitors are recommended since the bleeding risk is elevated in burn injuries and may be life-threatening. Antacids have been associated with an increased risk of hemorrhage and mortality; thus, they are contraindicated for this purpose.

20.3.4.1 Liver

Severe burns cause numerous metabolic alterations, including hyperglycemia, lipolysis, and protein catabolism [4, 8, 104]. These changes can induce multiorgan failure and sepsis leading to significant morbidity and mortality [104–106]. The liver plays a significant role in mediating survival and recovery in burn patients, and preexisting liver disease is directly associated with adverse clinical outcomes following severe burn [87, 107, 108]. In the study by Price et al. in 2007, they demonstrated that preexisting liver disease increased mortality risk from 6 to 27%, indicating that liver impairment worsens the prognosis in patients with thermal injury. Severe burn also directly induces hepatic dysfunction and damage, delaying recovery. More recently, work by Jeschke et al. (2009) and Song et al. (2009) has shed light on the mechanism of the hepatic dysfunction following thermal injury, mainly by the upregulation of the ER stress response, and increased cell death contributing to compromised hepatic function post burn [109–114]. Severe burns alter the liver mitochondria, resulting in increased respiratory capacity and function, and ultimately increasing ATP production [115]. Thus, one must be cognizant of the significant deleterious effects of hepatic dysfunction in the thermally injured patient as it has significant consequence in terms of multiorgan failure, morbidity, and the subsequent mortality of these patients; one can focus therapeutic modalities to alter this response and possibly improve outcome.

20.3.4.2 Pancreas

Insulin resistance is commonplace in burn patients, with an incidence as high as 43%. This resistance decreases with time [116]. There is no prospective adult trial addressing glucose management in major burns, but retrospective studies suggest that toxic levels of hyperglycemia (>10 mmol/L) should be avoided and treated to prevent graft failure and infections (both increase with hyperglycemia) [117], sarcopenia, and mortality. In contrast, data are available on children in whom tight glucose control (90–120 mg/dL) was shown to reduce infections and mortality [118]. Despite the demonstrated benefit of insulin administration on the maintenance of skeletal muscle mass, it is unknown if this effect translates to improved clinical outcomes in the thermally injured patient. Optimal glycemic level remains uncertain; indeed, feeding interruptions due to the procedures expose the patients to the risk of hypoglycemia. A good compromise is probably to opt for a glucose target of 130–150 mg/dL [119].

20.3.4.3 Micronutrients and Antioxidants

Critically ill burned patients are characterized as having a strong oxidative stress, an intense inflammatory response, and a hypermetabolic state that can last for months. Trace element (TE) deficiencies have repeatedly been described. The complications observed in major burns, such as infections and delayed wound healing, can be partly attributed to TE deficiencies [120, 121]. Plasma TE concentrations are low as a result of TE losses in biological fluids, low intakes, dilution by fluid resuscitation, and the redistribution from plasma to tissues mediated by the inflammatory response. The large exudative losses cause negative TE balances. Copper, which plays an essential role in collagen synthesis, wound repair, and immunity, is strongly depleted in burns [122]; this is unique among medical conditions. Intravenous supplementation trials show that early substitution improves recovery (IV doses: Cu 3.5 mg/day, Se 400–500 μg/day, Zn 40 mg/day), reduces infectious complications (particularly nosocomial pneumonia), normalizes thyroid function, improves wound healing, and shortens hospital length of stay. The mechanisms underlying these improvements are a combination of antioxidant effects (particularly of selenium through the restoration of glutathione peroxidase activity), but also immune (Cu, Se, Zn) and anabolic effects (Zn particularly).

High vitamin C requirements after major burns were identified already in the 1940s, and have been confirmed since. Studies by Tanaka et al. in 2000 and Kremer in 2010 demonstrated that high doses of vitamin C administered during the first 24 h after a major injury reduced the capillary leak, probably through antioxidant mechanisms, resulting in significant reductions in fluid resuscitation requirements [123, 124]. The use of high-dose vitamin C has been linked to calcium oxalate nephropathy [125]; nonetheless, current data still favor its use as an aid during the resuscitation phase.

20.3.5 Renal

Acute kidney injury (AKI) is a major complication of burn injury. The incidence of AKI in burned patients ranges from 1.2 to 20% and the incidence of acute renal failure requiring renal replacement therapy (RRT) is from 0.7 to 14.6% [15, 126–128]. Although AKI is relatively rare, early diagnosis is important, as the mortality of burn patients who manifest AKI has been reported around 50% [126]. Applying the RIFLE (risk, injury, failure, loss, and end-stage kidney disease) classification to burn patients, Coca et al. found that the incidence of AKI was 27%, and it carried with it a mortality rate of 73% in patients who received renal replacement therapy (RRT).

Different classifications systems have been developed to define the presence of AKI. The RIFLE and AKIN (Acute Kidney Injury Network) classifications have been validated in multiple studies, inclusive of burn patients. Both show a direct correlation between the severity of AKI and adverse outcomes [129]. The KDIGO (Kidney Disease: Improving Global Outcomes) guidelines incorporate smaller serum creatinine changes and are less restrictive on the time AKI takes to develop, both of which are significant differences from prior classification systems. Unfortunately, the experience in burn patients using this classification has been limited.

The use of biomarkers early after injury has been proposed to predict the development of AKI. The use of plasma and urine neutrophil gelatinase-associated lipocalin within 48 h of admission have been associated with AKI development and mortality in burn patients.

Burn-related AKI can be divided into early and late AKI, depending on the time of onset, with each having different etiologies [128, 130]. Early AKI occurs during the first 5 days post burn and its main causes are hypovolemia, hypotonia, increased inflammatory mediators, cardiac dysfunction, and myoglobinuria. Its prevention focuses on early aggressive fluid resuscitation and escharotomies or fasciotomies. Late AKI begins more than 5 days post burn and is usually multifactorial (generally caused by sepsis and/or nephrotoxic antibiotics) [130].

Rhabdomyolysis caused by direct thermal or electrical injury results in the dissolution of muscle fibers. Muscle edema, the release of inflammatory mediators, and the release of myoglobin in the systemic circulation contribute to the pathophysiology of burn-related AKI. Intravenous fluids are the main component of management. Supportive measures include correcting acidosis and treating any further muscle damage, such as compartment syndrome. The use of sodium bicarbonate and mannitol remains controversial.

Regardless of the cause of the kidney injury, there is strong evidence that RRT should be instituted as early as possible in burn patients with renal dysfunction before the traditional criteria for RRT have been established. Patients with preexisting chronic kidney disease with superimposed AKI might benefit from early RRT, minimizing episodes of volume overload [129]. Added to the discussion of RRT is the choice in mode of delivery. CRRT offers several potential advantages in the management of severe acute renal failure in burn patients. It is slow and continuous, consequently allowing for very efficient metabolic clearance and the ultra-filtration of fluids, while minimizing hemodynamic compromise, thus allowing for ongoing optimization of fluid and metabolic management. The weakness of CRRT is the need for anticoagulation, antibiotic dosing, and close monitoring. The RESCUE trial (Randomized Controlled Evaluation of Hemofiltration in Adult Burn Patients With Septic Shock and Acute Renal Failure trial; ClinicalTrials.gov ID: NCT01213914) is expected to be completed in late 2017 and will help assess if high-volume hemofiltration in addition to standard of care will result in improved outcomes when compared to standard of care alone in the treatment of critically ill patients with AKI secondary to septic shock. Hemodialysis is surely a viable option if the patient tolerates it. In children, an alternative is peritoneal dialysis with placement of a Tenckhoff catheter.

20.3.6 Endocrine (Adrenal, Thyroid, Gonadal)

20.3.6.1 Adrenal

In the post-burn state, pronounced hormonal and metabolic changes take place [4, 8], starting immediately after injury. There is a tremendous increase in stress hormones after major burns, the increase being particularly marked during the first 2–3 weeks, but the alterations will persist for months and even years [87]. In response to the afferent stimuli from the burn wound, an intense sympathico-adrenal response is elicited. Catecholamine secretion contributes to arterial pressure maintenance but also to a massive increase in cardiac afterload. The concentration of epinephrine and norepinephrine remains elevated for several days after injury and contributes to the integrated neuroendocrine stress response. Cortisol increases markedly, and the intensity of the response is modulated by the optimization of pain control with good analgesia [8, 87].

Burn patients are at an increased risk for adrenal insufficiency and this risk appears to be greatest with older patients, large burns, and inhalation injury. Severely burned patients frequently are intubated for airway protection. A rapid-sequence intubation protocol includes etomidate, which has been associated with a higher risk of developing adrenal insufficiency, even as a single dose [131]. The correlation between the severity of thermal trauma and probability of developing adrenal insufficiency during the course of the injury has been documented [132].

As with many hormonal changes, the circadian rhythm also changes. Aldosterone levels increase for several days. ACTH response frequently parallels the cortisol levels and tends to be elevated for a few weeks. The increase is proportional to the burn size. An increase in plasma rennin activity and aldosterone persists for several weeks.

A patient suffering from infection/sepsis or persistent hypotension should be considered for possible adrenal insufficiency. The current guidelines call for a baseline cortisol level and if that level is low an ACTH challenge test should be performed to rule out insufficiency. If an adrenal insufficiency is present, low-dose cortisol should be given. Despite the apparent lack of consensus, the Surviving Sepsis Campaign guidelines recommend (grade C) 7 days of treatment with low-dose (200–300 mg/day) intravenous corticosteroids for all septic patients requiring vasopressor support despite adequate fluid resuscitation.

Glucagon concentration is also increased after burn injury, contributing heavily to the hypermetabolic response, while insulin tends to remain within normal values, being paradoxically normal while plasma glucose concentration is elevated.

20.3.6.2 Thyroid

The thyroid axis exhibits major abnormalities in patients with major burns, and these changes are thought to be related to metabolic adaptation. The use of exogenous dopamine can suppress TSH pulse release though this effect is reversible a day after discontinuation [133]. The most constant finding is a "low T3 syndrome": TSH is generally normal, with low T3 levels, and T4 levels in the low-normal values, with elevated rT3 levels reflecting an altered de-iodination at the hepatic level. Low T3 might be a result of selenium deficiency, which should be replete. There are no conclusive data that the biochemical changes in the acute phase correspond with a clinical disorder [116] but low levels of T3 have been independently associated with mortality in burn patients [133].

20.3.6.3 Gonadal

The gonadal axis is depressed in any patient with major burns. In men, changes following severe burn in testosterone and 17β-estradiol are greater than in females, even during the first days. Plasma testosterone also decreases steeply in limited burn injuries. The alterations last at least 4–5 weeks, but may persist for months in critically ill burned patients. The changes seem proportional to the severity of burns. A decreased pituitary stimulation causes lowered hormonal secretions from the testes. This change contributes to the low anabolic response and opens substitution perspectives. LH is generally normal, LH-RH is decreased, FSH is low, and prolactin is low to elevated.

In premenopausal females, amenorrhea is a nearly universal phenomenon, despite a near-normal 17β-estradiol plasma concentration. Progesterone levels remain very low for many months after injury. The testosterone response is very different from that of males, with nearly normal concentrations in young females, and a normal response to ACTH, which elicits an increase in testosterone, while it decreases in men. Prolactin levels are also higher than seen in men.

In children, despite adequate nutritional support, severe thermal injury leads to decreased anabolic hormones over a prolonged period (Jeschke et al. 2005). These changes contribute to a stunting of growth observed after major burns. Female patients have significantly increased levels of anabolic hormones, which are associated with decreased pro-inflammatory mediators and hypermetabolism, leading to a significantly shorter ICU length of stay compared with male patients.

20.3.7 Metabolic Modulation

In burned patients, a continued catabolic state results in weight loss, a decrease in lean body mass, immunologic compromise, and poor or delayed wound healing with prolonged recovery times. Various efforts have been made to promote anabolism in the thermally injured patient.

20.3.7.1 Propranolol

The massive catecholamine production associated with thermal injury heavily contributes to the intense catabolic response in major burn patients. The effects are the result of intense stimulation of both alpha and beta receptors and subsequent cardiovascular thermogenic and metabolic changes. Studies have shown that nonselective beta blockers efficiently reduce the metabolic rate and protein catabolism, particularly in children and young adults, and reduce the risk of liver steatosis [134, 135]. The metabolic advantages are observed with a 15–20% reduction of heart rate. Propranolol treatment attenuates muscle wasting in severely burned patients mainly by increasing protein synthesis and muscle protein synthesis efficiency, while protein breakdown remains unchanged [134]. The limitations are the usual contraindications to beta blockade. Treatment should be initiated as soon as resuscitation is completed (after 3–10 days depending on the severity of burns), as it reduces the hypermetabolic response [136]. For adults, starting doses are 10 mg TID until achieving a 20% reduction in heart rate.

20.3.7.2 Oxandrolone

Oxandrolone is a testosterone analog that can revert sarcopenia and improve nitrogen homeostasis. It has been successfully used in chronic wasting syndromes. The pharmacologic modulation of anabolism to counteract loss of lean body mass is beneficial in children with major burns [137]. A recent systematic review that included children and adults showed that the use of oxandrolone results in a reduction in net weight loss, lean body mass loss, nitrogen loss, donor-site healing time, and length of stay in the catabolic and rehabilitative phases, without any increase in mortality, infection, metabolic rate, hyperglycemia, or liver dysfunction rate. Over the long term, the use of oxandrolone can lead to an additional gain in lean body mass after 6–12 months of up to 11%, with additional improvements in height and weight, as well as bone mineral content and muscle strength [138]. Usual dosing corresponds to 20 mg/day in adults and 0.2 mg/kg/day in pediatric patients. Patients often receive the medication for 6–12 months. Its use should be adapted in case of renal failure and monitoring of liver function. The limited androgenic effects make its use possible in women.

20.3.7.3 Recombinant Human Growth Hormone

Recombinant human growth hormone (rhGH) therapy has been extensively investigated in GH-deficient children, where rhGH therapy improves nitrogen balance, increases body cell mass, and promotes bone formation [139]. These effects make rhGH a candidate for anabolism stimulation. Supplementation studies in burned pediatric patients have shown a decrease in donor-site healing times and length of stay relative to the percentage of TBSA burns, and the attenuation of hypermetabolism and inflammation, particularly when used in combination with propranolol [140]. While safe in children, the use of rhGH in critically ill adult patients is not proven, as it has been linked to hyperglycemia and increased metabolism and a doubling of mortality, mainly due to multiple organ dysfunction and septic shock [141, 142].

20.3.7.4 Insulin

Insulin is an anabolic hormone, promoting protein synthesis. High-dose intravenous glucose along with insulin has been shown to reduce the donor-site healing time of adolescent patients by 2 days [143]. However, recent data show that high loads of glucose promote de novo lipogenesis in the critically ill patient [144], questioning the rationale of providing large glucose loads along with insulin. This data, in combination with data showing increased liver fat deposits on postmortem evaluation in patients receiving large glucose loads [145], indicate that using high glucose loads along with insulin should be restricted until further studies prove its safe use. Total glucose administration (nutritional and delivered with drugs) should probably not exceed 6 g/kg BW/day, i.e., its maximal oxidation capacity.

20.3.7.5 Metformin

Severely burned patients exhibit periods of hyperglycemia and insulin insensitivity associated with increased muscle breakdown. Metformin lowers blood glucose levels by decreasing hepatic glucose production, reducing glucose absorption from the intestines, and increasing glucose uptake and utilization to peripheral tissues. The anabolic effect of metformin is based on decreased insulin resistance in the setting of the stress response in burn injury. Gore et al. showed that metformin treatment followed by 7-day insulin infusion increased the rate of muscle protein synthesis [146]. Though metformin has potential benefits, more data are needed to determine its safety and efficacy. Lactic acidosis is a known complication of the use of metformin, especially in critically ill patients with impaired renal function.

20.3.8 Electrolyte Disorders

In severely burned patients, nearly any electrolyte abnormality can be observed. The causes for these disturbances are many and include fluid resuscitation with crystalloids, exudative and evaporative losses, impaired renal regulation, and responses to counter-regulatory hormones.

20.3.8.1 Sodium

During the first 24 h, patients receive major amounts of sodium with their fluid resuscitation. Sodium accumulates in the interstitial space with edema. Despite this, hypernatremia occurring during the first 24 h reflects under-resuscitation and should be treated with additional fluid. Thereafter, mobilization of this fluid during the first weeks frequently results in hypernatremia and its resolution requires free water. Hypernatremia may also result from persistent evaporative losses from the wounds, particularly in case of treatment on a fluidized bed (contraindicated with severe hypernatremia) or in case of fever. Hypernatremia may also herald a septic episode.

20.3.8.2 Chloride

During the early resuscitation and the surgical debridements of the burn wound, patients tend to receive significant amounts of NaCl resulting in hyperchloremic acidosis. The excess chloride is difficult to handle for the kidney, but the condition generally resolves without further intervention.

20.3.8.3 Phosphate and Magnesium

Burns have high requirements for phosphate and magnesium in the absence of renal failure. Those requirements start early, and are largely explained by two mechanisms: large exudative losses and increased urinary excretion associated with acute protein catabolism and stress response. Stimulation of sodium excretion is usually required and can usually be achieved by the simultaneous administration of free water (D5W IV or enteral water) along with furosemide with or without thiazide diuretics.

20.3.8.4 Calcium

Cytokines such as IL-1 and TNF-α can cause upregulation of the parathyroid calcium-sensing receptor, resulting in calcium metabolism and bone matrix disturbances. These changes are thought to be partially responsible for burn-related hypocalcemia, hypercalciuria, and hyperparathyroidism [147].

Total plasma calcium concentration consists of three fractions: 15% is bound to multiple anions (sulfate, phosphate, lactate, citrate), about 40% is bound to albumin (in a ratio of 0.2 mmol/L of calcium per 10 g/L of albumin), and the remaining 45% circulates as physiologically active ionized calcium. Calcium metabolism is tightly regulated. As albumin levels vary widely in burns and only ionized calcium is biologically active, only ionized calcium is a true indicator of status, as total plasma calcium determination is not a reliable indicator of calcium status. The calcium correction for albumin formula:

$$\text{Corrected Ca} = \text{Total Ca Measured} + \left(0.8 \times \left[\text{Normal albumin - Patient's Albumin}\right]\right)$$

Hypocalcemia may occur during the early resuscitation phase, or in the context of massive perioperative blood transfusion and requires intravenous supplementation using any form of available intravenous calcium formulation. Hypercalcemia remains a poorly recognized cause of acute renal failure in patients with major burns that occurs as early as 3 weeks after injury. The triad of hypercalcemia, arterial hypertension, and acute renal failure is well known in other critical illnesses, while the association of hypercalcemia and renal failure in patients with major burns is much less reported in the literature. In a recent retrospective study, hypercalcemia was shown to occur in 19% of burned patients with hospital lengths of stay of more than 28 days and was associated with an increased mortality [148]. Hypercalcemia may also occur in patients with smaller burns requiring a stay of more than 20 days in the ICU. Ionized calcium determination enabled earlier detection, while using total calcium determination "with albumin correction" was only slightly sensitive, as shown by normal corrected values in 15 cases with ionized hypercalcemia.

The treatment of hypercalcemia includes hydration, volume expansion, and early mobilization. As most causes of severe hypercalcemia depend on increased osteoclast activation, drugs that decrease bone turnover are effective. The treatment of choice in cases that do not resolve with the simple measures relies on the bisphosphonates, pamidronate disodium and zoledronic acid, which are available in intravenous forms. In burned children, acute intravenous pamidronate administration has been shown to help to preserve bone mass, achieving a sustained therapeutic effect on bone [149]. An alternative treatment of the latter in burns includes anabolic agents such as oxandrolone [150]. Bisphosphonates, specifically etidronate, have been advocated in the management of heterotopic ossification, a complication that occurs in 1.2% of burn patients [151, 152].

20.3.9 Bone Demineralization and Osteoporosis

Due to the substantial alterations of calcium and phosphorus metabolism, bone formation is reduced both in adults and children when burns exceed 40% TBSA. Bone mineral density is significantly lower in burned children compared with the same age normal children [8, 153, 154]. The consequences are increased risk of fractures, decreased growth velocity, and stunting.

The bone is affected by various means: alteration of mineral metabolism, elevated cytokine and corticosteroid levels, decreased growth hormone, nutritional deficiencies (vitamin D), and immobilization. Cytokines contribute to the alterations, particularly interleukin-1beta and interleukin-6, both of which are greatly increased in burns and stimulate osteoblast-mediated bone resorption. The increased cortisol production in thermal injury leads to decreased bone formation, and the low growth hormone levels fail to promote bone formation [155], further exacerbating the situation. Various studies suggest that immobilization plays a significant role in the pathogenesis of burn-associated bone disease. Alterations of magnesium and calcium homeostasis constitute another cause. Hypocalcemia and hypomagnesemia are constant findings, and ionized calcium levels remain low for weeks. The alterations are partly explained by large exudative magnesium and phosphorus losses. Serial measurement of bone markers might not be useful but [156] close monitoring of ionized calcium, magnesium, and inorganic phosphate levels is recommended since burn patients usually require substantial supplementation by intravenous or enteral routes.

Osteoporosis is a complication related to burn injury. Burn patients have a lower bone density when matched to healthy individuals. This effect seems to be more significant in the lumbar vertebrae. The effect is proportional to the

TBSA [157]. Biphosphonates, such as pamidronate, have been used in severely burned children during the acute phase, showing promising results in preserving bone mass [158, 159]. Children are particularly susceptible to the long-term effects of low bone density. Vitamin D has also been studied, with patients showing a reduced incidence of bone fractures at 22 months after injury [160]. The supplementation of vitamin D to maintain normal physiological levels improves bone health and muscle strength, deterring the effects of sarcopenia related to burn injury [161]. Moreover, cholecalciferol supplementation to those critically ill patients with severe vitamin deficiency decreases hospital mortality [162].

20.3.10 Coagulation and Thrombosis Prophylaxis

The coagulation and hematologic system is profoundly affected by a burn and the associated changes vary from consumption coagulopathy to overproduction. Alterations in coagulation pathways have been explained by the release of tissue factor and acute phase reactants, consumption coagulopathy, platelet dysfunction, and platelet-specific microparticles [163]. The degree of these changes correlates with a patient's age and body mass index, TBSA burned, presence of inhalation injury, and higher number of invasive procedures.

Alterations of the clotting factors associated with disseminated intravascular coagulation have been demonstrated in several studies in burn-injured patients [164]. Disseminated intravascular coagulation occurs more frequently in patients with greater than 40% TBSA burns, and aggressive crystalloid resuscitation has been postulated as a significant contributor [163, 165]. Microvascular emboli have been noted in the capillaries of major organs after severe burn injury, and these could account for the multiple organ dysfunction syndrome seen in burn-injured patients [166]. Hematological alterations observed after burns are complex and can last for several months and can be summarized as follows:

- Fibrin split products increase during the early phase after burns.
- Dilution and consumption explain early low prothrombin time values.
- The coagulation cascade is activated.
- Fibrin factors V and VIII increase as part of the acute phase response.
- Antithrombin deficiency is frequent.
- Alpha angle and mean amplitude are increased on TEG and ROTEM
- Early thrombocytopenia and subsequent thrombocytosis take place as the process of wound closure occurs.

The risk of deep venous thrombosis and of pulmonary embolism is at least as high as in any other surgical condition. Incidence is highly variable, ranging from 0.3% to as high as 23%. Specific risk factors include central venous lines, prolonged bed rest, multiple transfusions, repeated surgical interventions, and an intense inflammatory state.

Prophylaxis should be started from admission. The American College of Chest Physicians recommend routine thromboprophylaxis in all burn patients with advanced age, morbid obesity, extensive or lower extremity burns, concomitant lower extremity trauma, the use of a femoral venous catheter, and/or prolonged immobility (grade 1A). For burned patients who have additional risk factors for venous thromboembolism, if there are no contraindications, they recommend the use of either low molecular weight heparin or low-dose unfractionated heparin starting as soon as it is considered safe to do so (grade 1C). For burn patients who have a high bleeding risk, they recommend mechanical thromboprophylaxis with compression stockings and/or intermittent pneumatic compression until the bleeding risk decreases (grade 1A) [167].

Factors that are known to exacerbate or induce coagulopathy should be limited. Prompt and aggressive burn shock treatment, aimed at achieving a normal cardiac output and a normal blood pressure, is important to avoid tissue hypoperfusion and its associated detrimental effects on hemostasis. Furthermore, adequate body temperature conservation should be applied to avoid hypothermia, especially during fluid resuscitation and the perioperative period. On the other hand, as hemodilution may also trigger a dilutional coagulopathy, restrictive fluid therapy has also been suggested. Early and aggressive use of plasma transfusion has been suggested for coagulopathic patients with severe burn injury undergoing burn wound excisions [168, 169]. Interruptions in surgery should be reduced to a minimum and discussed with the surgical team.

Summary Box

The management of the critically ill thermally injured patient can be very complex. The treatment modalities remain at times controversial, as there is a lack of high-level evidence for them. There have been many advances in the field of critical care of the thermally injured patient, which would benefit from large-scale multicenter trials. This chapter highlights a few of the important nuances in the care of these patients and places emphasis on the need for intricate support for all organ systems in order to improve morbidity and mortality.

References

1. National Hospital Ambulatory Medical Care Survey: 2013 Emergency Department Summary tables. In The Ambulatory and Hospital Care Statistics Branch, Editor. National Hospital Ambulatory Medical Care Survey. Centers for Disease Control and Prevention; 2013.
2. McDermott KW, Weiss AJ, Elixhauser A. Burn-related hospital inpatient stays and Emergency Department visits, 2013: statistical brief #217, in Healthcare Cost and Utilization Project (HCUP) statistical briefs. Rockville: Agency for Healthcare Research and Quality (US); 2006.
3. Herndon DN, editor. Total burn care. 3rd ed. Philadelphia: Saunders Elsevier; 2007.
4. Herndon DN, Tompkins RG. Support of the metabolic response to burn injury. Lancet. 2004;363(9424):1895–902.
5. Jeschke MG, et al. Handbook of burns, vol. 1. Wien: Springer; 2012.
6. Kraft R, et al. Burn size and survival probability in paediatric patients in modern burn care: a prospective observational cohort study. Lancet. 2012;379(9820):1013–21.
7. Jeschke MG, et al. Morbidity and survival probability in burn patients in modern burn care. Crit Care Med. 2015;43(4):808–15.
8. Jeschke MG, et al. Pathophysiologic response to severe burn injury. Ann Surg. 2008;248(3):387–401.
9. Shirani KZ, Pruitt BA Jr, Mason AD Jr. The influence of inhalation injury and pneumonia on burn mortality. Ann Surg. 1987;205(1):82–7.
10. Chen MC, et al. The impact of inhalation injury in patients with small and moderate burns. Burns. 2014;40(8):1481–6.
11. Enkhbaatar P, et al. Pathophysiology, research challenges, and clinical management of smoke inhalation injury. Lancet. 2016;388(10052):1437–46.
12. ABA. 2011 National burn repository: report of data from 2001-2010. American Burn Association; 2011.
13. Maan ZN, et al. Burns ITU admissions: length of stay in specific levels of care for adult and paediatric patients. Burns. 2014;40(8):1458–62.
14. Williams FN, et al. The leading causes of death after burn injury in a single pediatric burn center. Crit Care. 2009;13(6):R183.
15. Barrow RE, Jeschke MG, Herndon DN. Early fluid resuscitation improves outcomes in severely burned children. Resuscitation. 2000;45(2):91–6.
16. Greenhalgh DG. Burn resuscitation. J Burn Care Res. 2007;28(4):555–65.
17. Greenhalgh DG. Burn resuscitation: the results of the ISBI/ABA survey. Burns. 2010;36(2):176–82.
18. Kraft R, et al. Optimized fluid management improves outcomes of pediatric burn patients. J Surg Res. 2013;181(1):121–8.
19. Wolf SE, et al. Mortality determinants in massive pediatric burns. An analysis of 103 children with > or = 80% TBSA burns (> or = 70% full-thickness). Ann Surg. 1997;225(5):554–65; discussion 565–9
20. Wiggins-Dohlvik K, et al. Tissue inhibitor of metalloproteinase-2 inhibits burn-induced derangements and hyperpermeability in microvascular endothelial cells. Am J Surg. 2016;211(1):197–205.
21. Lund T, Onarheim H, Reed RK. Pathogenesis of edema formation in burn injuries. World J Surg. 1992;16(1):2–9.
22. Arturson G, Jakobsson OP. Oedema measurements in a standard burn model. Burns Incl Therm Inj. 1985;12(1):1–7.
23. Kremer T, et al. Burn plasma transfer induces burn edema in healthy rats. Shock. 2008;30(4):394–400.
24. Rae L, Fidler P, Gibran N. The physiologic basis of burn shock and the need for aggressive fluid resuscitation. Crit Care Clin. 2016;32(4):491–505.
25. Horton JW, et al. Postburn cardiac contractile function and biochemical markers of postburn cardiac injury. J Am Coll Surg. 1995;181(4):289–98.
26. Klein MB, et al. The association between fluid administration and outcome following major burn: a multicenter study. Ann Surg. 2007;245(4):622–8.
27. Pham TN, Cancio LC, Gibran NS. American Burn Association practice guidelines burn shock resuscitation. J Burn Care Res. 2008;29(1):257–66.
28. Salinas J, et al. Computerized decision support system improves fluid resuscitation following severe burns: an original study. Crit Care Med. 2011;39(9):2031–8.
29. Cancio LC, Salinas J, Kramer GC. Protocolized resuscitation of burn patients. Crit Care Clin. 2016;32(4):599–610.
30. Ivy ME, et al. Intra-abdominal hypertension and abdominal compartment syndrome in burn patients. J Trauma. 2000; 49(3):387–91.
31. Bittner EA, et al. Acute and perioperative care of the burn-injured patient. Anesthesiology. 2015;122(2):448–64.
32. Greenhalgh DG, et al. American Burn Association consensus conference to define sepsis and infection in burns. J Burn Care Res. 2007;28(6):776–90.
33. Latenser BA. Critical care of the burn patient: the first 48 hours. Crit Care Med. 2009;37(10):2819–26.
34. Baxter CR, Shires T. Physiological response to crystalloid resuscitation of severe burns. Ann N Y Acad Sci. 1968;150(3):874–94.
35. Rivers E, et al. Early goal-directed therapy in the treatment of severe sepsis and septic shock. N Engl J Med. 2001;345: 1368–77.
36. Hodgman EI, et al. Future therapies in burn resuscitation. Crit Care Clin. 2016;32(4):611–9.
37. Saffle JI. The phenomenon of "fluid creep" in acute burn resuscitation. J Burn Care Res. 2007;28(3):382–95.
38. Faraklas I, et al. Colloid normalizes resuscitation ratio in pediatric burns. J Burn Care Res. 2011;32(1):91–7.
39. Cochran A, et al. Burn patient characteristics and outcomes following resuscitation with albumin. Burns. 2007;33(1):25–30.
40. Navickis RJ, Greenhalgh DG, Wilkes MM. Albumin in burn shock resuscitation: a meta-analysis of controlled clinical studies. J Burn Care Res. 2016;37(3):e268–78.
41. O'Mara MS, et al. A prospective, randomized evaluation of intra-abdominal pressures with crystalloid and colloid resuscitation in burn patients. J Trauma. 2005;58(5):1011–8.
42. Huzar TF, et al. Admission Rapid Thrombelastography (rTEG(R)) values predict resuscitation volumes and patient outcomes after thermal injury. J Burn Care Res. 2018;39(3):345.
43. Perel P, Roberts I, Ker K. Colloids versus crystalloids for fluid resuscitation in critically ill patients. Cochrane Database Syst Rev. 2013;(2):CD000567.
44. Bunn F, Trivedi D. Colloid solutions for fluid resuscitation. Cochrane Database Syst Rev. 2012;(7):CD001319.
45. Cartotto R, Callum J. A review of the use of human albumin in burn patients. J Burn Care Res. 2012;33(6):702–17.
46. Snell JA, et al. Clinical review: the critical care management of the burn patient. Crit Care. 2013;17(5):241.
47. Palmieri TL, et al. Transfusion Requirement in Burn Care Evaluation (TRIBE): a multicenter randomized prospective trial of blood transfusion in major burn injury. Ann Surg. 2017;266(4):595–602.
48. Evans AE, et al. Cardiovascular responsiveness to vasopressin and alpha1-adrenergic receptor agonists after burn injury. J Burn Care Res. 2017;38(2):90–8.
49. Andel D, et al. Base deficit and lactate: early predictors of morbidity and mortality in patients with burns. Burns. 2007;33(8):973–8.
50. Jeng JC, et al. Serum lactate, not base deficit, rapidly predicts survival after major burns. Burns. 2002;28(2):161–6.
51. Husain FA, et al. Serum lactate and base deficit as predictors of mortality and morbidity. Am J Surg. 2003;185(5):485–91.
52. Guillory AN, et al. Cardiovascular dysfunction following burn injury: what we have learned from rat and mouse models. Int J Mol Sci. 2016;17(1):E53.

53. Branski LK, et al. Transpulmonary thermodilution for hemodynamic measurements in severely burned children. Crit Care. 2011;15(2):R118.
54. Kuntscher MV, et al. Transcardiopulmonary vs pulmonary arterial thermodilution methods for hemodynamic monitoring of burned patients. J Burn Care Rehabil. 2002;23(1):21–6.
55. Etherington L, Saffle J, Cochran A. Use of transesophageal echocardiography in burns:a retrospective review. J Burn Care Res. 2010;31(1):36–9.
56. Paratz JD, et al. Burn resuscitation--hourly urine output versus alternative endpoints: a systematic review. Shock. 2014;42(4):295–306.
57. Kuntscher MV, Germann G, Hartmann B. Correlations between cardiac output, stroke volume, central venous pressure, intra-abdominal pressure and total circulating blood volume in resuscitation of major burns. Resuscitation. 2006;70(1):37–43.
58. Ivy ME, et al. Abdominal compartment syndrome in patients with burns. J Burn Care Rehabil. 1999;20(5):351–3.
59. Hershberger RC, et al. Abdominal compartment syndrome in the severely burned patient. J Burn Care Res. 2007;28(5):708–14.
60. Balogh ZJ, et al. Postinjury abdominal compartment syndrome: from recognition to prevention. Lancet. 2014;384(9952):1466–75.
61. Milner SM, et al. Cody. Eplasty. 2015;15:e35.
62. Birman C, Beckenham E. Acquired tracheo-esophageal fistula in the pediatric population. Int J Pediatr Otorhinolaryngol. 1998;44(2):109–13.
63. Chung KK, et al. High-frequency percussive ventilation and low tidal volume ventilation in burns: a randomized controlled trial. Crit Care Med. 2010;38(10):1970–7.
64. Kennedy JD, et al. ECMO in major burn patients: feasibility and considerations when multiple modes of mechanical ventilation fail. Burns Trauma. 2017;5:20.
65. Smailes ST, Martin RV, McVicar AJ. The incidence and outcome of extubation failure in burn intensive care patients. J Burn Care Res. 2009;30(3):386–92.
66. Palmieri TL, et al. Inhalation injury in children: a 10 year experience at Shriners Hospitals for Children. J Burn Care Res. 2009;30(1):206–8.
67. Nayyar A, Charles AG, Hultman CS. Management of pulmonary failure after burn injury: from VDR to ECMO. Clin Plast Surg. 2017;44(3):513–20.
68. Sutton T, et al. Severity of inhalation injury is predictive of alterations in gas exchange and worsened clinical outcomes. J Burn Care Res. 2017;38:390–5.
69. Sheridan RL, Hess D. Inhaled nitric oxide in inhalation injury. J Burn Care Res. 2009;30(1):162–4.
70. Endorf FW, Gamelli RL. Inhalation injury, pulmonary perturbations, and fluid resuscitation. J Burn Care Res. 2007;28(1):80–3.
71. Kealey GP. Carbon monoxide toxicity. J Burn Care Res. 2009;30(1):146–7.
72. Erdman AR. Is hydroxocobalamin safe and effective for smoke inhalation? Searching for guidance in the haze. Ann Emerg Med. 2007;49(6):814–6.
73. Nguyen L, et al. Utility and outcomes of hydroxocobalamin use in smoke inhalation patients. Burns. 2017;43(1):107–13.
74. Finnerty CC, Herndon DN, Jeschke MG. Inhalation injury in severely burned children does not augment the systemic inflammatory response. Crit Care. 2007;11(1):R22.
75. Bai C, et al. Application of flexible bronchoscopy in inhalation lung injury. Diagn Pathol. 2013;8:174.
76. Weaver LK. Clinical practice. Carbon monoxide poisoning. N Engl J Med. 2009;360(12):1217–25.
77. Holm C, et al. Effect of crystalloid resuscitation and inhalation injury on extravascular lung water. Chest. 2002;121(6):1956–62.
78. Barrow RE, et al. Mortality related to gender, age, sepsis, and ethnicity in severely burned children. Shock. 2005;23(6):485–7.
79. Miller AC, Elamin EM, Suffredini AF. Inhaled anticoagulation regimens for the treatment of smoke inhalation-associated acute lung injury: a systematic review. Crit Care Med. 2014;42(2):413–9.
80. Glas GJ, et al. HEPBURN - investigating the efficacy and safety of nebulized heparin versus placebo in burn patients with inhalation trauma: study protocol for a multi-center randomized controlled trial. Trials. 2014;15:91.
81. Enkhbaatar P, et al. Inducible nitric oxide synthase dimerization inhibitor prevents cardiovascular and renal morbidity in sheep with combined burn and smoke inhalation injury. Am J Physiol Heart Circ Physiol. 2003;285(6):H2430–6.
82. Foncerrada G, et al. Safety of nebulized epinephrine in smoke inhalation injury. J Burn Care Res. 2017;38(6):396–402.
83. Tabrizi MB, et al. Inhaled epoprostenol improves oxygenation in severe hypoxemia. J Trauma Acute Care Surg. 2012;73(2):503–6.
84. Carlson DL, Horton JW. Cardiac molecular signaling after burn trauma. J Burn Care Res. 2006;27(5):669–75.
85. Marano MA, et al. Serum cachectin/tumor necrosis factor in critically ill patients with burns correlates with infection and mortality. Surg Gynecol Obstet. 1990;170(1):32–8.
86. Kim HS, et al. Changes in the levels of interleukins 6, 8, and 10, tumor necrosis factor alpha, and granulocyte-colony stimulating factor in Korean burn patients: relation to burn size and postburn time. Ann Lab Med. 2012;32(5):339–44.
87. Jeschke MG, et al. Long-term persistance of the pathophysiologic response to severe burn injury. PLoS One. 2011;6(7):e21245.
88. Hung TY, et al. Increased risk of ischemic stroke in patients with burn injury: a nationwide cohort study in Taiwan. Scand J Trauma Resusc Emerg Med. 2016;24:44.
89. Cubitt JJ, et al. Intensive care unit-acquired weakness in the burn population. J Plast Reconstr Aesthet Surg. 2016;69(5):e105–9.
90. de Jonge E, Bos MM. Patients with cancer on the ICU: the times they are changing. Crit Care. 2009;13(2):122.
91. Gore DC, et al. Influence of fever on the hypermetabolic response in burn-injured children. Arch Surg. 2003;138(2):169–74; discussion 174.
92. Hogan BK, et al. Correlation of American Burn Association sepsis criteria with the presence of bacteremia in burned patients admitted to the intensive care unit. J Burn Care Res. 2012;33(3):371–8.
93. Murray CK, et al. Evaluation of white blood cell count, neutrophil percentage, and elevated temperature as predictors of bloodstream infection in burn patients. Arch Surg. 2007;142(7):639–42.
94. Davis SL, et al. Sustained impairments in cutaneous vasodilation and sweating in grafted skin following long-term recovery. J Burn Care Res. 2009;30(4):675–85.
95. Bernal E, Wolf S, Cripps M. New-onset, postoperative tachyarrhythmias in critically ill surgical patients. Burns. 2018;44(2):249–55.
96. Goff DR, et al. Cardiac disease and the patient with burns. J Burn Care Rehabil. 1990;11(4):305–7.
97. Bouadma L, Wolff M, Lucet JC. Ventilator-associated pneumonia and its prevention. Curr Opin Infect Dis. 2012;25(4):395–404.
98. Sen S, et al. Ventilator-associated pneumonia prevention bundle significantly reduces the risk of ventilator-associated pneumonia in critically ill burn patients. J Burn Care Res. 2016;37(3):166–71.
99. Bassetti M, et al. Management of ventilator-associated pneumonia: epidemiology, diagnosis and antimicrobial therapy. Expert Rev Anti Infect Ther. 2012;10(5):585–96.
100. Mosier MJ, et al. Early enteral nutrition in burns: compliance with guidelines and associated outcomes in a multicenter study. J Burn Care Res. 2011;32(1):104–9.
101. Lam NN, Tien NG, Khoa CM. Early enteral feeding for burned patients--an effective method which should be encouraged in developing countries. Burns. 2008;34(2):192–6.
102. Raff T, Hartmann B, Germann G. Early intragastric feeding of seriously burned and long-term ventilated patients: a review of 55 patients. Burns. 1997;23(1):19–25.

103. Markell KW, et al. Abdominal complications after severe burns. J Am Coll Surg. 2009;208(5):940–7; discussion 947–9
104. Williams FN, et al. Modulation of the hypermetabolic response to trauma: temperature, nutrition, and drugs. J Am Coll Surg. 2009;208(4):489–502.
105. Pereira C, Murphy K, Herndon D. Outcome measures in burn care. Is mortality dead? Burns. 2004;30(8):761–71.
106. Pereira CT, et al. Age-dependent differences in survival after severe burns: a unicentric review of 1,674 patients and 179 autopsies over 15 years. J Am Coll Surg. 2006;202(3):536–48.
107. Jeschke MG. The hepatic response to thermal injury: is the liver important for postburn outcomes? Mol Med. 2009;15(9-10):337–51.
108. Price LA, et al. Liver disease in burn injury: evidence from a national sample of 31,338 adult patients. J Burns Wounds. 2007;7:e1.
109. Jeschke MG, et al. Insulin protects against hepatic damage postburn. Mol Med. 2011;17(5-6):516–22.
110. Gauglitz GG, et al. Post-burn hepatic insulin resistance is associated with endoplasmic reticulum (ER) stress. Shock. 2010;33(3):299–305.
111. Song J, et al. Severe burn-induced endoplasmic reticulum stress and hepatic damage in mice. Mol Med. 2009;15(9–10):316–20.
112. Jeschke MG, et al. Calcium and Er stress mediate hepatic apoptosis after burn injury. J Cell Mol Med. 2009;13:1857–65.
113. Jeschke MG, Micak RP, Finnerty CC, Herndon DN. Changes in liver function and size after a severe thermal injury. Shock. 2007;28:172–7.
114. Jeschke MG, et al. Changes in liver function and size after a severe thermal injury. Shock. 2007;28(2):172–7.
115. Bohanon FJ, et al. Burn trauma acutely increases the respiratory capacity and function of liver mitochondria. Shock. 2018;49(4):466–73.
116. Senel E, et al. The evaluation of the adrenal and thyroid axes and glucose metabolism after burn injury in children. J Pediatr Endocrinol Metab. 2010;23(5):481–9.
117. Gore DC, et al. Association of hyperglycemia with increased mortality after severe burn injury. J Trauma. 2001;51(3):540–4.
118. Pham TN, et al. Impact of tight glycemic control in severely burned children. J Trauma. 2005;59(5):1148–54.
119. Jeschke MG. Clinical review: glucose control in severely burned patients - current best practice. Crit Care. 2013;17(4):232.
120. Baxter CR. Metabolism and nutrition in burned patients. Compr Ther. 1987;13(1):36–42.
121. Medlin S. Nutrition for wound healing. Br J Nurs. 2012;21(12):S11–2, S14–5
122. Berger M. Acute copper and zinc deficiency due to exudative losses - substitution versus nutritional requirements - [Burns 2005;31(6): 711-6]. Burns. 2006;32(3):393.
123. Kremer T, et al. High-dose vitamin C treatment reduces capillary leakage after burn plasma transfer in rats. J Burn Care Res. 2010;31(3):470–9.
124. Tanaka H, et al. Reduction of resuscitation fluid volumes in severely burned patients using ascorbic acid administration: a randomized, prospective study. Arch Surg. 2000;135(3):326–31.
125. Buehner M, et al. Oxalate nephropathy after continuous infusion of high-dose vitamin C as an adjunct to burn resuscitation. J Burn Care Res. 2016;37(4):e374–9.
126. Chrysopoulo MT, et al. Acute renal dysfunction in severely burned adults. J Trauma. 1999;46(1):141–4.
127. Jeschke MG, et al. Mortality in burned children with acute renal failure. Arch Surg. 1998;133(7):752–6.
128. Kallinen O, et al. Multiple organ failure as a cause of death in patients with severe burns. J Burn Care Res. 2012;33(2): 206–11.
129. Clark A, et al. Acute kidney injury after burn. Burns. 2017;43(5):898–908.
130. Holm C, et al. Acute renal failure in severely burned patients. Burns. 1999;25(2):171–8.
131. Mosier MJ, Lasinski AM, Gamelli RL. Suspected adrenal insufficiency in critically ill burned patients: etomidate-induced or critical illness-related corticosteroid insufficiency?-A review of the literature. J Burn Care Res. 2015;36(2):272–8.
132. Fuchs P, et al. Cortisol in severely burned patients: investigations on disturbance of the hypothalamic-pituitary-adrenal axis. Shock. 2007;28(6):662–7.
133. Gangemi EN, et al. Low triiodothyronine serum levels as a predictor of poor prognosis in burn patients. Burns. 2008;34(6):817–24.
134. Herndon DN, et al. Reversal of catabolism by beta-blockade after severe burns. N Engl J Med. 2001;345(17):1223–9.
135. Morio B, et al. Propranolol decreases splanchnic triacylglycerol storage in burn patients receiving a high-carbohydrate diet. Ann Surg. 2002;236(2):218–25.
136. Breitenstein E, et al. Effects of beta-blockade on energy metabolism following burns. Burns. 1990;16(4):259–64.
137. Jeschke MG, et al. The effect of oxandrolone on the endocrinologic, inflammatory, and hypermetabolic responses during the acute phase postburn. Ann Surg. 2007;246(3):351–60; discussion 360–2
138. Li H, et al. The efficacy and safety of oxandrolone treatment for patients with severe burns: a systematic review and meta-analysis. Burns. 2016;42(4):717–27.
139. Klein GL. Burn-induced bone loss: importance, mechanisms, and management. J Burns Wounds. 2006;5:e5.
140. Jeschke MG, et al. Combination of recombinant human growth hormone and propranolol decreases hypermetabolism and inflammation in severely burned children. Pediatr Crit Care Med. 2008;9(2):209–16.
141. Takala J, et al. Increased mortality associated with growth hormone treatment in critically ill adults. N Engl J Med. 1999;341(11):785–92.
142. Diaz EC, et al. Effects of pharmacological interventions on muscle protein synthesis and breakdown in recovery from burns. Burns. 2015;41(4):649–57.
143. Pierre EJ, et al. Effects of insulin on wound healing. J Trauma. 1998;44(2):342–5.
144. Tappy L, et al. Effects of isoenergetic glucose-based or lipid-based parenteral nutrition on glucose metabolism, de novo lipogenesis, and respiratory gas exchanges in critically ill patients. Crit Care Med. 1998;26(5):860–7.
145. Burke JF, et al. Glucose requirements following burn injury. Parameters of optimal glucose infusion and possible hepatic and respiratory abnormalities following excessive glucose intake. Ann Surg. 1979;190(3):274–85.
146. Gore DC, et al. Influence of metformin on glucose intolerance and muscle catabolism following severe burn injury. Ann Surg. 2005;241(2):334–42.
147. Murphey ED, et al. Up-regulation of the parathyroid calcium-sensing receptor after burn injury in sheep: a potential contributory factor to postburn hypocalcemia. Crit Care Med. 2000;28(12):3885–90.
148. Sam R, et al. Hypercalcemia in patients in the burn intensive care unit. J Burn Care Res. 2007;28(5):742–6.
149. Przkora R, et al. Body composition changes with time in pediatric burn patients. J Trauma. 2006;60(5):968–71; discussion 971
150. Przkora R, Herndon DN, Suman OE. The effects of oxandrolone and exercise on muscle mass and function in children with severe burns. Pediatrics. 2007;119(1):e109–16.
151. Peterson SL, et al. Postburn heterotopic ossification: insights for management decision making. J Trauma. 1989;29(3):365–9.

152. Vanden Bossche L, Vanderstraeten G. Heterotopic ossification: a review. J Rehabil Med. 2005;37(3):129–36.
153. Jeschke MG, et al. Endogenous anabolic hormones and hypermetabolism: effect of trauma and gender differences. Ann Surg. 2005;241(5):759–67; discussion 767–8
154. Jeschke MG, et al. Gender differences in pediatric burn patients: does it make a difference? Ann Surg. 2008;248(1):126–36.
155. Przkora R, et al. Beneficial effects of extended growth hormone treatment after hospital discharge in pediatric burn patients. Ann Surg. 2006;243(6):796–801; discussion 801–3
156. Rousseau AF, et al. Bone markers during acute burn care: relevance to clinical practice? Burns. 2017;43(1):176–81.
157. Roshanzamir S, Partovi A, Dabbaghmanesh A. Prevalence and severity of bone loss in burned patients. Burns. 2017;43(4):766–70.
158. Klein GL, et al. The efficacy of acute administration of pamidronate on the conservation of bone mass following severe burn injury in children: a double-blind, randomized, controlled study. Osteoporos Int. 2005;16(6):631–5.
159. Przkora R, et al. Pamidronate preserves bone mass for at least 2 years following acute administration for pediatric burn injury. Bone. 2007;41(2):297–302.
160. Mayes T, et al. Investigation of bone health subsequent to vitamin D supplementation in children following burn injury. Nutr Clin Pract. 2015;30(6):830–7.
161. Rousseau AF, et al. Effects of cholecalciferol supplementation and optimized calcium intakes on vitamin D status, muscle strength and bone health: a one-year pilot randomized controlled trial in adults with severe burns. Burns. 2015;41(2):317–25.
162. Amrein K, et al. Effect of high-dose vitamin D3 on hospital length of stay in critically ill patients with vitamin D deficiency: the VITdAL-ICU randomized clinical trial. JAMA. 2014;312(15):1520–30.
163. Midura EF, et al. Impact of platelets and platelet-derived microparticles on hypercoagulability following burn injury. Shock. 2016;45(1):82–7.
164. Lippi G, Ippolito L, Cervellin G. Disseminated intravascular coagulation in burn injury. Semin Thromb Hemost. 2010;36(4):429–36.
165. King DR, Namias N, Andrews DM. Coagulation abnormalities following thermal injury. Blood Coagul Fibrinolysis. 2010;21(7):666–9.
166. Garcia-Avello A, et al. Degree of hypercoagulability and hyperfibrinolysis is related to organ failure and prognosis after burn trauma. Thromb Res. 1998;89(2):59–64.
167. Geerts WH, et al. Prevention of venous thromboembolism: American College of Chest Physicians Evidence-Based Clinical Practice Guidelines (8th Edition). Chest. 2008;133(6 Suppl):381S–453S.
168. Palmieri TL, Greenhalgh DG, Sen S. Prospective comparison of packed red blood cell-to-fresh frozen plasma transfusion ratio of 4: 1 versus 1: 1 during acute massive burn excision. J Trauma Acute Care Surg. 2013;74(1):76–83.
169. Sherren PB, et al. Acute burn induced coagulopathy. Burns. 2013;39(6):1157–61.

Nutrition Support for the Burn Patient

21

Audra Clark, Jonathan Imran, Tarik Madni, and Steven E. Wolf

21.1 Background

Nutritional support remains an important aspect in the care of critically ill patients, especially those with severe burns. The unique hypermetabolic state occurring after a severe burn can cause metabolic rates to double and is accompanied by severe catabolism. The hypermetabolic state persists for more than a year after severe injury, and if nutritional support does not meet the increased energy expenditures, patients experience significant loss of lean muscle mass, impaired wound healing and immune dysfunction [1, 2]. The goal of nutritional support in the burn patient is to ameliorate and optimize the deranged metabolism and avoid nutritional complications.

This chapter reviews the current state of knowledge of metabolism and nutrition after burn. At this time, our understanding of the complicated physiology of nutrition is incomplete, and nutritional treatments differ widely among burn centers. Much of our information on nutritional support is inferred from studies in other patient populations, especially trauma and critical care. Many questions still exist regarding the ideal volume, composition, and route of dietary provision for burned patients.

A. Clark · J. Imran · T. Madni
Department of Surgery, University of Texas—Southwestern Medical Center, Dallas, TX, USA
e-mail: audra.clark@phhs.org; jonathan.imran@phhs.org; tarik.madni@phhs.org

S. E. Wolf (✉)
Department of Surgery, University of Texas Medical Branch, Galveston, TX, USA
e-mail: swolf@utmb.edu

21.2 Initial Assessment of Nutritional Status

During acute burn treatment, primary concerns are centered on fluid resuscitation, hemodynamic monitoring, and respiratory care; however, nutritional assessment and support must not be overlooked. Completing an initial assessment of the patient's prior nutritional status is challenging but important. A baseline nutritional assessment should begin with a focused history from the patient or family to determine the presence of preexisting conditions or dietary habits such as diabetes mellitus and alcoholism. Some may be malnourished prior to the inciting event, while others become malnourished during prolonged hospitalization. Vitamin and mineral deficiencies and conditions such as obesity should also be elucidated when possible.

In obese patients, the nutritional assessment can be difficult, and despite an excess of fat, these patients can still be malnourished. Using actual body weight to estimate caloric needs may then lead to overestimation and overfeeding. Contrary to the reduced mortality observed in obese patients receiving care in medical and surgical intensive care units, obese burn patients have been shown to have higher mortality compared to normal weight burn patients [3]. Moreover, in the pediatric burn population, those who were obese were more likely to require ventilator support and had longer duration of hospitalization [4, 5]. A few enteral formulas have been created specifically for obese patients, but they are not well studied. Some clinicians advocate for hypocaloric feeding which involves low-calorie, high-protein diets to maintain lead body mass while encouraging weight loss and glycemic control [6]. Data for this strategy is limited, and more studies will be needed before it can be recommended [7, 8].

21.3 Metabolic Response to Burn Injury

Severe burns cause an intense stress response leading to a drastically amplified metabolic rate that can last for years after burn. Patients have a similar state of hypermetabolism

M. G. Jeschke et al. (eds.), *Handbook of Burns Volume 1*, https://doi.org/10.1007/978-3-030-18940-2_21

after traumatic injury and sepsis, but not nearly to the degree and duration of burned patients [9]. Hypermetabolism after burn is not entirely understood, and the underlying mechanisms of this immense inflammatory, metabolic, and hormonal dysregulation are still being studied. The classic "ebb" and "flow" physiology was originally described by Cuthberson in 1982 and is characterized by decreased metabolism and tissue perfusion immediately after severe injury (the "ebb" phase) followed by increased metabolism and hyperdynamic circulation (the "flow" phase) [10]. This prolonged hypermetabolic response is proportional to the extent of the burn wound, and in patients with greater than 40% total body surface area (TBSA) burn can have resting energy expenditures from 40% to 100% above normal [11, 12]. The importance of nutrition to support the increased metabolic needs and mitigate the stress response cannot be overstated. Unchecked hypermetabolism leads to massive loss of lean muscle mass, immune dysfunction, and poor wound healing.

21.4 Timing and Route of Nutritional Therapy

Despite improvements in burn care, resuscitation of the severely burned patient can have profound detrimental effects on the gastrointestinal tract. Large volume crystalloid resuscitation can cause intestinal edema, potentially leading to paralytic ileus [13]. In addition, intestinal permeability increases within 24 h after injury in patients with moderate to severe burns [14]. The mucosal damage and resultant increased intestinal permeability allows for bacterial translocation and decreased nutrient absorption [15].

Based on recent recommendations, enteral nutritional support should be initiated within 24 h of injury [13]. Early enteral nutrition has a number of advantageous effects including increased immune function and immunoglobulin production, reduction of hormones such as catecholamines, cortisol, and glucagon, improved intestinal mucosal integrity, motility, and blood flow, and a reduction in stress (Curling) ulceration [16, 17].

Providing early nutritional support can be challenging as burn patients are prone to ileus, and burn shock is associated with splanchnic hypoperfusion. Feedings are not always well tolerated, leading to repeated interruptions, insufficient nutrient delivery, and increased risk of complications such as aspiration [18, 19].

In the 1960s and 1970s, parenteral nutrition was regularly used for burn patients, but it has been almost entirely supplanted by enteral nutrition [20]. The superiority of enteral nutrition over parenteral nutrition is unanimously accepted, and a parenteral route should only be used in burn patients with contraindication to enteral feeding. Parenteral formulas are more expensive and carry greater risks including complications with gaining central venous access, line infections, and poorer glycemic control [21]. Studies have also found that parenteral nutrition is associated with overfeeding, liver and immune dysfunction, and a threefold increase in mortality [22, 23].

For enteral feedings, either a gastric tube or a post-pyloric tube may be used effectively. The advantages of gastric feeding are larger diameter tubes, which have less clogging, and the ability to give bolus feeds. Providers can place them easily at bedside. Smaller post-pyloric tubes are more prone to clogging and malposition, but these are often more comfortable, and post-pyloric feedings can be safely continued even during operative procedures to maintain caloric aims [24]. The stomach often develops dysmotility after burn, and some argue that patients do not tolerate gastric feedings well and are put at a higher risk for aspiration. However, a large meta-analysis found no difference in mortality or aspiration rates between gastric and small bowel feedings [25]. The small bowel feedings, however, did take longer to initiate and experienced more frequent interruptions. Either route can be successfully utilized in the burn population.

21.5 Estimating Energy Expenditure

Successful nutritional management relies on accurate estimate of energy expenditure which can be particularly challenging after burn due to the profound hypermetabolic response that these patients experience [26]. Underestimation can lead to malnutrition which is associated with pneumonia development and impaired wound healing [27]. Overestimating energy expenditure leads to overfeeding, which can cause numerous adverse effects including fatty infiltration of the liver and difficulty with glycemic control and ventilator weaning [28, 29].

Many formulas to estimate the energy expenditure and caloric needs of burn patients have been developed and employed [30]. One of the first, the Curreri formula was developed in the 1970s by retrospectively calculating the calories that would have been needed in nine patients to account for weight loss. This and other older formulas often overestimate current metabolic needs, and as such more sophisticated formulas have been proposed (Table 21.1) [28]. Highlighting the difficultly of predicating nutritional utilization, a study of 24 burn patients found that out of 46 different formulas to predict caloric needs, none correlated well with the measured energy expenditure [31]. Energy expenditure after burn fluctuates and static formulas often lead to underfeeding during times of high energy consumption and to overfeeding later in the course.

Indirect calorimetry is currently the gold standard for energy expenditure measurement, but it is difficult to perform

Table 21.1 Common formulas used to calculate caloric needs of burn patients

	kcal/day	Comments
Adult formulas		
Harris Benedict	Men: 66.5 + 13.8 (weight in kg) + 5 (height in cm) − 6.76 (age in years) Women: 655 + 9.6 (weight in kg) + 1.85 (height in cm) − 4.68 (age in years)	Estimates basal energy expenditure; can be adjusted by both activity and stress factor, multiply by 1.5 for common burn stress adjustment
Toronto Formula	−4343 + 10.5 (TBSA) + 0.23 (calorie intake in last 24 h) + 0.84 (Harris Benedict estimation without adjustment) + 114 (temperature) − 4.5 (number of postburn days)	Useful in acute stage of burn care; must be adjusted daily
Davies and Lilijedahl	20 (weight in kg) + 70 (TBSA)	Often overestimates caloric needs for large injuries
Ireton-Jones	Ventilated patient: 1784 − 11 (age in years) + 5 (weight in kg) + (244 if male) + (239 if trauma) + (804 if burn) Non-ventilated patient: 629 − 11 (age in years) + 25 (weight in kg) − (609 if obese)	Complex formula that integrates variables for ventilation and injury status
Curreri	Age 16–59: 25 (weight in kg) + 40 (TBSA) Age >60: 20 (weight in kg) + 65 (TBSA)	Commonly overestimates caloric needs
Pediatric formulas		
Galveston	0–1 years: 2100 (body surface area) + 1000 (body surface area × TBSA) 1–11 years: 1800 (body surface area) + 1300 (body surface area × TBSA) 12–18 years: 1500 (body surface area) + 1500 (body surface area × TBSA)	Goal focuses on maintaining body weight
Curreri junior	<1 year: recommended dietary allowance + 15 (TBSA) 1–3 years: recommended dietary allowance + 25 (TBSA) 4–15 years: recommended dietary allowance + 40 (TBSA)	Commonly overestimates caloric needs

and as such is not practical on a routine basis. Indirect calorimetry measurement calculates oxygen consumption and carbon dioxide production and therefore metabolic rate by measuring the volume of expired gas and the oxygen and carbon dioxide concentration of the inhaled and exhaled gas via a face mask or ventilator. Under or overfeeding can be detected by calculating the ratio of carbon dioxide produced to oxygen consumed, known as the respiratory quotient (RQ) [30]. RQ is dependent on metabolism of specific substrates. Fat is the major energy source during unstressed starvation which gives an RQ of approximately 0.7. Normal metabolism of mixed substrates gives an RQ between 0.75 and 0.90. Overfeeding is characterized by the creation of fat from carbohydrate and leads to an RQ greater than 1.0, which explains why overfeeding can cause difficultly in weaning a patient from the ventilator [32]. It is important to note that despite this concern, one study found that in a group of pediatric burn patients, a high-carbohydrate diet did not result in an RQ over 1.05 or any other respiratory complications but did have the positive effect of decreased muscle wasting [33].

21.6 Nutrient Metabolism

Carbohydrates, lipids, and proteins are the three macronutrients that provide energy and biological building blocks to fuel complex metabolic processes. They provide energy via different pathways, and the ratios of these nutrients must be considered for the burn patient after a caloric goal has been determined.

Carbohydrates are the preferred source of energy for burn patients, and high carbohydrate diets improve wound healing and have a protein sparing effect. In a randomized study of severely burned children, those who were fed a high carbohydrate diet had significantly less muscle protein degradation than those on a high-fat diet [34]. These positive effects are, however, limited by the ability to oxidize and utilize glucose. Glucose administration more than 9 mg/kg/min cannot be oxidized at the upper limit, and therefore, this strategy cannot be used above this range. Unfortunately, this maximum rate can be less than the estimated caloric expenditure, inferring some burned patients may have greater glucose needs than can be given safely. If glucose is given at a higher rate than this, it leads to hyperglycemia, glycosuria, dehydration, conversion of glucose to fat, and respiratory problems [35, 36].

Protein is also an important macronutrient after burn and must be carefully considered in the development of a nutritional support plan. Protein needs are greatly increased in these patients because of the catabolic response to burn, and protein supplementation is vital to meet the ongoing demands and supply substrate for wound healing and immune function and to mitigate the loss of leady body mass [37]. Giving supra-normal protein doses does not decrease catabolism of endogenous protein stores, but it does promote protein synthesis and improved nitrogen balance [38]. Predicted protein requirements are 1.5–2.0 g/kg/day for burned adults and

2.5–4.0 g/kg/day for burned children. Protein should always be provided in addition to considerable calories from carbohydrates and fat; otherwise, the protein will be used only as an energy source instead of as a specific nutrient to provide substrate for wound healing and maintenance of muscle mass. Optimal non-protein to nitrogen ratio is a function of burn size and should be around 150:1 for smaller burn up to 100:1 for larger burns [39]. Despite high rates of protein supplementation, burn patients will experience some loss of muscle protein because of the hormonal and proinflammatory reaction to severe burn.

Two specific amino acids have been studied and found to play unique roles after burn. Glutamine provides direct energy for lymphocytes and enterocytes and is crucial for preserving small bowel integrity and sustaining gut-associated immune function [40, 41]. It also portends some degree of cellular protection after stress via increased production of heat shock proteins, and it is a precursor of an important antioxidant, glutathione [42, 43]. Supplementation of 25 g/kg/day of glutamine has shown to reduce mortality and length of stay in burn patients [44, 45]. Arginine is another important amino acid with significant effects on the immune system. Arginine supplementation in burn patients led to improvement in wound healing and immune responsiveness; however, data from critically ill nonburn patients suggest that it is potentially harmful [46–49]. For this reason, arginine supplementation is not currently recommended in burn patients, but further investigations are underway.

Lipids are necessary to prevent essential fatty acid deficiency, but fat supplementation is only recommended in limited doses [50]. Lipolysis and lipid mobilization are increased after burn, while at the same time, utilization of lipids as an energy source is decreased [51, 52]; most free fatty acids are not used and lead to lipid accumulation in the liver. Increased fat intake has also been shown to worsen immune function, and because of these effects, burn patients should have no more than 15% of their calories from lipids. Many forego lipid emulsions completely for patients receiving parenteral nutrition for less than 10 days. The composition of administered fat must also be considered. Many of the commonly used enteral formulas contain omega-6 fatty acids which create proinflammatory cytokines during metabolism. Lipids with a high proportion of omega-3 fatty acids do not promote proinflammatory mediators and have been associated with improved immune response, less hyperglycemia, and improved outcomes [53, 54]. Omega-3 fatty acids are a component of "immune-enhancing diets" because of these effects. Most formulas have an omega 6:3 ratio ranging from 2.5:1 to 6:1, but the "immune-enhancing diets" have a ratio closer to 1:1. The optimal composition and volume of fat in the diet of burn patients is still controversial and deserves further investigation.

21.7 Micronutrients

Vitamins and trace elements supplementation is also crucial after burn, as these are important for immunity and wound healing. Reduced levels of vitamins A, C, and D, Fe, Cu, Se, and Zn have been found to impair wound healing and skeletal and immune functions [55–57]. Vitamin A improves epithelial growth and accelerates wound healing. Vitamin C supports in the formation and cross-linking of collagen [58]. Vitamin D is important in maintaining bone density, and the levels are often deficient after burn, leading to bone demineralization and even spontaneous fractures [59]. Other trace elements including Fe, Cu, Se, and Zn are vital for cellular and humoral immunity, but they are lost in significant amounts with exudative burn wound losses [55]. Zn is needed for protein synthesis, wound healing, lymphocyte function, and DNA replication [60]. Se promotes cell-mediated immunity, and Fe is a cofactor for oxygen-carrying proteins [61, 62]. Cu is vital for collagen creation and wound healing, and its deficiency has been associated with arrhythmias and immune dysfunction in burn patients [63]. These micronutrients are therefore important to supplement [64, 65]. Table 21.2 shows the recommended micronutrient supplementation for burned patients.

21.8 Enteral and Parenteral Formulas

A multitude of enteral formulas with varied amounts of substrates and micronutrients are commercially available. Table 21.3 includes a few of the commonly used formulas, but it is far from exhaustive. A formula with a high carbohydrate concentration should be used as glucose in the pre-

Table 21.2 Recommended micronutrient supplementation

Age, years	Vit A, IU	Vit D, IU	Vit E, IU	Vit C, IU	Vit K, μg	Folate, μg	Cu, mg	Fe, mg	Se, μg	Zn, mg
0–13										
Nonburned	1300–2000	600	6–16	15–50	2–60	65–300	0.2–0.7	0.3–8	15–40	2–8
Burned	2500–5000			250–500		1000	0.8–2.8		60–140	12.5–25
≥13										
Nonburned	200–3000	600	23	75–90	75–120	300–400	0.9	8–18	40–60	8–11
Burned	10,000			1000		1000	4		300–500	25–40

Table 21.3 Selected adult enteral nutrition formulas [79]

Formula	kcal/mL	Carbohydrate, g/L (% calories)	Protein, g/L (% calories)	Fat, g/L (% calories)	Comments
Impact	1.0	130 (53)	56 (22)	28 (25)	IED with arginine, glutamine fiber
Crucial	1.5	89 (36)	63 (25)	45 (39)	IED with arginine, hypertonic
Osmolite	1.06	144 (54)	44 (17)	35 (29)	Inexpensive, isotonic
Glucerna	1.0	96 (34)	42 (17)	54 (49)	Low carbohydrate, for diabetic patients
Nepro	1.8	167 (34)	81 (18)	96 (48)	Concentrated, for patients with renal failure

ferred energy source for burn patients [33, 66]. Parenteral formulas typically consist of 25% dextrose, 5% crystalline amino acids, and maintenance electrolytes. Essential fatty acids are supplemented with infusions of 250 mL of 20% lipid emulsions three times per week, although some clinicians forego this supplementation in courses of parenteral nutrition that are less than a week [67, 68].

Recently, much attention has been given to immune-enhancing diets or immunonutrition. These are formulas that have been fortified with micronutrients in hopes of improving immune function and wound healing. A study in burned children found that those receiving nutrition containing omega-3-fatty acid, arginine, histidine, and vitamins A and C had shorter length of stay, less wound infections, and trended toward better survival [69]. A small study of burned adults found no difference in major outcomes between immune-enhancing diet and a traditional formula [70]. Studies in nonburn patients have been contradictory with some even suggesting that immune-enhancing diets could be harmful [49, 71, 72]. Some suggest that immune-enhancing diets are not indicated in the burn population because they likely receive a satisfactory dose of the immune-enhancing nutrients due to the high volume of feeds they receive. A variety of formulas and multiple methods for calculating nutritional needs are successfully used for burn patients, suggesting that no formula or calculation is perfect, but most are satisfactory to support the patient and prevent nutritional complications.

21.9 Monitoring Nutritional Support

Monitoring the adequacy of nutritional support after severe burn can be difficult as there is no one variable or endpoint that fully communicates nutritional status. Serial weight measurement, nitrogen balance, the serum proteins prealbumin and albumin, and imaging of lean body mass are commonly used, and functional measures such as exercise tolerance can also be helpful in assessment.

Nitrogen inputs and losses can be used to study protein metabolism as nitrogen is an essential component of amino acids. Positive nitrogen balance represents growth and increases in the total body protein, while negative nitrogen balance occurs with fasting, trauma, and burns. Calculation of nitrogen balance requires urine collection for the determination of urea nitrogen (UUN) as well as a determination of dietary nitrogen intake. Nitrogen balance can be approximated with the following formula:

$$\text{Nitrogen balance} = \text{Nitrogen intake in 24 h} - \left[1.25 \times (\text{UUN} + 4)\right]$$

Nitrogen losses may be underestimated by this formula as the constants are simply approximations of the nitrogen losses in burn patient's urine and burn wound exudates [73, 74].

The serum proteins albumin and prealbumin are also commonly used to assess nutritional status, but these also have limitations. After severe burn, metabolic pathways as a ratio function are shifted away from creation of these proteins. Even with adequate nutrition, serum albumin levels are reduced making it an unreliable marker [75]. Prealbumin is often considered to be ore reactive to nutritional changes due to its short half-life of 2 days, but in actuality, prealbumin levels fall rapidly after burn injury and recover slowly and may not correspond well with current nutritional status [76]. Serum protein makers should be interpreted in context with the patient's clinical state and with global trend in mind.

Nutritional monitoring can also be aided with a few imaging techniques, but these are typically used only in research due to cost and availability. Bioimpedence analysis is a method that measures the body's resistance to electrical currents to calculate total body water and the body's fat-free cell mass. There is a concern that the significant fluid shifts that occur after burn might confound this measurement. Dual X-ray absorptiometry (DEXA) scanning is another imaging option which measures bone density and lean body mass [77], but is only a static measure that is best considered in series.

A survey of burn centers in 2007 revealed that the most commonly used parameters for nutritional monitoring were prealbumin (86% of centers), body weight (75%), calorie count (69%), serum albumin (45.8%), nitrogen balance (54%), and transferrin (16%) [78]. No single method is completely reliable or appropriate for the nutritional motoring of burn patients, and the overall clinical picture must be incorporated into the assessment.

Summary Box

Nutritional support is an essential element of burn care, and the principal goal is purely to avoid nutritional complications. Successful nutritional assessment and management can augment wound healing and decrease various complications as well as mortality. Enteral nutrition with formulas high in carbohydrate is beneficial, although nutritional support must be individualized and continually monitored and adjusted. Accurate nutritional endpoints and goals need to be established and corroborated before the optimum nutritional treatment can be determined.

References

1. Suri MP, Dhingra VJS, Raibagkar SC, Mehta DR. Nutrition in burns: need for an aggressive dynamic approach. Burns. 2006;32(7):880–4.
2. Goran MI, Broemeling L, Herndon DN, Peters EJ, Wolfe RR. Estimating energy requirements in burned children: a new approach derived from measurements of resting energy expenditure. Am J Clin Nutr. 1991;54(1):35–40.
3. Carpenter AM, Hollett LP, Jeng JC, Wu J, Turner DG, Jordan MH. How long a shadow does epidemic obesity cast in the burn unit? A dietitian's analysis of the strengths and weaknesses of the available data in the National Burn Repository. J Burn Care Res. 2008;29(1):97–101.
4. Gottschlich MM, Mayes T, Khoury JC, Warden GD. Significance of obesity on nutritional, immunologic, hormonal, and clinical outcome parameters in burns. J Am Diet Assoc. 1993;93(11):1261–8.
5. Patel L, Cowden JD, Dowd D, Hampl S, Felich N. Obesity: influence on length of hospital stay for the pediatric burn patient. J Burn Care Res. 2010;31(2):251–6.
6. Berger MM, Chiolero RL. Hypocaloric feeding: pros and cons. Curr Opin Crit Care. 2007;13(2):180–6.
7. McCowen KC, Friel C, Sternberg J, et al. Hypocaloric total parenteral nutrition: effectiveness in prevention of hyperglycemia and infectious complications--a randomized clinical trial. Crit Care Med. 2000;28(11):3606–11.
8. Dickerson RN, Boschert KJ, Kudsk KA, Brown RO. Hypocaloric enteral tube feeding in critically ill obese patients. Nutrition. 2002;18(3):241–6.
9. Cuthbertson DP, Angeles Valero Zanuy MA, Leon Sanz ML. Postshock metabolic response. 1942. Nutr Hosp. 2001;16(5):176–82, discussion 185–6
10. Cuthbertson DP. The metabolic response to injury and other related explorations in the field of protein metabolism: an autobiographical account. Scott Med J. 1982;27(2):158–71.
11. Porter C, Herndon DN, Borsheim E, et al. Long-term skeletal muscle mitochondrial dysfunction is associated with hypermetabolism in severely burned children. J Burn Care Res. 2016;37(1):53–63.
12. Hart DW, Wolf SE, Mlcak R, et al. Persistence of muscle catabolism after severe burn. Surgery. 2000;128(2):312–9.
13. Rousseau A-F, Losser M-R, Ichai C, Berger MM. ESPEN endorsed recommendations: nutritional therapy in major burns. Clin Nutr. 2013;32(4):497–502.
14. Deitch EA. Intestinal permeability is increased in burn patients shortly after injury. Surgery. 1990;107(4):411–6.
15. Magnotti LJ, Deitch EA. Burns, bacterial translocation, gut barrier function, and failure. J Burn Care Rehabil. 2005;26(5):383–91.
16. Lam NN, Tien NG, Khoa CM. Early enteral feeding for burned patients--an effective method which should be encouraged in developing countries. Burns. 2008;34(2):192–6.
17. Chiarelli A, Enzi G, Casadei A, Baggio B, Valerio A, Mazzoleni F. Very early nutrition supplementation in burned patients. Am J Clin Nutr. 1990;51(6):1035–9.
18. Gottschlich MM, Jenkins ME, Mayes T, Khoury J, Kagan RJ, Warden GD. The 2002 Clinical Research Award. An evaluation of the safety of early vs delayed enteral support and effects on clinical, nutritional, and endocrine outcomes after severe burns. J Burn Care Rehabil. 2002;23(6):401–15.
19. Wasiak J, Cleland H, Jeffery R. Early versus late enteral nutritional support in adults with burn injury: a systematic review. J Hum Nutr Diet. 2007;20(2):75–83.
20. Ireton-Jones CS, Baxter CR. Nutrition for adult burn patients: a review. Nutr Clin Pract. 1991;6(1):3–7.
21. Gramlich L, Kichian K, Pinilla J, Rodych NJ, Dhaliwal R, Heyland DK. Does enteral nutrition compared to parenteral nutrition result in better outcomes in critically ill adult patients? A systematic review of the literature. Nutrition. 2004;20(10):843–8.
22. Herndon DN, Barrow RE, Stein M, et al. Increased mortality with intravenous supplemental feeding in severely burned patients. J Burn Care Rehabil. 1989;10(4):309–13.
23. Herndon DN, Stein MD, Rutan TC, Abston S, Linares H. Failure of TPN supplementation to improve liver function, immunity, and mortality in thermally injured patients. J Trauma. 1987;27(2):195–204.
24. Jenkins ME, Gottschlich MM, Warden GD. Enteral feeding during operative procedures in thermal injuries. J Burn Care Rehabil. 1994;15(2):199–205.
25. Ho KM, Dobb GJ, Webb SA. A comparison of early gastric and post-pyloric feeding in critically ill patients: a meta-analysis. Intensive Care Med. 2006;32(5):639–49.
26. Yu YM, Tompkins RG, Ryan CM, Young VR. The metabolic basis of the increase of the increase in energy expenditure in severely burned patients. JPEN. J Parenter Enteral Nutr. 1999;23(3):160–8.
27. Martindale RG, McClave SA, Vanek VW, et al. Guidelines for the provision and assessment of nutrition support therapy in the adult critically ill patient: Society of Critical Care Medicine and American Society for Parenteral and Enteral Nutrition: executive summary. Crit Care Med. 2009;37(5):1757–61.
28. Saffle JR, Medina E, Raymond J, Westenskow D, Kravitz M, Warden GD. Use of indirect calorimetry in the nutritional management of burned patients. J Trauma. 1985;25(1):32–9.
29. Barret JP, Jeschke MG, Herndon DN. Fatty infiltration of the liver in severely burned pediatric patients: autopsy findings and clinical implications. J Trauma. 2001;51(4):736–9.
30. Ireton-Jones CS, Turner WW Jr, Liepa GU, Baxter CR. Equations for the estimation of energy expenditures in patients with burns with special reference to ventilatory status. J Burn Care Rehabil. 1992;13(3):330–3.
31. Dickerson RN, Gervasio JM, Riley ML, et al. Accuracy of predictive methods to estimate resting energy expenditure of thermally-injured patients. JPEN. J Parenter Enteral Nutr. 2002;26(1):17–29.
32. Graf S, Pichard C, Genton L, Oshima T, Heidegger CP. Energy expenditure in mechanically ventilated patients: the weight of body weight! Clin Nutr. 2017;36(1):224–8.
33. Hart DW, Wolf SE, Zhang XJ, et al. Efficacy of a high-carbohydrate diet in catabolic illness. Crit Care Med. 2001;29(7):1318–24.
34. Hart DW, Wolf SE, Herndon DN, et al. Energy expenditure and caloric balance after burn: increased feeding leads to fat rather than lean mass accretion. Ann Surg. 2002;235(1):152–61.
35. Rodriguez NA, Jeschke MG, Williams FN, Kamolz LP, Herndon DN. Nutrition in burns: Galveston contributions. JPEN. J Parenter Enteral Nutr. 2011;35(6):704–14.

36. Burke JF, Wolfe RR, Mullany CJ, Mathews DE, Bier DM. Glucose requirements following burn injury. Parameters of optimal glucose infusion and possible hepatic and respiratory abnormalities following excessive glucose intake. Ann Surg. 1979;190(3):274–85.
37. Wolfe RR. Metabolic response to burn injury: nutritional implications. Semin Nephrol. 1993;13(4):382–90.
38. Patterson BW, Nguyen T, Pierre E, Herndon DN, Wolfe RR. Urea and protein metabolism in burned children: effect of dietary protein intake. Metabolism. 1997;46(5):573–8.
39. Isbi Practice Guidelines C. ISBI practice guidelines for burn care. Burns. 2016;42(5):953–1021.
40. Souba WW. Glutamine: a key substrate for the splanchnic bed. Annu Rev Nutr. 1991;11:285–308.
41. Wischmeyer PE. Can glutamine turn off the motor that drives systemic inflammation? Crit Care Med. 2005;33(5):1175–8.
42. Peng X, Yan H, You Z, Wang P, Wang S. Clinical and protein metabolic efficacy of glutamine granules-supplemented enteral nutrition in severely burned patients. Burns. 2005;31(3):342–6.
43. Garrel D, Patenaude J, Nedelec B, et al. Decreased mortality and infectious morbidity in adult burn patients given enteral glutamine supplements: a prospective, controlled, randomized clinical trial. Crit Care Med. 2003;31(10):2444–9.
44. Gore DC, Jahoor F. Glutamine kinetics in burn patients. Comparison with hormonally induced stress in volunteers. Arch Surg. 1994;129(12):1318–23.
45. Windle EM. Glutamine supplementation in critical illness: evidence, recommendations, and implications for clinical practice in burn care. J Burn Care Res. 2006;27(6):764–72.
46. Yan H, Peng X, Huang Y, Zhao M, Li F, Wang P. Effects of early enteral arginine supplementation on resuscitation of severe burn patients. Burns. 2007;33(2):179–84.
47. Marin VB, Rodriguez-Osiac L, Schlessinger L, Villegas J, Lopez M, Castillo-Duran C. Controlled study of enteral arginine supplementation in burned children: impact on immunologic and metabolic status. Nutrition. 2006;22(7–8):705–12.
48. Wibbenmeyer LA, Mitchell MA, Newel IM, et al. Effect of a fish oil and arginine-fortified diet in thermally injured patients. J Burn Care Res. 2006;27(5):694–702.
49. Heyland DK, Samis A. Does immunonutrition in patients with sepsis do more harm than good? Intensive Care Med. 2003;29(5): 669–71.
50. Demling RH, Seigne P. Metabolic management of patients with severe burns. World J Surg. 2000;24(6):673–80.
51. Mochizuki H, Trocki O, Dominioni L, Ray MB, Alexander JW. Optimal lipid content for enteral diets following thermal injury. JPEN. J Parenter Enteral Nutr. 1984;8(6):638–46.
52. Garrel DR, Razi M, Lariviere F, et al. Improved clinical status and length of care with low-fat nutrition support in burn patients. JPEN. J Parenter Enteral Nutr. 1995;19(6):482–91.
53. Alexander JW, Gottschlich MM. Nutritional immunomodulation in burn patients. Crit Care Med. 1990;18(2 Suppl):S149–53.
54. Alexander JW, Saito H, Trocki O, Ogle CK. The importance of lipid type in the diet after burn injury. Ann Surg. 1986;204(1):1–8.
55. Berger MM, Shenkin A. Trace element requirements in critically ill burned patients. J Trace Elem Med Biol. 2007;21(Suppl 1):44–8.
56. Gottschlich MM, Mayes T, Khoury J, Warden GD. Hypovitaminosis D in acutely injured pediatric burn patients. J Am Diet Assoc. 2004;104(6):931–41, quiz 1031
57. Berger MM, Binnert C, Chiolero RL, et al. Trace element supplementation after major burns increases burned skin trace element concentrations and modulates local protein metabolism but not whole-body substrate metabolism. Am J Clin Nutr. 2007;85(5):1301–6.
58. Rock CL, Dechert RE, Khilnani R, Parker RS, Rodriguez JL. Carotenoids and antioxidant vitamins in patients after burn injury. J Burn Care Rehabil. 1997;18(3):269–78, discussion 268
59. Klein GL. Burns: where has all the calcium (and vitamin D) gone? Adv Nutr. 2011;2(6):457–62.
60. Selmanpakoglu AN, Cetin C, Sayal A, Isimer A. Trace element (Al, Se, Zn, Cu) levels in serum, urine and tissues of burn patients. Burns. 1994;20(2):99–103.
61. Hunt DR, Lane HW, Beesinger D, et al. Selenium depletion in burn patients. JPEN. J Parenter Enteral Nutr. 1984;8(6):695–9.
62. Berger MM. Antioxidant micronutrients in major trauma and burns: evidence and practice. Nutr Clin Pract. 2006;21(5):438–49.
63. Sampson B, Constantinescu MA, Chandarana I, Cussons PD. Severe hypocupraemia in a patient with extensive burn injuries. Ann Clin Biochem. 1996;33(Pt 5):462–4.
64. Meyer NA, Muller MJ, Herndon DN. Nutrient support of the healing wound. New Horiz. 1994;2(2):202–14.
65. Berger MM, Baines M, Raffoul W, et al. Trace element supplementation after major burns modulates antioxidant status and clinical course by way of increased tissue trace element concentrations. Am J Clin Nutr. 2007;85(5):1293–300.
66. Bouletreau P, Chassard D, Allaouchiche B, et al. Glucose-lipid ratio is a determinant of nitrogen balance during total parenteral nutrition in critically ill patients: a prospective, randomized, multicenter blind trial with an intention-to-treat analysis. Intensive Care Med. 2005;31(10):1394–400.
67. Chen Z, Wang S, Yu B, Li A. A comparison study between early enteral nutrition and parenteral nutrition in severe burn patients. Burns. 2007;33(6):708–12.
68. Berger M. Basics in clinical nutrition: nutritional support in burn patients. e-SPEN Eur e-J Clin Nutr Metab. 2009;4(6):e308–12.
69. Gottschlich MM, Jenkins M, Warden GD, et al. Differential effects of three enteral dietary regimens on selected outcome variables in burn patients. JPEN J Parenter Enteral Nutr. 1990;14(3):225–36.
70. Saffle JR, Wiebke G, Jennings K, Morris SE, Barton RG. Randomized trial of immune-enhancing enteral nutrition in burn patients. J Trauma. 1997;42(5):793–2.
71. Heys SD, Walker LG, Smith I, Eremin O. Enteral nutritional supplementation with key nutrients in patients with critical illness and cancer: a meta-analysis of randomized controlled clinical trials. Ann Surg. 1999;229(4):467–77.
72. Bower RH, Cerra FB, Bershadsky B, et al. Early enteral administration of a formula (Impact) supplemented with arginine, nucleotides, and fish oil in intensive care unit patients: results of a multicenter, prospective, randomized, clinical trial. Crit Care Med. 1995;23(3):436–49.
73. Konstantinides FN, Radmer WJ, Becker WK, et al. Inaccuracy of nitrogen balance determinations in thermal injury with calculated total urinary nitrogen. J Burn Care Rehabil. 1992;13(2 Pt 1):254–60.
74. Milner EA, Cioffi WG, Mason AD, McManus WF, Pruitt BA Jr. A longitudinal study of resting energy expenditure in thermally injured patients. J Trauma. 1994;37(2):167–70.
75. Rettmer RL, Williamson JC, Labbe RF, Heimbach DM. Laboratory monitoring of nutritional status in burn patients. Clin Chem. 1992;38(3):334–7.
76. Cynober L, Prugnaud O, Lioret N, Duchemin C, Saizy R, Giboudeau J. Serum transthyretin levels in patients with burn injury. Surgery. 1991;109(5):640–4.
77. Thomas SJ, Morimoto K, Herndon DN, et al. The effect of prolonged euglycemic hyperinsulinemia on lean body mass after severe burn. Surgery. 2002;132(2):341–7.
78. Graves C, Saffle J, Cochran A. Actual burn nutrition care practices: an update. J Burn Care Res. 2009;30(1):77–82.
79. Saffle JR, Graves C, Cochran A. Chapter 29 - Nutritional support of the burned patient A2. In: Herndon DN, editor. Total burn care. 4th ed. London: W.B. Saunders; 2012. p. 333–53.e335.

Anabolic and Anticatabolic Agents in Burns

22

Roohi Vinaik, Eduardo I. Gus, and Marc G. Jeschke

22.1 Introduction

Traumatic injuries such as burns result in a substantial release of inflammatory mediators, which leads to significant metabolic derangements and the introduction of a post-injury stress environment. This hypermetabolic response is characterized by accelerated lipolysis, glycolysis, insulin resistance, organ dysfunction, and proteolysis [1, 2]. If untreated in the acute phase, the net effect of these post-burn changes is physiological exhaustion and organ failure. Long-term alterations and entry into a hypermetabolic state result in immunodeficiency, compromised wound healing, loss of total and lean body mass, and growth retardation in pediatric patients [3].

Particularly, an important feature of the post-burn hypermetabolic response is generalized catabolism. Hypercatabolism can be attributed to a shift in the production of anabolic to catabolic factors. Increased levels of pro-inflammatory cytokines (e.g., tumor necrosis factor (TNF) and interleukin-6 (IL-6)) occur immediately after injury and are intimately associated with augmented catabolic hormones, principally cortisol and catecholamines [4]. Furthermore, hypermetabolism is associated with a suppression of the endocrine axis, which can result in a substantial decrease in serum levels of endogenous anabolic hormones. Indeed, burn patients exhibit diminished levels of hormones such as human growth hormone (hGH), IGF-I, and testosterone post-trauma [5].

Several non-pharmacologic interventions such as exercise, appropriate nutrition, and heating the environment have been employed to manage post-trauma hypermetabolism. While they improve hypermetabolic catabolism, pharmacologic interventions appear critical for clinical efficacy. Various pharmacological strategies have been used to prevent catabolism and promote anabolism in thermally injured patients. This chapter analyzes the anticatabolic and anabolic pharmacologic interventions currently utilized. It covers propranolol, growth hormone (GH), insulin growth factor 1 (IGF-1), insulin growth factor binding protein 3 (IGFBP-3), insulin, metformin, testosterone, oxandrolone, and thyroid hormones. Furthermore, novel therapeutics utilized in other conditions, such as cancer-related cachexia, are discussed. These agents may potentially be used to mitigate post-injury catabolism and bolster anabolic responses, ultimately improving morbidity and mortality in burn and critically ill patients.

22.2 Propranolol

Substantial catecholamine production occurs after burns, with sustained increases persisting for months after the inciting injury [1, 2]. Prolonged elevation in catecholamine levels is a major contributor to the post-burn hypermetabolic response. Elevated catecholamine levels result in a hyperdynamic circulation, increased resting energy expenditure (REE), lipolysis, and muscle catabolism, to list a few downstream effects [6]. Additionally, catecholamines contribute to the generalized catabolic response seen in burn patients via stimulation of both α and β receptors.

Propranolol, which is a non-selective β-blocker, attenuates this hyperactive sympathetic response. Ideally, it should

R. Vinaik · E. I. Gus
Faculty of Medicine, University of Toronto, Toronto, ON, Canada
e-mail: roohi.vinaik@sri.utoronto.ca

M. G. Jeschke (✉)
Faculty of Medicine, University of Toronto, Toronto, ON, Canada

Faculty of Medicine, Institute of Medical Science, University of Toronto, Toronto, ON, Canada

Biological Sciences, Sunnybrook Research Institute, Toronto, ON, Canada

Ross Tilley Burn Centre, Sunnybrook Health Sciences Centre, Sunnybrook Hospital, Toronto, ON, Canada

Division of Plastic and Reconstructive Surgery, Department of Surgery, Faculty of Medicine, University of Toronto, Toronto, ON, Canada

Department of Immunology, Faculty of Medicine, University of Toronto, Toronto, ON, Canada
e-mail: Marc.Jeschke@sunnybrook.ca

M. G. Jeschke et al. (eds.), *Handbook of Burns Volume 1*, https://doi.org/10.1007/978-3-030-18940-2_22

be administered post-resuscitation (3–10 days after burn) to mitigate the hypermetabolic response and aid in recovery [7]. In adults, starting doses are 10 mg TID until a 20% reduction in heart rate is achieved. In pediatric patients, propranolol is given at 1 mg/kg/day and escalated to ~4 mg/kg/day to achieve a 20% reduction in heart rate [8]. Recent studies demonstrated that propranolol use was associated with improved wound healing, decreased healing time and blood loss during skin grafting, and shorter hospital length of stay (LOS) [9]. Manzano-Nunez et al. conducted a systematic review and meta-analysis of propranolol therapy in severely burned (TBSA > 20%) adults and children. The included studies demonstrated decreased requirements for blood transfusions and decreased heart rate in propranolol-treated patients [10]. Administration of propranolol to severely burned patients reduces cardiac work by a 15–20% reduction in heart rate [11–13]. Similarly, use of other beta blockers that are comparable to propranolol, such as esmolol, demonstrates beneficial sympathetic effects in critically ill patients in septic shock with post-resuscitation tachycardia. In these patients, propranolol decreases cardiac workload, which reduces mortality by 40% [14].

In addition to its direct sympathetic effects, propranolol prevents peripheral lipolysis and proteolysis by mitigating catecholamine signaling and reducing resting energy expenditure [1, 2, 15, 16]. Hart and colleagues further elucidated the anticatabolic effect of propranolol during the early post-burn hypercatabolic stage. They compared treatment with propranolol to a combination of propranolol and recombinant human growth hormone (rhGH) in severely burned (TBSA > 40%) children, demonstrating that propranolol is a potent anticatabolic agent. Additionally, association with rhGH did not produce a synergistic positive effect [15]. Furthermore, Jeschke and colleagues compared the outcomes with rhGH with propranolol versus rhGH alone. They demonstrated that combination therapy mitigates hypermetabolism and inflammation and ameliorates the deleterious effects found with rhGH monotherapy [16]. In addition to its anticatabolic function, propranolol has anabolic effects as well. Herndon et al. previously demonstrated that propranolol therapy in severely burned (>40% TBSA) children increases net muscle–protein balance by 82% over baseline, with a significant upregulation in genes involved in muscle metabolism [11]. Also, propranolol does not compromise exercise-induced enhancements in muscle mass, strength, and peak aerobic capacity in children with >30% TBSA [17].

Moreover, prolonged administration of propranolol has multiple beneficial effects. Patients receiving propranolol for 1 year post-injury demonstrated significant reductions in bone loss, decreased predicted heart rate, and REE [18]. Prolonged therapy is safe and does not increase incidence of infections or sepsis, highlighting the benefit of long-term therapy with this anticatabolic agent [18–21].

However, Martinez et al. recently proposed in a small series of cases that use of propranolol with vasopressors in septic shock could predispose patients to intestinal ischemia. They postulated that endogenous catecholamine release during hypotensive and septic periods in concert with β-blockade could lead to unopposed α-adrenergic activity. This in turn would impair circulation via severe splanchnic vasoconstriction and lead to bowel ischemia [22]. Taken together, these results highlight the potential risks of propranolol. Other potential side effects include hypotension and bradycardia; however, both can easily be diagnosed and managed in a burn intensive care unit.

Despite these potential negative effects, there is ample evidence for the benefits of propranolol therapy. However, this evidence is primarily limited to pediatric patients, and there is insufficient published data demonstrating these effects in adults and elderly patient [23, 24]. Currently, there is no published randomized controlled data in adult burn patients indicating metabolic benefits of non-selective β-blocker therapy. Further studies are needed to establish propranolol therapy as an effective means to improve outcomes in adult burn patients [25–27]. Ongoing randomized control trials sponsored by the American Burn Association are currently investigating efficacy of propranolol on burn outcomes in these patients.

Summary: While there is limited evidence in adult and elderly burn patients, current studies suggest that propranolol could effectively decrease stress responses and be a useful anticatabolic agent in pediatric burn patients, as well as adult burn patients. The dose range is in children: 1–4 mg/kg/day and in adults 10–40 mg QID P.O.

22.3 Recombinant Human Growth Hormone

Human growth hormone (hGH) is an endogenous anabolic hormone produced by the pituitary gland in children and young adults. The pituitary gland produces approximately 0.5–0.8 mg of hGH daily, which associates with a variety of GH binding proteins and receptors in various tissues [28]. In GH-deficient children, recombinant human growth hormone (rhGH) therapy has been employed to increase body cell mass and stimulate bone formation [29]. Disruption in the GH/insulin-like growth factor-1 (IGF-1)/IGF binding protein-3 (IGFBP-3) hormone axis are known to occur after burn, potentially due to the inhibitory effects of proinflammatory cytokines, which are overexpressed post-burn [30]. In these cases, daily intramuscular injection of the anabolic agent rhGH is an attractive option to counteract the catabolic effects of burn injury.

Treatment outcomes with rhGH have been comprehensively studied in children and adult burn patients. As mentioned earlier, Hart and colleagues investigated the effects of up to 1 year post-injury treatment with 0.05 mg/kg/day rhGH in children with burns >40% TBSA. This study showed more pronounced weight and height gain, higher lean body weight, and bone mineral density with rhGH treatment compared to placebo [15]. An adult study by Kim et al. demonstrated that a 3-month rhGH treatment in patients with full thickness burns greater than 20% TBSA had a positive effect on fitness, muscle power, and other metabolic processes [31]. Similarly, Branski and colleagues demonstrated improved growth and lean body mass with rhGH treatment, while hypermetabolism was significantly diminished [32]. Additional studies by Jeschke et al. also demonstrated attenuated post-burn hypermetabolic and hyperinflammatory responses, notably when utilized as a combination with propranolol [16].

Long-term treatment with rhGH has multiple putative effects; for example, it can increase thyroid hormone-binding sites, which may be involved in the growth arrest seen in post-burn children [33]. Other studies have shown that rhGH ceases growth arrest in thermally injured children, decreases REE, and decreases cortisol levels and the acute phase proteins, TNF-α and IL-1. Also, rhGH is not a risk factor for hypertrophic scar formation; Branski and colleagues showed that rhGH treatment significantly improved scarring 1 year post-burn [32].

A Cochrane systematic review published in 2012 on the implementation of rhGH in thermally injured patients appraised 13 randomized controlled trials (totally 701 adult and pediatric patients). Primary outcomes included healing of the burn wound and donor sites and rates of wound infection, and secondary outcomes were mortality, hospital LOS, scar assessment, and adverse events such as hyperglycemia or septicemia. The review demonstrated that there is evidence that rhGH use in large burns (>40% TBSA) could induce more rapid wound healing in adults and children and reduced hospital LOS without an increase in mortality [34].

However, the 2012 Cochrane review showed that rhGH treatment is associated with increased hyperglycemia. While the conclusions of this review were based on studies with smaller sample sizes, which introduces the risk of bias, increased hyperglycemia is a potential concern. Additionally, the beneficial outcomes seen with rhGH treatment in burn patients, such as improvement in muscle protein kinetics, donor site healing, and REE, are not translatable in critically ill, non-burned patients. A prospective, multicenter, double-blind, randomized, placebo-controlled trial of 0.10 ± 0.02 mg/kg rhGH in 285 critically ill non-burned patients was associated with a 40% increase in morbidity and mortality, hyperglycemia, and insulin resistance [35]. So, while rhGH does seem to have a positive anabolic effect, the concern for hyperglycemia, decreased effectiveness in non-burned, critically ill patients, and lack of an oral formulation limit its use.

Summary: While it may have some beneficial effects, rhGH should be very carefully considered and is currently not a standard of care in burn or critically ill patients. RhGH should not be administered in the state of infection or sepsis.

22.4 Insulin Growth Factor 1 (IGF-1) and Insulin Growth Factor Binding Protein 3 (IGFBP-3)

The anabolic effects of hGH are mostly modulated by IGF-1, which is produced by the liver in response to GH. IGF-1 is a polypeptide with a sequence similarity to proinsulin. More than 95% of IGF-1 is bound to an IGFBP 1–6; its principle binding protein is IGFB-3 [36].

Critically ill burn patients characteristically have reduced circulating IGF-1, which could be attributed to alterations in IGF-1 clearance. Indeed, IGF-1 has a shorter half-life when administered to patients after a major surgery compared to healthy controls [37]. This is potentially due to lower levels of IGFBPs, especially reductions in IGFBP-3 levels. During traumatic injuries and in hypermetabolic states, IGF-1 improves the metabolic rate, gut mucosal function, and wound healing and attenuates protein loss by mediating GH [38].

For up to 3 years post-burn, pediatric patients have persistently lower serum IGF-1 and IGFBP-3 levels, which is associated with severe growth arrest [39]. Thus, anabolic agents such as IGF-1 are putatively beneficial in these patients. Wolf and colleagues investigated the effects of exogenous IGF-1 treatment on Th1/Th2 cytokine profiles in mononuclear cells. Compared to controls, they found depressed Th1 and exaggerated Th2 cytokine responses in all burn patients. Interestingly, exogenous IGF-1/IGFBP-3 treatment can partly reverse this response [40]. Likely, the IGF-1/IGFBP-3 complex balances pro- and anti-inflammatory cytokines, which results in improved organ function. This treatment can also attenuate the type I and type II hepatic acute phase response, improving serum levels of constitutive proteins that modify hypercatabolic responses [30, 41–43].

However, while both rhGH and IGF-1 could mediate post-burn hypermetabolism and generalized catabolism in burn patients, their use has been limited due to side effects, namely hyperglycemia with rhGH and hypoglycemia with IGF-I [44]. Additionally, IGF-1 as a monotherapy should be avoided as Langouche and Van den Berghe showed that IGF-1 alone lacks efficacy in critically ill, non-burned patients [45]. However, since the effects of GH are mediated by IGF-1 and IGFBP-3, IGF-1 combined with equimolar doses of IGFBP-3 is another potential treatment option. Combination therapy of IGF-1/IGFBP-3 at doses of 1–4 mg/kg/day in severely burned children was shown to improve protein fractional synthetic rate and net protein balance. Debroy et al. showed a similar effect in severely burned adult patients and concluded that dual therapy may be effective in reducing catabolism [46]. Importantly, improvement in protein synthesis with combination therapy occurs with fewer hyperglycemic incidences than patients given rhGH and with fewer hypoglycemic incidences than IGF-1 treatment alone [1, 2, 41, 42, 47]. However, the IGF-1/IGFBP-3 complex used in the study by Debroy et al. was associated with adverse events such as neuropathies, currently precluding their use in a clinical setting.

Summary: There is limited evidence in favor of IGF-1 monotherapy or IGF-1/IGFB-3 complex therapy.

22.5 Insulin

Insulin is an effective anabolic and anticatabolic hormone that is utilized as an antihyperglycemic in severely burned patients. Jeschke et al. conducted a large cohort study demonstrating that insulin should be given at doses that achieve a glucose target of 130 mg/ds in pediatric burn patients [48, 49]. In general, critical care literature recommends doses that maintain a blood glucose range of 90–140 mg/dL in burn patients [50]. In addition to its glucose regulating effects, insulin is an attractive agent due to its added ability to increase muscle protein synthesis, accelerate donor site healing, and mitigate lean body mass loss [12, 13]. While its capability of reducing protein degradation is unequivocal, there is still debate regarding the underlying mechanism and the dose required to produce these anticatabolic effects. Insulin likely mitigates protein breakdown at lower doses and stimulates protein synthesis at higher doses [51].

Van den Berghe et al. suggest that this suppression of proteolysis and activation of protein synthesis is at least partly facilitated by an increase in serum IGF-1 levels [52]. However, intensive insulin therapy (IIT) in critically ill non-burned patients results in further suppression of serum IGF-1, IGFBP-3, and other GH-binding protein levels, with a corresponding increase in circulating GH [53]. Presumably, insulin primarily exerts its anabolic effects by suppressing IGFBP-1, thereby increasing the bioavailability of IGF-1. Thus, the fact that IIT did not affect IGFBP-1 levels in critically ill patients could explain why the anabolic effects of insulin did not appear to have a major positive effect on outcomes [52]. Additionally, IIT does not counteract catabolism associated with critical illness; however, it can improve the overall outcomes in pediatric ICU patients [54, 55]. In a subpopulation of critically ill pediatric cardiac surgical patients, insulin administration to achieve normoglycemia similarly did not significantly impact skeletal muscle degradation [56]. Contrarily, high doses of insulin or insulin with amino acid supplementation can restore anabolism in cardiac surgical patients [57].

In critically ill burn patients, Jeschke et al. demonstrated that insulin increases the anabolic factor IGF-1 and IGFBP-3 and mitigates hypermetabolism [19–21, 58]. Gore et al. studied the effects of insulin on skeletal muscle in patients with burns greater than 40% TBSA, demonstrating that hyperinsulinemia increases leg blood flow and the rate of muscle protein synthesis [59, 60]. Additionally, similar work by Ferrando et al. showed that a submaximal insulin dose, which would minimize the risk of hypoglycemic episodes, could actually elicit muscle anabolic effects [61]. Fram et al. aimed to elucidate the mechanism by which IIT is beneficial in an acute pediatric burn unit setting. Their results suggested that IIT treatment decreases REE and improves mitochondrial oxidative capacity and insulin sensitivity in these patients [62].

Despite its utility as an anabolic agent, several studies that were conducted to establish a clear survival benefit with insulin presented conflicting mortality data in both pediatric and adult burn patients. However, there is a consensus that insulin treatment decreases infection rates, sepsis, and organ failure [48, 49, 63–65]. While it lacks a significant survival benefit, insulin improves secondary outcomes such as serum glucose levels and seems to be beneficial as an anabolic agent in burn patients. It is more cost effective than GH or IGF-1 and has a well-established side effect profile, which is only limited to hypoglycemia. However, the risk of hypoglycemia needs to be carefully considered prior to initiating insulin therapy in susceptible patients.

Summary: Insulin is a safe and cheap anabolic agent with a clear side effect profile. While insulin-induced hypoglycemia is associated with adverse outcomes, insulin currently appears to be an effective agent in regulating muscle catabolism. Insulin can be given to target glucose levels or as a therapy approach to reduce hypermetabolism but glucose levels need to be carefully monitored and/or considered to be given simultaneously.

22.6 Metformin

Metformin is a biguanide that has recently emerged as the primary alternative to insulin for hyperglycemia management in severely injured patients [66]. Metformin is administered daily *per os* with a maximum daily dose of 35 mg/kg (2.5 g/day) body weight [67]. Standard formulations require multiple dosing, while metformin XR (extended release) is administered once daily, resulting in better medication regimen adherence [68].

Although the underlying mechanisms are complex and still debated, the downstream effects of metformin are known. It has a dual role in enhancing peripheral insulin sensitivity and regulating gluconeogenesis. Metformin suppresses hepatic glucagon production and thus hyperglycemia by mitigating the synthesis of cyclic AMP [69]. Cyclic AMP is elevated after thermal injury and is one of the potential mechanisms in the development of post-burn hyperglycemia and insulin resistance. As a result, metformin counters the underlying processes and is an attractive option in managing burn-induced hyperglycemia.

Similar to insulin, metformin may be applicable as both an antihyperglycemic and a muscle protein anabolic agent in critically injured patients. However, the mechanism by which metformin mediates muscle protein balance is still unclear. According to Gore and colleagues, there is a relationship between elevated glucose levels and net muscle protein catabolism. Gore et al. conducted a double-blind, randomized study focusing on peripheral metabolic effects of insulin versus metformin after a severe burn injury. The results showed an increased fractional synthetic rate of muscle protein and improvement in net muscle protein balance in metformin-treated patients [70, 71]. Metformin, therefore, functions as a muscle protein anabolic agent in critically ill patients, likely due to its ability to improve insulin receptor sensitivity and attenuate hyperglycemia. Given that metformin augments insulin sensitivity, it is plausible that metformin and insulin may synergistically function in regulating glucose levels and ameliorating skeletal muscle catabolism.

However, a possible metformin side effect is lactic acidosis or potential worsening of renal failure in susceptible patients [72]. As a result, metformin should not be given in patients with impaired lactate elimination, including those with renal and hepatic failure [73]. In severely burned patients a recent safety and efficacy clinical trial demonstrated no worsening of renal or hepatic function and no incidences of lactic acidosis in burn patients treated with metformin. Additionally, a review of clinical trials on type II diabetic patients also did not have any cases, highlighting the low incidence of lactic acidosis [74]. While no patients had lactic acidosis in the previously mentioned studies, this condition can be effectively managed in the burn ICU setting, making careful administration of metformin a safe alternative to insulin.

Compared to insulin, metformin demonstrates non-inferiority in terms of glycemic regulation and anabolic effects and superiority in terms of its antilipolytic effects [75]. Beyond clinical efficacy, there are other benefits such as cost-effectiveness and ease of administration. Metformin is given *per os*, and glucose levels need to be checked less frequently versus insulin once glucose and medication levels are stabilized. Given the clinical benefits and minimal side effects, metformin is an attractive treatment option and an integral component of post-burn care.

Summary: Metformin effects and its application as an anabolic agent are yet to be comprehensively studied. A recent safety however indicated the efficacy and safety of metformin in burn patients. Dosing should be 500–1000 mg BIP or even TID if no hepatic or renal concern.

22.7 Testosterone

Under the conditions of severe stress, the hypothalamic–pituitary–gonadal axis functions by reducing the signal for the production of testosterone. Burn patients have significant reductions in total and free testosterone levels such that severely burned men have comparable levels of serum testosterone to women [5]. This deficit persists after discharge.

Ideally, restoration of testosterone levels by exogenous therapy should facilitate skeletal muscle anabolism. Ferrando et al. investigated the effects of testosterone treatment at a dose of 200 mg/week IM for 2 weeks in severely burned (>70% TBSA) male patients. They demonstrated that normalizing testosterone levels results in a twofold reduction in muscle protein catabolism with normal feedings [76]. As the protein synthetic rate is maintained, the primary mechanism of action seems to be due to the reduction in skeletal muscle breakdown. Interestingly, while short-term testosterone treatment has similar anabolic outcomes in adult and pediatric burn patients, there is a marked difference in the mechanism of action. As mentioned above, testosterone therapy regulates catabolism in adult burn patients. Alternatively, pediatric patients demonstrate greater muscle protein synthesis rather than decreased catabolism [77, 78].

An important consideration that limits the use of testosterone in burn patients is its side effect profile. Side effects of testosterone therapy include increased risk of cardiovascular events, such as myocardial infarction, coronary artery disease and deep vein thrombosis, hepatotoxicity, erythrocytosis, and prostatic and dermatologic disorders [79]. Additionally, the use of this agent may be limited in women due to its androgenic effects. Owing to its broad side effect profile and the lack of oral methods of administration, alternative agents are preferred to testosterone. This includes its synthetic derivative, oxandrolone, which has a more favorable pharmacological profile.

Summary: While testosterone may have some beneficial anabolic effects in burn patients, its use is limited due to the risk of adverse events and limited applicability to male patients.

22.8 Oxandrolone

Oxandrolone, which is a synthetic derivative of testosterone, has been successfully implemented in pediatric patients with constitutional delays in growth, cachexia associated with alcoholic hepatitis, and HIV-related catabolic syndrome [80]. Studies in non-burn patients demonstrated enhanced weight and muscle mass gain, which is optimally augmented with administration of appropriate nutrition.

Previous work in adult burn patients studied the effects of 20 mg/day oxandrolone *per os* a minimum of 2 days post-burn [81]. As outlined in the previous section on testosterone, the mechanism of action differs between pediatric and adult patients. Oxandrolone has primarily an anticatabolic effect in adults and anabolic effect in children [82]. Barrow et al. analyzed the gene expression patterns in skeletal muscle obtained from pediatric burn patients treated with oxandrolone. Interestingly, the authors showed altered expression of 21 genes and increased muscle protein net balance, which was corroborated by muscle biopsies [83]. Similar findings have been seen in other studies as well [84].

Tuvdendorj et al. showed reduced acute phase and increased constitutive protein levels during the acute phase in pediatric patients with burns greater than 20% TBSA [85]. Jeschke et al. conducted a large, prospective, double-blind, randomized single-center study on burn patients to assess the effects of oxandrolone during the acute phase post-burn. The authors demonstrated that oxandrolone shortened hospital LOS, maintained lean body mass, and augmented hepatic protein synthesis [19–21]. Wolf et al. demonstrated similar findings in a multicenter, prospective, randomized, double-blind trial enrolling 81 adults with burns 20–60% TBSA. In this trial and other similar studies, oxandrolone therapy also shortened the hospital LOS [86, 87]. Wolf et al. also showed that oxandrolone effectively restored lean body mass in the acute and rehabilitation phase post-burn. Importantly, oxandrolone therapy may potentially be associated with improved survival, theoretically due to its prolonged beneficial effects in the acute and rehabilitation phase [88]. In the latter, 1 year oxandrolone treatment exhibited long-term improvements in lean body mass, bone mineral content, and bone mineral density, significant increases in height and weight, and a decrease in REE. There is further evidence that oxandrolone may also have long-term effects that can persist for up to 5 years post-burn [89].

To provide a consensus, recent meta-analyses have evaluated the use of oxandrolone in thermally injured patients. Real et al. demonstrated decreased lean body mass loss, less negative nitrogen balance, and shorter hospital LOS. However, this meta-analysis excluded pediatric patients and included few studies. Most recently, Li et al. conducted a meta-analysis that included 15 randomized controlled trials. While the authors showed that oxandrolone treatment does not affect mortality or the risk of infection, it does shorten hospital LOS, donor-site healing time, and time between surgical procedures. Additionally, oxandrolone mitigates weight and nitrogen loss, resulting in an accrual of lean body mass 6–12 months post-burn [90].

While it is equally as effective in decreasing weight loss and has similar benefits to other anticatabolic agents such as rhGH, oxandrolone has an improved side effect profile. Demling demonstrated this in a randomized, prospective study comparing rhGH and oxandrolone after severe thermal injury. The authors showed that rhGH results in significant hyperglycemia and accentuated hypermetabolism compared to oxandrolone. Additionally, oxandrolone, which is available as an oral formulation, has a similar but more favorable pharmacologic profile to testosterone; it has ten times greater anabolic effects and only 10% of the androgenic effects [91]. However, reversible sexual changes have been noted during oxandrolone therapy in pediatric patients. The most common side effect reported is hepatotoxicity. Previous studies compared liver dysfunction, assessed by liver transaminase levels, in thermally injured pediatric and adult patients [19–21, 92]. However, McCullough et al. demonstrated no significant differences in liver dysfunction between treatment and control groups in adult burn patients, and Miller and Btaiche similarly showed only a mild increase in transaminase levels in pediatric patients [91]. While oxandrolone therapy in severely burned patients during the acute phase and long-term is beneficial, liver function monitoring during treatment is recommended.

Summary: Oxandrolone is an effective alternative to testosterone therapy. The improved side effect profile and availability of an oral formulation make it an attractive option. Currently recommended as an anabolic agent. Dosing 10 mg BID in pediatrics or adults and 5 mg BID in elderly.

22.9 Thyroid Hormones

Thyroid hormones have overarching effects on growth and energy expenditure. The hypothalamic–pituitary–thyroid axis consists of hypothalamic thyrotropin-releasing hormone (TRH), thyroid-stimulating hormone (TSH) at the pituitary level, and peripheral thyroxine (T4), tri-iodothyronine (T3), and reverse T3. Alterations in the hypothalamic–pituitary–thyroid axis during illness results in a condition known as euthyroid sick syndrome whereby serum levels of thyroid hormones are low in patients without thyroid disease [93]. This is distinct from patients who simply present with hypothyroidism.

In critical care settings, thyroid hormone levels are inversely correlated with biochemical markers of catabolism such as urea production and markers of bone degradation. Moreover, administration of thyroid hormones was shown to reduce markers of catabolism. This challenges the notion that low thyroid hormone levels are an adaptive, protective response to hypercatabolism in prolonged critical illness [94]. Currently, clinical benefits of the active hormone T3 or the prohormone T4 during critical illness remains controversial. In critically ill patients admitted to an ICU for at least 14 days, TRH therapy with GH release peptide has been used [95]. This study utilized a 1 µg/kg GHRP-2 plus 1 µg/kg TRH bolus followed by a continuous infusion of 1 µg/kg/h GHRP-2 plus 1 µg/kg/h TRH. Potentially, this may stimulate and maintain pulsatility, responsiveness, and feedback inhibition of GH and TSH secretion, inducing a shift toward anabolic metabolism.

However, there is limited data on the utility of thyroid hormone replacement in burn patients. In fact, giving T3 has little to no effect on recovery rate or rates of deaths from pneumonia and sepsis in these patients. Additionally, thyroid hormone replacement does not mitigate hypermetabolism or the elevated catecholamine levels seen after burn injury. This suggests that in burn patients, hypermetabolic responses are primarily under sympathetic regulation rather than thyroidal adaptive mechanisms. Additionally, there is a concern that administering T3 can increase the incidence of arrhythmias because of the known association between hyperthyroidism and tachyarrhythmias [96].

Summary: At this time, there is insufficient data to demonstrate efficacy with exogenous thyroid hormone therapy in euthyroid critically ill patients. Thyroid hormones can be considered when low thyroid levels are present.

22.10 Novel Treatment Strategies

Currently, there are alternative novel anticatabolic agents available. However, it is important to note that their indication as anabolic agents have been tested in very specific patient populations; for example, patients with cancer cachexia and other muscle wasting disorders. Importantly, none of these medications have been tested for thermally injured or critically ill patients. Therefore, they require further investigation prior to implementation as anticatabolic agents in these patients.

Enobosarm is a nonsteroidal selective androgen receptor modulator that was first developed in 1998. It functions directly by activating muscle androgen receptors and indirectly through non-muscle androgen receptor pathways, which are mediated by muscle fibroblasts [97]. Preliminary studies suggest that treatment with enobosarm at a dose of 3 mg/day induces significant improvements in lean body mass [98]. When tested in healthy elderly men and menopausal women, enobosarm showed a substantial enhancement in physical function [99]. Potentially, it can be utilized in muscle wasting and cachexia secondary to cancer, COPD, heart failure, AIDS, and end-stage liver and renal diseases [100–102]. Clinical trials suggest that the drug is well tolerated, with no difference in the incidence of adverse events between placebo and treatment groups. Adverse events are mild and most commonly include back pain, fatigue, nausea, diarrhea, and flu-like illness.

Ghrelin, which is a peptide hormone primarily produced by the gastrointestinal mucosa, induces release of GH from the pituitary gland. Production of ghrelin stimulates energy intake and inhibits expenditure, which creates a positive net energy balance and results in weight gain. A potent, selective ghrelin receptor agonist, *anamorelin*, is an alternative option to exogenous ghrelin. It has a longer half-life than ghrelin and comes in oral formulations as well, with doses typically ranging from 50 to 100 mg daily [103]. Anamorelin was previously tested in cancer-related cachexia, and it showed a positive clinical response profile. Specifically, these patients had sustained increases in lean body mass and appendicular lean body mass (a surrogate of muscle mass), improved measures of muscle strength, and a better quality of life. However, common adverse effects associated with anamorelin include hyperglycemia, nausea, and dizziness. While the previously mentioned trials are promising, further investigation into efficacy and safety are still needed [97, 104–108].

Another important target in the management of skeletal muscle cachexia is the β-adrenergic signaling pathway, which has a crucial role in regulating protein synthesis and degradation. A newer generation β-agonist, *formoterol*, elicits an anabolic response even when given at very low doses of 80 µg daily. Additionally, medications such as formoterol have reduced collateral effects on the cardiovascular system compared with older generation β-agonists (e.g., fenoterol and clenbuterol). However, these agents may still possess some adverse cardiovascular side effects common to β-agonists, highlighting the importance of further research and refinement [109, 110].

22.11 Conclusion

Critically ill and thermally injured patients exhibit common aspects during the course of their illness, which are primarily components of hypermetabolism. These clinical features include hyperglycemia and insulin resistance, hyperinflammation, catecholamine surges, and generalized catabolism. Importantly, these injury-related consequences can occur years after the acute phase, necessitating the implementation of pharmacological interventions. Currently, many pharmacological agents have been studied to improve morbidity and mortality in these patients. This chapter focuses on anticatabolic and anabolic medications, which function through a variety of mechanisms to shift the balance from muscle breakdown to muscle synthesis.

Of the drugs reviewed, insulin is the primary one that is widely utilized in burn patients. There is a plethora of studies demonstrating its safety and efficacy both as an antihyperglycemic and as an anabolic agent. Metformin is an alternative antihyperglycemic to insulin that has the potential as an anabolic agent. However, the mechanism by which metformin mediates muscle protein balance is still unclear. Additionally, trials investigating adverse outcomes in burn patients are limited in size, warranting additional studies prior to broad implementation.

Propranolol is another promising anabolic agent with additional anticatabolic features. Namely, it prevents peripheral lipolysis and proteolysis by mitigating catecholamine signaling. Importantly, dual therapy with propranolol and rhGH diminishes hypermetabolism and inflammation and ameliorates the deleterious effects found with rhGH monotherapy. There is currently ample evidence for the benefits of propranolol therapy in pediatric patients. However, there is insufficient published data demonstrating similar effects in adult and elderly burn patients.

Outcomes of rhGH treatment have been comprehensively studied in children and adult burn patients, with higher lean body weight and bone mineral density compared to placebo. Additionally, rhGH treatment attenuates the post-burn hypermetabolic and hyperinflammatory responses, particularly when combined with propranolol. However, rhGH is associated with hyperglycemia, and the beneficial outcomes seen in burn patients are not translatable in critically ill, non-burned patients. Combination therapy of IGF-1/IGFBP-3 in severely burned children similarly improves net protein balance, with an analogous effect in severely burned adult patients. However, the IGF-1/IGFBP-3 complex is associated with adverse events such as neuropathies, currently precluding their clinical use.

Testosterone also demonstrates some beneficial anabolic effects in burn patients, but its use is limited due to the risk of adverse events and limited applicability to male patients. Oxandrolone is an attractive alternative to testosterone therapy with an improved side effect profile. Treatment is beneficial during acute phase and rehabilitative phase, and long-term treatment can increase lean body mass 6–12 months post-burn. However, while oxandrolone shows great promise, it is currently not a gold standard therapy.

While many of the drugs discussed in this chapter are encouraging, they require additional investigation. Thyroid hormones and the other novel therapeutics have some favorable results, but many of the recent studies using these drugs are in non-burned patients. As a result, they cannot be implemented in burn and critically ill patients at this time. Future studies are necessary to expand the repertoire of anticatabolic and anabolic agents in use in burn management.

Conflicts of Interest and Source of Funding This study was supported by National Institutes of Health R01-GM087285-01, CFI Leader's Opportunity Fund: Project #25407, and Canadian Institutes of Health Research (CIHR) grant #123336. The authors have no conflicts of interest to declare.

Summary Box

The anabolic and anticatabolic agents have entered the clinical arena to treat hypermetabolic and catabolic responses after burn. Frustratingly, there is a very little evidence on what to do and what to use. Human growth hormone and IGF-1 have somewhat failed to substantiate initial findings. Insulin and metformin seemed to be novel avenues that have endocrine as well as paracrine effects that could improve systemic metabolic responses. Testosterone and oxandrolone are quite impactful, and at this time, oxandrolone should be preferred over testosterone, due to testosterone side effects. We believe that novel avenues, including thyroid hormones or other anabolic agents, may be introduced to effectively treat hypermetabolic and hyperinflammatory, as well as hypercatabolic, responses. Some of those agents may be even very much upstream, for example, centrally acting.

References

1. Williams FN, Herndon DN, Jeschke MG. The hypermetabolic response to burn injury and interventions to modify this response. Clin Plast Surg. 2009;36(4):583–96.
2. Williams FN, Jeschke MG, Chinkes DL, et al. Modulation of the hypermetabolic response to trauma: temperature, nutrition, and drugs. J Am Coll Surg. 2009;208:489–502.
3. Ipaktchi K, Arbabi S. Advances in burn care. Crit Care Med. 2006;34(9S):S239–44.
4. Rojas Y, Finnerty CC, Radhakrishnana RS, Herndon DN. Burns: and update on current pharmacotherapy. Expert Opin Pharmacother. 2012;13(17):2485–94.
5. Ferrando AA, Sheffield-Moore M, Wolf SE, et al. Testosterone administration in severe burn patients ameliorates muscle catabolism. Crit Care Med. 2001;29:1936–42.
6. Pereira C, Murphy K, Jeschke MG, Herndon DN. Post burn muscle wasting and the effects of treatment. Int J Biochem Cell Biol. 2005;37(10):1948–61.
7. Breitenstein E, Chioléro RL, Jéquier E, et al. Effects of beta-blockade on energy metabolism following burns. Burns. 1990;16:259–64.
8. Finnerty CC, Herndon DN. Is propranolol of benefit in pediatric burn patients? Adv Surg. 2013;47:177–97.
9. Mohammadi AA, Bakhshaeekia A, Alibeigi P, et al. Efficacy of propranolol in wound healing for hospitalized burn patients. J Burn Care Res. 2009;30(6):1013–7.
10. Manzano-Nunez R, García-Perdomo HA, Ferrada P, et al. Safety and effectiveness of propranolol in severely burned patients: systematic review and meta-analysis. World J Emerg Surg. 2017;12:11.
11. Herndon DN, Hart DW, Wolf SE, et al. Reversal of catabolism by beta-blockade after severe burns. N Engl J Med. 2001;345:1223–9.
12. Williams FN, Herndon DN, Kulp GA, Jeschke MG. Propranolol decreases cardiac work in a dose-dependent manner in severely burned children. Surgery. 2011;149:231–9.

13. Williams FN, Branski LK, Jeschke MG. What, how and how much should burn patients be fed. Surg Clin North Am. 2011;91(3):609–29.
14. Wischmeyer PE, San-Millan I. Winning of the war against ICU-acquired weakness: new innovations in nutrition and exercise physiology. Crit Care. 2015;19:S6.
15. Hart DW, Wolf SE, Chinkes DL, et al. β-Blockade and growth hormone after burn. Ann Surg. 2002;236(4):450–7.
16. Jeschke MG, Finnerty CC, Kulp GA, et al. Combination of recombinant human growth hormone and propranolol decreases hypermetabolism and inflammation in severely burned children. Pediatr Crit Care Med. 2008;9(2):209–16.
17. Peña R, Ramirez LL, Crandall CG, et al. Effects of community-based exercise in children with severe burns: a randomized trial. Burns. 2016;42(1):41–7.
18. Herndon DN, Rodriguez NA, Diaz EC, et al. Long-term propranolol use in severely burned pediatric patients: a randomized controlled study. Ann Surg. 2012;256(3):402–11.
19. Jeschke MG, Boehning DF, Finnerty CC, Herndon DN. Effect of insulin on the inflammatory and acute phase response after burn injury. Crit Care Med. 2007;35(9S):S519–23.
20. Jeschke MG, Norbury WB, Finnerty CC, et al. Propranolol does not increase inflammation, sepsis, or infectious episodes in severely burned children. J Trauma. 2007;62:676–81.
21. Jeschke M, Finnerty CC, Suman OE, et al. The effect of oxandrolone on the endocrinologic, inflammatory, and hypermetabolic responses during the acute phase postburn. Ann Surg. 2007;246:351–62.
22. Martinez R, Rogers A, Numanoglu A, Rode H. Fatal non-occlusive mesenteric ischemia and the use of propranolol in pediatric burns. Burns. 2016;42:e70–3.
23. Arbabi S, Ahrns KS, Wahl WL, et al. Beta-blocker use is associated with improved outcomes in adult burn patients. J Trauma. 2004;56(2):265–9.
24. Flores O, Stockton K, Robers JA, et al. The efficacy and safety of adrenergic blockade after burn injury: a systematic review and meta-analysis. J Trauma Acute Care Surg. 2016;80(1):146–55.
25. Brown DA, Gibbons J, Honari S, et al. Propranolol dosing practices in adult burn patients: implications for safety and efficacy. J Burn Care Res. 2016;37:e218–26.
26. LeCompte MT, Rae L, Kahn SA. A survey of the use of propranolol in burn centers: who, what, when, why. Burns. 2017;34:121–6.
27. Nuñez-Villaveirán T, Sánches M, Millán P, García-de-Lorenzo A. Systematic review of the effect of propranolol on hypermetabolism in burn injuries. Med Intensiva. 2015;39(2):101–13.
28. Demling RH. The role of anabolic hormones for wound healing in catabolic states. J Burns Wounds. 2007;4:46–62.
29. Klein GL. Burn-induced bone loss: importance, mechanisms, and management. J Burns Wounds. 2006;1:32–8.
30. Jeschke MG, Barrow RE, Suzuki F, et al. IGF-1/IGFBP-3 equilibrates ratios of pro- to anti-inflammatory cytokines, which are predictors for organ function in severely burned pediatric patients. Mol Med. 2002;8(5):238–46.
31. Kim JB, Cho YS, Jang KU, et al. Effects of sustained release growth hormone treatment during the rehabilitation of adult severe burn survivors. Growth Horm IGF Res. 2016;27:1–6.
32. Branski LK, Herndon DN, Barrow RE, et al. Randomized controlled trial to determine the efficacy of long-term growth hormone treatment in severely burned children. Ann Surg. 2009;250:514–23.
33. Connolly CM, Barrow RE, Chinkes DL, et al. Recombinant human growth hormone increases thyroid hormone-binding sites in recovering severely burned children. Shock. 2003;19(5):399–402.
34. Breederveld RS, Tuinebreijer WE. Recombinant human growth hormone for treating burns and donor sites (Cochrane Systematic Review). Cochrane Database Syst Rev. 2014;(9):CD008990.
35. Takala J, Ruokonen E, Webster NR, et al. Increased mortality associated with growth hormone treatment in critically ill adults. N Engl J Med. 1999;341(11):785–92.
36. Lang CH, Frost RA. Role of growth hormone, insulin-like growth factor-I, and insulin-like growth factor binding proteins in the catabolic response to injury and infection. Curr Opin Clin Nutr Metab Care. 2002;5:271–9.
37. Carroll PV. Treatment with growth hormone and insulin-like growth factor-I in critical illness. Best Pract Res Clin Endocrinol Metab. 2001;15(4):435–51.
38. Froesch ER, Schmid C, Schwander J, Zapf J. Actions of insulin-like growth factors. Annu Rev Physiol. 1985;47:443–67.
39. Gauglitz GG, Herndon DN, Kulp GA, et al. Abnormal insulin sensitivity persists up to three years in pediatric patients post-burn. J Clin Endocrinol Metab. 2009;94:1656–64.
40. Wolf SE, Woodside KJ, Ramirez RJ, et al. Insulin-like growth factor-1/insulin-like growth factor binding protein-3 alters lymphocyte responsiveness following severe burn. J Surg Res. 2004;117:255–61.
41. Jeschke MG, Barrow RE, Herndon DN. Recombinant human growth hormone treatment in pediatric burn patients and its role during the hepatic acute phase response. Crit Care Med. 2000;28:1578–84.
42. Jeschke MG, Barrow RE, Herndon DN. Insulin-like growth factor I plus insulin-like growth factor binding protein 3 attenuates the proinflammatory acute phase response in severely burned children. Ann Surg. 2000;231(2):246–52.
43. Spies M, Wolf SE, Barrow RE, et al. Modulation of types I and II acute phase reactants with insulin-like growth factor-1/binding protein-3 complex in severely burned children. Crit Care Med. 2002;30:83–8.
44. Hasselbren PO. Burns and metabolism. J Am Coll Surg. 1999;188(2):98–103.
45. Van den Berghe G. On the neuroendocrinopathy of critical illness. Am J Respir Crit Care Med. 2016;194(11):1337–48.
46. Debroy MA, Wolf SE, Zhang XJ, et al. Anabolic effects of insulin-like growth factor in combination with insulin-like growth factor binding protein-3 in severely burned adults. J Trauma. 1999;47(5):904.
47. Heszele MF, Price SR. Insulin-like growth factor 1: the yin and yang of muscle atrophy. Endocrinology. 2004;145:4803–5.
48. Jeschke MG, Kraft R, Emdad F, et al. Glucose control in severely thermally injured pediatric patients: what glucose range should be the target? Ann Surg. 2010;252(3):521–7.
49. Jeschke MG, Kulp GA, Kraft R, et al. Intensive insulin therapy in severely burned pediatric patients – a prospective randomized trial. Am J Respir Crit Care Med. 2010;182:352–9.
50. Jeschke MG. Clinical review: glucose control in severely burned patients – current best practice. Crit Care. 2013;17(4):232.
51. Diaz EC, Herndon DN, Porter C, et al. Effects of pharmacological interventions on muscle protein synthesis and breakdown in recovery from burns. Burns. 2015;41(4):649–57.
52. Van den Berghe G. How does blood glucose control with insulin save lives in intensive care? J Clin Invest. 2004;114(9):1187–25.
53. Mesotten D, Wouters PJ, Peeters RP, et al. Regulation of the somatotropic axis by intensive insulin therapy during protracted critical illness. J Clin Endocrinol Metab. 2004;89(7):3105–13.
54. Branco RG, Garcia PC, Piva JP, et al. Pilot mechanistic study of insulin modulation of somatotrophic hormones, inflammation, and lipid metabolism during critical illness in children. Pediatr Crit Care Med. 2017;18:e35–41.

55. Marijke G, Mesotten D, Brugts M, et al. Effect of intensive insulin therapy on the somatotropic axis of critically ill children. Clin Endocrinol Metab. 2011;96:2558–66.
56. Fisher JG, Sparks EA, Khan FA, et al. Tight glycemic control with insulin does not affect skeletal muscle degradation during the early post-operative period following pediatric cardiac surgery. Pediatr Crit Care Med. 2015;16(6):515–21.
57. Codère-Maruyama T, Schricker T, Shum-Tim D, et al. Hyperinsulinemic-normoglycemic clamp administered together with amino acids induces anabolism after cardiac surgery. Am J Physiol Regul Integr Comp Physiol. 2016;311:1085–92.
58. Jeschke MG, Klein D, Herndon DN. Insulin treatment improves the systemic inflammatory reaction to severe trauma. Ann Surg. 2004;239:553–60.
59. Gore DC, Wolf SE, Herndon DN, Wolfe RR. Relative influence of glucose and insulin on peripheral amino acid metabolism in severely burned patients. JPEN J Parenter Enteral Nutr. 2002;26(5):272–7.
60. Gore DC, Wolf SE, Sanford AP, et al. Extremity hyperinsulinemia stimulates muscle protein synthesis in severely injured patients. Am J Physiol Endocrinol Metab. 2004;286:E529–34.
61. Ferrando AA, Chinkes DL, Wolf SE, et al. A submaximal dose of insulin promotes net skeletal muscle protein synthesis in patients with severe burns. Ann Surg. 1999;229(1):11–8.
62. Fram RY. Intensive insulin therapy improves insulin sensitivity and mitochondrial function in severely burned children. Crit Care Med. 2010;38(6):1475–83.
63. Gibson BR, Galiatsatos P, Rabiee A, et al. Intensive insulin therapy confers a similar survival benefit in the burn intensive care unit to the surgical intensive care unit. Surgery. 2009;146:922–30.
64. Hemmila MR, Taddonio MA, Arbabi S, et al. Intensive insulin therapy is associated with reduced infectious complications in burn patients. Surgery. 2008;144(4):629–37.
65. Pham TN, Warren AJ, Phan HH, et al. Impact of tight glycemic control in severely burned children. J Trauma. 2005;59:1148–54.
66. Gore DC, Wolf SE, Herndon DN, Wolfe RR. Metformin blunts stress-induced hyperglycemia after thermal injury. J Trauma. 2003;54:555–61.
67. Kanto K, Ito H, Noso S, et al. Effects of dosage and dosing frequency on the efficacy and safety of high-dose metformin in Japanese patients with type 2 diabetes mellitus. J Diabetes Investig. 2018;9:587–93.
68. Ali S, Fonseca V. Overview of metformin: special focus on metformin extended release. Drug Eval. 2012;13:1797–805.
69. Miller RA, Chu Q, Xie J, et al. Biguanides suppress hepatic glucagon signaling by decreasing production of cyclic AMP. Nature. 2013;494(7436):256–60.
70. Gore DC, Herndon DN, Wolfe RR. Comparison of peripheral metabolic effects of insulin and metformin following severe burn injury. J Trauma. 2005;59:316–23.
71. Gore DC, Wolf SE, Sanford A, et al. Influence of metformin on glucose intolerance and muscle catabolism following severe burn injury. Ann Surg. 2005;241:334–42.
72. Salpeter SR, Greyber E, Pasternak GA, Salpeter EE. Risk of fatal and nonfatal lactic acidosis with metformin use in type 2 diabetes mellitus: systematic review and meta-analysis. Arch Intern Med. 2003;163:2594–02.
73. Riesenman PJ, Braithwaite SS, Cairns BA. Metformin-associated lactic acidosis in a burn patient. J Burn Care Res. 2007;28:342–7.
74. Sears B, Perry M. The role of fatty acids in insulin resistance. Lipids Health Dis. 2015;14:121.
75. Auger C, Samadi O, Jeschke MG. The biochemical alterations underlying post-burn hypermetabolism. Biochim Biophys Acta. 2016;10:2633–44.
76. Ferrando AA. Anabolic hormones in critically ill patients. Curr Opin Clin Nutr Metab Care. 1999;2(2):171–5.
77. Ferrando AA, Wolfe RR. Restoration of hormonal action and muscle protein. Crit Care Med. 2007;35:S630–4.
78. Spratt DI. Altered gonadal steroidogenesis in critical illness: is treatment with anabolic steroids indicated? Best Pract Res Clin Endocrinol Metab. 2001;15(4):479–94.
79. Basaria S, Coviello AD, Travison TG, et al. Adverse events associated with testosterone administration. N Engl J Med. 2010;363(2):109–22.
80. Hart DW, Wolf SE, Ramzy PI, et al. Anabolic effects of oxandrolone after severe burn. Ann Surg. 2001;233(4):556–64.
81. Real DS, Reis RP, Piccolo MS, et al. Oxandrolone use in adult burn patients. Systematic review and meta-analysis. Acta Cir Bras. 2014;29(3):68–76.
82. Di Girolamo FG, Situlin R, Biolo G. What factors influence protein synthesis and degradation in critical illness? Curr Opin Clin Nutr Metab Care. 2017;20:124–30.
83. Barrow RE, Dasu MR, Ferrando AA, et al. Gene expression patterns in skeletal muscle of thermally injured children treated with oxandrolone. Ann Surg. 2003;237(3):422–8.
84. Wolf SE, Thomas SJ, Dasu MR, et al. Improved net protein balance, lean mass, and gene expression changes with oxandrolone treatment in the severely burned. Ann Surg. 2003;237(6):801–11.
85. Tuvdendorj D, Zhang X-J, Chinkes DL, et al. Intensive insulin treatment increases donor site wound protein synthesis in burn patients. Surgery. 2011;149(4):512–8.
86. Cochran A, Thuet W, Holt B, et al. The impact of oxandrolone on length of stay following major burn injury: a clinical practice evaluation. Burns. 2013;39:1374–9.
87. Wolf SE, Edelman LS, Kemalyan N, et al. Effects of oxandrolone on outcome measures in the severely burned: a multicenter prospective randomized double-blind trial. J Burn Care Res. 2006;27:131–9.
88. Pham TN, Klein MB, Gibran NS, et al. Impact of oxandrolone treatment on acute outcomes after severe burn injury. J Burn Care Res. 2008;29(6):902–6.
89. Porro LJ, Herndon DN, Rodriguez NA, et al. Five-year outcomes after oxandrolone administration in severely burned children: a randomized clinical trial of safety and efficacy. J Am Coll Surg. 2012;214(4):489–502.
90. Li H, Guo Y, Yang Z, et al. The efficacy and safety of oxandrolone treatment for patients with severe burns: a systematic review and meta-analysis. Burns. 2016;42:717–27.
91. Miller JT, Btaiche IF. Oxandrolone treatment in adults with severe thermal injury. Pharmacotherapy. 2009;29(2):213–26.
92. McCullough MC, Namias N, Schulman C, et al. Incidence of hepatic dysfunction is equivalent in burn patients receiving oxandrolone and controls. J Burn Care Res. 2007;28:412–20.
93. Ellger B, Debaveye Y, Van den Berghe G. Endocrine interventions in the ICU. Eur J Intern Med. 2005;16:71–82.
94. Van den Berghe G. Novel insights into the neuroendocrinology of critical illness. Eur J Endocrinol. 2000;143:1–13.
95. Van den Berghe G, Wouters P, Weekers F, et al. Reactivation of pituitary hormone release and metabolic improvement by infusion of growth hormone-releasing peptide and thyrotropin-releasing hormone in patients with protracted critical illness. J Clin Endocrinol Metab. 1999;84:1311–23.
96. Stathatos N, Levetan C, Burman KD, Wartofsky L. The controversy of the treatment of critically ill patients with thyroid hormone. Best Pract Res Clin Endocrinol Metab. 2001;15(4):465–78.
97. Molfino A, Amabile MI, Rossi Fanelli F, Muscaritoli M. Novel therapeutic options for cachexia and sarcopenia. Expert Opin Biol Ther. 2016;16(10):1239–44.
98. Dobs AS, Boccia RV, Croot CC, et al. Effects of enobosarm on muscle wasting and physical function in patients with cancer: a double-blind, randomised controlled phase 2 trial. Lancet Oncol. 2013;14(4):335–45.

99. Dalton JT. The selective androgen receptor modulator GTx-024 (enobosarm) improves lean body mass and physical function in healthy elderly men and postmenopausal women: results of a double-blind, placebo-controlled phase II trial. J Cachexia Sarcopenia Muscle. 2011;2:153–61.
100. Crawford J, Prado CM, Johnston MA, et al. Study design and rationale for the phase 3 clinical development program of enobosarm, a selective androgen receptor modulator, for the prevention and treatment of muscle wasting in cancer patients (POWER Trials). Curr Oncol Rep. 2016;18:37–48.
101. Srinath R, Dobs A. Enobosarm (GTx024, S22): a potential treatment for cachexia. Future Oncol. 2014;10:187.
102. Von Haehling S, Anker SD. Treatment of cachexia: an overview of recent developments. Int J Cardiol. 2015;184:736–42.
103. Esposito A, Criscitiello C, Gelao L, et al. Mechanisms of anorexia–cachexia syndrome and rational for treatment with selective ghrelin receptor agonist. Cancer Treat Rev. 2015;41:793–7.
104. Bai Y, Hu Y, Zhao Y, et al. Anamorelin for cancer anorexia-cachexia syndrome: a systematic review and meta-analysis. Support Care Cancer. 2017;25:1651–9.
105. Ebner N, Steinbeck L, Doehner W, et al. Highlights from the 7th Cachexia Conference: muscle wasting pathophysiological detection and novel treatment strategies. J Cachexia Sarcopenia Muscle. 2014;5:27–34.
106. Garcia JM. Therapeutic potential of anamorelin, a novel, oral ghrelin mimetic, in patients with cancer-related cachexia: a multicenter, randomized, double-blind, crossover, pilot study. Support Care Cancer. 2013;21:129–37.
107. Garcia JM, Boccia RV, Graham CD, et al. Anamorelin for patients with cancer cachexia: an integrated analysis of two phase 2, randomised, placebo-controlled, double-blind trials. Lancet Oncol. 2015;16:108–16.
108. Su J, Geng J, Bao J, et al. Two ghrelin receptor agonists for adults with malnutrition: a systematic review and meta-analysis. Nutr J. 2016;15:97.
109. Greig CA, Johns N, Gray C, et al. Phase I/II trial of formoterol fumarate combined with megestrol acetate in cachectic patients with advanced malignancy. Support Care Cancer. 2014;22:1269–75.
110. Ryall JG, Lynch GS. The potential and the pitfalls of β-adrenoreceptor agonists for the management of skeletal muscle wasting. Pharmacol Ther. 2008;120:219–32.

Diagnosis and Treatment of Infections in Burns

23

Kaitlin A. Pruskowski, Kevin S. Akers, and Kevin K. Chung

23.1 Introduction

Infection is a frequent complication for patients with thermal injury and is a leading cause of death in burn patients [1, 2]. Wound infection, bacterial pneumonia, and bloodstream infections are cited as the leading causes of mortality among burn patients [3].

The skin is a barrier against infection; damage to the skin leaves patients at high risk for both local and systemic infections [1]. Topical antimicrobials have led to the decline of burn wound infections but have not completely eliminated this complication [3].

In addition to physical injury, burn patients experience profound and sustained physiologic and metabolic alterations. Additionally, dysregulation of the host immune function and inflammatory response put patients at increased risk for both local and systemic infections. These changes also alter the way infections declare and present, making its prompt recognition challenging. Finally, the distribution, metabolism, and elimination of antimicrobial medications can be significantly altered, thereby complicating drug dosing [4].

The goal of this chapter is to describe diagnostic criteria and treatment of infections in burn patients. Early recognition of infection and optimal antimicrobial dosing are keys to optimal outcomes.

K. A. Pruskowski · K. S. Akers
Burn Center, United States Army Institute of Surgical Research, Fort Sam Houston, TX, USA

Department of Medicine, Uniformed Services University, Bethesda, MD, USA
e-mail: kaitlin.a.pruskowski.civ@mail.mil; kevin.s.akers.mil@mail.mil

K. K. Chung (✉)
Department of Medicine, Uniformed Services University, Bethesda, MD, USA
e-mail: kevin.k.chung.mil@mail.mil

23.2 Sepsis in the Burn Patient

Because of the unique physiologic changes and chronic systemic inflammation that accompany burn injury, the typical systemic inflammatory response syndrome (SIRS) criteria lack specificity and sensitivity to accurately diagnose burn sepsis (Table 23.1). Most burn patients would have at least one component of SIRS, and this definition would not carry much meaning in the burn population. The American Burn Association (ABA) has developed a consensus definition for sepsis in the burn patient. This consensus statement defines burn sepsis as any change in the burn patient that triggers the concern for sepsis plus a documented infection [5]. Changes in the burn patient that trigger concern for sepsis include hyper- or hypothermia, progressive tachycardia, progressive tachypnea, thrombocytopenia, hyperglycemia, and the inability to continue enteral feedings for at least 24 h. In addition to the presence of any of these triggers, the patient must have a documented infection, defined as a culture-positive infection, pathologic tissue source, or a clinical response to antibiotics [5]. Patients who have shock-like hemodynamic parameters and require the initiation of vasopressors in addition to meeting the above criteria for sepsis are considered to have septic shock [5].

The Third International Consensus Definitions for Sepsis and Septic Shock (SEPSIS-3) has recently refined the definition for sepsis in the general medical population. According to SEPSIS-3, sepsis is life-threatening organ dysfunction caused by a dysregulated host response to infection [7]. More objectively, an acute change in the Sequential Organ Failure Assessment (SOFA) score of 2 or more points would indicate the development of sepsis [7]. Patients are considered to have septic shock when they meet the above criteria for sepsis and also have underlying circulatory and metabolic abnormalities that are sufficiently profound to substantially increase mortality [7]. Objectively, these patients have persistent hypotension and require vasopressors to maintain a mean arterial pressure (MAP) of at least 65 mmHg. These patients also have a serum lactate persistently greater than

M. G. Jeschke et al. (eds.), *Handbook of Burns Volume 1*, https://doi.org/10.1007/978-3-030-18940-2_23

Table 23.1 Diagnostic criteria for the systemic inflammatory response syndrome (SIRS) [6]

Temperature	>38 °C <36 °C
Heart rate	>90 beats per minute
Respiratory	Respiratory rate >20 breaths/min $PaCO_2$ <32 torr
White blood cell count (WBC)	WBC >12,000 cells/mm^3 WBC <4000 cells/mm^3 >10% immature (band) forms

Table 23.2 Criteria triggering concern for sepsis in the burn patient [5]

Criteria	Definition
Hyper or hypothermia	Temperature >39 or <36.5 °C
Progressive tachycardia	Heart rate >110 beats per minute in adult burn patients
Progressive tachypnea	Respiratory rate >25 breaths per minute in non-ventilated adult patients Minute ventilation >12 L per minute in ventilated patients
Thrombocytopenia	Platelets <100,000 cells/mm^3 (Not applicable until 3 days after initial resuscitation)
Hyperglycemia	Blood glucose >200 mg/dL Resistance to >7 units/h of regular insulin >25% increase in insulin requirement over 24 h
Inability to continue enteral feedings for >24 h	Abdominal distension Residuals at least two times the enteral feeding rate Uncontrollable diarrhea (>2.5 L per day)

2 mmol/L, despite adequate fluid resuscitation [7]. The SEPSIS-3 definitions of sepsis, as well as the SOFA score, have not yet been evaluated in burn patients.

The Surviving Sepsis Campaign recommends that combinations of clinical interventions ("bundles") be performed within 3 and 6 h of the development of sepsis or patient presentation to the healthcare facility. The sepsis bundles have been key in promoting timely recognition and treatment of sepsis, as well as decreasing mortality due to sepsis and septic shock [10]. Within the first 3 h of presentation, providers should measure the patient's serum lactate, provide fluid resuscitation with at least 30 mL/kg of crystalloid if the patient is hypotensive or has a serum lactate of at least 4 mmol/L, obtain blood cultures prior to antibiotic administration, and initiate broad-spectrum antibiotics [9]. The 2016 Surviving Sepsis Guidelines recommend that appropriate microbiologic cultures be drawn and empiric broad-spectrum antibiotics be initiated within the first hour following recognition of sepsis or septic shock [10]. These guidelines further recommend that antimicrobial therapy be revised to culture-directed therapy once organism and antimicrobial susceptibility data are available and recommend against the use of sustained systemic antimicrobial therapy in patients with severe inflammatory states (which would include burn injury) [10].

Within 6 h of the development of sepsis, lactate levels should be re-measured and the patient's fluid status should be re-assessed if they remain hypotensive. Fluid status can be re-assessed with a focused physical exam, CVP measurement, $SCVO_2$ measurement, cardiovascular ultrasound, or dynamic assessment of fluid response [9]. If the patient remains hypotensive (MAP less than 65 mmHg) despite ade-

Table 23.3 Sequential Organ Failure Assessment (SOFA) Scoring System [8]

Points assigned	1	2	3	4
Variable				
Respiratory				
PaO_2/FiO_2	≤400	≤300	≤200	≤100
Coagulation				
Platelets, $10^3/\mu L$	<150	<100	<50	<20
Hepatic				
Bilirubin, mg/dL	1.2–1.9	2.0–5.9	6.0–11.9	≥12.0
Cardiovascular				
Hypotension	MAP <70 mmHg	Dopamine ≤5 or dobutamine (any dose)[a]	Dopamine >5 or epinephrine ≤0.1 or norepinephrine ≤0.1	Dopamine >15 or epinephrine >0.1 or norepinephrine >0.1
Central nervous system				
Glasgow Coma Score	13–14	10–12	6–9	<6
Renal				
Creatinine, mg/dL	1.2–1.9	2.0–3.4	3.5–4.9	>5.0
Urine output			<500 mL/day	<200 mL/day

[a]Infusion rates are displayed in μg/kg/min

quate intravascular volume repletion, vasopressors should be initiated [10].

23.3 Sites of infection

23.3.1 Burn Wound Infection

Burn wound infection is one of the most common types of infection in burn patients [3]. The burn wound should always be considered as a potential source of infection.

Burn wound surfaces are sterile immediately after thermal injury but subsequently become colonized with bacteria. Colonization can be loosely defined as positive bacterial growth from surface swab cultures in the absence of clinical concern for infection. Gram-positive cocci, such as *Staphylococci*, that survive the initial insult are usually the first organisms to heavily colonize the burn wound. These organisms, including methicillin-resistant *Staphylococcus aureus* (MRSA) and coagulase-negative *Staphylococci*, are usually the most common pathogens in burn wound infections [1]. Other common causes of burn wound infection include *Enterococcus*, *Pseudomonas aeruginosa*, *Escherichia coli*, and *Klebsiella pneumoniae* [1].

Colonization should not be treated with systemic antimicrobials. For this reason, surface swab cultures are not recommended as a routine practice without clinical concern for infection. However, colonization can lead to burn wound infection, which should be treated [5].

Burn wound infection can be further classified into cellulitis, invasive infection, impetigo, and burn-related surgical wound infection. Each of these is further described in Table 23.4.

Table 23.4 Types and clinical characteristics of burn wound infections [1, 5]

Invasive infection	• Invasion or destruction of burned and unburned skin and tissue • Causes separation of eschar or graft loss, invasion of adjacent separation of eschar or graft loss, invasion of adjacent unburned tissue, or cause the systemic response of sepsis syndrome • Usually life-threatening
Cellulitis	• Advancing erythema, induration, swelling, warmth, tenderness in surrounding tissues • Extension of infection into the healthy, uninjured skin and soft tissues surrounding the burn wound or donor site • Not associated with other signs of wound infection
Impetigo	• The loss of epithelium from previously re-epithelialized surface
Burn-related surgical wound infection	• Includes both excised burn and donor sites that have not yet epithelialized • Wounds produce purulent exudate that is culture-positive • May have loss of synthetic or biological covering of the wound, changes in wound appearance, and erythema in uninjured skin surrounding the wound

23.3.2 Pneumonia

The diagnosis of pneumonia relies upon clinical criteria. In order to meet the criteria for pneumonia, a patient must have a chest radiograph showing a new or persistent infiltrate, consolidation, or cavitation; recent change in sputum or new purulence in the sputum; and/or meet the criteria for sepsis, as defined earlier [5]. The diagnosis of pneumonia can be confirmed with positive microbiologic data [5]. Pneumonia-causing pathogens commonly include *Staphylococcus aureus, Pseudomonas aeruginosa, Escherichia coli, Klebsiella pneumonia,* and *Serratia marcescens* [3].

Empiric treatment for ventilator-associated or hospital-acquired pneumonia should include agents with activity against MRSA and against *Pseudomonas aeruginosa.* Anaerobic coverage is not generally required given the rarity of anaerobes as a cause of nosocomial pneumonia. While some broad-spectrum empiric therapies used for pneumonia include anaerobic activity (piperacillin/tazobactam), others do not (cefepime). Antibiotic therapy should be tailored based on culture results as they become available, and the treatment should generally be continued for a total of 7 days, although a longer course can be considered for multidrug-resistant organisms [11].

23.3.3 Bloodstream Infection

Bacteremia in the burn patient can be due to usual causes, such as intravenous catheters, but can also be secondary to burn care-related factors. Burn wound colonization or infection can lead to transient bacteremia, which is often culture-negative. In the early stages after thermal injury, intestinal blood flow and perfusion are decreased, which can allow for translocation of normal gut flora into the bloodstream. Early enteral nutrition can help preserve the gut-barrier function and prevent bacterial translocation [1].

Patients are considered to have bloodstream infections if they have recognized pathogens cultured from at least two blood cultures or at least one positive blood culture in the presence of sepsis (as defined earlier in this chapter). Patients who have common skin contaminants from at least two blood cultures drawn on separate occasions and clinical signs of sepsis can also be considered to have a bloodstream infection [5]. *Staphylococcus aureus* (including MRSA), *Pseudomonas aeruginosa, Escherichia coli, Klebsiella pneumoniae, Enterobacter* species, *Serratia marcescens, Acinetobacter* species, *and Enterococcus faecalis* are some of the most common causative pathogens [3].

Management of bloodstream infections should begin with removing any indwelling catheters and the initiation of systemic antimicrobial therapy. Empiric antibiotic coverage for bloodstream infections should include an agent with activity against MRSA. Patients with femoral catheters should also receive coverage for gram-negative bacilli and *Candida* [12]. Antimicrobial therapy should be continued for 14 days after the first negative blood culture (day 1 of antibiotic therapy is the first day where negative blood culture results are obtained) [12].

23.3.4 Invasive Fungal Wound Infection

Invasive fungal wound infections are more likely to affect patients later in their course of burn wound treatment. The repeated and long-term use of antibacterial agents can create an environment where fungi and yeast can thrive, thus promoting fungal colonization [1]. Additionally, critically ill burn patients commonly experience relative immune suppression that allows fungal pathogens to result in invasive infections [4].

In a retrospective autopsy series of severely burned patients, the most common sites of fungal infections that were associated with attributable mortality included the burn wound, pulmonary system, abdomen, urinary system, and bloodstream [13]. In 13 of 14 cases (93%) included in this retrospective review, mortality was attributed to *Aspergillus* [13]. This retrospective review also found that larger burn injury and greater length of hospital stay were associated with fungal infection and attributable mortality from fungal infection [13].

The most common pathogens associated with fungal wound infection and invasive fungal infection include *Candida*, *Aspergillus*, *Mucor*, and *Fusarium* [1, 13].

Fungal endophthalmitis is an infection of the internal eye structures most often caused by *Candida* species, and resulting from fungemia with this organism. Because the treatment of this infection requires prolonged and potentially high-dose antifungal therapy, fundus examination with a dilated retinal exam is considered compulsory following candidemia in non-burn patients. Ideally, this examination is performed by an ophthalmologist within the first week of therapy [14]. Candidemia has been documented in burn populations at rates of 2–5% [15, 16]. The prevalence of endophthalmitis among burn patients with candidemia is unknown.

23.3.5 Other Infections

In addition to the above disease states, other infections may develop in the burn population. *Clostridium difficile*-associated diarrhea (CDAD) may affect up to 8% of burn patients and should be suspected in patients with unexplained diarrhea or in patients with diarrhea and other signs or symptoms of sepsis [17]. Development of CDAD has been associated with longer hospital length of stay and increased mortality, thus early recognition and treatment of this disease is imperative to reduce morbidity and mortality [18]. Endocarditis, though only seen in 0.4% of burn patients, has been associated with a mortality rate of 100%. Even though endocarditis is seen in a small percentage of the overall burn population, it affects up to 9% of patients with bacteremia [19]. Gram-negative organisms, including *Pseudomonas aeruginosa*, *Acinetobacter*, and *Klebsiella*, are the most common pathogens in the burn population [19]. Any patient with recurrent or persistent bacteremia should further evaluated for endocarditis. Viral infections, including herpes simplex (HSV) and cytomegalovirus (CMV), are associated with morbidity (including increased risk for bacterial sepsis) and mortality in burn patients [20]. In a recent autopsy series, 5% of deaths were attributed to viral infections [3]. Diagnosis of these infections in burn patients is difficult; the risks and benefits of empiric treatment must be weighed before antivirals are initiated.

23.4 Pharmacokinetic and Pharmacodynamic Changes in Critically Ill Patients

Increasing data from multiple patient populations support the growing recognition that manufacturer-recommended doses may not be universally applicable across all patient populations, particularly the critically ill. In order to understand the pharmacokinetic changes that occur in burn patients, it is imperative to know the basic pharmacokinetic parameters and definitions. Table 23.5 defines the basic pharmacokinetic parameters.

23.4.1 Changes in Absorption

Critically ill patients have many physiologic derangements that affect absorption of medications. During sepsis and/or shock, blood is shunted to the most vital organs, including the brain and the heart, and away from the gastrointestinal tract, muscle, and skin, thus reducing the absorption and bioavailability of medications that are given via these routes. Medications given intramuscularly or subcutaneously can fail to distribute away from the site of administration due to lack of regional blood flow, thus resulting in a drug depot. When regional blood flow is restored, the medication contained within the depot can be rapidly released, potentially leading to adverse drug events. Because of these changes, it is ideal to give most medications intravenously [21, 23].

Table 23.5 Pharmacokinetic definitions [21–23]

Pharmacokinetics (PK)	Describes the movement of drugs throughout the body
Pharmacodynamics (PD)	Describes the pharmacologic response that results when a drug reaches its receptor or site of action
Absorption	Rate and extent to which a medication leaves its site of administration and moves to systemic circulation
Bioavailability	Fraction of a medication dose that reaches systemic circulation
Distribution	Process by which drug molecules move through the bloodstream and pass through organs and tissues
Volume of distribution	Describes the relationship between a dose of a medication and the resulting serum concentration
Metabolism	Chemical conversion of drug molecules to active or inactive metabolites
Elimination	Removal of drug from the body
Elimination rate constant (k_e)	Fraction of the total amount of drug in the body eliminated per unit time
Clearance	Volume of serum or blood completely cleared of the drug per unit time

23.4.2 Changes in Distribution

Once a medication is absorbed into the bloodstream, it must travel throughout the body and distribute into the interstitial and intracellular fluids in order to reach its site of action. Large-volume fluid resuscitation, capillary leakage, and extravascular fluid sequestration ("third-spacing") can dramatically increase the volume of distribution, especially for hydrophilic drugs. Higher than usual doses and/or the use of loading doses of these medications may be needed to achieve therapeutic concentrations in critically ill patients.

Proteins which bind and transport drugs in humans (primarily albumin and alpha-1 acid glycoprotein) are considered to be acute phase reactants; albumin production drastically decreases in the setting of systemic inflammation. Medications that are highly bound to albumin may have increased concentrations of the unbound active drug, potentially leading to associated toxicities [21, 23].

Table 23.6 Dosing recommendations for antimicrobial agents

Drug	Usual dose	CVVH[a]	IHD
Vancomycin	20–25 mg/kg loading dose, 15 mg/kg maintenance, titrate to trough 15–20 μg/mL (for *S. aureus*)	15–20 mg/kg loading dose; titrate to trough 15–20 μg/mL (for *S. aureus*) Clearance increased at CVVH dose >40 mL/kg/h (cont. infusion may be helpful)	1000–1750 mg loading dose, then 500–1000 mg after IHD sessions, titrate to trough 15–20 μg/mL
Daptomycin	10 mg/kg (or 750 mg) q24h	8 mg/kg q48h	4–6 mg/kg q48h (administer after IHD sessions on IHD days)
Imipenem-cilastatin	500–1000 mg q6–8h	1000 mg loading dose, then 500 mg q6–8h	500 mg q12h
Meropenem	1000 mg q8h (3 h infusion recommended for organisms MIC ≥2 μg/mL)	1000 mg q8h (or by cont. infusion)	500–1000 mg q24h (administer after IHD sessions on IHD days)
Piperacillin-tazobactam	2.25 g q8h–4.5 g q6h (4.5 g q6h with 4 h infusion recommended for *Pseudomonas* with MIC = 16 μg/mL, assuming normal renal function)	3.375 g q6h (3 h or cont. infusion may increase levels)	2.25 g q6–8h
Cefepime	2 g q8h (4 h infusion recommended for *Pseudomonas* with MIC ≥8 μg/mL)	2 g loading dose, then 1–2 g q12h	1 g loading dose, then 0.5–1 g q24h or 2 g after IHD sessions
Levofloxacin	250–750 mg q24h (depending on renal function)	500–750 mg loading dose, then 250 mg q24h (from non-burn data)	500–750 mg loading dose, then 250–500 mg after IHD sessions
Ciprofloxacin	400 mg q8h (for *Pseudomonas*)	200 mg q12h or 400 mg q24h (from non-burn data)	200–400 mg q24h
Amikacin	20 mg/kg q24h; titrate peak:MIC ≥10 and/or AUC_{24}:MIC >150:1 with low troughs	Usual dose; MICs have greater impact than CVVH clearance; titrate peak:MIC ≥10 with low troughs	5–7.5 mg/kg/dose; redose when pre-IHD level <10 μg/mL; titrate to peak 15–40 μg/mL (depending on severity of infection)
Amphotericin B (liposomal)	3–5 mg/kg q24h	No change	No change
Voriconazole	6 mg/kg q12h for 1 day, then 4 mg/kg q12h	No change; cyclodextrin is removed	IV formulation is not recommended
Micafungin	150 mg q24h (consider up to 300 mg q24h for *C. parapsilosis*)	No change	No change

[a]Assumes effluent rate (sum of dialysate, replacement fluid and ultrafiltration rates) of 25 mL/kg/h or 2 L/h. Filter clearance of unbound drugs generally depends on effluent rate and fluid replacement configuration; PK/PD optimization may require customized dose adjustment for specific circumstances

23.4.3 Changes in Metabolism

Changes in drug metabolism are affected by both changes in hepatic blood flow and alterations in hepatic enzymatic activity. The hepatic extraction ratio ranges from 0 to 1 and indicates the fraction of the drug removed after one pass through the liver. For drugs that have high hepatic extraction ratios, such as fentanyl and midazolam, circulating levels are very sensitive to changes in hepatic blood flow. Hepatic blood flow can be reduced in the late stages of sepsis, secondary to decreased cardiac output and vasopressor use. Conversely, hepatically metabolized drugs with low hepatic extraction ratios, such as phenytoin, are sensitive to changes in hepatic function, rather than hepatic blood flow [23].

Enzymes involved in drug metabolism, particularly the cytochrome P 450 (CYP 450) system, can either be induced or inhibited (or both) during critical illness. Medications that cause drug interactions through competitive inhibition are also an important source of variability, to which clinicians should remain attentive. Understanding the underlying disease state in the critically ill patient can help to predict how these enzymes, and consequently drug metabolism, can be affected.

23.4.4 Changes in Elimination

During the hyperdynamic phase of sepsis, patients may have increased drug clearance, as renal blood flow is increased during this time [23]. Higher doses or more frequent dosing of antibiotics may be required to optimize pharmacokinetic and pharmacodynamic (PKPD) parameters during this time. As sepsis progresses, renal blood flow decreases, and up to 70% of patients may develop acute kidney injury or acute renal failure, which can drastically decrease drug elimination [21]. Extending dosing intervals may be required to prevent drug accumulation and potential adverse drug events.

23.4.5 PK-PD Changes in Burn Patients

Within the first 48 h after burn injury, patients experience burn shock and severe hypovolemia. Local and systemic inflammatory processes lead to vasodilation, vascular permeability, and negative interstitial pressure, causing a fluid and albumin shift from the intravascular space into the interstitial space. During this time, cardiac output and glomerular filtration are decreased. These physiologic changes lead to changes in distribution and elimination; patients tend to have a slower rate of drug distribution and lower renal elimination [24].

The resuscitative phase typically occurs within 12 h after burn injury and lasts up to 72 h. During this time, multiple physiologic changes occur. Increased capillary permeability and decreased interstitial oncotic pressure result in hypovolemia, decrease in effective circulating volume, decreased myocardial contractility, and edema formation in burned and non-burned tissues. Prolonged drug distribution, increased volume of distribution, delay in onset of action, and slower elimination are consequences of these physiologic alterations [4].

The hypermetabolic phase follows the resuscitative phase. The hypermetabolic phase usually begins by post-injury day 5 and can last up to 3 years post-injury [4]. Increases in catecholamines, cortisol, glucagon, and prostaglandins lead to increased cardiac output and hyperdynamic circulation. This also increases blood flow to the liver and kidneys, which can increase the rate of metabolism and elimination. As a result of burn injury, hepatic enzymes, including enzymes in the cytochrome P 450 system, are induced, enhancing drug metabolism [24]. Increased blood flow to the kidneys increases creatinine clearance/glomerular filtration rate. Additionally, non-renal clearance is increased, as exudate leaks from partial- and full-thickness burns. During the hypermetabolic phase, increased doses or more frequent dosing of medications may be required to optimize the PKPD parameters of the agents.

Early in the hypermetabolic phase, synthesis of alpha-1 acid glycoprotein increases, while albumin production drastically decreases. The former is the predominant carrier of antimicrobial agents in humans. The free fraction of drugs that are highly albumin-bound, such as phenytoin, is increased, which could potentially lead to adverse drug effects. It is important to recognize that in contrast to single stated values found in the literature, protein binding is a dynamic process with substantial within- and between-patient variability. As a heteroscedastic process, protein binding can vary even within a single dose interval of an antimicrobial agent.

Recovery from burn injury is a dynamic process. Throughout their hospital course, burn patients tend to move between the resuscitative and hypermetabolic phases. Clinicians should be attentive to their patients' overall clinical picture and consider how this will affect PK-PD parameters.

23.5 Discussion of Drug Classes

As previously discussed, early recognition and treatment of burn sepsis is key to preventing morbidity and mortality in the burn patient. Because mortality increases hourly in untreated sepsis, early and aggressive antimicrobial therapy is a cornerstone of sepsis treatment. Antimicrobial agents must be dosed in a manner that optimizes their pharmacodynamic effects in order to optimally treat underlying infection. Generally accepted optimization parameters (T > MIC, AUC:MIC, Cmax:MIC) derive from studies of experimental infection in immunocompromised animals, thereby removing the influence of the immune system in order to isolate the effects of the antimicrobial agent against a pathogen in vivo. A simple linear regression is performed between pathogen burden and one of the three parameters above in which the ratio of the numerator is varied (exposure time above MIC, AUC or peak concentration), with the best curve fit determining which parameter is most predictive of antimicrobial activity. Some antimicrobials may share two parameters sufficiently comparable that neither is clearly superior. Further studies are then required to determine what should be the minimum acceptable target reached for the relevant parameter in order to optimize treatment of the infection. Limitations to this approach include failure to account for the influence of the immune system and its basis in an animal-based experimental model rather than from human infection. Also, this numerical approach to PK-PD optimization can in some cases be discordant from empiric observation, as in the case of colistin, where clinical cures are observed despite the impossibility of achieving optimal targets from recommended doses. Finally, the primary determinant of whether numerical PK-PD parameters can be achieved is the pathogen MIC, which can vary significantly by region and/or institution.

As continuous renal replacement therapy (CRRT) is becoming more widely available in burn centers, an increasing number of patients may be placed on this therapy. Drug dosing for patients on CRRT will need to be adjusted based on CRRT mode and dose. Replacement fluid configuration and efficiency will also need to be considered. To optimize drug dosing, it is essential that a clinical pharmacist, who has experience in both burn and critical care, be included on multidisciplinary burn team.

23.5.1 B-lactams

Beta-lactam antibiotics exhibit bactericidal activity by inhibiting bacterial cell wall synthesis. With respect to pharmacodynamics, this class of antibiotics exhibits the most bactericidal activity when the time above the minimum inhibitory concentration (MIC) is optimized. This can be done by increasing the dose or frequency of dosing or by administering extended-interval or continuous infusions. In general, systemic drug concentrations should be greater than the MIC for at least 50% of the dosing interval to deliver optimal pharmacodynamic efficacy. However, specific optimization targets vary depending on the specific drug and severity of illness.

Of all the penicillin antibiotics, piperacillin/tazobactam has the most literature regarding pharmacokinetic changes in burn patients. A recent review has shown that piperacillin/tazobactam dosed at 4.5 g intravenously (IV) infused over 4 h and administered every 6 h optimized PK-PD parameters and eradicated most susceptible organisms [4].

The third-generation cephalosporins, ceftazidime and cefepime, are often used to treat infections due to Gram-negative organisms, including *Pseudomonas aeruginosa*. Serum concentrations of ceftazidime have been shown to be up to 43% lower in patients with burn injury, as compared to healthy patients. As a result, it has been recommended that higher doses (up to 6 g per day) and prolonged infusion times (at least 3 h) be used to optimize PKPD parameters [4, 25]. Similarly, the infusion time for cefepime should be prolonged to at least 4 h to optimize its effects [4].

Newer generation cephalosporins, including ceftaroline, ceftazidime/avibactam, and ceftolozane/tazobactam, provide alternative options for treating multidrug-resistant organisms. However, these agents have not yet been studied in the burn population, and dosing recommendations for these medications are not available at this time.

Carbapenems exert optimal bactericidal activity when serum concentrations are above the MIC for at least 40% of the dosing interval. Imipenem and meropenem have pharmacokinetic data available specifically in the burn population. For these agents, PK-PD parameters are not significantly different in patients with burn injury, as compared with non-burn patients [25]. However, in burn patients who are infected with organisms that have an MIC greater than 2 μg/mL, extending the infusion time to 3 h may be required to achieve adequate concentrations for at least 40–50% of the dosing interval [4].

23.5.2 Aztreonam

Aztreonam is a monobactam which inhibits bacterial cell wall synthesis. There is much debate about whether aztreonam pharmacodynamics are best described by the time above the MIC or the area under the curve (AUC)-to-MIC ratio (≥184:1). Treatment for most infections with aztreonam will not require a dose adjustment. However, for patients with *Pseudomonas* isolates that have an MIC greater than 8 μg/mL, it is recommended that an extended infusion of aztreonam 2 g IV every 8 h or a standard infusion of aztreonam 2 g IV every 6 h be given [4].

23.5.3 Aminoglycosides

Aminoglycosides inhibit bacterial protein synthesis and exhibit concentration-dependent killing. The highest bactericidal potential occurs when the maximum concentration (C_{max}) is at least ten times the MIC of the infecting organism. Because of high-volume resuscitation and resulting edema, burn patients have larger volumes of distribution for aminoglycosides; higher doses may be required to achieve the goal peak concentration. Due to augmented renal function, aminoglycosides can be eliminated more quickly, so increased dosing frequency may be needed. In this population, once-daily dosing of aminoglycosides is unlikely to provide optimal bactericidal activity. It is recommended that drug levels be drawn frequently and dose adjustments be made to avoid drug concentrations that are undetectable for more than 10 h [4].

23.5.4 Fluoroquinolones

The fluoroquinolones prevent the unwinding of bacterial DNA, thus preventing transcription. These agents are optimally bactericidal when the AUC-to-MIC ratio is greater than 125 to 1. In order to achieve this, it is recommended to administer ciprofloxacin 400 mg IV every 8 h or levofloxacin 750 mg IV every 24 h, with appropriate adjustments for renal insufficiency [4, 25].

23.5.5 Polymyxins

Recently, the polymyxins have re-emerged as treatments of last resort for multidrug-resistant organisms. These agents damage the bacterial cytoplasmic membranes, resulting in cell death.

Polymyxin E (colistin) is delivered in humans as a methanesulfonated prodrug (colistin methanesulfonate, also known as colistimethate). Although the PK-PD properties are still being elucidated, optimizing colistin's AUC-to-MIC ratio to be greater than 30 to 1 causes the greatest bactericidal effect. However, due to physiologic and pharmacologic changes of burn injury, usual doses of colistin are unlikely to result in such concentrations, and increased doses expose patients to an increased risk of nephrotoxicity. Due to concerns regarding dose adequacy from a PK-PD perspective, colistimethate should not be administered as monotherapy for the treatment of multidrug-resistant Gram-negative organisms [4]. Colistin methanesulfonate can also be delivered by nebulization for the treatment of pneumonia. Because nebulized colistin is absorbed at a low level across the alveoli, there is a theoretical risk for promotion of resistance if used without concurrent systemic colistin.

To date, the PK-PD changes of polymyxin B have not been evaluated in patients with burn injury. Thus, no dosing changes can be recommended at this time.

23.5.6 Vancomycin

Vancomycin is a glycopeptide that inhibits bacterial wall synthesis. This agent has become a mainstay of empiric antibiotic therapy, providing coverage against methicillin-resistant *Staphylococcus aureus* (MRSA). Historically, vancomycin's pharmacodynamics have been optimized by targeting a goal trough level of 15–20 μg/mL, although newer literature shows that targeting an AUC-to-MIC ratio of at least 400 to 1 can provide similar effects. In patients with burn injury, dosing vancomycin to achieve a goal trough between 15 and 20 μg/mL is likely to achieve an AUC-to-MIC ratio of at least 360 to 1 [26].

Patients with burn injury tend to have a higher volume of distribution of vancomycin, as well as enhanced elimination. Because of this, patients will likely need 40–70 mg/kg per day to optimize the PKPD properties of vancomycin. In some cases, continuous infusions of vancomycin may be needed to achieve this. When dosing vancomycin, one must carefully weigh the risks of nephrotoxicity with the benefits of optimizing this agent [4].

23.5.7 Linezolid

Linezolid is an alternative option for the treatment of pneumonia or wound infections caused by MRSA. It is a bacteriostatic oxazolidinone that inhibits bacterial protein synthesis. Because of its bacteriostatic activity, this agent is not the ideal choice for the treatment of bacteremia. Pharmacodynamic effects are optimized when the AUC-to-MIC ratio is greater than 80 to 1 [4]. In patients with severe burn injury, the AUC may be decreased by as much as 50%, as compared to non-burn patients [27]. Due to this decrease, higher doses of linezolid may be warranted to achieve optimal pharmacodynamics; however, such doses are yet to be evaluated and cannot be recommended at this time.

23.5.8 Daptomycin

Daptomycin exerts its bactericidal effects by inhibiting the synthesis of bacterial DNA, RNA, and proteins. Daptomycin is active against MRSA. However, this agent is inactivated by surfactant produced by type II pneumocytes, rendering it ineffective for the treatment of pneumonia. Daptomycin exerts its effects in a dose-dependent manner, although optimizing the AUC-to-MIC ratio may lead to better outcomes. A pharmacokinetic study of daptomycin showed that AUC decreased, while volume of distribution and clearance were increased in burn patients, and suggested that doses of 12 mg/kg may be warranted [28]. A recent review found that daptomycin given at a fixed dose of 750 mg daily may achieve similar clinical responses as the weight-based dosing of 10 mg/kg [4]. More studies are needed to determine the optimal dosing strategy for patients with burn injury.

23.5.9 Antifungals

As previously mentioned, burn patients are at high risk for developing fungal infections. Despite this, there is a paucity of literature on antifungal pharmacokinetics in patients with burn injury.

23.5.10 Azoles

Of the azoles, fluconazole has the most narrow spectrum against common burn pathogens, having activity only against *Candida* and *Coccidioides* species. Posaconazole has a broader spectrum of activity, as compared to fluconazole and has activity against *Candida* species, *Aspergillus* species, *Cryptococcus neoformans*, *Fusarium* species, *Coccidioides* species, and *Mucor* species. Voriconazole is also a potential option for the treatment of fungal infections due to *Aspergillus*, *Candida*, *Fusarium*, *Penicillium*, and *Coccidioides* but is known to have various problematic toxicities and non-linear PK leading to erratic levels; thus, therapeutic drug monitoring is recommended. Isavuconazole is the newest azole antifungal to come to market and covers infections caused by *Aspergillus* and *Mucor*. These agents have not been extensively studied in the burn population, and empiric dose adjustments cannot be recommended at this time [4].

23.5.11 Echinocandins

The echinocandins exhibit concentration-dependent activity with post-antifungal effects against *Candida* and *Aspergillus*. Of the echinocandins, micafungin has literature available specific to the burn population. The standard dose of micafungin (100 mg daily) has been shown to have lower peak concentrations and higher clearance in critically ill burn patients; higher doses of micafungin may be needed to achieve optimal levels [29, 30]. However, very little data has been published on the safety and efficacy of high-dose micafungin, and no recommendations can be made at this time.

23.5.12 Amphotericin

Amphotericin alters fungal cell membrane permeability and is a broad-spectrum antifungal agent that exhibits activity against *Candida* and *Aspergillus*, among other fungi. Due to the lack of available data, no dosing changes can be recommended at this time.

23.6 Conclusion

Infection is a frequent complication of burn injury. Due to physiologic changes after burns, infection may present in an atypical manner. Early recognition and appropriate treatment are likely to reduce morbidity and mortality. Patients with burn injury are subject to continuously fluctuating alterations in drug absorption, distribution, metabolism, and elimination that must be considered when designing an optimal antimicrobial dosing regimen.

Summary Box

- Infection is one of the most frequent complications for patients with thermal injury.
- Early recognition of infection and sepsis are imperative but extremely challenging.
- Dosing of antibacterials and antifungals must be individualized.
- The clinician must understand these changes and make the appropriate drug adjustments to optimize treatment and outcomes.

References

1. Church D, Elsayed S, Reid O, et al. Burn wound infections. Clin Micro Rev. 2006;19(2):403–34.
2. Gomez R, Murray CK, Hospenthal DR, et al. Causes of mortality by autopsy findings of combat casualties and civilian patients admitted to a burn unit. J Am Coll Surg. 2009;208:348–54.
3. D'Avignon LC, Hogan BK, Murray CK, et al. Contribution of bacterial and viral infections to attributable mortality in patients with severe burns: an autopsy series. Burns. 2010;36:773–9.
4. Cota JM, Fakhri Ravari A, Rowan MP, Chung KK, Murray CK, Akers KS. Intravenous antibiotic and antifungal agent pharmacokinetic-pharmacodynamic dosing in adults with severe burn injury. Clin Ther. 2016;38(9):2016–31.
5. Greenhalgh DG, Saffle JR, Holmes JH, et al. American Burn Association consensus conference to define sepsis and infection in burns. J Burn Care Res. 2007;28(6):776–90.
6. Bone RC, Balk RA, Cerra FB, et al. American College of Chest Physicians/Society of Critical Care Medicine Consensus Conference: definitions for sepsis and organ failure and guidelines for the use of innovative therapies in sepsis. Crit Care Med. 1992;20(6):864–74.
7. Singer M, Deutschman CS, Seymour CW, et al. The third international consensus definitions for sepsis and septic shock (Sepsis-3). JAMA. 2016;315(8):801–10.
8. Vincent JL, Moreno R, Takala J, et al. The SOFA (sepsis-related organ failure assessment) score to describe organ dysfunction/failure. Inten Care Med. 1996;22:707–10.

9. Surviving Sepsis Campaign. Updated bundles in response to new evidence [Internet]. Mount Prospect: Society of Critical Care Medicine; 2015. 2 p. http://www.survivingsepsis.org/Bundles/.
10. Rhodes A, Evans LE, Alhazzani W, et al. Surviving Sepsis Campaign: international guidelines for management of sepsis and septic shock: 2016. Crit Care Med. 2017;45(3):486–552.
11. Kalil AC, Metersky ML, Klompas M, et al. Management of adults with hospital-acquired and ventilator-associated pneumonia: 2016 clinical practice guidelines by the Infectious Diseases Society of America and the American Thoracic Society. Clin Infect Dis. 2016;63(5):e61–e111.
12. Mermel LA, Allon M, Bouza E, et al. Clinical practice guidelines for the diagnosis and management of intravascular catheter-related infection: 2009 Updated by the Infectious Diseases Society of America. Clin infect Dis. 2009;49(1):1–45.
13. Murray CK, Loo FL, Hospenthal DR, et al. Incidence of systemic fungal infection and related mortality following severe burns. Burns. 2008;34(8):1108–12.
14. Pappas PG, Kaufman CA, Andes DR, Clancy CJ, Marr KA, Ostrosky-Zeichner L, Reboli AC, Schuster MG, Vazquez JA, Walsh TJ, Zaoutis TE, Sobel JD. Clinical practice guideline for the management of Candidiasis: 2016 update by the Infectious Diseases Society of America. Clin Infect Dis. 2016;62(4):e1–50.
15. Ha JF, Italiano CM, Heath CH, Shih S, Rea S, Wood FM. Candidemia and invasive candidiasis: a review of the literature for the burns surgeon. Burns. 2011;37(2):181–95.
16. Pedrosa AF, Rodrigues AG. Candidemia in burns patients: figures and facts. J Trauma. 2011;70(2):498–506.
17. Crabtree SJ, Robertson JL, Chung KK, et al. *Clostridium difficile* infections in patients with severe burns. Burns. 2011;37:42–8.
18. Finnerty CC, Herndon DN, Lee JO, et al. Morbidity and mortality in severely burned children with *Clostridium difficile*-associated diarrhea. Surgery. 2016;159:1631–7.
19. Regules JA, Glasser JS, Wolf SE, et al. Endocarditis in burn patients: clinical and diagnostic considerations. Burns. 2008;34:610–6.
20. Kagan RJ, Naraqi S, Matsuda T, et al. Herpes simplex virus and cytomegalovirus infections in burned patients. J Trauma. 1985;25(1):40–5.
21. Boucher BA, Wood GC, Swanson JM. Pharmacokinetic changes in critical illness. Crit Care Clin. 2006;22:255–71.
22. Bauer LA. Applied clinical pharmacokinetics. 3rd ed. Chicago: McGraw Hill Medical; 2001. p. 3–27. Chapter 1, Clinical pharmacokinetic and pharmacodynamics concepts.
23. Smith BS, Yogaratnam D, Levasseur-Franklin KE, et al. Introduction to drug pharmacokinetics in the critically ill patient. Chest. 2012;141(5):1327–36.
24. Blanchet B, Jullien V, Vinsonneau C, Tod M. Influence of burns on pharmacokinetics and pharmacodynamics of drugs used in the care of burn patients. Clin Pharmacokinet. 2008;47(10):635–54.
25. Weinbren MJ. Pharmacokinetics of antibiotics in burn patients. J Antimicrob Chemother. 1999;44:319–27.
26. Akers KS, Cota JM, Chung KK, et al. Serum vancomycin levels resulting from continuous or intermittent infusion in critically ill burn patients with or without continuous renal replacement therapy. J Burn Care Res. 2012;33:e254–62.
27. Lovering AM, Le Floch R, Hovsepian L, et al. Pharmacokinetic evaluation of linezolid in patients with major thermal injuries. J Antimicrob Chemother. 2009;63(3):553–9.
28. Mohr JF, Ostrosky-Zeichner L, Wainright DJ, et al. Pharmacokinetic evaluation of single-dose intravenous daptomycin in patients with thermal burn injury. Antimicrob Agents Chemother. 2008;52(5):1891–3.
29. Asensio MJ, Sanchez M, Galvan B, et al. Micafungin at a standard dosage of 100 mg/day achieves adequate plasma exposure in critically ill patients with severe burn injuries. Intensive Care Med. 2015;41(2):371–2.
30. Neofytos D, Huang YT, Cheng K, et al. Safety and efficacy of intermittent intravenous administration of high-dose micafungin. Clin Infect Dis. 2015;61(Suppl 6):S652–61.

Perioperative Care of the Burned Patient

24

Jamie L. Sparling, J. A. Jeevendra Martyn, and Erik S. Shank

24.1 Introduction

Each year, approximately 486,000 people seek treatment for burn injury in the United States, including 40,000 patients who are hospitalized and 3275 patients who die from burn injuries.[1] Approximately 60% of these patients are cared for in 1 of 128 national burn centers. Anesthesiologists, in both burn centers and other hospitals, play a critical role in addressing the early challenges of treating acute burn injury, including leveraging expertise in airway management, vascular access, and hemodynamic and pulmonary support. Additionally, many anesthesiologists will care for burn patients in the operating theater during both acute and chronic phases of burn injury. Thus, it is critical that anesthesiologists understand the pathophysiology of major burn injury and resuscitation. A brief overview of these topics is presented here, but several specific areas including inhalation injury and fluid resuscitation will be discussed in a more detailed fashion elsewhere. Non-anesthesiologists can benefit from applying many of these same principles in the intensive care unit during acute perioperative care.

[1]American Burn Association: Burn incidence and treatment in the US: 2016 fact sheet. Available at: http://ameriburn.org/who-we-are/media/burn-incidence-fact-sheet/. Accessed June 14, 2017.

J. L. Sparling
Department of Anesthesiology, Critical Care and Pain Medicine, Harvard Medical School, Massachusetts General Hospital, Boston, MA, USA
e-mail: jlsparling@partners.org

J. A. J. Martyn (✉)
Clinical and Biochemical Pharmacology Laboratory, Harvard Medical School, Massachusetts General Hospital, Shriners Hospital for Children, Boston, MA, USA
e-mail: jmartyn@mgh.harvard.edu

E. S. Shank
Harvard Medical School, Massachusetts General Hospital, Shriners Hospital for Children, Boston, MA, USA
e-mail: esshank@mgh.harvard.edu

24.2 Anesthetic Considerations by System

24.2.1 Cardiovascular

Immediately following a major burn injury (>20–25% total body surface area [TBSA]), cardiac output is significantly reduced due to the burn size-dependent decline in effective blood volume, a decrease in cardiac contractility, and often the compressive effects of circumferential burns of chest and abdomen which impair venous return [1, 2]. During this period, patients may require inotropic support to improve cardiac output while avoiding volume overload. Transesophageal echocardiography (TEE) may be used to guide supportive care during this initial phase [3]. In many cases, cardiac output may remain depressed despite adequate volume resuscitation; this is hypothesized to be due to myocardial depression from inflammatory mediators released as a result of the burn injury, as well as the increased systemic vascular resistance secondary to the release of antidiuretic hormone (vasopressin) and pain- and anxiety-induced catecholamines [4]. The hemoconcentration and the associated increase in viscosity add to the increased systemic vascular resistance.

Within 3–5 days following an acute burn injury, the hypermetabolic/hyperdynamic phase begins, and the cardiac output increases greater than two- to threefold; this persists for weeks to months, particularly in previously healthy patients with burns involving more than 40% of total body surface area (TBSA) [2]. If decreased cardiac output is observed, investigation should be made to rule out sepsis or hypovolemia. A reversible cardiomyopathy may also occur. Hypertension may occur during this phase, but pain is a common cause. In the setting of adequate pain control, hypertension can be due to increased levels of catecholamines, atrial natriuretic factor, endothelin-1, and vasopressin and activation of the renin–angiotensin system (RAS) [5, 6]. Propranolol may be used to decrease cardiac work and mitigate the systemic vascular response during this period [7]. Cardiac output usually declines with the decrease in metabolic demand associated with wound closure, but elevations may persist for up to 2 years [8].

M. G. Jeschke et al. (eds.), *Handbook of Burns Volume 1*, https://doi.org/10.1007/978-3-030-18940-2_24

24.2.2 Pulmonary

Burn injury may affect the entire respiratory tract, from the upper airways to the terminal alveoli, with upper airway damage generally a result of thermal injury, whereas lower airway damage generally because of chemical injury from inhalation of toxic gases and smoke. Inhalation injury should be suspected in all house (non-open) fires, particularly in the presence of singed nasal hairs or nasal passages, and may occur even in the absence of any external injury. The presence of inhalation injury compounds the prognosis from a cutaneous burn and markedly increases mortality rate.

Cooling of inspired superheated air may cause thermal injury to the larynx and result in massive edema formation, which can lead to airway obstruction, sometimes resembling epiglottitis. More distally, the thermal insult affects the ciliated epithelium and mucosa of the proximal bronchi. The distal bronchi and alveoli are injured from nitric acid and sulfuric acid, which are formed from the reaction of water vapor with inhaled nitrogen dioxide and sulfur dioxide, respectively. Additionally, hydrochloric acid, sulfuric acid, and phosgene travel to the distal tracheobronchial tree as aerosols where they cause direct injury to the alveolar membrane and disrupt surfactant. Aldehydes formed from the combustion of cotton and wool can cause pulmonary edema in concentrations as low as 10 ppm [9]. Cyanide formed from the combustion of synthetic materials (such as insulation and wall paneling) can cause histotoxic hypoxia and death and may be a cause of immediate death [10]. Carbon monoxide (CO) poisoning must always be suspected in house fires.

The net result of inhalation injury is a bronchopneumonia characterized by necrotizing bronchitis, bronchial swelling, alveolar destruction, loss of surfactant, and bronchospasm. Mechanical obstruction can also occur due to inhalation of particulate matter or denudation of bronchial mucosal epithelium. The loss of integrity of the pulmonary capillary endothelium can cause non-cardiogenic pulmonary edema, and this together with bronchial edema reduces pulmonary compliance. Chest wall compliance can be also reduced in cases of circumferential chest burns [1]. The result is ventilation–perfusion mismatch and increase in intrapulmonary shunting, which may be mitigated by the optimization of the functional residual capacity (FRC) through application of positive end expiratory pressure (PEEP) and recruitment maneuvers in ventilated patients. Insult to the respiratory system alone may cause hypoxemia, but other factors including the aforementioned changes in cardiac output together with pericapillary leak may play a role in the development of cardiogenic pulmonary edema and resultant hypoxemia. The P_aO_2/F_iO_2 ratio and baseline carboxyhemoglobin levels are predictive of mortality. Inhaled heparin and acetylcysteine are controversial therapies, with initial trials demonstrating a reduction in airway cast formation and mucus plugging, while subsequent studies have failed to demonstrate efficacy [11].

At the cellular level, not only does CO inhalation reduce the oxygen carrying capacity of hemoglobin, it also impairs cellular respiration. CO binds to hemoglobin with 200–250 times greater affinity, compared with oxygen. The result is a leftward-shift of the oxyhemoglobin dissociation curve, and reduced oxygen delivery to the tissues. The deleterious effects of CO inhalation are further amplified in pregnant women; fetal hemoglobin undergoes an exaggerated left shift and the minimal competition from oxygen to displace CO because of lower placental p_aO_2 and results in less CO being driven from hemoglobin and worsened tissue hypoxia in the fetus.

24.2.3 Renal

Both myoglobinuria and hemoglobinuria may play a role in renal injury following an acute burn. Myoglobinuria is more common after electrical burns, while hemoglobinuria is more common following cutaneous burns. Acute tubular necrosis may occur secondary to the hypovolemia, hypotension, and hypoxemia common in acute injuries, as described above. Further, a surge of catecholamines, activation of the renin–angiotensin system, upregulation of vasopressin receptors, and release of vasoactive peptides such as endothelin-1 and vasopressin together produce systemic vasoconstriction and worsening pre-renal injury [12]. As a result of this, fluid retention is commonly seen in the first 2–5 days following an acute burn, which is then followed by a diuresis. After this acute stage, glomerular filtration rate (GFR) increases in conjunction with increased cardiac output and basal metabolic rate. The GFR is high even in hypovolemic states, resulting in continued urine output. This will be reflected by an elevation in the blood urea nitrogen (BUN) to creatinine ratio greater than 20. Throughout an acute burn injury, compromised renal function (due to inadequate fluid resuscitation or sepsis) may delay excretion of many drugs and their active metabolites; as GFR improves, care must be taken to accurately dose medications during rapid changes in renal function. Assessment of laboratory values including the BUN, creatinine, and urine electrolytes, as well as ratios including the BUN/creatinine ratio and fractional excretion of sodium and/or urea (FE_{Na} and FE_{Urea}, respectively) may help to distinguish pre-renal versus intrinsic renal dysfunction. However, care must be taken in interpreting these values during periods of rapid evolution. Renal tubular dysfunction may persist, resulting in poor renal concentrating ability; thus, as indicated above, urine output may be a poor indicator of volume status. Additionally, hypertension may persist following burn injuries, due to prolonged activation of the renin–angiotensin system and increased catecholamine release; this should prompt treatment to reduce episodes of hypertensive encephalopathy and prevent longer term stress on the heart due to elevated afterload.

24.2.4 Hepatic

Early liver damage may occur due to "shock liver" as a result of hypoperfusion, due to direct toxic injury from inhaled toxins, or as a consequence of reperfusion injury once adequate circulation is reestablished. The increased gut permeability associated with burn injury allows bacterial translocation and inflammatory responses in the liver with aberrant metabolic function. Later liver dysfunction may occur from iatrogenic drug toxicity, blood transfusions, sepsis, or the hypermetabolic response to burns, which entails increased protein synthesis and degradation, as well as increased hepatic gluconeogenesis [13]. Sepsis can dramatically reduce hepatic glucose output and alanine uptake, while hepatic blood flow and oxygen consumption remain elevated [14]. Fatty liver infiltration can also occur due to the marked increase in peripheral lipolysis during the hypermetabolic response, even in the absence of total parental nutrition [15].

With transition to the hypermetabolic phase, increased hepatic blood flow and enzyme induction together may decrease the half-life of perfusion-dependent (e.g., lidocaine, fentanyl) and enzyme-dependent (methadone, diazepam) drugs, respectively [16]. Clinical studies of the same drugs, however, may be conflicting, due to variation in the magnitude of burns, timeframe following a burn, co-administration of drugs, protein-binding, and volume of distribution.

24.2.5 Central Nervous System

Injury to the central nervous system (CNS) may occur from inhalation of neurotoxic chemicals, hypoxic encephalopathy, sepsis, hyponatremia, or hypovolemia. Such injury, together with side effects from pharmacologic therapy, may manifest as coma, delirium, seizures, focal neurologic symptoms, hallucinations, or personality changes. As many burn patients are unresponsive at the scene of injury, a neurologic "baseline" exam is essential prior to administration of sedation or anesthesia. Cerebral edema and elevated intracranial pressure may contribute to CNS dysfunction during the initial phase; should this be suspected, prompt neurologic and/or neurosurgical consultation should be sought and treatment to decrease ICP instituted immediately. Severely burned patients appear to be especially susceptible to central pontine myelinolysis when rapid overcorrection of hyponatremia occurs [17]. Extensive burn injury also appears to confer patients with significant anorexia, which is thought to be related to regional aberration of the central amine neurotransmitters (serotonin, norepinephrine, and dopamine) [18].

24.2.6 Hematologic

Prior to adequate fluid resuscitation, hemoconcentration may occur, as well as alteration in plasma protein content, the net effect of which is an increase in blood viscosity. About 48 h following the injury and subsequent resuscitation, anemia may occur secondary to both microangiopathic hemolytic anemia and a decline in hematopoiesis [19], as well as iatrogenically due to multiple blood withdrawals. The role of recombinant erythropoietin is controversial, with one study suggesting a lower transfusion rate for those who received erythropoietin, but no randomized controlled trial to date demonstrates any impact on mortality [20].

Initially, thrombocytopenia often occurs due to platelet aggregation and trapping of platelets in the lungs. This is usually followed by in an increase in platelets 10–14 days following the burn, but in some cases the thrombocytopenia persists for months. Both a lower nadir of platelet count and a longer period of thrombocytopenia are associated with increased mortality [21]. Patients are at increased risk for disseminated intravascular coagulopathy (DIC) for the first 3–5 days. In patients with elevated platelet counts, the sudden onset of thrombocytopenia has been associated with the onset of sepsis [22]; while fibrinogen concentrations can likewise fluctuate, they do not appear to herald an increase in thrombotic events [23].

24.2.7 Gastrointestinal

Gastric stasis and intestinal ileus begin to occur immediately following the initial injury, which should trigger prompt decompression of the stomach and appropriate gastric acid ulcer prophylaxis. As generalized edema, as well as bowel edema, begins to resolve at approximately 2–3 days following an injury, gastrointestinal function should improve, and enteral feeding should be established. Early enteral feeding not only provides caloric intake but also blunts the hypermetabolic response, attenuates gluconeogenesis, prevents stress ulceration, diminishes muscle catabolism, and reduces bacteria translocation into the systemic circulation. The net result of early enteral feeding is a reduction in mortality and decreased catabolic state [24]. If nasogastric feeding is not tolerated, alternatives such as nasojejunal feeds should be pursued [25]; if, however, enteral feeding is not possible, parental nutrition should be initiated promptly [26]. Although Curling's ulcers, or stress ulcers, are classically associated with burn injury, their incidence has declined substantially due to improved pharmacologic prophylaxis and better resuscitation methods. In burn patients, larger or more frequent doses of H_2-receptor antagonists or proton pump inhibitors may be required due to increased clearance of these drugs in this population [27]. Some institutions continue enteral feeding even during anesthesia and surgery, provided the enteral tube is post-pyloric.

24.2.8 Endocrine

The stress associated with thermal injury, as well as the subsequent fluid shifts, induces endocrine responses as seen with other critical illnesses. Triiodothyronine (T3), dehydroepiandrosterone (DHEA), and testosterone levels decline, while levels of antidiuretic hormone (ADH), the renin–angiotensin system (RAS), cortisol, and catecholamines increase [28]. Replacement of testosterone with analogs, such as oxandrolone, has been shown to reduce hospital length of stay, reduce lean body mass loss, improve body composition, and increase hepatic protein synthesis [29]. Hyperglycemia may result from both the increased cortisol levels and associated insulin resistance. Tight glucose control is shown to decrease the rate of urinary tract infections and may improve survival, as well as reduce the muscle catabolic state [30]. Insulin resistance may persist for some time following initial injury, as long as 6–9 months.

Many burn patients develop hypocalcemia due to abnormalities in both calcium and magnesium metabolism, as well as hypoparathyroidism due to a reduced set point for calcium suppression of PTH secretion [31]. Pamidronate, a bisphosphonate, has been shown to preserve bone mass after burn injury, thought to be due to inhibition of glucocorticoid-induced apoptosis of osteoblasts and osteocytes [32]. While hypophosphatemia and hypermagnesemia tend to resolve in the latter phase of recovery, hypocalcemia often persists, and the usual reciprocal relationship between calcium and phosphate is disrupted. Calcium replacement is vital, particularly with rapid colloid infusions intraoperatively (especially fresh frozen plasma), which may cause citrate toxicity and resultant hypocalcemia. Ionized hypocalcemia can severely impair cardiovascular function and manifest as severe hypotension or even cardiac arrest. Calcium chloride or calcium gluconate are shown to produce equivalent increases in calcium concentration; small, frequent boluses are safer than intermittent large boluses [33].

24.2.9 Skin

Severe burns can impair the skin's ability to regulate body heat, block bacterial entry, and maintain fluid and electrolyte homeostasis. The number of tissue layers injured correlates directly with the permeability of burned tissues. Mechanisms to preserve body heat include elevating the ambient temperature, use of radiant warmers, plastic coverings around the extremities, reflective insulated blankets, hot-air warming blankets, and in-line heat-and-moisture exchangers in breathing circuits. Contractures may result as a late complication, which may impair respiratory excursion, limit mouth opening (microstomia), and create difficult vascular access [1]. Topical antimicrobial therapies have been shown to play an important role in the prevention of sepsis secondary to wound infection [34].

24.2.10 Metabolic

Acute burn victims have increased oxygen demand and carbon dioxide production secondary to increased metabolism of glucose, fat, and protein. These changes are mediated by interleukin-1 (IL-1), tumor necrosis factor (TNF), catecholamines, prostanoids, and other stress hormones. Hyperthermia from sepsis or centrally mediated hyperthermia will further increase oxygen consumption and carbon dioxide production. This hypermetabolic period can persist even beyond complete closure of the wounds. Parenteral nutrition rich in carbohydrates may also contribute to increased carbon dioxide production, thereby requiring a higher minute ventilation to adequately maintain normocapnia [35]. Fever or shivering due to cold environment can further increase energy expenditure and muscle protein catabolism, suggesting a benefit to treatment with antipyretics in such patients. Postoperatively, the use of meperidine will help mitigate the shivering.

24.2.11 Psychiatric

Psychological trauma may accompany the physical trauma sustained by burn patients. As many as 35% of children sustaining a significant burn injury may develop an acute stress disorder or posttraumatic stress disorder (PTSD) [36]. Increased size of the burn, increased pain, higher pulse rates, and the presence of parental stress symptoms directly correlate with the rate of development of PTSD [37]. Anesthesia providers must be aware of and plan for associated anxiety relief in burn patients who present for repeated procedures to the operating theater.

24.2.12 Specific Pediatric Considerations

Children represent a large proportion of patients presenting with severe burns injuries. The rule of nines applied to adult patients cannot be directly applied to pediatric patients as the surface area for different parts of the body are different. As discussed above, maintenance of body temperature is made difficult by the compromise in the skin's integrity. Because children have a much greater ratio of body surface area to mass compared with adults, they are even more likely to become hypothermic. Because of the greater baseline oxygen consumption in infants and children, as compared to adults, the increase in oxygen demand due to hypermetabolism is accentuated. As a result, pediatric burn patients may desaturate quickly necessitating the need for swift airway management. Fluid requirements are also increased in children, with evaporative fluid losses exceeding 4000 mL/m^2 of burned surface daily, compared with 2500 mL/m^2 in an adult [38]. Further, intravenous access in children may be already difficult, and it is often further complicated by burns affecting a large TBSA. Children may require general anesthetics in order to tolerate dressing and line changes during the acute period, as well as for laser therapy to treat contractures and scarring in the long-term. Both children and their caregivers may present with heightened anxiety in the perioperative setting. Pediatric patients may particularly benefit from oral premedication or intravenous premedication if an intravenous line is already present. In addition to burn-induced pathophysiological changes, the altered physiology and pharmacology of pediatric patients compared to adults must be kept in mind.

Pediatric burn patients may require repeat general anesthetics in both the acute and chronic phases of burn injury (e.g., for debridement, excision and grafting, and scar revisions). There is concern for negative neurocognitive impact from repeated exposure to general anesthetics in early childhood development, based upon multiple animal studies demonstrating cumulative dose-dependent neurotoxicity. Because of this growing body of evidence, the SmartTots and the American Academy of Pediatrics (AAP) released a statement in 2012 recommending deferring elective anesthetics in children under 3 years of age [39]. This research has also prompted randomized controlled trials in humans to further elucidate the safety of general anesthesia in pediatric patients, notably the GAS trial (General Anesthesia compared to Spinal Anesthesia). To date, the GAS trial has demonstrated no increase in the risk of adverse neurodevelopmental outcomes at 2 years of age for patients exposed to a single general anesthetic in infancy [40]. Clinical trials in humans examining this impact for repeat exposure, however, have not been conducted.

24.2.13 Specific Geriatric Considerations

The elderly are also at increased risk for burn injury due to both physical and cognitive limitations. These patients may present with a number of significant comorbidities. In the geriatric patient, the hypermetabolic phase, which normally begins about 72 h after injury, may be delayed or not occur. When it does occur, the increase in cardiac output may be poorly tolerated by patients with underlying ischemic heart disease; further, patients with pre-existing diastolic dysfunction are at heightened risk for pulmonary edema as a result of fluid resuscitation and pericapillary leak in the immediate post-burn period. Impaired renal and hepatic functions at baseline may limit clearance of anesthetics, analgesics, and sedatives administered during the acute injury. The elderly are also at increased risk of postoperative delirium that may persist even after discharge from hospital [41]. Strategies to mitigate the risk of postoperative delirium include non-pharmacologic interventions to reorient patients, maximization of non-opioid analgesics, avoidance of benzodiazepines, and use of processed EEG monitoring to tailor depth of anesthesia.

24.3 Pharmacologic Considerations in the Burn Patient

Following a major burn injury (>40% TBSA), a number of physiological derangements exist affecting both pharmacodynamics (i.e., the effect a drug has on the body) and pharmacokinetics (i.e., the effect the body has on the drug). During the initial phase, clearance may be compromised due to impaired organ perfusion as a result of hypovolemia, depressed cardiac function, decreased systemic vascular resistance secondary to the release of vasoactive substances, and increased blood viscosity [16, 42]. The subsequent hypermetabolic phase is characterized by enhanced clearance secondary to hepatic enzyme induction and increased hepatic and renal blood flow [14, 16, 27].

For drugs which are bound to plasma proteins, their activity depends on the unbound portion, so small changes in the unbound fraction may result in a large clinical effect. Plasma protein concentrations are altered during burn injury, with the serum albumin concentrations decreased, while the α_1-acid glycoprotein concentration, an acute phase reactant, increased. Thus, the free concentration of albumin-bound drugs, including benzodiazepines and antiepileptics, is effectively increased, while α_1-acid glycoprotein-bound drugs (e.g., neuromuscular relaxants, tricyclic antidepressants) are more highly bound with a decreased free fraction [16, 43]. The volume of distribution may also be increased due to edema, requiring increased bolus doses and higher maintenance infusion rates of many medications.

24.3.1 Tolerance and Contraindications

The effects of receptor-mediated drug effects may be altered due to the up- or downregulation of receptors during acute burn injury and the subsequent hormonal response. For example, there is an increased sensitivity to succinylcholine

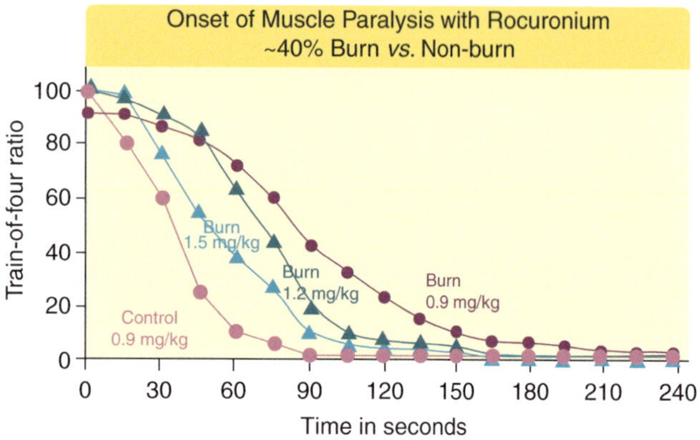

Fig. 24.1 Dose–response curves for rocuronium in burned and non-burned adults. On the *y*-axis, the train-of-four (TOF) ratio is represented as the percentage of twitch suppression between the fourth and first twitch at 2 Hz. Burned adults with mean 40% TBSA burns, at least 1 week following the burn injury, were studied at 0.9, 1.2, and 1.5 mg/kg rocuronium. In controls (non-burned adults), rocuronium administration is shown at a dose of 0.9 mg/kg, resulting in a 95% twitch suppression in ≤60 s. In the burned adults, a similar dose required >120 s for 95% twitch suppression. A dose of 1.5 mg/kg still required >90 s for 95% twitch suppression

at the neuromuscular junction due to de novo expression of extrajunctional acetylcholine receptors, and it is well studied that use of a depolarizing neuromuscular blocker greater than 72 h after a burn injury may result in life-threatening hyperkalemia [44]. The presence of upregulated extrajunctional receptors, particularly the expression of α-7 acetylcholine receptors, plays an important role in the resistance to the neuromuscular effects of non-depolarizing blockers [44]. Figure 24.1 demonstrates tolerance to the effect of rocuronium in patients with a mean 40% TBSA burn. While normal patients achieve >95% twitch suppression in ≤90 s at a dose of 0.9 mg/kg, the burn patients studied had onset >120 s with the same dose. Further, even at a dose of 1.5 mg/kg, onset is still >90 s [45]. Severe burns are also associated with an increased sensitivity to dopamine in the pulmonary circulation [46]. Clearance of aminoglycosides, such as gentamicin, is increased resulting in inadequate serum concentrations unless larger and more frequent doses are administered [47]. Despite a greater free fraction of diazepam in burn patients, the clearance is reduced and repeated administrations may result in significant accumulation [48]. The clearance of lorazepam is increased in major burns. Clearance of H_2-receptor antagonists, such as cimetidine and ranitidine, which are renally cleared, is increased [27]. Thus, patients require increased doses to adequately achieve prophylaxis against stress ulcers. Both the volume of distribution and the clearance of fentanyl and propofol are increased, thus increasing the dosage required to produce adequate analgesia. However, high bolus doses may cause hypotension in the hypovolemic patient. These pharmacologic changes are summarized in Table 24.1.

Table 24.1 Pharmacokinetic alterations in burn injury

Medication class	Pharmacokinetic alteration in burn injury
Depolarizing neuromuscular blockers	Increased sensitivity (contraindicated after 72 h)
Non-depolarizing neuromuscular blockers	Resistance (seen usually after 72 h)
Aminoglycosides	Increased clearance
Benzodiazepines	Variable clearance depending on metabolic pathway
H_2-antagonists	Increased clearance
Opioids	Increased clearance, increased volume of distribution (morphine and fentanyl) and unknown for methadone

Dexmedetomidine, a selective α_2-antagonist, may be used for sedation and analgesia in critically ill burn patients, as well as an adjunct agent during or premedication prior to a general anesthetic, particularly in opioid tolerant patients. A recent meta-analysis concludes that dexmedetomidine may provide deeper sedation and prevent hypertension in burn patients, but due to the known hypotensive potential, it is important to ensure euvolemia and limit total dosage administered to prevent hypotension [49]. Because the alterations in pharmacokinetics make the response to any medication somewhat unpredictable, clinical effects should be closely monitored, and guided by laboratory analysis of plasma concentration whenever possible.

24.3.2 Multimodal Sedation and Analgesia Guidelines

Critically ill burned patients will often require a multimodal approach to address both pain and anxiety, and this approach may need modulation over time due to changes in sensitivity threshold and development of tolerance. Continuous opioid infusions may cause opioid-induced hyperalgesia, tolerance, and thus compounding the need for subsequent opioids. Treatment of opioid tolerance may include opioid rotation and co-administration of non-opioid analgesics including acetaminophen, NMDA-antagonists (i.e., ketamine), α_2-antagonists (i.e., dexmedetomidine or clonidine), gabapentanoids, and/or local anesthetics. Many burn centers utilize a standardized, protocol-based approach to provide appropriate care of pain and sedation [50]. It is important that such guidelines meet the following criteria: (1) safety and efficacy over a broad range of age and injury severity, (2) establish explicit recommendations for drug choice, initial dose selection, and dose titration, (3) a limited formulary to promote familiarity, and (4) regular assessment of pain and anxiety. An example of such guidelines is shown in Table 24.2. Daily interruption of analgesics/sedatives allows patients to be awake, allows better assessment and treatment of pain, and is associated with fewer ventilator days.

Table 24.2 Examples of sedation and analgesia guidelines

Stage of injury	Baseline anxiolysis	Baseline analgesia	Procedural anxiolysis	Procedural analgesia
Acute burn, mechanically ventilated	1. Midazolam infusion 2. Dexmedetomidine infusion 3. Antipsychotics 4. Propofol infusion (use for <48 h)	Morphine or fentanyl infusion	1. Midazolam boluses 2. Higher dexmedetomidine infusion 3. Slow haloperidol boluses 4. Propofol boluses	Morphine or fentanyl boluses
Acute burn, not mechanically ventilated	Dexmedetomidine (IV) or scheduled lorazepam (IV or PO)	Morphine (IV or PO) or fentanyl (IV)	Lorazepam (IV or PO)	Morphine (IV or PO) or fentanyl (IV) or ketamine (IV)
Chronic acute burn	Scheduled lorazepam (PO) or antipsychotics	Scheduled morphine or methadone	Lorazepam or antipsychotics	Morphine (PO) or oxycodone

24.4 Anesthetic Care of the Burn Patient

24.4.1 Airway Management

Both acute injuries and chronic sequelae following burns may make airway management difficult. Factors that contribute to this difficulty include macroglossia or direct thermal injury to the glottis and airways during the acute phase, as well as limited mouth opening and neck motion due to contractures in the subacute to chronic phase [51]. Burn victims who sustained injury in a closed space have increased likelihood of airway injury. Signs of inhalational injury include vocal changes, stridor, or hoarseness, and these may be an important predictor of difficult intubation. Fiberoptic intubation may be used on the "awake" but sedated patient. Dexmedetomidine may be used to provide sedation without respiratory depression, while preventing large sympathetic responses to the procedure. For patients with macroglossia secondary to edema, manual distraction of the tongue and jaw lift can be helpful. Suction or gauze may be utilized to aid with grasping the tongue for such a maneuver [52]. Laryngeal mask airway may also be placed once general anesthesia is induced and used to ventilate the patient while the bronchoscope is guided through the LMA lumen. LMA-aided intubation may be especially useful in the case of perioral edema. Additional techniques include the use of retrograde wires following tracheotomy or tracheostomy, fiber-optic "stylets" that can fit through narrow mouth openings, as well as light-wand-guided intubations. In cases with a severe neck or oral contractions, the patient may be induced with an agent, such as ketamine, that will maintain spontaneous ventilation; following induction, the surgeon may release the contracture facilitating airway instrumentation. Since awake or moderate sedation intubation is not possible in children, ketamine seems the best choice for intubation in pediatric patients, since the pharyngeal tone is well maintained while also maintaining spontaneous breathing efforts.

24.4.2 Vascular Access

Vascular access in burned patients may be technically difficult due to large TBSA affected by the burn itself, peripheral edema resulting from massive fluid resuscitation, and multiple graft harvest sites occupying much of the unaffected skin. Both peripheral and central venous access, as well as arterial cannulation, may be achieved more safely and rapidly under ultrasonic guidance [53]. Although internal jugular cannulation is preferred for central venous access to minimize the risk of pneumothorax, alternate sites could include the subclavian or femoral veins. At times, it may be necessary to place catheters through burn wounds; in such cases, it is extremely important to meticulously prepare the area with antiseptic solutions just prior to placement of the catheter. Additionally, venous cannulation in burn patients comes with increased risks of bloodstream infection, as well as deep venous thrombosis due to prior venous cannulations, prolonged immobility, and hypercoagulability. Ultrasound guidance may help to diagnose the presence of an in situ clot, thereby avoiding futile attempts at cannulation at that site. Placement of central venous and arterial catheters under controlled conditions in the operating room is associated with a low rate of mechanical (0.3%) and thrombotic (0.6%) complications [53]. If no intravenous access can be obtained, patients of any age may receive a temporary intraosseous (IO) line until an alternative is available. Additionally, IO is our preferred method for emergent access should IV access be needed urgently or lost intraoperatively. One such scenario would be laryngospasm in a burned patient with no IV access.

24.4.3 Evaluation of Volume Status/Fluid Resuscitation

Prompt intravascular volume resuscitation is necessary to address acute shock in severe burn injury, in order to prevent hypovolemia and subsequent tissue hypoperfusion and multiple organ failure. Additionally, lung microvascular permeability changes seen with smoke inhalation are made

Burn Estimate and Diagram
Age and Area

Initital evaluation*

Signature: ______________________

Date of burn: ______________________

Date completed: ______________________

*To be completed by the admitting physician or Licensed Independent Practitioner on admission

This is a working burn estimate diagram only, and is not as accurate as photography.

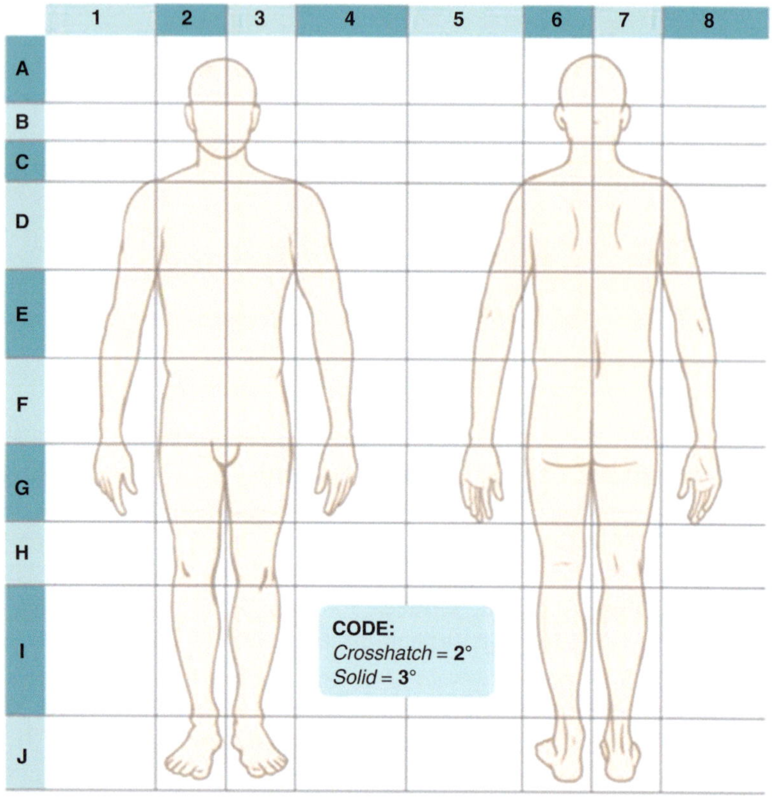

Area	Birth-1 yr.	1-4 yrs.	5-9 yrs.	10-14 yrs.	15 yrs.	Adult	2°	3°	TOTAL
Head	9	17	13	11	9	7			
Neck	2	2	2	2	2	2			
Anterior trunk	13	13	13	13	13	13			
Posterior trunk	13	13	13	13	13	13			
Right buttock	2.5	2.5	2.5	2.5	2.5	2.5			
Left buttock	2.5	2.5	2.5	2.5	2.5	2.5			
Genitalia	1	1	1	1	1	1			
Right upper arm	4	4	4	4	4	4			
Left upper arm	4	4	4	4	4	4			
Right lower arm	3	3	3	3	3	3			
Left lower arm	3	3	3	3	3	3			
Right hand	2.5	2.5	2.5	2.5	2.5	2.5			
Left hand	2.5	2.5	2.5	2.5	2.5	2.5			
Right thigh	5.5	6.5	8	8.5	9	9.5			
Left thigh	5.5	6.5	8	8.5	9	9.5			
Right lower leg	5	5	5.5	6	6.5	7			
Left lower leg	5	5	5.5	6	6.5	7			
Right foot	3.5	3.5	3.5	3.5	3.5	3.5			
Left foot	3.5	3.5	3.5	3.5	3.5	3.5			
***Only 2° and 3° burns are included in the total TBSA burn percent*						*TOTAL*			

Fig. 24.2 Lund–Browder burn diagram and table. The Lund–Browder burn diagram and table indicate the varying proportions in surface area across different ages. A diagram such as this one should be completed at the initial presentation to document the estimated size, location, and depth of a burn

worse by inadequate fluid resuscitation. However, overly aggressive fluid resuscitation may result in pulmonary, intestinal, and peripheral edema.

In order to guide adequate fluid resuscitation, it is necessary to estimate the percentage total body surface area (TBSA) affected by the burn. In adults, the "rules of nines" may be used, but because body proportions vary with age, the Lund–Browder burn diagram (see Fig. 24.2) may be a useful aid in estimating the % TBSA in children [54]. This can then be applied using the fluid resuscitation formulae below.

Table 24.3 Indicators of adequate fluid resuscitation

Parameter	Target
Urine output	0.5–1 mL/kg/h
Blood pressure	Within normal limits (adjusted for age in children)
Heart rate	Within normal limits (when pain and anxiety are adequately addressed)
Central venous pressure	3–8 mmHg
Fractional excretion of sodium (FE_{Na})	>1% (lower values suggest pre-renal injury and hypovolemia)
BUN/Cr ratio	<20 (ratio >20 suggests maximal resorption of BUN and hypovolemia)
Base deficit	<5 (larger values suggest hypoperfusion in the absence of carbon monoxide or cyanide poisoning)

Several methods are available for guiding initial fluid resuscitation; however, these are estimates and require modification based on clinical and laboratory parameters, the most important of which is an adequate urine output (see Table 24.3). It is important to note, however, that urine output may be deceivingly low owing to the elevated level of antidiuretic hormone seen in acute burn injury [55].

Conversely, high urine output has been seen in spite of hypovolemia, because of the osmotic effects of breakdown products and the increased GFR with tubular dysfunction. Often serum BUN to creatinine ratio of >20 indicates hypovolemia. In patients in whom these traditional measures are difficult to interpret, novel methods may aid in assessing fluid status. In addition to transthoracic echocardiography (TTE) or transesophageal echocardiography (TEE) [3], technetium-99m ventriculography has been used in burn patients to diagnose and treat low cardiac output states [56]. More recently, esophageal Doppler monitoring has been applied to burn shock resuscitation [57]. Noninvasive ultrasound-based cardiac output monitors (applied via a suprasternal or pulmonary window) have been piloted in other critically ill patients and may hold promise in burn patients, but their applicability will be limited in patients with burns affecting the chest and thorax [58].

Burns less than 15% TBSA may be treated with either oral or IV fluids administered at a rate 50% greater than the maintenance rate. For larger burns, the Parkland (Baxter) and Brooke formulae are the most commonly used guides. Both formulae may underestimate fluid needs in infants less than 10 kg. In these children, one may calculate the maintenance fluid requirements and add this to the amount suggested by either the Parkland or Brooke formulas, or one may modify the infusion volumes based on clinical responses.

When using crystalloid, often Lactated Ringer's is chosen over normal saline given the hyperchloremic metabolic acidosis that may occur with massive administration of the latter solution. Alternatively, use of colloid may reduce the degree of peripheral edema that occurs with massive fluid resuscitation. Traditionally, the Parkland formula advocated a transition to colloid after the initial 24 h, but many burn centers have begun colloid administration earlier in burn wound resuscitation [59]. These may be particularly advantageous in very young children and in the elderly. While a recent Cochrane review found no difference in morbidity or mortality with the use of hypertonic saline versus isotonic saline, hypertonic saline did reduce overall fluid requirements, but with an accompanying transient increase in the serum sodium [60]. Currently most burn centers do not use hypertonic saline for resuscitation. After approximately 36–48 h, the permeability of the capillary wall returns to normal in non-burned areas, and peripheral edema begins to resolve over the subsequent 1–2 weeks. During this period, fluid requirements decrease and diuretics administered as needed to help mobilize the edema.

Severe burn patients are at increased risk for hyperosmolar, hyperglycemic non-ketotic coma, which is characterized by severe dehydration, marked hyperglycemia, and coma in the absence of ketoacidosis. Because of this, and in light of the insulin resistance and resultant hyperglycemia seen in acute burns, glucose-containing solutions are typically avoided, though they may be used in young infants and other patients at risk for hypoglycemia.

No clear, validated transfusion threshold exists across all burn patients. In each, it is most important to maintain adequate circulation and metabolic homeostasis. A national survey of burn centers revealed that the hemoglobin level below which clinicians would transfuse increases with increased % TBSA, history of cardiac disease, presence of ARDS, and age [61]. Blood products may be used in anticipation of continued blood loss, for example, during excision and grafting procedures. In addition to packed red blood cells, it may be appropriate to administer fresh frozen plasma in anticipation of the development of coagulopathy in patients undergoing massive blood loss intraoperatively, particularly when blood transfusion approximates one blood volume.

24.4.4 Temperature Regulation

The maintenance of normal body temperature is critical in both the operating room and the intensive care unit. Particularly susceptible periods include both the initial volume resuscitation and when dressings are removed for assessment and treatment. The initial inflammatory response to severe burns causes an increase in the hypothalamic core temperature set point, and hypermetabolism occurs (as above) to maintain this increased temperature. Hypothermia causes an increase in oxygen consumption due to shivering, which can exacerbate the catabolism seen with burn injuries. The shivering also causes dislodgement of grafted tissues. In addition, hypothermia during excisions can increase blood loss secondary to coagulopathy and has been shown to increase the risk of acute lung injury [62]. Maintenance of normothermia is made more difficult by the loss of the thermal regulatory function of intact skin. Efforts to maintain adequate body temperature are essential and may include increasing the ambient temperature (often as high as 80–100 °F), use of warming blankets and radiant warmers, administration of fluids and blood products via fluid warmer, minimization of exposed skin, and wrapping exposed skin in plastic insulation.

24.4.5 Pain Management and Opioid Sparing Techniques

Pain management in burn patients can be especially challenging, as nearly all aspects of burn treatment are associated with pain, including dressing changes, excision and grafting procedures, physical and occupational therapy, daily weighing, and vascular access procedures. In general, the severity of pain is proportional to the magnitude of TBSA burned, but it is important to recognize that psychosocial factors affect the individual's experience of pain, as well. Poorly treated background pain can provoke anxiety which will exacerbate pain and lead to anticipatory procedural anxiety in a viscous cycle. Additionally, burn patients are shown to suffer from both hyperalgesia and allodynia.

Opioid administrations have been the cornerstone of pain therapy for many decades. While there has been significant fear of promoting long-term opioid addiction, treatment of adult burn patients with opioids has revealed a very low rate of addiction, and no reports of children developing addiction after therapeutic use of opioids for burn pain have been published. This research has led to some liberalization in opioid dosing to provide adequate analgesia in burn patients, but other concerns remain with respect to opioid use including opioid-induced hyperalgesia and immunosuppression. Patient-controlled analgesia (PCA) is one safe and effective mode of delivering opioids in burn injuries [63]. The presence of bandages on the hand may preclude the use of PCA. It is important to recognize that opioid tolerance will develop and appropriate dose adjustments made. Opioid requirements tend to decrease dramatically following successful closure of the thermal wounds. The most effective analgesic and anxiolytic strategy is to ensure that definitive wound closure happens as expeditiously as possible. Counter to the acute effects of sedatives, which potentiate the effects of opiates, a rodent study suggests that prolonged administration of midazolam with morphine accelerates the development of hyperalgesia [64].

Alternative or adjunct analgesics include ketamine, dexmedetomidine, gabapentin, and acetaminophen and methadone. Ketamine may have particular utility in counteracting the hyperalgesic effects of upregulated *N*-methyl-D-aspartate (NMDA) receptors seen after burn; it may be used as an adjunct analgesic intraoperatively, as a continuous infusion in the intensive care unit, or bolused for painful bedside procedures, such as dressing changes. Ketamine may also possess anti-inflammatory effects in patients with burns and/or sepsis [65] and mitigate opioid-induced hyperalgesia [66]. Dexmedetomidine is a parentally administered α_2-agonist with sedative, anxiolytic, and analgesic effects. It has been demonstrated to reduce opioid requirements postoperatively in adults [67], but while it appears to provide good sedation for pediatric burn patients, it consistently decreases mean arterial pressure and may not diminish opioid requirements in children particularly with long-term use due to the development of tolerance to dexmedetomidine [68]. Gabapentin reduces opioid consumption and lowers pain scores, with these effects extending beyond the duration of pharmacologic action, indicating a likely role in the mitigation of opioid-induced hyperalgesia [69]. While acetaminophen has a ceiling effect and is generally insufficient to adequately control burn-related pain on its own, it has proven opioid-sparing effects and should be considered in conjunction with the analgesics described above. Because of the potential for bleeding, NSAIDs (including ketorolac) are generally avoided in the acute phase of burn. Methadone, in addition to being an opioid. has multiple other sites of action enhancing analgesia. Its main downside is the variable half-life influenced by genetic and co-administered drugs [70].

Finally, the potential for a regional anesthetic should be considered in all burn cases, especially when adequate analgesia is expected to be a challenge. The benefits of regional anesthesia include not only superior intraoperative and postoperative analgesia but also facilitation of earlier rehabilitation via participation in physical and occupational therapies. Pain from a split-thickness donor site often exceeds that from the actual grafted burn wound. In cases where the size of the donor site is not excessive, the surgeon may inject tumescent local anesthesia into the donor site prior to harvesting; the size of site that may be covered with such a technique is limited by the accepted maximal local anesthetic dose (e.g., lidocaine 7 mg/kg or bupivacaine 2.5 mg/kg maximum) [71]. The placement of subcutaneous catheters to the donor sites has also been described and provided postoperative analgesia for a mean of 3.1 days [72]. Traditional peripheral nerve blocks, with or without continuous infusions via a catheter, improve postoperative pain control versus local anesthetic infiltration alone [73]. Neuraxial techniques (i.e., spinals and epidurals) may also be used with good effect, as well as truncal blocks, such as paravertebral and transversus abdominis place (TAP). The lateral femoral cutaneous block is particularly useful as the lateral thigh is frequently chosen as a donor site for split-thickness skin graft, and the block offers the advantage of being purely sensory. In cases where coverage of the anterior and medial thigh is also desired, the lateral femoral cutaneous block may be combined with a fascia iliaca block [74].

24.5 Conclusion

The perioperative care of burn patients involves complex pathophysiologic changes, which evolve throughout the course of injury and recovery. The anesthesiologist must face these challenges, anticipate alterations in pharmacodynamics and pharmacokinetics, and address the procedural complexities of airway management and obtaining venous access. Pediatric and geriatric patients require special consideration, as well. New advances in regional anesthesia/analgesia and multimodal therapies are allowing for opioid sparing while optimizing pain control. These factors are best addressed through a multidisciplinary collaboration, so that the patient may be cared for in a streamlined, coordinated fashion throughout the perioperative period.

Summary Box

Anesthesiologists often play a critical role in the initial stabilization of acute burn patients, as well as in the perioperative care of both acute and chronic burn injuries. Thus, they must understand the pathophysiological impact of large total body surface area burns on each system and adjust their anesthetic management accordingly. Both pediatric and geriatric patients are at increased risk of burn injury and merit special attention to psychologic and comorbid medical conditions. Appropriate anesthetic and analgesic medication dosing will require consideration of the stage of burn injury in order to accommodate for changes in pharmacokinetics. Tolerance is also a frequent problem with severe burn injury, prompting the anesthesiologist to pursue alternative pain and sedation regimens, incorporating multimodal and regional analgesia techniques. Finally, anesthesia providers must be prepared to address the specific challenges to airway management and vascular access posed by severe burn injuries.

References

1. Turbow ME. Abdominal compression following circumferential burn: cardiovascular responses. J Trauma. 1973;13:535–41.
2. Williams FN, et al. Changes in cardiac physiology after severe burn injury. J Burn Care Res. 2011;32(2):269–74.
3. Etherington L, Saffle J, Cochran A. Use of transesophageal echocardiography in burns: a retrospective review. J Burn Care Res. 2010;31:36–9.
4. Barret JP, Herndon DN. Modulation of inflammatory and catabolic responses in severely burned children by early burn wound excision in the first 24 hours. Arch Surg. 2003;138:127–32.
5. Murton SA, Tan ST, Prickett TC, Frampton C, Donald RA. Hormone responses to stress in patients with major burns. Br J Plast Surg. 1998;51:388–92.
6. Kulp GA, Herndon DN, Lee JO, Suman OE, Jeschke MG. Extent and magnitude of catecholamine surge in pediatric burned patients. Shock. 2010;33:369–74.
7. Williams FN, Herndon DN, Kulp GA, Jeschke MG. Propranolol decreases cardiac work in a dose-dependent manner in severely burned children. Surgery. 2011;149:231–9.
8. Lalonde C, Demling RH. The effect of complete burn wound excision and closure on postburn oxygen consumption. Surgery. 1987;102:862–8.
9. Fein A, Leff A, Hopewell PC. Pathophysiology and management of the complications resulting from fire and the inhaled products of combustion: review of the literature. Crit Care Med. 1980;8:94–8.
10. Barillo DJ, Goode R, Esch V. Cyanide poisoning in victims of fire: analysis of 364 cases and review of the literature. J Burn Care Rehabil. 1994;15:46–57.
11. Oremus M, Hanson MD, Whitlock R, et al. A systematic review of heparin to treat burn injury. J Burn Care Res. 2007;28:794–804.
12. Aikawa N, Wakabayashi G, Ueda M, Shinozawa Y. Regulation of renal function in thermal injury. J Trauma. 1990;30:S174–8.
13. Jeschke MG, Barrow RE, Herndon DN. Extended hypermetabolic response of the liver in severely burned pediatric patients. Arch Surg. 2004;139:641–7.
14. Wilmore DW, Goodwin CW, Aulick LH, et al. Effect of injury and infection on visceral metabolism and circulation. Ann Surg. 1980;192:491–504.
15. Barret JP, Jeschke MG, Herndon DN. Fatty infiltration of the liver in severely burned pediatric patients: autopsy findings and clinical implications. J Trauma. 2001;51:736–9.
16. Martyn J. Clinical pharmacology and drug therapy in the burned patient. Anesthesiology. 1986;65:67–75.
17. McKee AC, Winkelman MD, Banker BQ. Central pontine myelinolysis in severely burned patients: relationship to serum hyperosmolality. Neurology. 1988;38:1211–7.
18. Chance WT, Berlatzky Y, Minnema K, et al. Burn trauma induces anorexia and aberrations in CNS amine neurotransmitters. J Trauma. 1985;25:501–7.
19. Wallner SF, Vautrin R. The anemia of thermal injury: mechanism of inhibition of erythropoiesis. Proc Soc Exp Biol Med. 1986;181:144–50.
20. Lundy JB, Hetz K, Chung KK, et al. Outcomes with the use of recombinant human erythropoietin in critically ill burn patients. Am Surg. 2010;76:951–6.
21. Warner P, Fields AL, Braun LC, et al. Thrombocytopenia in the pediatric burn patient. J Burn Care Res. 2011;32:410–4.
22. de Macedo JL, Rosa SC, Castro C. Sepsis in burned patients. Rev Soc Bras Med Trop. 2003;36:647–52.
23. Levin GY, Egorihina MN. The role of fibrinogen in aggregation of platelets in burn injury. Burns. 2010;36:806–10.
24. Khorasani EN, Mansouri F. Effct of early enteral nutrition on morbidity and mortality in children with burns. Burns. 2010;36:1067–71.
25. Sefton EJ, Boulton-Jones JR, Anderton D, Teahon K, Knights DT. Enteral feeding in patients with major burn injury: the use of nasojejunal feeding after the failure of nasogastric feeding. Burns. 2002;28:386–90.
26. Williams FN, Branski LK, Jeschke MG, Herndon DN. What, how, and how much should patients with burns be fed? Surg Clin North Am. 2011;91:609–29.

27. Martyn JA, Greenblatt DJ, Hagen J, Hoaglin DC. Alteration by burn injury of the pharmacokinetics and pharmacodynamics of cimetidine in children. Eur J Clin Pharmacol. 1989;36:361–7.
28. Matsui M, Kudo T, Kudo M, Ishihara H, Matsuki A. The endocrine response after burns. Agressologie. 1991;32:233–5.
29. Jeschke MG, Finnerty CC, Suman OE, et al. The effect of oxandrolone on the endocrinologic, inflammatory, and hypermetabolic responses during the acute phase postburn. Ann Surg. 2007;246:351–60.
30. Fram RY, Cree MG, Wolfe RR, et al. Intensive insulin therapy improves insulin sensitivity and mitochondrial function in severely burned children. Crit Care Med. 2010;38:1475–83.
31. Szyfelbein SK, Drop LJ, Martyn JAJ, Martyn JA. Persistent ionized hypocalcemia in patients during resuscitation and recovery phases of body burns. Crit Care Med. 1981;9:454–8.
32. Klein GL, Wimalawansa SJ, Kulkarni G, et al. The efficacy of acute administration of pamidronate on the conservation of bone mass following severe burn injury in children: a double-blind, randomized, controlled study. Osteoporos Int. 2005;16:631–5.
33. Coté CJ, Drop LJ, Daniels AL, Hoaglin DC. Calcium chloride versus calcium gluconate: comparison of ionization and cardiovascular effects in children and dogs. Anesthesiology. 1987;66:465–70.
34. Greenhalgh DG. Topical antimicrobial agents for burn wounds. Clin Plast Surg. 2009;36:597–606.
35. Childs C, Little RA. Acute changes in oxygen consumption and body temperature after burn injury. Arch Dis Child. 1994;71:31–4.
36. De Young AC, Kenardy JA, Cobham VE, Kimble R. Prevalence, comorbidity and course of trauma reactions in young burn-injured children. J Child Psychol Psychiatry. 2012;53:56–63.
37. Giannoni-Pastor A, Eiroa-Orosa FJ, Fidel Kinori SG, Arguello JM, Casas M. Prevalence and predictors of posttraumatic stress symptomatology among burn survivors: a systematic review and meta-analysis. J Burn Care Res. 2016;37(1):e79–89.
38. Sun B-W, Zhou X-Q, Xia C-L, et al. Management of severe burn injuries in neonates. J Burn Care Rehabil. 2004;25:219–23.
39. Rappaport BA, Suresh S, Hertz S, Evers AS, Orser BA. Anesthetic neurotoxicity—clinical implications of animal models. N Engl J Med. 2015;372(9):796–7.
40. Davidson AJ, et al. Neurodevelopmental outcome at 2 years of age after general anaesthesia and awake-regional anaesthesia in infancy (GAS): an international multicentre, randomised controlled trial. Lancet. 2016;387(10015):239–50.
41. American Geriatrics Society Expert Panel on Postoperative Delirium in Older Adults. American Geriatrics Society abstracted clinical practice guideline for postoperative delirium in older adults. J Am Geriatr Soc. 2015;63(1):142–50.
42. Bittner EA, Shank E, Woodson E, Martyn JA. Acute and perioperative care of the burn-injured patient. Anesthesiology. 2015;122:448–64.
43. Martyn JA, Abernethy DR, Greenblatt DJ. Plasma protein binding of drugs after severe burn injury. Clin Pharmacol Ther. 1984;35:535–9.
44. Martyn J, Goldhill DR, Goudsouzian NG. Clinical pharmacology of muscle relaxants in patients with burns. J Clin Pharmacol. 1986;26:680–5.
45. Han TH, Martyn JA. Onset and effectiveness of rocuronium for rapid onset of paralysis in patients with major burns: priming or large bolus. Br J Anaesth. 2009;102:55–60.
46. Martyn J, Wilson RS, Burke JF. Right ventricular function and pulmonary hemodynamics during dopamine infusion in burned patients. Chest. 1986;89:357–60.
47. Glew RH, Moellering RC Jr, Burke JF. Gentamicin dosage in children with extensive burns. J Trauma. 1976;16:819–23.
48. Martyn JA, Greenblatt DJ, Quinby WC. Diazepam kinetics in patients with severe burns. Anesth Analg. 1983;62:293–7.
49. Asmussen S, Maybauer DM, Fraser JF, Jennings K, George S, Maybauer MO. A meta-analysis of analgesic and sedative effects of dexmedetomidine in burn patients. Burns. 2013;39(4):625–31.
50. Faucher L, Furukawa K. Practice guidelines for the management of pain. J Burn Care Res. 2006;27:659–68.
51. Fuzaylov G, Fidkowski CW. Anesthetic considerations for major burn injury in pediatric patients. Paediatr Anaesth. 2009;19:202–11.
52. Haastrup AA, Mendez P, Coté CJ. Suction the tongue: a new adjunct for improving the laryngeal view for fiberoptic intubation. Anesth Analg. 2011;112:1512–3.
53. Wait M, Hunt JL, Purdue GF. Duplex scanning of central vascular access sites in burn patients. Ann Surg. 1990;211:499–503.
54. Hettiaratchy S, Papini R. ABC of burns: initial management of a major burn: II—assessment and resuscitation. BMJ. 2004;329(7457):101–3.
55. Morgan RJ, Martyn JA, Philbin DM, Coggins CH, Burke JF. Water metabolism and antidiuretic hormone (ADH) response following thermal injury. J Trauma. 1980;20:468–72.
56. Martyn JA, McKusick K, Strauss HW, Burke JF. Ventricular volume and ejection fraction in the diagnosis of the aetiology of low cardiac output in burned patients. Anaesthesia. 1986;41:511–5.
57. Wang GY, Ma B, Tang HAT, Zhu SH, Lu J, Wie W, et al. Esophageal echo-Doppler monitoring in burn shock resuscitation: are hemodynamic variables the critical guiding fluid therapy? J Trauma. 2008;65:1396–401.
58. Knobloch K. Non-invasive hemodynamic monitoring in burn shock resuscitation. Burns. 2010;36(7):1135–6.
59. Lawrence A, Faraklas I, Watkins H, et al. Colloid administration normalizes resuscitation ratio and ameliorates “fluid creep”. J Burn Care Res. 2010;31:40–7.
60. Shrum B, Church B, McArthur E, Burns KE, Znajda T, McAlister V. Hypertonic salt solution for peri-operative fluid management. Cochrane Database Syst Rev. 2016;6:CD005576.
61. Palmieri TL, Greenhalgh DG. Blood transfusion in burns: what do we do? J Burn Care Rehabil. 2004;25(1):71–5.
62. Oda J, Kasai K, Noborio M, Ueyama M, Yukioka T. Hypothermia during burn surgery and postoperative acute lung injury in extensively burned patients. J Trauma. 2009;66:1525–9.
63. Gaukroger PB, Chapman MJ, Davey RB. Pain control in paediatric burns—the use of patient-controlled analgesia. Burns. 1991;17:396–9.
64. Song L, Wang S, Zuo Y, Chen L, Martyn JA, Mao J. Midazolam exacerbates morphine tolerance and morphine-induced hyperactive behaviors in young rats with burn injury. Brain Res. 2014;20(1564):52–61.
65. Hofbauer R, Moser D, Hammerschmidt V, Kapiotis S, Frass M. Ketamine significantly reduces the migration of leukocytes through endothelial cell monolayers. Crit Care Med. 1998;26:1545–9.
66. Joly V, Richebe P, Guignard B, Fletcher D, Maurette P, Sessler DI, Chauvin M. Remifentanil-induced postoperative hyperalgesia and its prevention with small-dose ketamine. Anesthesiology. 2005;103(1):147–55.
67. Unlugenc H, Gunduz M, Guler T, Yagmur O, Isik G. The effect of pre-anaesthetic administration of intravenous dexmedetomidine on postoperative pain in patients receiving patient-controlled morphine. Eur J Anaesthesiol. 2005;22:386–91.
68. Shank ES, Sheridan RL, Ryan CM, Keaney TJ, Martyn JA. Hemodynamic responses to dexmedetomidine in critically ill intubated pediatric burned patients: a preliminary study. J Burn Care Res. 2013;34(3):311–7.
69. Cuignet O, Pirson J, Soudon O, Zizi M. Effects of gabapentin on morphine consumption and pain in severely burned patients. Burns. 2007;33:81–6.
70. Kharasch ED. Current concepts in methadone metabolism and transport. Clin Pharmacol Drug Dev. 2017;6:125–34.

71. Bussolin L, Busoni P, Giorgi L, Crescioli M, Messeri A. Tumescent local anesthesia for the surgical treatment of burns and postburn sequelae in pediatric patients. Anesthesiology. 2003;99:1371–5.
72. Hernandez JL, Savetamal A, Crombie RE, Cholewczynski W, Atweh N, Possenti P, Schulz JT 3rd. Use of continuous local anesthetic infusion in the management of postoperative split-thickness skin graft donor site pain. J Burn Care Res. 2013;34:e257–62.
73. Shank ES, Martyn JA, Donelan MB, Perrone A, Firth PG, Driscoll DN. Ultrasound-guided regional anesthesia for pediatric burn reconstructive surgery; a prospective study. J Burn Care Res 2014. 2016;37(3):e213–7.
74. Cuignet O, Pirson J, Boughrouph J, Duville D. The efficacy of continuous fascia iliaca compartment block for pain management in burn patients undergoing skin grafting procedures. Anesth Analg. 2004;98:1077–81.

Treatment and Prevention of Pain in Children and Adults with Burn Injuries

25

Stefan J. Friedrichsdorf

25.1 Introduction

Pain is one of the most distressing symptoms children and adults are experiencing following a burn injury [1]. The severity of burn pain is difficult to predict from the wound depth, location, or extend alone. The initial painful stimulation of nerve endings by the burn injury with continued painful stimuli results in peripheral and central sensitization causing up-regulation of painful stimuli, and the eventual development of persistent pain syndromes that can be difficult to treat [2]. Inadequate pain treatment in the hospital immediately after the burn trauma results in a much higher risk of post-traumatic stress disorder (PTSD) [3–6]. Also, parents watching their children experiencing unrelieved pain following burn trauma including procedural pain are more likely to develop PTSD themselves [7]. Poor pain and anxiety management can contribute to delayed wound healing [8], and good pain management results in faster healing and better patient care [9, 10]. Despite advances in burn care, inadequate pain management continues to exist during both the acute and rehabilitation phases of care [11], and burn patients often suffer needless pain. Especially in hospitalized children pain is common, under-recognized, and under-treated [12–15].

Clinical Practice Guidelines and protocols for burn care commonly recommend the use of scheduled analgesia to address background pain and acute treatments in the prevention and relief of pain associated with burn care procedures [16, 17]. Several state-of-the-art pain treatment modalities are utilized to help prevent and treat the pain of a burn injury, and when used concurrently, pain can usually be prevented or minimized. This chapter will discuss evidence-based safe multi-modal (i.e., opioid-sparing) analgesia [18], which may include one, several, or all of the following approaches in the effective treatment of pediatric or adult burn patients: pharmacology (e.g., simple analgesia and/or opioids and/or adjuvant analgesia), anesthetic interventions (e.g., neuroaxial analgesia, nerve blocks), rehabilitation (e.g., physical therapy, occupational therapy, sleep hygiene), psychology (e.g., cognitive behavioral therapy), and age-appropriate positioning and integrative ("non-pharmacological") therapies, such as breathing techniques, self-hypnosis, and distraction.

Following a description of different pain pathophysiologies, this chapter will review the use of basic analgesics, opioids, and adjuvant analgesics for all age groups from infants to adults, as well as rehabilitative, integrative ("non-pharmacological") modalities.

25.2 Burn Pain Pathophysiology

The majority of burn patients experience different distinct and at times overlapping entities of pain pathophysiology concurrently and/or subsequently, explaining the need of advanced protocols providing multi-modal analgesia. The most common pain entities burn patients are experiencing include acute somatic pain, procedural pain, neuropathic pain, psycho-spiritual-emotional pain, and/or chronic persistent pain and will be discussed in more detail below.

25.3 Acute Somatic Pain

Acute somatic nociceptive pain is caused by the actual skin and tissue injury of the burn trauma as well as by the repetitive trauma (such as debridement, graft, or inflammation) during the initial hospitalization. The key to preventing long-lasting pain appears to initiate "multi-modal analgesia" [18] pain protocols on day one of the burn injury. Studies have shown that if pain is not adequately controlled right after the burn trauma, there is an increased risk of post-traumatic stress disorder (PTSD) in infants, children, and adults [3–6].

S. J. Friedrichsdorf (✉)
Department of Pain Medicine, Palliative Care and Integrative Medicine, Children's Hospitals and Clinics of Minnesota, University of Minnesota Medical School, Minneapolis, MN, USA
e-mail: stefan.friedrichsdorf@childrensMN.org; https://www.childrensmn.org/painpalliativeintegrativemed

M. G. Jeschke et al. (eds.), *Handbook of Burns Volume 1*, https://doi.org/10.1007/978-3-030-18940-2_25

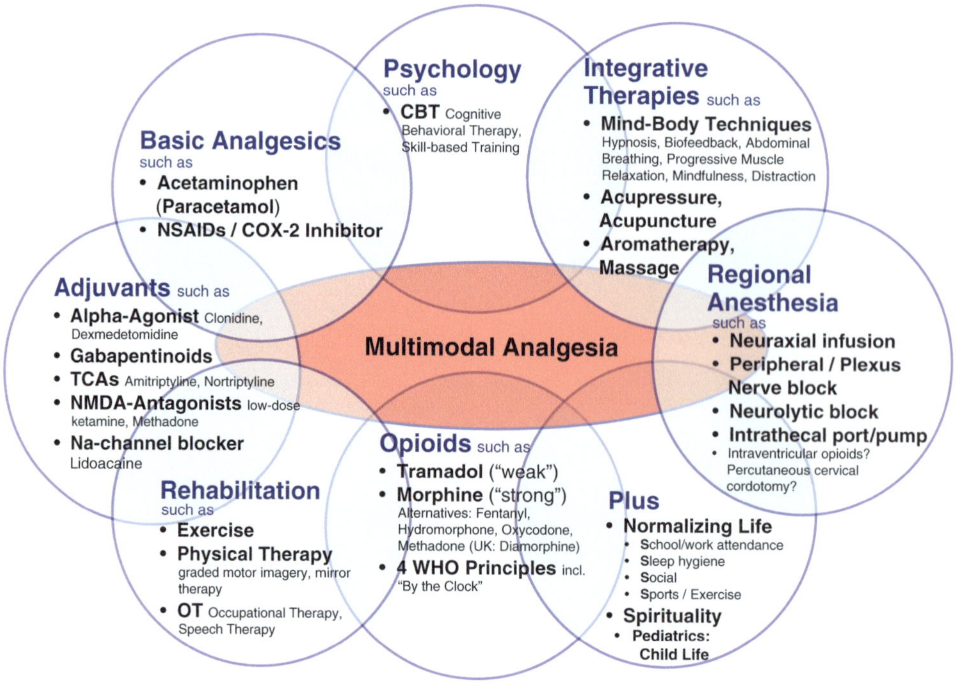

Fig. 25.1 Multimodal analgesia

Acute pain management usually requires scheduling pain medications around-the-clock with the addition of "as-needed" (or "breakthrough," "rescue," or pro re nata "PRN") medication. A combination of the following seven strategies may be most effective with the least side-effects:

1. *Basic analgesia*: acetaminophen (paracetamol) plus a non-steroidal-anti-inflammatory drug (NSAIDs), such as ibuprofen or ketorolac. If bleeding side-effects or stomach discomfort occurs, another option might be a COX-2 inhibitor, such as celecoxib.
2. *Opioids*: include medications such as tramadol, morphine, fentanyl, hydromorphone, oxycodone, or methadone carefully titrated to effect. However, "If Coke doesn't work, switch to Pepsi"—in other words, a significant number of children or adults may experience opioid-induced side-effect (which might be mitigated by a low-dose naloxone infusion) or poor analgesia on one opioid and then need to be "rotated" or switched to another strong opioid for better control. After discharge to home we wean slowly the opioids completely off and in the absence of new tissue trauma hardly ever expect patient to be on opioids for a long time (e.g., not longer than 1–2 months at home).
3. *Adjuvant Analgesia*: such as gabapentinoids (e.g., gabapentin, pregabalin), alpha-agonist (e.g., dexmedetomidine, clonidine), NMDA-channel blocker (low-dose ketamine, methadone), sodium-channel blocker (e.g., lidocaine), tricyclic antidepressants (e.g., low-dose amitriptyline).
4. *Interventional modalities* or neuroaxial analgesia (e.g., nerve blocks, paravertebral blocks, or epidural pain pumps).
5. *Rehabilitation*: Physical therapy, occupational therapy, speech therapy.
6. *Psychology*, stress-reduction.
7. *Active integrative ("non-pharmacological") therapies*—treatments/remedies that do not involve the use of medications, such as active mind–body techniques (deep breathing, biofeedback, self-hypnosis, etc.)

Procedural pain might be caused by dressing changes, intravenous (IV) access, blood draws, injections, etc. Patients report that in addition to dressing changes especially repetitive needle pokes are among the worst kind of pain they experience during their hospitalization [12]. Although this kind of pain can be completely prevented or significantly reduced by simple strategies, many hospitals may not be offering these strategies to all their patients yet.

Successful examples of providing system-wide pain management include the Children's Hospitals and Clinics of Minnesota "*Children's Comfort Promise: We promise to do everything to prevent and treat pain*" [19–21] where painful procedures are performed under mild, moderate, or deep sedation as needed. In addition, for pain caused by elective needle procedures, such as blood draws, injections, vaccinations, and intravenous cannulation, the hospital always offer "Four Non-Negotiables"

- "*Numb the skin*" (for children 36 weeks corrected gestational age and older) 4% lidocaine cream [22] or needleless lidocaine application via a J-tip® (sterile, single-use, disposable injector that uses pressurized gas to propel medication through the skin) [23, 24] as topical anesthetics.
- *Sucrose* [25, 26] or *breastfeeding* [27] for infants 0–12 months [28].
- *Comfort positioning*. Restraining children for procedures is never supportive and creates a negative experience. Children restrained for painful procedures reported they felt ashamed, humiliated, powerless, and described the loss of the right to control their own body [29]. For infants swaddling, warmth, skin-to-skin contact, or facilitated tucking. For children who are 6 months and older offer them to sit upright, including on their parent's lap.
- *Age-appropriate distraction* [30], such as toys, books, blowing bubbles or pinwheels, stress balls, and using apps, videos, or games on electronic devices.

Neuropathic pain is defined by the International Association for the Study of Pain (IASP) as pain arising as a direct consequence of a lesion or disease affecting the "somatosensory" (i.e., nervous) system [31]. A significant number of burn patients develop neuropathic pain as a result of nerve damage caused by the burn trauma and the treatment [32]. In addition to NSAIDs and opioids (for the initial post-traumatic hospitalization only), several "adjuvant" pain medications, including gabapentinoids, low-dose tricyclic antidepressants; alpha-agonists and/or NMDA-channel blocker are commonly administered to mitigate pain. Although several medications may assist with controlling neuropathic pain, physical therapy, and psychology (and for some patients: nerve blocks) are usually required components of excellent pain control and should not be omitted.

Psycho-spiritual-emotional pain. The psychological and emotional impact of a burn injury [33] results in real existing measurable pain—however, this pain cannot be treated by opioids (or other pain medications), but rather by addressing those needs through family and social support as well as an interdisciplinary care team which includes team members such as a social worker, chaplain, and/or psychologist.

Chronic or persistent pain: Pain can persist after healing, with many patients after severe burns reporting ongoing burn-related pain many years later. In one large study [34], 358 burn survivors with injuries covering an average of 59% of their bodies were asked about their pain experience on average 12 years after the trauma: The majority (52%) described ongoing burn-related pain, two-thirds (66%) reported that pain interfered with their rehabilitation, and 55% reported that pain interfered with their daily lives.

Common chronic pain locations include the injury site, but also primary pain disorders (formerly functional pain syndromes) which includes primary headaches (incl. tension headaches and migraines), centrally mediated abdominal pain syndromes (formerly functional abdominal pain), and/or wide-spread pain in muscles, joints, and bones [incl. fibromyalgia] as well as Complex Regional Pain Syndrome or CRPS (formerly Reflex Sympathetic Dystrophy) [35]. Effective treatments of these common pain disorders usually do not rely on medications, but rather on four rehabilitative strategies utilized concurrently. A common misconception is to spend a lot of time and energy on just one or two of these modalities, and when found to be ineffective, patients may become frustrated "I have done it all, and nothing worked" when in fact usually they have not been done at the same time over a few months. Also patients may need to be reminded that sometimes pain even gets worse, before it gets better, especially when they are deconditioned. An effective rehabilitative pain program should offer concurrently:

- *Physical therapy/exercise*: Many patients with chronic pain are deconditioned and exercise may even cause worsening of pain. A thoughtful daily (at home) training program then is required to improve movement and normalize function as much as possible.
- *Active integrative therapies*, such as daily practicing of deep breathing, biofeedback (a technique using a videogame that trains people to improve their pain by controlling relaxing bodily processes that normally happen involuntarily, such as heart rate, blood pressure, muscle tension, and skin temperature.), self-hypnosis, mindfulness, progressive muscle relaxation, and/or yoga can reduce pain by stimulating "endorphins" (the body's own pain medication that makes us to feel good) in the pain center of the brain.
- *Psychology*: Pain can cause stress, and stress usually worsens pain. Worsened pain then worsens mood, which may affect anxiety and depression. Effective strategies include cognitive behavioral therapy (CBT), or play therapy for children, and stress-reduction offered by a licensed therapist.
- *Normalizing Life*: Key to effective pain control appears to normalize function first, and then the pain gets better (unfortunately not the other way around), including returning to school or work, normalizing sleep, normalizing exercise and social life.

Medications are usually ineffective for a large number of patients with chronic and persistent pain, if not accompanied by the above four strategies. Opioids are usually not indicated for chronic persistent pain (unless there is repetitive new tissue injury) [36]. Some adjuvant analgesia, especially for nerve pain, however appear to be well tolerated and might be effective, as described below.

25.4 Regional Anesthesia

The majority of burn pain patients to date unfortunately do not receive one of the most effective analgesic modalities, which would prevent and treat unrelieved pain with the least amount side-effects: Regional or neuroaxial anesthesia [37–42]. Patients often have more intense postoperative pain from the split-thickness skin donor site than from the grafted burn wound [42, 43]. Especially if a burn injury of an extremity or the trunk requires hospitalization on a burn unit, it must now be expected standard of care to ensure assessment the infant, child, adolescent, or adult by an anesthesiologist for potential regional anesthesia. Blocking pain nociception using a local anesthetic such as bupivacaine, in some cases in conjunction with an opioid and/or alpha-agonist can provide complete analgesia, without any of the opioid-induced side-effects. Pain pathways can be blocked, when anesthesiologist trained in regional anesthesia utilize central neuraxial infusions, peripheral nerve and plexus blocks or infusions, or neurolytic blocks [44]. Occasionally, implanted intrathecal ports and pumps for baclofen, opioids, local anesthetics, and other adjuvants might be considered.

Benefits of regional anesthesia include [45]

- significantly reduce or eliminated need for opioids
- no systemic side-effects
- no sedation
- no nausea
- minimal side-effects with epidural (itching, urinary retention)
- improved gastrointestinal motility
- less postoperative cardiac arrhythmias
- significantly reduced pulmonary complications
- significantly reduced delirium
- improved mobility that reduces rates of deep vein thrombosis (DVTs)
- extremely high patient satisfaction
- patient is awake and can remember conversations with clinicians and family
- evidence for reduction of development of chronic pain and phantom pain

Central neuraxial techniques (spinal and epidural catheters) have been utilized with good effect as both primary anesthetics and postoperative adjuncts in burn-injured patients [43]. Epidural abscesses are not more common in burn patients, but there might be an increased risk that intravascular catheters are more likely to become infected if placed in or near burned tissue [42], so similarly caution is likely reasonable in selecting appropriate burn patients for central neuraxial techniques [43].

Because the nociceptive nerves cannot be numbed independent of all the other nerves that receive local anesthesia ("what wires together, fires together"), there are side-effects such as motor weakness, hypotension, pruritus, or urinary retention [45]. If the patient has breakthrough pain that breaks through a low continuous infusion of the local anesthetic, a patient-controlled analgesia (PCA) bolus allows the patient to give him- or herself additional medication as needed, called patient-controlled regional analgesia (PCRA). Similar to an opioid PCA, the patient can use their PCRA button for breakthrough pain, but without the side-effects caused by opioids. Patients can be sent home with a nerve block catheter, connected to a disposable pump or one that is returned to the hospital. There are no opioids in the infusion, eliminating misuse potential. That may lead to less adverse events, including sedation, delirium, sleep disturbances, and opioid-induced hyperalgesia.

25.5 Pharmacological Considerations

Large burns in children and adults result in altered pharmacokinetic and pharmacodynamic responses to many medications. Plasma protein loss through injured skin and further dilution of plasma proteins by resuscitation fluids decrease the concentration of albumin, an important drug-binding protein [43]. There is an increase in volume of distribution in most studied medications, including opioids such as fentanyl, the general anesthetic propofol, and muscle relaxants [46]. During the acute injury (resuscitation), phase of large burns in the first 48 h cardiac output, and subsequently renal and hepatic blood flow is decreased, possibly increasing half-life of opioids and other analgesics and requiring somewhat lower starting doses or frequency of administration. However, around day three during the hyperdynamic phase elevated renal and hepatic blood flow results in increased clearance, and doses of analgesics (and sedatives) commonly need to be increased significantly [43].

Morphine, for instance, is metabolized by the liver glucuronyl-transferase into morphine-6 glucuronide (M6G) and morphine-3 glucuronide (M3G). M6G is a much stronger analgesic (40–100 times stronger) and displays adverse effects including nausea, vomiting, sedation, and respiratory depression. M3G is not an analgesic but is a μ-opioid antidote with unique adverse effects, especially hyperexcitability

Table 25.1 Basic analgesia for children (>6 months) and adults

Drug	Route	Pediatric dose	Maximal dose	Dosing interval
Ibuprofen	PO	5–10 mg/kg	400–600 mg	6–8 h
Ibuprofen-sodium[a] (Advil®) 256 mg tablet = 200 mg ibuprofen	PO	5–10 mg/kg	200–400mg	6–8 h
Acetaminophen	PO, PR	10–15 mg/kg	60 mg/kg/day <2 years 90 mg/kg/day >2 years	4–6 h
Acetaminophen[b]	IV	<10 kg = 7.5 mg/kg;	30 mg/kg/day	6 h
		1–2 years = 15 mg/kg;	60 mg/kg/day	6 h
		>2 years (<50 kg) = 15 mg/kg;	75 mg/kg/day	6 h
		>13 years (>50 kg) = 1000 mg	4000 mg/day	6 h
Ketorolac[c] (Toradol)	IV	<2 years = 0.25 mg/kg >2 years = 0.5 mg/kg	30 mg	6–8 h
Celecoxib[d]	PO	1–2 mg/kg	100 mg	12–24 h

[a]Fast-Acting, compared to regular ibuprofen: onset after 10 min, last longer, and only half the dose required
[b]ONLY if rectal or oral administration contraindicated; re-evaluate daily
[c]Recommend dosing no longer than 5 days
[d]If classical NSAIDs contraindicated; safety and efficacy has been established only in children 2 years of age or older and for a maximum of 6 months of treatment in JRA

and neurotoxicity. The ratio of M6G/M3G thereby defines the analgesia to adverse effect profile in individual patients. Both metabolites need to be excreted by the kidney, and patients in renal failure, and/or during low cardiac output of the resuscitation phase 0–48 h with subsequently decreased renal and hepatic blood, have a higher risk of unwanted side-effects. Fentanyl or methadone, neither of which is excreted renally, might be a better choice in this scenario.

25.6 Pharmacology Step 1: Basic Analgesia

Acetaminophen (Paracetamol) (10–15 mg/kg p.o./p.r./i.v. every 4–6 h; dose limit: <2 years: 40 mg/kg/day, >2 years: 75 mg/kg/day, max. 650 mg every 6 h) is generally well tolerated by children and adults and lacks gastrointestinal and hematological side-effects. Significant hepatoxicity [47] is rare, but careful attention to dosing is paramount.

Ibuprofen (5–10 mg/kg p.o. every 6 h; dose limit 2400 mg/day) has the least gastrointestinal side-effects among non-steroidal anti-inflammatory drugs (NSAIDs) that are nonselective for cyclooxygenase-2 (COX-2). It should be used with caution in individuals with hepatic or renal impairment, or a history of gastrointestinal bleeding or ulcers, and it inhibits platelet aggregation.

Ibuprofen-sodium Meta-analysis showed that NSAID-salts display far more rapid absorption, faster initial pain reduction, good overall analgesia in more patients at the same dose, and probably evoke longer-lasting analgesia, without reports of adverse events [48]. When compared to ibuprofen, ibuprofen-sodium (available over the counter in the United States and many countries) produces significantly greater analgesia over 6 h, and required fewer re-medications than standard formulations [49]. In addition, 200 mg fast-acting ibuprofen (Numbers-needed-to-treat [NNT] 2.1; 95% confidence interval (CI) 1.9–2.4) was as effective as 400 mg standard ibuprofen (NNT 2.4; 95% CI 2.2–2.5), and produced a faster onset of analgesia.

Ketorolac has the advantage of i.v. administration, but it should be rotated to oral ibuprofen, as soon as tolerated (<2 years: 0.25 mg/kg every 6 h; >2 years: 0.5 mg/kg every 6 h; max. 30 mg/dose; recommended dosing no longer than 3–5 days).

Celecoxib (a COX-2 > COX-1 inhibitor) might be considered if classical NSAIDs are contraindicated (e.g., owing to bleeding risks, or gastrointestinal side-effects). It does not display less renal toxicity compared to classic NSAIDs. Safety and efficacy have been established only in children 2 years of age or older and for a maximum of 6 months of treatment in juvenile rheumatoid arthritis (1–2 mg/dose [max. 100 mg] every 12 h).

25.7 Pharmacology Step 2: Opioids

Opioids remain a mainstay in the analgesic treatment of acute somatic pain cause by the tissue injury as well as subsequent interventions, including pain at skin donor site and the grafted burn wound. Opioid rotation may be necessary, if tolerance develops or dose-limiting opioid toxicity occurs. A switch from one opioid to another is often accompanied by a change in the balance between analgesia and side-effects [50]. A favorable change in opioid side-effect profile may be experienced if there is less cross-tolerance at the opioid receptors mediating analgesia than at those mediating adverse effects. If rotating opioids because of decreasing effectiveness or limiting side-effects (i.e., because of incomplete cross-tolerance), it can be considered to begin at around 50% of the equianalgesic dose and titrate to effect. However, the required decrease for incomplete cross-tolerance may be

Table 25.2 Opioid analgesics: usual starting doses for children (>6 months) and adults

Drug (route of administration)	Equianalgesic dose (parenteral)	Starting dose IV	IV:PO ratio	Starting dose PO (transdermal)
Morphine (PO, SL, IV, SC, PR)	10 mg	*Bolus dose*: 0.05–0.1 mg/kg (max. 5 mg) every 2–4 h *Continuous infusion*: 0.01–0.03 mg/kg/h (max. 0.5–1.5 mg/h)	1:3	0.15–0.3 mg/kg (max. 7.5–15 mg) every 4 h
Fentanyl (IV, SC, SL, transdermal, buccal)	**100–250 μg**	**Bolus dose: 1–3 μg/kg (max. 25–75 μg) (slowly over 3–5 min—fast bolus of higher doses may cause thorax rigidity)** **Continuous infusion: 1–2 μg/kg/h (max. 50–100 μg/h)**	**1:1 (IV to trans dermal)**	**12 μg/h patch** (must be on the equivalent of at least 30 mg oral morphine/24 h, before switched to patch)
Hydromorphone (PO, SL, IV, SC, PR)	**1.5–2 mg**	**Bolus dose: 15–20 μg/kg (max. 1 mg) every 4 h** **Continuous infusion: 5 μg/kg/h (max. 250 μg/h)**	**1:5**	**60 μg/kg (max. 2000–3000 μg or 2–3 mg) every 3–4 h**
Oxycodone (PO, SL, PR)	**5–10 mg**	**n/a**	**n/a**	**0.1–0.2 mg/kg (max. 5–10 mg) every 4 h *or* 0.15–0.3 mg/kg (max. 7.5–15 mg) every 6 h**
Tramadol (PO, PR)	**100 mg**	**IV not available in the United States** ***[Bolus dose: 1 mg/kg every 3–4 h Continuous infusion: 0.25 mg/kg/h]***	**1:1**	**1–2 mg/kg every 3–4 h, max. of 8 mg/kg/day (>50 kg: max. of 400 mg/day)**
Methadone (PO, PR, SL, IV)	**Nonlinear conversion (see** Table 25.5)	**0.04–0.08 mg/kg (max. 2–4 mg) IV Q8h**	**1:1 to 1:2** (in adults usually IV usually 50% of PO dose; in pediatrics usually IV = 80% of PO dose)	**0.05–0.1 mg/kg (max. 2.2–5 mg) PO Q8h**

1. Above doses represent starting doses, which then need to be titrated to effect and may be significantly higher
2. Maximum per kg dose capped at 50 kg body weight
3. Calculated rescue (breakthrough) dose: 10–16% of 24-h opioid dose to be given every 1–2 h as needed

IV intravenous, *PO* by mouth, *SL* sublingual, *SC* subcutaneous, *PR* rectal, *n/a* not applicable

higher or lower, depending on the clinical context of the individual patient [51]. Opioid-associated side-effects (e.g., constipation, pruritus, and nausea) should be anticipated and treated accordingly.

Morphine For recommended starting doses, see Tables 25.2 and 25.3. Morphine undergoes a first-pass metabolism: The currently accepted oral-to-i.v. potency ratio for morphine is 1:3 [1 mg i.v. morphine equals 3 mg oral morphine]. Routes of administration include oral, sublingual, intravenous, intramuscular, subcutaneous, intrathecal, and epidural. Morphine is also effective topically in open wounds [52].

Morphine appears safe and efficacious in full-term neonates; however, starting doses are usually lower compared to those used in older children (see Table 25.3). Long-term neurodevelopmental outcome years after former preterm or term babies are exposed to continuous morphine or fentanyl infusion displayed no adverse effects of the opioids on intelligence, motor function, or behavior [53–56].

Fentanyl is a popular opioid for analgesia prior to painful procedures owing to its rapid onset (about 1 min) and its brief duration of action (30–45 min). Intranasal fentanyl for dressing changes in burn patients [57]. Fentanyl provides a good alternative to morphine when tolerance or dose-limiting side-effects mandate opioid rotation [58, 59].

Hydromorphone, like morphine and fentanyl, is another selective μ-opioid receptor agonist. Unlike morphine metabolism, there is no hydromorphone-6-glucuronide (H6G), but metabolism of the parent compound does result in hydromorphone-3-glucoronide (H3G). Opioid hyperexcitability has been reported in patients with renal failure taking hydromorphone [60, 61]. The normal H3G to hydromorphone plasma ratio is 27:1, but in renal failure it is 100:1 [62].

Oxycodone is a selective μ-opioid receptor agonist although some animal studies suggest κ-receptor agonist activity as well [63] The oral potency ratio of oral oxycodone to morphine is between 1:1 and 2:1 [64]. One advantage of oxycodone over morphine is the slightly longer half-life, frequently 6-h dosing (as oppose to 4-h with morphine). Renal and hepatic impairment increase oxycodone serum levels [65].

Methadone is an excellent opioid choice in advanced pediatric and adult analgesia, but it remains under-utilized [66–68]. In the United States, it is available as an intravenous

Table 25.3 Analgesia for neonates and infants 0–6 months of age [1]

Drug	Route	Pediatric Dose (age)	Maximal Dose	Dosing Interval
Basic Analgesia				
Ibuprofen[a]	PO	5–10 mg/kg (infants 3–6 months)	40 mg/kg/day	6–8 h
Acetaminophen	PO, PR	5–10 mg/kg (neonates 0–30 days) 10 mg/kg (infants 1–3 months) 10–15 mg/kg (infants 3–6 months)	20–40 mg/kg/day 40 mg/kg/day 40–60 mg/kg/day	4–6 h (maximum 4 doses/day)
Acetaminophen[b]	IV	<10 kg = 7.5 mg/kg	30 mg/kg/day	6 h
Opioids				
Morphine	PO/PR/SL	0.075–0.15 mg (neonates 0–30 days)		6 h
		0.08–0.2 mg (infants 1–6 months)		4–6 h
Morphine[c]	IV/SC[d]	0.025–0.05 mg/kg (neonates 0–30 days)		6 h
		0.1 mg/kg (infants 1–6 months)		6 h
		Infusion (with PCA bolus of same dose): 0.005–0.01 mg/kg/h (neonates 0–30 days) 0.01–0.03 mg/kg/h(infants 1–6 months)		
Fentanyl[c]	IV/SC[d]	1–2 μg/kg (neonates and infants 0–12 months)		2–4 h
		Infusion (with PCA bolus of same dose): 0.5–1 μg/kg/h (neonates and infants 0–6 months)		
Oxycodone	PO/PR/SL	0.05–0.125 mg/kg (infants 1–6 months)		4 h
Adjuvant Analgesics				
Gabapentin	PO	4.5 mg/kg (neonates and infants 0–6 months)	15 mg/kg	6 h
Dexmedetomidine (Precedex®)	IV	Infusion:	Slowly titrate to max. of	Cont. infusion
		0.2 μg/kg/h (neonates and infants 0–6 months)	2 μg/kg/h	
Clonidine	PO	1–3 μg/kg		4–6 h
Amitriptyline[e]	PO	0.1 mg/kg (infants 3–12 months)	0.4 mg/kg	QHS (once at night)

[a]For infants <3 months consult Pain Service
[b]ONLY if rectal or oral administration contraindicated; re-evaluate daily
[c]Administer IV slowly over at least 5 min
[d]The intravenous doses for neonates are based on acute pain management and sedation dosing information. Lower doses are required for non-ventilated neonates
[e]EKG to rule out QTc-prolongation/Torsade des Pointes

Table 25.4 Usual starting doses for patient (or nurse)-controlled analgesia (PCA) pumps—dose escalation usually in 50% increments both for continuous and PCA bolus dose (Department of Pain Medicine, Palliative Care & Integrative Medicine, Children's Hospitals and Clinics of Minnesota, USA)

	Continuous infusion [μg/kg/h]	PCA bolus [μg]	Lock-out time [min]	Maximum number of boluses/hour
Morphine	20 (max. 1000)	20 (max. 1000)	5–10	4–6
Hydromorphone	3–5 (max. 250)	3–5 (max. 250)	5–10	4–6
Fentanyl	1 (max. 50)	1 (max. 50)	5	4–6

Doses for children >6 months of age and are capped at 50 kg body weight

formulation also (with commonly used conversion ratios of adults: 1 mg PO = 0.5 mg IV and 1 mg IV = 1 mg PO; however in Pediatrics: 1 mg PO = 0.8 mg IV and 1 mg IV = 1.2 mg PO). Early methadone initiation may reduce the development of opioid tolerance (i.e., reducing the need to increase opioids rapidly to achieve analgesia) and thereby have a significant effect on ventilator outcomes in critically injured patients with burn injury [69].

This multi-mechanistic analgesic is a μ (δ, κ)-opioid receptor agonist, an NMDA-channel blocker, and a presynaptic blocker of serotonin and norepinephrine re-uptake. Advantages include methadone's long half-life (allowing every 8–12 h dosing), high effectiveness in complex pain conditions, including the management of neuropathic pain, decreased incidence of constipation, lack of active metabolites, and safe usage in renal failure and in stable liver disease.

Table 25.5 Adjuvant analgesics used in pediatric and adult pain management (Pain Medicine and Palliative Care, Children's Hospitals and Clinics of Minnesota) [2]

Class	Medication	Dose	Route of administration	Comments/side effects (see text for further details)
Tricyclic antidepressants (TCA)	Amitriptyline	Starting dose 0.1 mg/kg QHS, usually slowly titrated up to 0.5 mg/kg (max. 20–25 mg)	PO	Tertiary amine TCA; stronger anticholinergic side effects (including sedation) than nortriptyline
	Nortriptyline	Starting dose 0.1 mg/kg QHS, usually titrated up to 0.5 mg/kg (max. 20–25 mg)	PO	Secondary amine TCA; anticholinergic side effects
Gabapentenoids	Gabapentin	Starting dose 2 mg/kg QHS, usually slowly titrated up to initial target dose of 6 mg/kg/dose TID (max. 300 mg/dose TID). Max. dose escalation to 24 mg/kg/dose TID (max. 1200 mg/dose TID)	PO	Slow dose increase required; side effects: ataxia, nystagmus, myalgia, hallucination, dizziness, somnolence, aggressive behaviors, hyperactivity, thought disorder, peripheral edema
	Pregabalin	Starting dose 0.3 mg/kg QHS, usually slowly titrated up to initial target dose of 1.5 mg/kg/dose BID (max. 75 mg/dose BID). Max. dose escalation to 6 mg/kg/dose BID (max. 300 mg/dose BID)	PO	Switch from gabapentin, if distressing side effects or inadequate analgesia. Side effects: ataxia, nystagmus, myalgia, hallucination, dizziness, somnolence, aggressive behaviors, hyperactivity, thought disorder, peripheral edema; associated with weight gain
Sodium-channel blocker/local anesthetic	Lidocaine 5%	Max. of 4 patches (in patients >50 kg) 12 h on/12 h off	Transdermal patch	Not for severe hepatic dysfunction
Alpha-agonist	Clonidine	1–3 μg/kg [max 50–150 μg] QHS to Q4–6h	PO/ transdermal	
	Dexmedetomidine	Infusion: 0.2 μg/kg/h (max. 10 μg/h); titrate to max. 2 μg/kg/h (max. 100 μg/h)	IV	
Hormone	Melatonin	0.06–0.2 mg/kg (max. 3–10 mg) QHS	PO	Sleep induction, use extended-release, if interrupted sleep, possible analgesic effect

QHS every night at bedtime; *PO* per os, oral administration; *IV* intravenous administration; *BID* bis in die, twice a day; *TID* ter in die, three times a day; *Q4–6h* every 4–6 h

There are several disadvantages, however, including wide dosing variation, a long half-life (which may lead to accumulation, making quick titration difficult), and a more complex equianalgesic conversion, which requires longer and closer patient observation than with other opioids. Safe use requires that the effects of methadone should be closely monitored for several days, particularly when it is first started and after any dosing change. Methadone has been effectively used in burn patients [6, 70].

There are significant problems with applying adult-based opioid conversion tables to children [51] and data supporting pediatric conversion rates from short-acting opioids to methadone remain unclear [66, 71–73]. This lack of data may put children at risk for under-medication (with resulting unrelieved pain and/or withdrawal) or over-medication (with resulting over-sedation and/or respiratory depression). Despite an increase in methadone administration in children, the appropriate pediatric methadone equianalgesic dose remains unknown [66]. There are multiple adult dosing strategies for methadone conversion [74–86], but their application in the pediatric population has not been evaluated. See Table 25.5 for conversion ratios used in pediatrics and adult medicine.

25.8 Opioids for Chronic Pain

Opioids should *not* be administered to pediatric or adult patients with primary pain disorders [87], i.e., chronic pain defined that extends beyond the expected time of healing which hence lacks the acute warning function of physiological nociception. Opioids may be more likely to cause more harm than benefit in the treatment of "primary pain disorders,", which include conditions such as tension headaches/migraines, chronic musculoskeletal pain/fibromyalgia, "chronic sickle cell pain" (pain that extends beyond the expected time of acute vaso-occlusive crisis) and, functional abdominal pain/centrally mediated abdominal pain syndrome. Opioids administered for primary pain disorders have low long-term efficacy, a poor safety profile, and commonly a worse clinical outcome [88–94].

25.9 Pharmacology: Step 3—Adjuvant Analgesics

Adjuvant analgesics (such as low-dose tricyclic antidepressants, gabapentinoids, and α-agonists) commonly serve as valuable adjuncts in the treatment of burn pain. Most data for this heterogeneous class of medications is derived from adult neuropathic and acute pain conditions [95–101]. For a comprehensive systematic review of pharmacotherapy for neuropathic pain, including numbers-needed-to-treat (NNT) and numbers needed to harm (NNH), see Finnerup et al. [98] See Table 25.5 for recommended starting doses.

Gabapentinoids: A recent meta-analysis showed gabapentinoids to be efficacious in the control of neuropathic pain of various etiologies with a NNT of 2.9–3.9 [25]. Gabapentinoids are alpha-2-delta ligands, locking on a voltage-gated calcium-channel at the presynaptic nerve terminal (first neuron) at the level of the dorsal horn, resulting in decreased release of pain transmitters, such as glutamate, norepinephrine, and substance P. Gabapentin (NNT: 6.3; NNH: 25.6) appears to be slightly more effective than pregabalin (NNT: 7.7; NNH: 13.9), which seems more effective than extended-release gabapentin (NNT 8.3; NNH 31.9) [98]. Adult data and pediatric experience suggest that a significant number of patients who experience inadequate analgesia from pregabalin benefit from gabapentin, and vice versa. Conversion from gabapentin to pregabalin is around 6:1, meaning 300 mg gabapentin TID (=900 mg/day) equals pregabalin 75 mg BID (=150 mg/day) [19]. To avoid pain or precipitating seizures, these anticonvulsants should be weaned over a period of 1–2 weeks.

Gabapentin: An initial low starting dose is 2 mg/kg/dose (max 100 mg/dose) once at night titrated to 6 mg/kg/dose (max. 300 mg/dose) three times/day (TID). For mild to medium neuropathic pain, the titration may take up to 2 weeks to avoid side-effects. For severe pain, the titration may be significantly faster (1–3 days). If analgesia is inadequate, the dose may be titrated in steps up to 12 mg/kg/dose (max. 600 mg/dose) TID, then up to 18 mg/kg/dose (max. 900 mg/dose) TID, and finally up to 24 mg/kg/dose (max. 1200 mg/dose) TID. Gabapentin (as oppose to pregabalin) has a non-linear bioavailability, meaning dose increases close to the maximum dose may have less of an effect. Side-effects include lethargy, ataxia, nystagmus, dizziness, thought disorder, hallucinations, headache, peripheral edema, and myalgia; these side-effects appear to be mitigated by slow dose escalation. Especially gabapentin, and to a lesser degree pregabalin, are commonly used in pediatric chronic pain management. There have been no pediatric RCTs and only a few case reports published [99, 100].

Pregabalin should be considered a second choice, if gabapentin is ineffective or displays side-effects. Safety and efficacy are not established in pediatric patients and there is no accepted pediatric dosing. Experience and anecdotal evidence suggests the following for older children and teenagers: Initial starting dose 0.5 mg/kg/dose (max 50 mg/dose) q HS slowly titrated to 1.5 mg/kg/dose (max. 75 mg/dose) BID. For mild to medium neuropathic pain, the titration may take up to 2 weeks to avoid side-effects. For severe pain, the titration may be significantly faster (2–3 days). If analgesia is inadequate, the dose may be titrated in steps up to 3 mg/kg/dose (max. 150 mg/dose) BID, then up to 4.5 mg/kg/dose (max. 225 mg/dose) BID, and finally up to 6 mg/kg/dose (max. 300 mg/dose) BID.

Possible side-effects of pregabalin include blurred vision, life-threatening angioedema (take precautions if prescribing ACE inhibitors concurrently), dizziness, somnolence, and weight gain.

Tricyclic antidepressants (TCAs) are among the best-studied antidepressant class that show efficacy in treating neuropathic pain. Amitriptyline and nortriptyline, which have been extensively studied, block re-uptake of serotonin and norepinephrine, which possibly stimulates descending inhibiting pathways stemming from the periaqueductal grey, and they may also block the NMDA-receptor. In addition, opioid analgesia might be improved with concurrent TCA administration via a serotonergic mechanism at the brainstem. Adverse effects of all TCAs include arrhythmia and anticholinergic/antihistamine effects, such as dry mouth, constipation, urinary retention, blurred vision, and sedation. Nortriptyline (a secondary amine) may be better tolerated than amitriptyline (a tertiary amine) because it has fewer anticholinergic side-effects.

Amitriptyline and nortriptyline show some efficacy in treating adult neuropathic pain [98]; however, despite the fact that they are commonly used in children, there are no pediatric RCTs [102, 103]. Amitriptyline has NNT of 3.6 and a NNH of 13.4, and has not shown a dose–response effect [98].

Dose recommendations are the same for both amitriptyline and nortriptyline. Both are available in liquid form and are usually started at 0.1 mg/kg by mouth at bedtime (adult dose 5 mg) and increased to a max of 0.4–0.5 mg (max. 20–25 mg once at night). Experience has shown that increasing beyond that dose does not appear to result in increased analgesic effect. It may take 1–2 weeks to titrate up to an effective dose and to determine if the analgesic therapy is working; however, the induction of sleep will start much sooner. An EKG to rule out QTc-prolongation/WPW-Syndrome prior to initiation is recommended.

Overall, the efficacy of TCAs and gabapentinoids appears equal [98]. If a single adjuvant appears ineffective and there are no contraindications in the individual pediatric or adult patient, a combination of a medication from each group is recommended since their mechanism of action is synergistic.

NMDA-Channel Blocker: *N*-methyl-D-aspartate (NMDA) channels may be involved in the spinal neural circuitry that leads to a neuropathic pain state of resistance to higher dose opioids. At a normal resting level, the NMDA-channel is blocked by magnesium. Increased excitation, including strong pain stimuli, may open the NMDA-channel, producing hyperexcitability of dorsal root neurons, leading to central sensitization (i.e., amplification of neural signaling

Table 25.6 Methadone Conversion Table

Total daily oral morphine dose	Estimated daily oral methadone requirement: Gazelle G, Fine PG. Methadone for the treatment of pain #75. J Palliat Med. 2003;6(4):620–1	*ROXANE LABORATORIES, INC. Columbus, OH 43216* http://www.accessdata.fda.gov/drugsatfda_docs/label/2006/006134s028lbl.pdf	Toombs JD (2005) American Family Physician 71(7):1353–8
<100 mg	3:1	20–30%	33%
101–300 mg	5:1	10–20%	20%
301–600 mg	10:1	8–12%	10%
601–800 mg	12:1	5–10%	8%
801–1000 mg	15:1	5–10%	7%
>1000 mg	20:1	<5%	5%

When rotating from another opioid to methadone, the initial maximum starting dose of methadone, decrease by 50% for incomplete cross-tolerance, should not be higher than 30 mg/day PO

1. World_Health_Organization. *WHO-Principles of Acute Pain Management for Children* http://whqlibdoc.who.int/publications/2012/9789241548120_Guidelines.pdf. 2012; Available from: http://whqlibdoc.who.int/publications/2012/9789241548120_Guidelines.pdf
2. Friedrichsdorf, S.J., *Prevention and Treatment of Pain in Hospitalized Infants, Children, and Teenagers: From Myths and Morphine to Multimodal Analgesia.*, in *Pain 2016: Refresher Courses. 16th World Congress on Pain.* 2016, International Association for the Study of Pain, IASP Press: Washington, D.C. p. 309–319

within the CNS that elicits pain hypersensitivity), wind-up phenomenon, and memory of pain. NMDA-receptor antagonists, such as ketamine, methadone, and levorphanol (possibly dextrometorphane and amantadine)—which block the channel—can help prevent this phenomenon, leading to decreased opioid resistance, improved hyperalgesia and improved allodynia.

Ketamine is an NMDA-receptor antagonist, but it possesses other actions which may contribute to its analgesic effect, including a mu-, delta-, and kappa-opioid like effect, interactions with calcium and sodium channels, cholinergic transmission, and noradrenergic and serotonergic re-uptake inhibition. Ketamine is effective for pediatric neuropathic pain in low (i.e., sub-anesthetic) doses, both alone or in combination with opioids. Ketamine is unique among anesthetic agents in that it does not depress respiratory and cardiovascular systems. In low analgesic doses, the typical anesthetic-dose side-effects of ketamine (nystagmus, lacrimation, tachycardia, and altered sensorium) are not usually seen though pediatric data is limited. Many centers schedule a low-dose benzodiazepine during the ketamine administration to avoid psychotomimetic side-effects. There is evidence of significant opioid reduction and improved analgesia following initiation of low-dose ketamine [104, 105]. Low-dose ketamine has been described as effective in burn patients [106].

Analgesic (sub-anesthetic) ketamine dosing includes the following: IV: 1–5 μg/kg/min [=0.06–0.3 mg/kg/h]; with maximum of 3–15 mg/h. IV; PO: 0.2–0.5 mg/kg TID-QID and PRN. Ketamine may also be administered by sc, sl, intranasal, pr, or spinal route. In the United States, ketamine is only available as a racemic mixture [*S*(+)-enantiomer (providing analgesia, general anesthesia); *R*(−)-enantiomer (causing bronchodilatation, nightmares)]. In most other countries, ketamine-S [*S*(+)-enantiomer] is also available, reducing the required dose by 40–50%.

Sodium-channel blocker: Other adjuvant analgesia that appears to be effective for neuropathic pain in selective patients includes intravenous lidocaine [107, 108], including for the treatment of background or procedural burn pain [109]. Side-effects of intravenous lidocaine include allergic reaction (serious, but rare), and dose-related numbness around the mouth, dizziness, slurring of speech, hallucinations, muscle twitches, and seizures [110].

Alpha-2-adrenergic agonists such as clonidine or dexmedetomidine can be effective adjuvant analgesics for both nociceptive and neuropathic pain [111–117]. They act at the spinal cord in two ways. First, they act on the same neurons in the cord and lead to the same intracellular events as opioids, but act through a different receptor; 2-adrenergic and-opioid receptors activate the same potassium channel via inhibitory G proteins. Thus, it is likely that they enhance the anti-nociceptive effects of opioids. Second, alpha-2-adrenergic agonists decrease sympathetic outflow involved with neuropathic pain and hyperarousal [118]. Clonidine can be given orally, transdermally, or intraspinally. Side-effects include lethargy, dry mouth, and hypotension. Dexmedetomidine can also be an effective adjuvant, leading to opioid-sparing. It carries the advantage of not affecting respiration. However, potential side-effects include hypotension and bradycardia, leading most institutions to restrict its use to intensive care units. Dose recommendations: Dexmedetomidine (0.2–2 μg/kg/h IV), max. 100 μg/h; Clonidine (starting dose 1–3 μg/kg [max 50–150 μg] per dose QHS to q4–6h titrated to effect PO or transdermal).

Marijuana: There are no published pediatric studies, and adult studies lack evidence to support its use for acute or chronic pain [119, 120]. The updated American Academy of Pediatrics policy opposes marijuana use [121], citing lack of research and potential harms including correlation with mental illness [122], testicular cancer [123–125], decline in IQ [126, 127], and increase risk of addiction [128].

25.9.1 Nitrous Gas Analgesia Sedation

Nitrous gas has been shown to be effective for procedural pain such as dressing changes in burn patients [129]. Data reveals that children receiving nitrous gas before and during painful procedures have lower levels of distress, lower pain scores, were more relaxed, and many have no recollection of the procedure afterwards [130–133]. It has been well documented that poorly managed pain has serious short- and long-term consequences. Inadequate analgesia and the memory of previous painful experience for procedures in children diminish the effects of adequate analgesia in subsequent procedures [134] and unrelieved pain increases the risk of post-traumatic stress disorder even in very young children [6]. Alternatively, many centers are achieving excellent results in eliminating procedural pain and decreasing stress and anxiety using moderate to deep sedation, usually with help of the general anesthetic propofol, often with the addition of an opioid such as fentanyl [135].

25.10 Physical Therapy

Physical therapy and exercise are key modalities in the treatment of patients with chronic pain and primary pain disorder [136–143]. Patients with chronic pain usually have a lower physical activity level [144] and physical activity has been shown to reduce the risk for depression [145]. In patients participating in a rehabilitative pain program, the rate of improvement in function was significantly more rapid than the decrease in pain [140].

25.11 Integrative Medicine: Active Mind–Body Techniques

Integrative modalities (sometimes referred to as complementary and alternative medicine) that have been described as effective in the management of pediatric pain include hypnosis, yoga, acupuncture, and massage [146–154]. Active mind–body techniques, such as guided imagery, hypnosis, biofeedback, yoga, and distraction each and all evoke pain modulation by engaging a number of mechanisms within the analgesic neuraxis. Techniques such as distraction and guided imagery appear to modulate the release of endogenous opioids from the periaqueductal and periventricular gray regions to disinhibit descending inhibitory pathways of the brainstem to suppress pain transmission in the dorsal horn of the spinal cord [155–159]. As well, distraction has been shown to increase activity of the orbitofrontal and perigenual anterior cingulate cortex, as well as periaqueductal gray and the posterior thalamus to modulate pain at the supraspinal level [160, 161].

25.12 Psychological Intervention

Anxiety, depressive, and behavioral disorders are early risk factors of chronic pain (rather than vice versa) [162]. At low levels of anxiety, higher pain is predictive of greater disability; however, highly anxious adolescents tend to function poorly regardless of level of pain [163]. Psychological treatments significantly reduce pain intensity that is reported by children and adolescents with headache, abdominal pain, and musculoskeletal/joint pain [164, 165]. Cognitive behavioral therapy (CBT) led to significant improvements in pain coping, catastrophizing, and efficacy that were sustained over time in adolescents with chronic pain [166]. CBT has been shown to increase gray matter in the prefrontal cortex of patients with chronic pain, and this increase in prefrontal cortical gray matter has been associated with reduced pain catastrophizing [167].

25.13 Conclusion

The effective prevention and treatment of pain in children and adults after burn injuries requires intensive "multi-modal" pain control starting within the first minutes following the admission to the hospital. It is inappropriate to perform elective painful procedures in children or adults without evidence-based treatments to avoid or minimize pain. Equally important to medications are physical therapy and regular exercise as well as integrative therapies, psychology, and normalizing life. Unfortunately in 2019, pain management is still not taught sufficiently in most medical training programs to clinicians and a large number of hospital leaderships have grossly neglected to invest in state-of-the-art pain programs. Insurance companies are often unwilling to pay for evidence-based excellent pain control (namely physical therapy and psychology). The majority of burn pain patients unfortunately do not receive one of the most effective analgesic modalities, which would prevent and treat their unrelieved pain with far less side-effects: Regional anesthesia.

Several state-of-the-art pain treatment modalities are utilized to help prevent and treat the pain of a burn injury, and when used concurrently, pain can usually be prevented or significantly minimized. Safe multi-modal, i.e., opioid-sparing, analgesia [18], may include one, several, or all of the following approaches in the effective treatment of pediatric or adult burn patients: Pharmacology (e.g., simple analgesia and/or opioids and/or adjuvant analgesia), anesthetic interventions (e.g., neuroaxial analgesia, nerve blocks), rehabilitation (e.g., physical therapy, occupational therapy, sleep hygiene), psychology (e.g., cognitive behavioral therapy), and age-appropriate positioning and integrative ("non-pharmacological") therapies, such as breathing techniques, self-hypnosis, and distraction.

Summary Box

The prompt prevention and treatment of pain in children and adults after burn injuries is a pillar of evidence-based clinical care and must not omitted. State-of-the-art analgesia requires intensive "multimodal" pain control commencing within the first minutes following the admission to the clinical setting. Multi-modal analgesia are utilized to help prevent and treat the pain of a burn injury, and when used concurrently, pain can usually be prevented or significantly minimized. Safe multi-modal, i.e., opioid-sparing, analgesia often require several or all of the following approaches in the effective treatment of pediatric or adult burn patients: Pharmacology (e.g., simple analgesia and/or opioids and/or adjuvant analgesia), anesthetic interventions (e.g., neuroaxial analgesia, nerve blocks), rehabilitation (e.g., physical therapy, occupational therapy, sleep hygiene), psychology (e.g., cognitive behavioral therapy), and age-appropriate positioning and integrative ("nonpharmacological") therapies, such as breathing techniques, self-hypnosis, and distraction. The majority of burn pain patients unfortunately do not receive regional anesthesia, one of the most effective analgesic modalities, which would prevent and treat their unrelieved pain with far less side-effects. Furthermore, it is inappropriate and unethical to perform elective painful procedures in children or adults without evidence-based treatments to avoid or minimize pain. Equally important to medications are physical therapy and regular exercise as well as integrative therapies, psychology, and normalizing life.

References

1. Mendoza A, Santoyo FL, Agullo A, Fenandez-Canamaque JL, Vivo C. The management of pain associated with wound care in severe burn patients in Spain. Int J Burns Trauma. 2016;6(1):1–10.
2. Gallagher G, Rae CP, Kinsella J. Treatment of pain in severe burns. Am J Clin Dermatol. 2000;1(6):329–35.
3. Saxe G, Stoddard F, Courtney D, Cunningham K, Chawla N, Sheridan R, et al. Relationship between acute morphine and the course of PTSD in children with burns. J Am Acad Child Adolesc Psychiatry. 2001;40(8):915–21.
4. Saxe GN, Stoddard F, Hall E, Chawla N, Lopez C, Sheridan R, et al. Pathways to PTSD, part I: children with burns. Am J Psychiatry. 2005;162(7):1299–304.
5. Hall E, Saxe G, Stoddard F, Kaplow J, Koenen K, Chawla N, et al. Posttraumatic stress symptoms in parents of children with acute burns. J Pediatr Psychol. 2006;31(4):403–12.
6. Stoddard FJ Jr, Sorrentino EA, Ceranoglu TA, Saxe G, Murphy JM, Drake JE, et al. Preliminary evidence for the effects of morphine on posttraumatic stress disorder symptoms in one- to four-year-olds with burns. J Burn Care Res. 2009;30(5):836–43.
7. Rizzone LP, Stoddard FJ, Murphy JM, Kruger LJ. Posttraumatic stress disorder in mothers of children and adolescents with burns. J Burn Care Rehabil. 1994;15(2):158–63.
8. Brown NJ, Kimble RM, Gramotnev G, Rodger S, Cuttle L. Predictors of re-epithelialization in pediatric burn. Burns. 2014;40(4):751–8.
9. Thomas SH, Shewakramani S. Prehospital trauma analgesia. J Emerg Med. 2008;35(1):47–57.
10. Thomas SH, Silen W. Effect on diagnostic efficiency of analgesia for undifferentiated abdominal pain. Br J Surg. 2003;90(1):5–9.
11. Patterson DR, Hofland HW, Espey K, Sharar S. Nursing Committee of the International Society for Burn I. Pain management. Burns. 2004;30(8):A10–5.
12. Friedrichsdorf SJ, Postier A, Eull D, Weidner C, Foster L, Gilbert M, et al. Pain outcomes in a US Children's Hospital: a prospective cross-sectional survey. Hosp Pediatr. 2015;5(1):18–26.
13. Taylor EM, Boyer K, Campbell FA. Pain in hospitalized children: a prospective cross-sectional survey of pain prevalence, intensity, assessment and management in a Canadian pediatric teaching hospital. Pain Res Manag. 2008;13(1):25–32.
14. Zhu LM, Stinson J, Palozzi L, Weingarten K, Hogan ME, Duong S, et al. Improvements in pain outcomes in a Canadian Pediatric Teaching Hospital following implementation of a multifaceted knowledge translation initiative. Pain Res Manag. 2012;17(3):173–9.
15. Stevens BJ, Harrison D, Rashotte J, Yamada J, Abbott LK, Coburn G, et al. Pain assessment and intensity in hospitalized children in Canada. J Pain. 2012;13(9):857–65.
16. Briggs M, Ferris FD, Glynn C, Harding K, Hofman D, Hollinworth H, et al. Assessing pain at wound dressing-related procedures. Nurs Times. 2004;100(41):56–7.
17. Gamst-Jensen H, Vedel PN, Lindberg-Larsen VO, Egerod I. Acute pain management in burn patients: appraisal and thematic analysis of four clinical guidelines. Burns. 2014;40(8):1463–9.
18. Friedrichsdorf SJ. Prevention and treatment of pain in hospitalized infants, children, and teenagers: from myths and morphine to multimodal analgesia. Pain 2016: Refresher Courses 16th World Congress on Pain. Washington, D.C. IASP Press: International Association for the Study of Pain; 2016. p. 309–19.
19. Minnesota CsHaCo. Children's Comfort Promise 2017. http://www.childrensMN.org/comfortpromise.
20. Friedrichsdorf SJ, Eull D, Weidner CA. Children's Comfort Promise: how can we do everything possible to prevent and treat pain in children using quality improvement strategies? (Commentary). Pediatr Pain Lett. 2016;18(3):26–30.
21. Council CsMYA. The Comfort Promise: The Youth Advisory Council highlights children's unique approach to help patients prevent and treat pain. 2016. https://vimeo.com/128990829.
22. Taddio A, Riddell RP, Ipp M, Moss S, Baker S, Tolkin J, et al. Relative effectiveness of additive pain interventions during vaccination in infants. CMAJ. 2017;189(6):E227–34.
23. Lunoe MM, Drendel AL, Levas MN, Weisman SJ, Dasgupta M, Hoffmann RG, et al. A randomized clinical trial of jet-injected lidocaine to reduce venipuncture pain for young children. Ann Emerg Med. 2015;66(5):466–74.
24. Lunoe MM, Drendel AL, Brousseau DC. The use of the needle-free jet injection system with buffered lidocaine device does not change intravenous placement success in children in the emergency department. Acad Emerg Med. 2015;22(4):447–51.
25. Stevens B, Yamada J, Ohlsson A, Haliburton S, Shorkey A. Sucrose for analgesia in newborn infants undergoing painful procedures. Cochrane Database Syst Rev. 2016;(7):CD001069.
26. Gao H, Gao H, Xu G, Li M, Du S, Li F, et al. Efficacy and safety of repeated oral sucrose for repeated procedural pain in neonates: a systematic review. Int J Nurs Stud. 2016;62:118–25.

27. Shah PS, Herbozo C, Aliwalas LL, Shah VS. Breastfeeding or breast milk for procedural pain in neonates. Cochrane Database Syst Rev. 2012;(12):CD004950.
28. Nursing CsBStBrtatUoOsSo. Be Sweet to Babies. 2014. http://www.cheo.on.ca/en/BeSweet2Babies.
29. Karlson K, Darcy L, Enskär K. The use of restraint is never supportive (poster). Nordic Society of Pediatric Hematology/Oncology (NOPHO) 34th Annual Meeting 2016 and 11th Biannual Meeting of Nordic Society of Pediatric Oncology Nurses (NOBOS); May 27–31, 2016; Reykjavik, Iceland 2016.
30. Uman LS, Birnie KA, Noel M, Parker JA, Chambers CT, McGrath PJ, et al. Psychological interventions for needle-related procedural pain and distress in children and adolescents. Cochrane Database Syst Rev. 2013;(10):CD005179.
31. (IASP) IAftSoP. IASP taxonomy. https://www.iasp-pain.org/Taxonomy.
32. Portilla AS, Bravo GL, Miraval FK, Villamar MF, Schneider JC, Ryan CM, et al. A feasibility study assessing cortical plasticity in chronic neuropathic pain following burn injury. J Burn Care Res. 2013;34(1):e48–52.
33. Bronson M. Psychological and emotional impact of a burn injury. The Phoenix Society for Burn Survivors. 2014. https://www.phoenix-society.org/resources/entry/psychological-and-emotional-impact.
34. Dauber A, Osgood PF, Breslau AJ, Vernon HL, Carr DB. Chronic persistent pain after severe burns: a survey of 358 burn survivors. Pain Med. 2002;3(1):6–17.
35. Friedrichsdorf SJ, Giordano J, Desai-Dakoji K, Warmuth A, Schulz CA. Chronic pain in children and adolescents: diagnosis and treatment of primary pain disorders in head, abdomen, muscles and joints. Children (Basel). 2016;3(4):E42.
36. Dowell D, Haegerich TM, Chou R. CDC guideline for prescribing opioids for chronic pain—United States, 2016. MMWR Recomm Rep. 2016;65(1):1–49.
37. Sen IM, Sen RK. Regional anesthesia for lower limb burn wound debridements. Arch Trauma Res. 2012;1(3):135–6.
38. Cuignet O, Mbuyamba J, Pirson J. The long-term analgesic efficacy of a single-shot fascia iliaca compartment block in burn patients undergoing skin-grafting procedures. J Burn Care Rehabil. 2005;26(5):409–15.
39. Bussolin L, Busoni P, Giorgi L, Crescioli M, Messeri A. Tumescent local anesthesia for the surgical treatment of burns and postburn sequelae in pediatric patients. Anesthesiology. 2003;99(6):1371–5.
40. Hernandez JL, Savetamal A, Crombie RE, Cholewczynski W, Atweh N, Possenti P, et al. Use of continuous local anesthetic infusion in the management of postoperative split-thickness skin graft donor site pain. J Burn Care Res. 2013;34(4):e257–62.
41. Shank ES, Martyn JA, Donelan MB, Perrone A, Firth PG, Driscoll DN. Ultrasound-guided regional anesthesia for pediatric burn reconstructive surgery: a prospective study. J Burn Care Res. 2016;37(3):e213–7.
42. Cuignet O, Pirson J, Boughrouph J, Duville D. The efficacy of continuous fascia iliaca compartment block for pain management in burn patients undergoing skin grafting procedures. Anesth Analg. 2004;98(4):1077–81, table of contents.
43. Bittner EA, Shank E, Woodson L, Martyn JA. Acute and perioperative care of the burn-injured patient. Anesthesiology. 2015;122(2):448–64.
44. Rork JF, Berde CB, Goldstein RD. Regional anesthesia approaches to pain management in pediatric palliative care: a review of current knowledge. J Pain Symptom Manage. 2013;46(6):859–73.
45. Burns DA. Using regional anesthesia to manage pediatric acute pain. In: 10th Pediatric Pain Master's Class; Minneapolis, MN 2017.
46. Blanchet B, Jullien V, Vinsonneau C, Tod M. Influence of burns on pharmacokinetics and pharmacodynamics of drugs used in the care of burn patients. Clin Pharmacokinet. 2008;47(10):635–54.
47. Heubi JE, Barbacci MB, Zimmerman HJ. Therapeutic misadventures with acetaminophen: hepatoxicity after multiple doses in children. J Pediatr. 1998;132(1):22–7.
48. Moore RA, Derry S, Straube S, Ireson-Paine J, Wiffen PJ. Faster, higher, stronger? Evidence for formulation and efficacy for ibuprofen in acute pain. Pain. 2014;155(1):14–21.
49. Peloso PM. Faster, higher, stronger: to the gold medal podium? Pain. 2014;155(1):4–5.
50. Drake R, Longworth J, Collins JJ. Opioid rotation in children with cancer. J Palliat Med. 2004;7(3):419–22.
51. Friedrichsdorf SJ. From Coke to Pepsi to Mountain Dew? Rotating opioids in advanced pediatric palliative care. AAHPM Winter Quart Clin Pearls. 2014;15(4):8–9.
52. Jacobsen J. Topical opioids for pain #185. J Palliat Med. 2009;12(4):380–1.
53. McPherson C, Haslam M, Pineda R, Rogers C, Neil JJ, Inder TE. Brain injury and development in preterm infants exposed to fentanyl. Ann Pharmacother. 2015;49(12):1291–7.
54. Steinhorn R, McPherson C, Anderson PJ, Neil J, Doyle LW, Inder T. Neonatal morphine exposure in very preterm infants-cerebral development and outcomes. J Pediatr. 2015;166(5):1200–7.. e4.
55. MacGregor R, Evans D, Sugden D, Gaussen T, Levene M. Outcome at 5-6 years of prematurely born children who received morphine as neonates. Arch Dis Child Fetal Neonatal Ed. 1998;79(1):F40–3.
56. de Graaf J, van Lingen RA, Valkenburg AJ, Weisglas-Kuperus N, Groot Jebbink L, Wijnberg-Williams B, et al. Does neonatal morphine use affect neuropsychological outcomes at 8 to 9 years of age? Pain. 2013;154(3):449–58.
57. Borland ML, Bergesio R, Pascoe EM, Turner S, Woodger S. Intranasal fentanyl is an equivalent analgesic to oral morphine in paediatric burns patients for dressing changes: a randomised double blind crossover study. Burns. 2005;31(7):831–7.
58. Cherny NJ, Chang V, Frager G, Ingham JM, Tiseo PJ, Popp B, et al. Opioid pharmacotherapy in the management of cancer pain: a survey of strategies used by pain physicians for the selection of analgesic drugs and routes of administration. Cancer. 1995;76(7):1283–93.
59. Goodarzi M. Comparison of epidural morphine, hydromorphone and fentanyl for postoperative pain control in children undergoing orthopaedic surgery. Paediatr Anaesth. 1999;9(5):419–22.
60. Babul N, Darke AC. Putative role of hydromorphone metabolites in myoclonus. Pain. 1992;51(2):260–1.
61. Davis M, Wilcock A. Modified release opioids. Europ J Palliative Care. 2001;(8):142–6.
62. Babul N, Darke AC, Hagen N. Hydromorphone metabolite accumulation in renal failure. J Pain Symptom Manage. 1995;10(3):184–6.
63. Nielsen CK, Ross FB, Lotfipour S, Saini KS, Edwards SR, Smith MT. Oxycodone and morphine have distinctly different pharmacological profiles: radioligand binding and behavioural studies in two rat models of neuropathic pain. Pain. 2007;132(3):289–300.
64. Kalso E. How different is oxycodone from morphine? Pain. 2007;132(3):227–8.
65. Kaiko R, Benziger D, Cheng C, Hou Y, Grandy R. Clinical pharmacokinetics of controlled-release oxycodone in renal impairment. Clinical Pharm Ther. 1996;59(1):130.
66. Fife A, Postier A, Flood A, Friedrichsdorf SJ. Methadone conversion in infants and children: retrospective cohort study of 199 pediatric inpatients. J Opioid Manag. 2016;12(2):123–30.
67. Friedrichsdorf S, Kang T. The management of pain in children with life-limiting illnesses. Pediatr Clin North Am. 2007;54(5):645–72.
68. Altier N, Dion D, Boulanger A, Choiniere M. Successful use of methadone in the treatment of chronic neuropathic pain arising from burn injuries: a case-study. Burns. 2001;27(7):771–5.

69. Jones GM, Porter K, Coffey R, Miller SF, Cook CH, Whitmill ML, et al. Impact of early methadone initiation in critically injured burn patients: a pilot study. J Burn Care Res. 2013;34(3):342–8.
70. Williams PI, Sarginson RE, Ratcliffe JM. Use of methadone in the morphine-tolerant burned paediatric patient. Br J Anaesth. 1998;80(1):92–5.
71. Siddappa R, Fletcher JE, Heard AM, Kielma D, Cimino M, Heard CM. Methadone dosage for prevention of opioid withdrawal in children. Paediatr Anaesth. 2003;13(9):805–10.
72. Anghelescu DL, Faughnan LG, Hankins GM, Ward DA, Oakes LL. Methadone use in children and young adults at a cancer center: a retrospective study. J Opioid Manag. 2011;7(5):353–61.
73. Davies D, DeVlaming D, Haines C. Methadone analgesia for children with advanced cancer. Pediatr Blood Cancer. 2008;51(3):393–7.
74. Gudin JA. The changing landscape of opioid prescribing: long-acting and extended-release opioid class-wide Risk Evaluation and Mitigation Strategy. Ther Clin Risk Manag. 2012;8:209–17.
75. Mercadante S, Caraceni A. Conversion ratios for opioid switching in the treatment of cancer pain: a systematic review. Palliat Med. 2011;25(5):504–15.
76. Pereira J, Lawlor P, Vigano A, Dorgan M, Bruera E. Equianalgesic dose ratios for opioids. a critical review and proposals for long-term dosing. J Pain Symptom Manage. 2001;22(2):672–87. Review. PMID: 11495714.
77. Toombs JD, Kral LA. Methadone treatment for pain states. Am Fam Physician. 2005;71(7):1353–8.
78. von Gunten C. Methadone: starting dosing information no. 86. J Palliat Med. 2004;7(2):304–5.
79. Jacox A, Carr D, Payne R. New clinical-practice guidelines for the management of pain in patients with cancer. N Engl J Med. 1994;330(9):651–5.
80. Patanwala AE, Duby J, Waters D, Erstad BL. Opioid conversions in acute care. Ann Pharmacother. 2007;41(2):255–66.
81. Moryl N, Santiago-Palma J, Kornick C, Derby S. Pitfalls of opioid rotation: substituting another opioid for methadone in patients with cancer pain. Pain. 2002;96(3):325–8.
82. Johnson P, Boyles K, Miller J. Selection of the initial methadone regimen for the management of iatrogenic opioid abstinence syndrome in critically ill children. Pharmacotherapy. 2012;32(2):148–57.
83. Walker P, Palla S, Pei B-L, Kaur G, Zhang K, Hanohano J, et al. Switching from methadone to a different opioid: what is the equianalgesic dose ratio? J Palliat Med. 2008;11(8):1103–8.
84. Weschules DJ, Bain KT. A systematic review of opioid conversion ratios used with methadone for the treatment of pain. Pain Med. 2008;9(5):595–612.
85. Gazelle G, Fine PG. Methadone for the treatment of pain #75. J Palliat Med. 2003;6(4):620–1.
86. ROXANE LABORATORIES IC, OH 43216. DOLOPHINE® HYDROCHLORIDE CII (Methadone Hydrochloride Tablets, USP) [cited 2015 June 19, 2015]. http://www.accessdata.fda.gov/drugsatfda_docs/label/2006/006134s028lbl.pdf.
87. Schechter NL. Functional pain: time for a new name. JAMA Pediatr. 2014;168(8):693–4.
88. Chapman CR, Lipschitz DL, Angst MS, Chou R, Denisco RC, Donaldson GW, et al. Opioid pharmacotherapy for chronic non-cancer pain in the United States: a research guideline for developing an evidence-base. J Pain. 2010;11(9):807–29.
89. Chapman CR, Davis J, Donaldson GW, Naylor J, Winchester D. Postoperative pain trajectories in chronic pain patients undergoing surgery: the effects of chronic opioid pharmacotherapy on acute pain. J Pain. 2011;12(12):1240–6.
90. Elliott JA, Horton E, Fibuch EE. The endocrine effects of long-term oral opioid therapy: a case report and review of the literature. J Opioid Manag. 2011;7(2):145–54.
91. Chaparro LE, Furlan AD, Deshpande A, Mailis-Gagnon A, Atlas S, Turk DC. Opioids compared with placebo or other treatments for chronic low back pain: an update of the Cochrane Review. Spine (Phila Pa 1976). 2014;39(7):556–63.
92. Ashworth J, Green DJ, Dunn KM, Jordan KP. Opioid use among low back pain patients in primary care: is opioid prescription associated with disability at 6-month follow-up? Pain. 2013;154(7):1038–44.
93. Scherrer JF, Salas J, Lustman PJ, Burge S, Schneider FD. Residency Research Network of Texas I. Change in opioid dose and change in depression in a longitudinal primary care patient cohort. Pain. 2015;156(2):348–55.
94. Chen L, Vo T, Seefeld L, Malarick C, Houghton M, Ahmed S, et al. Lack of correlation between opioid dose adjustment and pain score change in a group of chronic pain patients. J Pain. 2013;14(4):384–92.
95. Friedrichsdorf SJ, Nugent AP. Management of neuropathic pain in children with cancer. Curr Opin Support Palliat Care. 2013;7(2):131–8.
96. Vidor LP, Torres IL, Custodio de Souza IC, Fregni F, Caumo W. Analgesic and sedative effects of melatonin in temporomandibular disorders: a double-blind, randomized, parallel-group, placebo-controlled study. J Pain Symptom Manage. 2013;46(3):422–32.
97. Schwertner A, Conceicao Dos Santos CC, Costa GD, Deitos A, de Souza A, de Souza IC, et al. Efficacy of melatonin in the treatment of endometriosis: a phase II, randomized, double-blind, placebo-controlled trial. Pain. 2013;154(6):874–81.
98. Finnerup NB, Attal N, Haroutounian S, McNicol E, Baron R, Dworkin RH, et al. Pharmacotherapy for neuropathic pain in adults: a systematic review and meta-analysis. Lancet Neurol. 2015;14(2):162–73.
99. Hauer JM, Solodiuk JC. Gabapentin for management of recurrent pain in 22 nonverbal children with severe neurological impairment: a retrospective analysis. J Palliat Med. 2015;18(5):453–6.
100. Edwards L, DeMeo S, Hornik CD, Cotten CM, Smith PB, Pizoli C, et al. Gabapentin use in the neonatal intensive care unit. J Pediatr. 2016;169:310–2.
101. Derry S, Wiffen PJ, Moore RA, Quinlan J. Topical lidocaine for neuropathic pain in adults. Cochrane Database Syst Rev. 2014;(7):CD010958.
102. Bahar RJ, Collins BS, Steinmetz B, Ament ME. Double-blind placebo-controlled trial of amitriptyline for the treatment of irritable bowel syndrome in adolescents. J Pediatr. 2008;152(5):685–9.
103. Saps M, Youssef N, Miranda A, Nurko S, Hyman P, Cocjin J, et al. Multicenter, randomized, placebo-controlled trial of amitriptyline in children with functional gastrointestinal disorders. Gastroenterology. 2009;137(4):1261–9.
104. Assouline B, Tramer MR, Kreienbuhl L, Elia N. Benefit and harm of adding ketamine to an opioid in a patient-controlled analgesia device for the control of postoperative pain: systematic review and meta-analyses of randomized controlled trials with trial sequential analyses. Pain. 2016;157(12):2854–64.
105. Finkel J, Pestieau S, Quezado Z. Ketamine as an adjuvant for treatment of cancer pain in children and adolescents. J Pain. 2007;8(6):515–21.
106. Norambuena C, Yanez J, Flores V, Puentes P, Carrasco P, Villena R. Oral ketamine and midazolam for pediatric burn patients: a prospective, randomized, double-blind study. J Pediatr Surg. 2013;48(3):629–34.
107. Peixoto RD, Hawley P. Intravenous lidocaine for cancer pain without electrocardiographic monitoring: a retrospective review. J Palliat Med. 2015;18(4):373–7.
108. Krane E, Leong M, Golianu B, Leong Y. Treatment of pediatric pain with nonconventional analgesics. In: Schechter N, Berde

C, Yaster M, editors. Pain in infants, children, and adolescents. Philadelphia: Lippincott Williams & Wilkins; 2003. p. 225–40.

109. Wasiak J, Mahar PD, McGuinness SK, Spinks A, Danilla S, Cleland H, et al. Intravenous lidocaine for the treatment of background or procedural burn pain. Cochrane Database Syst Rev. 2014;(10):CD005622.

110. Ferrini R, Paice JA. How to initiate and monitor infusional lidocaine for severe and/or neuropathic pain. J Support Oncol. 2004;2(1):90–4.

111. Brummett CM, Trivedi KA, Dubovoy AV, Berland DW. Dexmedetomidine as a novel therapeutic for postoperative pain in a patient treated with buprenorphine. J Opioid Manag. 2009;5(3):175–9.

112. Roberts SB, Wozencraft CP, Coyne PJ, Smith TJ. Dexmedetomidine as an adjuvant analgesic for intractable cancer pain. J Palliat Med. 2011;14(3):371–3.

113. O'Mara K, Gal P, Wimmer J, Ransom JL, Carlos RQ, Dimaguila MA, et al. Dexmedetomidine versus standard therapy with fentanyl for sedation in mechanically ventilated premature neonates. J Pediatr Pharmacol Ther. 2012;17(3):252–62.

114. Chrysostomou C, Schulman SR, Herrera Castellanos M, Cofer BE, Mitra S, da Rocha MG, et al. A phase II/III, multicenter, safety, efficacy, and pharmacokinetic study of dexmedetomidine in preterm and term neonates. J Pediatr. 2014;164(2):276–82 e1-3.

115. O'Neil T, Rodgers PE, Shultz C. Dexmedetomidine as adjuvant therapy for acute postoperative neuropathic pain crisis. J Palliat Med. 2014;17(10):1164–6.

116. Horvath R, Halbrooks EF, Overman DM, Friedrichsdorf SJ. Efficacy and safety of postoperative dexmedetomidine administration in infants and children undergoing cardiac surgery: a retrospective cohort study. J Pediatr Intensive Care. 2015;(3):138–45.

117. Aydogan MS, Korkmaz MF, Ozgul U, Erdogan MA, Yucel A, Karaman A, et al. Pain, fentanyl consumption, and delirium in adolescents after scoliosis surgery: dexmedetomidine vs midazolam. Paediatr Anaesth. 2013;23(5):446–52.

118. Funai Y, Pickering AE, Uta D, Nishikawa K, Mori T, Asada A, et al. Systemic dexmedetomidine augments inhibitory synaptic transmission in the superficial dorsal horn through activation of descending noradrenergic control: an in vivo patch-clamp analysis of analgesic mechanisms. Pain. 2014;155(3):617–28.

119. Hill KP. Medical marijuana for treatment of chronic pain and other medical and psychiatric problems: a clinical review. JAMA. 2015;313(24):2474–83.

120. Deshpande A, Mailis-Gagnon A, Zoheiry N, Lakha SF. Efficacy and adverse effects of medical marijuana for chronic noncancer pain: systematic review of randomized controlled trials. Can Fam Physician. 2015;61(8):e372–81.

121. Pediatrics AAo. Updated AAP policy opposes marijuana use, citing potential harms, lack of research. 2015. http://aapnews.aappublications.org/content/early/2015/01/26/aapnews.20150126-1.

122. Casadio P, Fernandes C, Murray RM, Di Forti M. Cannabis use in young people: the risk for schizophrenia. Neurosci Biobehav Rev. 2011;35(8):1779–87.

123. Daling JR, Doody DR, Sun X, Trabert BL, Weiss NS, Chen C, et al. Association of marijuana use and the incidence of testicular germ cell tumors. Cancer. 2009;115(6):1215–23.

124. Trabert B, Sigurdson AJ, Sweeney AM, Strom SS, McGlynn KA. Marijuana use and testicular germ cell tumors. Cancer. 2011;117(4):848–53.

125. Lacson JC, Carroll JD, Tuazon E, Castelao EJ, Bernstein L, Cortessis VK. Population-based case-control study of recreational drug use and testis cancer risk confirms an association between marijuana use and nonseminoma risk. Cancer. 2012;118(21):5374–83.

126. Meier MH, Caspi A, Ambler A, Harrington H, Houts R, Keefe RS, et al. Persistent cannabis users show neuropsychological decline from childhood to midlife. Proc Natl Acad Sci U S A. 2012;109(40):E2657–64.

127. Moffitt TE, Meier MH, Caspi A, Poulton R. Reply to Rogeberg and Daly: no evidence that socioeconomic status or personality differences confound the association between cannabis use and IQ decline. Proc Natl Acad Sci U S A. 2013;110(11):E980–2.

128. Meier MH, Hall W, Caspi A, Belsky DW, Cerda M, Harrington HL, et al. Which adolescents develop persistent substance dependence in adulthood? Using population-representative longitudinal data to inform universal risk assessment. Psychol Med. 2016;46(4):877–89.

129. Tourtier JP, Raynaud L, Murat I, Gall O. Audit of protocols for treatment of paediatric burns in emergency departments in the Ile de France. Burns. 2010;36(8):1196–200.

130. Hockenberry MJ, McCarthy K, Taylor O, Scarberry M, Franklin Q, Louis CU, et al. Managing painful procedures in children with cancer. J Pediatr Hematol Oncol. 2011;33(2):119–27.

131. Pedersen RS, Bayat A, Steen NP, Jacobsson ML. Nitrous oxide provides safe and effective analgesia for minor paediatric procedures—a systematic review. Dan Med J. 2013;60(6):A4627.

132. Tobias JD. Applications of nitrous oxide for procedural sedation in the pediatric population. Pediatr Emerg Care. 2013;29(2):245–65.

133. Friedrichsdorf SJ. Nitrous gas analgesia and sedation for lumbar punctures in children: has the time for practice change come? Pediatr Blood Cancer. 2017;64(11).

134. Weisman SJ, Bernstein B, Schechter NL. Consequences of inadequate analgesia during painful procedures in children. Arch Pediatr Adolesc Med. 1998;152(2):147–9.

135. Anghelescu DL, Burgoyne LL, Faughnan LG, Hankins GM, Smeltzer MP, Pui CH. Prospective randomized crossover evaluation of three anesthetic regimens for painful procedures in children with cancer. J Pediatr. 2013;162(1):137–41.

136. Logan DE, Carpino EA, Chiang G, Condon M, Firn E, Gaughan VJ, et al. A day-hospital approach to treatment of pediatric complex regional pain syndrome: initial functional outcomes. Clin J Pain. 2012;28(9):766–74.

137. Eccleston C, Malleson PN, Clinch J, Connell H, Sourbut C. Chronic pain in adolescents: evaluation of a programme of interdisciplinary cognitive behaviour therapy. Arch Dis Child. 2003;88(10):881–5.

138. Maynard CS, Amari A, Wieczorek B, Christensen JR, Slifer KJ. Interdisciplinary behavioral rehabilitation of pediatric pain-associated disability: retrospective review of an inpatient treatment protocol. J Pediatr Psychol. 2010;35(2):128–37.

139. Palermo TM, Scher MS. Treatment of functional impairment in severe somatoform pain disorder: a case example. J Pediatr Psychol. 2001;26(7):429–34.

140. Lynch-Jordan AM, Sil S, Peugh J, Cunningham N, Kashikar-Zuck S, Goldschneider KR. Differential changes in functional disability and pain intensity over the course of psychological treatment for children with chronic pain. Pain. 2014;155(10):1955–61.

141. Sherry DD, Wallace CA, Kelley C, Kidder M, Sapp L. Short- and long-term outcomes of children with complex regional pain syndrome type I treated with exercise therapy. Clin J Pain. 1999;15(3):218–23.

142. Odell S, Logan DE. Pediatric pain management: the multidisciplinary approach. J Pain Res. 2013;6:785–90.

143. Lee BH, Scharff L, Sethna NF, McCarthy CF, Scott-Sutherland J, Shea AM, et al. Physical therapy and cognitive-behavioral treatment for complex regional pain syndromes. J Pediatr. 2002;141(1):135–40.

144. Wilson AC, Palermo TM. Physical activity and function in adolescents with chronic pain: a controlled study using actigraphy. J Pain. 2012;13(2):121–30.

145. Jerstad SJ, Boutelle KN, Ness KK, Stice E. Prospective reciprocal relations between physical activity and depression in female adolescents. J Consult Clin Psychol. 2010;78(2):268–72.
146. Bussing A, Ostermann T, Ludtke R, Michalsen A. Effects of yoga interventions on pain and pain-associated disability: a meta-analysis. J Pain. 2012;13(1):1–9.
147. Evans S, Moieni M, Taub R, Subramanian SK, Tsao JC, Sternlieb B, et al. Iyengar yoga for young adults with rheumatoid arthritis: results from a mixed-methods pilot study. J Pain Symptom Manage. 2010;39(5):904–13.
148. Vas J, Santos-Rey K, Navarro-Pablo R, Modesto M, Aguilar I, Campos MA, et al. Acupuncture for fibromyalgia in primary care: a randomised controlled trial. Acupunct Med. 2016;34(4):257–66.
149. Verkamp EK, Flowers SR, Lynch-Jordan AM, Taylor J, Ting TV, Kashikar-Zuck S. A survey of conventional and complementary therapies used by youth with juvenile-onset fibromyalgia. Pain Manag Nurs. 2013;14(4):e244–50.
150. Friedrichsdorf S, Kuttner L, Westendorp K, McCarty R. Integrative pediatric palliative care. In: Culbert T, Olness K, editors. Integrative pediatrics. New York: Oxford University Press; 2010.
151. Kuttner L, Friedrichsdorf SJ. Hypnosis and palliative care. Therapeutic hypnosis with children and adolescents. 2nd ed. Bethel: Crown House Publishing Limited; 2013. p. 491–509.
152. Hunt K, Ernst E. The evidence-base for complementary medicine in children: a critical overview of systematic reviews. Arch Dis Child. 2011;96(8):769–76.
153. Evans S, Tsao JC, Zeltzer LK. Complementary and alternative medicine for acute procedural pain in children. Altern Ther Health Med. 2008;14(5):52–6.
154. Richardson J, Smith JE, McCall G, Pilkington K. Hypnosis for procedure-related pain and distress in pediatric cancer patients: a systematic review of effectiveness and methodology related to hypnosis interventions. J Pain Symptom Manage. 2006;31(1):70–84.
155. Hemington KS, Coulombe MA. The periaqueductal gray and descending pain modulation: Why should we study them and what role do they play in chronic pain? J Neurophysiol. 2015;114(4):2080–3. https://doi.org/10.1152/jn.00998.2014.
156. Valet M, Sprenger T, Boecker H, Willoch F, Rummeny E, Conrad B, et al. Distraction modulates connectivity of the cingulo-frontal cortex and the midbrain during pain—an fMRI analysis. Pain. 2004;109(3):399–408.
157. Tracey I, Ploghaus A, Gati JS, Clare S, Smith S, Menon RS, et al. Imaging attentional modulation of pain in the periaqueductal gray in humans. J Neurosci. 2002;22(7):2748–52.
158. Derbyshire SW, Osborn J. Modeling pain circuits: how imaging may modify perception. Neuroimaging Clin N Am. 2007;17(4):485–93, ix.
159. Bingel U, Wanigasekera V, Wiech K, Ni Mhuircheartaigh R, Lee MC, Ploner M, et al. The effect of treatment expectation on drug efficacy: imaging the analgesic benefit of the opioid remifentanil. Sci Transl Med. 2011;3(70):70ra14.
160. Yu R, Gollub RL, Spaeth R, Napadow V, Wasan A, Kong J. Disrupted functional connectivity of the periaqueductal gray in chronic low back pain. Neuroimage Clin. 2014;6:100–8.
161. Giordano J. The neurobiology of nociceptive and anti-nociceptive systems. Pain Physician. 2005;8(3):277–90.
162. Tegethoff M, Belardi A, Stalujanis E, Meinlschmidt G. Comorbidity of mental disorders and chronic pain: chronology of onset in adolescents of a national representative cohort. J Pain. 2015;16(10):1054–64.
163. Cohen LL, Vowles KE, Eccleston C. The impact of adolescent chronic pain on functioning: disentangling the complex role of anxiety. J Pain. 2010;11(11):1039–46.
164. Palermo TM, Eccleston C, Lewandowski AS, Williams AC, Morley S. Randomized controlled trials of psychological therapies for management of chronic pain in children and adolescents: an updated meta-analytic review. Pain. 2010;148(3):387–97.
165. Eccleston C, Palermo TM, Williams AC, Lewandowski Holley A, Morley S, Fisher E, et al. Psychological therapies for the management of chronic and recurrent pain in children and adolescents. Cochrane Database Syst Rev. 2014;(5):CD003968.
166. Kashikar-Zuck S, Sil S, Lynch-Jordan AM, Ting TV, Peugh J, Schikler KN, et al. Changes in pain coping, catastrophizing, and coping efficacy after cognitive-behavioral therapy in children and adolescents with juvenile fibromyalgia. J Pain. 2013;14(5):492–501.
167. Seminowicz DA, Shpaner M, Keaser ML, Krauthamer GM, Mantegna J, Dumas JA, et al. Cognitive-behavioral therapy increases prefrontal cortex gray matter in patients with chronic pain. J Pain. 2013;14(12):1573–84.
168. Stefan J. Friedrichsdorf, Donna Eull, Christian Weidner, Andrea Postier, A hospital-wide initiative to eliminate or reduce needle pain in children using lean methodology. PAIN Reports 3:e671

Psychological Factors During Acute Hospitalization: Delirium, Anxiety, and Acute Stress Disorder

26

Shelley A. Wiechman

26.1 Introduction

The focus of this section is on identifying common issues during the ICU and acute phase of recovery that can impact quality of life long after discharge. The major psychological issues characteristic of this phase of recovery are delirium, anxiety, acute stress disorder, and depression [1–4]. Pain is also a primary issue and can interact with and exacerbate all of these issues and lead to long-term distress. Specifically, high inpatient pain levels predict higher rates of depression and suicidality up to 2 years following the burn injury [4–6]. High inpatient pain levels also predict rates of PTSD following the injury and many patients report that the trauma that they are re-experiencing is not the initial burn trauma, but the subsequent painful wound care [4]. Please see Chap. 27 for a more thorough discussion of pain. Ultimately, optimizing long-term quality of life following a burn injury starts in the ICU.

Screening for delirium, anxiety, acute stress disorder, and depression should be conducted as soon patient is alert enough to participate in an assessment. Early identification and intervention is key to reducing the likelihood of long-term negative effects. Knowing established risk factors for these disorders can help to identify those patients who are a high priority for screening and intervention. Some studies have shown that the strongest predictor of emotional distress in the hospital is a premorbid history of mental health issues. Further, there are higher rates of premorbid mental health issues in the burn population and these issues can significantly impact burn recovery [7]. It is important to note that delirium, anxiety, acute stress disorder, and depression are all DSM-V disorders, but many patients do not meet the full criteria for an actual diagnosis. However, the symptoms that they do have may be so severe that they are interfering with care and quality of life and should be treated.

S. A. Wiechman (✉)
Department of Rehabilitation Medicine, Harborview Burn Center, University of Washington, Seattle, WA, USA
e-mail: wiechman@u.washington.edu

Nonpharmacological interventions are critical adjuncts to medications in treating these symptoms. Hypnosis, meditation, progressive relaxation, imagery, mindfulness, and environmental interventions have all been shown to be effective in managing these symptoms [8, 9].

26.2 Delirium

The environment of the intensive care unit can be both overstimulating with its bright lights, machines, and multiple health care providers, yet also extremely monotonous, as patients are forced to lie in a hospital bed, often immobile for weeks at a time. These conditions, along with the multiple medications and the actual trauma itself, can lead to delirium. Delirium is defined by the DSM-V as a disturbance in attention and awareness and cognitive function that develops over a short period of time and is a change from baseline attention and awareness [10]. These disturbances cannot be better explained by another neurocognitive disorder, such as a traumatic brain injury, anoxia, or stroke. A hallmark feature of delirium that defines it from other forms of brain injury is that it tends to fluctuate in severity over the course of the day. Delirium is further defined as being hyperactive (mood lability, agitation, hyperactive motor activity), hypoactive (sluggishness, lethargy), or a mixed level of activity where the person has normal psychomotor activity even though attention and awareness are disturbed. Hypoactive delirium has been associated with more negative long-term outcomes than hyperactive delirium [11]. The pathophysiology of delirium is still not fully understood but some point to a neurotransmitter imbalance and neuroinflammation [12, 13]. Although 80% of ICU patients develop delirium, it is often thought that it resolves before discharge; however, a systematic review on hospital delirium showed that it can persist at hospital discharge in 45% of patients and in 33% of patients it was present 1 month later. This was particularly true for those with predisposing factors, such as older age [14].

M. G. Jeschke et al. (eds.), *Handbook of Burns Volume 1*, https://doi.org/10.1007/978-3-030-18940-2_26

Much of our knowledge of delirium in the ICU is from research on non-burn trauma and medical populations, and it is unclear how those with burn injuries may differ. One recent study by Agarwal and colleagues sought to identify the prevalence and risk factors of delirium in patients in the burn ICU by using the CAM-ICU [15]. Across two sites, they found the prevalence of delirium to be 77% with a median duration of 3 days. This is similar to that found in the general ICU population. Risk factors identified were exposure to benzodiazepines. Exposure to IV opiates and methadone were associated with a lower risk of delirium. In fact, higher doses of IV opiates reduced the odds of developing delirium by almost half. They hypothesized that this was due to better pain reduction as high pain levels are also a cause of delirium. Finally, they found that hypoactive delirium was much more prevalent than the hyperactive subtype and advocated for routine screening of delirium since the majority of those with hypoactive delirium will be missed given the absence of the more noticeable positive symptoms (i.e., agitation).

In 2012–2013, The American College of Critical Care Medicine (ACCM) established a multidisciplinary task force to develop evidence-based clinical practice guidelines for the management of pain, agitation, and delirium in the intensive care unit. Their focus included patients admitted to both trauma and medical conditions [16]. After a thorough review of the literature and lengthy discussion, they concluded that delirium was associated with increased mortality, longer lengths of stay, and impairments after discharge. Risk factors for the development of delirium in the ICU included, preexisting dementia, history of hypertension, alcoholism, and increased injury severity on admission. Other studies have found that old age, poor vision, and poor hearing to contribute to delirium [17, 18]. Precipitating factors include medications (particularly benzodiazepines and anticholinergic agents), surgery/anesthesia, anemia, infections, and acute illness [17, 18]. The task force found that the strongest evidence for intervening to prevent delirium was early mobilization. They found that atypical antipsychotics may reduce the duration of delirium but there was no published evidence for the use of Haldol.

Delirium is typically assessed by the bedside nurse. It is important to conduct this assessment throughout the day (typically once per shift) as the hallmark of delirium is that it is transient and the medical team needs a sense of the percentage of the day that the patient is delirious to better inform treatment. Several measures exist for assessing delirium. The ACCM Task force on delirium also recommended routine monitoring by using either the Confusion Assessment Method for the ICU [19] or the Intensive Care Delirium Checklist [20]. Once a person has screened positive for delirium given these measures, a more thorough evaluation should be conducted.

Delirium Management. A memorable mnemonic (DELIRIUM) has been established for a thorough review of all contributing factors to delirium that should be ruled out. This table can be found elsewhere [21]. All possible contributing factors to delirium should be addressed and it is important to note that small, multidimensional interventions can lead to substantial improvement. A 2015 meta-analysis of nonpharmacological interventions for delirium found a significant reduction in the incidence of delirium with an odds ratio of 0.47, CI, 0.38–0.58 [22]. These interventions are listed below.

- Minimize medications that can contribute to delirium when possible.
- Assess medical factors that could contribute to delirium (e.g., infections).
- Continuously reorient the patient and place reorientation cues in the room (e.g., calendar, pictures of family).
- Announce when you walk into the room and tell the patient what you will be doing.
- Put the patient on a regularly sleep/wake cycle and differentiate days and nights.
- Minimize nighttime interruptions.
- Limit overstimulation (too much light, too many people in the room, TV).
- Speak to the patient in a direct, calm manner using easy-to-understand language and short sentences.
- Allow the patient extra time to respond to questions.
- Consider a medication to reduce delirium.

26.3 Anxiety

The ICU is universally considered a stressful event. The injury itself and treatment of the injury, the acute stress reaction, the environment, and the presence of endotracheal tubes can all cause discomfort and lead to anxiety. Several studies have examined patients' experience of anxiety in the ICU setting. Upwards of 80% of ICU patients report anxiety during their ICU stay. The majority of these patients then report delusional memories of the ICU and put them at risk for the development of PTSD after discharge [23].

Patients report that thirst, fear, sleep disturbances, nightmares, and hallucinations are anxiety provoking and commonly occurred during their ICU stay [23]. Traditionally, when a patient has mechanical ventilation, they are sedated. However, deep sedation can lengthen an ICU stay and interfere with early mobility and increase delirium. Recently, practice has been to reduce or eliminate sedation and to have periods of no sedation to improve delirium and decrease ICU stay. It is unclear what effect this lighter sedation will have on a patient's anxiety or long-term outcomes. One study looked at 206 ventilated patients and compared their ICU experiences to the depth of sedation [24]. They found that 82% of patients recalled at least one stressful experience while ventilated. These experiences included motion restriction by lines and tubes, being thirsty, inability to speak, and being in pain. These reported stressful experiences were significantly related to the depth of sedation, whereas those who were more awake recalled more stressful experiences. When the same investigators looked at the patient at 2 months post ICU, those who experienced more agitation and extreme fear in the ICU were at greater risk of developing high levels of PTSD symptoms [25]. Further, perception of stressful experiences was also related to a longer length of stay in the ICU and more nightmares. In this study, those more heavily sedated also reported more nightmares and were more commonly sedated with midazolam. Nightmares under sedation are not necessarily of the traumatic injury. Midazolam is also more likely to lead to amnesia for the events and this is associated with higher rates of PTSD [26].

Lengthy assessments of anxiety can be avoided. Anxiety can be quickly assessed by asking patients to rate their anxiety on a 0–10 scale. For nonverbal patients, a strong indicator of anxiety is whether or not they show pain behaviors or agitation prior to any painful procedures.

Anxiety Management. Both procedural and baseline anxiety can increase a patient's perception of pain and should be treated as aggressively as we treat pain. Unfortunately, pharmacologic treatment of both pain and anxiety with opiates and benzodiazepines will also lead to delirium. In addition, high pain and anxiety levels can also lead to delirium. The complex relationship between mechanical ventilation, sedation, anxiety, and delirium underscores the importance of nonpharmacological management and the bedside staff. These patients will need constant reorientation, frequent and clear communication, sympathetic reassurance, and coordination of care to minimize disturbance.

Helping the patient to feel more control over their environment can also be effective in managing anxiety. The hospital setting strips control from both adults and children. Having the patient work with the nurse in devising a plan for the day, having a predictable daily routine, constant reorientation to time, date, place, and caregivers, and some choice over daily decisions help a patient to feel more in control and experience less anxiety.

It is also important to introduce a relaxation technique at this phase of recovery. A wide range of techniques have been shown to be effective and include deep breathing, muscle relaxation, music, meditation, and hypnosis [27–33]. One study even found that the simple technique of jaw relaxation that is practiced 20 min prior to dressing changes can significantly reduce pain and anxiety during and after the procedure [34].

Hypnosis involves a blend of relaxation, imagery, and cognitive restructuring. Tightly controlled studies with reliable measures of pain and anxiety have supported hypnosis as an effective nonpharmacologic approach to burn pain and anxiety [34–40]. The hypnosis protocol used by Patterson and colleagues [41] is to provide hypnosis prior to wound care and have nurses provide standard post-hypnotic suggestions during wound care. This approach is efficient for both the therapist and the nurses. It is important to note that hypnosis used in this fashion be an adjunct to, rather than replacement for, pain and anxiety medication. Finally, hypnosis should not be used if patients are still in delirium.

- Calming reassurance
- Giving patient more control over their environment
- Introducing a relaxation technique—deep breathing imagery, music, hypnosis, meditation

26.4 Acute Stress Disorder (ASD)

Acute Stress Disorder (ASD) and Post-Traumatic Stress Disorder (PTSD) are terms that are often used casually to encompass all emotional symptoms that occur after a trauma. But in fact, ASD/PTSD is a constellation of symptoms that make up an actual DSM-V diagnosis [10]. ASD occurs between 3 days and 1 month following the injury and is then diagnosed as Post-Traumatic Stress Disorder (PTSD) 1 month or more following injury. The primary diagnostic symptom that differentiates it from PTSD is dissociation, or the feeling of an altered sense of reality or seeing oneself from another's perspective. Other symptoms applying to both diagnoses include exposure to actual or threatened death or serious injury by directly experiencing the trauma, witnessing the trauma in others, or learning that the event occurred to a close family member or friend. There must also be the presence of nine or more symptoms in the broad categories of intrusion (nightmares, flashbacks), negative mood, dissociation avoidance, and arousal (sleep disturbance, agitation, hypervigilance) [10]. Untreated ASD can increase agitation and pain levels [42, 43]. Many studies have now shown that the strongest predictor of the onset of PTSD is the presence of ASD early in the hospitalization. Other risk factors include female gender and a past history of traumatic events. In fact, if a person has experienced PTSD in the past, the current trauma may trigger these past symptoms and they may begin to have nightmares and flashbacks of their prior trauma. In non-trauma populations, the use of benzodiazepines, such as midazolam and lorazepam, and higher doses of opiates, are associated with higher rates of

PTSD following hospitalization. However, high pain and anxiety levels during wound care are also associated with high rates of PTSD and depression years later.

It is important to screen, and treat ASD as early in the hospital stay as is feasible. Screening for ASD can be done by asking patients if they are having any nightmares or flashbacks of the injury, or if they are observed to have disturbed and restless sleep. If so, a consultation from the mental health team is warranted for further assessment. No gold standard screening tools exist for ASD so behavioral indicators such as nightmares, flashbacks, and hypervigilance or agitation should be used as an indication for further assessment and intervention, particularly in those with the aforementioned risk factors. There are many screening tools for PTSD but they are quite lengthy for bedside nurses or social workers. Similarly to the screening of ASD mentioned above, patients can simply be asked if they are having nightmares or flashbacks of the injury or if their sleep is disturbed and restless. If they indicate they are, consult the mental health provider for further assessment.

ASD Management. The treatments that have the most evidence base for PTSD are the exposure-based treatments that expose the patient to the trauma, either by talking about it repeatedly or writing about it, while simultaneously teaching them relaxation techniques to manage dysregulation and cognitive restructuring to change the way the patient views the trauma. This is a difficult treatment and patients who are still in the ICU or acute care phase of recovery are not appropriate for this treatment as their cognitive and emotional energy is going towards survival and managing the painful treatments. Patients can engage in this treatment once they are outpatients. While inpatients, ASD is best treated by managing each symptom. For hypervigilance, the same techniques can be used to treat anxiety: teaching a patient a relaxation technique and providing the patient as much control over their environment as possible. It is also important to help the patient to stop reinforcing any unwanted memories of the trauma by refusing to tell details of the accident repeatedly and by stopping flashbacks. Avoiding memories of the trauma and avoiding talking about the trauma is appropriate at this phase of recovery.

- Psychoeducation about the fight-or-flight response and instinctual nature of ASD.
- Normalize the response and give expectation of recovery over time.
- Teach a thought stopping technique to avoid engaging in flashbacks of the trauma.
- Support patient in telling visitors that they do not wish to repeat details of the trauma.
- Teach patient a relaxation technique to regulate anxiety.

For nightmares, the American Academy of Sleep Medicine published Best Practice Guidelines for the treatment of nightmares [44]. First-line treatments included the medication, prazosin, and a type of cognitive behavior therapy known as imagery rehearsal therapy. A recent meta-analysis of both prazosin and IRT for nightmares, sleep quality, and posttraumatic stress symptoms found moderate effect sizes for both treatments and no difference between the two treatments. When adding traditional CBT focused on insomnia was added to IRT, treatment outcomes were enhanced [45].

26.5 Depression

The term "depression" is often used to describe a variety of states, such as low mood sadness, general distress, and a syndrome or collection of symptoms that frequently occur together and qualify for a diagnosis of Major Depressive Disorder (MDD). The Diagnostic and Statistical Manual of Mental Disorders V (DSM-V) [10] defines MDD on the basis of the presence of a minimum number of symptoms that impact daily functioning and quality of life. The diagnosis of MDD requires the presence of at least one of the two hallmark features, sad mood or loss of interest or pleasure (anhedonia), and five of nine cognitive and somatic symptoms (feelings of worthlessness or guilt, fatigue, changes in sleep, inability to focus or concentrate, appetite changes, and suicidality). The symptoms must be consistently present for at least 2 weeks and cause clinically significant impairment in daily functioning [10].

One of the primary challenges to diagnosing depression in persons who have sustained burn injuries is determining whether somatic symptoms are attributable to the effects of the injury, secondary medical conditions, environmental factors, or to depression itself. Obviously, this challenge is not restricted to those with burn injuries, but is present among medical and other trauma patients, and persons with disabilities [46]. Williams and colleagues [47] propose two primary approaches to handling the effect of traumatic injury on the diagnosis of depression. The *inclusive approach* counts depressive symptoms towards the diagnosis of depression regardless of whether the symptom is thought to be due to medical causes. The *etiologic approach* reflects the DSM's criteria that count symptoms towards a diagnosis unless the symptom is clearly accounted for by a medical condition. The inclusive approach reflects the belief that there is no evidence to suggest that somatic symptoms of depression are not a meaningful dimension of depressive symptoms in the burn population. Therefore, clinically, we recommend the inclusive approach to understand depression in this population. Regardless of whether a diagnosis of major depressive disorder can be made, patients should be treated for depression if symptoms are interfering with their ability to participate in treatment and affecting quality of life [48].

Screening should be done early in the ICU. If there is a positive screen and the patient's depressive symptoms are interfering with care, such as showing decreased motivation to participate in care, intervention should be implemented. The quality consensus committee convened by the ABA has recommended several screening tools for depression [49]. The Patient Health Questionnaire, either 9-item or 2-item (PHQ-9 or 2) [50] can be easily used by the bedside nurse or social worker and is free of charge. Screening for depression is only effective once the person's mental status has cleared. The committee recommends screening for depression at least once after admission when mental status clears, once prior to discharge, and at least once in the outpatient clinic visit. A positive screen should lead to consultation with the mental health provider for further assessment and treatment.

Depression Management. Behavioral activation such as getting the patient up, groomed, dressed, and out of bed and having one positive activity or event that they can look forward to everyday is particularly effective in the inpatient setting. As the patients mental status clears, the nature of both the emotional impact of the injury and the interventions that can be done changes as they become more alert and oriented to their situation. Supportive counseling might be effective to provide safety and reassurance and to give patients a safe place to process the impact of their injury and plan for the future. This must be done in a way that is comfortable for the patient and fits into their own pre-injury coping style. Some patients will want to talk about what has happened to them and be more emotional in their processing while others will want to focus on concrete problem-solving strategies to get on with their future with little expressed emotion or discussion of the nature of their injury. Either style is effective and attempting to change a person's coping style in the midst of a crisis such as a critical injury is rarely successful. Successful processing of the injury can promote posttraumatic growth and resiliency long after discharge. Peer visitors can be especially effective in providing support, as they are usually that one voice who can truly understand what the patient is going through. Most burn centers have utilized the Phoenix Society's SOAR program and those peer visits can be useful in providing support and hope to both the patient and the family and establishing this relationship early in the hospitalization.

Family support is also important during this time. The patient's coping ability is often influenced by cues from significant others. As family members express high levels of anxiety and sadness, the patient may detect these cues and behave accordingly. It is important to help family members understand this process and encourage them to convey a sense of optimism, hope, and calmness that may be transmitted to the patient. Keeping the family informed of the patient's current condition and the long-term plan for recovery is crucial. Going over the plan or goals of the day, informing them of any changes in condition, and periodically holding family meetings can ease the family's anxiety. Family should be encouraged to engage in their own self-care (e.g., giving them permission to leave the hospital to take care of other matters, sleeping and eating regularly, and exercising). The relationship that all members of the burn team form with the family at this stage is critical for the long-term partnership that is needed to care for the patient for years to come.

26.6 Sleep

Sleep disturbance is common in both the ICU and acute floor and can exacerbate anxiety, ASD, and delirium [51]. Oftentimes, a patient's days and nights go undifferentiated and they may sleep much of the day and then find it difficult to sleep at night. Behavioral interventions for sleep are highly effective and can include designing a daily schedule for the patient so that they know what to expect throughout the day and evening. Keeping lights on and shades up with activities throughout the day is important, as is turning the TV off and pulling the shades at night when it is time to sleep. Minimizing nighttime interruptions for nursing care is also critical to promoting prolonged sleep. Napping during the day should be discouraged if possible. Pharmacological sleep aides, such as melatonin, should also be considered if behavioral interventions are not adequate. Other medications typically used for sleep may put a patient at risk for delirium, especially in the elderly.

26.7 Adherence to Treatment

Adherence to painful treatments, such as range of motion and wound care can arise as patients move along in their hospitalization. Oftentimes as patients move out of the ICU, they are weaned from opiate medication. This makes for more painful range of motion and therapy. Patients can suddenly "hit a wall" and lose motivation to continue aggressive participation in their physical and occupational therapy, particularly if they have had a long ICU stay. They will be more focused on discharge and getting out of the hospital, despite not being independent enough in wound care and therapies. Strategies to enhance motivation include helping a patient feel more in control of their own care and outcome. The team should engage the patient in setting their own functional goals and having input into their daily routines and discharge planning. Setting up a quota system where the focus is on increasing their performance goals by 10% every day and working towards that goal versus stopping when there is pain can also be effective [52]. Again, SOAR visitors can often exemplify, "the light at the end of the tunnel" and help the patient to overcome these temporary barriers to treatment.

26.8 Post-Intensive Care Syndrome

In this chapter, we have talked about delirium, anxiety, ASD/PTSD, depression, and sleep issues. The term Post-Intensive Care Syndrome (PICS) has been coined to explain the impact of an ICU stay on long-term outcomes [53]. The syndrome is characterized by multiple domains of functioning following a critical illness, including physical, cognitive, and psychological. The psychological domain includes anxiety, PTSD, depression, and cognitive deficits. Treating symptoms associated with PICS is critical as patients with higher levels of depression, PTSD, and anxiety have lower levels of health-related quality of life and can impact functional outcomes of burn recovery [54–57]. Recent research has shown that these issues can continue long after discharge if not managed properly in the inpatient hospitalization. For example, depression and PTSD at 3 months post-ICU discharge were associated with a greater risk of additional hospitalizations in the year following discharge [58]. Further, inpatient delirium can lead to decreased cognitive function and increases in rates of depression after discharge [54].

Prevalence rates of these disorders are much higher in patients following an ICU stay than in the general population. For example, prevalence rates of PTSD following an ICU stay range from 10 to 44% where the identified trauma is the ICU stay itself. This is higher than the 6.8% lifetime prevalence rate of PTSD found in the general population. There have been over 5 systematic reviews of PTSD associated with PICS that included 30 studies. Modifiable risk factors include symptoms of acute stress, depression, and anxiety in the ICU. Sedation, extreme agitation, physical restraints, and traumatic or delusional memories of the ICU are also risk factors. Factual memories of the ICU stay are less likely to cause PTSD post-ICU [58].

A systematic review of depression after an ICU stay found 14 studies (one in the trauma population) and reported rates were 28–35%, higher than the 7% found in the general population [59]. Modifiable risk factors for the onset of depression include early depressive symptoms in the ICU, traumatic or delusional memories of the ICU, sedation, psychiatric symptoms at discharge, and impairment of physical function at discharge. Non-modifiable risk factors include female gender and younger age.

26.9 Conclusion

Patients with burn injuries present a unique challenge in that the management of some constellation of symptoms has a negative impact on other symptoms. For example, the painful procedures that are required for burn care necessitate the need for higher doses of opiates and anxiolytics not needed for other conditions in the ICU. However, these medications can cause delirium and can exacerbate acute stress symptoms. It is a difficult balance to achieve as high pain levels can also cause delirium and high anxiety levels exacerbate pain. Delirium needs to be distinguished from agitation and acute stress disorder and depression so appropriate interventions can be applied, but this can be a challenge when patients are not able to accurately report symptoms due to mental status or communication challenges. It is safer to rule out delirium before attributing a patient's agitation and confusion to either anxiety, ASD, or depression since overlooking delirium and leaving it untreated can cause more severe consequences [60]. All of these challenges point to the importance of nonpharmacological interventions for these conditions. Early screening and nonpharmacological management can alleviate the severity of these disorders and possibly prevent long-term consequences while maximizing functional and emotional outcomes after the burn injury.

Summary Box

Delirium, anxiety, and acute stress disorder are the major psychological issues characteristic of the critical and acute phase of recovery. Pain is also a primary physical challenge and can interact with and exacerbate all of these issues and lead to long-term distress. Patients with burn injuries present a unique challenge in that the management of some constellation of symptoms has a negative impact on other symptoms. For example, the painful procedures that are required for burn care necessitate the need for higher doses of opiates and anxiolytics not needed for other conditions in the ICU. However, these medications can cause delirium and can exacerbate acute stress symptoms. It is a difficult balance to achieve as high pain levels can also cause delirium and high anxiety levels exacerbate pain. All of these challenges point to the importance of nonpharmacological interventions for these conditions. Early screening and nonpharmacological management can alleviate the severity of these disorders and possibly prevent long-term consequences while maximizing functional and emotional outcomes after the burn injury.

References

1. Corry NH, Klick B, Fauerbach JA. Posttraumatic stress disorder and pain impact functioning and disability after major burn injury. J Burn Care Res. 2010;31(1):13–25. PMID: 20061832.
2. Thombs BD, Bresnick MG, Magyar-Russel G. Depression in survivors of burn injury: a systematic review. Gen Hosp Psychiatry. 2006;28(6):494–502.
3. Wiechman Askay S, Patterson D. What are the psychiatric sequelae of burn pain? Curr Pain Headache Rep. 2008;12(2):94–7.

4. Edwards RR, Smith MT, Klick B, et al. Symptoms of depression and anxiety as unique predictors of pain-related outcomes following burn injury. Ann Behav Med. 2007;34(3):313–22.
5. Edwards RR, Magyar-Russell G, Thombs B, Smith MT, Holavanahalli RK, Patterson DR, Blakeney P, Lezotte DC, Haythornthwaite JA, Fauerbach JA. Acute pain at discharge from hospitalization is a prospective predictor of long-term suicidal ideation after burn injury. Arch Phys Med Rehabil. 2007;88(12 Suppl 2):S36–42.
6. Thombs BD, Bresnick MG, Magyar-Russell G, Lawrence JW, McCann UD, Fauerbach JA. Symptoms of depression predict change in physical heath after burn injury. Burns. 2007;33(3):292–8.
7. Patterson DR, Finch CP, Wiechman SA, Bonsack R, Gibran NS, Heimbach DM. Premorbid mental health status of adult burn patients: comparisons with a normative sample. J Burn Care Rehabil. 2003;24(5):347–50.
8. Patterson DR, Hoffman HG, Wiechman SA, Jensen MP, Sharar SR. Optimizing control of pain from severe burns: a literature review. Am J Clin Hypn. 2004;47(1):43–54.
9. Wiechman Askay S, Patterson D. A randomized controlled trial of hypnosis for burn wound care. Rehabil Psychol. 2007;52(3):247–53.
10. American Psychiatric Association. Diagnostic and statistical manual of mental disorders. 5th ed. Washington, DC: American Psychiatric Association; 2013.
11. Meagher DJ, Trzepacz PT. Motoric subtypes of delirium. Semin Clin Neuropsychiatry. 2000;5:75–85.
12. Inouye SK, Westendorp RG, Saczynski JS. Delirium in elderly people. Lancet. 2014;383:911–22.
13. Marcantonio ER. Postoperative delirium: a 76-year-old woman with delirium following surgery. JAMA. 2012;308:73–81.
14. Cole MG, Ciampi A, Belzile E, Zhong L. Persistent delirium in older hospital patients: a systematic review of frequency and prognosis. Age Ageing. 2009;38(1):19–26.
15. Argawal V, O'Neill PJ, Cotton BA, et al. Prevalence and risk factors for development of delirium in burn intensive care unit patients. J Burn Care Res. 2010;31:70–715.
16. Barr J, Gilles LF, Puntillo K, et al. Clinical practice guidelines for the management of pain, agitation and delirium in adult patients in the intensive care unit. Crit Care Med. 2013;41:263–306.
17. Inouye SK, Charpentier PA. Precipitation factors for delirium in hospitalized elderly persons: predictive model and interrelationship with baseline vulnerability. JAMA. 1996;275:852–7.
18. Marcantonio ER, Juarez G, Goldman L, et al. The relationship of postoperative delirium with psychoactive medications. JAMA. 1994;272:1518–22.
19. Ely EW, Margolin R, Francis J, et al. Evaluation of delirium in critically ill patients: validation of the confusion assessment method for the intensive care unit (CAM-ICU). Crit Care Med. 2001;29:1370–9.
20. Bergeron N, Dubois MJ, Dumont M, Dial S, Skrobik Y. Intensive care delirium screening checklist: evaluation of a new screening tool. Intensive Care Med. 2001;27:859–64.
21. Marcantonio ER. Delirium in hospitalized older patients. N Engl J Med. 2017;377:1456–66.
22. Hsieh TT, Yue J, Oh E, et al. Effectiveness of multicomponent nonpharmacological delirium interventions: a meta-analysis. JAMA Intern Med. 2015;175:512–20.
23. Rotondi AJ, Chelluri L, Sirio C, Mendelsohn A, Schulz R, Belle S, Im K, Donahoe M, Pinsky MR. Patients' recollections of stressful experiences while receiving prolonged mechanical ventilation in an intensive care unit. Crit Care Med. 2002;30:746–52.
24. Samuelson KAM, Lundberg D, Fridlund B. Stressful experiences in relation to depth of sedation in mechanically ventilated patients. Nurs Crit Care. 2007;12(2):93–104.
25. Samuelson KAM, Lundberg D, Fridlund B. Stressful memories and psychological distress in adult mechanically ventilated intensive care patients—a 2 month follow up study. Acta Anaesthesiol Scand. 2007;51:671–8.
26. Rundshagen I, Schnabel K, Wegner C, Schulte am Esch J. Incidence of recall, nightmares, and hallucinations during analgosedation in intensive care. Intensive Care Med. 2002;28:38–43.
27. Park E, Oh H, Kim T. The effects of relaxation breathing on procedural pain and anxiety during burn care. Burns. 2013;39(6):1101–6.
28. Wernick RL, Jaremko ME, Taylor PW. Pain management in severely burned adults: a test of stress inoculation. J Behav Med. 1981;4:103–9.
29. Whitehead-Pleaux AM, Baryza MJ, Sheridan RL. The effects of music therapy on pediatric patients' pain and anxiety during donor site dressing change. J Music Ther. 2006;43:136–53.
30. Elliott CH, Olson RA. The management of children's distress in response to painful medical treatment for burn injuries. Behav Res Ther. 1983;21:675–83.
31. Foertsch CE, O'Hara MW, Stoddard FJ, Kealey GP. Treatment resistant pain and distress during pediatric burn dressing changes. J Burn Care Rehabil. 1998;19:219–24.
32. Presner JD, Yowler CJ, Smith LF, Steele AL, Fratianne RB. Music therapy for assistance with pain and anxiety management in burn treatment. J Burn Care Rehabil. 2001;22(1):83–8; discussion 82–3.
33. Tan X, Yowler CJ, Super DM, Fratianne RB. The efficacy of music therapy protocols for decreasing pain, anxiety, and muscle tension levels during burn dressing changes: a prospective randomized crossover trial. J Burn Care Res. 2010;31(4):590–7.
34. Mohammadi Fakhar F, Rafii F, Jamshidi Orak R. The effect of jaw relaxation on pain anxiety during burn dressings: randomized clinical trial. Burns. 2013;39(1):61–7.
35. Patterson DR, Questad KA, Boltwood MD. Hypnotherapy as a treatment for pain in patients with burns: research and clinical considerations. J Burn Care Rehabil. 1987;8:263–8.
36. Patterson DR, Everett JJ, Burns GL, Marvin JA. Hypnosis for the treatment of burn pain. J Consult Clin Psychol. 1992;60:713–7.
37. Patterson DR, Ptacek JT. Baseline pain as a moderator of hypnotic analgesia for burn injury treatment. J Consult Clin Psychol. 1997;65:60–7.
38. Patterson DR, Jensen M. Hypnosis and clinical pain. Psychol Bull. 2003;129:495–521.
39. Patterson DR, Questad KA, DeLateur BJ. Hypnotherapy as an adjunct to narcotic analgesia for the treatment of pain for burn debridement. Am J Clin Hypn. 1989;31:156–63.
40. Shakibaei F, Harandi AA, Gholamrezaei A, Samoei R, Pejman S. Hypnotherapy in management of pain and reexperiencing of trauma in burn patients. Int J Clin Exp Hypn. 2008;56(2):185–97.
41. Askay SW, Patterson DR, Jensen MP, Sharar SR. A randomized controlled trial of hypnosis for burn wound care. Rehabil Psychol. 2007;52:247–53.
42. Ehde DM, Patterson DR, Wiechman SA, Wilson LG. Post-traumatic stress symptoms and distress 1 year after burn injury. J Burn Care Rehabil. 2000;21:105–11.
43. McKibben J, Bresnick M, Wiechman Askay S, Fauerbach J. Acute stress disorder and posttraumatic stress disorder: a prospective study of prevalence, course and predictors in a sample with major burn injuries. J Burn Care Res. 2008;29(1):22–35.
44. Aurora RN, Zak RS, Auerbach SH, et al. Best practice guide for the treatment of nightmare disorder in adults. J Clin Sleep Med. 2010;6:389–401.
45. Seda GS, Sanchez-Ortuno MM, Welsh CH, Halbower AC, Edinger JD. Comparative meta-analysis of prazosin and imagery rehearsal therapy for nightmare frequency, sleep quality, and posttrauamtic stress. J Clin Sleep Med. 2015;11(1):11–22.
46. Stewart DE. Physical symptoms of depression: unmet needs in special populations. J Clin Psychiatry. 2003;64:12–6.
47. Williams JW, Noel PH, Cordes JA, Ramirez G, Pignone M. Is this patient clinically depressed? JAMA. 2002;287(9):1160–70.

48. Wiechman SA, Kalpakjian CZ, Johnson KL. Measuring depression in adults with burn injuries: a systematic review. J Burn Care Res. 2016;37(5):e415–26.
49. Gibran NS, Wiechman SA, Meyer WM, et al. American Burn Association consensus statement. J Burn Care Res. 2013;34(4):361–85.
50. Kroenke K, Spitzer RL, Williams JB, Lowe B. The patient health questionnaire somatic, anxiety and depressive symptom scales: a systematic review. Gen Hosp Psychiatry. 2010;32(4):345–59.
51. Jaffe SE, Patterson DR. Treating sleep problems in patients with burn injuries: practical considerations. J Burn Care Rehabil. 2004;25(3):294–305.
52. Ehde DM, Patterson DR, Fordyce WE. The quota system I burn rehabilitation. J Burn Care Rehabil. 1998;19(5):436–40.
53. Svenngsen H, Langhorn L, Agard AS, Dreyer P. Post-ICU symptoms, consequences, and follow-up: an integrative review. Nurs Crit Care. 2015;22:212–20. https://doi.org/10.1111/nicc.12165.
54. Davidow DS, Hough CL, Zatzick D, Katon WJ. Psychiatric symptoms and acute scare service utilization over the course of the year following medical-surgical ICU admission: a longitudinal investigation. Crit Care Med. 2014;42(12):2473–81.
55. Davidow DS, Hough CL, Levine DA, Langa KM, Iwashyna TJ. Functional disability, cognitive impairment, and depression after hospitalization for pneumonia. Am J Med. 2013;126(7):615–24.e5.
56. Davidow D. The burden of adverse mental health outcomes in critical illness survivors. Crit Care. 2010;14(1):125.
57. Davidow D. Posttraumatic stress disorder in critical illness survivors: too many questions remain. Crit Care Med. 2015;43(5):1151–2.
58. Jones C, Griffiths RD, Humphris G, Skirrow PM. Memory, delusions and the development of acute posttraumatic stress disorder-related symptoms after intensive care. Crit Care Med. 2001;29(3):573–80.
59. Hashem MD, Nallaqanqula A, Nalamalapu S, et al. Patient outcomes after critical illness: a systematic review of qualitative studies following hospital discharge. Crit Care. 2016;20(1):345.
60. Walder B, Tramer MR. Analgesia and sedation in critically ill patients. Swiss Med Wkly. 2004;134:333–46.

27 Nursing Management of the Burn Patient

Judy Knighton

27.1 Introduction

Nursing the burn-injured patient is simultaneously challenging, complex, and professionally rewarding. The repertoire of necessary skills is varied and includes comprehensive clinical assessment and monitoring, pain management, wound care, and psychosocial support. The burn nurse may care for the burn survivor throughout all phases of care, from entry into the hospital through to discharge home and re-integration into the community. Ongoing research into the practice of burn nursing is encouraged in order to identify new knowledge to guide best practices. This chapter is intended to assist the nurse in providing comprehensive care to the burn patient and his/her family.

27.2 General Definition and Description

27.2.1 Incidence

Each year, an estimated 486,000 people seek care for burns in the United States and approximately 40,000 require hospitalization, three-quarters of whom die from their injuries [1]. In Canada, about 55,000 people are injured and required some medical care [2]. Around the world, nearly 11 million people needed medical attention for burn injuries, and about 180,000 died as a result of burns, the majority from low- and middle-income countries [3].

27.2.2 Prevention

Most burn injuries are preventable and nurses have ample opportunity to serve as advocates and educators in the area of burn and fire prevention. Worldwide, there has been a slow, but steady, decrease in the number of burns occurring annually. The focus of burn prevention programs has shifted from concentrating on individual blame and changing individual behaviors to include more legislative changes. Attention continues to be focused on "at risk" groups, such as infants, toddlers, and the elderly [4–7]. Additional effort includes those attempts aimed at having a positive impact upon government legislation for items, such as safe temperature levels for hot water heaters, children's flame-retardant sleepwear, self-extinguishing cigarettes, and "child-proof" cigarette lighters. There is also increased awareness and use of fire sprinklers, along with hard-wired smoke alarms and carbon monoxide detectors [8, 9]. Safer new home construction and stricter workplace safety standards are additional factors contributing to the decrease in burn injuries [10].

27.2.3 Classification

Burn complexity can range from a relatively minor, uncomplicated injury to a life-threatening, multi-system trauma. The American Burn Association (ABA) has a useful classification system that rates burn injury magnitude from minor to moderate, uncomplicated to major (Table 27.1). This system takes into account the depth and extent of the injury, the location of burns on the body, and the patient's overall medical history. With advances in burn care over the years and the establishment of specialized facilities staffed by skilled, multidisciplinary burn team members, more patients with severe injuries are surviving. However, survival is no longer enough. The ultimate challenge for the burn team is to support and guide the burned person and his/her family towards a complete and optimal level of recovery, both physically and psychosocially.

J. Knighton (✉)
Burn Care, Sunnybrook Health Sciences Centre, Toronto, ON, Canada
e-mail: knighton@burnresource.com

M. G. Jeschke et al. (eds.), *Handbook of Burns Volume 1*, https://doi.org/10.1007/978-3-030-18940-2_27

Table 27.1 American Burn Association Adult Burn Classification

Classification	Assessment criteria
Minor burn injury	<15% TBSA burn in adults <40 years age <10% TBSA burn in adults >40 years age <2% TBSA full-thickness burn without risk of functional or esthetic impairment or disability
Moderate uncomplicated burn injury	15–25% TBSA burn in adults <40 years age 10–20% TBSA burn in adults >40 years age <10% TBSA full-thickness burn without functional or esthetic risk to burns involving the face, eyes, ears, hands, feet, perineum, or major joints
Major burn injury	>25% TBSA burn in adults <40 years age >20% TBSA burn in adults >40 years age OR >10% TBSA full-thickness burn (any age) OR injuries involving the face, eyes, ears, hands, feet perineum, or major joints, likely to result in functional or esthetic disability OR high-voltage electrical burn OR all burns with inhalation injury or major trauma

Table 27.2 Causes of burn injuries

Home and leisure	Workplace
• Hot water heaters set too high (140 °F or 60 °C) • Overloaded electrical outlets • Frayed electrical wiring • Carelessness with cigarettes, lighters, matches, candles • Pressure cookers • Microwaved foods and liquids • Hot grease or cooking liquids • Open space heaters • Gas fireplace doors • Radiators • Hot water bottles and heating pads • Hot sauna rocks • Improper use of flammable liquids: – Starter fluids – Gasoline – Kerosene • Electrical storms • Overexposure to sun	• Electricity: – Power lines – Outlet boxes • Chemicals: – Acids – Alkalis • Tar • Hot steam sources: – Boilers – Pipes – Industrial cookers • Hot industrial presses • Flammable liquids: – Propane – Acetylene – Natural gas

27.2.4 Etiology and Risk Factors

The causes of burn injuries are numerous and found in both the home and leisure and workplace settings (Table 27.2). People are most frequently burned in their own kitchen and bathroom, while involved in activities such as cooking, bathing, or smoking. Campfires, trailers, and boats serve as recreational sources for burn injuries, while industrial settings are common sites for workplace injuries, involving electricity, chemicals, and explosions. Burn injuries occur throughout the world, but predominantly to women in the developing world, among all cultures and across all age ranges. In the developed world, about two-thirds of those injured are male and about one-third are less than 16 years of age. A number of identifiable factors place someone at greater risk for sustaining a burn injury such as involvement in risk-prone activities at home or work, inattention, carelessness, lack of knowledge and resources, a sense of invincibility, lower socioeconomic status, histories of substance abuse, and mental health illness. Some incidents, however, are the result of unfortunate circumstances or medical illness, such as epilepsy or diabetes. Burn prevention programs aim to identify these risk factors, educate and heighten awareness of individual risk, and encourage people to practice safe strategies in order to decrease their level of risk at home, work, or play.

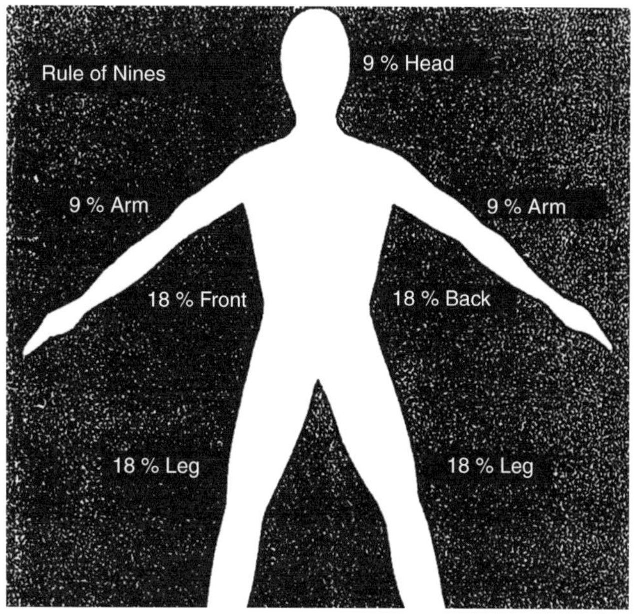

Fig. 27.1 Rule of Nines method for estimating extent of burn

Box 27.1 Burn Severity Factors
1. Extent of body surface area burned
2. Depth of tissue damage
3. Age of person
4. Part of body burned
5. Past medical history

27.3 Pathophysiology

27.3.1 Severity Factors

There are five factors to be considered when determining the severity of a burn injury (Box 27.1).

1. **Extent**—There are several, paper-based methods available to accurately calculate the percentage of body surface area involved. The simplest and most easily recalled is the Rule of Nines (Fig. 27.1). **However, it is only for**

LUND AND BROWDER EXTENT OF BURN DIAGRAM

AREA	AGE–YEARS							
	0-1	1-4	5-9	10-15	ADULT	% 2°	% 3°	% TOTAL
HEAD	19	17	13	10	7			
NECK	2	2	2	2	2			
ANT TRUNK	13	13	13	13	13			
POSTTRUNK	13	13	13	13	13			
R BUTTOCK	2.5	2.5	2.5	2.5	2.5			
L BUTTOCK	2.5	2.5	2.5	2.5	2.5			
GENITALIA	1	1	1	1	1			
RU ARM	4	4	4	4	4			
LU ARM	4	4	4	4	4			
RL ARM	3	3	3	3	3			
LL ARM	3	3	3	3	3			
R HAND	2.5	2.5	2.5	2.5	2.5			
L HAND	2.5	2.5	2.5	2.5	2.5			
R THIGH	5.5	6.5	8.5	8.5	9.5			
L THIGH	5.5	6.5	8.5	8.5	9.5			
R LEG	5	5	5.5	6	7			
L LEG	5	5	5.5	6	7			
R FOOT	3.5	3.5	3.5	3.5	3.5			
L FOOT	3.5	3.5	3.5	3.5	3.5			
					TOTAL			

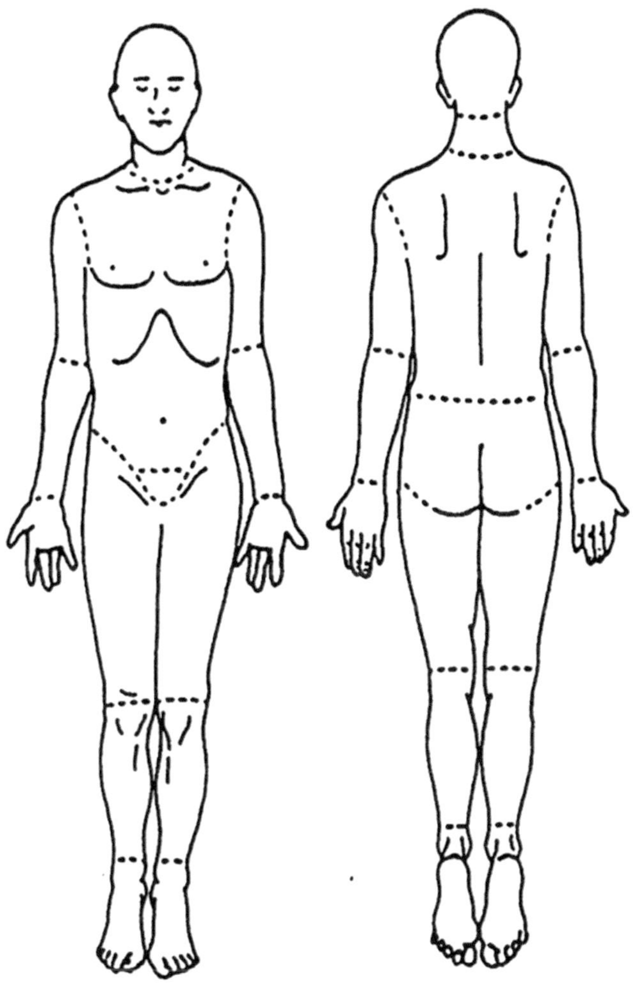

Fig. 27.2 Lund and Browder method for estimating extent of burn

use with the adult burn population. The Lund and Browder method (Fig. 27.2) is useful for all age groups, but is more complicated to use. For the pediatric population, there is a modified version of the Lund and Browder method (Fig. 27.3). If the burned areas are small and irregularly shaped, the Rule of Palm can be used. The palmer surface of the burned person's hand, **including the extended fingers,** represents 1% body surface area.

Fig. 27.3 Pediatric estimation of burn area using modified Lund and Browder

ESTIMATION OF BURN AREA

Name ________ Age ________ Ward ________

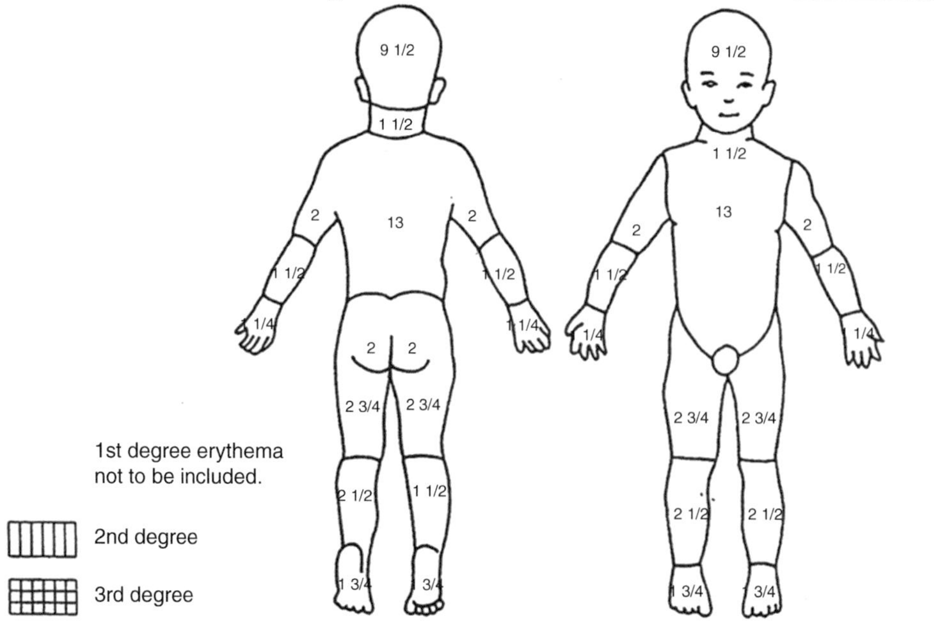

Area	Age in years					
	0	1	5	10	15	Adult
Head area	19	17	13	11	9	7
Trunk area	26	26	26	26	26	26
Arm area	7	7	7	7	7	7
Thigh area	5 1/2	6 1/2	8 1/2	8 1/2	9 1/2	9 1/2
Leg area	5	5	5	6	6	7

Total 3rd degree burn ________ Total 2nd degree burn ________ TOTAL BURNS ________

Reliability of the palmar surface area tool for obese patients has been questioned and alternative methods suggested [11]. There are also a number of internet-based or mobile technologies available to calculate the extent of the body burn, which might help to decrease the problems with both over- and under-estimation of burn size by pre-hospital, hospital, and burn team personnel [12–16].

2. **Depth**—Two factors determine the depth of a burn wound—temperature of the burning agent and duration of exposure time. Previously, the terminology used to describe burn depth was first, second, and third degree. In recent years, these terms have been replaced by those more descriptive in nature: superficial partial-thickness, deep partial-thickness, and full-thickness (Table 27.3). The skin is divided into three layers, which include the epidermis, dermis, and subcutaneous tissue (Fig. 27.4). The dermis, which is about 30–45 times thicker that the epidermis, contains connective tissue, blood vessels, hair follicles, nerve endings, sweat glands, and sebaceous glands. Skin-reproducing cells are located along the shafts of the hair follicles, sweat glands, and sebaceous glands. The sufficient presence or absence of these re-epithelializing cells determines whether the wound will heal on its own or require skin grafting. At the present time, visualization with the naked eye, by experienced burn practitioners, is used to determine burn depth. However, there is ongoing research exploring the use of newer laser technologies to determine burn depth [17].
3. **Age**—In patients less than 2 years of age and greater than 50, there is a higher incidence of morbidity and mortality. Infants, toddlers, and the elderly have thinner skin, making the risk of a deeper burn greater in these age groups. Persons of this age also have weaker physical resources to mount a resistance against the debilitating effects brought on by a burn [18, 19].
4. **Part of the body burned**—Patients with burns to the face, eyes, neck, hands, feet, joints, or perineum have greater functional and esthetic challenges to overcome and require the specialized care offered by a burn center.
5. **Past medical history**—A burn injury will exacerbate pre-existing conditions. Persons with diabetes or peripheral vascular disease have a more difficult time with wound healing, a central factor in burn recovery, particularly if the

Table 27.3 Classification of burn injury depth

Degree of burn	Cause of injury	Depth of injury	Appearance	Treatment
First degree	Superficial sunburn Brief exposure to hot liquids or heat flash	Superficial damage to epithelium Tactile and pain sensations intact	Erythematous, blanching on pressure, no blisters, sensate	Complete healing within 3–5 days with no scarring
Superficial partial-thickness (second degree)	Brief exposure to flame, flash, or hot liquids	Destruction of epidermis, superficial damage to papillary layer of dermis, epidermal appendages intact	Moist, weepy, blanching on pressure, blisters, pink or red color, sensate	Complete healing within 14–21 days with no scarring
Deep partial-thickness (deep second degree)	Exposure to flame, scalding liquids, or hot tar	Destruction of epidermis, damage to reticular layer of dermis, some epidermal appendages intact	Pale and less moist; no blanching or prolonged, deep pressure sensation intact, pinprick sensation absent	Prolonged healing time usually >21 days with scarring. Skin grafting may be necessary for improved functional and esthetic outcome
Full-thickness (third degree)	Prolonged contact with flame, steam, scalding liquids, hot objects, chemicals, or electrical current	Complete destruction of epidermis, dermis and, epidermal appendages; injury through most of the dermis	Dry, leathery, pale, mottled brown or red in color; visible thrombosed vessels insensitive to pain and pressure	Requires skin grafting
Full-thickness (fourth degree)	Major electrical current, prolonged contact with heat source (i.e., unconscious patient)	Complete destruction of epidermis, dermis, and epidermal appendages; injury involving connective tissue, muscle, and bone	Dry, black, mottled brown, white or red; no sensation and limited movement of burned limbs or digits	Requires skin grafting and likely amputation

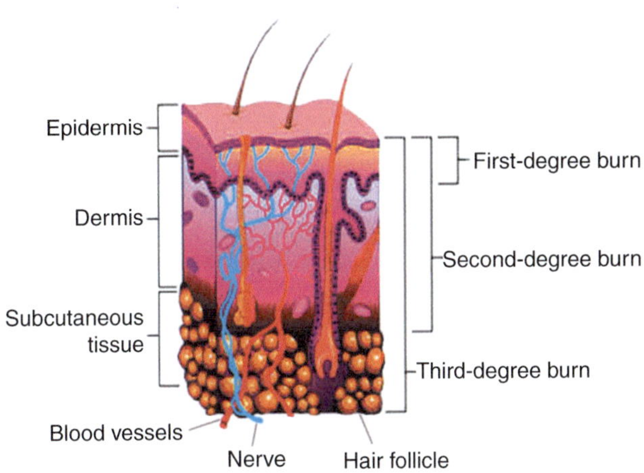

Fig. 27.4 Anatomy of burn tissue depth

burns are on the legs and/or feet [20, 21]. Burn patients with poor nutritional status pre-burn or with previous drug and/or alcohol abuse patterns have fewer physical reserves to draw from and, as such, require more resources for a prolonged period of time.

27.3.2 Local Damage

Local, burn wound damage varies, depending upon the temperature of the agent, duration of contact time, and the type of tissue involved. The deepest zone of damage, *coagulation* (full-thickness), is the site of irreversible cell death, where blood vessels and re-epithelializing cells have been completely destroyed. These areas require skin grafting for permanent coverage. The middle layer, or zone of *stasis*, is the area of deep, partial-thickness injury where there are some skin-reproducing cells present in the dermis and circulation to the area is partially intact. Healing will occur generally within 14–21 days, as long as infection or desiccation is prevented. The outermost zone of *hyperemia* is the area of least damage. This superficial, partial-thickness wound has minimal cell involvement and will generally recover spontaneously within 7–10 days. Areas of partial-thickness injury, devoid of infection and desiccation, will heal by primary intention from the edges of the wound and from below. Full-thickness wounds require early excision and skin grafting. Over time, the collagen fibers and re-epithelializing cells continue to heal and add strength to the newly formed tissue. The healed areas initially look pale and flat. However, as the blood supply increases to those areas over the next month or so, they become red and raised. In addition to these scars forming, there is a natural tendency for burned tissue to shorten and contractures to develop. Over the next year to 18 months, the burn scars will fully mature and become less red and less raised [22, 23].

27.3.3 Fluid and Electrolyte Shifts

The immediate post-burn period is marked by dramatic circulation changes, producing what is known as “burn shock”

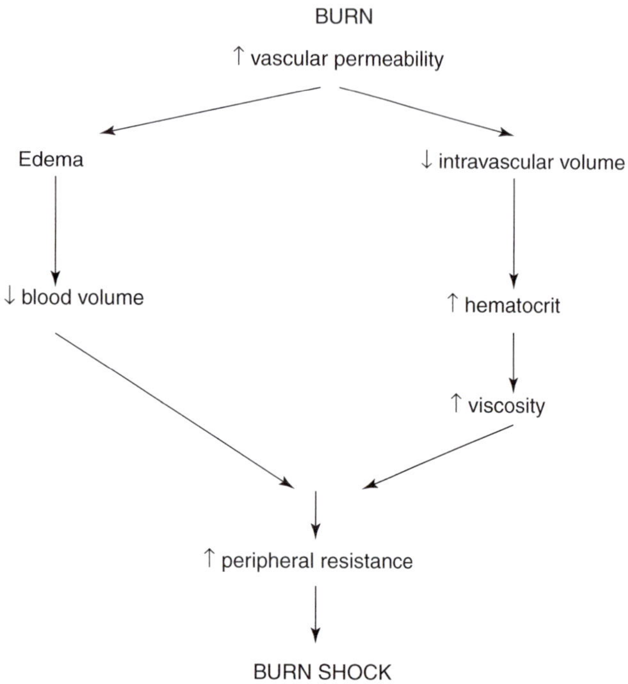

Fig. 27.5 Burn shock

(Fig. 27.5). Blood flow increases to the area surrounding the wound. The burned tissue then releases vasoactive substances, which results in increased capillary permeability. As early as 15 min post-injury, there is a shift of fluid from the intravascular compartment to the interstitial space, producing edema, decreased blood volume, and hypovolemia. There is also insensible fluid loss through evaporation from large, open body surfaces. A non-burned individual loses about 30–50 mL/h. A severely burned patient experiences intravascular volume depletion, with fluid loss anywhere from 200 to 400 mL/h. Following successful completion of the fluid resuscitation phase, capillary membrane permeability is restored. Fluids gradually shift back from the interstitial space to the intravascular space. The patient is no longer grossly edematous and diuresis is ongoing.

27.4 Types of Burn Injuries

Burns can be grouped into numerous categories: thermal, chemical, electrical, and smoke/inhalation. The causative agent does influence both the management and outcome of each injury.

27.4.1 Thermal

Thermal injuries are caused by dry heat, such as flame and flash, moist heat, such as steam and hot liquids, and direct contact, such as hot surfaces and objects (Table 27.4). Thermal burns are a major source of morbidity and mortality across all age groups (Figs. 27.6 and 27.7).

Table 27.4 Causes of thermal burns

Cause	Examples
Dry heat—Flame	• Clothing catches on fire • Skin exposed to direct flame
Dry Heat—Flash	• Flame burn associated with explosion (combustible fuels)
Moist Heat—Hot liquids (scalds)	• Bath water • Beverages—coffee, tea, soup • Cooking liquids or grease
Moist Heat—Steam	• Pressure cooker • Microwaved food • Overheated car radiator
Contact—Hot surfaces	• Oven burner and door • Barbecue grill
Contact—Hot objects	• Tar • Curling iron • Cooking pots/pans • Heating pad • Hot water bottle

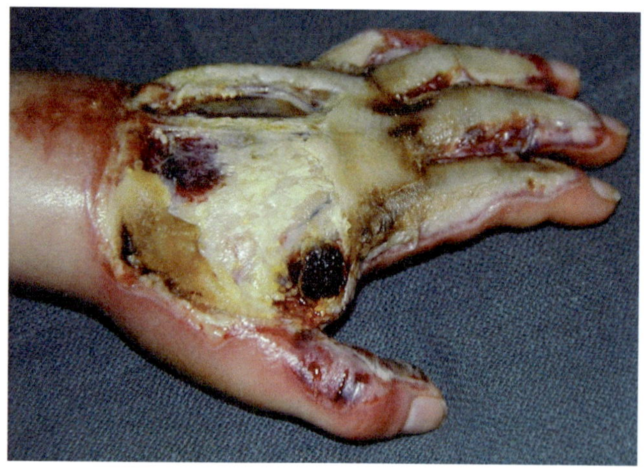

Fig. 27.6 Flame burn

27.4.2 Chemical

The types of chemical injuries seen are usually related to the geography, industry, and culture of the local population. There are more than 25,000 chemicals in the world and most can be divided into two major groups: acids and alkalis. Necrotizing substances in the chemicals cause tissue injury and destruction (Fig. 27.8). Acids, in general, cause coagulation necrosis with protein precipitation. Alkalis produce liquefaction necrosis with loosening of the tissue, which allows the alkali to diffuse more deeply into the tissues. Therefore, on a volume-to-volume basis, alkaline material can produce far more tissue damage than acids. The extent and depth of a

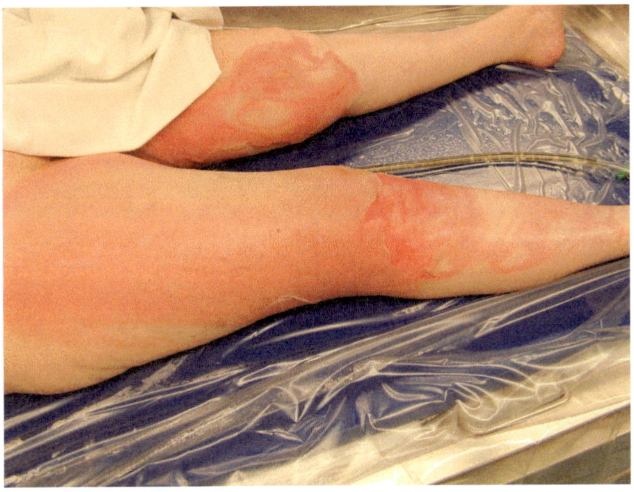

Fig. 27.7 Scald burn

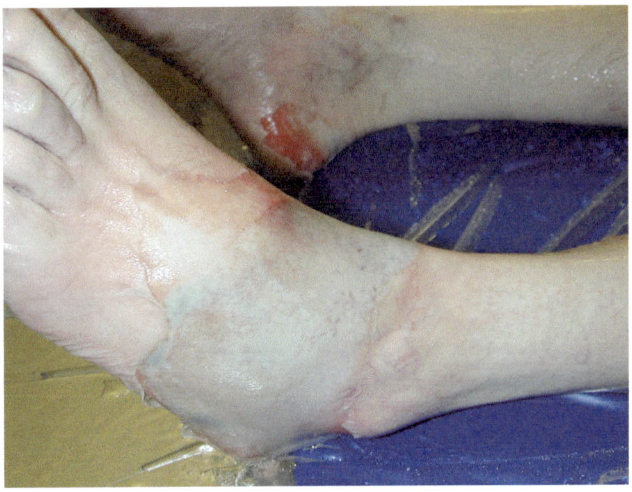

Fig. 27.8 Chemical burn

chemical injury is directly proportional to the amount, type and strength of the agent, its concentration, extent of penetration, mechanism of action, and length of contact time with the skin. Chemicals will continue to destroy tissue until they are inactivated by reaction with tissues, are neutralized, or are diluted with water. The burning process may continue for variable and, often prolonged, periods of time (i.e., up to 72 h) after the initial contact with the chemical agent. It is important to remove the person from the burning agent as soon as possible and to begin copiously flushing the area with water—the solution to the pollution is dilution [24]. Neutralizing agents should not be used as they may produce additional tissue damage through heat production. Dry chemicals should be gently brushed off the skin before flushing begins. Most industries have detailed information on the chemicals their workers are exposed to and are required, by Occupational Health and Safety law, to have portable eyewash and shower stations for first aid use. Chemical burns to the eye require an ophthalmology consult, on admission, and late complications, such as corneal ulceration, secondary glaucoma, and cataracts, are fairly common and require follow-up. Ingestion of caustic materials may cause chemical burns to the oropharynx, tongue, esophagus, stomach, and duodenum. The patient should be given nothing by mouth, closely monitored and fluid resuscitated. Laryngeal edema may occur, producing upper airway obstruction. Endotracheal intubation or tracheostomy may be required to maintain airway patency.

27.4.3 Electrical

Electrical injuries comprise a small portion of the burn population, but the outcomes can be devastating, including deep tissue damage and potential loss of one or more limbs (Fig. 27.9). Injuries occur mainly in males and are usually occupation related. When electrical current passes through the body, intense heat is generated and coagulation necrosis results. The severity of the electrical injury is determined by the type and voltage of the circuit (whether alternating current—AC or direct current—DC), amperage of the current, resistance of the body, pathway of the current, and duration of contact. Electrical current takes the path of least resistance through the body. Least resistance is offered by nerves and blood vessels, whereas bone and fat offer the most resistance. If major body organs, such as the heart, brain, or kidneys are involved, the damage is more profound than if the current only passed through tissue. In some situations, electrical sparks may ignite the person's clothing, causing a flame burn, in addition to the electrical injury. If there is an explosion at an electrical panel and the clothing catches fire, but no electricity passes through the body, it is termed an electrical flash burn, **not** an electrical burn. It is an important distinction to make in the early hours post-injury. The severity of an

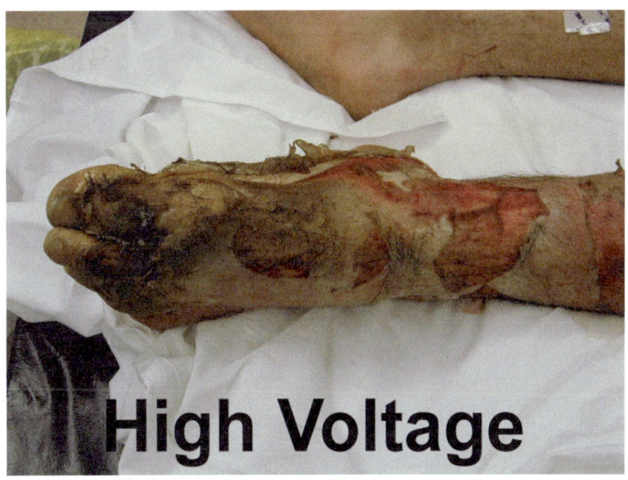

Fig. 27.9 Electrical burn

electrical injury can be difficult to determine as most of the damage may be below the skin at the level of muscle, fat, and bone. This phenomenon is referred to as the "iceberg" effect. Contact points, produced at the time of the injury, may help determine the probable path of the current and potential areas of injury. The history of the event can provide valuable clues as to what actually transpired at the accident scene. Many electrical injuries occur when a worker is suspended from an aerial basket or ladder and makes contact with a live wire. If the person has fallen post-injury, precautions to protect the head and cervical spine must be taken during transport. Spinal X-rays and neurological assessment are necessary, following admission to hospital. Contact with electrical current can cause tetanic muscle contractions that may produce long bone and vertebral fractures.

The person, who has sustained an electrical burn injury, may have also experienced cardiac arrhythmias or asystole post-injury. Immediate CPR is essential following cardiac arrest. He/she then continues to be at risk for cardiac arrhythmias for 24 h post-burn and must be monitored and have an electrocardiogram performed on admission to hospital.

Severe metabolic acidosis develops shortly after the injury occurs because of extensive tissue destruction and cell rupture. Assessment includes arterial blood gas analysis and, if needed to maintain normal serum pH levels, infusions of sodium bicarbonate. The kidneys also need to be closely monitored because of potentially high circulating levels of hemoglobin from damaged red blood cells and myoglobin from damaged muscle. In small amounts, the kidney tubules can filter them sufficiently. In larger concentrations, however, there is a significant risk of developing acute tubular necrosis and possible renal failure. Treatment consists of the early initiation of Lactated Ringer's solution at a rate that maintains a good urinary output of between 75 and 100 mL/h until the color of the urine is sufficient to suggest adequate dilution. In addition, an osmotic diuretic (e.g., mannitol) is usually given to establish and maintain acceptable urinary output.

27.4.4 Smoke and Inhalation Injury

In combination with a major burn, the presence of an inhalation injury can seriously increase mortality rates. Signs and symptoms of suspected, smoke inhalation include deep facial burns, history of being trapped in an enclosed space, and a laryngoscopic examination showing vocal cord swelling (Fig. 27.10). The most critical period for patients with inhalation injuries is 24–48 h post-burn. The airway becomes edematous and there is increased airway resistance. The respiratory mucosa sloughs, along with loss of ciliary function and poor diffusion of gases.

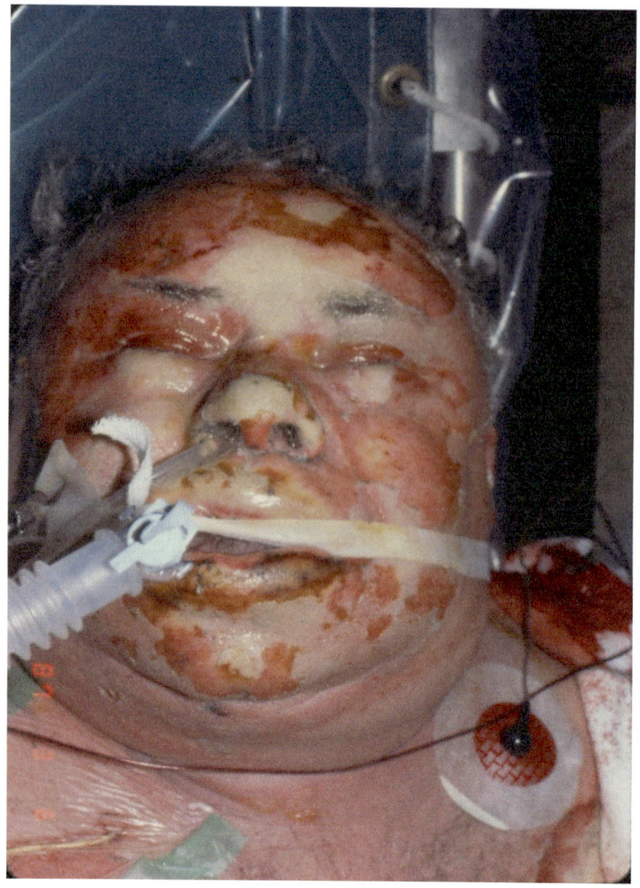

Fig. 27.10 Inhalation injury

Smoke and inhalation injuries can be divided into three types:

1. *Inhalation injury above the glottis.* Most smoke/inhalation injury damage (60%) is limited to the upper airway (pharynx, larynx, vocal cords) since the vocal cords and glottis close quickly as a protective mechanism following exposure to smoke or thermal agents, such as hot air or steam. There is redness and blistering. Edema and the onset of rapid airway obstruction, resulting in a respiratory emergency, are the primary concerns with this type of inhalation injury.
2. *Inhalation injury below the glottis.* Most injuries below the glottis are chemically produced through the inhalation of noxious products of combustion, resulting in tracheobronchitis. Major airway involvement (tracheobronchial tree) occurs about 30% of the time, with bronchopneumonia being the chief concern. Patients may not show symptoms until 12–24 h post-burn. Since gases are usually cooled before they reach the lung parenchyma, there is only a 10% injury occurrence at the level of the terminal bronchioles and alveoli. Primary concerns are pulmonary edema and adult respiratory distress syndrome (ARDS).

Table 27.5 Signs and symptoms of carbon monoxide poisoning

Carboxyhemoglobin saturation (%)	Signs and symptoms
5–10	Visual acuity impairment
11–20	Flushing, headache
21–30	Nausea, impaired dexterity
31–40	Vomiting, dizziness, syncope
41–50	Tachypnea, tachycardia
>50	Coma, death

3. *Carbon monoxide and hydrogen cyanide poisoning.* Most fatalities at a fire scene are caused by carbon monoxide, hydrogen cyanide poisoning, or asphyxiation. Carbon monoxide is produced by the incomplete combustion of burning materials. It then displaces the oxygen being carried by the hemoglobin molecules, resulting in less oxygen being delivered throughout the body. Carboxyhemoglobin and hydrogen cyanide levels should be measured, following admission of the person to an emergency department or burn center (Table 27.5). Treatment consists of aggressive fluid resuscitation and the administration of 100% humidified oxygen.

27.5 Clinical Manifestations

Recovery from a burn injury involves successful passage through three phases of care: emergent, acute, and rehabilitative. Principles of care for the emergent period involve resolution of the immediate problems resulting from the burn injury. The time required for this to occur is usually 1–2 days. The emergent phase ends with the onset of spontaneous diuresis. Principles of care for the acute period include avoidance, detection and treatment of complications, and wound care. This second phase of care ends when the majority of burn wounds have healed. During the third, and final, phase of rehabilitative care, the goals are for the burn patient to return to an optimal place in society and to accomplish any remaining functional and cosmetic reconstruction. This phase ends when there is complete resolution of any outstanding clinical problems resulting from the burn injury.

27.5.1 Subjective Symptoms

It is essential, throughout all phases of a burn patient's recovery, to seek out his/her perspective, when possible, and attempt to incorporate individual wishes into the plan of care. During the emergent period, patients and their families are likely in a state of physical and psychological shock. As a result of hypoxia, patients may also be disoriented or not able to recall what happened. Others remain very lucid throughout the ordeal and recall events with remarkable clarity. Some may not realize how serious their injuries are and be unrealistic about the care they require. Others may be intubated and sedated and not be aware for weeks to come. Pain may be a concern, while some may experience little discomfort. Thirst may be a symptom, depending upon the degree of fluid loss.

Some may complain of feeling cold or shiver as a result of heat loss, anxiety, and pain. The combination of hypovolemic shock, facial edema, intubation, and analgesics/sedative agents may alter a patient's sensory perception significantly over the first few days post-injury. If he/she is able to talk, common themes include "Will I die? What happened? Why me? I can't believe this is happening." In the acute phase, patients may experience varying levels of pain during dressing changes and physical/occupational therapy and might describe significant muscular discomfort, resulting from functional positioning and use of splinting materials. Unable to do any number of self-care activities, patients may become very frustrated about how dependent they have become on others. Concerns may be expressed regarding finances, family, and work obligations. Adaptation to the hospital environment and necessary treatments may absorb a considerable amount of the patient's physical and emotional energy. Adjustment to a variety of losses (personal and property), feelings of grief, guilt and blame, a need for information about what to expect over the coming weeks, and a search for meaning behind the event, are also experienced. Patients may feel angry or depressed post-injury. Relationships with family may become strained as everyone seeks to readjust and cope with this unexpected and traumatic event. During the rehabilitative phase of care, patients come to realize that they have completed the most difficult part of their recovery. However, many experience impatience with the time required for complete healing and physical rehabilitation. There is usually a desire to resume as much independence as possible, sometimes coupled with slight fear and hesitation about leaving the protective environment of the burn center. Questions, such as "What will it be like when I leave the hospital? How will I manage when the nurses and therapists are no longer around to help?" reflect the primary concerns for patients and family members at this time. There may be concerns about resumed sexual intimacy with a partner and self-acceptance of an altered body image. A request may be made to speak with a recovered burn survivor, who can offer words of support and advice based on personal experience. Over time, burn patients express feelings of pride at having overcome such tremendous physical and emotional challenges and begin to reflect on the path their lives will take post-burn as they move from burn "victim" to "survivor" and, perhaps, burn "thriver."

27.5.2 Objective Signs

The initial assessment of the burn patient is like that of any trauma patient and can best be remembered by the simple acronym "**ABCDEF**" (Box 27.2). Recently, recommendations for burn care management have been published to address the educational needs of both non-burn and burn specialists around the world [25, 26]. During the emergent period, burn patients quickly begin to exhibit signs and symptoms of hypovolemic shock (Box 27.3). Lack of circulating fluid volumes will also result in minimal urinary output and absence of bowel sounds. The patient may also be shivering due to heat loss, pain, and anxiety. If inhalation injury is a factor, the patient may demonstrate a number of physical findings upon visual assessment, laryngoscopy, and fiberoptic bronchoscopy (Box 27.4). The patient likely experiences pain, as exhibited by facial grimacing, withdrawing, and moaning when touched, particularly if the injuries are partial-thickness in nature. Some areas of full-thickness burn may be anesthetic to pain and touch, if the nerve endings have been destroyed. The loss of sensation may be temporary if the nerves have been compressed by resulting edema in the hypovolemic shock phase. It is important to examine areas of circumferential full-thickness burn for signs and symptoms of vascular compromise, particularly the extremities (Box 27.5).

Box 27.2 Primary Survey Assessment
- **A**—**A**irway
- **B**—**B**reathing
- **C**—**C**irculation
  - **C**-spine immobilization
  - **C**ardiac status
- **D**—**D**isability
  - Neurological **D**eficit
- **E**—**E**xpose and **e**valuate
- **F**—**F**luid resuscitation

Box 27.3 Signs and Symptoms of Hypovolemic Shock
- Restlessness, anxiety
- Skin—pale, cold, clammy
- Temperature below 37 °C
- Pulse is weak, rapid, ↓ systolic BP
- Urinary output <20 mL/h
- Urine specific gravity >1.025
- Thirst
- Hematocrit <35; BUN ↑

Box 27.4 Physical Findings of Suspected Inhalation Injury
- Deep facial burns
- History of being trapped in an enclosed space/exposed to smoke
- Laryngoscopic examination shows vocal cord swelling

Box 27.5 Signs and Symptoms of Vascular Compromise
- Pallor
- Deep tissue pain
- Progressive paresthesias
- Diminished or absent pulses
- Sensation of cold extremities

Areas of partial-thickness burn appear reddened, blistered, and edematous. Full-thickness burns may be dark red, brown, charred black, or white in color. The texture is tough, leathery, and no blisters are present.

If the patient is confused, health care professionals need to determine if it is the result of hypovolemic shock, inhalation injury, substance abuse, pre-existing history or, more rarely, head injury sustained at the time of the trauma. It is essential to immobilize the c-spines until a full assessment can be performed and the c-spines cleared. At this time, a secondary survey assessment is performed (Box 27.6). Additional objective data can then be collected, analyzed, and a plan of care developed, which includes a set of Admission Orders. In the acute phase, the focus is on wound care and prevention/management of complications. At this point, the burn wounds should have declared themselves as partial-thickness or full-thickness in nature. Eschar on partial-thickness wounds is thinner and, with dressing changes, it should be possible to see evidence of eschar separating from the viable wound bed. Healthy, granulation tissue is apparent on the clean wound bed, re-epithelializing cells are seen to migrate from the wound edges, and the dermal bed will slowly close the wound within 10–14 days. Full-thickness wounds have a thicker, leathery eschar, which does not separate easily from the viable wound bed. Those wounds require surgical excision and grafting. Continuous assessment of the patient's systemic response to the burn injury is an essential part of an individualized plan of care. Subtle changes, quickly identified by the burn team, can prevent complications from occurring or worsening over time. Physical examination by burn team staff and specialist consultants, laboratory tests, and diagnostic procedures will assist in the rapid identification and treatment of complications.

Box 27.6 Secondary Survey Assessment

- Head-to-toe examination
- Rule out associated injuries
- Pertinent history
  - circumstances of injury
  - medical history

During the final, rehabilitative phase, attention turns to scar maturation, contracture development, and functional independence issues [27–29]. The areas of burn, which heal either by primary intention or skin grafting, initially appear red or pink and are flat. Layers of re-epithelializing cells continue to form and collagen fibers in the lower scar tissue add strength to a fragile wound. Over the next month, the scars may become more red from increased blood supply and more raised from disorganized whorls of collagen and fibroblasts/myofibroblasts. The scars are referred to as hypertrophic in nature. If oppositional forces are not applied through splinting devices, exercises, or stretching routines, this new tissue continues to heal by shortening and forming contractures. A certain amount of contracture development is unavoidable, but the impact can be lessened through prompt and aggressive interventions.

The scar maturation process takes anywhere from 6 to 18 months. During this time, the scars will progress from a dark pink/red to a pale pink/whitened appearance. The final color is usually lighter than the surrounding unburned skin. For people with darkly pigmented skin, the process of color return may be prolonged as the melanocytes work to produce pigment in the areas where it has been lost [30]. Increasing amounts of pressure may be necessary to gently and continually flatten the scars which, in turn, push the extra blood from the area, making them lighter in color. Custom-fitted pressure garments and/or acrylic face masks apply constant pressure over a gradual wearing period of up to 23½ h a day [31]. Extra pressure over concave and difficult-to-fit areas can be provided through elastomer inserts or silicone sheeting under the garments or face mask [32]. The length of time a person might have to wear the garments varies, but is in the range of 1–1½ years, depending upon the intensity of the scarring and the body's response to pressure therapies. Patients will often experience itchiness and dry skin [33]. One of the best ways to decrease the itchiness is to get at the source of the problem: the dry skin. However, burned skin is different from healthy skin. Once the skin has been damaged by a burn injury, there are less natural oils available since the oil-reproducing glands have been destroyed, in whole or in part. In other words, the skin is "internally" dry as opposed to "externally" dry, such as when hands get chapped in the cold weather. Burned skin benefits from products that will be absorbed through the outer layer of the epidermis into the dry, dermal tissues. Water-based products do this. The more predominant products available are oil-based and contain mineral oil, petrolatum or paraffin. These ingredients coat the surface of the skin and, in essence, block the pores. This prevents loss of natural oils from the dermis, oils which burned skin is lacking. These ingredients are not absorbed into the dry dermis and do not bring moisture back into the skin. Mineral oil also breaks down elastic fibers in pressure garments and should be avoided. Suggested water-based products include Vaseline® Intensive Care Advanced Repair or Smith and Nephew's Professional Care®. Medications, such as diphenhydramine (<Atarax>, <Benadryl>), gabapentin (<Neurontin>), or pregabalin (<Lyrica>) can also be ordered to help with moderate to severe itchiness on a short-term basis, as can massage therapy.

27.6 Diagnostic Findings

There are a number of baseline diagnostic studies used to monitor a patient's clinical condition at the time of the injury and evaluate responses to care throughout the recovery period. They include laboratory tests, such as complete blood cell count (CBC), hemoglobin and hematocrit, group and screen, serum electrolyte levels, blood glucose, blood urea nitrogen (BUN), serum creatinine, calcium profile, serum lactate, liver function tests, and coagulation studies (PT, PTT, INR). Drug and alcohol screens may be indicated, upon admission, if the circumstances of the accident and/or patient's clinical presentation warrant it. If inhalation injury is suspected, a serum carboxyhemoglobin, serum cyanide, and arterial blood gas should be obtained, along with a chest X-ray. Laryngoscopy and/or fiberoptic bronchoscopy may also be indicated for inhalation-injured patients. Routine urinalysis, along with urine for hemoglobin and myoglobin in cases in electrical injury, also need to be collected. For patients with pre-existing cardiac disease or those sustaining electrical injuries, a 12-lead electrocardiogram (ECG) should be performed. For patients with suspected, head or spinal injury, fractures or internal trauma, X-rays or scans are indicated. Antibiotic resistant organism (MRSA and VRE) screening and wound swabs for culture and sensitivity (C + S) monitor the microbiological organisms present on admission. Blood cultures, along with urine and sputum for C + S, are helpful when investigating patients who become febrile or who may be developing sepsis. As the patient's condition changes, medical specialists from various services may be consulted and they may order various diagnostic tests, such as ultrasound, magnetic resonance imaging (MRI), or computerized axial tomography (CAT) scans to rule out or confirm diagnoses. Placement and monitoring of transduced, invasive central and arterial lines provide the team with information on a patient's cardiac and pulmonary functioning. Access to this wide variety of diagnostic information allows for timely clinical interventions by members of the burn team.

27.7 Possible Complications

Complications can arise throughout all phases of burn care although the potential for development is greater in the acute stage of recovery. Prompt identification and management are essential in order to reach the best possible patient outcome. The systems most commonly affected are cardiovascular, respiratory, gastrointestinal, and renal.

Cardiovascular system—Cardiovascular system complications include hypovolemic shock and arrhythmias. When the intravascular volume is reduced immediately post-burn, the cardiac output decreases dramatically and blood flow through the tissues and coronary artery is reduced. Prompt and adequate fluid resuscitation can effectively address the decrease in circulating volumes. Circulation to the extremities can also be impaired by the decreased volumes, the presence of circumferential burns and the formation of edema. Incisions through the leathery, devitalized burned tissue may be necessary in order to restore circulation to these limbs. That procedure is called an **escharotomy** (Fig. 27.11). Deeper burns (severe electrical or prolonged flame exposure) may require a **fasciotomy**. Patients with pre-existing cardiac disease may be more prone to the development of arrhythmias, brought on by the stress of a major burn injury. Direct cardiac damage may have also occurred from the passage of electrical current through the heart. All moderate to major burns should be monitored, using an external cardiac monitor, and invasive lines transduced. Hemodynamic parameters, such as heart rate, central venous pressure, and blood pressure/mean arterial pressure, are set within targeted ranges. Attention should also be paid to electrolyte levels, especially sodium and potassium. Early post-burn, sodium shifts into the interstitial spaces, only to return at the end of the hypovolemic shock phase. Potassium is initially released into the extracellular spaces by hemolyzed red blood cells and those cells injured by the burn. As fluids are mobilized, potassium levels increase in the vascular spaces. As plasma leaks into the interstitial space, there is a temporary increase in blood viscosity. Appropriate fluid resuscitation can correct that situation satisfactorily. Arrhythmia management may require a collaborative consultation with cardiology and medication on either a short-term or long-term basis. Evidence-based, venous thromboembolism prophylaxis should also be instituted and medications, such as enoxaparin, commenced as the incidence of DVTs in burns is estimated to be between 1 and 23%.

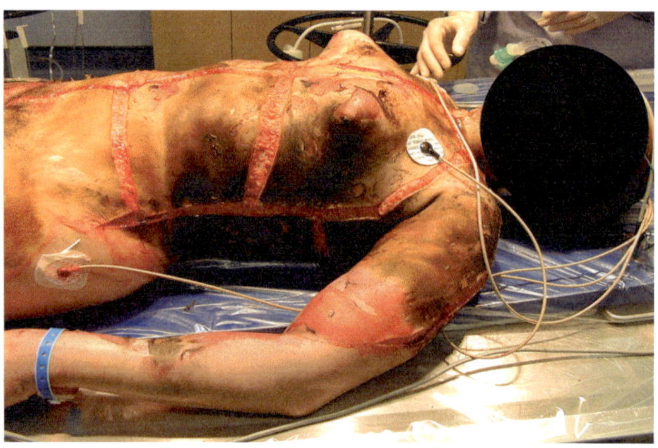

Fig. 27.11 Chest escharotomy

Respiratory system—There are, generally, two ways in which the respiratory system can be affected by a burn injury. One involves mechanical, upper airway obstruction due to heat injury and edema formation and/or constricting circumferential burns to the neck and chest. The other involves inhalation of noxious products of combustion, which produces a chemical irritation reaction to the middle and lower airways. Early in the emergent phase of care, the upper airway can close off very quickly because of massive facial and neck edema. Upon initial assessment, if there is any indication that the patient has a pharyngeal burn, is hoarse or has stridor, the patient should be nasally or, preferably, orally intubated with an **uncu**t endotracheal tube. This action serves to splint the airway open and maintain patency. Arterial blood gases (ABGs) should then be drawn and oxygen saturation levels monitored. If necessary, the patient may need to be mechanically ventilated in order to maintain sufficient levels of oxygenation. Mechanical ventilation protocols should be instituted and ventilator settings titrated to maintain desired $PaCO_2$, PaO_2, and SaO_2 readings.

When the edema subsides and/or ventilation parameters improve, the patient can be appropriately assessed and extubated safely. In most clinical settings, tracheostomies are performed if the patient is intubated for longer than 3 weeks. Patients, who do not have inhalation injury, may benefit from a face mask or nasal cannula to maintain oxygen saturations >92%. If there are circumferential flame burns to the chest and back, escharotomies of the chest and/or abdomen may need to be performed in order to release the constricting eschar, decrease respiratory distress, and improve chest expansion and ventilation. With an inhalation injury, it is not as obvious that there is damage to the middle or lower airways. At times, patients may present with bronchial and bronchiolar injury, such as bronchorrhea and/or expiratory wheezing. Examination of the lower respiratory tract, using fiberoptic bronchoscopy, should be performed. However, some may have an invisible injury at the level of respiratory gas exchange. This condition is often delayed and diagnosed by arterial blood gas analysis, rather than a chest X-ray.

Impaired gas exchange may be related to carbon monoxide poisoning. Carboxyhemoglobin levels should be drawn on admission (Table 27.5). Treatment of inhalation injury includes aggressive chest physiotherapy, tracheobronchial suctioning, administration of nebulized heparin and acetylcysteine, use of bronchodilators (ipratropium) to treat severe bronchospasm, and mechanical ventilation with positive end expiratory pressure (PEEP). PEEP prevents collapse of the alveoli and the development of progressive respiratory failure. If the patient's condition deteriorates and conventional ventilation strategies prove to be inadequate, newer forms of ventilation have been utilized in recent years and include strategies such as high frequency oscillation and implementation of prone positioning techniques. Patients, who have pre-existing respiratory problems, such as a history of frequent pneumonia or chronic obstructive pulmonary disease, are more likely to succumb to respiratory infection. Pneumonia is commonly seen in these patients since they are relatively immobile, may be debilitated, and have an abundance of microbial organisms that can settle in the lungs and require aggressive therapy to eradicate. Bundled, preventative measures may reduce the risk and incidence of ventilator-associated pneumonia (VAP) [34]. Older, more debilitated patients are also more prone to the development of pulmonary edema as a consequence of the fluid resuscitation required by inhalation-injured patients.

Maintaining the airway is crucial in these patients and frequent assessments of tube placement and stability are an essential part of care. Before patients are extubated, there is a weaning process which involves adjusting ventilator settings, so the machine is doing less of the work associated with breathing and patients are essentially breathing on their own. If they meet certain criteria, patients are extubated, placed in high Fowler's position, and given 100% oxygen. In addition, they require chest physiotherapy, suctioning, frequent repositioning, and deep breathing and coughing exercises. Mobilization at the bedside and in the hallways is also helpful in moving secretions from the upper and lower airways. Sometimes, patients tire too easily post-extubation and need to be reintubated. In situations where a patient cannot be weaned in the near distant future, a decision is made to perform a tracheostomy until such time as he/she can breathe unaided.

Gastrointestinal system—The gastrointestinal system is initially affected in the emergent phase by a lack of circulation to the splanchnic area. This hypoperfusion, secondary to hypovolemic shock, causes paralytic ileus and an absence of bowel sounds. The stress response post-burn causes a decrease in mucous production and an increase in gastric acid secretion, resulting in stress (Curling's) ulcers. Prompt and effective fluid resuscitation and a restoration of circulation to the gastrointestinal region result in a return of bowel sounds and indicate a functional gut. Bladder pressures should be measured q4h for 72 h in body surface area burns >30% and pressures >20 mmHg reported. Abdominal compartment syndrome is a life-threatening complication of high-volume fluid resuscitation. Management includes keeping the patient NPO for a few hours post-admission until things stabilize and then, beginning early enteral feeds to address the profound hypermetabolic effects of a burn injury. Anti-catabolic, anabolic agents, such as oxandralone and propanolol, may also prove to valuable adjuncts to therapy. Enteral feeding also maintains the integrity of the gut and avoids bacterial translocation. The hourly rate of feeds is increased, in a timely manner, to the desired goal rate, usually arrived at in consultation with the burn center dietitian. A nasogastric (NG) tube, connected to either straight drainage or wall suction, can be inserted for the purposes of gastric decompression and medication administration. Water flushes pre- and post-medication help ensure the tubes remain patent. Medications include prophylactic use of intravenous H_2 antagonists (i.e., ranitidine) to decrease hydrochloride secretion. During the acute phase of care, patients frequently become constipated as a result of codeine-containing pain medication received during their hospitalization and immobility. Prompt institution of a bowel regimen, upon admission, and attention to diet and/or choice of tube feedings can prevent or rectify the situation before it causes the patient unnecessary discomfort. Patients may also develop diarrhea, caused by certain tube feedings or antibiotics. Excessive diarrhea may warrant Clostridium difficile testing. Recommendations from the dietitian or pharmacist should be sought to correct the problem. A bowel management system may need to be inserted if loose stools interfere with optimal wound care. Sepsis is the most common cause of gastric ileus occurring in the acute phase of care and should be monitored closely [35]. Some burn centers are administering an anti-oxidant protocol, which includes selenium, acetylcysteine, ascorbic acid, vitamin E, zinc, and a multivitamin [36]. It is also important to monitor and, if necessary, institute potassium, calcium, magnesium, and phosphate replacements, and administer thiamine and folic acid, particularly if the patient has a history of alcohol abuse. Blood glucose point-of-care testing should be performed and an insulin nomogram commenced, as per ICU protocol, in order to maintain strict glucose control of 80–110 mg/dL [37].

Renal System—With the renal system post-burn, an early warning sign of complications is an increase in the specific gravity, which usually occurs before the urinary output falls. Acute tubular necrosis is the most frequent emergent phase complication and is due to hypovolemic shock. Fluid resuscitation is usually sufficient to correct such problems. Careful attention to trends in urinary output and specific gravity is a more helpful strategy than haphazardly increasing or decreasing the intravenous fluids. Insertion of a urinary catheter should occur, upon admission, to allow for accurate intake/output. If the injury is deep to the tissue and/or muscle, there is the additional complication of high circulating levels of hemoglobin (red blood cell breakdown) or myoglobin (muscle cell breakdown) pigments blocking the renal tubules. This situation is so common in electrical burns that the fluid resuscitation formula requires very aggressive resuscitation and the infusion of an osmotic diuretic (i.e., mannitol). In the acute phase of care, a decrease in urinary output or the development of high output renal failure, with rising levels of BUN and creatinine, may be indicative of a septic episode. Consultation with the renal service is essential if the patient doesn't respond to fluid challenges or diuretics. In the most serious of situations, the patient may require dialysis as a life-saving measure. Rising glucose levels indicate stress response, due to catecholamine release, and sepsis. High levels lead to compensatory osmotic diuresis, which means the burn patient needs more fluid.

Infection—Burn patients are at risk for the development of infection due to both the high bacterial loads on their devitalized, burn eschar and the loss of their primary barrier against infection—the skin. Infection is the leading cause of morbidity and mortality in burn patients. The degree of risk is increased due to the presence of devitalized burn eschar, which serves as an excellent breeding ground for organisms, invasive catheters and tubes, and a state of immunosuppression that continues long after the wounds have healed. The larger the burn wound, the greater the risk of infection. However, the advent of early burn excision and prompt wound closure has decreased the overall incidence of burn wound infection and, consequently, the incidence of sepsis and death. Evidence-based procedures for the insertion of central lines have resulted in impressive reductions in central line bloodstream infection rates. Ventilator-acquired pneumonia (VAP) rates have also declined since the advent of evidence-based practice bundles, such as chlorhexidine mouth rinse, head-of-bed elevation to 30°, gastrointestinal prophylaxis and turning patients, from side to side, q2h.

The primary sites for organisms are the burn wound, oral and pulmonary secretions, perineal and anal regions. Gram-negative organisms, such as E. coli, Klebsiella, Pseudomonas, and Serratia, are largely responsible for more than 50% of all septic episodes. They release endotoxins, which serve as key triggers for the sepsis cascade. All burn wounds are colonized with bacteria, which can be identified through qualitative wound swabs. More specific determinations can be made using quantitative, burn wound biopsies. If the bacterial count on a wound rises above 1×10^5/g of tissue, the wound is said to be infected, with the organisms having invaded into viable tissue. Local signs of burn wound infection include a change in wound exudate, alteration in wound appearance, increase in wound pain, erythema, edema, cellulitis, and induration at the wound edges. In the presence of a burn wound infection, a partial-thickness wound can convert to a full-thickness wound. If the organisms enter the lymphatic system, the patient can develop septicemia. Sepsis accounts for about 70% of deaths post-burn. Multisystem organ failure, often secondary to sepsis, is a serious and frequently fatal consequence of septicemia. Signs and symptoms of sepsis include an elevated temperature, increased pulse and respiratory rate, and decreased blood pressure and urinary output. The patient may become confused, feel and look unwell, have a diminished appetite and experience chills. It is important to identify and treat the source of sepsis as quickly as possible before multiple organ systems begin to fail. Cultures should be obtained from the blood, urine, sputum, invasive device sites and wounds. Multi-lumen catheters should be inserted in order to provide multiple access ports [38, 39]. Intravenous antibiotics may then be ordered by the burn center physicians, in consultation with the Infectious Disease service in the hospital. Initially, antibiotics can be ordered on speculation, pending culture and sensitivity reports from the lab. If necessary, the antibiotics may be changed to provide coverage specific to the organisms cultured. If the burn wounds, grafted areas or donor sites appear infected, topical antimicrobial coverage on the burn wound may need to be changed or instituted in order to provide treatment at a local level. In general, a patient's antibiotics can be discontinued when his/her WBC count is normal, when he/she is afebrile and when source control is obtained.

27.8 Clinical Management

27.8.1 Non-surgical Care

Therapeutic management of the burned person is conducted within these same three phases of burn recovery—emergent, acute, and rehabilitative. The *emergent* phase priorities include airway management, fluid therapy, and initial wound care. The goals of care are initial assessment, management, and stabilization of the patient during the first 48 h post-burn.

Assessment: During the rapid, primary survey, performed soon after admission, the airway and breathing assume top priority. Particularly with a large body surface area burn admission, some staff may feel a tendency to be overwhelmed by the sight and smell of the burn wound. The wounds are, however, a much lower priority than the airway. A compromised airway requires prompt attention and breath sounds verified in each lung field. If circumferential, full-thickness burns are present on the upper trunk and back, ventilation must be closely monitored as breathing might be impaired and releasing escharotomies necessary. The spine must be stabilized until c-spines are cleared. The circulation is assessed by examining skin color, sensation, peripheral pulses, and capillary filling. Circumferential, full-thickness burns to the arms or legs need to be assessed via palpation or Doppler for evidence of adequate circulation. Escharotomies might be required. Typically, burn patients are alert and oriented during the first few hours post-burn. If that is not the case, consideration must be given to associated head injury, (including a complete neurological assessment), substance abuse, hypoxia, or pre-existing medical conditions. All clothing and jewelry need to be removed in order to visualize the entire body and avoid the "tourniquet-like" effect of constricting items left in place as edema increases. Adherent clothing needs to be gently soaked off with normal saline to avoid further trauma and unnecessary pain. Attention then turns to prompt fluid resuscitation to combat the hypovolemic shock. The secondary, head-to-toe survey then rules out any associated injuries. A thorough assessment ensures all medical problems are identified and managed in a timely fashion. Circumstances of the injury should be explored as care can be influenced by the mechanism, duration, and severity of the injury. The patient's pertinent medical history includes identification of pre-existing disease or associated illness (cardiac or renal disease, diabetes, hypertension), medication/alcohol/drug history, allergies, and tetanus immunization status. A handy mnemonic can be used to remember this information (Box 27.7).

Box 27.7 Secondary Survey Highlights

A—**a**llergies
M—**m**edications
P—**p**revious illness, **p**ast medical history
L—**l**ast meal or drink
E—**e**vents preceding injury

Management: The top priority of care is to *stop the burning process* (Box 27.8). During the initial first aid period at the scene, the patient must be removed from the heat source, chemicals should be brushed off and/or flushed from the skin, and the patient wrapped in a clean sheet and blanket ready for transport to the nearest hospital. Careful, local cooling of the burn wound with saline-moistened gauze can continue as long as the patient's core temperature is maintained and he/she does not become hypothermic. Upon arrival at the hospital, the burned areas can be cooled further with normal saline, followed by a complete assessment of the patient and initiation of emergency treatment (Box 27.9). In a burn center, the cooling may take place, using a cart shower system, in a hydrotherapy room (Fig. 27.12). The temperature of the water is adjusted to the patient's comfort level, but tepid is usually best, while the wounds are quickly cleaned and dressings applied.

Airway management includes administration of 100% oxygen if burns are 20% body surface area or greater. Suctioning and ventilatory support may be necessary. If the patient is suspected of having or has an inhalation injury,

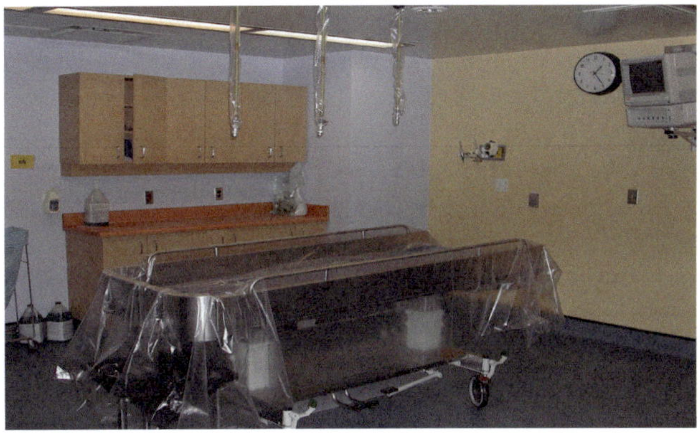

Fig. 27.12 Cart shower for hydrotherapy

Box 27.8 First Aid Management at the Scene

Steps	Action
Step 1	Stop the burning process—remove patient from heat source
Step 2	Maintain airway—resuscitation measures may be necessary
Step 3	Assess for other injuries and check for any bleeding
Step 4	Flush chemical burns copiously with cool water
Step 5	Flush other burns with cool water to comfort
Step 6	Protect wounds from further trauma
Step 7	Provide emotional support and have someone remain with patient to explain help is on the way
Step 8	Transport the patient as soon as possible to nearby emergency department

Box 27.9 Treatment of the Severely Burned Patient on Admission

Steps	Action
Step 1	Stop the burning process
Step 2	Establish and maintain an airway; inspect face and neck for singed nasal hair, soot in the mouth or nose, stridor, or hoarseness
Step 3	Administer 100% high flow humidified oxygen by non-rebreather mask. Be prepared to intubate if respiratory distress increases
Step 4	Establish intravenous line(s) with large bore cannula(e) and initiate fluid replacement using Lactated Ringer's solution
Step 5	Insert an indwelling urinary catheter
Step 6	Insert a nasogastric tube
Step 7	Monitor vital signs including level of consciousness and oxygen saturation
Step 8	Assess and control pain
Step 9	Gently remove clothing and jewelery
Step 10	Examine and treat other associated injuries
Step 11	Assess extremities for pulses, especially with circumferential burns
Step 12	Determine depth and extent of the burn
Step 13	Provide initial wound care—cool the burn and cover with large, dry gauze dressings
Step 14	Prepare to transport to a burn center as soon as possible

intubation needs to be performed quickly. *Circulatory management* includes intravenous infusion of fluid to counteract the effects of hypovolemic shock for adult patients with burns >15% body surface area and children with burns >10% body surface area. Upon admission, two large bore, intravenous catheters should be inserted, preferably into unburned tissue. However, if the only available veins are in a burned area, they should be used. Patients who have large burns, where intravenous access will be necessary for a number of days, benefit from a central venous access device inserted into either the subclavian, jugular, or femoral vein. The overall goal is to establish an access route that will accommodate large volumes of fluid for the first 48 h post-burn. The aim of fluid resuscitation is to maintain vital organ function, while avoiding the complications of inadequate or excessive therapy. Fluid calculations are based on the extent of the burn, the weight and age of the patient, pre-burn conditions (dehydration), or pre-existing chronic illnesses (respiratory, renal). The most commonly used fluid resuscitation regimen is the Parkland (Baxter) formula (Box 27.10). It involves the use of crystalloid (Lactated Ringer's) solution. **Fluids are calculated for the first 24 h post-burn with "0" hours being the time of the burn, *not* the time of admission to hospital**. One-half of the 24 h total needs to be administered over the first 8 h post-burn as this is the period during which extravasation of fluid into the interstitial space is greatest, along with the risk of renal tubule blockage from hemoglobin and myoglobin pigments. The remaining half of the estimated resuscitation volume should be administered over the subsequent 16 h of the first post-burn day. It is important to remember that **the formula is only a guideline**. The infusion needs to be adjusted based on the patient's clinical response, which includes vital signs, sensorium, and urinary output. For adults, 30–50 mL urine per hour is the goal and 1 mL/kg/h in children weighing less than 30 kg. An indwelling urinary catheter needs to be inserted at the same time as the IVs are established in order to reliably measure the adequacy of the fluid resuscitation. Vital signs should be trending around a systolic BP of ≥90–100 mgHg, a pulse rate of ≤120 for the older child/adult, <140 bpm in the child between 2 and 5 years of age and <160 bpm in the child under 2 years of age, with respirations at 16–20 breaths/min. The patient's sensorium should be such that he/she is alert and oriented to time, person, and place. An exception is made regarding the sensorium assessment for the intubated patient. During the second 24 h post-burn, the need for aggressive fluid resuscitation is generally less as capillary permeability begins to return to normal. Colloids, such as albumin, can be given as volume expanders to replace lost protein and minimize ongoing fluid requirements. Earlier administration of colloid would result in leakage out of the vascular space because of the increased capillary permeability. Some patients require extra fluid above and beyond the formula guidelines in order to produce satisfactory urinary output, stabile vital signs, and an adequate sensorium. They include those with (a) high-voltage injury, (b) inhalation injury, (c) delayed resuscitation, or (d) prior dehydration. Those patients with a high-voltage injury require administration of a diuretic to produce a urinary output of 75–100 mL/h in order to clear the tubules of hemoglobin and myoglobin pigments. The usual choice is Mannitol 12.5 g/L of fluid. Since the heme pigments are more soluble in an alkaline medium, sodium bicarbonate can be added to the resuscitation fluid as needed to maintain a slightly alkaline urine. Patients with severe inhalation injury and body surface area burns may require 40–50% more fluid in order to achieve adequate tissue perfusion. The need for extra fluid must be balanced against the risk of pulmonary edema and "fluid creep"/overload. There are others who are considered "volume sensitive." They are (a) ≥50 years of age, (b) ≤2 years of age, or (c) have pre-existing cardiopulmonary or renal disease. Particular caution must be exercised with these patients.

Box 27.10 Fluid Resuscitation Using the Parkland (Baxter) Formula

Formula	Administration	Example
4 mL Lactated Ringer's solution per kg body weight per % total body surface area (TBSA) burn = total fluid requirements for the first 24 h post-burn (0 h = time of injury)	½ total in first 8 h ¼ total in second 8 h ¼ total in third 8 h	For a 65 kg patient with a 40% burn injured at 1000 h: 4 mL × 65 kg × 40% burn = 10,400 mL in first 24 h ½ total in first 8 h (1000–1800 h) = 5200 mL (650 mL/h) ¼ total in second 8 h (1800–0200 h) = 2600 mL (325 mL/h) ¼ total in third 8 h (0200–1000 h) = 2600 mL (325 mL/h)

N.B. Remember that the formula is only a guideline. Titrate to maintain urinary Output at 30–50 mL/h, stable vital signs, and adequate sensorium

Wound care. Once a patent airway, adequate circulation, and fluid replacement have been established, attention can turn to wound care and the ultimate long-term goal of wound closure. Such closure will halt or reverse the various fluid/electrolyte, metabolic and infectious processes associated with an open burn wound. The burns are gently cleansed with normal saline, if the care is being provided on a stretcher or

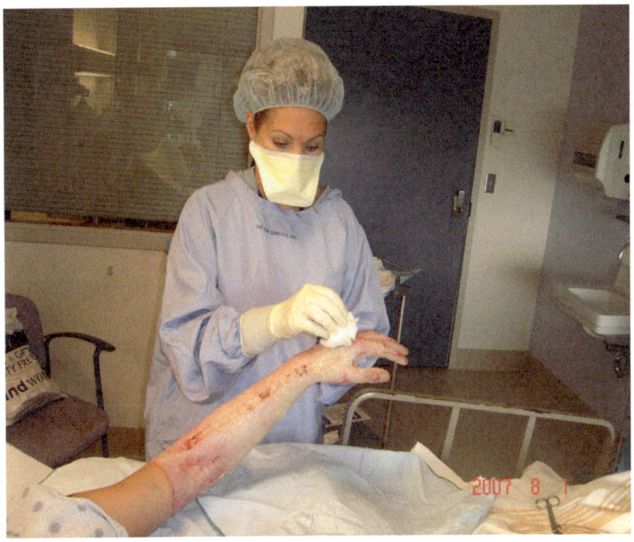

Fig. 27.13 Initial wound care post-admission

Table 27.6 Objectives of burn wound care

Objective	Rationale
Prevention of conversion	Wounds that dry out or develop an infection can become deeper. A partial-thickness wound could then convert to full-thickness and require skin grafting
Removal of devitalized tissue	Debridement, either through dressing changes or surgery, is necessary to clean the wounds and prepare for spontaneous healing or grafting
Preparation of healthy granulation tissue	Healthy tissue, free of eschar and nourished by a good blood supply, is essential for new skin formation
Minimization of systemic infection	Eschar contains many organisms. Removal is essential in order to decrease the bacterial load and reduce the risk of burn wound infection
Completion of the autografting process	Full-thickness wounds require the application of autologous skin grafts from available donor sites
Limitation of scars and contractures	Wounds that heal well the first time tend to have fewer scars and contractures. Some degree of scar and contracture formation are, however, part of the healing process and cannot be entirely prevented

bed. If a hydrotherapy cart shower or immersion tank are used, tepid water cleans the wounds of soot and loose debris (Fig. 27.13).

Sterile water is not necessary. Chemical burns should be flushed copiously for at least 20 min, preferably longer. Tar cannot be washed off the wound. It requires numerous applications of an emulsifying agent, such as mineral oil, Tween 80®, Medisol®, or Polysporin® ointment. After several applications, the tar will have been removed without unnecessary trauma to healthy tissue. During hydrotherapy, loose, necrotic tissue (eschar) may be gently removed (debrided) using sterile scissors and forceps. Hair-bearing areas that are burned should be carefully shaved, with the exception of the eyebrows. This serves to minimize the accumulation of organisms. Showering or bathing should be limited to 20 min in order to minimize patient heat loss and physical/emotional exhaustion. More aggressive debridement should be reserved for the operating room, unless the patient receives conscious or deep sedation. After the initial bath or shower, further decisions are made regarding wound care. There are three methods of treatment used in caring for burn wounds. The goals of any topical agent should include: elimination of pain from environmental factors, barrier to environmental flora, reduction in evaporative losses, absorption/containment of drainage, delay/minimization of wound colonization, ability to penetrate eschar, and provision of splinting to maintain a position of function. In the *open method*, the wound remains exposed, with only a thin layer (2.0–4.0 mm) of topical antimicrobial ointment spread on the wound surface using a sterile gloved hand or applicator. With the *closed method*, a dressing is left intact for 2–7 days. The frequency of dressing changes depending on the condition of the wound and the properties of the dressing employed. The choice of treatment method varies among institutions and also according to the severity of the burn wound. All treatment approaches have certain objectives in common (Table 27.6). In the emergent phase, wounds may be treated with a thin layer of topical antimicrobial cream. Topical coverage is selected according to the condition of the wound, desired results, properties of the topical agent (Table 27.7), availability and familiarity by the burn team.

Assessment criteria have been established for choosing the most appropriate agent (Box 27.11). In the past, the most commonly selected topical antimicrobial agent was silver sulfadiazine, which can be applied directly to saline-moistened gauze, placed on the wound, covered with additional dry gauze or a burn pad, and secured with gauze wrap or flexible netting (Fig. 27.14). These dressings are usually changed twice a day. If the hydrotherapy room is used for the morning dressing change, the evening dressing is done in the patient's room as it is too physically and emotionally exhausting to shower the burned person twice daily. It is preferred that the antimicrobial be applied directly to the gauze as opposed to being spread on the wound for two reasons: it is less likely that organisms will be spread from one part of a burn wound to another and it is generally less painful for the patient. After having been regarded for the past 40 years of use as a "gold standard in burn patient care," silver sulfadiazine cream has been noted to have a number of clinical disadvantages. Those disadvantages include the formation of a pseudo-eschar layer post-application, which interferes with evaluation of burn depth and rate of healing. Dressing changes need to be performed at least once, but generally twice, daily. Cytotoxic effects have also been noted, which slow down the healing process. A number of newer, burn wound products are becoming increasingly

Table 27.7 Topical antimicrobial agents used on burn wounds

Product	Preparation	Antimicrobial action	Applications
Silver sulfadiazine (SSD®, Silvadene®, Flamazine®)	1% water-soluble cream	Gram-positive and Gram-negative organisms, yeast Poor solubility with limited diffusion into eschar	Applied using the open or closed dressing method of wound care
Mafenide acetate (Sulfamylon®)	8.5% water-soluble cream 5% solution	Gram-positive and Gram-negative organisms Highly soluble and diffuses through the eschar Same as above	Applied using either the open (exposure) or closed (occlusive) dressing method
Silver nitrate	0.5% solution	Gram-positive and Gram-negative organisms, yeast, fungi Hypotonic solution	Saturated dressings are applied to the wound or grafted surface
Petroleum and mineral oil-based antimicrobial ointments (e.g., Neosporin®, Bacitracin®, Polysporin®)	Neosporin® (neomycin, bacitracin, polymyxin B); Bacitracin® (bacitracin zinc); Polysporin® (bacitracin, polymyxin B sulfate)	Gram-positive and Gram-negative organisms Ointments have limited ability to penetrate eschar	Applied to wound in a thin (1 mm) layer. Should be reapplied as needed to keep ointment in contact with wound
Acetic acid	0.5 and 2% solutions	Gram-positive and Gram-negative organisms, pseudomonas at higher concentration	Saturated dressings are applied and covered with dry gauze
Mupirocin (Bacitracin®)	2% cream and ointment	Gram-positive and Gram-negative organisms	Can be applied to an open face burn; can be applied to a body burn and covered with a dry dressing
Prontosan®	Gel Solution	Cleansing, decolonization, moisturizing, and prevention of biofilm	Can be applied to an open face burn; can be applied to body burn and covered with a dry dressing
Dakin's	Sodium hypochlorite 0.25–0.5%	Gram-positive and Gram-negative organisms, yeast, fungi	Can be used as a wound cleansing solution or applied as a dressing and covered a dry dressing
Dakin's 1:10	Sodium hypochlorite 0.05%	As above	As above

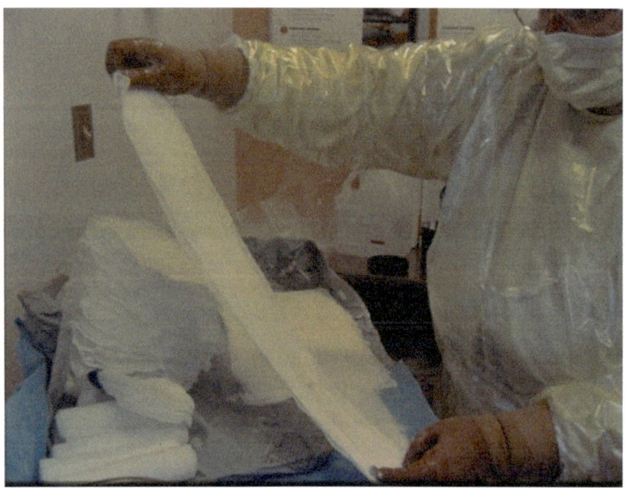

Fig. 27.14 Applying silver sulfadiazine cream to saline-moistened gauze

utilized, studied, and reported upon in the burn literature, thus providing burn care providers with a number of alternative options [40]. Patients lose a lot of body heat during dressing changes, so it is advised that the temperature of the room be elevated slightly and that only small to moderate-sized areas of the body be exposed at any one time. Cartilaginous areas, such as the nose and ears, are usually covered with mafenide acetate (Sulfamylon®), which has greater eschar penetration ability. Face care includes the application of warmed, saline-moistened gauze to the face for 20 min, followed by a gentle cleansing and re-application of a thin layer of ointment, such as polymyxin B sulfate (Polysporin®) (Fig. 27.15). Other alternatives include Prontosan® gel and mupirocin ointment/cream. A number of silver-impregnated dressings (Acticoat®/Acticoat® Flex, Aquacel® Ag, Mepilex Ag™) have also been commonly used in the emergent and acute phases of burn wound care [41]. These dressings are moistened with sterile water, placed on a burn wound and left intact anywhere from 3 to 4 days to as long as 21 days, depending on the patient's individual clinical status and particular product. More recently, negative pressure wound therapy (NPWT) manufacturers have incorporated an automated topical wound solution instillation and removal technology (V.A.C Veraflo™, KCI), which is being trialed in a number of burn centers, in addition to the traditional foam dressings [42–44]. It is generally recommended that silver dressings be used to reduce bioburden in acute burns that might be infected or are being prevented from healing by

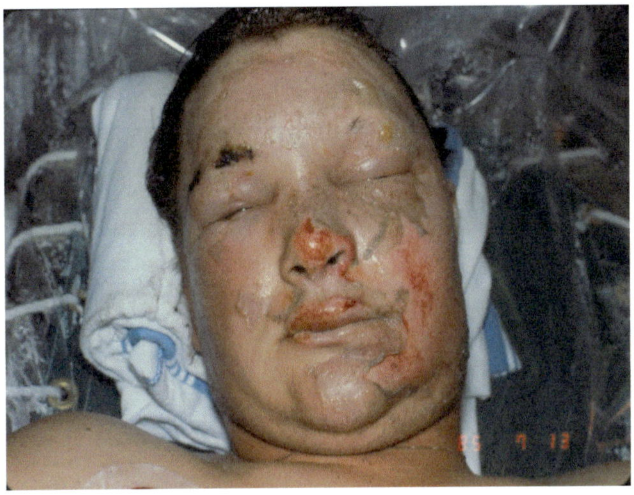

Fig. 27.15 Facial burn wound care

microorganisms or to act as an antimicrobial barrier for acute burns at high risk of infection or re-infection. When choosing a silver dressing, the needs of the patient and the wound, the characteristics of the wound environment, and burn team preferences are taken into consideration. Where bioburden is not a problem, silver dressings are not necessary. In those situations, petrolatum or paraffin-based, greasy gauze dressings are commonly applied to clean, partial-thickness wound beds during spontaneous wound healing.

Box 27.11 Properties of Topical Antimicrobial Agents

- Readily available
- Pharmacologic stability
- Sensitivity to specific organisms
- Non-toxic
- Cost-effective
- Non-painful on application
- Capacity for eschar penetration
- Familiarity of burn team with product

Infection may develop under the eschar as a result of organisms that were present deep in ducts or on adjacent areas which were not destroyed at the time of the burn. Topical antimicrobial coverage is selected according to the condition of the wound, desired results, properties of the topical agent, availability, and familiarity by the burn team. Whatever topical and dressing strategies are chosen, basic aseptic wound management techniques should be followed. Personnel generally wear isolation gowns over scrub suits, masks, head covers and clean, disposable gloves to remove soiled dressings or cleanse wounds. Sterile gloves should be used when applying inner dressings to the body or ointment to the face. The choice of dressings should take into consideration the condition of the wound, desired clinical results, properties of the particular dressing, physician preference, and availability in each burn center. There are currently a number of biologic, biosynthetic, and synthetic wound coverings available. The ideal dressing should possess particular criteria (Box 27.12). During the first few days post-burn, the wounds are examined to determine actual depth. It usually takes a few days for deep, partial-thickness wounds to "declare" themselves. Some wounds are deeper than they initially appear on admission. Scald injuries are almost always deeper than they appear on admission and need to be closely monitored. A treatment plan is then developed to ultimately close the burn wound, either through surgical or non-surgical means.

Box 27.12 Criteria for Burn Wound Coverings

- Absence of antigenicity
- Tissue compatibility
- Absence of local and systemic toxicity
- Water vapor transmission similar to normal skin
- Impermeability to exogenous microorganisms
- Rapid and sustained adherence to wound surface
- Inner surface structure that permits ingrowth of fibrovascular tissue
- Flexibility and pliability to permit conformation to irregular wound surface; elasticity to permit motion of underlying body tissue
- Resistance to linear and shear stresses
- Prevention of proliferation of wound surface flora and reduction of bacterial density of the wound
- Tensile strength to resist fragmentation and retention of membrane fragments when removed
- Biodegradability (important for "permanently" implanted membranes)
- Low cost
- Indefinite shelf life
- Minimal storage requirements and easy delivery

The focus of therapy in the *acute* phase is the management of any complications which might arise during the recovery period and closure of the burn wound. This phase can have a duration of anywhere from a week to several months. Commencement of this phase begins with the onset of spontaneous diuresis and return of fluid to the intravascular space.

Assessment: The focus of attention is on the continued need for fluid therapy, wound care, physiotherapy and occupational therapy, pain and anxiety management. *Fluid therapy* is administered in accordance with the patient's fluid losses and medication administration. *Wounds* are examined on a daily basis and adjustments made to the plan of care. The wound type, drainage, odor, appearance, and amount of pain are generally recorded on a wound assessment and treatment record. If a wound is full-thickness, arrangements need to be made to take the patient to the operating room for surgical excision and grafting.

The *physiotherapist and occupational therapist* will see patients daily and revise their plan of care on an ongoing basis [44]. The plan of care is understandably different if the patient is critically ill versus acutely ill but ambulatory. Efforts are made to adapt the care around major treatments, such as ORs, when the patient will be on bed-rest for a number of days. The patient's level of *pain and anxiety* need to be measured and responded to on a regular basis. A variety of pharmacologic strategies are available (Table 27.8) and require the full commitment of the burn team in order to be most effective. It is helpful to have multiple modalities of medications to handle both the background discomfort from the burn injury itself and pain/anxiety experienced during procedural, surgical, and rehabilitative activities [45–47].

Management: Selecting the best method to close the burn wound is by far the most important task in the acute period. However, the team needs to continually monitor for a change in the patient's status as a consequence of systemic complications, such as sepsis. Common *fluid replacement* choices include intravenous normal saline, glucose in saline or water, or Lactated Ringer's solution. On occasion, albumin, plasma, and packed red blood cells might be given. Central lines, with multiple lumens, are essential when administering fluids and multiple medications simultaneously.

Wound care is performed daily and treatments adjusted according to the changing condition of the wounds (Table 27.9). During the dressing changes, nurses may debride small amounts of loose, necrotic tissue for a short period of time, ensuring that the patient is receiving adequate analgesia and sedation. Enzymatic debriding agents can also be used to facilitate eschar removal [48]. A constant dialogue needs to take place between the nursing and medical staff to ensure the right medication in the right amount is available for each and every patient. As the eschar is removed from the areas of partial-thickness burn, the type of dressing selected is based on its ability to promote moist wound healing. There are biologic, biosynthetic, and synthetic dressings and skin substitutes available today (Table 27.10) [49, 50]. Areas of full-thickness damage require surgical excision and skin grafting. There are specific dressings appropriate for grafted areas and donor sites [51–54].

Physiotherapy and occupational therapy are an essential component of a patient's daily plan of care. Depending on the patient's particular needs and stage of recovery, there

Table 27.8 Sample burn pain management protocol

Recovery phase	Treatment	Considerations
Critical/acute with mild to moderate pain experience	IV morphine/hydromorphone – Continuous infusion – Bolus for breakthrough, i.e., 1/3 continuous infusion hourly dose – Bolus for acutely painful episodes/mobilization, i.e., 3× continuous infusion hourly dose;	– Assess patient's level of pain q1h using VAS (0-10) – Assess patient's response to medication and adjust as necessary – Assess need for anti-anxiety agents, i.e., lorazepam, midazolam – Relaxation exercises – Music distraction
Critical/acute with severe pain experience	1. IV morphine/hydromorphone – Continuous infusion for background pain – Bolus for breakthrough – IV fentanyl – Bolus for painful dressing changes/mobilization 2. IV midazolam or ketamine – Bolus for extremely painful dressing change/mobilization 3. Propofol infusion – Consult with Department of Anesthesia for prolonged and extremely painful procedures, i.e., major staple/dressing removal	– Consider fentanyl infusion for short-term management of severe pain – Assess level of pain q1h using VAS – Assess level of sedation using SASS score – Relaxation exercises – Music distraction – Assess need for anti-anxiety/sedation agents, i.e., lorazepam, midazolam
Later acute/rehab with mild to moderate pain experience	– Oral continuous release morphine or hydromorphone—for background pain BID – Oral morphine or hydromorphone for breakthrough pain and dressing change/mobilization – Consider adjuvant analgesics such as gabapentin, pregabalin, amitriptyline, ketoprofen, ibuprofen, acetaminophen	– Assess level of pain q1h using VAS – Consult equianalgesic table for conversion from I.V. to P.O. – Assess for pruritis

Table 27.9 Sample burn wound management protocol

Wound status	Treatment	Considerations
Early acute; partial or full—thickness; eschar/ blisters present	– Silver sulfadiazine cream – Mupirocin (Bactroban®) ointment/cream – Prontosan gel – Dakin's 0.05%–0.25–0.5% solution – Mafenide acetate (Sulfamylon®) to cartilaginous areas of face, i.e., nose, ears – Polymyxin B® sulfate (Polysporin®) to face	– Apply thin layer (2–3 mm) of silver sulfadiazine to avoid excessive build-up (pseudo-eschar) and facilitate removal, cleansing, and re-application – Prontosan gel prevents biofilm formation – Monitor for local signs of infection, i.e., purulent drainage, odor, and Notify the responsible physician if there is a potential need for alternative topical agents, i.e., acetic acid, mafenide acetate
Mid-acute; partial or full-thickness; leathery or cheesy eschar remaining	– Normal saline gauze – Mupirocin (Bactroban®) ointment/cream – Prontosan® gel – Dakin's (sodium hypochlorite) 0.05%–0.25–0.5% solution – Full-thickness wounds to be excised surgically	– Saline dressings to be applied to a relatively small area due to potentially painful nature of treatment – Potential use of enzymatic debriding agents (Collagenase Santyl®, Elase®, Accuzyme®) – Monitor for local signs of infection and notify M.D.
Late acute; clean partial-thickness wound bed	– Non-adherent greasy gauze dressing (Jelonet®, Adaptic®)	– Monitor for local signs of infection and notify M.D.
Post-op graft site	– Non-adherent greasy gauze dressing (Jelonet®, Adaptic®) → saline—moistened gauze → dry gauze → outer wrap – Leave intact ×2 days – Post-op day 2, gently debulk to non-adherent gauze layer →redress once daily – Post-op day 5, gently debulk to grafted area → redress once daily	– Select appropriate pressure-relieving sleep surface – Monitor for local signs of infection and notify M.D.
Early rehab; healed partial-thickness or graft site	– Polymyxin B sulfate (Polysporin®) until wound stable BID – When stable, moisturizing cream applied BID and prn	– Apply thin layer (2 mm) of polymyxin B sulfate (Polysporin®) to avoid excessive build-up – Avoid lanolin and mineral oil containing creams which clog epidermal pores and don't reach dry, dermal layer
Post-op donor site	– Hydrophilic foam dressing (i.e., Allevyn®, Mepilex®) or medicated greasy gauze dressing (i.e., Xeroform®) – Cover foam with transparent film dressing and pressure wrap ×24 h – Remove wrap and leave dressing intact until day 4; replace on day 4 and leave intact until day 8. Remove and inspect – If wound unhealed, reapply a second foam dressing – If healed, apply polymyxin B sulfate (Polysporin®) BID – When stable, apply moisturizing cream BID and prn – Cover Xeroform® with dry gauze and secure. Leave intact for 5 days – Remove outer gauze on day 5 and leave open to air. Apply light layer of polymyxin B sulfate (Polysporin®) ointment. If moist, reapply gauze dressing for 2–3 more days – When Xeroform® dressing lifts up as donor site heals, trim excess and apply polymyxin B sulfate (Polysporin®) ointment	– Monitor for local signs of infection and notify M.D.
Face	– Normal saline-moistened gauze soaks applied to face ×15 min – Remove debris gently using gauze – Apply thin layer of polymyxin B sulfate (Polysporin®) or Prontosan® gel – Repeat soaks q 4–6 h – Apply light layer of mafenide acetate (Sulfamylon®) cream to burned ears and nose cartilage	– For male patients, carefully shave beard area on admission and as necessary to avoid build-up of debris. Scalp hair may also need to be clipped carefully on admission to inspect for any burn wounds

Table 27.10 Temporary and permanent skin substitutes

Biological	Biosynthetic	Synthetic
Temporary	**Temporary**	**Temporary**
>Allograft/Homograft (cadaver skin) – clean, partial, and full-thickness burns >Amniotic membrane – clean, partial-thickness burns >Xenograft (pigskin) – clean, partial, and full-thickness burns	>Nylon polymer bonded to silicone membrane with collagenous porcine peptides (Biobrane™) – Clean, partial-thickness burns, donor sites >Calcium alginate from brown seaweed (Curasorb®, Kalginate®) – exudative wounds, donor sites >Mesh matrix of oat beta-glucan and collagen attached to gas-permeable polymer (BGC Matrix®) – clean, partial-thickness burns, donor sites	>Polyurethane and polyethylene thin film (OpSite®, Tegaderm®, Omiderm®, Bioclusive®) >Composite polymeric foam (Allevyn®, Mepilex®, Curafoam®, Lyofoam®) – clean, partial-thickness burns, donor sites >Non-adherent gauze (Jelonet®, Xeroform®, Adaptic®) – clean, partial-thickness burns, skin grafts, donor sites
Semi-permanent	**Semi-permanent**	
>Mixed allograft seeded onto widely meshed autograft – clean, full-thickness burns	>Bilaminar membrane of bovine collagen and glycosaminoglycan attached to Silastic layer (Integra®) – clean, full-thickness burns	
Permanent		
>Cultured epithelial autografts (CEA) grown from patient's own keratinocytes (Epicel®) – clean, full-thickness burns >Allograft dermis decellularized, freeze-dried and covered with thin autograft or cultured keratinocytes (AlloDerm®) – clean, full-thickness burns		

are certain range-of-motion exercises, ambulation activities, chest physiotherapy, stretching, and splinting routines to follow. The program adjusts on a daily/weekly basis as the patient makes progress towards particular goals and as his/her clinical condition improves or worsens.

Pain and anxiety management are critical in the acute period of care. Many of the activities a patient is required to do in order to get well cause him/her a degree of discomfort. The ongoing nature of the pain and the unfamiliar world of burn care can quickly exhaust a patient's pre-burn coping strategies. Establishment of unit-based protocols that can be adjusted to meet each patient's individual needs assists greatly in managing the pain and anxiety so often associated with burn care.

The focus of therapy during the *rehabilitative* phase is directed towards enabling the patient to return to a state of optimal physical and psychosocial functioning.

Assessment: The clinical focus in on ensuring all open wounds eventually close, observing and responding to the development of scars and contractures, and ensuring that there is a plan for future reconstructive surgical care, if the need exists. The transition from hospital to home or to a rehabilitation facility is a difficult one for most burn survivors and their family members to make. Although they are likely given information as to what to expect on a number of occasions by various members of the burn team and constantly reassured that support will be ongoing, pre-discharge anxiety levels can run high. As the burn patient prepares to leave the protective environment of the burn center, numerous feelings may be experienced. Burn team members need to be sensitive to and encourage patients to verbalize concerns and questions. The burned person may experience feelings of uncertainty, fear, and anxiety about what lies ahead, decreased confidence following weeks and, perhaps, months of dependence on hospital staff, along with concerns about coping with treatment protocols and impaired physical mobility. Some may have to re-enter society with an altered body image and decreased sense of self-esteem.

Management: Wound care is generally fairly simple at this time. Dressings should be minimal or non-existent. Most of the wounds should have healed or be very small. Frustration may result, however, when the patient realizes that his healed skin in still quite fragile and can break down with very little provocation. The need to moisturize the skin with water-based creams is emphasized in order to keep the skin supple and to decrease the itchiness that may be present. Ongoing counseling to assist with adjusting to an altered appearance and a dramatic change in one's life plan is a very necessary part of post-discharge care [55, 56]. Nervousness about returning home after a prolonged absence and concerns about resumption of previous roles and responsibilities may also be experienced. If the burn survivor is being transferred to a rehabilitation facility, concerns are often expressed about adjusting to an unfamiliar environment, staff, and routines. Anticipating these concerns and talking with patients and families before the transition occurs is an important part of the plan of care. Support to family is also important as they will assume the primary caretaker role once held by members of the burn team [57, 58]. Home care may need to be arranged and those health team members can bear some of the burden of care until the patient is more self-sufficient. Community-based caregivers can also alleviate some of the anxieties of family members. Visits to clinic serve as important connections for staff, patients, and family and provide an opportunity to have questions and concerns answered, to receive feedback on progress to date, and to talk about changes in the treatment plan. The occupational therapist plays an important role in the rehabilitation period for this is the time when scar maturation begins and contractures may worsen. Scar management techniques, including pressure garments, inserts, massage and stretching exercises, need to be taught to patients and their importance reinforced with each and every visit. Encouragement is also essential in order to keep patients and families motivated, particularly during the times when progress is slow and there seems to be no end in sight to the months of therapy. The burn surgeon can also plan future reconstructive surgeries for the patient, taking into consideration what improvements the burn patient wishes to achieve first. For many, the wish is for functional improvements before esthetic enhancements.

27.9 Surgical Care

Full-thickness burn wounds do not have sufficient numbers of skin-reproducing cells in the dermis to satisfactorily heal on their own. The area may slowly fill in with granulation and fibrous scar tissues, migrating in from the wound margins and underlying connective tissue. However, the process is very slow and the results unacceptable from a functional wound closure and esthetic outcome perspective. Common practice in surgical burn management is to begin surgically removing (excising) full-thickness burn wounds within a week of admission. This technique of early excision has had a significant positive impact on survival, especially for those patients with moderate to large-sized burn wounds. In the past, patients with extensive burns frequently died of overwhelming sepsis and/or malnutrition while awaiting surgery to remove the devitalized burn tissue. Most patients undergo excision and grafting in the same operative procedure. In some instances, if there is concern that the wound bed may not be clean enough for a graft to take, the wounds are excised and covered with topical antimicrobials, followed by a temporary biologic or synthetic dressing. The donor skin (skin graft), which is harvested in this first OR, is then wrapped up in sterile fashion and placed in a skin fridge for later application. Two days later, the patient returns to the OR to have the excised wounds (recipient bed) examined and the donor skin laid as a skin graft on the clean recipient bed. With large burn areas, it is necessary to serially excise and graft over a period of days to several weeks. Concern over blood loss, anesthetic and operative time, and lack of sufficient donor sites are the two limiting factors when attempting to excise and graft patients with extensive wounds.

Burn surgery involves excision of the non-viable eschar down to the point of punctate bleeding at the level of subcutaneous tissue or fascia (Fig. 27.16). Harvesting of donor sites for skin grafts is performed using a dermatome (Fig. 27.17). Hemostasis of both surgical sites must then be achieved and the donor skin placed onto the freshly excised recipient bed. Attempts are made to match skin thickness and color as closely as possible between donor sites and recipient sites. Grafts can be split-thickness or full-thickness in depth, meshed or unmeshed in appearance, temporary or permanent in nature (Table 27.11). The skin grafts are very thin (about .017 of an inch thick), but may be thicker, depending on the location of the recipient bed. For example, skin for an upper eyelid site would be much thinner than that intended for the back or a leg. Grafts should be left as unmeshed sheets for application to highly visible areas, such as the face, neck, or back of the hand (Fig. 27.18). Sheet grafts to the face are generally left open and frequently observed for evidence of serosanguinous exudate under the skin. In order to encourage a good blood supply from the recipient site to the donor site, the exudate needs to be removed. Two strategies frequently recommended include aspirating the exudate using a small gauge needle and syringe, or creating a small slit in the blister and gently using normal saline-soaked, cotton-tipped applicators to roll the fluid from the center of the "bleb" to the opening. On other parts of the body, grafts can be meshed using a dermatome mesher (Fig. 27.19). The mesher is set to an expansion ratio chosen by the surgeon. If there are sufficient donor sites to cover the excised areas, a 1½: 1 ratio is chosen. This expansion ratio allows for exudate to come through and be wicked

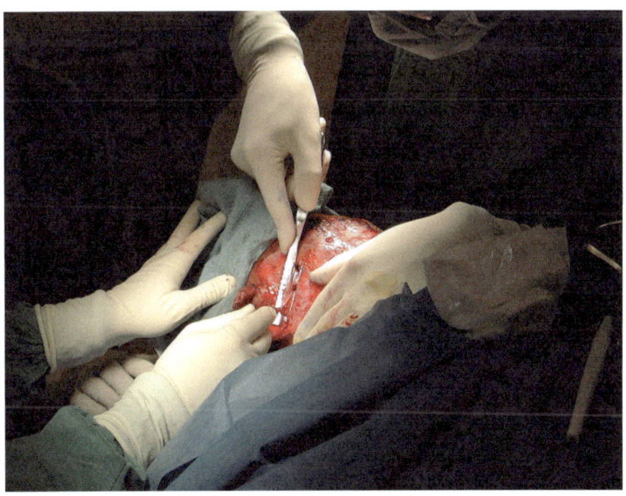

Fig. 27.16 Surgical excision of full-thickness burn wound

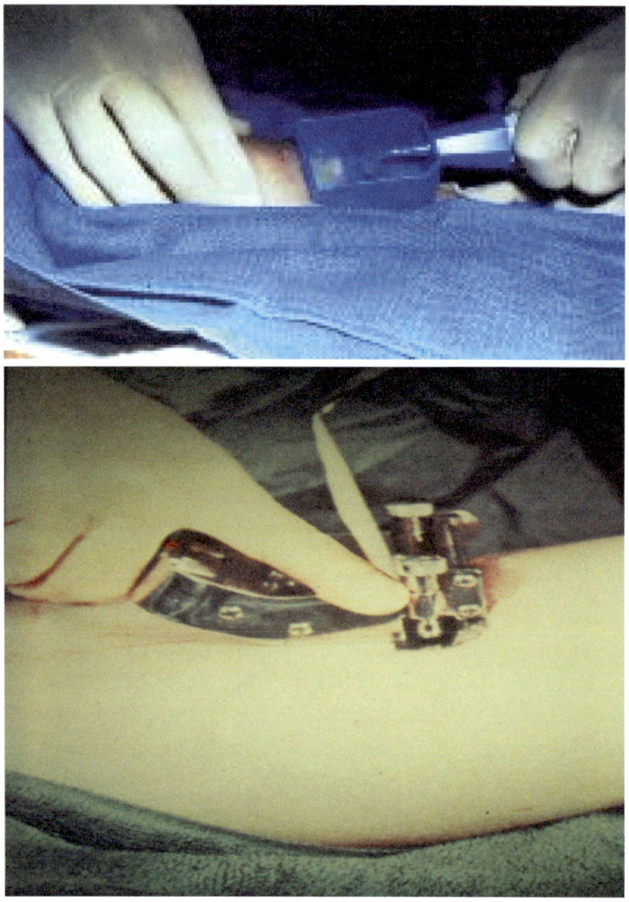

Fig. 27.17 Harvesting a split-thickness skin graft

Table 27.11 Sources of skin grafts

Type	Source	Coverage
Autograft	Patient's own skin	Permanent
Isograft	Identical twin's skin	Permanent
Allograft/homograft	Cadaver skin	Temporary
Xenograft/heterograft	Pigskin, amnion	Temporary

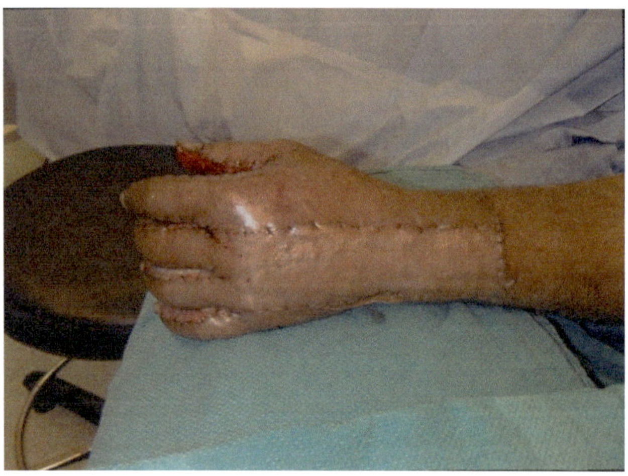

Fig. 27.18 Unmeshed split-thickness sheet graft

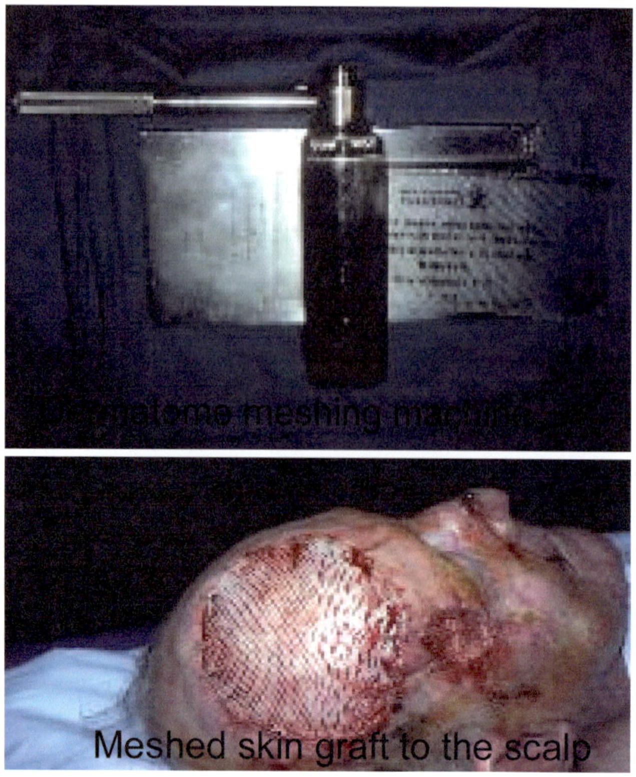

Fig. 27.19 Putting a skin graft through a dermatome mesher

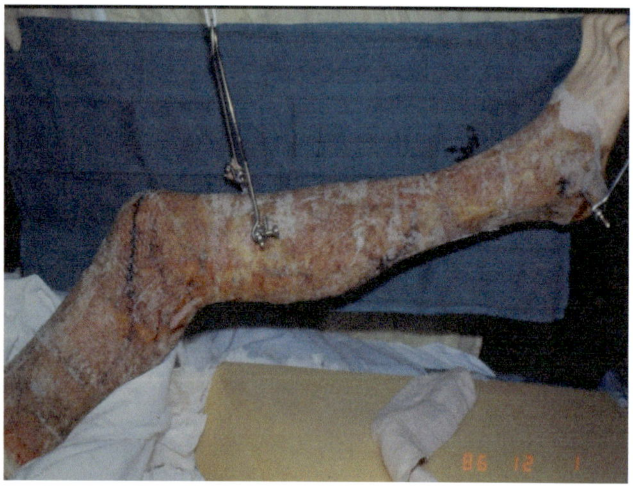

Fig. 27.20 Meshed split-thickness skin graft

into a protective dressing, while at the same time be cosmetically acceptable (Fig. 27.20). Wider expansion ratios (3:1, 6:1) allow for increased coverage when there are limited donor sites. However, the long-term appearance is less acceptable as the mesh pattern is more visible after healing and scar maturation are complete. Meshed skin grafts are generally covered with one of a number of possible options, including silver-impregnated, vacuum-assisted closure, greasy gauze, or cotton gauze dressings. Most dressings are left intact for 5 days to allow for good vascularization between the recipient bed and the skin graft. Following the initial "take-down" at post-op day 5, the dressings are changed every day until the graft has become adherent and stable, usually around post-op day 8. It is possible to gradually determine the percentage of "graft take" during these dressing changes. If necessary, "touch-up" surgeries can be arranged over the next few weeks. For the next year or so post-burn, the skin grafts mature and their appearance improves (Fig. 27.21). Once hemostasis has been assured through the application of pressure and saline/adrenalin soaks, the donor site can be dressed with either a transparent occlusive, hydrophilic foam, greasy gauze and, more recently, silver dressings (Fig. 27.22). To encourage moist wound healing, the dressing should be left intact for several days, inspected and reapplied if indicated. Donor sites generally heal in 12–14 days and can be reharvested, if necessary,

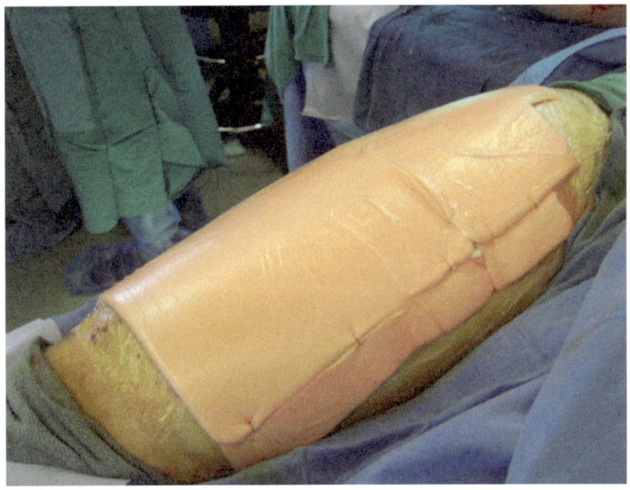

Fig. 27.22 Harvested donor site

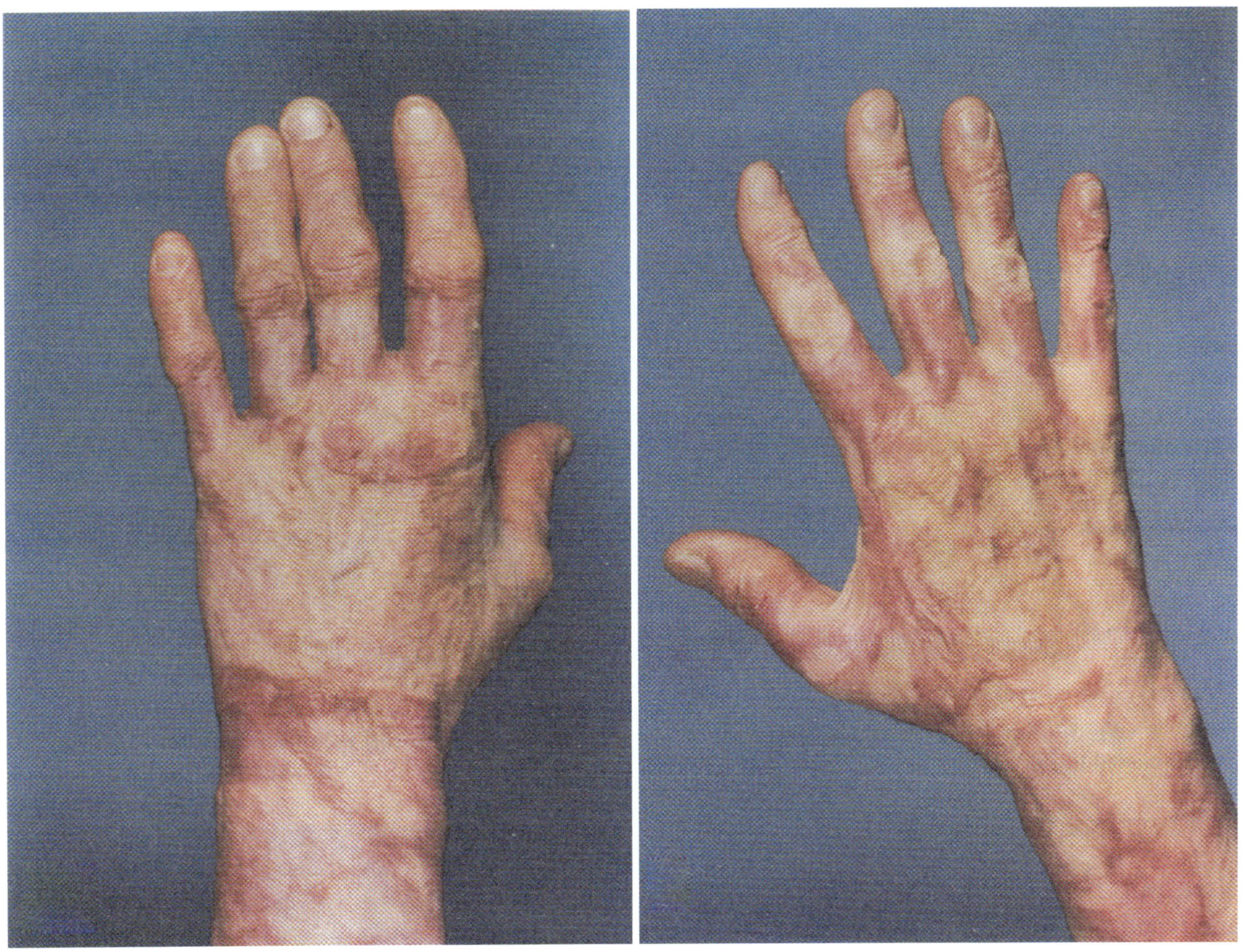

Fig. 27.21 Mature split-thickness skin graft

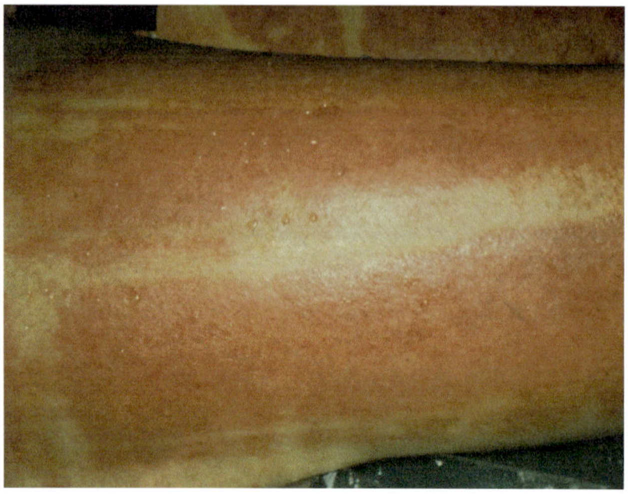

Fig. 27.23 Healed donor site

at subsequent operative procedures (Fig. 27.23). Surgical excision, skin grafting, and creation of donor sites can cause the patient's pain level to increase. A careful examination of the effectiveness of medications and delivery schedule is a necessary part of post-op patient care.

Blood loss during burn excisions can be a concern. The burn surgeon must carefully gauge how much excision and grafting can be performed in a single operation and be prepared to conclude earlier if the blood loss is too great. From the anesthetist's perspective, it is a challenge to estimate blood loss during a burn excision and then to know what blood replacement to give intraoperatively. From the patient's point of view, he/she may not wish to receive donated blood unless it is absolutely necessary. Today, with modern operative techniques, blood loss is less of a problem. The application of pressure, saline/adrenalin soaks, use of surgical tourniquets, and the newer tumescent technique have decreased blood loss significantly for burn excision procedures.

Over the past 10 years, there have been major advancements in the development, manufacture and clinical application of a number of temporary and permanent, biologic skin substitutes. Most of these products were initially developed in response to the problems faced when grafting the massive (i.e., >70%) burn wound where donor sites are limited (Table 27.12). As experience increases with these products, alternate applications are also being explored in both the burn patient and wound care populations. The search for a permanent skin substitute continues.

Table 27.12 Biologic skin replacements

Source	Product	Description
Cultured epithelial autograft (CEA)	Epicel® (Genzyme Corporation, Massachusetts)	– Cultured, autologous keratinocytes grown from patient's donated skin cells – 6–8 cells thick, 2–3 weeks culture time – Lacks dermal component; susceptible to infection – Lacks epidermal cell-to-connective tissue attachment and is, therefore, very fragile
Dermal replacement	Integra® (Johnson & Johnson, Texas)	– Synthetic, dermal substitute – Neodermis formed by fibrovascular ingrowth of wound bed into 2 mm thick glycosaminoglycan matrix dermal analog – Epidermal component, Silastic, removed in 2–3 weeks and replaced with ultrathin autograft—functional burn wound cover – Requires 2 ORs: 1 for dermal placement, 1 for epidermal graft
Dermal replacement	AlloDerm® (LifeCell Corporation, Texas)	– Cadaver allograft dermis rendered acellular and nonimmunogenic – Covered with autograft in same OR procedure

27.10 Coordination of Care: Burn Nursing's Unique Role

Burn nursing offers many challenges and rewards. To be burned is to sustain one of the worst injuries possible. The complex physical and psychosocial demands challenge patients for weeks to months. The one constant health care professional through all stages of recovery is the burn nurse. While the patient and family are the central focus of care around which all activities of the burn team revolve, it is the burn nurse who serves as the central coordinator of patient care.

27.10.1 Nursing Interventions: Emergent Phase

During the *emergent phase* of care, the nurse is present for the admission procedure and is a participant-observer during the head-to-toe assessment and stabilization procedures. In collaboration with the burn physician, a wound care plan is decided upon and implemented by the nurse. The bedside nurse closely monitors the patient, which includes *maintaining effective airway clearance and gas exchange*, assessing the *adequacy of fluid resuscitation*, and monitoring *adequate perfusion to vital organs and extremities. Supportive care to the patient and family* are key features of the nursing role at this time.

Thorough assessments and prompt interventions are important as the patient's clinical condition can change quite rapidly. Documenting and interpreting trends in objective patient data, along with keen subjective observations and guided clinical intuition alert the nurse to subtle changes in the patient's condition that might require intervention. Interpreting the complex environment and required treatments to patients and families is very important. Preparing the family for their first glimpse of the patient since admission requires careful thought and sensitivity. If the patient's face is burned, edema from the injury, compounded by the fluid resuscitation, may change the appearance dramatically. The eyes may swell shut and the head become enormously swollen. Reassuring the patient that the edema is only temporary and that his/her eyesight will return to normal is very important during the first 24 h or so post-injury. If there is concern about the eyesight, the patient should be reassured that ophthalmology will conduct a thorough examination as soon as the swelling subsides. Concerns about disfigurement are often high at this time, particularly with family members who worry about the patient's edematous, burned face. It is so very helpful if the nurse can instill in the family the importance of taking 1 day at a time and cautioning them that circumstances can change quickly and often in the first days post-burn.

Burn wounds are not uniform in depth and may need various wound care techniques. During the first few dressing changes, the nurse may notice changes in the wound appearance, indicating a deeper or lesser injury than initially diagnosed. Wounds should be assessed for their color, size, odor, depth, drainage, bleeding, edema, eschar separation, possible infection, cellulitis, epithelial budding, and altered sensation. Clean technique can be utilized for dressing removal and wound cleansing, with sterile technique reserved for the inner, sterile cream/ointment/dressing application. Loose, necrotic, and broken blister tissue can be removed with scissors and forceps as bacteria proliferate in burned tissue. Burn wounds can be cleansed using tap water, such as in a Home Care or Burn Clinic setting, or when using a cart shower system in a burn center.

Normal saline can be used for wound cleansing at the bedside on a nursing unit. Some burn centers utilize a mild soap solution to cleanse the wound of debris and reduce the microbial count. Consultation with the burn surgeon may result in an alteration in wound care or plan for surgery. Nursing's role would include informing and explaining the change in care to the patient and family, and appropriate documentation in the nursing plan of care. Face care is conducted about every 6 h with special attention paid to cartilaginous areas. Tie tapes used to secure endotracheal and/or nasogastric tubes should be inspected every hour to ensure they are not pressing into the burned skin or nose/ear cartilage, cutting off circulation, and deepening the tissue damage. Eye drops or lubricating ointments are gently administered to protect the eye from further damage. Pulses to circumferentially burned extremities need to be monitored closely, in the event the patient needs a releasing escharotomy or fasciotomy to restore circulation. Peripheral pulses should be palpated hourly in the emergent phase, when the onset of edema is profound. A hand-held audible, Doppler may also be needed, if palpation is ineffective. Signs of impaired circulation include progressive decrease or absence of pulses, progressive paresthesias, pallor and deep tissue pain. For burn-injured patients at risk for thromboembolism (i.e., those with lower extremity burns, obesity) and if there are no contraindications, low molecular weight heparin (enoxaperin <Lovenox>), or low dose fractionated heparin might be indicated. Burned arms and hands should be elevated, above the heart, on pillows or wedges to minimize edema. Patients with neck burns should not have pillows in order to prevent contractures. Burned ears must also be protected from external pressure as the blood supply to the cartilage is poor and infection can occur quite quickly. Patients should be positioned appropriately, i.e., anticontracture positioning, and assessed regularly for comfort and warmth. Moist dressings and prolonged dressing changes can increase the incidence of hypothermia and hypermetabolism. Care must be taken to continually monitor the patient's temperature and hypothermia avoided or minimized by increasing the ambient temperature of the room, using overbed heat lamps and covering the patient with a hypothermia blanket. Intravenous fluids can also be warmed using a specially designed infusion device. In concert with the rehabilitation staff, the patient's range of motion should be assessed at least twice a day. Rehabilitative or orthopedic devices should be inspected for appropriate application and specific instructions written in the patient's plan of care or posted in the patient's room for easy visibility and reference. The patient should also be turned frequently, i.e., q 2h, assessed for his/her susceptibility to pressure sores and appropriate preventive or therapeutic interventions.

For the critically ill, ventilated patient, the nurse pays close attention to the security of the airway—that the endotracheal tube is placed correctly, secured adequately to prevent accidental dislodgement during care or transport, and providing appropriate ventilation to the patient. The respiratory rhythm and character need to be monitored closely, along with signs of respiratory distress including nasal flaring, wheezes, stridor, intracostal/sternal retraction, tachypnea, and triggering the ventilator. When suctioning the patient, attention should be focused on the color (especially if there is soot from an inhalation injury), odor, and amount of sputum. For non-intubated patients, the same assessment takes place when the patient coughs up sputum on his/her own. Chest excursion needs also to be monitored to ensure good expansion and quality of respirations and, whether or not a releasing escharotomy is needed or requires revision. The nurse also ensures the patient is receiving adequate amounts of analgesia to control pain and anxiolytics/sedating agents to minimize anxiety and agitation. Patients may become extremely disoriented, withdrawn, combative, or have hallucinations and nightmare-like episodes. Pre-burn dementia and delirium are more acute at night and occur most often, but not exclusively, in older adults [59]. Consultation with psychiatry or gerontology services is helpful in quickly diagnosing and treatment delirium or similar behaviors. Nursing strategies to assist with care include frequent verbal re-orientation and reassurance, lights on/window blinds open in the day, sitting up in bed/wheelchair, and facing areas of activity to observe social interactions. Background pain (pain that is continuously present) and procedural pain (intermittent pain related to activity, clinical procedures or surgery) must be continually assessed, through the use of evidence-based pain scales [60]. Unrelieved pain can have long lasting effects, including stress-related immunosuppression, increased potential for infection, delayed wound healing, and depression. The patient's level of responsiveness to his/her surroundings, family members and stimuli in the room should also be assessed each hour. The use of neuromuscular/paralytic agents and sedatives must be carefully documented, along with the use of an evidence-based sedation scale.

Peripheral and central lines must be inspected frequently to ensure they are patent and secure as access is usually very limited in burn patients and so very necessary during the emergent phase. Fluid resuscitation, vasoactive drugs, pain and anxiety medications, along with numerous other intravenous drugs, require this method of access. Great care is taken not to pull them out during the admission procedure, dressing changes, or transport. The urinary catheter should also be examined routinely for patency and the perineal area kept clean and dry. The bladder should be palpated for distention. Hourly urinary output is a crucial indicator of the success of emergent period fluid resuscitation, in addition to its color, clarity, odor, and sediment. During daily team rounds, it is important to determine when a patient can be extubated, have IVs and urinary catheters removed, and paralytic/analgesic/sedative agents weaned.

27.10.2 Nursing Interventions: Acute Phase

As the patient progresses to the *acute phase* of care, the focus of nursing expertise is on *wound management*, *psychosocial interventions*, *pain management,* and *promotion of physical/occupational therapy initiatives*. Wound care focuses on time-limited debridement of loose tissue, evacuation of blisters, and gentle removal of exudate from the wound surface. A variety of dressings and/or biological/biosynthetic/synthetic skin substitutes are available and may be incorporated into the patient's plan of care. If the patient requires surgery, the nurse can explain the procedures and care required. Patients are frequently too overwhelmed to remember the burn surgeon's explanations pre-operatively.

Patient and family education about wound care procedures, rationale for particular dressings, and pre- and post-op care can be provided verbally and enhanced through booklets, articles, and videos. Incorporating cultural and learning styles into the educational process increases the likelihood the knowledge will be retained by the patient and family.

A hypermetabolic state, proportional to the size of the burn wound, occurs after a major burn injury. Resting metabolic expenditure may be increased by 50–100% above normal. Core temperature and catecholamine levels become elevated. Massive catabolism can occur, leading to protein breakdown and increased gluconeogenesis. Burn patients continue to be hypermetabolic long after their wounds have healed [61]. Proper nutrition plays a key role in their recovery. Increased caloric and protein requirements are usually met through nasogastric or nasojejunal tube feeding to maintain mucosal integrity. Calorie-containing nutritional supplements, milkshakes, and protein powder can also be administered. Nursing assessment includes frequent inspection of tube placement and patency. Placement is initially confirmed through radiographic confirmation. The involved are should be assessed for pressure necrosis and the feeding tube secured to avoid premature removal. The tube may also be used for free water flushes, if the patient has high sodium levels, and for medication administration. Ensuring continued nutrition, once a patient is extubated, his/her nurse can contact the burn team speech language pathologist to ensure safety of oral feeding [62]. The patient should also be assessed for a daily bowel movement and a bowel regimen implemented. Tissue ischemia/wound breakdown should be prevented/minimized through frequent repositioning and pressure-redistribution surfaces. Progress during the acute phase can be slow. It may be a very frustrating time for patients and families when the efforts being put forward seem to result in such small, daily gains. The nurse can play an important role as trusted coach and cheerleader, bringing to the patient's attention the progress that he/she observes. Nursing can also reinforce the rehabilitation therapists' plans of care by ensuring exercises are performed and splints are worn according to schedule. Encouraging the patient to sit up in a chair for periods at a time and to ambulate to/from hydrotherapy and around the nursing unit, not only brings physical benefit, but emotional rewards as well. Frequently, staff and visitors alike comment on how well a patient is doing and how much improvement they see, which boosts morale and is very encouraging.

Families may need to be encouraged to take care of themselves now that their loved one is out of immediate danger. For some, that may mean spending more time taking care of things at home and less time at the hospital. Out-of-town families may return home for a few days. Upon their return, they may also be encouraged to participate in their loved one's care to the extent they feel comfortable. Activities include assisting with hygiene and skin care, helping apply splints, and coaching through the exercise routines. As the patient is able to demonstrate increasing levels of self-care, family may need to be advised when to help and when to hold back and offer verbal encouragement. Emotional support to family members may be appreciated as patients can verbally lash out in angry frustration when having difficulty doing something and family are advised not to intervene. It may also be helpful for family to see the patient's wounds, from time to time, as it helps to put the recovery process into perspective. From then on, they have a reference point to compare how far the patient has come and what might lie ahead in the next phase.

27.10.3 Nursing Interventions: Rehabilitative Phase

Patients and families alike eagerly anticipate the final, *rehabilitative phase* of care. The focus for nursing is on *psychosocial interventions* and *discharge planning.* But for some, the reality is harder to accept than they had imagined [63]. Some patients have magical expectations about how things will be once they return home. Others express frustration at not being able to go home just yet and of the need to be transferred to a rehabilitation facility. Some patients may not want to participate in their exercise routines or wear their pressure garments and splints as often as is considered optimal. Nursing staff can play an important role of supportive listener/coach, acknowledging how hard it must be to keep going, day after day, knowing all the patient has been through and how long and difficult the recovery period may be. Short-term compromises can be negotiated in order to get the patient back on track, including a day off to recharge one's energy and renew a personal commitment to the plan of care.

Wound care during the rehabilitation period is usually minimal. The healed skin, fresh grafts, and donor sites are fragile and require a thin layer of polymyxin B sulfate (Polysporin®) ointment until they have "toughened" up a bit. At that point, water-based moisturizers are applied to reduce the dryness, flakiness, and itchiness [64–68]. The gentle act of applying the cream serves as a form of beneficial massage during the scar maturation process. Nursing staff can also point out to patients that the act of applying creams is a useful, non-threatening way to both desensitize the skin and to familiarize oneself with the parts of one's body that are burned. Nurses can respond to cues from the patient and uses the opportunity to explore how the patient views his/her altered appearance [69, 70]. It can be a helpful strategy for family members also. For couples, it may be a helpful adjunct to restoring intimacy back into their relationship, as the spouse makes the slow transition from caregiver to lover [71].

During this final phase of care, patients are encouraged by their rehabilitation therapists and nurses to perform as many self-care activities as possible. Rehabilitation routines are adjusted as the patient's abilities improve. There may be periods, however, when patients are fatigued, depressed, frustrated, and angry, and don't want to participate in care [72]. These very normal feelings need to be acknowledged and worked through in order to be able to move forward. Perhaps for the first time, patients are able to acknowledge the losses they have experienced since the burn injury. Now that physical survival is ensured, the body seems to shift its energies to the psychological impact of the trauma. Some of this realization begins in the acute phase, but the majority of the work begins now. Nurses can provide patients with opportunities to verbalize their feelings in a non-judgmental atmosphere. Discussing and acknowledging fears and anxieties is an important first step in overcoming them [73–76]. Many therapeutic conversations take place between nurses and patients if the nurse is responsive to the sometimes subtle cues the patient gives out indicating a readiness to talk. In general, patients benefit from having someone to listen to and reflect back what they are feeling, and to validate that other burn patients have felt the same things and successfully returned to a productive life. Burn nurses can see the possibility of a new and rewarding life at a time when the burn patient sees nothing but endless adjustments, physical and emotional. The transition from seeing oneself not as a "burn victim" but as a "burn survivor" takes time and helpful encouragement from people who know that things will get better. In recent years, post-traumatic growth has been identified in the burn patient population, whereby improvements in particular life domains can exceed pre-burn levels [77]. Nurses can encourage patients to link up with burn survivor support groups and seek support from a social worker, clinical nurse specialist, psychologist or psychiatrist. Family therapy may be helpful if there are issues between husband and wife, parents, and children. Couples therapy may assist in overcoming difficulties with sexuality post-burn. In most instances, these problems correct themselves, with love and patience, as both partners need time to adjust to the burn survivor's altered body image, fragile tissues, and stiff joints.

Adapting to a facial difference can pose a significant hurdle to patients and families. The biggest challenge is posed by responses from the general public. A patient can no longer blend into the crowd anonymously. Preparing the burn survivor to see him/herself for the first time requires careful thought and preparation. Nurses can assist patients to identify their pre-burn coping strategies and help apply them to the present situation. Social re-entry and communication skills need to be learned and practiced in order for patients to be able to move about in public with as much self-confidence as possible. Burn survivor, Barbara Kammerer Quayle has developed the BEST program that teaches simple, effective ways to improve communication and create positive relationships, using STEPS to Self-Esteem (Fig. 27.24). REACH OUT is based on "Changing Faces" founder, James Partridge's work on how communication skills can be used to help people cope with feelings of self-consciousness and others' reactions (Fig. 27.25). More recently, his "3-2-1-GO" program has given burn survivors another useful skill to develop, while navigating through the challenges of communicating and interacting with the public when you have a facial difference.

Nurses can begin to explore such opportunities with patients before and after discharge. Post-discharge, nursing care is provided in a burn clinic setting that may be staffed by burn center nurses, a clinic nurse and/or a clinical nurse specialist. Follow-up during this time is extremely important as the transitions from hospital to home can be difficult and complex. The need for support and guidance may continue for several years post-burn [78–81]. From a professional nursing perspective, the opportunity to work among the burned through months and years of recovery is a challenge and a privilege [82–84]. The courage and perseverance displayed by burned people and their families is truly a testament to the resilience of the human spirit.

27.11 Ongoing Care

In addition to the care already discussed, there are a number of areas that require ongoing attention. They include infection prevention and control, rehabilitation medicine, nutrition, pharmacology, and psychosocial supports.

27.11.1 Infection Prevention and Control

Infection prevention and control is a major focus in burn care and multifactorial in nature. Since 70% of patients who die do so from sepsis, the onus lies with all members of the burn team to eliminate potential reservoirs and prevent transfer wherever possible. Broad strategies include suppression of infection transfer, elimination of reservoirs of infection, use of antimicrobials, and support of immune mechanisms.

Suppression of infection transfer. In simple terms, all burn patients have organisms on their contaminated burn wounds. Certain organisms, normally located in the gut, can migrate to other areas of the body, such as the lungs. If one considers that everything in a patient's room becomes contaminated to him/her, then the focus is on environmental controls. Activities would include reducing items in that environment to strictly those considered essential, scrupulously cleaning items that come in and out of the room, such as shared equipment, X-ray and ECG machines, wearing isolation gowns and disposable gloves before entering a patient's room and scrupulous hand washing technique by all those entering and leaving the room. Appropriate use of personal protective equipment and individual patient risk assessment can dramatically reduce the potential for spread

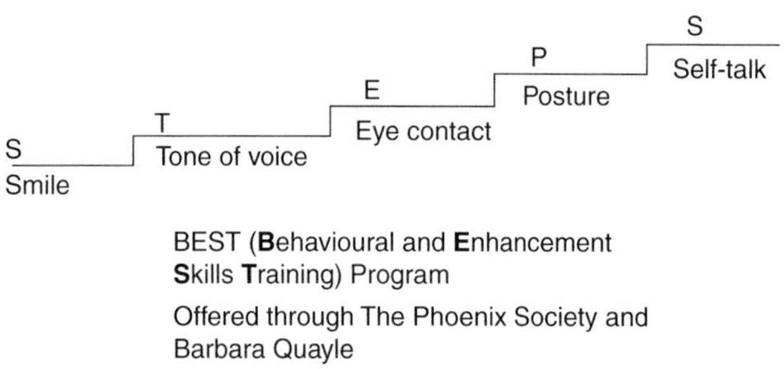

Fig. 27.24 STEPS to self-esteem

Fig. 27.25 REACH OUT communication skills

R **R**eassurance
E **E**nergy and effort
A **A**ssertive
C **C**ourage
H **H**umour

O **O**ut
U **U**nderstanding
T **T**ry again

(James Partridge, 1998)

"3 – 2 – 1 GO" Program

- 3 things to do when someone stares at you
- 2 things to say when someone asks what caused your scars/facial difference
- 1 thing to think if someone turns away from you

(James Partridge in Blakeney, 2008)

of an organism from one patient to another by a variety of vectors, the most frequent source being hands of caregivers. Common patient-care areas, such as hydrotherapy, dressing and operating rooms, need to be scrupulously cleaned after each patient use. Those patients, who have been identified as carriers of resistant or "difficult-to-treat" organisms, should be placed in strict isolation, not taken to the common patient-care areas or scheduled last in the OR schedule. Particular concern centers around hydrotherapy rooms and the risk that water-borne-resistant organisms could reside in the hose system or water supply.

Elimination of reservoirs of infection. Such practices include frequent dressing changes and surgical excision of eschar to reduce the bacterial load at the wound site. This also decreases the opportunity for invasive burn wound infections and systemic sepsis to develop. Another important practice is the physical handling and removal of soiled dressings and linen, and rapid, effective cleanup of body substance spills, such as urine and blood.

Use of antimicrobials. Most burn wounds are covered with a broad-spectrum antimicrobial in either a cream/gel format (silver sulfadiazene, mafenide acetate, mupirocin, Prontosan®), soaks (sodium hypochlorite—Dakin's; mafenide acetate, acetic acid, Prontosan®), or silver-impregnated dressings (Acticoat®, Acticoat® Flex, Aquacel® Ag, Mepilex™ Ag). The bacterial load is, therefore, controlled until such time as the eschar is physically debrided through dressing changes or surgical excision. As the bacterial load is reduced, the patient's clinical condition is more likely to improve.

Support of immune mechanisms. Burn patients are immunosuppressed until such time as their burn wounds have completely healed. The immune system can be enhanced by maintaining the integrity of unburned skin, proper nutrition, including antioxidants, and administration of fresh frozen plasma.

27.11.2 Rehabilitation Medicine

Although the formal rehabilitative phase of burn care begins when the wounds have closed, rehabilitation begins shortly after the patient is admitted to hospital. The physiotherapist and occupational therapist are key members of the burn team and work hard to engage the patient's participation in a long-term plan of care. The focus of this plan is aimed at regaining and maintaining function and independence. Interventions include edema management, positioning, splinting, passive/active-assisted/active range-of-motion (ROM) exercises, and ambulation. Attention is also directed towards functional activities, including activities of daily living (ADL), stretching, strengthening and endurance exercises, work hardening and conditioning activities, and burn scar management [85, 86]. Particular areas of the body pose greater rehabilitation challenges and require care in specialized burn treatment facilities. They include the face, neck, axillae, feet, hands, and burns across joints.

Physical therapy: The main goals are to: (a) *regain and maintain normal range of motion to all the joints.* Range can be achieved through passive, active, or active-assisted means; (b) *prevent/reduce contractures.* Wounds heal by the process of contraction and vigorous efforts must be made to position and/or splint patients into positions of function as opposed to comfort (anti-function). Joints and limbs must be moved and stretched numerous times a day to overcome the powerful forces attempting to reduce full range; (c) *increase muscle strength.* Patients need to continue to use muscles unaffected by the burn to avoid muscle wasting. In addition, a program to learn to reuse and regain strength and endurance of those muscles affected by the burn needs to be set up for each patient; and finally, (d) *restore/maintain cardiorespiratory function.* Chest physiotherapy, suctioning, deep breathing and coughing, and early ambulation are essential to the plan of care. Physiotherapy can take place in the patient's room, during hydrotherapy, in the operating room while the patient is under anesthesia, and in a burn center rehabilitation room. The patient then receives the benefits of a varied and intensive program. Progress can be evaluated, activities altered to meet the patient's changing needs and future surgical scar/contracture releases scheduled [87].

Occupational therapy: The primary goals of occupational therapy are to assist the patient in returning to as functional an ability level as possible, to maximize his/her independence, and to assist with burn scar management. In order to enhance personal motivation and to encourage active participation, the occupational therapist helps the patient to record and celebrate progress through wall charts and personal diaries. Encouraging participation in activities that are meaningful to the patient and journaling as a means of personal reflection are two strategies to engage a patient in long-term and often painful therapy. Early active involvement in activities of daily living is very important both from a physical and psychological perspective. Making a conscious effort to maximize independence is one of the major keys to successful rehabilitation. Use of adaptive devices, such as padded handles for cutlery and button hooks, should be restricted to such time as the patient can perform the activities unassisted.

The occupational therapist also fabricates custom-fitted splints to maintain appropriate positioning for burned hands, feet, neck, and axillae. These splints are essential during the early post-burn period (for antideformity/anticontracture positioning), immediately post-op (to preserve function), and during rehabilitation/post-burn reconstructive surgery periods (to maintain or increase elongation of scar tissue). Splints need to be reassessed and remolded frequently as the patient's edema increases or decreases, the contours of the wound change or range of motion improves. A very important part of the occupational therapist's role is the application of pressure devices to flatten burn scars. Conventional goals for the treatment of burn scars include minimizing hypertrophy, increasing pliability, preventing or minimizing contracture, maximizing the formation of scar to normal anatomic contours, and optimizing cosmetic outcomes. Application of pressure during the early to mid-phases of wound healing is useful in treating edema. Products include elastic bandages, self-adherent wraps, such as Coban® and tubular, cotton-elasticized bandages like Tubigrip®. Later, when the skin is less fragile, patients are measured for custom-fitted pressure garments to be worn 23½ h a day for anywhere from 1 to 1½ years. It is essential to provide patients with much support and encouragement during this difficult period of adapting to these garments [88]. It is exceptionally difficult for patients to adjust to facial masks, whether they be fabric or rigid, transparent plastic in nature. In order to provide extra support to contoured areas on the central face, in finger/toe web spaces, on the palm of the hand or interscapular area, inserts made from a variety of foam, rubberized materials, or thermoplastic splinting materials can be used. Silicone gel sheets have recently been used to treat smaller areas of the body where adequate pressure cannot be achieved, such as the face, arm, or hand.

Other physical agents commonly used as part of occupational therapy include hydrotherapy, paraffin, ultrasound, electrical stimulation, and continuous passive motion machines. Laser therapy to treat burn scars is an emerging area of clinical practice and research [89–91].

27.11.3 Nutrition

During the early hypovolemic shock phase, there is decreased perfusion to the gastrointestinal system, resulting in temporary paralytic ileus. Patients are generally kept NPO until their bowel sounds return. In recent years, there has been some movement towards feeding patients enterally soon after admission in order to preserve gut function, reduce bacterial translocation, and prevent stress ulcers. A nasogastric tube is inserted and connected to low intermittent suction to decompress the area. Intravenous fluid replacement is begun and the patient assessed for nutritional/metabolic needs by the burn center dietitian. When bowel sounds return, the patient can be fed using the most appropriate route, based on stage of recovery and size of burn. Nutrition plays an important role in burn recovery [92]. Patients require a diet high in calories and protein to counteract the hypermetabolic response noted post-burn and to support the growth of healthy tissue. A burn patient's metabolic rate increases in proportion to the size of the injury. Burns are considered the most extreme example of hypermetabolic stress. Inadequate nutrition can negatively impact upon an individual's immune response, wound healing, metabolic function, and survival. Metabolic expenditures can be calculated using a metabolic cart. Most caloric requirements now are based on a formula of 1.4 × basal energy expenditure (BEE). A volume-based feeding approach ensures patients receive their daily caloric requirements, despite interruptions in tube feedings throughout the day [93].

After the burn injury occurs, catecholamines are released and there is an increase in the patient's metabolic rate. In fact, there is a direct relationship between the size of the burn, the increase in metabolic rate and urinary catecholamine excretion. The metabolic rate returns to normal, but it may be several years after the burn wounds have completely healed. In addition to hypermetabolism, the patient experiences a state of hypercatabolism in which lean body mass is broken down to provide amino acids for gluconeogenesis. Nitrogen loss through urine and wounds is a concern, as are the heightened requirements for protein necessary for anabolism, wound repair, and improved immune response. Burn patients require fat in the form of lipids, vitamins, and trace minerals.

In order to determine each patient's caloric needs, the dietitian assesses his/her energy requirements using indirect calorimetry. A decision is then made as to what product should be given at what rate and by which route of enteral access. For burns less than 20%, many patients are well enough to consume sufficient calories and protein by mouth in the form of diet trays and oral supplements. If the oral intake doesn't meet metabolic demands, supplementation is required. The enteral route is preferred in order to maintain the functional integrity of the gut. If patients don't receive food early enough in their post-burn recovery period, it can result in intolerance to later feeding, diarrhea, greater likelihood bacteria will translocate from the gut to another part of the body, and increased risk of infectious complications. Challenges in the commencement and ongoing delivery of nutrition do occur and vigilant nursing support is required [94]. Patients can be fed enterally by both noninvasive and invasive procedures. The least complex method is nasogastric feeding, which can be administered continuously or by bolus feeds. Critically ill patients may have a gastric ileus and can't be fed by the gastric route. A small-bore, feeding tube, with a weighted end to facilitate passage, can then be passed beyond the pylorus into the small intestine. This approach is also safer for patients with altered levels of consciousness, artificial airways, ineffective cough reflexes, and altered swallowing ability.

Duodenal feeding tubes can be placed, endoscopically or via fluoroscopy, if the specialized equipment and staff are available. This allows for quicker absorption of nutrients and a decrease in the nausea and vomiting that may occur with large volume tube feedings into the stomach. If long-term placement is required, percutaneous endoscopic gastrostomy (PEG) or percutaneous endoscopic jejunostomy (PEJ) tubes are available. The position of any feeding tube must be checked at frequent intervals and attempts made to secure it safely into position. Some disadvantages associated with these tubes include displacement and blockage. The feeds may also give patients diarrhea although that may have more to do with medications, particularly antibiotics. Less common nutrition-related complications include abdominal distention and delayed gastric emptying, both of which can be assessed by a general surgery or internal medicine consultant. Patients also require monitoring for hyperglycemia and electrolyte imbalances associated with enteral feeding. As the patient's wounds heal, the metabolic demands are decreased and a reassessment is performed at least weekly by the dietitian to determine the optimal nutritional plan of care. Tube feedings are generally reduced, then tapered, as oral intake increases. Adaptive devices to feeding utensils, such as padded handles, can assist patients with burned hands to feed themselves. Families are also encouraged to bring in favorite foods from home to stimulate their loved one's appetite. Before discharge, the burn patient is advised on dietary requirements at home by the dietitian to avoid unnecessary weight gain once the burn injury has completely healed.

27.11.4 Pharmacology

Throughout burn recovery, patients may require medication. Some are admitted with a past medical history that includes drugs for pre-existing conditions. A number of patients have a drug and/or alcohol abuse history. The role of the burn team pharmacist is an important one in order to ensure patients receive appropriate medications in the correct amount for the most appropriate time period.

When burn patients are first admitted, they are assessed for tetanus toxoid, because of the risk of anaerobic burn wound contamination. Tetanus immunoglobulin is given to those patients who have not been actively immunized within the previous 10 years. They are also given pain medication, which should be administered intravenously during the hypovolemic shock phase as gastrointestinal function is impaired and intramuscular (IM) medications would not be absorbed adequately. There is a risk that the IM medications would pool in the edematous tissue and the patient would be overdosed when fluid mobilization begins. The medication of choice for moderate to severe pain management is an opioid, such as morphine or hydromorphone, as they are generally quite effective for most patients, can be given intravenously and orally, and are available in fast-acting and slow-release forms. Continuing education of health care professionals, regarding the use of such medications, remains an ongoing issue [95]. There are a number of other analgesics that have been identified as very effective with the burn patient population (Table 27.8). It is essential that burn patients' pain be acknowledged and treated from the time of admission until that point in their rehabilitation when the physical discomforts have lessened to the point they don't require medication [96]. A combination of analgesics for background pain (resting) and acute episodes (dressing changes, therapy) is most effective and gives team members flexibility to use the medication that is best for a variety of painful situations. As the burn wounds close and the patient's pain level increases, reductions in analgesic therapy should occur by careful taper, rather than abrupt discontinuation, of opioids [97]. If tapering does not occur, acute opioid withdrawal syndrome can occur. Burn patients, understandably, may be highly anxious and agitated. Sedative agents, along with analgesics, are necessary and can be very effective (Table 27.13). Non-pharmacologic approaches to pain management (hypnosis, relaxation, imagery) can serve as useful adjuncts to opioid-based approaches [98].

Topical antimicrobial therapy is an important part of burn wound care. Most centers have agents of choice and alternate/exchange them if a resistance pattern emerges. For many years in burn care, the most widely used, broad-spectrum antimicrobial agent, was silver sulfadiazine. Its role is to reduce the bacterial load on the burn wound until the eschar can be removed. Local application on the burn wound is necessary, as systemic antibiotics would not be able to reach the avascular burn wound. Mafenide acetate is indicated for burned ears and noses as it has a greater ability to penetrate through cartilage. It is, however, more painful upon application than silver sulfadiazine and its use is restricted to small areas of the body. Alternative agents include acetic acid, mupirocin (Bactroban®) ointment/cream, and Prontosan® gel/solution. Systemic antibiotics are added when a burn wound infection, such as MRSA, has been clinically diagnosed or other indicators of sepsis are present, such as pneumonia or uncontrolled fever [99, 100].

Table 27.13 Anxiolytics commonly used in burn care

Generalized anxiety	Situational anxiety (dressing changes, major procedures)	Delirium
Lorazepam (<Ativan>) I.V	Midazolam (<versed>) and ketamine (<Ketalar>) I.V.	Quetiapine (<Seroquel>) or haloperidol (<Haldol>) I.V.
– Works nicely in combination with analgesics for routine dressing changes and care	– Works nicely in combination with analgesics when very painful and prolonged procedures are performed; short-acting amnestic effect	– Works nicely for patients who appear agitated or disoriented; anti-psychotic and sedative effect

Table 27.14 Medications commonly used in burn care

Types and names	Rationale
Gastrointestinal care	
Ranitidine (<Zantac>) Domperidone (<Pantaloc>) Esomeprazole (<Nexium>)	Decreases incidence of stress (Curling's) ulcers
Nystatin (<Mycostatin>)	Prevents overgrowth of *Candida albicans* in oral mucosa
Milk of magnesia, lactulose, docusate sodium, sennosides, glycerin, or bisacodyl suppository	Prevents/corrects opioid-induced constipation
Nutritional care	
Vitamins A, C, E, and multivitamins	Promotes wound healing, immune function
Minerals: selenium, zinc sulfate, iron (ferrous gluconate and sulfate), folic acid, thiamine	Hemoglobin formation and cellular integrity
Anticoagulation therapy	
Enoxaperin (<Lovenox>) Heparin	Prevents venous thromboembolism

Medications may be prescribed to manage gastrointestinal complications, treat antiobiotic-induced superinfections and boost the patient's metabolic and nutritional status (Table 27.14). Because they receive pain medications that are constipating, patients benefit from a bowel routine, commencing upon admission. Attention must also be paid to reviewing and possibly ordering medications the patient was on before the burn injury, and arranging follow-up with a family physician upon discharge.

27.12 Psychosocial Supports

Psychosocial support to burn survivors and their family members is essential. Caring attention to family provides them with necessary comfort so they, in turn, can be the patient's single most important social support. Family frequently keep vigil by their loved one's bedside throughout a potentially lengthy recovery period and become primary caregivers once the patient returns home. The burn team social worker provides ongoing counseling and emotional support to patients and family members. Specific examples include assistance with financial concerns, finding alternative accommodation if elderly patients cannot return home, navigating hospital insurance coverage, preparing to return to work or school, and strategies to handle ongoing problems at work or home [101–104]. Chaplains offer spiritual support during times of crisis and at various points along the road to recovery. For some, the burn injury is a tremendous test of spiritual faith and may raise questions for which there are no easy answers, such as "Why did this happen to me? How to I move forward? What can I learn from this crisis?" Coming to terms with this traumatic event could move the patient forward in a positive way. Some burn patients are troubled psychologically pre-burn. They may have formal psychiatric diagnoses and/or histories of drug and/or alcohol abuse. For others, the psychological trauma begins with the burn injury. Referral to a burn team psychiatrist or psychologist for supportive psychotherapy and/or medication, such as antidepressants (i.e., venlafaxine <Effexor>, citalopram <Celexa>) can be very helpful. It is important, however, before such referrals are made, to discuss the situation with the patient (if he/she is considered mentally competent). This disclosure provides the team with an opportunity to share their interpretation of the patient's behaviors and to listen to how the patient views his/her coping abilities and behaviors. The burn patient and his family need to feel supported and not stigmatized by the recommendation to seek psychological support.

In recent years, the role of patient and family burn support groups has been examined and encouraged as the power of the lived experience is profound [105, 106]. The advice and caring that comes from one who truly knows what it is like to survive a burn injury or the family member of one who has been burned are valuable beyond measure. Many burn centers are fortunate to have a burn survivor's support group affiliated with them. Based in the United States, but with members from around the world, the Phoenix Society has hundreds of area coordinators and volunteers, through the SOAR (Survivors Offering Assistance in Recovery), who meet with burn survivors in their communities and help however they can http://www.phoenix-society.org or email info@phoenix-society.org or call 1-800-888-2876 (BURN). School re-entry programs and burn camps are also widely available through most pediatric burn centers. There are also work re-entry programs available in many rehabilitation centers and insurance programs. Additional information can be obtained from the Phoenix Society. Similar peer support systems exist globally.

27.13 Conclusion

Few injuries require the full repertoire of skills possessed by nurses of today as much as the burn patient. The demands are challenging, both intellectually and emotionally, but the rewards are immeasurable. Many burn nurses come to realize that they played a key role in helping their patients, not only to survive a critical life event, but to triumph over it and to thrive in the future. This chapter is intended to provide those working among the burned with a comprehensive review of theoretical and practical knowledge, aimed at promoting the delivery of evidence-based burn nursing practice. The author dedicates this chapter to burn nursing colleagues around the world.

Summary Box

Nursing the burn-injured patient and his/her family, throughout a potentially lengthy recovery period, requires a complex combination of clinical skills and nursing theory. It is the intention of this book chapter to explore the following areas of content, essential to the comprehensive care of the adult burn patient: critical care, acute care, burn wound care, pain and anxiety management, support throughout rehabilitation, and psychosocial community re-integration. Nurses employed in community emergency departments, critical/acute care units in general/trauma hospitals, rehabilitation hospitals, outpatient wound care clinics, and mental health support services can benefit from the knowledge shared in this comprehensive review. Burn nursing care continues to be driven by evidence-based practices in burn care and improved upon by both quantitative and qualitative nursing research. This book chapter aims to provide both evidence-based care currently in clinical practice and suggest areas for future nursing research to serve burn patients in the future.

References

1. Burn incidence and treatment in the United States: 2016. Chicago: American Burn Association; 2017. http://www.ameriburn.org/resources_factsheet.php. Accessed 6 Mar 2018.
2. Injuries in Ontario ICES Atlas. Institute for Clinical and Evaluative Sciences (ICES); 2005. http://ices.on.ca/publications/Atlases-and-Reports/2005/Injuries-in-Ontario. Accessed 3 July 2017.
3. Burns fact sheet number 365. WHO International; 2014. http://www.Who.int/mediacentrefactsheets/fs365/en. Accessed 3 July 2017.
4. Ramirez JI, Ridgway CA, Lee JG, Potenza BM, Sen S, Palmieri TL, et al. The unrecognized epidemic of electronic cigarette burns. J Burn Care Res. 2017;38:220–4. https://doi.org/10.1097/BCR.0000000000000472.
5. Lehna C, Coty MB, Fahey E, Williams J, Scrivener D, Wishnia G, Myers J. Intervention study for changes in home fire safety knowledge in urban older adults. Burns. 2015;41:1205–11. https://doi.org/10.1016/j.burns.2015.02.012.
6. Lehna C, Fahey E, Janes EG, Rengers S, Williams J, Scrivener D, Myers J. Home fire safety education for parents of newborns. Burns. 2015;41:1199–204. https://doi.org/10.1016/j.burns.2015.02.009.
7. Riedlinger DI, Jennings PA, Edgar DW, Harvey JG, Cleland HJ, Wood FM, Cameron PA. Scald burns in children aged 14 and younger in Australia and New Zealand—an analysis based on the Burn Registry of Australia and New Zealand (BRANZ). Burns. 2015;41:462–8. https://doi.org/10.1016/j.burns.2014.07.027.
8. Debinski B, McDonald E, Frattaroli S, Shields W, Omaki E, Gielen AC. Predictors of participation in a fire department community canvassing program. J Burn Care Res. 2017;38:225–9. https://doi.org/10.1097/BCR0000000000000484.
9. Banfield J, Rehou S, Gomez M, Redelmeier DA, Jeschke MG. Healthcare costs of burn patients from homes without fire sprinklers. J Burn Care Res. 2015;36:213–7. https://doi.org/10.1097/BCR.0000000000000194.
10. Alonso-Pena D, Arnaiz-Garcia ME, Valero-Gasalla JL, Arnaiz-Garcia AM, Campillo-Campana R, Alonso-Pena J, et al. Feet sunk in molten aluminium: the burn and its prevention. Burns. 2015;41:1122–5. https://doi.org/10.1016/j.burns.2014.12.003.
11. Butz DR, Zach Collier BA, O'Connor A, Magdziak M, Gottlieb LJ. Is palmar surface area a reliable tool to estimate burn surface areas in obese patients? J Burn Care Res. 2015;36:87–91. https://doi.org/10.1097/BCR.0000000000000146.
12. Thom D. Appraising current methods for preclinical calculation of burn size—a pre-hospital perspective. Burns. 2017;43:127–36. https://doi.org/10.1016/j.burns.2016.07.003.
13. Parvizi D, Girezlehner M, Wurzer P, Klein LD, Shoham Y, Bohanon FJ, et al. BurnCare 3D software validation study; burn size measurement accuracy and inter-rater reliability. Burns. 2016;42:329–35. https://doi.org/10.1016/j.burns.2016.01.008.
14. Godwin Z, Tan J, Bockhold J, Ma J, Tran NK. Development and evaluation of a novel smart device-based application for burn assessment and management. Burns. 2015;41:754–60. https://doi.org/10.1016/j.burns.2014.10.006.
15. Goverman J, Bittner EA, Friedstat JS, Moore M, Nozari A, Ibrahim AE. Discrepancy in initial pediatric burn estimates and its impact on fluid resuscitation. J Burn Care Res. 2015;36:574–9. https://doi.org/10.1097/BCR.0000000000000185.
16. Wurzer P, Parvizi D, Lumenta DB, Giretzlehner M, Branski LK, Finnerty CC, et al. Smartphone applications in burns. Burns. 2015;41:977–89. https://doi.org/10.1016/j.burns.2014.11.010.
17. Crouzet C, Nguyen JQ, Ponticorvo A, Bernal NP, Durkin AJ, Choi B. Acute discrimination between superficial-partial and deep-partial thickness burns in a preclinical model with laser speckle imaging. Burns. 2015;41:1058–63. https://doi.org/10.1016/j.burns.2014.11.018.
18. Jeschke MG, Pinto R, Costford SR, Amini-Nik S. Threshold age and burn size associated with poor outcomes in the elderly after burn injury. Burns. 2016;42:276–81. https://doi.org/10.1016/j.burns.2015.12.008.
19. Wearn C, Hardwicke J, Kitsios A, Siddons V, Nightingale P, Moiemen N. Outcomes of burns in the elderly: revised estimates from the Birmingham Burn Centre. Burns. 2015;41:161–8. https://doi.org/10.1016/j.burns.2015.04.008.
20. Duke JM, Randall SM, Fear MW, Boyd JH, O'Halloran E, Rea S, Wood FM. Increased admissions for diabetes mellitus after burn. Burns. 2016;42:1734–9. https://doi.org/10.1016/j.burns.2016.06.005.
21. Sayampanathan AA. Systematic review of complications and outcomes of diabetic patients with burn trauma. Burns. 2016;42:1644–51. https://doi.org/10.1016/j.burns.2016.06.023.
22. Tredget EE, Shupp JW, Schneider JC. Scar management following burn injury. J Burn Care Res. 2017;38:146–7. https://doi.org/10.1097/BRC.0000000000000548.
23. Finnerty CC, Jeschke MG, Branski LK, Barret JP, Dziewulski P, Herndon DN. Hypertrophic scarring: the greatest unmet challenge after burn injury. Lancet. 2016;388:1427–36.
24. Tan T, Wong DSY. Chemical burns revisited: what is the most appropriate method of decontamination? Burns. 2015;41:761–3. https://doi.org/10.1016/j.burns.2014.10.004.
25. ISBI Guidelines Committee. ISBI practice guidelines for burn care. Burns. 2016;42:953–1021. https://doi.org/10.1016/j.burns.2016.05.013.
26. Egro FM. Basic burns management e-learning: a new teaching tool. J Burn Care Res. 2017;38:715–21. https://doi.org/10.1097/BRC.0000000000000462.
27. Anthonissen M, Daly D, Janssens T, Van den Kerckhove E. The effects of conservative treatments on burn scars: a systematic review. Burns. 2016;42:508–18. https://doi.org/10.1016/j.burns.2015.12.006.
28. Holavanahalli RK, Helm PA, Kowalske KJ. Long-term outcomes in patients surviving large burns: the musculoskeletal system.

J Burn Care Res. 2016;37:243–54. https://doi.org/10.1097/BRC.0000000000000257.
29. Grice KO, Barnes KJ, Vogel KA. Influence of burn injury on activity participation of children. J Burn Care Res. 2015;36:414–20. https://doi.org/10.1097/BCR.0000000000000105.
30. Greenhalgh DG. A primer on pigmentation. J Burn Care Res. 2015;36:247–57. https://doi.org/10.1097/BCR.0000000000000224.
31. Sharp PA, Pan B, Yakuboff KP, Rothchild P. Development of a best evidence statement for the use of pressure therapy for management of hypertrophic scarring. J Burn Care Res. 2016;37:255–64. https://doi.org/10.1097/BCR.0000000000000253.
32. Nedelec B, Carter A, Forbes L, Hsu SCC, McMahon M, Parry I, et al. Practice guidelines for the application of non-silicone or silicone gels and gel sheets after burn injury. J Burn Care Res. 2015;36:345–74. https://doi.org/10.1097/BCR.0000000000000124.
33. Nedelec B, Carrougher GJ. Pain and pruritus post-burn injury. J Burn Care Res. 2017;38:142–5. https://doi.org/10.1097/BCR.0000000000000534.
34. Sen S, Johnston C, Greenhalgh D, Palmieri T. Ventilator-associated pneumonia prevention bundle significantly reduces the risk of ventilator-associated pneumonia in critically ill burn patients. J Burn Care Res. 2016;37:166–71. https://doi.org/10.1097/BCR.0000000000000228.
35. Ng JWG, Cairns SA, O'Boyle CP. Management of the lower gastrointestinal system in burns: a comprehensive review. Burns. 2016;42:728–37. https://doi.org/10.1016/j.burns.2015.08.007.
36. Kurmis R, Greenwood J, Aromataris E. Trace element supplementation following severe burn injury: a systematic review and meta-analysis. J Burn Care Res. 2016;37:143–59. https://doi.org/10.1097/BCR.0000000000000259.
37. Stoecklin P, Delodder F, Pantet O, Berger MM. Moderate glycemic control safe in critically ill adult burn patients: a 15 year cohort study. Burns. 2016;42:63–70. https://doi.org/10.1016/j.burns.2015.10.025.
38. Friedman BC, Mian MAH, Mullins RF, Hassan Z, Shaver JR, Johnston KK. Five-lumen antibiotic-impregnated femoral central venous catheters in severely-burned patients: an investigation of device utility and catheter-related bloodstream infection rates. J Burn Care Res. 2015;36:493–9. https://doi.org/10.1097/BCR.0000000000000186.
39. Austin RE, Shahrokhi S, Bolourani S, Jeschke MG. Peripherally-inserted central venous catheter safety in burn care: a single-center retrospective cohort review. J Burn Care Res. 2015;36:111–7. https://doi.org/10.1097/BCR.0000000000000207.
40. Heyneman A, Hoeksema H, Vandekerckhove D, Pirayesh A, Monstrey S. The role of silver sulphadiazine in the conservative treatment of partial-thickness burn wounds: a systematic review. Burns. 2016;42:1377–86. https://doi.org/10.1016/j.burns.2016.03.029.
41. Gee Kee EL, Kimble RM, Cuttle L, Khan A, Stockton KA. Randomized controlled trial of three burns dressings for partial-thickness burns in children. Burns. 2015;41:946–55. https://doi.org/10.1016/j.burns.2014.11.005.
42. Kantak NA, Mistry R, Halvorson EG. A review of negative-pressure wound therapy in the management of burn wounds. Burns. 2016;42:1623–33. https://doi.org/10.1016/j.burns.2016.06.011.
43. Mushin OP, Bogue JT, Esquenazi MD, Toscano N, Bell DE. Use of a home vacuum-assisted closure device in the burn population is both cost-effective and efficacious. Burns. 2017;43:490–4. https://doi.org/10.1016/j.burns.2016.03.038.
44. Serghiou MA, Niszczak J, Parry I, Richard R. Clinical practice recommendations for positioning of the burn patient. Burns. 2016;42:267–75. https://doi.org/10.1016/j.burns.2015.10.007.
45. Hylan EJ, D'Cruz R, Harvey JG, Moir J, Parkinson C, Holland AJA. An assessment of early child life therapy pain and anxiety management: a prospective randomized controlled trial. Burns. 2015;41:1642–52. https://doi.org/10.1016/j.burns.2015.05.017.
46. Singleton A, Preston RJ, Cochran A. Sedation and analgesia for critically ill pediatric burn patients: the current state of practice. J Burn Care Res. 2015;36:440–5. https://doi.org/10.1097/BCR.0000000000000165.
47. Wibbenmeyer L, Eid A, Kluesner K, Heard J, Zimmerman B, Kealey GP, Brennan T. An evaluation of factors related to postoperative pain control in burn patients. J Burn Care Res. 2015;36:580–6. https://doi.org/10.1097/BCR.0000000000000199.
48. Schulz A, Shoham Y, Rosenberg L, Rothermund I, Perbix W, Fuchs C, Lipensky A, Schiefer JL. Enzymatic versus traditional surgical debridement of severely burned hands: a comparison of selectivity, efficacy, healing time and three month scar quality. J Burn Care Res. 2017;38:745–55. https://doi.org/10.1097/BCR.00000000000047.
49. Austin RE, Merchant N, Shahrokhi S, Jeschke MG. A comparison of Biobrane™ and cadaveric allograft for temporizing the acute burn wound: cost and procedural time. Burns. 2015;41:749–53. https://doi.org/10.1016/j.burns.2014.10.003.
50. Tan H, Wasiak J, Paul E, Cleland H. Effective use of Biobrane™ as a temporary wound dressing prior to definitive split-skin graft in the treatment of severe burn: a retrospective analysis. Burns. 2015;41:969–76. https://doi.org/10.1016/j.burns.2014.07.015.
51. Fischer S, Wall J, Pomahae B, Riviello R, Halvorson EG. Extra-large negative pressure wound therapy dressings for burns—initial experience with technique, fluid management and outcomes. Burns. 2016;42:457–65. https://doi.org/10.1016/j.burns.2015.08.034.
52. Schulz A, Depner C, Lefering R, Kricheldorff J, Kastner S, Fuchs PC, Demir E. A prospective clinical trial comparing Biobrane™ Dressilk and PolyMem® dressings on partial-thickness skin donor sites. Burns. 2016;42:345–55. https://doi.org/10.1016/j.burns.2014.12.016.
53. Haith LR, Stair-Buchmann ME, Ackerman BH, Herder D, Reigart CL, Stoering M, et al. Evaluation of Aquacel® Ag for autogenous skin donor sites. J Burn Care Res. 2015;36:602–6. https://doi.org/10.1097/BCR.0000000000000212.
54. Nguyen TQ, Franczyk M, Lee JC, Grieves MR, O'Connor A, Gottlieb LJ. Prospective randomized controlled trial comparing two methods of securing skin grafts using negative pressure wound therapy: vacuum-assisted closure and gauze suction. J Burn Care Res. 2015;36:324–8. https://doi.org/10.1097/BCR.0000000000000089.
55. Dahl O, Wickman M, Bjornhagen V, Friberg M, Wengstrom Y. Early assessment and identification of posttraumatic stress disorder, satisfaction with appearance and coping in patients with burns. Burns. 2016;42:1678–85. https://doi.org/10.1016/j.burns.2016.09.012.
56. Simons M, Price N, Kimble R, Tyack Z. Patient experiences of burn scars in adults and children and development of a health-related quality of life conceptual model: a qualitative study. Burns. 2016;42:620–32. https://doi.org/10.1016/j.burns.2015.11.012.
57. Bond S, Gourlay C, Desjardins A, Bodson-Clermont P, Boucher M-E. Anxiety, depression and PTSD-related symptoms in spouses and close relatives of burn survivors: when the supporter needs to be supported. Burns. 2017;43:592–601. https://doi.org/10.1016/j.burns.2016.09.025.
58. Reimer RB, Bay RC, Alam NB, Sadler IJ, Richey KJ, Foster KN, et al. Measuring the burden of pediatric burn injury for parents and caregivers: informed burn center staff can help to lighten the load. J Burn Care Res. 2015;36:421–7. https://doi.org/10.1097/BCR.0000000000000095.
59. Harvey L, Mitchell R, Brodaty H, Draper B, Close J. Dementia: a risk factor for burns in the elderly. Burns. 2016;42:282–90. https://doi.org/10.1016/j.burns.2015.10.023.
60. Perez-Boluda MT, Morales Asencio JM, Carrera Vela A, Garcia Mayor S, Leon Campos A, Lopez Leiva I, et al. The dynamic experience of pain in burn patients: a phenomenological study. Burns. 2016;42:1097–104. https://doi.org/10.1016/j.burns.2016.03.008.

61. Jeschke MG. Post-burn hypermetabolism: past, present and future. J Burn Care Res. 2016;37:86–96. https://doi.org/10.1097/BCR.0000000000000265.
62. Rumbach AF, Clayton NA, Muller MJ, Maitz PKM. The speech-language pathologist's role in multidisciplinary burn care: an international perspective. Burns. 2016;42:863–71. https://doi.org/10.1016/j.burns.2016.01.011.
63. Johnson RA, Taggart SB, Gullick JG. Emerging from the trauma bubble: redefining "normal" after burn injury. Burns. 2016;42:1223–32. https://doi.org/10.1016/j.burns.2016.03.016.
64. McGarry S, Burrows S, Ashoorian T, Pallathil T, Ong K, Edgar DW, Wood F. Mental health and itch in burns patients: potential associations. Burns. 2016;42(4):763–8. https://doi.org/10.1016/j.burns.2016.01.016.
65. Van Loey NE, Hofland HW, Hendrickx H, Van de Steenoven J, Boekelaar A, Nieuwenhuis MK. Validation of the burns itch questionnaire. Burns. 2016;42:526–34. https://doi.org/10.1016/j.burns.2015.08.001.
66. Everett T, Parker K, Fish J, Pehora C, Budd D, Kelly C, et al. The construction and implementation of a novel post-burn pruritus scale for infants and children aged five years or less: introducing the Toronto itch scale. J Burn Care Res. 2015;36:44–9. https://doi.org/10.1097/BCR.0000000000000129.
67. Gauffin E, Oster C, Gerdin B, Ekselius L. Prevalence and prediction of prolonged pruritus after severe burns. J Burn Care Res. 2015;36:405–13. https://doi.org/10.1097/BCR.0000000000000152.
68. Schneider JC, Nadler DL, Herndon DN, Kowalske K, Matthews K, Wiechman SA, et al. Pruritus in pediatric burn survivors: defining the clinical cause. J Burn Care Res. 2015;36:151–8. https://doi.org/10.1097/BCR.0000000000000145.
69. Martin L, Byrnes M, McGarry S, Rea S, Wood F. Social challenges of visible scarring after severe burn: a qualitative analysis. Burns. 2017;43:76–83. https://doi.org/10.1016/j.burns.2016.07.027.
70. Martin C, Bonas S, Shepherd L, Hedges E. The experience of scar management for adults with burns: an interpretative phenomenological analysis. Burns. 2016;42:1311–22. https://doi.org/10.1016/j.burns.2016.03.002.
71. Oster C, Sween J. Is sexuality a problem? A follow-up of patients with severe burns 6 months to 7 years after injury. Burns. 2015;41:1572–8. https://doi.org/10.1016/j.burns.2015.04.017.
72. Toh C, Li M, Finlay V, Jackson T, Burrows S, Wood FM, Edgar DW. The brief fatigue inventory is reliable and valid for the burn patient cohort. Burns. 2015;41:990–7. https://doi.org/10.1016/j.burns.2014.11.014.
73. Cockerham ES, Cili S, Stopa L. Investigating the phenomenology of imagery following traumatic burn injuries. Burns. 2016;42:853–62. https://doi.org/10.1016/j.burns.2015.02.020.
74. Attoe C, Pounds-Cornish E. Psychosocial adjustment following burns: an integrative literature review. Burns. 2015;41:1375–84. https://doi.org/10.1016/j.burns.2015.02.020.
75. Cukor J, Wyka K, Leahy N, Yurt R, Difede J. The treatment of posttraumatic stress disorder and related psychosocial consequences of burn injury: a pilot study. J Burn Care Res. 2015;36:184–92. https://doi.org/10.1097/BCR.0000000000000177.
76. Hobbs K. Which factors influence the development of posttraumatic stress disorder in patients with burn injuries? A systematic review of the literature. Burns. 2015;41:421–30. https://doi.org/10.1016/j.burns.2014.10.018.
77. Martin L, Byrnes M, McGarry S, Rea S, Wood F. Posttraumatic growth after burn in adults: an integrative literature review. Burns. 2017;43:459–70. https://doi.org/10.1016/j.burns.2016.09.021.
78. Abrams TE, Ogletree RJ, Ratnapradipa D, Newmeister MW. Adult survivors' lived experience of burns and post-burn health: a qualitative analysis. Burns. 2016;42:152–62. https://doi.org/10.1016/j.burns.2015.09.011.
79. Ryan CM, Lee AF, Kazis LE, Shapiro GD, Schneider JC, Goverman J. Is real-time feedback of burn-specific patient-reported outcome measures in clinical settings practical and useful? A pilot study implementing the young adult burn outcome questionnaire. J Burn Care Res. 2016;37:64–74. https://doi.org/10.1097/BCR.0000000000000287.
80. Murphy ME, Holzer CE, Richardson LM, Epperson K, Ojeda S, Martinez M, et al. Quality of life of young adult burn survivors of pediatric burns using WHO disability assessment scale II and burn specific health scale-brief: a comparison. J Burn Care Res. 2015;36:521–33. https://doi.org/10.1097/BCR.0000000000000156.
81. Pan R, Egberts ME, Castanheira Nascimento L, Aparecida Rossi L, Vandermeulen E, Geesen R, Van Loey NE. Health-related quality of life in adolescent survivors of burns: agreement on self-reported and mothers' and fathers' perspectives. Burns. 2015;41:1107–13. https://doi.org/10.1016/j.burns.2014.12.011.
82. Christiansen M, Wallace A, Newton J, Caldwell N, Mann-Salinas E. Improving teamwork and resilience of burn center nurses through a standardized staff development program. J Burn Care Res. 2017;38:708–14. https://doi.org/10.1097/BCR.0000000000000299.
83. Olszewski A, Yanes A, Stafford J, Greenhalgh DG, Palmieri TL, Sen S, Tran N. Development and implementation of an innovative burn nursing handbook for quality improvement. J Burn Care Res. 2016;37:20–4. https://doi.org/10.1097/BCR.0000000000000299.
84. Shoham DA, Mundt MP, Gamelli RL, McGaghie WC. The social network of a burn unit team. J Burn Care Res. 2015;36:551–7. https://doi.org/10.1097/BCR.0000000000000218.
85. Voon K, Silberstein I, Eranki A, Phillips M, Wood FM, Edgar DW. Xbox Kinect™ based rehabilitation as a feasible adjunct for minor upper limb burns rehabilitation: a pilot RCT. Burns. 2016;42:1797–804. https://doi.org/10.1016/j.burns.2016.06.007.
86. Parry I, Painting L, Bagley A, Lawada J, Molitor F, Sen S, et al. A pilot prospective randomized control trial comparing exercises using videogame therapy to standard physical therapy: 6 months follow-up. J Burn Care Res. 2016;36:534–44. https://doi.org/10.1097/BCR.0000000000000165.
87. Orchard GR, Paratz JD, Blot S, Roberts JA. Risk factors in hospitalized patients with burn injuries for developing heterotopic ossification—a retrospective analysis. J Burn Care Res. 2015;36:465–70. https://doi.org/10.1097/BCR.0000000000000123.
88. Coghlan N, Copley J, Aplin T, Strong J. Patient experience of wearing compression garments post-burn injury: a review of the literature. J Burn Care Res. 2017;38:260–9. https://doi.org/10.1097/BCR.0000000000000506.
89. Issler-Fisher AC, Fisher OM, Smialkowski AO, Li F, VanSchalkwyk CP, Haertsch P, Maitz PKM. Ablative fractional CO_2 laser for burn scar reconstruction: an extensive subjective and objective short-term outcome analysis of a prospective treatment cohort. Burns. 2016;43:573–82. https://doi.org/10.1016/j.burns.2016.09.014.
90. Blome-Eberwein S, Gogal C, Weiss MJ, Boorse D, Pagella P. Prospective evaluation of fractional CO_2 laser treatment of mature burn scars. J Burn Care Res. 2016;37:379–87. https://doi.org/10.1097/BCR.0000000000000383.
91. Levi B, Ibrahim A, Mathews K, Wojcik B, Gomez J, Fagan S, et al. The use of CO_2 fractional photothermolysis for the treatment of burn scars. J Burn Care Res. 2016;37:106–14. https://doi.org/10.1097/BCR.0000000000000285.
92. Czapran A, Headdon W, Deane AM, Lange K, Chapman MJ, Heyland DK. International observational study of nutritional support in mechanically ventilated patients following burn injury. Burns. 2015;41:510–8. https://doi.org/10.1016/j.burns.2014.09.013.

93. Sudenis T, Hall K, Cartotto R. Enteral nutrition: what the dietitian prescribes is not what the burn patient gets! J Burn Care Res. 2015;36:297–305. https://doi.org/10.1097/BCR.0000000000000069.
94. Kurmis R, Heath K, Ooi S, Munn Z, Forbes S, Young V, et al. A prospective multi-center audit of nutrition support parameters following burn injury. J Burn Care Res. 2015;36:471–7. https://doi.org/10.1097/BCR.0000000000000125.
95. Bayuo J, Agbenorku P. Nurses' perceptions and experiences regarding morphine usage in burn pain management. Burns. 2015;41:864–71. https://doi.org/10.1016/j.burns.2014.10.031.
96. Retrouvey H, Shahrokhi S. Pain and the thermally injured patient—a review of current therapies. J Burn Care Res. 2015;36:315–23. https://doi.org/10.1097/BCR.0000000000000073.
97. Wibbenmeyer L, Oltrogge K, Kluesner K, Zimmerman MB, Kealey PG. An evaluation of discharge opioid prescribing practices in a burn population. J Burn Care Res. 2015;36:329–35. https://doi.org/10.1097/BCR.0000000000000110.
98. Parker M, Delahunty B, Heberlein N, Devenish N, Wood FM, Jackson T, et al. Interactive gaming consoles reduced pain during acute minor burn rehabilitation: a randomized, pilot trial. Burns. 2016;42:91–6. https://doi.org/10.1016/j.burns.2015.06.022.
99. Carter BL, Damer KM, Walroth TA, Buening NR, Foster DR, Sood R. A systematic review of vancomycin dosing and monitoring in burn patients. J Burn Care Res. 2015;36:641–50. https://doi.org/10.1097/BCR.0000000000000191.
100. Issler-Fisher AC, McKew G, Fisher OM, Harish V, Gottlieb T, Maitz PKM. Risk factors for and the effect of MRSA colonization on the clinical outcomes of severely burnt patients. Burns. 2015;41:1212–20. https://doi.org/10.1016/j.burns.2015.03.003.
101. Nguyen NT, Lorrain M, Pognon-Hanna JN, Elfassy C, Calva V, de Oliveira A, Nedelec B. Barriers and facilitators to work reintegration and burn survivors' perspectives on educating work colleagues. Burns. 2016;42:1477–86. https://doi.org/10.1016/j.burns.2016.05.014.
102. Arshad SN, Gaskell SL, Baker C, Ellis N, Potts J, Concill T, et al. Measuring the impact of a burns school reintegration program on the time taken to return to school: a multi-disciplinary team intervention for children returning to school after a significant burn injury. Burns. 2015;41:727–34. https://doi.org/10.1016/j.burns.2014.10.015.
103. Palmu R, Partonen T, Suiminen K, Vuola J, Isometsa E. Return to work six months after burn: a prospective study at the Helsinki burn centre. Burns. 2015;41:1152–60. https://doi.org/10.1016/j.burns.2015.06.010.
104. Pham TN, Carrougher GJ, Martinez E, Lezotte D, Rietschel C, Holavanahalli R, et al. Predictors of discharge disposition in older adults with burns: a study of the burn model systems. J Burn Care Res. 2015;36:607–12. https://doi.org/10.1097/BCR.0000000000000216.
105. Barnett BS, Mulenga M, Kisa MM, Charles AG. Qualitative analysis of a psychological supportive counseling group for burn survivors and families in Malawi. Burns. 2017;43:602–7. https://doi.org/10.1016/j.burns.2016.09.027.
106. Papamikrouli E, Van Schie CMH, Schoenmaker J, Boekelaar-vd Berge A, Gebhardt WA. Peer support needs among adults with burns. J Burn Care Res. 2017;38:112–20. https://doi.org/10.1097/BCR.0000000000000424.

28 Rehabilitation Management During the Acute Phase

Matthew Godleski and Nisha Chopra Umraw

28.1 Overview

28.1.1 Burn Rehabilitation

The overarching goals of burn rehabilitation are the restoration of function, independence, and quality of life following burn injury. Reaching this goal requires a detailed understanding of the impact of burn injury and the application of early interventions to prevent and treat complications that would impact recovery. In addition, burn rehabilitation providers must also be mindful of longer term complications associated with scar maturation as well as psychological and social consequences that may arise at later stages of recovery as survivors attempt to return to pre-morbid activities. In many cases, the impact of these late-stage factors can be mitigated by early interventions, planning, and patient education on the part of rehabilitation staff.

28.1.2 Defining Burn Therapy

Resources are available to guide rehabilitation providers towards the knowledge base, skills, and experience that are associated with burn injury recovery. The Burn Rehabilitation Therapist Competency Tool (BRTCT) project has worked to define the key areas of competence and best practice and exists to assist burn centers in developing center-specific standards for orientation and professional development of burn therapists [1, 2]. In many cases, these skill sets are largely outside of the routine training of occupational therapists, physiotherapists, and speech-language pathologists, and it can be argued that a burn rehabilitation therapist can evolve from a number of backgrounds with sufficient experience and education.

Burn treatment and rehabilitation require the dedicated effort of the entire interdisciplinary team. The core team consists of physicians, nurses, respiratory therapists, occupational therapists, physiotherapists, social workers, pharmacists, dieticians, speech-language pathologists, psychologists, child-life therapists as well as the patient and their families. It is important for everyone to work together to help the patient maximize their recovery. Many rehabilitation efforts must be coordinated with nursing, such as patient positioning, splinting, and encouraging functional use of the involved extremities. For example, range of motion (ROM) interventions can be done in conjunction with dressing changes to maximize windows if increased analgesia and sedation.

28.1.3 Patient Assessment and Goals

For any significant burn injury, early assessments should incorporate a functional history that includes an understanding of the patient's baseline activities and any pre-existing medical conditions that altered function, their social background and responsibilities, and patient-specific goals and concerns. Ongoing treatment should consider these goals and background as the plan of care is determined, and should be mindful of the potential psychological impact and quality of life. Concomitant injuries may also be present, particularly for instances of trauma.

Specific to the burn injury itself, multiple factors should be considered. Characteristics such as burn size (total body surface area), depth of injury, inhalational injury, and pre-existing medical conditions can predict hospital length of stay, surgical needs, and associated general immobility from hospitalization [3–5]. Typically, superficial and superficial partial burn injuries will heal spontaneously and do not have

M. Godleski (✉)
Department of Physical Medicine and Rehabilitation, Sunnybrook Health Sciences Centre, University of Toronto, Toronto, ON, Canada
e-mail: matthew.godleski@sunnybrook.ca

N. C. Umraw
Honors BSc Occupational Therapy, Sunnybrook Health Sciences Centre, Toronto, ON, Canada
e-mail: nisha.umraw@sunnybrook.ca

M. G. Jeschke et al. (eds.), *Handbook of Burns Volume 1*, https://doi.org/10.1007/978-3-030-18940-2_28

the same concerns associated with deeper injuries. However, pain and edema often still require management to aid in short-term functional recovery. Most of the consequences detailed within this chapter are specific to deep partial and full thickness burn injuries in which the body's capacity to heal spontaneously is compromised, skin grafting is frequently necessary, and more profound scarring and metabolic changes are triggered [6]. The location of burn injury must also be considered—particularly for areas of high function such as the hands and face and skin approximating bony joints. Finally, the source of burn injury can play a role in anticipated rehabilitation needs, particularly in the case of electrical injuries.

28.1.4 The Impact of Burn Rehabilitation

The impairments of burn injury have features that distinguish them from many other diagnoses with functional consequences. First, the base impairments such as edema, contracture, and hypertrophy can frequently be reduced or eliminated with consistent treatment. As a result, the goals of care are often directed at reducing the impairment (e.g., lack of full hand closure) rather than focusing on long-term adaptations or modified techniques to reduce disability. Second, burn injury impairments are recurrent for a period of months, requiring sustained treatment efforts to avoid ongoing development of scarring complications [7, 8]. As a result, patient and therapy efforts—whether through formal treatment, home exercises, or therapeutic activity—must often continue for long periods of time to prevent development of disability. If successful, many burn survivors have the capacity to return to most if not all pre-morbid activities [9, 10].

Therapy should begin at the time of hospital admission and typically will be ongoing until discharge unless medically contraindicated by specific conditions or concerns regarding early skin graft fragility. Early mobility training including transfer training and progressive ambulation has been found to improve functional outcomes such as ROM and hospital length of stay over more passive approaches focusing on positioning and splinting [11], however, approaches need to be customized case-by-case depending on the specific patient and burn injury. Many patients can discharge from the hospital once wound care can be managed in an outpatient setting if the patient is able to mobilize safely, carry out key aspects of self-care, and perform the required home therapy exercises independently [12]. Consideration should also be made for factors such as the size, location, and functional impact of the wounds, psychological health, social support, transportation to key services, and anticipated compliance with home exercise programs.

Patients with more severe injuries and/or those heavily impacting function may benefit from admission to a dedicated inpatient rehabilitation unit. Inpatient rehabilitation has been found to improve length of stay, ROM, function, and balance specific to burn recovery [13–16].

28.1.5 Quality of Life and Long-Term Recovery

A full review of the impact of burn injury long-term on quality of life, psychological factors, and body image is outside the scope of this chapter. However, when treating patients in an acute setting it is important to consider longer term outcomes. While quality of life is impacted by major burn injury, most survivors can return to a high level of health satisfaction even when injuries are present catastrophic [9, 10]. Many patients with burn injury will be able to return to work [10, 17–19]. A number of factors may influence their success such as the size, severity, and locations of injury (such as the hands), psychosocial factors, and job-specific factors. As a result of these issues, approximately a quarter of major burn survivors will not return to employment in long-term recovery and many return to alternate employment than their original career [20].

In the immediate period following discharge, it is important to note that at least one longitudinal study has found an association between mental health emergencies and the post-burn period, and mental health support should be considered in all cases of major burn injury [21]. Adjustment and coping with body image changes should also be considered as patients' transition through stages of care.

28.2 Functional Complications of Burn Injury

28.2.1 Contracture

Contracture is defined as a loss of ROM or malalignment of anatomical structures such as joints due to the development of scar tissue and the loss of normal soft tissue length and extensibility. By convention, contracture in burn injury is referred to by the direction of resistance; for example, an elbow flexion contracture impairs elbow extension [22].

Contracture is a common complication of burn injury and is associated with normal processes of healing, wound contracture, and scarring leading to a loss of normal skin elasticity [7]. A 38.7% incidence of shoulder, elbow, hip, and knee contractures has been reported among survivors of major burn injury at the time of acute care discharge [23]. Relative incidence was related to factors such as length of stay, skin grafting, and the size of burn injury, while the severity of contracture was associated with graft size, amputation, and the presence of inhalational injury [23]. In burn recovery, ROM is measured primarily through goniometry though additional tools have been validated for thumb opposition and compound finger flexion that facilitate tracking the movement of smaller joints less amenable to goniometry use (Fig. 28.1) [24–26].

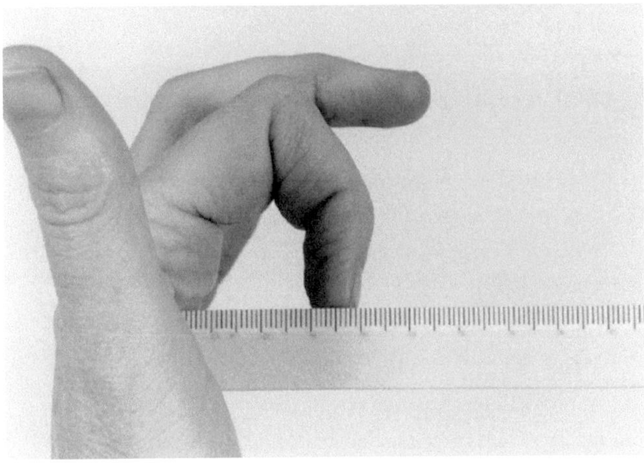

Fig. 28.1 Compound finger flexion using distance between the fingertip and palmar crease as a measurement of finger ROM at the metacarpophalangeal and interphalangeal joints. Source: Ellis and Bruton, 2002 [25]

One highly useful concept in understanding the potential impact of scar contracture is that of cutaneous functional units (CFUs) [27]. Under normal circumstances, uninjured skin allows for joint motion through a process of elongation and recoil. Intuitively, skin directly overlying a bony joint undergoes this process of stretching during motion; however, the research of Richard et al. has skin is recruited from a wide field surrounding the joint. For example, in the majority of individuals, full shoulder abduction is associated with skin movement and stretching to the level of the umbilicus in the majority of individuals (Fig. 28.2). The serial recruitment of this available pool of normal soft tissue segments—or CFUs—allows for full joint motion without skin trauma and is critical to normal function.

Following burn injury, this pliable skin is replaced with scar tissue with reduced elasticity. Not surprisingly, the volume of CFUs affected by burn injury has shown value in predicting the development of burn scar contracture in survivors [28]. As a result, burn rehabilitation providers should be mindful of not only the impact of local injury to a joint, but the compound effect of scarring to the pool of soft tissue surrounding the joint in a wider area involved in full joint motion. The risks of developing specific issues must also be considered, such as webbing between digits, microstomia

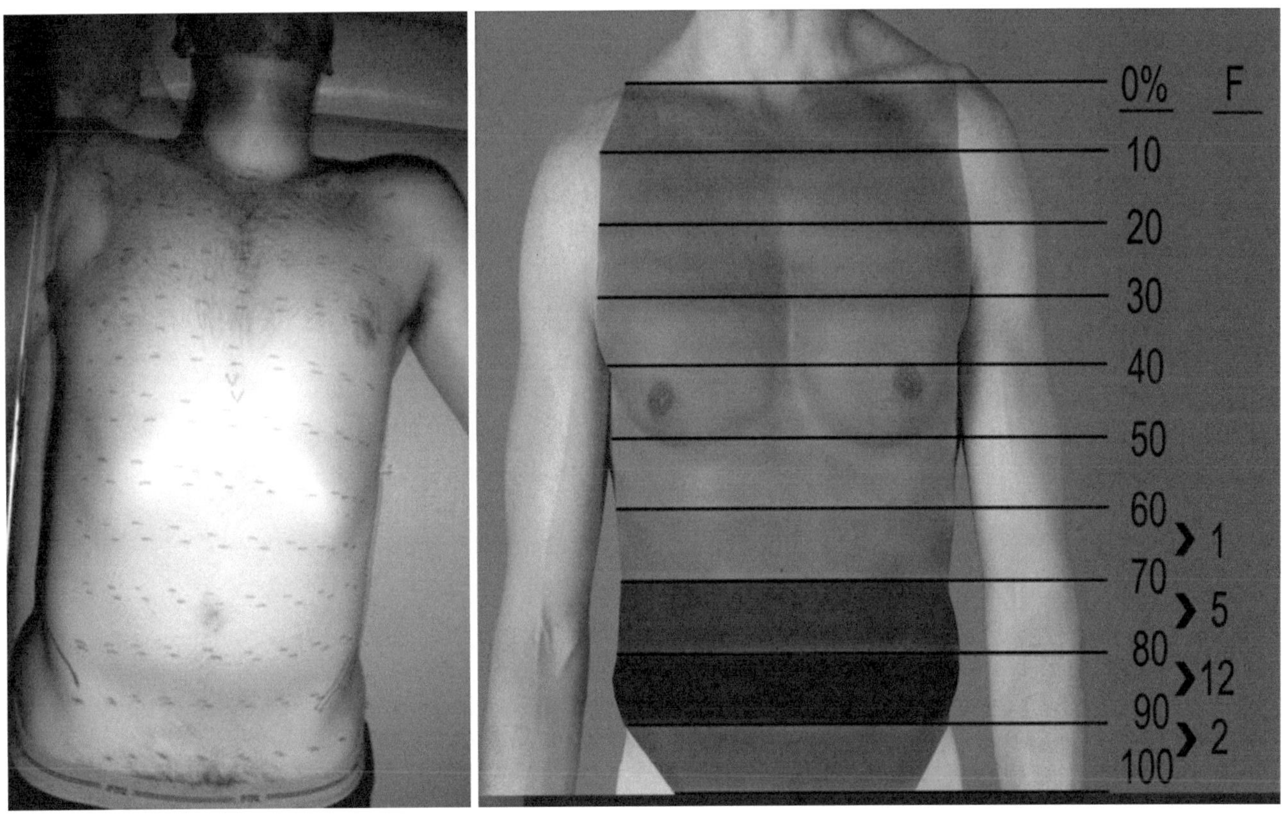

Fig. 28.2 Cutaneous functional units. Skin markings are spaced at 2 in. increments on the anterior torso. The image to the left is a double exposure photograph demonstrating the movement of markings indicating skin recruitment during shoulder abduction. The image on the right identifies the size of the soft tissue recruitment in normal individuals; the majority of the individuals tested (14 of 20) recruited soft tissue to at least the umbilicus. Source: Richard et al., 2009 [27]

(loss of opening volume of the mouth), ectropion (inversion of the eye lid), and lagophthalmos (incomplete eyelid closure) [6, 29].

Frequently, the methods employed for patients at varying stages of recovery need to evolve over time from the onset of injury. In early stages, techniques must accommodate bulky dressings, acute pain, ongoing medical interventions such as central lines, and patients with impaired level of consciousness and deconditioning. In later stages, these factors lessen, however, as patients regain independence contracture prevention methods may become more difficult to tolerate and may compete with functional use of limbs, but can be replaced with more active and functional techniques of restoring and maintaining ROM.

28.2.1.1 Mobilization

Early mobilization is key to limit the impact of bed rest, reduce adverse events, and to begin the process of functional recovery and contracture prevention. Specific to the post-grafting period, mobilization must balance concerns for early graft loss with the areas above. In many cases, surgeons will require a period of immobilization prior to resuming activity. Early post-operative mobilization has been proposed, but medical literature to guide specific decision-making are limited [30, 31]. Recent practice guidelines have been proposed from the burn rehabilitation community regarding early ambulation for patients with smaller grafts (less than 300 cm^2) which are not overlying joints and that can be effectively braced and have pressure dressings applied and can serve as a starting point for team decisions regarding early post-operative therapy [30].

28.2.1.2 Positioning

Patient positioning can be an important tool in the prevention of contracture during the acute phase of care. The body area affected by the burn should be positioned opposite the direction of potential burn scar contracture. Positioning must also consider the expected "position of comfort" in a setting of trauma and pain—most often the fetal position—as well as the impact of immobility and bed rest. Practice guidelines exist to serve as an effective starting point for considering positioning though individual scenarios and injury patterns should be considered in all cases for specific prescriptions of care [32] (Fig. 28.3).

28.2.1.3 Splinting

Splinting is frequently used to provide prolonged low-load stretching, particularly during periods of early graft fragility, reduced level of consciousness, but also with focused application in later care. A large range of splints have been employed in burn recovery to prevent and treat losses in ROM through prolonged, passive stretching, though scientific data supporting use of specific splint designs is limited, as are outcomes studies evaluating specific approaches and prescriptions of use [33–36]. While there are theoretical concerns regarding the influence of prolonged stretch on the development of contracture during wound healing, recent analyses have found substantially decreased odds ratios of developing contracture through splint usage as a therapy tool [37, 38].

- **Head:** the head should be positioned above the level of the heart.
- **Neck:** the neck should be positioned in the midline (no rotation or side bend) between neutral (0°) and 15° extension.
- **Shoulder:** the shoulder should be positioned in about 90° abduction and 15–20° horizontal flexion.
- **Elbow:** the elbow should be positioned in extension. Care should be given not to lock the elbow in full extension (about 5–10° from full extension) in order to prevent further joint trauma.
- **Forearm:** the forearm should be positioned in neutral (zero degrees) or in about 10° supination.
- **Wrist:** the wrist should be positioned in neutral to about 10–15° extension.
- **Hand:** the metacarpophalangeal (MCP) joints of digits 2–5 should be positioned in about 70–90 flexion, the interphalangeal (IP) joints should be positioned in full extension. The thumb should be positioned in a combination of palmar and radial abduction at the carpometacarpal (CMC) with the MCP and IP joints in full extension.
- **Hip:** the hip should be positioned in neutral (zero degrees), no rotation and approximately 10–15° abduction.
- **Knee:** the knee should be positioned in extension. Care should be given not to lock the knee in full extension (about 3–5° from full extension) in order to prevent joint capsular tightness.
- **Foot and Ankle:** the foot and ankle should be positioned in the neutral position (zero degrees plantarflexion/dorsiflexion flexion and zero degrees inversion/eversion).

Fig. 28.3 Clinical practice guidelines for joint positioning following burn injury. Source: Serghiou et al., 2016 [32]

28.2.1.4 Stretching and Scar Massage

Mechanical stretching and massage of scar tissue to improve extensibility are also traditional approaches to burn-associated contracture. Like other interventions, specific medical literature to guide technique and outcomes are limited but suggest benefit for burn recovery [39, 40]. Stretching has the theoretical advantages of being focused on specific areas of ROM losses, progressive throughout a treatment to continually advance ROM gains, and can be integrated into functional or recreational activities over time. Scar massage is typically deferred for a few weeks following skin grafting to prevent early graft shearing or superficial injury, but a number of techniques exist as potential tools once skin resilience has improved.

28.2.1.5 Functional Impact of Contracture

The specific functional impairment from contracture remains a complex issue. At face value, the basic relationship is simple—as ROM decreases, impairment is expected to increase. However, injuries of some locations on the body (e.g., hands) have much larger functional implications than a simple size and depth of burn for another location (e.g., torso). Predicting the impact of specific contractures is also challenged by the potential for multi-joint ROM losses leading to compound movement issues [41]. Finally, the functional needs of individual patients and baseline ROM may also vary.

28.2.2 Edema

Inflammation and wound healing lead to formation of edema particularly in the acute phase of care. Functionally, this can hinder mobility and cause pain particularly in dependent areas and can factor into contracture [42]. Elevation of dependent limbs above the heart can reduce edema and can be initiated early post-injury, and edema in the head and face can be managed by elevating the head of the bed. Compressive dressings and splinting can reduce edema while preventing contracture and become increasingly important for the lower extremities as patients mobilize [43]. Edema can be particularly limiting in the setting of hand injuries, and early graded pressure approaches can improve pain and ROM. In later stages, compression gloves can be employed. Active muscle contraction and functional use of the hand should be encouraged to promote edema mobilization.

28.2.3 Scar Hypertrophy

Scar formation is common following burn injury and is associated with many factors ranging from depth of injury, complications, age, and genetic background [44]. In many cases, scarring becomes hypertrophic, with progressive increases in scar height and thickness, altered pigmentation, erythema, and reduced pliability. During the acute phase of care, hypertrophic scarring is typically not present given the timeframe of development, however, acute care rehabilitation team members should be aware of the fundamentals of burn scar hypertrophy and its management.

Multiple measurement tools are available though serial measurements may be challenging due to the slow rate of change and the need to establish reproducible locations for measurement particularly in the setting of larger burn injuries [44, 45]. The Vancouver Scar Scale is one of the most studied in the setting of burn (Fig. 28.4) [46, 47].

Skin Characteristics	Parameters
Pliability	
0	Normal
1	Supple
2	Yielding
3	Firm
4	Adherent
Height	
0	Normal
1	1–2 mm
2	3–4 mm
3	5–6 mm
4	>6 mm
Vascularity	
0	Normal
1	Pink
2	Red
3	Purple
Pigmentation (hyper or hypo)	
0	Normal
1	Slightly ↑/↓
2	Moderately ↑/↓
3	Severely ↑/↓

Fig. 28.4 The modified Vancouver scar scale. Source: Nedelec et al., 2008 [47]

The two primary means of treatment are custom pressure garments and silicone gels and sheets. Pressure garments influence the collagen remodeling phase of wound healing. While the exact mechanism of action is unknown, it may be related to impact on local hydration, circulation, or inflammation [48]. Recent reviews of the available medical literature have found that pressure therapy is effective for scar height and erythema, less clearly associated with improvements in scar pliability and joint range of motion, and less likely to impact pigmentation or scar maturation [8]. Pressure garments should be custom fitted, employed as soon as wound healing allows application without adverse effect on dressings or injury from shearing, and worn 23 h per day for 12 months or until scar is mature [8].

Silicone is hypothesized to mitigate hypertrophy through mechanisms such as occlusion and hydration of the skin [49]. Recent practice guidelines for the use of silicone gels and sheets have noted the following: silicone should be applied in cases likely to form hypertrophy scars once the wound has re-epithelialized, the benefit is likely only for immature scars, and silicone gels may have reduced adverse reactions compared to gel sheets [50].

28.3 Skin Physiology Following Burn Injury

The skin is the largest organ in the human body, and it plays a range of physiological roles including the sense of touch, temperature regulation, and moisturization of the skin. The majority of these functions occur through dermis-derived structures that are compromised with deep tissue injury and which typically remain impaired despite split thickness or sheet grafting. Long-term physiological skin changes from deep dermal injury should be considered in early recovery and patient education.

The loss of distal nerve endings in the dermis leads to an increased threshold for detecting light touch, cold, and heat and a subsequent loss of perceived skin sensation and these changes typically persist long term [51, 52]. Temperature regulation occurs through the skin both through vascular shunting of blood via vasodilation and constriction as well as sweating and piloerection. Following skin grafting, these processes remain impaired with consequent decreased heat and cold tolerance relative to the size of skin injured [51, 53] though heat acclimation exercises may improve heat tolerance over time [54]. This is of particular importance given the benefits of strength training and aerobic conditioning in burn recovery [55].

Superficially, the loss of sebaceous glands and oil production may seem trivial, but problems with pruritis, dry skin, and need for artificial lubrication through lotion remain some of the most common long-term complaints following major burn injury [52]. Beyond the need for early education, alterations in skin oil may need to be considered for activities and employment that are accompanied by exposure to chemical irritants, dry heat, or cleaning materials.

28.4 Burn-Specific Complications

28.4.1 Peripheral Nerve Injury

The incidence of peripheral nerve injury in burn injury ranges widely in the medical literature depending on the inclusion criteria regarding the severity of burn injury [56, 57]. In those categorized as major burn injury, research has found an incidence of 11% and associations with larger burns, more days on mechanical ventilation, increased surgical requirements, and longer periods of hospitalization [56].

Focal peripheral nerve injury typically occurs in the region of the burn injury, but can also arise as a consequence of critical illness, pressure from positioning or dressings, edema, or compartment syndrome. Focal injury incidence typically follows that of entrapment neuropathies, with the median, ulnar, and peroneal nerves most often at-risk and the upper extremity a more common site than the lower [56–58].

28.4.2 Heterotopic Ossification

Heterotopic ossification is the formation of pathological, ectopic bone in soft tissue and it is associated with a wide range of conditions ranging from spinal cord injury and traumatic brain injury to bony fractures and joint replacement surgeries. In the setting of burn, it is a rare complication associated with larger total body surface area of injury, and most often occurring adjacent to the elbow joint [59]. While rare, the rehabilitation implications of heterotopic ossification can be severe, with patients experiencing increased pain, loss of ROM, and nerve entrapment particularly involving the ulnar nerve. These changes may often be first noted during therapy interventions. Described medical interventions for prevention and treatment have included non-steroidal anti-inflammatory drugs, bisphosphonates, and radiation, and many patients require surgical resection of heterotopic ossification once the process has matured and the risk of recurrence has diminished months after onset.

Specific to rehabilitation, management of heterotopic ossification is ill defined. Early studies and scientific theories raised concerns that early, aggressive mobilization may be associated with the development and progression of heterotopic ossification [60]. However, in many cases the absence of early mobilization in the at-risk population would be expected to lead to soft tissue contracture and, once present, heterotopic ossification can cause severe upper extremity disability present for prolonged periods before patients can become candidates for surgery. Given these competing demands, there may be a role for ongoing mobilization despite concerns with heterotopic ossification, but the timing, intensity, and safety parameters of doing so remain unclear [60–62].

28.4.3 Electrical

Electrical injuries can cause all of the complications and therapy concerns discussed in this chapter, but due to the potential for deep tissue injury from electrical current travelling through the body can cause a wide range of additional pathology with functional implications. Electrical injury is associated with fourfold increased risk of peripheral nerve injury, spinal cord injury and dysfunction, increased rates of limb amputation, ophthalmological complications including cataract formation, and a wide range of neurological and psychological manifestations [56, 63–68].

Complicating these issues is the fact that in many cases development of complications can continue to progress for weeks or months following injury. This may be due to the varied nature of the injury itself, with trauma occurring not only from thermal energy, but also due to vascular injury and pathological changes at a cellular or subcellular level [69], such as lasting cell membrane damage and protein denaturation. In addition—and likely also due to the unusual nature of damage from electrical injury—routine medical testing may fail to identify focal pathology [70]. As a result, rehabilitation providers should have a low index of suspicion for electrical injury-associated complications both at onset and over time, and consider the wide range of potential areas of tissue injury when reviewing patient complaints.

28.5 Summary

Early rehabilitation efforts are a key component of acute burn management. Burn caregivers should be aware of the short- and long-term impact of wound maturation and scarring and the consequences for functional recovery and quality of life, as well as techniques for preventing and treating burn-associated impairments. Successful programs should consider an evolution of recovery from the intensive care unit to the community and incorporate support and planning for sustained prevention of complications and long-term activity goals.

Summary Box

Early rehabilitation efforts are a key component of acute burn management. Care providers must consider both short- and long-term implications of wound healing and scar maturation as well as specific complications of burn that carry functional and quality of life implications. This chapter provides an overview of acute care therapy and rehabilitation including topics such as:

- Patient assessment and goals
- The impact of burn rehabilitation
- Quality of life and long-term recovery
- Functional complications of burn injury: contracture, edema, and scar hypertrophy
- Skin physiology following burn injury
- Burn-specific complications: peripheral nerve injury, heterotopic ossification, electrical injury

References

1. Parry I, Esselman PC. Rehabilitation Committee of the American Burn A. Clinical competencies for burn rehabilitation therapists. J Burn Care Res. 2011;32:458–67.
2. Parry I, Forbes L, Lorello D, Benavides L, Calvert C, Hsu SC, et al. Burn rehabilitation therapists competency tool-version 2: an expansion to include long-term rehabilitation and outpatient care. J Burn Care Res. 2017;38(1):e261–e8.
3. Tredget EE, Shankowsky HA, Taerum TV, Moysa GL, Alton JD. The role of inhalation injury in burn trauma. A Canadian experience. Ann Surg. 1990;212(6):720–7.
4. Burton KR, Sharma VK, Harrop R, Lindsay R. A population-based study of the epidemiology of acute adult burn injuries in the Calgary Health Region and factors associated with mortality and hospital length of stay from 1995 to 2004. Burns. 2009;35(4):572–9.
5. Thombs BD, Singh VA, Halonen J, Diallo A, Milner SM. The effects of preexisting medical comorbidities on mortality and length of hospital stay in acute burn injury: evidence from a national sample of 31,338 adult patients. Ann Surg. 2007;245(4):629–34.
6. Esselman PC, Thombs BD, Magyar-Russell G, Fauerbach JA. Burn rehabilitation: state of the science. Am J Phys Med Rehabil. 2006;85:383–413.
7. Nedelec B, Ghahary A, Scott PG, Tredget EE. Control of wound contraction. Basic and clinical features. Hand Clin. 2000;16:289–302.
8. Sharp PA, Pan B, Yakuboff KP, Rothchild D. Development of a best evidence statement for the use of pressure therapy for management of hypertrophic scarring. J Burn Care Res. 2016;37(4):255–64.
9. Anzarut A, Chen M, Shankowsky H, Tredget EE. Quality-of-life and outcome predictors following massive burn injury. Plast Reconstr Surg. 2005;116(3):791–7.
10. Holavanahalli RK, Helm PA, Kowalske KJ. Long-term outcomes in patients surviving large burns: the musculoskeletal system. J Burn Care Res. 2016;37(4):243–54.
11. Deng H, Chen J, Li F, Li-Tsang CW, Liu Q, Ma X, et al. Effects of mobility training on severe burn patients in the BICU: a retrospective cohort study. Burns. 2016;42(7):1404–12.
12. Choo B, Umraw N, Gomez M, Cartotto R, Fish JS. The utility of the functional independence measure (FIM) in discharge planning for burn patients. Burns. 2006;32(1):20–3.
13. Schneider JC, Qu HD, Lowry J, Walker J, Vitale E, Zona M. Efficacy of inpatient burn rehabilitation: a prospective pilot study examining range of motion, hand function and balance. Burns. 2012;38:164–71.
14. Sliwa JA, Heinemann A, Semik P. Inpatient rehabilitation following burn injury: patient demographics and functional outcomes. Arch Phys Med Rehabil. 2005;86:1920–3.
15. Spires MC, Bowden ML, Ahrns KS, Wahl WL. Impact of an inpatient rehabilitation facility on functional outcome and length of stay of burn survivors. J Burn Care Rehabil. 2005;26:532–8.
16. DeSanti L, Lincoln L, Egan F, Demling R. Development of a burn rehabilitation unit: impact on burn center length of stay and functional outcome. J Burn Care Rehabil. 1998;19:414–9.
17. Schneider JC, Bassi S, Ryan CM. Barriers impacting employment after burn injury. J Burn Care Res. 2009;30:294–300.
18. Schneider JC, Bassi S, Ryan CM. Employment outcomes after burn injury: a comparison of those burned at work and those burned outside of work. J Burn Care Res. 2011;32:294–301.
19. Quinn T, Wasiak J, Cleland H. An examination of factors that affect return to work following burns: a systematic review of the literature. Burns. 2010;36(7):1021–6.
20. Mason ST, Esselman P, Fraser R, Schomer K, Truitt A, Johnson K. Return to work after burn injury: a systematic review. J Burn Care Res. 2012;33(1):101–9.
21. Mason SA, Nathens AB, Byrne JP, Ellis J, Fowler RA, Gonzalez A, et al. Association between burn injury and mental illness among burn survivors: a population-based, self-matched, longitudinal cohort study. J Am Coll Surg. 2017;225(4):516–24.
22. Richard R, Baryza MJ, Carr JA, Dewey WS, Dougherty ME, Forbes-Duchart L, et al. Burn rehabilitation and research: proceedings of a consensus summit. J Burn Care Res. 2009;30:543–73.
23. Goverman J, Mathews K, Goldstein R, Holavanahalli R, Kowalske K, Esselman P, et al. Adult contractures in burn injury: a burn model system National Database Study. J Burn Care Res. 2016;42:1067.
24. Edgar D, Finlay V, Wu A, Wood F. Goniometry and linear assessments to monitor movement outcomes: are they reliable tools in burn survivors? Burns. 2009;35:58–62.

25. Ellis B, Bruton A. A study to compare the reliability of composite finger flexion with goniometry for measurement of range of motion in the hand. Clin Rehabil. 2002;16:562–70.
26. Parry I, Walker K, Niszczak J, Palmieri T, Greenhalgh D. Methods and tools used for the measurement of burn scar contracture. J Burn Care Res. 2010;31(6):888–903.
27. Richard RL, Lester ME, Miller SF, Bailey JK, Hedman TL, Dewey WS, et al. Identification of cutaneous functional units related to burn scar contracture development. J Burn Care Res. 2009;30:625–31.
28. Parry I, Sen S, Sattler-Petrocchi K, Greenhalgh D, Palmieri T. Cutaneous functional units predict shoulder range of motion recovery in children receiving rehabilitation. J Burn Care Res. 2017;38(2):106–11.
29. Esselman PC. Burn rehabilitation: an overview. [Review] Arch Phys Med Rehabil. 2007;88:S3–6.
30. Nedelec B, Serghiou MA, Niszczak J, McMahon M, Healey T. Practice guidelines for early ambulation of burn survivors after lower extremity grafts. J Burn Care Res. 2012;33(3):319–29.
31. Lorello DJ, Peck M, Albrecht M, Richey KJ, Pressman MA. Results of a prospective randomized controlled trial of early ambulation for patients with lower extremity autografts. J Burn Care Res. 2014;35(5):431–6.
32. Serghiou MA, Niszczak J, Parry I, Richard R. Clinical practice recommendations for positioning of the burn patient. Burns. 2016;42(2):267–75.
33. Richard R, Staley M, Miller S, Warden G. To splint or not to splint—past philosophy and present practice: part I. [Review] J Burn Care Rehabil. 1996;17:444–53.
34. Richard R, Staley M, Miller S, Warden G. To splint or not to splint: past philosophy and current practice—part II. J Burn Care Rehabil. 1997;18:64–71.
35. Richard R, Staley M, Miller S, Warden G. To splint or not to splint—past philosophy and present practice: part III. J Burn Care Rehabil. 1997;18:251–5.
36. Richard R, Ward RS. Splinting strategies and controversies. [Review] J Burn Care Rehabil. 2005;26:392–6.
37. Schouten HJ, Nieuwenhuis MK, van Zuijlen PP. A review on static splinting therapy to prevent burn scar contracture: do clinical and experimental data warrant its clinical application?. [Review] Burns. 2012;38:19–25.
38. Richard R, Dewey S, Parry I, Jones J. Letter to the editor. Burns. 2013;39(3):539–41.
39. Zhang Y-T, Li-Tsang CWP, Au RKC. A systematic review on the effect of mechanical stretch on hypertrophic scars after burn injuries. Hong Kong J Occup Ther. 2017;29(Suppl. C):1–9.
40. Godleski M, Oeffling A, Bruflat AK, Craig E, Weitzenkamp D, Lindberg G. Treating burn-associated joint contracture: results of an inpatient rehabilitation stretching protocol. J Burn Care Res. 2013;34(4):420–6.
41. Korp K, Richard R, Hawkins D, Renz E, Blackbourne LH. Refining "functional" in burn recovery outcomes. J Burn Care Res. 2011;32:S160.
42. Barillo D, Paulsen SM. Management of burns to the hand. Wounds. 2003;15(1):4–9.
43. Staley MJ, Richard RL. Use of pressure to treat hypertrophic burn scars. Adv Wound Care. 1997;10(3):44–6.
44. Dunkin CS, Pleat JM, Gillespie PH, Tyler MP, Roberts AH, McGrouther DA. Scarring occurs at a critical depth of skin injury: precise measurement in a graduated dermal scratch in human volunteers. Plast Reconstr Surg. 2007;119(6):1722–32; discussion 33–4.
45. Tyack Z, Simons M, Spinks A, Wasiak J. A systematic review of the quality of burn scar rating scales for clinical and research use. Burns. 2012;38(1):6–18.
46. Nedelec B, Shankowsky HA, Tredget EE. Rating the resolving hypertrophic scar: comparison of the Vancouver Scar Scale and scar volume. J Burn Care Rehabil. 2000;21(3):205–12.
47. Nedelec B, Correa JA, Rachelska G, Armour A, LaSalle L. Quantitative measurement of hypertrophic scar: intrarater reliability, sensitivity, and specificity. J Burn Care Res. 2008;29(3):489–500.
48. Bloemen MC, van der Veer WM, Ulrich MM, van Zuijlen PP, Niessen FB, Middelkoop E. Prevention and curative management of hypertrophic scar formation. Burns. 2009;35(4):463–75.
49. Mustoe TA. Evolution of silicone therapy and mechanism of action in scar management. Aesthet Plast Surg. 2008;32(1):82–92.
50. Nedelec B, Carter A, Forbes L, Hsu SC, McMahon M, Parry I, et al. Practice guidelines for the application of nonsilicone or silicone gels and gel sheets after burn injury. J Burn Care Res. 2015;36(3):345–74.
51. Nedelec B, Quanzhi H, Ismahen S, Choiniere M, Beauregard G, Dykes RW. Sensory perception and neuroanatomical structures in normal and grafted skin of burn survivors. Burns. 2005;31:817–30.
52. Holavanahalli RK, Helm PA, Kowalske KJ. Long-term outcomes in patients surviving large burns: the skin. J Burn Care Res. 2010;31:631–9.
53. Davis SL, Shibasaki M, Low DA, Cui J, Keller DM, Wingo JE, et al. Sustained impairments in cutaneous vasodilation and sweating in grafted skin following long-term recovery. J Burn Care Res. 2009;30(4):675–85.
54. Schlader ZJ, Ganio MS, Pearson J, Lucas RA, Gagnon D, Rivas E, et al. Heat acclimation improves heat exercise tolerance and heat dissipation in individuals with extensive skin grafts. J Appl Physiol (1985). 2015;119(1):69–76.
55. Nedelec B, Parry I, Acharya H, Benavides L, Bills S, Bucher JL, et al. Practice guidelines for cardiovascular fitness and strengthening exercise prescription after burn injury. J Burn Care Res. 2016;37(6):e539–e58.
56. Kowalske K, Holavanahalli R, Helm P. Neuropathy after burn injury. J Burn Care Rehabil. 2001;22(5):353–7; discussion 2.
57. Khedr EM, Khedr T, el-Oteify MA, Hassan HA. Peripheral neuropathy in burn patients. Burns. 1997;23:579–83.
58. Gabriel V, Kowalske KJ, Holavanahalli RK. Assessment of recovery from burn-related neuropathy by electrodiagnostic testing. J Burn Care Res. 2009;30(4):668–74.
59. Evans EB. Heterotopic bone formation in thermal burns. Clin Orthop Relat Res. 1991;263:94–101.
60. Casavant AM, Hastings H 2nd. Heterotopic ossification about the elbow: a therapist's guide to evaluation and management. [Review] J Hand Ther. 2006;19:255–66.
61. Rachel K, Nichola F, Dale E, Denis V, Elad O, Josef H, et al. The development and impact of heterotopic ossification in burns: a review of four decades of research. Scars Burn Heal. 2017;3:2059513117695659.
62. Coons D, Godleski M. Range of motion exercises in the setting of burn-associated heterotopic ossification at the elbow: case series and discussion. Burns. 2013;39(4):e34–8.
63. Ko SH, Chun W, Kim HC. Delayed spinal cord injury following electrical burns: a 7-year experience. Burns. 2004;30(7):691–5.
64. Lammertse DP. Neurorehabilitation of spinal cord injuries following lightning and electrical trauma. NeuroRehabilitation. 2005;20(1):9–14.
65. Tarim A, Ezer A. Electrical burn is still a major risk factor for amputations. Burns. 2013;39(2):354–7.
66. Handschin AE, Vetter S, Jung FJ, Guggenheim M, Künzi W, Giovanoli P. A case-matched controlled study on high-voltage electrical injuries vs thermal burns. J Burn Care Res. 2009;30(3):400–7.
67. Hsueh YY, Chen CL, Pan SC. Analysis of factors influencing limb amputation in high-voltage electrically injured patients. Burns. 2011;37(4):673–7.
68. Singerman J, Gomez M, Fish JS. Long-term sequelae of low-voltage electrical injury. J Burn Care Res. 2008;29(5):773–7.
69. Lee RC. Injury by electrical forces: pathophysiology, manifestations, and therapy. Curr Probl Surg. 1997;34(9):677–764.
70. Fish JS, Theman K, Gomez M. Diagnosis of long-term sequelae after low-voltage electrical injury. J Burn Care Res. 2012;33(2):199–205.

Part IV

Specialized Burn Care

29 Pediatric Burns

Robert L. Sheridan

29.1 Introduction

The basic principles of burn care are similar in adults and children, but some of the specific physiologic and technical details vary substantially [1]. The objective of this chapter is not to repeat what is covered by other chapters in this textbook, but rather to briefly highlight specific practical components of burn care in which important differences between adults and children exist.

29.2 Physiologic, Anatomic, and Psychologic Differences

Driving many of the practical differences in care between adults and small children are various physiologic, anatomic, and psychologic factors (Table 29.1). Many of these differences are physiologic and are more pronounced in younger children and infants [2]. Bronchospasm seems more problematic and common in young children who are fluid overloaded or who have inhalation injury. Very young infants may have a lesser ability to concentrate urine than older children, making them more susceptible to dehydration. Young children also seem to be more susceptible to fluid overload, making accurate fluid administration essential. Young children have a higher metabolic rate and therefore energy requirements than adults, making accurate nutritional support an early priority. In some cases, young children may be more susceptible to hyponatremia when administered hypotonic fluid, resulting in cerebral edema and seizures. Young children have a higher surface area to body weight ratio, making them more susceptible to hypothermia (Fig. 29.1).

Table 29.1 Physiologic and anatomic differences of practical significance

Physiologic differences
• Children seem more susceptible to symptomatic bronchospasm than adults
• Young infants may have a less mature renal concentrating ability than adults
• Young children seem to handle fluid overload poorly in comparison to adults
• Children resuscitated with hypotonic fluid may develop cerebral edema and seizures
• Young children have a higher metabolic rate and energy requirements per unit body weight and will lose lean body mass more rapidly if fasted
• Young children have a higher surface area to body weight ratio which makes hypothermia more likely to occur
• Young children may form hypertrophic scar more readily than older adults
Anatomic differences
• Child's upper airway is narrower and therefore more susceptible to occlusion by soft-tissue swelling
• Child's trachea is shorter and therefore more susceptible to mainstem intubation
• Young children have thinner skin than older children and adults which makes burn healing and donor harvesting more problematic
• Young children have smaller blood vessels than adults which makes vascular access more challenging
• Young children grow, often outgrow, with an initially good surgical result and require revision
Psychologic differences
• Pain and anxiety assessment is more difficult in children than adults
• Family and school issues have a major impact on physical and emotional recovery in children
• Major changes in psychologic needs with developmental stage are predictable

Important anatomic differences also exist. The child's upper airway is narrow and more prone to occlusion from resuscitation-associated edema. The trachea is shorter in infants, and more susceptible to mainstem intubation. Young children have small caliber blood vessels, making vascular access more challenging. Children will often outgrow an ini-

R. L. Sheridan (✉)
Boston Shriners Hospital for Children, Boston, MA, USA

Division of Burns, Massachusetts General Hospital, Boston, MA, USA

Harvard Medical School, Boston, MA, USA
e-mail: rsheridan@mgh.harvard.edu

M. G. Jeschke et al. (eds.), *Handbook of Burns Volume 1*, https://doi.org/10.1007/978-3-030-18940-2_29

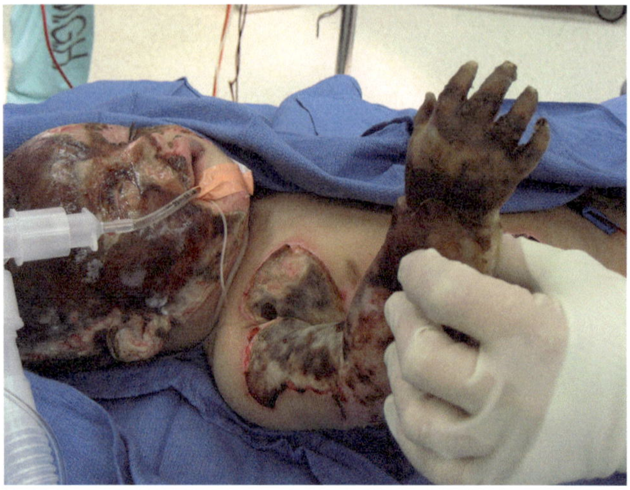

Fig. 29.1 Young children have a high surface area to mass ratio and often minimal subcutaneous fat, making them extremely prone to hypothermia

tial good surgical result, requiring more frequent reconstructive interventions. Anecdotally, young children more vigorously form hypertrophic scar than the elderly. Young children, like the elderly, have a much thinner skin, making burn healing and donor procurement more challenging.

Important emotional and psychologic differences also exist. Pain and anxiety are more difficult to assess in young children and adults. Emotional pitfalls and needs vary with development, with the middle school years being particularly difficult. Family and school issues have a major impact on the well-being of a recovering child.

29.3 Epidemiology and Mechanism Differences

The etiology and incidence of burns varies most with socioeconomic status and age [3]. In the developing world, legislative safety mandates are less frequently enforced resulting in both a higher incidence of injury and differing mechanisms. Electrical injuries are far more common in developing countries as are related cooking injuries. In the developed world, scald injuries predominate in infants and toddlers.

Safety and prevention are laudable efforts in this age group. Safety mandates are variably enforced and include legislation regarding fire retardant sleepwear, fire safe cigarettes, and hot water heater temperature set points. Prevention efforts focused on family education have been successful [4]. Constant repetition is essential.

Importantly, abuse and neglect as a mechanism of injury are more frequent in young children [5]. Burn providers are mandated reporters to their state child protective services.

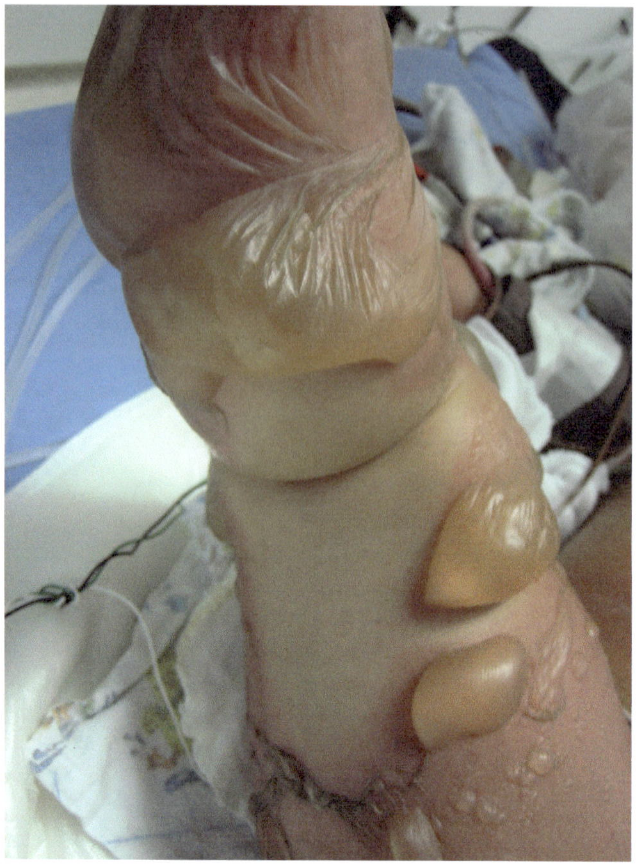

Fig. 29.2 When caring for children in whom abuse or neglect is suspected, detailed and non-judgmental documentation, careful wound diagrams, and quality wound photography are extremely important

When caring for such children, non-judgmental documentation, careful wound diagrams, and quality wound photography are extremely important (Fig. 29.2).

29.4 Outpatient Care Differences

Most burns in children are small and are quite competently managed in the outpatient setting by general pediatric practices [6]. Having a connection with a regional burn program is useful to such practices for the purpose of consultation and follow-up. Children selected for outpatient care should not need a fluid resuscitation, should have no airway embarrassment, should be taking adequate liquids by mouth, should have no circumferential burns, and should not have deep burns of critical areas, or deep burns clearly requiring early surgery. Very importantly, the child's family should be capable of dealing with the child's acute and ongoing follow-up needs [7]. Numerous topical management strategies exist that apply equally well to adults and not be repeated here, the reader referred to the outpatient burn chapter. As in adult out-

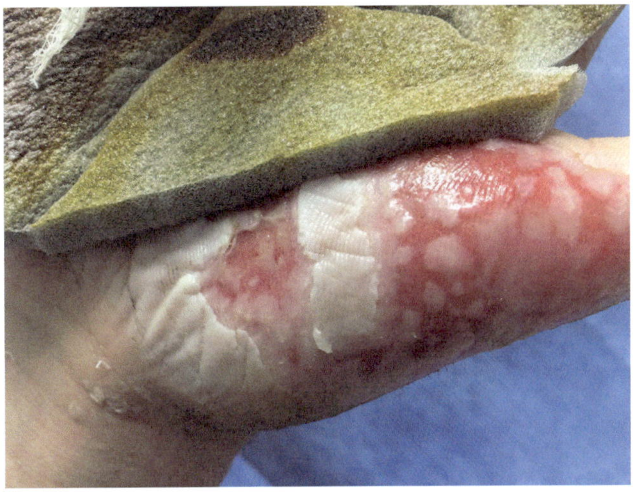

Fig. 29.3 As in adult outpatient care, membrane dressings of a variety of types have proven efficacious in extending the ability to provide comfortable outpatient burn care. This membrane dressing absorbs moisture while releasing silver ion. Many partial thickness wounds will epithelialize under such membranes, but monitoring for submembrane infection is important

patient care, membrane dressings of a variety of types have proven efficacious in extending the ability to provide comfortable outpatient burn care (Fig. 29.3).

29.5 Inpatient Care Differences

The general management strategy for children with large burns based on the early excision paradigm is not conceptually different than that for adult patients [8]. These principles are well outlined elsewhere in this book. However, some subtle but important differences in execution do exist. Engaging the family throughout the care process is important. Time should be budgeted in the busy provider's day to review progress and plans with the family frequently. Having the family as an ally is extremely helpful both short and long term.

Some critical care differences are of practical importance. Endotracheal tube security is a particularly important issue in mobile young children with facial edema. Reintubating children after unplanned extubation can be quite challenging and is best avoided through adequate sedation and mechanical tube security, one of which is a tube–tie harness system (Fig. 29.4). Uncuffed tubes are ideally avoided in all age groups [9]. Tracheostomy is needed in some children with injuries requiring long-term mechanical ventilation [10], but fairly long-term trans-laryngeal intubation is also associated with good outcomes [11]. Assessing and controlling pain and anxiety in young children with deep burns is very difficult, but should be done on a regular basis [12]. Children will predictably develop rapid tolerance to standard doses of opiates and benzodiazepines, and humane escalation is advised. Early use of a "third drug" is useful in blunting dose escalation. Dexmedetomidine is an excellent choice. Procedural interventions often generate additional sedation needs, which can generally be addressed with additional opiates and benzodiazepines or ketamine [13]. Good control of pain and anxiety may require high-dose pharmacotherapy but it has enduring positive psychologic benefit [14].

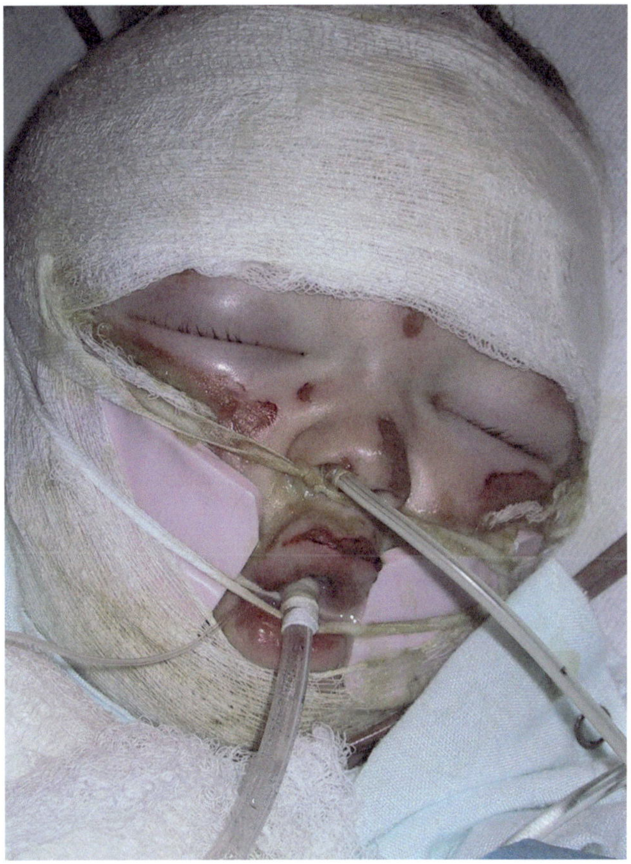

Fig. 29.4 Reintubating children after unplanned extubation can be quite challenging and is best avoided through adequate sedation and mechanical tube security, one of which is a tube–tie harness system as illustrated here

The hypermetabolic catabolic state is poorly tolerated by young children. Early tube feedings are advocated, generally beginning during resuscitation. Short-term parenteral nutrition is well tolerated and can be useful during periods of sepsis or hemodynamic instability [15]. Nutritional targets should include 2–2.5 g per kilogram of ideal body weight per day of protein and a caloric target of 1.5–1.7 times a basal metabolic rate [16]. The use of anabolic agents remains an area of some controversy in the field with good outcomes documented on both sides [17, 18].

Differentiating benign fever from sepsis in children can be challenging. Many young children have a propensity to manifest high fever in the absence of infection. In the current era of antibiotic stewardship, if a child looks toxic with a

Table 29.2 Suggested resuscitation endpoints in children

- Comfortable but easily arousable sensorium
- Warm distal extremities with easily palpable pulses
- Systolic blood pressure of 60 mmHg systolic in infants, 70–90 plus 2 times age in years in mmHg for older children, and mean arterial pressure over 60 mmHg for adolescents
- Pulse between 80 and 180 per minute (age dependent)
- Urine output of 0.5–1 cm^3 per kg per hour (glucose negative)
- Base deficit less than −2

fever, drawing blood cultures and starting antibiotics with a plan to stop them if the blood cultures are negative at 72 h is reasonable [19]. Children with inhalation injury and respiratory failure are ideally managed with lung protective strategies of mechanical ventilation, pulmonary toilet, and focused treatment for infection [20]. It was not that long ago that young age was an independent predictor of mortality in burns. However, that is no longer the case largely secondary to the evolution of pediatric critical care techniques with early wound excision, accurate individualized fluid resuscitation, lung protective strategies of ventilation, and focused treatment of infection [21].

29.6 Fluid Resuscitation Differences

Basic principles of burn resuscitation are similar in adults and children. Here again, this section will only present differences that have practical clinical consequences. Children with burns less than about 15% of the body surface generally need no formal resuscitation. Providing them fluid at about 150% of a maintenance rate via combined oral and intravenous route is generally sufficient. Adequacy of hydration can be monitored by urine output (weighing diapers and physical exam looking at mucous membranes and peripheral pulse quality).

As burns become larger, a calculated resuscitation is advisable. It has been the authors experience that over-resuscitation is quite common in young children which exacerbates the complications associated with anasarca. Resuscitation-associated anasarca can be minimized by refining resuscitation endpoints (Table 29.2) and by more liberal use of colloid early in resuscitation [22]. Extreme anasarca is associated with morbidity related to retrobulbar edema, compartment pressure elevations, impaired gas exchange, and abdominal visceral edema (Fig. 29.5). While acknowledging the success of crystalloid-only resuscitation, the author's personal practice has included early colloid for many years, and is detailed in Table 29.3 [23].

As in adults, inhalation injury, very deep burns, and resuscitation delay increase fluid needs. Enteral burn resuscitation can be successful, particularly in children with small and medium size burns [24]. In all injuries requiring fluid resuscitation, frequent monitoring and titration is the only way to ensure that resuscitation accurately meets individual patient needs.

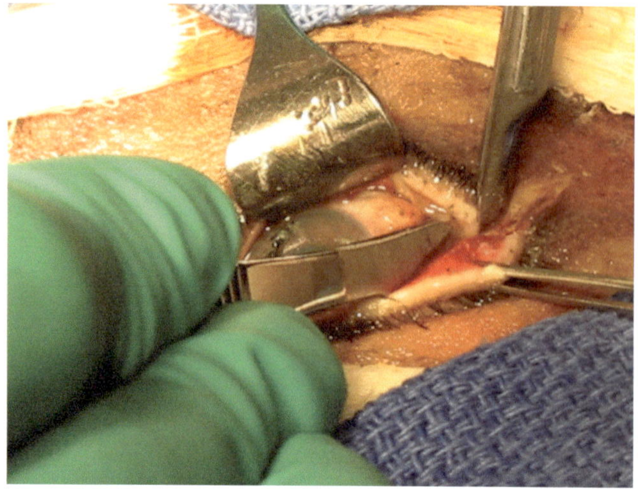

Fig. 29.5 Extreme anasarca contributes to retrobulbar edema, requiring decompression as illustrated here, as well as extremity compartment pressure elevations, impaired gas exchange, and abdominal visceral edema. It can be minimized with a careful individualized resuscitation emphasizing refined endpoints and early use of colloid

Table 29.3 Author's personal fluid resuscitation practice

Initial infusions		
Burn size	*LR*	*5% albumin*
1–20%	1.5M	None
20–50%	P minus 1M	1M
>50%	P minus 2M	2M
M = calculated maintenance rate based on weight		
P=Parkland calculation for crystalloid (4 cm^3/kg/%burn in first 24 h, half in first 8 post-injury hours—typically 0.25 cm^3/kg/%burn/h for first 8 h)		
Other points		
1. During first 24 h, fluid rate titrated hourly to resuscitation endpoints. For first 24 h, LR is titrated. At 24 h, LR and albumin are titrated in tandem. Typically, patients need about 1.5M at 24 h		
2. If patient is child less than 20 kg, 1M of initial LR is given as D5LR, with the remainder given as LR		
3. When needed, boluses are given as 10 cm^3/kg of 5% albumin		
4. Overall goal is to be "just on the dry side of normovolemia"		
5. Tube feedings can be started at trophic rate during first 24 h in stable patients. Tube feeding rate is subtracted from LR rate		

29.7 Acute Procedural and Operative Differences

Techniques of burn procedures and operations are covered elsewhere in this textbook. However, there are some important points to emphasize when managing young pediatric patients. When doing procedures on the burn unit, children are difficult to calm verbally. Child life interventions can be incredibly effective and should be used whenever available. If these are not adequate to make a bedside procedure safe and humane, ketamine is a safe and effective way to do make otherwise frightening and uncomfortable procedures safe and tolerable.

Certain intraoperative considerations are useful [25]. Preemptive temperature management is important when operating on young children who will rapidly become hypothermic unless the operating room temperature is kept high. They are generally quite easy to cool when necessary, but to perform a large excisional operation in a small child will require operating room temperatures approaching 120 °F to maintain normothermia and normal coagulation. Temperature monitors should be placed on induction. Well-trained pediatric anesthesia teams are essential. They best do their job when continuous communication is initiated by the surgical team regarding operative blood loss, temperature management, vascular access, fluid administration, urine output, and gas exchange. Comfortable and respectful collaboration is an important element of success.

The use of hemostatic techniques of excision should be absolutely routine in all patients. Careful operative planning facilitates swift execution of the procedures. Extremity exsanguination and proximal tourniquets are useful. Dilute epinephrine clysis is incredibly effective at limiting blood loss from excised wounds and donor sites [26].

29.8 Reconstruction and Rehabilitation Differences

The need to meet developmental milestones puts added pressure on the burn team to deliver a high quality functional result. Children will quickly outgrow an initially adequate result, mandating frequent follow-up with operative and rehabilitation interventions to meet these needs. The quality of a child's family and school environment has an enormous impact on both their emotional and physical recovery [27]. Burn teams should be prepared to train and guide families and help them meet their child's burn recovery needs. The burn team should also be prepared to help the child's school with reintegration. This may take the form of class education and input into individualized education plans.

29.9 Conclusion

Burn care for children has improved substantially in recent decades [28]. Concentration of care in high-volume pediatric centers has been shown to enhance survival outcomes [29]. Even children with massive burns can become happy and productive citizens when participants in a holistic recovery program [30]. The opportunity to follow a child through their growing years and help them to realize an optimal physical and emotional recovery is a rare and rewarding gift.

Summary Box

- Burns are common injuries in children.

  General management strategy for pediatric burns is similar to that for adult patients.
- Family involvement is an important component of inpatient and outpatient care.

  All phases of management are complicated by anatomic and physiologic differences unique to children.
- Critical acute management implications include age-specific resuscitation, vascular and airway access issues, nutritional support needs, and temperature control.
- Long-term follow-up is essential to ensure optimal results in growing children.

  Children have unique developmentally specific reintegration needs.

References

1. Sheridan RL. Burns at the extremes of age. J Burn Care Res. 2007;28(2):580–6.
2. Sheridan RL, Remensnyder JP, Prelack K, Petras L, Lydon M. Treatment of the seriously burned infant. J Burn Care Rehabil. 1998;19:115–8.
3. Shah A, Suresh S, Thomas R, Smith S. Epidemiology and profile of pediatric burns in a large referral center. Clin Pediatr (Phila). 2011;50(5):391–5.
4. Cox SG, Burahee A, Albertyn R, Makahabane J, Rode H. Parent knowledge on paediatric burn prevention related to the home environment. Burns. 2016;42:1854. pii: S0305-4179(16)30165-6.
5. Peck MD, Priolo-Kapel D. Child abuse by burning: a review of the literature and an algorithm for medical investigations. J Trauma. 2002;53(5):1013–22.
6. Warner PM, Coffee TL, Yowler CJ. Outpatient burn management. Surg Clin North Am. 2014;94(4):879–92.
7. Sheridan R. Outpatient burn care in the emergency department. Pediatr Emerg Care. 2005;21(7):449–56.
8. Cancio L, Lundy J, Sheridan RL. Burns and environmental injuries. In: Cannon J, editor. Injury care in deployed settings. Surg Clin North Am. 2012;92(4):959–86.
9. Sheridan RL. Uncuffed endotracheal tubes should not be used in seriously burned children. Pediatr Crit Care Med. 2006;7(3):258–9.
10. Kadilak PR, Vanasse S, Sheridan RL. Favorable short- and long-term outcomes of prolonged translaryngeal intubation in critically ill children. J Burn Care Rehabil. 2004;25(3):262–5.
11. Sen S, Heather J, Palmieri T, Greenhalgh D. Tracheostomy in pediatric burn patients. Burns. 2015;41(2):248–51.
12. Singleton A, Preston RJ, Cochran A. Sedation and analgesia for critically ill pediatric burn patients: the current state of practice. J Burn Care Res. 2015;36(3):440–5.
13. Owens VF, Palmieri TL, Comroe CM, Conroy JM, Scavone JA, Greenhalgh DG. Ketamine: a safe and effective agent for pain-

ful procedures in the pediatric burn patient. J Burn Care Res. 2006;27(2):211–6.
14. Sheridan R, Stoddard F, Hinson M, Lydon M, Tompkins R. Long-term post-traumatic stress symptoms vary inversely with early opiate dosing in children recovering from serious burns: effects durable at four years. J Trauma Acute Care Surg. 2014;76(3):828–32.
15. Dylewksi ML, Baker M, Prelack K, Weber JM, Hursey D, Lydon M, Fagan SP, Sheridan RL. The safety and efficacy of parenteral nutrition among pediatric patients with burn injuries. Pediatr Crit Care Med. 2013;14(3):e120–5.
16. Prelack K, Dwyer J, Dallal GE, Rand WM, Yu Y-M, Kehayuias JJ, Antoon A, Sheridan RL. Growth deceleration and restoration after serious burn injury. J Burn Care Res. 2007;28(2):262–8.
17. Prelack K, Dylewski M, Sheridan RL. Practical guidelines for nutritional management of burn injury and recovery. Burns. 2007;33(1):14–24.
18. Abdullahi A, Jeschke MG. Nutrition and anabolic pharmacotherapies in the care of burn patients. Nutr Clin Pract. 2014;29(5):621–30.
19. Sheridan RL. Sepsis in pediatric burn patients. Pediatr Crit Care Med. 2005;6(3):S112–9.
20. Sheridan RL. Fire-related inhalation injury. N Engl J Med. 2016;375(5):464–9.
21. Sheridan RL, Schnitzer JJ, Weber JM, Schulz JT, Ryan CM, Tompkins RG. Young age is not a predictor of mortality in burns. Pediatr Crit Care Med. 2001;2(3):223–4.
22. Müller Dittrich MH, Brunow de Carvalho W, Lopes Lavado E. Evaluation of the "early" use of albumin in children with extensive burns: a randomized controlled trial. Pediatr Crit Care Med. 2016;17(6):e280–6.
23. Sheridan R. Less is more-revisiting burn resuscitation. Pediatr Crit Care Med. 2016;17(6):578–9.
24. Kramer G, Michell MW, Oliveira H, Brown TLH, Herndon DN, Baker D, Muller M. Oral and enteral resuscitation of burn shock: the historical record and implications for mass casualty care. Eplasty. 2010;10:e56.
25. Sheridan RL, Chang P. Acute burn procedures. Surg Clin North Am. 2014;94(4):755–64.
26. Sheridan RL, Szyfelbein SK. Staged high-dose epinephrine clysis is safe and effective in extensive tangential burn excisions in children. Burns. 1999;25(8):745–8.
27. Sheridan R, Lee A, Kazis L, Shriners Pediatric Burn Outcome Group. Family characteristics impact long-term pediatric injury recovery. J Trauma. 2012;73(3):S205–12.
28. Sheridan RL. Burn care: results of technical and organizational progress. JAMA. 2003;290(6):719–22.
29. Palmieri TL, Taylor S, Lawless M, Curri T, Sen S, Greenhalgh DG. Burn center volume makes a difference for burned children. Pediatr Crit Care Med. 2015;16(4):319–24.
30. Sheridan RL, Hinson MM, Liang MM, Mulligan JL, Ryan CM, Tompkins RG. Long-term outcome of children surviving massive burns. JAMA. 2000;283(1):69–73.

Geriatric Burns

30

Holly B. Cunningham, Kathleen S. Romanowski, and Herb A. Phelan

30.1 Epidemiology and Risk Factors for Geriatric Burn Injury

The large majority of burns sustained by elders arise from one of three general mechanisms or activities: those sustained due to smoking, those suffered from mishaps while cooking, and scald injuries. The fact that elders are uniquely vulnerable to burn injury is borne out by the National Center for Health Statistics' 2010 finding that adults 65 years of age and older accounted for 35% of all national burn deaths while accounting for 13% of the population [1].

Mobility limitation is prevalent in 44% of elders [2] and by itself has been shown to lead to a loss of independence [3], decreased quality of life [3, 4], institutionalization [5], and mortality [6, 7]. While general age-related declines in mobility are multifactorial, they tend to funnel down into a common pathway for the risk for burn injury. Patients with limitations in mobility have difficulty evacuating themselves from a burning structure. Confinement to a wheel chair is problematic, as the difficulties of navigating a chair during an emergency require both upper body strength and a structure that is chair-compatible. Additionally, limitations in mobility make it difficult for elders to quickly remove an article of clothing which has ignited. Finally, difficulties with mobility and balance put patients at risk for a ground level fall during their reaction to the event which can lead to hip fractures or head injuries both of which complicate their prognosis..

Cognitive impairment with or without dementia is a very common comorbidity as it is seen in 3.4 million [8] and 5.4 million [9] Americans age 71 years or older, respectively. Cognitive impairment can also be iatrogenic since aging entails developing increasing numbers of chronic illnesses. Americans today are living longer with these comorbidities, and most of them are treated pharmacologically with regimens that each come with their own risk profile. Elders are known to commonly have adverse reactions due to differences in pharmacokinetics, and are at risk for poorly coordinated or duplicated care due to visiting multiple prescribers and pharmacies [10, 11]. These drug regimens can lead to episodes of hypotension, drowsiness, and impaired judgement. Alcohol and illicit drug use in the elderly is prevalent, and can by itself or in conjunction with prescribed medications exacerbate cognitive impairment [12]. Regardless of the etiology of impaired mental function, these conditions all put an elder at risk for burn injury due to their effect on the elder's ability to recognize behavior as dangerous, that hazards are present, or that certain solutions are logical or not. Additionally, a confused patient may have difficulty recognizing the severity of a given injury leading to a delay in seeking necessary medical attention.

While home oxygen therapy is common among the elderly, the proportion of those who continue to actively smoke is rarely commented upon in the literature. In the few studies that could be located which specifically addressed this issue, the proportions seen ranged from 20% [13] to 38% in the Nocturnal Oxygen Therapy Trial [14], and 43% in the British Medical Council's trial of home oxygen in COPD [15]. The risks entailed with this practice are clear, but the strength of addiction makes curtailing this activity difficult.

Age-related diminishing of sensory is a risk factor for burn injury. A decrease in auditory acuity results in an inability to hear smoke alarms, just as a loss of visual acuity increases the likelihood of not being able to see cues to the presence of a fire hazard or subtle signs of flames or smoke. Olfactory losses can make the detection of smoke or natural gas difficult. Finally, diminished sensation is a common

H. B. Cunningham · H. A. Phelan (✉)
Division of Burn, Trauma, and Critical Care, Department of Surgery, University of Texas Southwestern Medical Center, Dallas, TX, USA
e-mail: holly.cunningham@utsouthwestern.edu; herb.phelan@utsouthwestern.edu

K. S. Romanowski
Department of Surgery, University of Iowa Health Care, Iowa City, IA, USA
e-mail: kathleen-romanowski@uiowa.edu

M. G. Jeschke et al. (eds.), *Handbook of Burns Volume 1*, https://doi.org/10.1007/978-3-030-18940-2_30

finding in the elderly which can cause them to place their feet too close to heat sources or to have difficulty assessing water temperature [1].

Fixed incomes have been shown to be a risk factor for burn injury. According to the Social Security Administration's 2016 data, 21% of married Social Security Recipients and 43% of single recipients rely on Social Security for 90% of their gross monthly income [16]. Nine percent of the elderly live below the poverty line, with many more living close to it [17]. Living on a fixed income often lends itself to living in housing that is substandard with electrical and mechanical systems that are outdated or under-maintained. When central heating is absent or not dependable, the elderly will often turn to such heating sources as space heaters, fireplaces, and cooking ovens. Further, these environments may not have fire safety as a priority. A 2008 survey of homebound urban elders found that 37% had no functional smoke alarms, 82% had no access to a fire extinguisher, and 46% had hot tap water that exceeded 120 °F [18]. This association with fixed incomes is also reflected in racial and gender differences in fire-related mortality as African-American females age 85 years and older have an 11-fold increase in the relative risk of dying in a fire than the general population [1], and males 19-fold higher [1].

It is human nature to try to retain independence for as long as is possible, and for seniors maintaining independence is a significant feature of quality of life [19]. With functional adaptations, many caregivers are able to assist elders in safely staying in their own home. However, for a significant proportion despite warning signs such as escalating medical needs, caregiver strain, or concerns about safety, the stigma associated with skilled nursing facilities causes them to procrastinate on the decision to move their care to a less independent environment. Compounding this risk is the fact that as spouses die, many elders are left to live alone. In total, 28%, or 12.1 million, of non-institutionalized seniors live alone [20].

30.2 Burn Injury Prevention for the Elderly

Fire safety and burn prevention programs have historically been geared towards children and the general population [21]. This general lack of awareness regarding the importance of educating seniors is reflected in the fact that adults age 60 years and older are the least targeted demographic for burn prevention and fire safety [22]. Indeed, a 2008 survey of New York and New Jersey seniors revealed that less than 20% reported receiving fire safety within 5 years [23]. Additionally, when asked to rank where fire safety and burn prevention ranked in the order of 13 common health topics they discussed with their PCP, seniors reported fire safety and burn prevention to be last [23]. While there is a small body of literature assessing the effect of an educational program in the elderly which demonstrate an increase in seniors' burn prevention knowledge [24–28], all have a follow up.

Residential fire deaths due to unextinguished cigarettes have been addressed via an engineering solution in which a design standard has now been approved which requires that cigarettes self-extinguish when not actively being smoked. This has been accomplished by the placement of two to three thin bands of less-porous paper in the cigarette which causes an extinguish rate of 75% over 40 average cigarettes. In 2010, Wyoming became the 50th state to pass legislation requiring the use of the fire-safe cigarette design at the local point of sale. A subsequent study found that passage of the law was associated with a 19% reduction in overall residential fire mortality rates with a protective effect seen for every age, sex, race, and ethnicity strata that was analyzed [29].

Other burn injury preventions that lack evidence but which are safe, inexpensive, and possibly efficacious are to be recommended. For seniors with impaired cognition who insist on attempting to continue cooking, the use of a timer in the kitchen to remind them to turn off the stove or burners is an option. For those for whom cooking is no longer deemed to be safe by their caregiver, removal of the knobs from the stove is a solution. Special smoke alarms have been created for the hard of hearing. When activated these devices will flash, emit low-frequency audible alarms, and have bed-shaker attachments. The use of adaptive safety equipment such as bathtub stools and rails can help mitigate scald risk. Primary care physicians (PCPs) can potentially play a central role in burn prevention as these are the medical professionals with whom the elderly have the most frequent contact. Routine screening and counselling to assess fire risk and mitigation at office visits is to be recommended.

30.3 Resuscitation

Due to a lack of geriatric-specific evidence-based guidelines, resuscitation of the geriatric burn patient is treated the same as any other adult burn resuscitation. The ABA State of Science meeting identified this as an opportunity for improvement and tasked the research community with defining the special needs of the elderly population and determining the optimal instruments for measuring efficacy of resuscitation in this group [30].

The concept that geriatric burn patients may require special resuscitation is not novel. A 2009 article by Benicke et al. sought to alter the widely used Baxter-Parkland resuscitation formula in hopes of better suiting individual patient requirements. The new formula was created with the addition of several variables including inhalation injury (IHI) and high blood alcohol level (BAL), as well as a compensating factor for advanced age [31]. This formula was found to have a superior predictive value for the true volume of resuscitation fluids administered to patients; however, the study did not look at clinical outcomes, and the impact of age on actual resuscitation requirements remains unknown.

The discussion surrounding optimal monitoring techniques is not unique to geriatric burns. Monitoring circulatory shock and hemodynamics has also been a topic of interest for the Task Force of the European Society of Intensive Care Medicine. The group constructed a list of consensus guidelines, which argue against the requirement of hypotension for a diagnosis of shock and instead emphasize the importance of perfusion markers such as lactate, mixed venous oxygen saturation, and central venous oxygen saturation. The group recommended against the use of a single variable for the management of shock as best practice. In terms of measuring response to therapy, the best practice recommendation was to use more than one hemodynamic variable. Routine measurements of cardiac output for patients responding to therapy were not recommended [32]. A paper published in Burns in 2016 reviewed the literature on critical care in burns. With respect to hemodynamic monitoring, the concept of permissive hypotension and the importance of using multiple dynamic variables were highlighted [33].

30.4 Nutrition

There is a paucity of literature on the topic of nutritional support in the geriatric burn population. In fact, the lack of progress in this area was recently highlighted at an American Burn Association (ABA) State of Science meeting where developing a nutrition protocol for elderly patients was addressed [30]. Until more targeted studies are performed on this topic, we must apply existing knowledge of burn nutrition to geriatric burn patients, albeit with caution.

The physiological response to burn injury and the natural changes in nutritional status among the elderly have been extensively studied. Interestingly, some degree of protein-energy malnutrition is present in greater than 50% of older burn victims at admission, which results in increased morbidity and mortality [34]. Nutritional deficiencies can exacerbate the complications of burn injury including muscle catabolism, delayed wound healing, and infection.

30.4.1 Glucose Control

Elderly patients often suffer from multiple comorbidities, including diabetes. While glycemic control has been greatly studied in the critical care population, ideal glucose range recommendations for burn patients have yet to be established. For now, the European Society for Clinical Nutrition and Metabolism has endorsed recommendations for nutrition in major burns to support moderate glucose control [35]. This is to avoid the complication of hypoglycemia seen with intensive glucose control for which geriatric burn patients are at increased risk given their elevated nutritional requirements and comorbid diseases.

30.4.2 Glutamine

Classified among the immunomodulating agents, glutamine has been looked at for potential benefit in the hypermetabolic population of burn patients. A 2013 meta-analysis of four randomized controlled trials comparing glutamine supplementation and non-supplementation in 155 total adult burn patients showed a significant decrease in hospital mortality and gram-negative bacteremia [36]. There was no difference found with regard to wound infection or length of stay.

30.4.3 Trace Elements

The catabolic response to burn injury known to occur in younger cohorts is also seen in the elderly at a comparable rate; however, the possibility of preexisting malnutrition or lean mass deficits may complicate the picture and require more aggressive nutritional support [34]. The administration of trace elements (Cu, Se, Zn) is often a consideration. This is especially highlighted as these elements have been found to be acutely depleted post-severe burn injury. A recent systematic review and meta-analysis on this topic in burn patients revealed that a parenterally administered combination of trace elements decreased the rate of infectious complications [37].

30.4.4 Oxandrolone

As men and women age, they undergo a decline in skeletal muscle mass and strength due to a number of likely contributing factors, including malnutrition. Muscle catabolism is a known physiological response to severe burn injury and can be of special concern in the elderly population. Oxandrolone, an anabolic steroid, has been shown to induce muscle anabolism in children [38] and older men and women [39] and may be used to combat this catabolic response.

30.4.5 Enteral Versus Parenteral Feeding

Enteral feeding is considered the preferred method for all patients when available due to the widely accepted advantage of maintaining gut mucosal integrity. The decision for parenteral versus enteral nutritional support should be based on an individual patient's clinical picture. There is discussion in the literature of combined enteral and parenteral therapy as a means to provide adequate nutrition, considering that one of the disadvantages of enteral feeding is the sometimes frequent interruption of its administration due to surgical intervention or intolerance [40]. Again, this should be placed in the context of a patient's clinical history, course, and goals of care. There are no guidelines directed towards the feeding technique for nutritional support in the elderly burn population.

30.5 Delirium

The most recent edition of the Diagnosis and Statistical Manual of Mental Disorders (DSM-5) was published in 2013 with revisions to the criteria for delirium which is now defined as [41] a disturbance in attention and awareness, developing over a short period of time, representing a change from baseline and tending to fluctuate in severity during the course of a day. The condition may include an additional disturbance in cognition, and these changes cannot be explained by a preexisting neurocognitive disorder. There must be evidence that the disturbance is a direct physiological consequence of another medical condition, substance intoxication or withdrawal, exposure to a toxin, or multiple etiologies.

Delirium is a topic which, in general, has received much attention due to its association with poor clinical outcomes in diverse settings. The relevance of this diagnosis in elderly burn patients seems obvious; however, there has been very little work to identify and define the risk factors, optimal treatments, and outcomes in this particular population.

A 2017 study published in the Journal of Burn Care and Research aimed to address these points in 385 severely burned patients ranging in age from 18 to 65 years who underwent early escharotomy. The primary outcome was postoperative delirium (POD) as measured by the Confusion Assessment Method (CAM). The incidence of POD was 14.6% with 85.7% of those cases occurring within 24 h after surgery. Significant risk factors for developing POD included age greater than 50 years, history of alcohol consumption, preexisting pulmonary and cardiovascular diseases, larger total burn surface areas (TBSAs), intraoperative hypotension, and longer surgeries (>180 min), among others. More interesting perhaps were the findings of outcome differences between the POD and non-POD groups. The POD group exhibited increased rates of complications such as hepatic and renal impairment as well as increased lengths of stay and higher mortality rates [42].

It is important to note that patients older than 65 and those with preoperative diagnoses of cognitive dysfunction were excluded from the study described above. The incidence of delirium among these excluded patients is likely much higher and carries clinical implications. This significance was elucidated in a 2016 study of patients 65 years and older who were hospitalized for burn injury. In this population, a preexisting diagnosis of dementia was associated with a one in five chance of developing delirium or a urinary tract infection during a patient's hospitalization [43].

The development of delirium is likely multifactorial; however, medications certainly play a part. Some investigators have examined the role of postoperative pain treatment in the prevention of delirium. Lynch et al. discovered in a prospective, observational study of noncardiac surgical patients, ages 50 and up, a significant relationship between postoperative pain and the development of delirium such that patients with higher pain scores were at greatly increased risk of delirium [44]. This association persisted after controlling for other preoperative risk factors including baseline cognitive status. This study did not find significance when looking at method of analgesia, type of opioid, or cumulative opioid dose, leaving physicians to individualize pain regimens based on the clinical picture and the risks and benefits of therapy options. Adverse outcomes in mechanically ventilated patients have also been described [45], and there is literature which encourages the use of formal evaluation methods to identify delirium in these patients, and suggests changes in sedation protocols in an effort to promote better outcomes in these patients [46].

30.6 Wound Healing in the Elderly

Aging alters skin physiology and biology as well as slows the healing process [47, 48]. Due to these changes, burns which would be less severe in younger patients can have a devastating effect on the elderly patient. Aging affects all layers and components of the skin [49]. As skin ages, the epithelium in general becomes thinner, but there is also thickening of the epidermis due to sun exposure [50]. Overall the net effect is a thinning of the skin. Thinner skin means that burns which would be partial thickness in younger patients have a higher likelihood of presenting as or evolving into full thickness burns. Additionally, with aging of the skin, the junction between the epidermis and dermis flattens, reducing the size of the rete pegs. This ultimately leads to an increased risk of shearing of the skin, causing blisters of the epidermis to form. In the subdermal tissue, aging manifests as a decreased capability for angiogenesis leading to delayed revascularization [51, 52]. When revascularization does occur, the new vessels tend to have a greater tendency to leak. Both of these factors lead to impaired lymphatic drainage, predisposing the skin to increased edema, which further impairs wound healing.

For the burn victim, the most deleterious age-related skin change is the reduction in the number of skin adnexa: hair follicles, oil glands, sebaceous glands, and other adnexa [53]. It is well established that partial-thickness wounds re-epithelize from both the epithelial edge of the wound and the skin adnexa [54]. The keratinocytes in the basal layer of the epithelium migrate towards the center of the wound, covering 1–2 cm from the wound edge. Any wound that is larger than this, or is full thickness, or lacks skin appendages attempts to heal by contraction of the wound and ultimately scar formation. In partial-thickness wounds, the hair follicles or other skin adnexa are retained so that the keratinocytes migrate from the remaining adnexa to resurface the wound. The density of the skin adnexa in the wound influences the rate of healing such that skin areas with a higher density of adnexa heal faster. For example, a wound on the scalp will heal within 4–5 days as opposed to a wound on the lower leg which can take 2–3 weeks to heal. The decrease in skin adnexa related to age therefore increases time to healing and increases scar formation. Despite the increased time to healing and the fact that prolonged healing time promotes hypertrophic scarring, it is unclear if the same holds true in the elderly [55]. Skin gets looser as it ages, therefore reducing the risk of tension on the wound which leads to contracture and hypertrophic scar.

The numerous changes that occur to the skin related to aging are well documented; however, the exact effects that these changes have on burn wounds, and how these changes should affect our treatment of these wounds are unclear. Additionally, the ultimate outcomes for elderly burn-injured patients have not been well studied. More work is needed to understand the effects of aging on the production of growth factors, stem cell biology, and the specific biological differences between elderly burn patients and their younger counterparts. It is not clear whether the tenets of early excision and grafting are beneficial in the elderly or if they are better served by waiting. Additionally, it is unknown whether surgery should be done in one stage or across multiple trips to the operating room. We as a burn community need to investigate the wounds of elderly burn patients and their management to determine the best methods of treatment.

30.7 Frailty

Traditionally, the prediction of burn outcomes has been based on patient age and %TBSA burned. Updated prediction models include more variables such as the presence/amount of full-thickness burns, inhalation injury, and gender, but still rely heavily on patient age [56]. Unfortunately, individuals with the same chronologic age vary widely in their health and functional status, making age alone a poor predictor of patient outcomes [57]. Frailty is present in 10–20% of the population over the age of 65, potentially making it a good surrogate outcome measure for elderly patients [58].

30.7.1 Importance of Frailty

Multiple studies have been conducted across a variety of clinical services that have examined frailty and its relationship to outcomes [58–60]. Conroy and Dowsing studied frailty in patients admitted to a medical unit [59]. They found that frailty predicted mortality but did not predict length of stay or readmission. In patients undergoing elective surgery, increased frailty was independently predictive of postoperative complications, increased length of stay, and discharge to a skilled nursing facility [60, 61]. In trauma patients, higher preinjury frailty predicted an unfavorable discharge (skilled nursing facility or death) [62]. In general, frailty has been associated with an increased risk of falls, delirium, cognitive decline, iatrogenic complications, and death [57].

30.7.2 Measurements of Frailty

Frailty has been defined as an age-related vulnerability related to multiple physiologic systems that can coexist with disability and chronic disease or be independent of these conditions [57]. This definition of frailty is generally well accepted; however, the issue of how to measure frailty is still up for debate. There are over 70 tools in existence for measuring frailty, and there is no consensus on which tool is best, as most have been used only within one area of medicine and have not been widely tested across patient populations or against each other to determine if there is one superior test [63].

Frailty tools can range in length from a single item to more than 90 items and can be classified as objective, subjective, or mixed. The simplest objective measures are single-item assessment tools such as gait speed measurements and the timed up-and-go test [64, 65]. These single-item tests have been found to be independently predictive of morbidity and mortality in surgical patients, as well as quick and easy to administer; however, they lack the specificity and sensitivity of full frailty assessments. The most commonly studied objective scales are those created by Brown et al. [66] and Gill et al. [67]. The Modified Physical Performance Test (MPPT) [66] examined 107 community-dwelling elderly adults on nine functional tasks (Table 30.1). Each task is scored on a four-point scale with a higher score indicating a better functional status. No single task identified frailty as well as the MPPT as a whole. Gill et al. [67] tested participants for physical frailty by conducting a rapid gait test over 10 ft (covering the distance in greater than 10 s was considered frail) and a qualitative chair stand test (an inability to stand up from a chair with arms folded indicated frailty). Subjects who were considered frail on only one test were considered moderately frail, while those who failed both tests were frail [68].

Table 30.1 Items in the Modified Physical Performance Test (MPPT)

Lift a 7-lb book to a shelf from waist height
Put on and remove a jacket
Pick up a penny from the floor
Perform a 360-degree turn
50-ft walk test
Climb a flight of stairs
Climb up and down four flights of stairs
Stand up 5 times from a 16-in. chair
Progressive Romberg Test

Table 30.2 Canadian Study on Health and Aging rules-based definition of frailty

Score	Description
0	Walk without help, perform basic activities of daily living, is continent of bowel and bladder, and is not cognitively impaired
1	Bladder incontinence only
2	One (or two if incontinent) of the following: needing assistance with mobility or activities of daily living, has cognitive impairment, or has bowel or bladder incontinence
3	Two (or three if incontinent) of the following: needing assistance with mobility or activities of daily living, has cognitive impairment, or has bowel or bladder incontinence

Table 30.3 Canadian Study on Health and Aging clinical frailty scale

1—Very fit	Robust, active, energetic, well motivated and fit
2—Well	Without active disease, but less fit than people in category 1
3—Well with treated comorbid disease	Disease symptoms are well controlled compared with those in category 4
4—Apparently vulnerable	Although not frankly dependent, these people commonly complain of being "slowed up" or have disease symptoms
5—Mildly frail	With limited dependence on others for instrumental activities of daily living
6—Moderately frail	Help is needed with both instrumental and non-instrumental activities of daily living
7—Severely frail	Completely dependent on others for the activities of daily living, or terminally ill

Table 30.4 Phenotype of frailty scale

Unintentional weight loss
Self-reported exhaustion
Weakness (measured as grip strength)
Slow walking speed
Low physical activity

Each item is scored as 0 or 1. Total score: 0 = not frail; 1–2 = pre-frail; ≥3 = frail

Purely subjective frailty assessments are also available, the majority of which are products of the Canadian Study on Health and Aging (CSHA). The CSHA is a 10-year study of the epidemiology of dementia in Canada that followed patients from 1991 to 2001. The initial study was a 5-year prospective cohort trial that included 9008 people aged 65 and older [69]. While the study was aimed at studying dementia, they also developed a rules-based definition of frailty (Table 30.2). The rules-based definition was able to demonstrate a dose response relationship between frailty, institutionalization, and death. A secondary analysis of 2914 patients who were part of the initial cohort of CSHA participants was conducted. The patients were assessed for frailty using a 20-item frailty index of observed deficits [70]. The CSHA frailty index was found to be a sensitive predictor of survival in this population. On average, study authors found that the elderly without cognitive impairment accumulated functional deficits at a rate of 3% per year. In an effort to simplify the measurement of frailty, the CSHA Clinical Frailty Scale was developed [71]. It is a seven-point clinical opinion scale (Table 30.3) that was validated in the 2305 patients who participated in the second stage of the CSHA. The Clinical Frailty Scale was highly correlated with the previously developed frailty index and like its predecessors was predictive of institutionalization and death.

Many of the frailty scores that have been developed combine subjective and objective measures. The phenotype of frailty by Fried et al. is the most commonly studied scale that uses subjective and objective measures [72]. This scale looks at five variables that are scored as either 0 if absent or 1 if present (Table 30.4). The frail phenotype was independently predictive of falls, worsening mobility, or activities of daily living disability, hospitalization, and death. This scale also demonstrated that frailty is not synonymous with either comorbidity or disability, but comorbidity is a risk factor for, and disability is an outcome of, frailty. Another mixed assessment tool is the Edmonton Frail Scale [73]. This scale looks at a wide range of domains including cognition, general health status, functional independence, social support, medication use, nutrition, mood, continence, and functional performance. The benefit of this scale is the broad domains that it covers, including social support, and its ability to be administered by a non-geriatrician.

Researchers have moved beyond generic frailty indices to create scales that are designed to be used within a specific patient population. The Trauma-Specific Frailty Index (TSFI) is a 15-variable frailty index that looks at the domains of comorbidities, daily activities, health attitudes, and nutrition [62]. The TSFI has been validated in a trauma population and was found to predict unfavorable discharge (death or discharge to a skilled nursing facility). The TSFI was the only significant predictor of poor outcome in its validation study. A similar instrument has recently been created by this same group for emergency general surgery patients [74].

30.7.3 Frailty in Burn Patients

Thus far in burns the only scale that has been used in studies related to frailty and outcomes is the CSHA Clinical Frailty Scale [75–77]. These studies have demonstrated that patients who are frailer have higher mortality rates following burn injury and are more likely to be discharged to a skilled nursing facility. More research is warranted to determine the optimal scale for use in an elderly burn population to predict outcomes and for other decision-making.

30.8 Rehabilitation/Disposition

Long-term outcomes of geriatric burn patients are largely unknown as little data are available in this area. This was also discussed at the ABA State of Science meeting where the tasks of identifying elderly long-term outcomes and creating follow-up with multidisciplinary teams were prioritized [30].

30.8.1 Rehabilitation

Rehabilitation is an important part of many burn patient recoveries. In a study of patients with hand burns, a comprehensive rehabilitation program was superior to routine care in terms of physical function; more surprisingly, however, the rehabilitation arm also performed better on measures of psychological function, social function, and general health [78]. Early physical and occupational therapy, even in ventilated, critically ill patients, has been shown to improve outcomes as well [79].

Despite multidisciplinary data reinforcing the importance and impact of rehabilitation programs on patient outcomes, there is a wide variation in utilization rates of inpatient burn rehabilitation centers between states [80]. These differences persist when controlling for possible confounding factors and should be further investigated with the goal of standardizing the criteria for inpatient rehabilitation referrals.

30.8.2 Disposition

Not surprisingly, older patients often warrant higher levels of care such as skilled nursing after discharge from the hospital even when controlling for inpatient rehabilitation stay [81]. Post-hospital care for geriatric burns must be carefully planned and executed to achieve optimal outcomes. The process can prove to be complex with multiple patient factors, medical and social among others, playing a role. Some researchers are working to predict which patients would benefit from or even require a transitional facility with the goal of decreased hospital length of stay and improved patient satisfaction and outcomes.

The Comorbidity-Polypharmacy Score (CPS) has been identified as an independent predictor of need for transfer to extended care facilities in the older burn population [82]. This is useful because this variable can be measured on admission, and a treatment team may begin the planning process earlier in the patient's hospital course. The frailty score is another topic of interest in predicting outcomes and disposition in elderly trauma and burn patients. It has been found to be increased in those patients discharged to a skilled nursing facility when compared to those discharged to rehabilitation centers or to home [76, 83].

The Baux score is a tool which has been in use by burn physicians since the 1960s to predict prognosis after burn injury and has recently been applied by the Prognostic Assessment of Life and Limitations After Trauma in the Elderly (PALLiATE) Consortium to predict discharge disposition in geriatric burn patients (www.palliateconsortium.com). The authors reviewed data from the National Burn Repository on patients 65 years of age and older. Three discharge outcomes were studied in 8001 subjects, including death, discharge to home, and discharge to a non-home setting. Overall, 42.5% of patients were discharged to home with 13% transferred to a skilled nursing facility and 10% discharged to a rehabilitation center. There was an 18.9% mortality rate, and the remaining patient dispositions (15.6%) were mixed between needing home health services, being lost to follow-up, having left the hospital against medical advice, or having unavailable data. The conclusion after data analysis was that for Baux scores greater than 86, the return-to-home rate drops drastically. Additionally, mortality increases at a score greater than 93, with death almost always seen at a score greater than or equal to 130 [84]. This study's findings naturally lead into a discussion about end-of-life decisions and goals of care with patients and their families; however, this is out of the scope of the current section of text.

Of note, a 2017 study looking at discharge destination in older trauma patients found higher rates of readmission among those patients discharged to extended care facilities or rehabilitation centers, even when controlling for injury severity and comorbidities [85]. The reasons for this have not yet been elucidated.

30.8.3 Reintegration

The transition to reintegration after burn injury can be isolating and supporting resources scarce. In light of these findings, the Aftercare Reintegration Committee was formed to help burn patients, with emphasis on social skills training, peer support, and body image. While this group has ignited discussion at meetings on these topics, not much research into the interventions and implications for outcomes has been generated [86]. Any information from these discussions will likely apply, possibly in a more significant manner, to geriatric burn patients, although we will not know for certain until data are collected and analyzed.

30.9 Long-Term Outcomes for Elderly Burn Patients

There have been many studies that look at the short-term outcomes for elderly burn patients, but there have been few significant studies that look at long-term outcomes in the elderly. As we do not have any data on long-term outcomes, it is not clear if the elderly survive acute hospitalization only to die shortly thereafter. Despite this, there is some evidence that when elderly patients are admitted to a long-term facility, or admitted to a nursing home, they have a very poor long-term outcome and usually die within 2 years [87]. For elderly burn patients, it is currently not clear what long-term outcomes should be expected.

Currently, long-term follow-up for elderly burn patients is conducted primarily by burn surgeons and not by multidisciplinary teams. In the trauma literature, there has been a movement towards creating multidisciplinary teams for the care of the elderly trauma patient. The G-60 trauma unit is a multidisciplinary trauma unit that was developed at the Dallas Medical Center in an effort to improve the care of elderly trauma patients [88]. All patients aged 60 years and older with a traumatic injury were admitted to the G-60 unit under the care of the multidisciplinary G-60 team. The team consisted of a trauma surgeon, a medical hospitalist, a physical medicine and rehabilitation physician, and representatives from PT/OT, respiratory therapy, nursing, social work, nutrition, pharmacy, and palliative care. Patients who were treated in the G-60 unit by the multidisciplinary team had a decreased length of stay from 7 to 4.8 days ($p = 0.0002$) and a decreased ICU length of stay from 5.2 to 3 days. Additionally, there was a statistically significant decrease in urinary tract infections, respiratory failure, congestive heart failure, ventilator-associated pneumonia, and acute renal failure. There was no difference seen in mortality or discharge disposition. We have long utilized multidisciplinary teams in burn care; however, we need to consider the addition of team members when caring for elderly burn patients. Additionally, it seems imperative that long-term follow-up should be conducted by a team that specializes in elderly burn care.

30.10 Outcomes Prediction/Goals of Care/Futility

Outcomes following burn injury have been steadily improving over the last 70 years, and while outcomes for the elderly have also improved, they have not done so to the degree as other age groups [89–91]. This makes the use of accurate outcome prediction scores especially important in the elderly burn patient. Jeschke et al. [92] attempted to find a cutoff age that predicted survivability of a burn injury but were unable to do so. They did, however, identify that the risk of death is linearly related to age and that the LD50 (burn size that is lethal to 50% of patients) decreases from 45% TBSA to 25% TBSA from the age of 55 to 70 years. This increase in mortality occurs despite the implementation of modern protocolized burn care. Since its development in the 1960s, the Baux score has been the traditional model for predicting outcomes among burn-injured patients [93]. This score is made up of the patient's age and their percent TBSA burned, and a total score of more than 75 portended a poor prognosis. It was developed using data sets that were inclusive of all ages and therefore not specific to elderly burn patients. The Baux score was modified in 1979 by excluding patients younger than 20 years old from the analysis, as it was determined that mortality did not increase linearly with age in this group. The resulting model demonstrated that a score of greater than 95 was equivalent to poor prognosis or mortality [94]. Because outcomes in the elderly are not the same as their younger counterparts, there has been an attempt to improve the predictive ability of the Baux score in this population. Hodgman et al. [84] used the Baux score on geriatric patients within the National Burn Repository and found that a score greater than 86 resulted in significantly fewer patients discharging to home. When the score reached 93, there was a significant increase in mortality, and death was virtually unavoidable above a score of 130. Multiple other outcome prediction models have been developed to further refine our ability to predict mortality. In addition to the modified Baux score, the scores that have been used to evaluate outcomes in the elderly are the Abbreviated Burn Severity Index (ABSI) and the score developed by Ryan et al. [95, 96]. The ABSI is calculated as the weighted sum of age, gender, %TBSA, percentage of full thickness, and presence of inhalation injury. Ryan et al. reviewed the charts of 1665 patients and identified three variables available at admission (age, TBSA burn >40%, and inhalation injury) as predictors of mortality. These were incorporated into a simple logistic regression model to objectively predict mortality. Of the scores used in the elderly, the modified Baux score has been shown to be the best predictor of survival in this population. There have been two studies that demonstrated its prognostic value. Wibbenmeyer et al. evaluated the modified Baux score and the ABSI in a cohort of 308 elderly patients and showed that the modified Baux score was superior to the ABSI (area under curve = 0.932 ± 0.02 vs. 0.815 ± 0.03, respectively) [97]. Additionally, the modified Baux score was the superior outcome score when compared with the ABSI and the Ryan et al. score in a retrospective cohort of 265 elderly patients [98].

While care for the burn-injured patient has improved significantly, there are still patients who do not respond well to treatment or have injuries that are determined to be nonsurvivable. In the elderly, it is especially important to consider having goals-of-care discussions early. Few studies have been done looking at when and how goals-of-care discussions are conducted with elderly burn patients. Madni et al. [77] examined factors associated with having goals-of-care discussions and found that in only 25% of cases were goals-of-care conversations documented. They found that a patient appearance of frailty increased the likelihood that a goals-of-care discussion occurred. Another group examined the reasons cited by decision makers for withdrawal of life-extending therapy. They found that these decisions in elderly patients (≥65 years old) were closely tied to underlying comorbidities, while in younger patients the size of the burn was a much more important factor [99]. An international survey of burn care providers assessing their feelings on end-of-life decision-making identified that these providers were more comfortable with withholding care than withdrawing care [100]. In burn patients, treatment limitations accounted for a minority of deaths. The primary reasons that they gave for either withholding or withdrawing care were severity of burn (78%), medical condition/high probability of death (68%), and unresponsiveness to therapy (68%). End-of-life care remains an area in need of both study and education among burn practitioners. In situations where survival is unlikely, we owe it to our patients and their families to have the best information possible to aid them in making care decisions.

30.11 Special Considerations

30.11.1 Specialty Consults

The complex physiologic and sociologic changes associated with advancing age have resulted in a specialty dedicated to studying and providing care for the elderly community. Geriatricians are experts in the management of the special health issues that arise in this age group, and the trauma community has begun to explore whether routine inclusion of these professionals results in better outcomes for their older patients. Olujo et al. initiated mandatory geriatric consults for all admitted trauma patients 70 years of age or older with the goal of examining do-not-resuscitate orders, rates of delirium, referral for cognitive evaluation, and patient outcomes pre- and postintervention. The rate of preintervention geriatric consults was 3.26%. This increased to 100% postintervention and resulted in improved advanced care planning and reduced ICU readmission rates from 8.26 to 1.96% ($p = 0.06$). There were no changes in 30-day hospital readmission, length of stay, or mortality, although the study was underpowered for some of these analyses [101]. Of note, an audit of a burn unit in South Australia found that the appointment of a geriatrician did not significantly reduce length of stay in patients 70 years of age and older; however, the authors asserted that the geriatrician assisted greatly in the placement of their patients, and the authors planned to make the addition permanent [102]. Speech pathology consults are also employed throughout the world, most often for patients who have experienced dysphagia as a sequela of their burn injury [103].

30.11.2 Holistic Therapy

Multimodal therapy regimens have been proposed to help with some of the challenges experienced by burn patients. For example, playing music during dressing changes can be a helpful adjunct to pharmacologic interventions [104, 105]. Additionally, aromatherapy massage and inhalation aromatherapy have been shown to reduce both pain and anxiety in burn patients [106]. Given the potential in elderly patients for polypharmacy and adverse reactions to medications, alternative therapies should be considered as part of a well-rounded treatment plan.

30.11.3 Psychologic Effects

There has been an increased interest in the psychosocial impairments seen in burn patients in the literature. A large, longitudinal, multicenter study using the National Institute on Disability, Independent Living, and Rehabilitation Research Burn Model System database found that Satisfaction With Life Scale scores were significantly lower for burn patients compared with nonburn, healthy controls. This remained true at time intervals of 6, 12, and 24 months after injury and was associated with both medical and psychological variables [107].

Emotional trauma is a recognized phenomenon in the burn patient's experience and recovery, and it is important to address as part of a complete treatment plan. Patients can suffer from pain, anxiety, mental illnesses such as depression and post-traumatic stress disorder (PTSD), and have many stressors related to reintegration into the community surrounding their scars and other factors. A qualitative study conducted in 2016 explored the concept of a "new normal" for burn patients and emphasized the importance of family closeness and empowerment through self-care [108].

Along these lines, it is noteworthy that mental disorders, particularly depression, are significant predictors of levels of functioning after burn injury [109]. This is particularly striking when one study's results revealed that 20.5% of burn patients experience clinically significant PTSD at 6 months post injury. And while the presence of burn injury has not been found to increase the rate of mental health issues, burn patients tend to have higher rates of preexisting illness compared to controls [110].

In order to construct meaningful interventions and positively impact burn patient recovery, health care providers must continue to develop knowledge of the patient experience. A 2017 literature review focused on the postburn growth process and concluded that overall function, quality of life, social support and optimism, and new opportunities each contribute to the growth process after burn injury. The authors noted that each of these areas has potential for therapeutic intervention [111]. Interestingly, we are finding that the interventions with the most impact are not necessarily pharmacologic or medical and that teaching patients healthy, active coping strategies including positive reframing and humor may in fact improve the overall experience for the burn patient [112].

30.11.4 End of Life/Goals of Care

End-of-life conversations and goals-of-care discussions become of increased importance in elderly populations across all specialties. Communication regarding these issues between physicians and patients has become a hot topic of research in recent years. The Study to Understand Prognoses and Preferences for Outcomes and Risks of Treatments (SUPPORT) trial published in 1995 highlighted the shortcomings in care for severely ill adults. This trial found that only 47% of physicians knew when their patients preferred to avoid CPR and that 50% of patients who died while in the hospital were felt by family members to have suffered from severe pain for a large portion. The study's intervention provided physicians with estimates for 6-month survival, outcomes of CPR, and functional disability at 2 months; however, this was found to have no significant impact on patient care measures of communication [113].

Historically, surgeons have been thought to be less equipped to address these issues despite the potential morbidity and mortality inherent to surgical interventions. For this reason, an effort is being made to change the way surgeons interact with their patients during these encounters. One example is through training surgeons to use a framework which shifts the focus of conversation from isolated surgical problems to treatment alternatives and outcomes [114]. In the geriatric trauma population, prognostic indicators such as the Geriatric Trauma Outcome Score (GTOS) and Trauma and Injury Severity Score (TRISS) accurately predict probability of death [115]. Ongoing research projects will explore the utility of using newly developed frameworks along with validated outcome estimators to improve communication in both trauma and burn settings.

The impact of improved communication regarding these difficult issues extends beyond patient satisfaction. There is a recognized potential economic advantage associated with executing this interaction well. The care of burn patients is expensive in general; however, more health care dollars are spent on nonsurvivors than on survivors. Laboratory tests, imaging, nutritional support, renal support, and blood products make up a majority of these costs [116]. The identification of patients who favor comfort care measures over aggressive and life-prolonging interventions could lead to a drastic decrease in expenditures in this area and allow money to be reallocated to those patients with a potential for better outcomes.

Summary Box

Burn outcomes have improved over time for most demographic cohorts, but this cannot be said for thermal injuries in the elderly. This is especially problematic when one considers that seniors represent the fastest growing population in the United States and they possess characteristics which place them at higher risk for porr outcomes such as thinning skin, decreased sensation, mental alterations, pre-existing comorbidities and numerous other contributing factors. Despite these facts, little progress has been made over the last several decades in improving outcomes after thermal injury in the elderly as the LD50 for a burn in an elder has remained relatively constant at 30 to 35% TBSA. This chapter will review the medical and social aspects of burn care unique to seniors

References

1. Fire risk to older adults in 2010. Topical Fire Report Series. Vol. 14. Federal Emergency Management Agency; 2013.
2. Shumway-Cook A, Ciol MA, Yorkston KM, Hoffman JM, Chan L. Mobility limitations in the Medicare population: prevalence and sociodemographic and clinical correlates. J Am Geriatr Soc. 2005;53(7):1217–21. https://doi.org/10.1111/j.1532-5415.2005.53372.x.
3. Rubenstein LZ, Powers CM, MacLean CH. Quality indicators for the management and prevention of falls and mobility problems in vulnerable elders. Ann Intern Med. 2001;135(8 Pt 2):686–93.
4. Netuveli G, Wiggins RD, Hildon Z, Montgomery SM, Blane D. Quality of life at older ages: evidence from the English longitudinal study of aging (wave 1). J Epidemiol Community Health. 2006;60(4):357–63. https://doi.org/10.1136/jech.2005.040071.
5. von Bonsdorff M, Rantanen T, Laukkanen P, Suutama T, Heikkinen E. Mobility limitations and cognitive deficits as predictors of institutionalization among community-dwelling older people. Gerontology. 2006;52(6):359–65. https://doi.org/10.1159/000094985.

6. Hirvensalo M, Rantanen T, Heikkinen E. Mobility difficulties and physical activity as predictors of mortality and loss of independence in the community-living older population. J Am Geriatr Soc. 2000;48(5):493–8.
7. Lyyra TM, Leskinen E, Heikkinen E. A cohort study found good respiratory, sensory and motor functions decreased mortality risk in older people. J Clin Epidemiol. 2005;58(5):509–16. https://doi.org/10.1016/j.jclinepi.2004.08.015.
8. Plassman BL, Langa KM, Fisher GG, Heeringa SG, Weir DR, Ofstedal MB, Burke JR, Hurd MD, Potter GG, Rodgers WL, Steffens DC, Willis RJ, Wallace RB. Prevalence of dementia in the United States: the aging, demographics, and memory study. Neuroepidemiology. 2007;29(1–2):125–32. https://doi.org/10.1159/000109998.
9. Plassman BL, Langa KM, Fisher GG, Heeringa SG, Weir DR, Ofstedal MB, Burke JR, Hurd MD, Potter GG, Rodgers WL, Steffens DC, McArdle JJ, Willis RJ, Wallace RB. Prevalence of cognitive impairment without dementia in the United States. Ann Intern Med. 2008;148(6):427–34.
10. Linjakumpu T, Hartikainen S, Klaukka T, Veijola J, Kivela SL, Isoaho R. Use of medications and polypharmacy are increasing among the elderly. J Clin Epidemiol. 2002;55(8):809–17.
11. Golchin N, Frank SH, Vince A, Isham L, Meropol SB. Polypharmacy in the elderly. J Res Pharm Pract. 2015;4(2):85–8. https://doi.org/10.4103/2279-042X.155755.
12. McGill V, Kowal-Vern A, Gamelli RL. Outcome for older burn patients. Arch Surg. 2000;135(3):320–5.
13. Cornette A, Petitdemange I, Briancon S, Burlet C, Polu JM. [Evaluation of smoking in chronic severe respiratory insufficiency patients treated with long-term oxygen at home]. Rev Mal Respir. 1996;13(4):405–11.
14. McSweeny AJ, Grant I, Heaton RK, Adams KM, Timms RM. Life quality of patients with chronic obstructive pulmonary disease. Arch Intern Med. 1982;142(3):473–8.
15. Long term domiciliary oxygen therapy in chronic hypoxic cor pulmonale complicating chronic bronchitis and emphysema. Report of the Medical Research Council Working Party. Lancet. 1981;1(8222):681–6.
16. Fact Sheet. Social Security Administration; 2017.
17. U.S. Census Bureau, Income, Poverty, and Health Insurance Coverage in the United States: 2011. Current Population Reports; 2012.
18. Ehrlich AR, Bak RY, Wald-Cagan P, Greenberg DF. Risk factors for fires and burns in homebound, urban elderly. J Burn Care Res. 2008;29(6):985–7. https://doi.org/10.1097/BCR.0b013e31818ba1ab.
19. Fried TR, Bradley EH, Towle VR, Allore H. Understanding the treatment preferences of seriously ill patients. N Engl J Med. 2002;346(14):1061–6. https://doi.org/10.1056/NEJMsa012528.
20. A profile of older Americans. Administration on Aging; 2013.
21. Ta VM, Frattaroli S, Bergen G, Gielen AC. Evaluated community fire safety interventions in the United States: a review of current literature. J Community Health. 2006;31(3):176–97.
22. Gielen A, McDonald EM, Piver J. Fire and Life Safety Education in U.S. Fire Departments: Results of a National Survey, Final Report to the Home Safety Council. Johns Hopkins Center for Injury Research and Policy & Johns Hopkins Bloomberg School of Public Health, Baltimore, Maryland; 2007.
23. Leahy NEJL, Smith M. Senior burn safety: opportunities to send the message? J Burn Care Rehabil. 2008;29(2):S44–S169.
24. Tan J, Banez C, Cheung Y, Gomez M, Nguyen H, Banfield J, Medeiros L, Lee R, Cartotto R, Fish JS. Effectiveness of a burn prevention campaign for older adults. J Burn Care Rehabil. 2004;25(5):445–51.
25. Victor J, Lawrence P, Munster A, Horn SD. A statewide targeted burn prevention program. J Burn Care Rehabil. 1988;9(4):425–9.
26. Lehna C, Coty MB, Fahey E, Williams J, Scrivener D, Wishnia G, Myers J. Intervention study for changes in home fire safety knowledge in urban older adults. Burns. 2015;41(6):1205–11. https://doi.org/10.1016/j.burns.2015.02.012.
27. Lehna C, Merrell J, Furmanek S, Twyman S. Home fire safety intervention pilot with urban older adults living in Wales. Burns. 2017;43(1):69–75. https://doi.org/10.1016/j.burns.2016.06.025.
28. Leahy NE, Sessler KA, Baggott K, Laverde L, Rabbitts A, Yurt RW. Engaging older adults in burn prevention education: results of a community-based urban initiative. J Burn Care Res. 2012;33(3):e141–6. https://doi.org/10.1097/BCR.0b013e3182335a14.
29. Yau RK, Marshall SW. Association between fire-safe cigarette legislation and residential fire deaths in the United States. Inj Epidemiol. 2014;1(1):10. https://doi.org/10.1186/2197-1714-1-10.
30. Jeschke MG, Peck MD. Burn care of the elderly. J Burn Care Res. 2017;38(3):e625–8. https://doi.org/10.1097/BCR.0000000000000535.
31. Benicke M, Perbix W, Lefering R, Knam F, Ipaktchi KR, Tannapfel A, Neugebauer EA, Spilker G. New multifactorial burn resuscitation formula offers superior predictive reliability in comparison to established algorithms. Burns. 2009;35(1):30–5. https://doi.org/10.1016/j.burns.2008.06.006.
32. Cecconi M, De Backer D, Antonelli M, Beale R, Bakker J, Hofer C, Jaeschke R, Mebazaa A, Pinsky MR, Teboul JL, Vincent JL, Rhodes A. Consensus on circulatory shock and hemodynamic monitoring. Task force of the European Society of Intensive Care Medicine. Intensive Care Med. 2014;40(12):1795–815. https://doi.org/10.1007/s00134-014-3525-z.
33. Lavrentieva A. Critical care of burn patients. New approaches to old problems. Burns. 2016;42(1):13–9. https://doi.org/10.1016/j.burns.2015.04.009.
34. Porro LJ, Demling RH, Pereira CT, Herndon DN. Care of geriatric patients. 2012;415–9.e412. https://doi.org/10.1016/b978-1-4377-2786-9.00036-9.
35. Rousseau AF, Losser MR, Ichai C, Berger MM. ESPEN endorsed recommendations: nutritional therapy in major burns. Clin Nutr. 2013;32(4):497–502. https://doi.org/10.1016/j.clnu.2013.02.012.
36. Lin JJ, Chung XJ, Yang CY, Lau HL. A meta-analysis of trials using the intention to treat principle for glutamine supplementation in critically ill patients with burn. Burns. 2013;39(4):565–70. https://doi.org/10.1016/j.burns.2012.11.008.
37. Kurmis R, Greenwood J, Aromataris E. Trace element supplementation following severe burn injury: a systematic review and meta-analysis. J Burn Care Res. 2016;37(3):143–59. https://doi.org/10.1097/BCR.0000000000000259.
38. Hart DW, Wolf SE, Ramzy PI, Chinkes DL, Beauford RB, Ferrando AA, Wolfe RR, Herndon DN. Anabolic effects of oxandrolone after severe burn. Ann Surg. 2001;233(4):556–64.
39. Sheffield-Moore M, Paddon-Jones D, Casperson SL, Gilkison C, Volpi E, Wolf SE, Jiang J, Rosenblatt JI, Urban RJ. Androgen therapy induces muscle protein anabolism in older women. J Clin Endocrinol Metab. 2006;91(10):3844–9. https://doi.org/10.1210/jc.2006-0588.
40. Prelack K, Dylewski M, Sheridan RL. Practical guidelines for nutritional management of burn injury and recovery. Burns. 2007;33(1):14–24. https://doi.org/10.1016/j.burns.2006.06.014.
41. European Delirium Association, American Delirium Society. The DSM-5 criteria, level of arousal and delirium diagnosis: inclusiveness is safer. BMC Med. 2014;12:141. https://doi.org/10.1186/s12916-014-0141-2.
42. Guo Z, Liu J, Li J, Wang X, Guo H, Ma P, Su X, Li P. Postoperative delirium in severely burned patients undergoing early escharotomy: incidence, risk factors, and outcomes.

J Burn Care Res. 2017;38(1):e370–6. https://doi.org/10.1097/BCR.0000000000000397.
43. Harvey L, Mitchell R, Brodaty H, Draper B, Close J. Dementia: a risk factor for burns in the elderly. Burns. 2016;42(2):282–90. https://doi.org/10.1016/j.burns.2015.10.023.
44. Lynch EP, Lazor MA, Gellis JE, Orav J, Goldman L, Marcantonio ER. The impact of postoperative pain on the development of postoperative delirium. Anesth Analg. 1998;86(4):781–5.
45. Mehta S, Cook D, Devlin JW, Skrobik Y, Meade M, Fergusson D, Herridge M, Steinberg M, Granton J, Ferguson N, Tanios M, Dodek P, Fowler R, Burns K, Jacka M, Olafson K, Mallick R, Reynolds S, Keenan S, Burry L, SLEAP Investigators, Canadian Critical Care Trials Group. Prevalence, risk factors, and outcomes of delirium in mechanically ventilated adults. Crit Care Med. 2015;43(3):557–66. https://doi.org/10.1097/CCM.0000000000000727.
46. Riker RR, Fraser GL. Altering intensive care sedation paradigms to improve patient outcomes. Crit Care Clin. 2009;25(3):527–38., , viii–ix. https://doi.org/10.1016/j.ccc.2009.05.004.
47. Gerstein AD, Phillips TJ, Rogers GS, Gilchrest BA. Wound healing and aging. Dermatol Clin. 1993;11(4):749–57.
48. Jeschke MG, Patsouris D, Stanojcic M, Abdullahi A, Rehou S, Pinto R, Chen P, Burnett M, Amini-Nik S. Pathophysiologic response to burns in the elderly. EBioMedicine. 2015;2(10):1536–48. https://doi.org/10.1016/j.ebiom.2015.07.040.
49. Gosain A, DiPietro LA. Aging and wound healing. World J Surg. 2004;28(3):321–6. https://doi.org/10.1007/s00268-003-7397-6.
50. Wulf HC, Sandby-Moller J, Kobayasi T, Gniadecki R. Skin aging and natural photoprotection. Micron. 2004;35(3):185–91. https://doi.org/10.1016/j.micron.2003.11.005.
51. Sharma R. Skin age testing criteria: characterization of human skin structures by 500 MHz MRI multiple contrast and image processing. Phys Med Biol. 2010;55(14):3959–79. https://doi.org/10.1088/0031-9155/55/14/002.
52. Zouboulis CC, Makrantonaki E. Clinical aspects and molecular diagnostics of skin aging. Clin Dermatol. 2011;29(1):3–14. https://doi.org/10.1016/j.clindermatol.2010.07.001.
53. Birch MP, Messenger JF, Messenger AG. Hair density, hair diameter and the prevalence of female pattern hair loss. Br J Dermatol. 2001;144(2):297–304.
54. Greenhalgh DG. Wound healing. In: Herndon DN, editor. Total burn care. 3rd ed. Philadelphia: Elsevier Saunders; 2007. p. 578–95.
55. Deitch EA, Wheelahan TM, Rose MP, Clothier J, Cotter J. Hypertrophic burn scars: analysis of variables. J Trauma. 1983;23(10):895–8.
56. Hussain A, Choukairi F, Dunn K. Predicting survival in thermal injury: a systematic review of methodology of composite prediction models. Burns. 2013;39(5):835–50. https://doi.org/10.1016/j.burns.2012.12.010.
57. Robinson TN, Walston JD, Brummel NE, Deiner S, Brown CH, Kennedy M, Hurria A. Frailty for surgeons: review of a National Institute on Aging Conference on Frailty for Specialists. J Am Coll Surg. 2015;221(6):1083–92. https://doi.org/10.1016/j.jamcollsurg.2015.08.428.
58. McDonald VS, Thompson KA, Lewis PR, Sise CB, Sise MJ, Shackford SR. Frailty in trauma: a systematic review of the surgical literature for clinical assessment tools. J Trauma Acute Care Surg. 2016;80(5):824–34. https://doi.org/10.1097/TA.0000000000000981.
59. Conroy S, Dowsing T. The ability of frailty to predict outcomes in older people attending an acute medical unit. Acute Med. 2013;12(2):74–6.
60. Dasgupta M, Rolfson DB, Stolee P, Borrie MJ, Speechley M. Frailty is associated with postoperative complications in older adults with medical problems. Arch Gerontol Geriatr. 2009;48(1):78–83. https://doi.org/10.1016/j.archger.2007.10.007.
61. Makary MA, Segev DL, Pronovost PJ, Syin D, Bandeen-Roche K, Patel P, Takenaga R, Devgan L, Holzmueller CG, Tian J, Fried LP. Frailty as a predictor of surgical outcomes in older patients. J Am Coll Surg. 2010;210(6):901–8. https://doi.org/10.1016/j.jamcollsurg.2010.01.028.
62. Joseph B, Pandit V, Zangbar B, Kulvatunyou N, Tang A, O'Keeffe T, Green DJ, Vercruysse G, Fain MJ, Friese RS, Rhee P. Validating trauma-specific frailty index for geriatric trauma patients: a prospective analysis. J Am Coll Surg. 2014;219(1):10–17.e11. https://doi.org/10.1016/j.jamcollsurg.2014.03.020.
63. Rodriguez-Manas L, Feart C, Mann G, Vina J, Chatterji S, Chodzko-Zajko W, Gonzalez-Colaco Harmand M, Bergman H, Carcaillon L, Nicholson C, Scuteri A, Sinclair A, Pelaez M, Van der Cammen T, Beland F, Bickenbach J, Delamarche P, Ferrucci L, Fried LP, Gutierrez-Robledo LM, Rockwood K, Rodriguez Artalejo F, Serviddio G, Vega E, FOD-CC Group. Searching for an operational definition of frailty: a Delphi method based consensus statement: the frailty operative definition-consensus conference project. J Gerontol A Biol Sci Med Sci. 2013;68(1):62–7. https://doi.org/10.1093/gerona/gls119.
64. Abellan van Kan G, Rolland Y, Bergman H, Morley JE, Kritchevsky SB, Vellas B. The I.A.N.A Task Force on frailty assessment of older people in clinical practice. J Nutr Health Aging. 2008;12(1):29–37.
65. Savva GM, Donoghue OA, Horgan F, O'Regan C, Cronin H, Kenny RA. Using timed up-and-go to identify frail members of the older population. J Gerontol A Biol Sci Med Sci. 2013;68(4):441–6. https://doi.org/10.1093/gerona/gls190.
66. Brown M, Sinacore DR, Binder EF, Kohrt WM. Physical and performance measures for the identification of mild to moderate frailty. J Gerontol A Biol Sci Med Sci. 2000;55(6):M350–5.
67. Gill TM, Baker DI, Gottschalk M, Peduzzi PN, Allore H, Byers A. A program to prevent functional decline in physically frail, elderly persons who live at home. N Engl J Med. 2002;347(14):1068–74. https://doi.org/10.1056/NEJMoa020423.
68. Gill TM, Richardson ED, Tinetti ME. Evaluating the risk of dependence in activities of daily living among community-living older adults with mild to moderate cognitive impairment. J Gerontol A Biol Sci Med Sci. 1995;50(5):M235–41.
69. Rockwood K, Stadnyk K, MacKnight C, McDowell I, Hebert R, Hogan DB. A brief clinical instrument to classify frailty in elderly people. Lancet. 1999;353(9148):205–6. https://doi.org/10.1016/S0140-6736(98)04402-X.
70. Mitnitski AB, Graham JE, Mogilner AJ, Rockwood K. Frailty, fitness and late-life mortality in relation to chronological and biological age. BMC Geriatr. 2002;2:1.
71. Rockwood K, Song X, MacKnight C, Bergman H, Hogan DB, McDowell I, Mitnitski A. A global clinical measure of fitness and frailty in elderly people. CMAJ. 2005;173(5):489–95. https://doi.org/10.1503/cmaj.050051.
72. Fried LP, Tangen CM, Walston J, Newman AB, Hirsch C, Gottdiener J, Seeman T, Tracy R, Kop WJ, Burke G, McBurnie MA, Cardiovascular Health Study Collaborative Research Group. Frailty in older adults: evidence for a phenotype. J Gerontol A Biol Sci Med Sci. 2001;56(3):M146–56.
73. Rolfson DB, Majumdar SR, Tsuyuki RT, Tahir A, Rockwood K. Validity and reliability of the Edmonton Frail Scale. Age Ageing. 2006;35(5):526–9. https://doi.org/10.1093/ageing/afl041.
74. Orouji Jokar T, Ibraheem K, Rhee P, Kulavatunyou N, Haider A, Phelan HA, Fain M, Mohler MJ, Joseph B. Emergency general surgery specific frailty index: a validation study. J Trauma Acute Care Surg. 2016;81(2):254–60. https://doi.org/10.1097/TA.0000000000001120.
75. Masud D, Norton S, Smailes S, Shelley O, Philp B, Dziewulski P. The use of a frailty scoring system for burns in the elderly. Burns. 2013;39(1):30–6. https://doi.org/10.1016/j.burns.2012.03.002.

76. Romanowski KS, Barsun A, Pamlieri TL, Greenhalgh DG, Sen S. Frailty score on admission predicts outcomes in elderly burn injury. J Burn Care Res. 2015;36(1):1–6. https://doi.org/10.1097/BCR.0000000000000190.
77. Madni TD, Nakonezny PA, Wolf SE, Joseph B, Mohler MJ, Imran JB, Clark A, Arnoldo BA, Phelan HA. The relationship between frailty and the subjective decision to conduct a goals of care discussion with burned elders. J Burn Care Res. 2018;39(1):82–8. https://doi.org/10.1097/BCR.0000000000000594.
78. Li L, Dai JX, Xu L, Huang ZX, Pan Q, Zhang X, Jiang MY, Chen ZH. The effect of a rehabilitation nursing intervention model on improving the comprehensive health status of patients with hand burns. Burns. 2017;43(4):877–85. https://doi.org/10.1016/j.burns.2016.11.003.
79. Schweickert WD, Pohlman MC, Pohlman AS, Nigos C, Pawlik AJ, Esbrook CL, Spears L, Miller M, Franczyk M, Deprizio D, Schmidt GA, Bowman A, Barr R, McCallister KE, Hall JB, Kress JP. Early physical and occupational therapy in mechanically ventilated, critically ill patients: a randomised controlled trial. Lancet. 2009;373(9678):1874–82. https://doi.org/10.1016/S0140-6736(09)60658-9.
80. Greene NH, Pham TN, Esselman PC, Rivara FP. Variation in inpatient rehabilitation utilization after hospitalization for burn injury in the United States. J Burn Care Res. 2015;36(6):613–8. https://doi.org/10.1097/BCR.0000000000000200.
81. Pham TN, Carrougher GJ, Martinez E, Lezotte D, Rietschel C, Holavanahalli R, Kowalske K, Esselman PC. Predictors of discharge disposition in older adults with burns: a study of the burn model systems. J Burn Care Res. 2015;36(6):607–12. https://doi.org/10.1097/BCR.0000000000000216.
82. Justiniano CF, Coffey RA, Evans DC, Jones LM, Jones CD, Bailey JK, Miller SF, Stawicki SP. Comorbidity-polypharmacy score predicts in-hospital complications and the need for discharge to extended care facility in older burn patients. J Burn Care Res. 2015;36(1):193–6. https://doi.org/10.1097/BCR.0000000000000094.
83. Joseph B, Pandit V, Rhee P, Aziz H, Sadoun M, Wynne J, Tang A, Kulvatunyou N, O'Keeffe T, Fain MJ, Friese RS. Predicting hospital discharge disposition in geriatric trauma patients: is frailty the answer? J Trauma Acute Care Surg. 2014;76(1):196–200. https://doi.org/10.1097/TA.0b013e3182a833ac.
84. Hodgman EI, Joseph B, Mohler J, Wolf SE, Paulk ME, Rhodes RL, Nakonezny PA, Phelan HA. Creation of a decision aid for goal setting after geriatric burns: a study from the prognostic assessment of life and limitations after trauma in the elderly [PALLIATE] consortium. J Trauma Acute Care Surg. 2016;81(1):168–72. https://doi.org/10.1097/TA.0000000000000998.
85. Strosberg DS, Housley BC, Vazquez D, Rushing A, Steinberg S, Jones C. Discharge destination and readmission rates in older trauma patients. J Surg Res. 2017;207:27–32. https://doi.org/10.1016/j.jss.2016.07.015.
86. Holavanahalli RK, Badger K, Acton A. Community reintegration. J Burn Care Res. 2017;38(3):e632–4. https://doi.org/10.1097/BCR.0000000000000563.
87. Palmieri TL, Molitor F, Chan G, Phelan E, Shier BJ, Sen S, Greenhalgh DG. Long-term functional outcomes in the elderly after burn injury. J Burn Care Res. 2012;33(4):497–503. https://doi.org/10.1097/BCR.0b013e31825aeaac.
88. Mangram AJ, Mitchell CD, Shifflette VK, Lorenzo M, Truitt MS, Goel A, Lyons MA, Nichols DJ, Dunn EL. Geriatric trauma service: a one-year experience. J Trauma Acute Care Surg. 2012;72(1):119–22. https://doi.org/10.1097/TA.0b013e318241f0ba.
89. Wearn C, Hardwicke J, Kitsios A, Siddons V, Nightingale P, Moiemen N. Outcomes of burns in the elderly: revised estimates from the Birmingham Burn Centre. Burns. 2015;41(6):1161–8. https://doi.org/10.1016/j.burns.2015.04.008.
90. McGwin G Jr, Cross JM, Ford JW, Rue LW 3rd. Long-term trends in mortality according to age among adult burn patients. J Burn Care Rehabil. 2003;24(1):21–5. https://doi.org/10.1097/01.BCR.0000045649.18004.F1.
91. Forjuoh SN, Smith GS. Case-fatality rates by body part affected and trends in hospitalized burns in Maryland, 1981-90. Burns. 1993;19(5):387–91.
92. Jeschke MG, Pinto R, Costford SR, Amini-Nik S. Threshold age and burn size associated with poor outcomes in the elderly after burn injury. Burns. 2016;42(2):276–81. https://doi.org/10.1016/j.burns.2015.12.008.
93. Baux S. Contribution a l'Etude du traitement local des brulures thermigues etendues. Paris: These; 1961.
94. Stern M, Waisbren BA. Comparison of methods of predicting burn mortality. Scand J Plast Reconstr Surg. 1979;13(1):201–4.
95. Tobiasen J, Hiebert JM, Edlich RF. The abbreviated burn severity index. Ann Emerg Med. 1982;11(5):260–2.
96. Ryan CM, Schoenfeld DA, Thorpe WP, Sheridan RL, Cassem EH, Tompkins RG. Objective estimates of the probability of death from burn injuries. N Engl J Med. 1998;338(6):362–6. https://doi.org/10.1056/NEJM199802053380604.
97. Wibbenmeyer LA, Amelon MJ, Morgan LJ, Robinson BK, Chang PX, Lewis R 2nd, Kealey GP. Predicting survival in an elderly burn patient population. Burns. 2001;27(6):583–90.
98. Lumenta DB, Hautier A, Desouches C, Gouvernet J, Giorgi R, Manelli JC, Magalon G. Mortality and morbidity among elderly people with burns—evaluation of data on admission. Burns. 2008;34(7):965–74. https://doi.org/10.1016/j.burns.2007.12.004.
99. Ismail A, Long J, Moiemen N, Wilson Y. End of life decisions and care of the adult burn patient. Burns. 2011;37(2):288–93. https://doi.org/10.1016/j.burns.2010.08.009.
100. Metaxa V, Lavrentieva A. End-of-life decisions in Burn Intensive Care Units—an International Survey. Burns. 2015;41(1):53–7. https://doi.org/10.1016/j.burns.2014.05.018.
101. Olufajo OA, Tulebaev S, Javedan H, Gates J, Wang J, Duarte M, Kelly E, Lilley E, Salim A, Cooper Z. Integrating geriatric consults into routine care of older trauma patients: one-year experience of a level I trauma center. J Am Coll Surg. 2016;222(6):1029–35. https://doi.org/10.1016/j.jamcollsurg.2015.12.058.
102. Solanki NS, Greenwood JE, Wagstaff MJ, Franchi BF. Length of stay of elderly patients in an acute burns unit: has the pilot appointment of a geriatrician to the service made a difference? J Burn Care Res. 2012;33(3):e178. https://doi.org/10.1097/BCR.0b013e31823b262b.
103. Rumbach AF, Clayton NA, Muller MJ, Maitz PK. The speech-language pathologist's role in multidisciplinary burn care: an international perspective. Burns. 2016;42(4):863–71. https://doi.org/10.1016/j.burns.2016.01.011.
104. Hsu KC, Chen LF, Hsiep PH. Effect of music intervention on burn patients' pain and anxiety during dressing changes. Burns. 2016;42(8):1789–96. https://doi.org/10.1016/j.burns.2016.05.006.
105. Najafi Ghezeljeh T, Mohades Ardebili F, Rafii F, Haghani H. The effects of music intervention on background pain and anxiety in burn patients: randomized controlled clinical trial. J Burn Care Res. 2016;37(4):226–34. https://doi.org/10.1097/BCR.0000000000000266.
106. Seyyed-Rasooli A, Salehi F, Mohammadpoorasl A, Goljaryan S, Seyyedi Z, Thomson B. Comparing the effects of aromatherapy massage and inhalation aromatherapy on anxiety and pain in burn patients: a single-blind randomized clinical trial. Burns. 2016;42(8):1774–80. https://doi.org/10.1016/j.burns.2016.06.014.
107. Goverman J, Mathews K, Nadler D, Henderson E, McMullen K, Herndon D, Meyer W 3rd, Fauerbach JA, Wiechman S, Carrougher

G, Ryan CM, Schneider JC. Satisfaction with life after burn: a Burn Model System National Database Study. Burns. 2016;42(5): 1067–73. https://doi.org/10.1016/j.burns.2016.01.018.
108. Johnson RA, Taggart SB, Gullick JG. Emerging from the trauma bubble: redefining 'normal' after burn injury. Burns. 2016;42(6):1223–32. https://doi.org/10.1016/j.burns.2016.03.016.
109. Palmu R, Partonen T, Suominen K, Vuola J, Isometsa E. Functioning, disability, and social adaptation six months after burn injury. J Burn Care Res. 2016;37(3):e234–43. https://doi.org/10.1097/BCR.0000000000000258.
110. Logsetty S, Shamlou A, Gawaziuk JP, March J, Doupe M, Chateau D, Hoppensack M, Khan S, Medved M, Leslie WD, Enns MW, Stein MB, Asmundson GJ, Sareen J. Mental health outcomes of burn: a longitudinal population-based study of adults hospitalized for burns. Burns. 2016;42(4):738–44. https://doi.org/10.1016/j.burns.2016.03.006.
111. Martin L, Byrnes M, McGarry S, Rea S, Wood F. Posttraumatic growth after burn in adults: an integrative literature review. Burns. 2017;43(3):459–70. https://doi.org/10.1016/j.burns.2016.09.021.
112. Martin L, Byrnes M, McGarry S, Rea S, Wood F. Social challenges of visible scarring after severe burn: a qualitative analysis. Burns. 2017;43(1):76–83. https://doi.org/10.1016/j.burns.2016.07.027.
113. A controlled trial to improve care for seriously ill hospitalized patients. The study to understand prognoses and preferences for outcomes and risks of treatments (SUPPORT). The SUPPORT Principal Investigators. JAMA. 1995;274(20):1591–8.
114. Taylor LJ, Nabozny MJ, Steffens NM, Tucholka JL, Brasel KJ, Johnson SK, Zelenski A, Rathouz PJ, Zhao Q, Kwekkeboom KL, Campbell TC, Schwarze ML. A framework to improve surgeon communication in high-stakes surgical decisions: best case/worst case. JAMA Surg. 2017;152(6):531–8. https://doi.org/10.1001/jamasurg.2016.5674.
115. Madni TD, Ekeh AP, Brakenridge SC, Brasel KJ, Joseph B, Inaba K, Bruns BR, Kerby JD, Cuschieri J, Mohler MJ, Nakonezny PA, Clark A, Imran J, Wolf SE, Paulk ME, Rhodes RL, Phelan HA 3rd. A comparison of prognosis calculators for geriatric trauma: a Prognostic Assessment of Life and Limitations After Trauma in the Elderly consortium study. J Trauma Acute Care Surg. 2017;83(1):90–6. https://doi.org/10.1097/TA.0000000000001506.
116. Anami EH, Zampar EF, Tanita MT, Cardoso LT, Matsuo T, Grion CM. Treatment costs of burn victims in a university hospital. Burns. 2017;43(2):350–6. https://doi.org/10.1016/j.burns.2016.08.022.

31 Burns in Patients with Special Comorbidities

Kevin N. Foster

31.1 Introduction

Traditional determinants of morbidity and mortality in burn patients are the extent of burn injury and the age of the patient. The presence of smoke inhalation injury is a third determinant, although likely of lesser importance than the first two [1–3]. Comorbidities, or preexisting medical conditions, can also affect the outcomes in burn patients.

A recent review of over 31,000 adult burn patients in the American Burn Association National Burn Repository demonstrated that 26% of these patients had one or more comorbidities. The number of comorbidities was positively correlated with a greater hospital length of stay and with an increased risk of mortality. The most common comorbidities identified were hypertension, alcohol and drug abuse, pulmonary disease, diabetes, and psychiatric diagnoses [4]. Other studies have supported the idea that comorbidities can adversely affect the outcomes in burn patients [5, 6].

Comorbid pathologic conditions can complicate clinical management of the thermally injured patient in a number of ways. Initial fluid resuscitation, ongoing cardiopulmonary and renal support, operative management of the burn wound, wound healing, and rehabilitation are particularly sensitive to perturbation by comorbidities. This chapter briefly examines the effect of common comorbidities on the pathophysiology and clinical management of burn injury.

31.2 Nervous System Disorders

The incidence of the leading adult brain and neurologic disorders leading to loss of cognitive and functional abilities is shown below.

The incidence of brain and neurologic disorders in the United States [7]

Condition	Annual incidence (persons/year)
Stroke	600,000
Alzheimer's	250,000
Epilepsy	135,000
Parkinson's	55,000
Multiple sclerosis	10,000

Cerebrovascular injury (CVA), or stroke, is the fifth leading cause of death and the leading cause of preventable, serious long-term disability in the United States [8]. Parkinson's disease (PD) and multiple sclerosis (MS), while less common than stroke, still confer significant morbidity on those affected. PD tends to affect older patients, and MS tends to affect younger patients. While the pathophysiology of these three conditions differs considerably, the effect on burn patients is similar [5].

Cerebrovascular injury incidence appears to be greater in burn patients than in the general population. The effect seems to be greater for ischemic than hemorrhagic CVA. The risk is greatest during the inpatient stay but also persists after discharge from acute care. Risk factors include sepsis, age > 60 years, and increasing burn size, although the data supporting the latter are equivocal [9–13].

Cerebrovascular injury, whether premorbid or simultaneous, affects burn patients in several ways. Initial resuscitation and operative management are usually not impacted. However, pain control, particularly assessment of adequacy of analgesia and sedation, can be difficult depending upon the specific manifestations of the neurologic injury. Additionally, physical and occupational therapy and rehabilitation are complicated by less than full functionality of the patient. Finally, CVA and burn injury together may result in greater immune dysfunction than either condition alone [14].

Multiple sclerosis is an immune disorder resulting in loss of myelin and subsequent nerve dysfunction. The disease has a variable course, but is the leading cause of neurologic morbidity and mortality in young adults. Caring for MS patients who have suffered burns is challenging. Because of the highly variable neurologic involvement, burn care profes-

K. N. Foster (✉)
Department of Surgery, The Arizona Burn Center—Valleywise Health, Phoenix, AZ, USA
e-mail: kevin_foster@dmgaz.org

M. G. Jeschke et al. (eds.), *Handbook of Burns Volume 1*, https://doi.org/10.1007/978-3-030-18940-2_31

sionals should consider autonomic and neurologic dysfunction is all systems. Bowel and bladder autonomic dysfunctions are particularly common. MS patients are susceptible to temperature increase, and the increased metabolic response in burn injury can be expected to cause exacerbation or deterioration of symptoms. Thus a balance between keeping burn patients warm and yet not overheating MS patients must be achieved. Spinal nerve involvement is not uncommon, and spinal anesthesia should be approached with great care. General anesthesia and surgery do not specifically seem to have adverse effects on MS patients. Any change in neurologic symptoms should prompt a search for infection in MS patients who are burned. Finally, rehabilitation should avoid increasing body temperature; hydrotherapy and water exercise are particularly helpful for MS patients [15, 16].

Parkinson's disease is a degenerative disorder of unknown etiology caused primarily by decreased dopamine production in the substantia nigra in the midbrain. This results in the clinical manifestations of PD including hypokinesis, rigidity, tremor and shaking, and ambulatory difficulties. As the disease progresses, patients often develop dementia and other cognitive dysfunction as well as psychiatric disorders such as depression [17]. PD patients are frequently hospitalized and are more susceptible to accidental injury than the general population [18]. It is unclear whether PD is associated with an increased incidence of burn injury [5, 19]. Once admitted to the burn center, PD patients can be expected to deteriorate neurologically because of the metabolic impact of the burn [18]. Two known risk factors for exacerbation of PD symptoms are change in medication regimen and infection [18]. Thus, it is important not to disrupt PD patients' medication regimen. Additionally, any acute deterioration of symptoms should initiate a search for infection or sepsis. Rehabilitation of PD patients with burns is complicated, like that for CVA and MS patients.

Epilepsy is a diverse collection of neurologic disorders caused by pathologic electrical activity in the brain, typically resulting in abnormal movements and/or behavior called seizures. In most cases, the cause of epilepsy is unknown. Epilepsy can be caused secondarily by other conditions such as traumatic brain injury, stroke, infections, and others. Although seizures are a characteristic feature of epilepsy, not all seizures are due to epilepsy. Single, isolated seizures (provoked seizures) can be caused by fever, infection, blood chemistry abnormalities, etc. Indeed, although close to 10% of persons in the United States will experience a seizure at least once in their lifetimes, epilepsy will affect less than 1% of the population [20]. Epilepsy and seizures are a definitive risk factor for burns. Seizures during cooking and bathing/showering or seizures resulting in a fall onto hot pavement are common causes of thermal injury in this population of patients [21–25]. Some studies suggest patients who suffer burn injury as a result of a seizure do not have increased mortality, and their hospitalization can be expected to be similar to that of a burn patient without a seizure disorder [26]. Other studies suggest an increased mortality and/or length of stay [27]. Regardless, it is common to see neurologic decompensation and exacerbation of symptoms in epileptic patients secondary to burn injury. Fever, hypovolemia, pain, perturbation in sleep cycle, hyperventilation, and ambient stimulations (light and sound) can all reduce seizure threshold. Additionally, the hypermetabolic state can lead to alterations in anticonvulsant metabolism and in serum protein binding of anticonvulsants, both of which can predispose to increased seizure activity [28]. Therefore, key issues in caring for an epileptic patient with burns include vigilant monitoring of hemodynamics and metabolism including arterial blood gases, electrolytes, acid–base status, calcium magnesium and phosphorus levels, and infectious work-up including cultures and antibiotic sensitivities. It is important to maintain medication regimen and to check drug levels [29].

There are two additional aspects of neurologic dysfunction and burn injury that must be considered. The first is prevention. Almost all thermal injuries happening to patients with neurologic dysfunction are preventable. A crucial part of care is to work with the patient, family, and other care providers to ensure the patient's environment is safe and hazard free so that the burn injury is not repeated.

The second issue is end of life provisions. The neurologic diseases discussed above are chronic and often progressive. A significant burn injury in patients with one of these diseases can be fatal or result in long-term morbidity and diminution of functional status. Frank discussion of the effects of the burn injury and likely prognosis and outcome with the patient and family are mandatory.

31.3 Cardiovascular Disease

Cardiovascular disease (CVD) is a substantial health challenge in most parts of the world. CVD is the single largest contributor to overall global mortality. Although CVD mortality rates are declining in most high-income, industrialized nations, mortality rates are increasing in most middle- and low-income countries. Additionally, CVD deaths in developing countries tend to disproportionately affect younger patients compared to industrialized countries [30]. In the United States today, CVD is the leading cause of death for both men and women. Overall, one in four deaths in the United States is due to CVD [31].

Premorbid cardiac disease has been shown to adversely affect the outcomes in a variety of surgical patients. CVD is a major cause of hospital and perioperative morbidity and mortality [32]. Cardiac disease can manifest in multiple ways including atherosclerotic coronary artery disease (ASCAD), myocardial ischemia and infarction, congestive heart failure, dysrhythmias, cardiomyopathy, cardiac arrest, and hypertension. Cardiac disease likewise can be expected to impact patients with burn injury. It has been demonstrated that 13% of burn-injured patients develop a cardiac event including myocardial infarction, dysrhythmia, or cardiac arrest [33]. This rate is likely even higher in burn patients suffering an electrical injury [34]. The mechanisms by which premorbid cardiac disease impact burn patients are multifactorial [35].

Following burn injury, there is an initial depression of cardiac output and myocardial function that lasts 24–72 h following burn injury (the "ebb" phase of injury). Following this, there is an increase in all parameters of cardiac function including heart rate, contractility, myocardial consumption, and myocardial work (the "flow" phase of injury). These parameters are sustained until wound closure is achieved.

Large %TBSA injuries are characterized by the release of multiple inflammatory mediators, including those causing platelet aggregation and vasoconstriction. This biochemical milieu is similar to that seen in patients with myocardial infarction and/or unstable angina [33]. One might anticipate that these inflammatory mediators may contribute to cardiovascular dysfunction in the face of preexisting cardiac disease.

Diagnosing and treating myocardial infarction (MI) in a burn patient with premorbid CVD can be challenging. Although the incidence of premorbid CVD is high, the actual incidence of MI in burn patients appears to be low (<1%). Traditional methods of diagnosing MI can be confusing and misleading in burn patients. A study of cardiac function in electrical injury patients demonstrated that 56% of patients had abnormal elevations in CK-MB isoenzyme studies and 31% of patients had abnormal EKG findings. Subsequent assessment of cardiac function failed to reveal evidence of cardiac dysfunction or MI [36]. Two similar studies assessed the troponin-I (Tn-I) values in burn patients. One study found all patients with >18% TBSA burn had abnormally elevated Tn-I levels but only 5% of these patients had actual cardiac dysfunction [37]. The second study found all patients with burns >30% TBSA had abnormally elevated but none of these patients had EKG changes consistent with myocardial ischemia [38]. The authors noted a decrease in Tn-I levels with burn excision and hypothesized that the elevated Tn-I levels were associated with the generalized inflammatory response that accompanies burn injury. Gregg et al., in 2006, described a patient with a 50% TBSA flash burn who experienced an acute MI during burn resuscitation. The diagnosis was suggested by the patient's clinical picture and acute EKG changes of myocardial ischemia. The patient underwent emergency coronary angiography with balloon dilation and stenting, which was successful. The patient subsequently required anticoagulation and antiplatelet therapy and was able to undergo burn excision and autografting with incident [39]. In conclusion, MI appears to be a relatively rare occurrence in burn patients. Its diagnosis is difficult because enzyme levels are frequently elevated simply because of the burn. Diagnosis and intervention may require angiography with or without stenting and balloon dilation. Finally, patients who require anticoagulation and/or antiplatelet therapy can have effective surgical management of the burn wound.

With regard to dysrhythmias, 34–56% of burn patients can be expected to have dysrhythmias during their acute hospitalization. The most common dysrhythmias are sinus tachycardia and prolonged QT interval. Other dysrhythmias included premature atrial contractions (PACs), premature ventricular contractions (PVCs), and non-specific ST and T wave abnormalities. The cardiac dysrhythmias experienced by burn patients appear to be relatively benign and similar to those experienced by other hospitalized patients. The extent of the burn injury does not seem to be correlated with the incidence or severity of dysrhythmia [40, 41]. Most dysrhythmias have little or no hemodynamic consequences. Those that do can be treated appropriately with pharmacologic intervention, pacing, and/or cardioversion.

An interesting study by Loguidice et al., in 2016, assessed the utility of heart rate variability (HRV) via 24-h Holter monitoring to predict mortality in burn patients. Abnormal HRV is seen in a variety of pathologic cardiac and noncardiac conditions and has been shown to be associated with poor cardiac outcomes. Abnormal HRV was indeed predictive of mortality in burn patients. However, the cause of death was not specified, and it is thus unclear if these deaths were due to cardiac dysfunction [42].

Special consideration must be given to the patient in active congestive heart failure (CHF) who suffers a thermal injury and must be resuscitated with large volumes of intravenous fluid. This particular situation presents a challenge to burn care providers because this patient requires fluid to both avoid burn shock and maintain organ and tissue function and yet is at risk for fluid overload, decreasing cardiac function, pulmonary edema, and poor cardiac outcome [43]. Overall predictors of poor outcome for patients include left ventricular (LV) ejection fraction less than 30%, LV end-diastolic diameter greater than 7 cm, LV end-diastolic volume greater than 130 cc, elevated serum norepinephrine levels, narrowed pulse pressure, and New York Heart Association class 4 symptoms [44]. Early echocardiogram can identify patients at risk and the degree of CHF and myocardial function. Additionally, brain natriuretic peptide (BNP) can help to diagnose CHF and differentiate the pulmonary edema of CHF from acute lung injury (ALI) from other causes. Serum BNP levels are a sensitive indicator of LV dysfunction and are elevated in patients who are in active CHF. Normal or low levels of BNP essentially rule out CHF [45]. Once diagnosed with CHF, these patients require more intensive monitoring during fluid resuscitation that just implies following urine output. While noninvasive monitors of cardiac function may assist in guiding fluid administration, often invasive monitoring with pulmonary artery catheters, or serial or continuous echocardiogram assessment and close assessment of cardiac output/index, central venous pressure, mixed oxygen saturation, and oxygen delivery/consumption parameters are necessary. Intervention includes a delicate balance of judicious fluid administration and gentle diuresis, if necessary. Pharmacologic interventions include the use of angiotensin-converting enzyme (ACE) inhibitors to help off load the heart, and administration of inotropic agents such as dobutamine and/or milrinone. More advanced cases may require continuous renal replacement therapy (CRRT) and may even necessitate intra-aortic balloon pump use [44]. Key strategies in these complicated patients include correct diagnosis, prompt intervention, and close assessment and monitoring of cardiac function.

31.4 Pulmonary Disorders

Pulmonary disorders do not seem to be an independent risk factor for poor patient outcomes. However, burn patients with known pulmonary disease tend to do worse than burn patients without because pulmonary disorders are usually associated with one or more other comorbidities. And these additional comorbidities in conjunction with the pulmonary disorders can cause worse outcomes [4].

Chronic obstructive pulmonary disease (COPD) will likely soon be the third leading cause of death throughout the world and is the most significant respiratory condition impacting burn patients. COPD imposes a tremendous medical and economic burden on patients and society as a whole due to the serious and chronic nature of the disease process. Additionally, COPD both preferentially affects older patients and has a greater impact with increasing age [46]. There are several challenges in caring for the burn patient who has COPD.

The first challenge is airway management during resuscitation. COPD patients are more likely to require a definitive airway, because of increased sensitivity to smoke inhalation, lack of pulmonary reserve, and need for ventilator assistance due to the metabolic effect of the burn and smoke injury. Attaining a definitive airway may be more difficult because of lack of reserve. A difficult airway should be anticipated in these patients and the most experienced team member(s) should participate in this process.

Once intubated, mechanical ventilation of COPD patients may require different techniques than that used in patients with normal pulmonary function. Specifically, a characteristic of COPD patients is airflow obstruction caused by chronic inflammation, secretions, and/or bronchospasm. This obstruction impedes both inhalation and exhalation, but typically results in the need for prolonged exhalation. Failure to incorporate this in ventilator management may result in air trapping, auto-positive end-expiratory pressure (auto-PEEP), increased airway pressures, and resulting hypoxia and/or hypercarbia. Techniques to avoid this include support ventilation or synchronous intermittent mandatory ventilation modes, lower respiratory rates, and high inspiratory flow rates to decrease inspiratory:expiratory (I:E) ratio. A common pitfall in this situation is increasing respiratory rate in response to hypercarbia and/or acidosis which subsequently increases autoPEEP, exacerbates decreased ventilation, and worsens the respiratory failure [47, 48].

Another consideration in both intubated and non-intubated COPD patients is chronic, compensatory CO_2 retention that is seen in COPD patients who have lost their hypercarbic drive. Correcting hypoxia in these patients with high inspired oxygen therapy can improve hypoxia but simultaneously eliminate the hypoxic respiratory drive and inadvertently push the patients into respiratory failure.

COPD patients because of airflow obstruction, air trapping, and over-distention of alveoli, have a higher likelihood of barotrauma or volutrauma with mechanical ventilation, particularly if ventilator settings result in high inspiratory volumes or increased peak airway pressures. The risk of this can be minimized by utilizing the strategies discussed above and using lung-protective strategies. A sudden decompensation in a ventilated burn patient who also has COPD should prompt a search for an iatrogenic pneumothorax.

Intubated COPD patients are at greater risk for ventilator-associated pneumonia (VAP) than ventilated patients without COPD [49]. This is almost certainly true in burn patients and indeed may be more pronounced in the burn population because of the often long duration of ventilation, frequency of infectious processes elsewhere, immunosuppressive nature of the burn injury, and the presence of bacterial wound colonization. Signs and symptoms of infection and/or sepsis in a burn patient with COPD should prompt aggressive diagnostic and therapeutic maneuvers confirm, characterize, and treat a potential VAP. Development of a VAP in a burn patient can be expected to increase mortality and increase duration of ventilation and ICU stay.

Special consideration must be given to the patient who suffers a burn injury due to smoking while on chronic home oxygen therapy (HOT). The incidence of this injury has been increasing [50]. HOT is most commonly prescribed for COPD, but is also used for other pulmonary, cardiac, and neuromuscular diseases. HOT is a beneficial treatment, improving oxygenation and decreasing mortality [51]. However, patients who continue to smoke tobacco while using HOT (and often smoking is the reason necessitating HOT use in the first place) have a high risk for burn injury [52–58]. The mechanism of the injury is that the HOT acts as an accelerant for combustion, making hot objects or objects on fire, such as cigarettes, burn hotter and faster [51]. Because the injury typically occurs when the patient brings the cigarette toward his/her mouth, face and head burns are common. Fortunately, these flash burns are usually superficial partial thickness and can be managed with outpatient care, or after a brief overnight inpatient stay without intubation and without surgical intervention. However, the mortality associated with these injuries is not inconsequential and the cost is high.

31.5 Gastrointestinal Disorders

Gastrointestinal (GI) disorders, with one exception, generally do not play a great role in premorbid pathology associated with burn injury. Liver failure and cirrhosis can have a significant impact on outcome following burn injury; these are reviewed below. Other disorders to be considered are inflammatory bowel disease, irritable bowel syndrome, and pancreatitis.

Inflammatory bowel disease (IBD) is a group of several conditions (e.g., Crohn's disease and ulcerative colitis) that affect various areas of the GI tract causing diarrhea, vomiting, bleeding, pain, and weight loss. IBD may exhibit manifestations outside of the GI tract including arthritis, skin lesions, cholangitis, deep venous thrombosis, and other symptoms. The important considerations for IBD in patients with burn injury are diagnosis and management of an acute IBD exacerbation and maintaining nutritional status. Diagnosis is usually suspected by worsening of symptoms described above and by colonoscopy with or without biopsy. Treatment includes symptomatic care, and usually anti-inflammatory drugs such as mesalazine in combination with immunosuppression drugs such as corticosteroids or azathioprine [59].

Irritable bowel syndrome (IBS) is a condition characterized by abdominal pain and change in bowel habits without the anatomic changes seen in IBD. Other conditions associated with IBS include anxiety, depression, and chronic fatigue syndrome. IBS is more common in women and seems to decrease with age. There is no cure for IBS; treatment is symptomatic and supportive. Pain control for the burn injury may be complicated by the abdominal pain seen with IBS [60].

Acute pancreatitis is an inflammatory disorder caused by intracellular activation of caustic digestive enzymes leading to abdominal pain and nausea and vomiting. Pancreatitis is rarely seen as a complication of burn injury. It is associated with an increased mortality in burn patients [61]. Preexisting pancreatitis typically arising from alcohol abuse, gallstones, or medications is occasionally seen in burn patients. The biggest issue in these patients is pain control. Nutritional supplementation is a secondary concern if patients cannot tolerate enteral feeding.

31.5.1 Liver Failure and Cirrhosis

The liver is a gland essential in metabolism, substrate utilization, protein synthesis, and various aspects of immune function. As such, the liver plays a pivotal role in the inflammatory response in burn injury. The most frequent liver disease which impacts burn patients is cirrhosis. Cirrhosis is most commonly caused by alcohol, viruses (hepatitis C and B), autoimmune disease, or inherited defects in metabolism. It is characterized by gradual replacement of normal hepatic parenchyma with fibrotic scar accompanied by subsequent global functional failure of hepatocytes [62]. Two common scoring systems have been employed to stratify risk of patients with cirrhosis. The Child-Pugh-Turcotte classifies cirrhotic patients into three categories (A, B, and C) based on the likelihood of mortality for elective, non-hepatic surgery. The Model for End-Stage Liver Disease (MELD) score is used as a prognostic indicator for cirrhotic patients to prioritize graft allocation. It has also been shown to permit risk stratification for cirrhotic patients with acute traumatic injury. A recent study found that the MELD did not allow risk stratification for burn patients. However, the same study found that the mortality for cirrhotic patients with burns of 10–50% TBSA was 83% compared to 12% mortality for non-cirrhotic patients with equivalent burn size. The authors stated that patients with cirrhosis were rarely able to survive burn injury greater than 10% TBSA [63].

There is no specific treatment for cirrhosis short of liver transplantation. The clinical goals for the burn care team in caring for a cirrhotic patient with a burn are to preserve existing hepatic function, to avoid/treat the complications of cirrhosis such as coagulopathy, encephalopathy, and ascites, and to achieve burn wound closure as quickly as possible. It is not uncommon to see deterioration of hepatic function as a result of burn injury. Two particular problems faced by the burn care team are fluid resuscitation and operative coagulopathy.

Cirrhotic patients often are hyponatremic, fluid overloaded, and have a poor ability to handle a sodium load. This makes initial burn resuscitation challenging. Strategies include judicious fluid administration with close monitoring, the use of colloid, diuresis near the end of resuscitation, utilization of continuous renal replacement or conventional hemodialysis, and consideration for plasma exchange.

Cirrhotic patients are also often coagulopathic because of the liver's inability to synthesize coagulation factors and because of thrombocytopenia. This can make operative management of the burn wound challenging. Operative strategies include the use of tourniquets, facial rather than tangential excision, subeschar clysis, and topical hemostatic agents. Biochemical strategies included the administration of vitamin K, repletion of factors with infusion of fresh frozen plasma and platelets, and administration of anti-fibrinolytic agents such as aminocaproic acid. The use of prothrombin concentration complex and/or activated factor VII are limited by the current paucity of clinical data in this setting, but may be considered as rescue therapies.

Oxandrolone is an anabolic steroid that improves burn patient outcomes. It does not predispose to burn patients to hepatic dysfunction. However, it can augment liver impairment and should not be used in the face of any degree of hepatic dysfunction [64–67].

31.6 Renal Insufficiency and Failure

Acute renal insufficiency and renal failure are common complications of burn injury and contribute significantly to morbidity and mortality. Here we will briefly discuss the impact of preexisting renal failure on the clinical care of burn patients. The major concern is maintenance of fluid, electrolyte, and acid–base status during acute resuscitation and subsequent hospitalization. One can expect deterioration in renal function as a result of the burn injury. For a patient not already on hemodialysis, fluid and biochemical status may be maintained with judicious fluid administration with or without the use of diuretics. Often, the burn injury will push renal patients not requiring dialysis into oliguric or anuric renal failure. These patients, along with patients already requiring hemodialysis, are best managed with continuous renal replacement therapy (CRRT). This is especially important during acute resuscitation when fluid and electrolytes shifts and alterations are greatest. Once the patient has stabilized after the first 48–72 h, the patient can often be transitioned to conventional hemodialysis.

31.7 Endocrine Disorders: Diabetes

Diabetes is a common clinical disorder in burn patients and is a risk factor for increased length of stay and higher rates of infection [68, 69]. Additionally, diabetic complications such as retinopathy, neuropathy, and gait disturbances predispose diabetics to burn injury [70]. Diabetes manifests pathologically in burn patients in several ways. First and most obvious is glucose intolerance and poor blood sugar control. The stress and inflammatory response that accompanies thermal injury produces hyperglycemia and insulin resistance. This exacerbates diabetes and increases difficulty in glucose control. Studies have shown that an elevated admission glucose level $\geq$ 150 mg/dL correlates with increased infectious complications in burn patients. Many other studies have documented poorer outcomes in diabetic burn patients [71, 72]. Numerous studies have shown that aggressive and appropriate glucose control can reduce infections and improve outcomes [71, 73, 74]. The precise cutoff level for "tight glucose control" in burn patients remains to be elucidated.

Diabetes complications also affect burn patients in other ways. The associated neuropathy, foot deformities, and gait disturbances can make physical and occupational therapy more difficult than in nondiabetic burn patients. Neuropathy may also adversely affect healing of burn wounds, skin grafts, and donor sites. Additionally, associated vasculopathy may produce decreased blood flow and impair healing.

31.8 Psychological and Psychiatric Disorders

A well-known complication of burn injury in many patients is the development of acute psychological maladies such as posttraumatic stress disorder or acute stress disorder [75]. Less well-known is the incidence and characterization of preexisting and more chronic psychological diagnoses and the effect on the care and recovery of burn patients [76].

The incidence of preexisting mental illness in patients with burn injury has been reported to be as low as 6% and as high as 13% [76, 77]. The most common mental health diagnosis in burn patients was depression. Forty percent of patients with a psychiatric diagnosis have more than one mental health disorder diagnosis. Mental health disorders may contribute to the development of burn injury. Premorbid mental health disorders in burn patients are associated with a variety of poorer outcomes including pain issues, healing, readmissions, number of transfusions, and others. These patients tend to experience longer length of stays in the hospital and to demonstrate slower wound healing [78]. Additionally, burn patients with psychiatric disorders are more likely to be discharged to a facility other than home and are at greater risk for death. All burn patients should be screened for preexisting mental health disorders. Treatment of these disorders should be aggressive and multidisciplinary.

Substance abuse frequently accompanies and often is contributory to burn injury. A review of multiple studies demonstrated that positive alcohol intake was reported in 1–50% of burn admissions. Most studies typically show that 20–33% of patients admitted with burn injury had been drinking alcohol around the time of injury [79, 80]. Up to 20% of burn admissions may have consumed enough alcohol to impair cognition. This impairment may have contributed to the cause of the injury and/or contributed to the inability to avoid or escape the injury [80]. Alcohol-related burn injuries tend to have flame as the etiology more frequently than non-alcohol-related burns. And alcohol-related burn injuries tend to have worse outcomes. Specifically, intoxicated patients tend to have more associated injuries and infections, greater ventilator days and total hospital days (length of stay), and greater numbers of transfusions and operations [81, 82]. Substance abuse does not appear to be an independent risk factor for mortality [81, 82] and in several studies alcohol use/abuse was NOT an independent risk factor for mortality [81, 82].

Similarly, abuse of substances other than alcohol including legal and illegal opioids, methamphetamine, cocaine, marijuana, and others is often seen in burn patients and often contributes to the etiology and severity of the burn injury. These patients frequently have complicated hospital courses marked by acute withdrawal and detoxification, more difficult pain control, delayed wound healing, and prolonged hospital stays, among other issues. Burn patients should be screened for mental illness and alcohol and substance abuse, and treated aggressively positive.

Burn patients who test positive for methamphetamine, and/or who are injured by methamphetamine lab explosions present unique challenges for the burn care team. These patients are often violent because of acute intoxication. And they often go through methamphetamine withdrawal [83]. They tend to require more aggressive fluid resuscitation. They have greater incidence of inhalation injury, longer times on the ventilator, and greater tracheostomy rates [84].

Summary Box

Burn patients frequently have pre-existing medical conditions in addition to their burn injuries. These conditions can complicate care and can adversely affect patient outcomes. This chapter briefly reviews the impact that common comorbid medical conditions can have on the morbidity and mortality of burn injured patients. The focus of this review is on the pathophysiology of medical conditions with respect to the burn injury and on interventions to minimize negative impact.

References

1. Ryan C, Schoenfeld D, Thorpe W, et al. Objective estimates of the probability of death from burn injuries. N Engl J Med. 1998;338(6):362–6.
2. O'Keefe G, Hunt J, Purdue G. An evaluation of risk factors for mortality after burn trauma and the identification of gender-dependent differences in outcomes. J Am Coll Surg. 2001;192(2):153–60.
3. Smith D, Cairns B, Ramadan F, et al. Effect of inhalation injury, burn size, and age on mortality: a study of 1447 consecutive burn patients. J Trauma. 1994;37(4):655–9.
4. Thombs B, Singh V, Halonen J, et al. The effects of preexisting medical comorbidities on mortality and length of hospital stay in acute burn injury: evidence from a national sample of 31,338 adult patients. Ann Surg. 2007;245(4):629–34.
5. Backstein R, Peters W, Neligan P. Burns in the disabled. Burns. 1993;19(3):192–7.
6. Bozkurt M, et al. Impact of para-neurologic and para-mental premorbidities on burn injury patients. Ulus Travma Acil Cerrahi Derg. 2011;17(3):220–4.
7. Family Caregiver Alliance. Incidence and prevalence of the major causes of brain impairment. 2013. https://www.caregiver.org/incidence-and-prevalence-major-causes-brain-impairment.
8. American Heart Association. Impact of stroke. 2016. http://www.strokeassociation.org/STROKEORG/AboutStroke/Impact-of-Stroke-Stroke-statistics_UCM_310728_Article.jsp - .WrpZp2aZPVo.
9. Chen C, Huang C, Wang H, et al. Stroke after burn: population data analysis. Burns. 2014;40(2):230–4.
10. Hung T, et al. Increased risk of ischemic stroke in patients with burn injury: a nationwide cohort study in Taiwan. Scand J Trauma Resusc Emerg Med. 2016;24(44):1–8.
11. Chung S, Chen C, Lin H, et al. Increased risk for stroke in burn patients: a population-based one-year follow-up study. Burns. 2014;40(1):54–60.
12. Lee Y, Chen C, Pan S. Acute stroke in the burn patient. J Burn Care Res. 2007;28(2):351–4.
13. Cho S, Minn Y, Kwon K. Stroke after burn. Cerebrovasc Dis. 2007;24(2):261–3.
14. Menges P, Kessler W, Kloecker C, et al. Surgical trauma and postoperative immune dysfunction. Eur Surg Res. 2012;48(4):180–6.
15. Bronnum-Hansen H, Hansen T, Koch-Henriksen N, et al. Fatal accidents among Danes with multiple sclerosis. Mult Scler. 2006;12(3):329–32.
16. Edlich R, et al. Special considerations in the management of a patient with multiple sclerosis and burn injury. J Burn Care Rehabil. 1991;12(2):162–9.
17. Beitz J. Parkinson's disease: a review. Front Biosci. 2014;1(6):65–74.
18. Gerlach O, et al. Deterioration of Parkinson's disease during hospitalization: survey of 684 patients. BMC Neurol. 2012;12(13):1–6.
19. Wang H, et al. Risk of accidental injuries amongst Parkinson disease patients. Eur J Neurol. 2014;21(6):907–13.
20. Helmers S, Thurman D, Durgin T, et al. Descriptive epidemiology of epilepsy in the U.S. population: a different approach. Epilepsia. 2015;56(6):942–8.
21. Abedipour M, Tavasouli A, Sobouti B, et al. Frequency and causes of seizure among hospitalized burned children. Burns. 2014;40(4):737–43.
22. Rimmer R, Bay R, Foster K, et al. Thermal injury in patients with seizure disorders: an opportunity for prevention. J Burn Care Res. 2007;28(2):318–23.
23. Minn Y. Who burned and how to prevent? Identification of risk for and prevention of burns among epileptic patients. Burns. 2007;33(1):127–8.
24. Jang Y, et al. Burns in epilepsy: seven years of experience from the Hallym Burn Center in Korea. J Burn Care Res. 2006;27(6):877–81.
25. Al-Qattan M. Burns in epileptics in Saudi Arabia. Burns. 2000;26(6):561–3.
26. Othman D, et al. Paediatric burns with epilepsy or learning disabilities do not have increased risk of hospitalization of increased length of stay compared to the adulty burns. Burns. 2016;42(1):233–4.
27. Boschini L, et al. The role of seizure disorders in burn injury and outcome in sub-Saharan Africa. J Burn Care Res. 2014;35(6):e406–12.
28. Gragnani A, Muller B, Oliveira A, et al. Burns and epilepsy—review and case report. Burns. 2015;41(2):e15–8.
29. Mukhdomi G, Desai M, Herndon D. Seizure disorders in burned children: a retrospective review. Burns. 1996;22(4):316–9.
30. Institute of Medicine. Promoting cardiovascular health in the developing world. A critical challenge to achieve global health. Washington, DC: National Academies Press; 2010.
31. Centers for Disease Control and Prevention. Heart disease facts. 2017. https://www.cdc.gov/heartdisease/facts.htm.
32. Davenport D, Ferraris V, Hosokawa P, et al. Multivariable predictors of postoperative cardiac adverse events in surgery study. J Am Coll Surg. 2007;204(6):1199–210.
33. Goff D, Rurdue G, Hunt J, et al. Cardiac disease in the patients with burns. J Burn Care Res. 1990;11(4):305–7.
34. Guinard J, Chiolero R, Buchser E, et al. Myocardial injury after electrical burn: short and long term study. Scand J Plast Reconstr Surg Hand Surg. 1987;21:301–2.
35. Abu-Sittah G, Sarhane K, Ibrahim A. Cardiovascular dysfunction in burns: review of the literature. Ann Burns Fire Disasters. 2012;25(1):26–37.
36. Housinger T, Green L, Shahangian S, et al. A prospective study of myocardial damage in electrical injuries. J Trauma. 1986;25(2):122–4.
37. Murphy J, Horton J, Purdue G, et al. Evaluation of troponin-I as an indicator of cardiac dysfunction after thermal injury. J Trauma. 1998;45(4):700–4.
38. Chen Y, Luo Z, Zeng L, et al. Cardiac troponin-I: a marker for postburn cardiac injury. Ann Clin Biochem. 2000;37(Pt 4):447–51.

39. Gregg S, Fidler P, Atweh N. Coronary stenting during burn shock: diagnostic and treatment considerations. J Burn Care Res. 2006;27(6):905–9.
40. Iyah G, Reddy P, El-Amin O, et al. Electrocardiographic abnormalities in patients with acute burn injuries. J La State Med Soc. 2008;160(1):39–40.
41. Meyers D, Hoestje S, Korentager R. Incidence of cardiac events in burned patients. Burns. 2003;29(4):367–8.
42. Loguidice M, Schutt R, Horton J, et al. Heart rate variability as a predictor of death in burn patients. J Burn Care Res. 2016;37(3):e227–33.
43. Lin C, Wu C, Yeong E, et al. Prognostic significance of left ventricular diastolic function in burn patients. Shock. 2012;37(5):457–62.
44. Harrington D. Complicated burn resuscitation. Crit Care Clin. 2016;32(4):577–86.
45. Lansink-Hartgring A, Eshuis J, Nieuwenhuis M, et al. Adult respiratory distress syndrome or congestive heart failure in severe burn: a role for brain natriuretic peptide. Burns. 2010;36(6):e87–90.
46. Centers for Disease Control and Prevention. Chronic obstructive pulmonary disease (COPD). https://www.cdc.gov/copd/index.html. Accessed 8 Apr 2017.
47. Mah M. Mechanical ventilation and the COPD patient. http://www.rtmagazine.com/2007/02/mechanical-ventilation-and-the-copd-patient/. Accessed 2 July 2007.
48. O'Donnell D, Laveneziana P. Physiology and consequences of lung hyperinflation in COPD. Eur Respir Rev. 2006;15(100):61–7.
49. Rouze A, Cottereau A, Nseir S. Chronic obstructive pulmonary disease and the risk for ventilator-associated pneumonia. Curr Opin Crit Care. 2014;20(5):525–31.
50. Amani H, Lozano D, Blome-Eberwein S. Brother, have you got a light? Assessing the need for intubation in patients sustaining burn injury secondary to home oxygen therapy. J Burn Care Res. 2012;33(6):e280–5.
51. Assimacopoulos E, Liao J, Heard J, et al. The national incidence and resource utilization of burn injuries sustained while smoking on home oxygen therapy. J Burn Care Res. 2016;37(1):25–31.
52. Kayser J, Nault D, Ostiguy G. Resolving moral distress for patients who smoke while using home oxygen therapy. Home Healthc Nurse. 2012;30(4):208–15.
53. Lindford A, Tehrani H, Sassoon E, et al. Home oxygen therapy and smoking: a dangerous practice. Ann Burns Fire Disasters. 2006;19(2):99–100.
54. Litt E, Ziesche R, Happak W, et al. Burning HOT: revisiting guidelines associated with home oxygen therapy. Int J Burns Trauma. 2012;2(3):167–70.
55. Muelberger T, Smith M, Wong L. Domiciliary oxygen and smoking: an explosive combination. Burns. 1998;24(7):658–60.
56. Robb R, Hungess E, Hershko D, et al. Home oxygen therapy; adjunct or risk factor? J Burn Care Rehabil. 2003;24(6):402–6.
57. Murabir A, Tredger E. Review of burn injuries secondary to home oxygen. J Burn Care Res. 2012;33(2):212–7.
58. Vercruysse G, Ingram W. A rationale for significant cost savings in patients suffering home oxygen burns: despite many comorbid conditions, only modest care is necessary. J Burn Care Res. 2012;33(6):e268–74.
59. Abraham C, Cho J. Inflammatory bowel disease. NEJM. 2009;361:2066–78.
60. Ford A, Lacy B, Talley N. Irritable bowel syndrome. NEJM. 2017;376:2566–78.
61. Rivero H, Lee J, Herndon D, et al. The role of acute pancreatitis in pediatric burn patients. Burns. 2011;37(1):82–5.
62. Jeschke M. The hepatic response to thermal injury: is the liver important for postburn outcomes? Mol Med. 2009;15(9–10):337–51.
63. Burns C, Chung K, Aden J, et al. High risk but not always lethal: the effect of cirrhosis on thermally injured adults. J Burn Care Res. 2013;34(1):115–9.
64. Jeschke M, Finnerty C, Suman O, et al. The effect of oxandrolone on the endocrinologic, inflammatory, and hypermetabolic responses during the acute phase postburn. Ann Surg. 2007;246(3):351–60; discussion 360–2
65. Reeves P, Herndon D, Tanksley J, et al. Five-year outcomes after long-term oxandrolone administration in severely burned children: a randomized clinical trial. Shock. 2016;45(4):367–74.
66. Wolf S, Edelman L, Kemalyan N, et al. Effects of oxandrolone on outcome measures in the severely burned: a multicenter prospective randomized double-blind trial. J Burn Care Res. 2006;27(2):131–9; discussion 140–1
67. Li H, Guo Y, Yang Z, et al. The efficacy and safety of oxandrolone treatment for patients with severe burns: a systematic review and meta-analysis. Burns. 2016;42(4):717–27.
68. McCampbell B, Wasif N, Rabbits A, et al. Diabetes and burns: retrospective cohort study. J Burn Care Rehabil. 2002;23(3):157–66.
69. Memmel H, Kowal-Vern A, Latenser B. Infections in diabetic patients. Diabetes Care. 2004;27:229–33.
70. Murphy C, Coffery R, Wisler J, et al. The relationship between acute and chronic hyperglycemia and outcomes in burn injury. J Burn Care Res. 2013;34:109–14.
71. Ray J, Meizoso J, Allen C, et al. Admission hyperglycemia predicts infectious complications after burns. J Burn Care Res. 2017;38(2):85–9.
72. Sayampanathan A. Systematic review of complications and outcomes of diabetic patients with burn trauma. Burns. 2016;42(8):1644–51.
73. Hemmila M, Taddonio M, Arbabi S, et al. Intensive insulin therapy is associated with reduced infectious complications in burn patients. Surgery. 2008;144:629–37.
74. Low Z, Ng W, Fook-Chong S. Comparison of clinical outcomes in diabetic and non-diabetic burns patients in a National Burn Referral Centre in Southeast Asia: a 3-year retrospective review. Burns. 2017;43(2):435–44.
75. Palmu R, Suominen K, Vuola J, et al. Mental disorders after burn injury: a prospective study. Burns. 2011;37(4):601–9.
76. Hudson A, Al Youha S, Samargandi O, et al. Pre-existing psychiatric disorder in the burn patient is associated with worse outcomes. Burns. 2017;43(5):973–82.
77. Mahendraraj K, Durgan D, Chamberlain R. Acute mental disorders and short and long term morbidity in patients with third degree flame burn: a population-based outcome study of 96,451 patients from the Nationwide inpatient sample (NIS) database (2001-2011). Burns. 2016;42(8):1766–73.
78. Tarrier N, Gregg L, Edwards J, et al. The influence of pre-existing psychiatric illness on recovery in burn injury patients: the impact of psychosis and depression. Burns. 2005;31(1):45–9.
79. Anwar M, Majumder S, Austin O, et al. Smoking, substance abuse, psychiatric history, and Burns: trends in adult patients. J Burn Care Rehabil. 2005;26(6):493–501.
80. Barillo D. Substance abuse in victims of fire. J Burn Care Rehabil. 1996;17(1):71–6.
81. Grobmyer S, Maniscalco S, Purdue G, et al. Alcohol, drug intoxication, or both at the time of burn injury as a predict of complications and mortality in hospitalized patients. J Burn Care Rehabil. 1996;17(6):532–9.
82. Hodgman E, Subramanian M, Wolf S, et al. The effect of illicit drug use on outcomes following burn injury. J Burn Care Res. 2017;38(1):e89–94.
83. Danks R, Wibbenmeyer L, Faucher L, et al. Methamphetamine-associated burn injuries: a retrospective analysis. J Burn Care Rehabil. 2004;25(5):425–9.
84. Santos A, Wilson A, Hornung C, et al. Methamphetamine laboratory explosion: a new and emerging burn injury. J Burn Care Rehabil. 2005;26(3):228–32.

32 Wound Healing

Eleanor Curtis and Nicole S. Gibran

32.1 History of Wound Care

The study of wound healing occupies a central role in surgical history and continues to represent a common challenge for all surgical subspecialties. As early as 1550 BC, the Ebers Papyrus of ancient Egypt documents the use of many natural remedies in wound healing. The Egyptians observed that honey, now known to have antibacterial properties, proved an effective wound dressing. Mild antiseptics such as frankincense, date-wine, turpentine, and acacia gum also found a place in the Egyptian pharmacopeia. The Egyptians documented the use of sutures for primary wound closure, and in a strikingly early use of twentieth century medicines, there is documentation of the application of sour or moldy bread to wounds, now understood to harbor antibiotic-producing fungus [1].

Galen of Pergamon, the celebrated surgeon and anatomist, derived a wealth of wound care experience from serving as surgeon to the Roman gladiators. He emphasized the importance of maintaining a moist environment for wound healing, although we have only recently understood that wound epithelialization is greatly enhanced in sufficiently hydrated wound beds [2]. Further developments in wound care took millennia to arrive, often returning to old remedies. The sixteenth-century French barber surgeon, Amboise Paré, changed the practice of cauterizing gunshot wounds with hot oil, instead using a Roman salve of egg-white, rose-oil, and turpentine improving infection rates and pain control for wounded soldiers [3]. In 1607, Wilhelm Fabry's *De Combustionibus* first described the three stages of burns [4]. The idea of treating burns and other skin wounds surgically was not a mainstay of treatment until the late 1800s, after the advent of germ theory and anesthesia [5].

Ignaz Philipp Semmelweis, a Hungarian obstetrician, noted that the incidence of puerperal infections was significantly lower when medical students on the ward washed their hands with soap and hypochlorite after attending cadaver dissection. Louis Pasteur related natural phenomena such as the souring of milk to the fermentation of sugar by microorganisms. He developed a heat treatment (pasteurization) that prevented the transmission of microbes such as tuberculosis and typhoid. Robert Koch formulated a generalizable set of criteria for microbial infections, now known as Koch's postulates. First, microorganisms should be in abundance in those suffering (but not in healthy persons). Second, microorganisms isolated from the diseased should be able to be grown in pure culture. Third, cultured microorganisms should cause disease when introduced into a healthy organisms, and finally that the organism has not changed when re-isolated from the new host [6].

English surgeon, Joseph Lister is widely credited as the father of antiseptic surgery. Lister's use of carbolic acid for surgical sterilization is said to derive from his observation that sewage treated with the chemical was less murky than without. He began treating surgical instruments and instituted handwashing protocols with carbolic acid, which initially led to his suspension from practice, but eventually paved the way for institution of sterile technique in surgery [6].

32.2 Types of Wounds

The nature of the wound and the manner in which it may heal are fundamentally linked to the mechanism of insult. Injuries by physical agents may be broadly classified into groups: mechanical trauma, thermal injury, chemical injury, electrical injury, and injury caused by ionizing radiation. These are primary wounds; the category and subtypes are listed in Table 32.1 with typical characteristics of the wounds. In

E. Curtis · N. S. Gibran (✉)
Department of Surgery, University of Washington, Seattle, WA, USA

UW Medicine Regional Burn Center, Seattle, WA, USA
e-mail: nicoleg@uw.edu

M. G. Jeschke et al. (eds.), *Handbook of Burns Volume 1*, https://doi.org/10.1007/978-3-030-18940-2_32

Table 32.1 Categories of wounds and various subtypes

Category	Subtype	Wound characteristics
Mechanical	Abrasions Contusions Lacerations Incisions Puncture wounds	Removal of superficial skin layer(s) Disruption of blood vessels and extravasation of blood into tissue Tissue disruption caused by blunt or sharp instrument, usually irregular Tissue disruption caused by sharp instrument, usually linear Penetration of sharp instrument or projectile into tissue
Thermal	Superficial Partial thickness Full thickness	Burns confined to epidermis Burns involving papillary (superficial) or reticular (deep) dermis Burns extending through dermis into subcutaneous tissue
Chemical	Alkali Acid Hydrocarbons	Fat saponification, cellular dehydration, and deep tissue penetration Hard eschar, thermal injury, and electrolyte imbalances Dissolution of cell membranes, typically superficial erythema & blistering
Electrical	Complex	Degrees of cutaneous and deep tissue injury associated with systemic complications
Radiation	Complex	Basal skin layer damage with short- and long-term sequelae
Chronic	Complex	Persistent inflammation and matrix degradation leading to nonhealing

addition, chronic wounds are caused by any of the above insults.

Mechanical injuries take on a variety of forms. Abrasions are caused by a friction event such as scraping or rubbing and result in the removal of superficial skin layers. More severe forms of abrasions include avulsions, which involve detachment of skin and possibly underlying tissue. Degloving injuries are avulsions with compromised blood supply to the detached. Contusions, or bruises, are caused by blunt trauma and characteristically rupture blood vessels. Extravasation of blood into the affected tissue is evident by skin discoloration, which evolves over time as the hemoglobin degrades. Lacerations and incisions refer to tissue separation extending through the skin, with lacerations caused by accidental trauma and incisions caused by purposeful dissection. Puncture wounds result from sharp penetration through the skin by an instrument or a projectile. They may extend into deeper structures and/or produce a second wound at the exit site (through-and-through wounds).

In the mid twentieth century, Jackson described thermal injuries as demonstrating a characteristic cutaneous injury pattern, which is divided into three zones based on blood perfusion and tissue viability: zone of coagulation, zone of stasis, and zone of hyperemia. The innermost zone of coagulation represents the irreversibly damaged, necrotic tissue without perfusion. Surrounding the necrotic tissue is an area of moderately burned tissue that may survive or progress to coagulative necrosis depending on the wound environment. This so-called zone of stasis is characterized by increased capillary permeability and vascular damage. The final zone of hyperemia is an area of intense vasodilatation and inflammation that contains viable tissue and is not usually at risk of progression to necrosis [7, 8].

Electrical injuries produce a variety of cutaneous and extracutaneous damage that depend upon the strength (amperage), duration of contact, and path of transmission through the body. If the contact time is brief, damage is relatively restricted to the cell membrane and electrical mechanisms (e.g., heart arrhythmias), rather thermal mechanisms will dominate the injury pattern. With longer contact time, thermal injury dominates and the entire cell is affected. Higher amperage (charge per unit time) burns are associated with a greater degree of systemic complications such as ventricular fibrillation, rhabdomyolysis, compartment syndrome, and renal failure [9].

Chemical injuries are subdivided by causative agent into alkali and acid, with alkali burns generally considered the most severe. Alkali burns induce fat saponification (calcification) or liquefaction, profound cellular dehydration, and formation of alkaline proteinates (completely ionized proteins) that cause deeper tissue damage. Examples of alkalis include lime, cement, potassium hydroxide, and bleach. Acid injuries induce protein hydrolysis (tanning) and do not penetrate tissue as readily as alkalis. One notable acid burn results from hydrofluoric acid due to its unique mechanism of fluoride chelating calcium in the tissue and the risk of hypocalcemia; this is the only acid burn with a specific treatment with topical or systemic calcium. Finally, hydrocarbons such as organic solvents are capable of dissolving cell membranes and producing skin necrosis. Systemic absorption of hydrocarbons is associated with respiratory depression and hepatic toxicity [10].

Radiation with energy high enough to break up molecules is called ionizing radiation. Radiation injuries, which can be accidental or iatrogenic, are known to cause short- and long-term sequelae. Acute radiation syndrome describes the adverse effects of large doses of ionizing radiation on the skin. Basal skin layer damage results in inflammation, erythema, and desquamation. Blistering and ulceration may follow in days to weeks, and most wounds will heal normally, though larger doses may result in destruction of skin appendages, fibrosis, abnormal pigmentation, and ulceration or necrosis of exposed tissue. Acute ionizing radiation exposure is also associated with dysfunction of hematopoietic, gastrointestinal, and cerebrovascular, and systems [11].

32.3 Mechanisms of Wound Healing

Wound healing is classically divided into four phases: hemostasis, inflammation, proliferation, and remodeling. Considerable overlap exists between each phase, and a combination of biochemical and cellular events contributes to the natural continuum of tissue repair.

32.3.1 Hemostasis

The initial phase of wound healing is characterized by a coordinated effort between circulating platelets, soluble clotting factors, and vascular endothelium to stop hemorrhage by the formation of a clot. The key sequences of events are divided into (1) coagulation cascade and (2) platelet activation, although it is important to remember the fundamentally integrated nature of these processes.

Hemostasis is initiated by a chain reaction of soluble serum proteins to form an insoluble fibrin mesh. The coagulation cascade is grouped into the contact activation and tissue factor pathways (historically the intrinsic and extrinsic pathways, respectively). The initial reactions of the two enzyme cascades are unique with a final common pathway consisting of factors X, V, and thrombin. The primary pathway for blood coagulation is the tissue factor pathway, with the contact activation pathway playing a secondary role. The clotting cascade results in the generation of fibrin, which enhances platelet aggregation, and structurally reinforces the ensuing platelet plug [12]. Topical fibrin sealants promote hemostasis and skin graft adhesion in excised burn wounds [13].

Disruption of normal endothelium exposes subendothelial collagen and thrombogenic extracellular matrix molecules, most notably von Willebrand factor (vWF). Platelets adhere to vWF via the glycoprotein (GP) Ib receptor, which strengthens the interaction between platelets and underlying extracellular matrix. Patients with vWF deficiency or with mutations in the glycoprotein (GP) Ib receptor are known to have von Willebrand disease, which is the most common hereditary coagulation deficiency. Likewise, mutations in the GPIb receptor result in Bernard–Soulier syndrome. Both of these conditions result in bleeding tendencies because of altered platelet adhesion to exposed subendothelium [14].

Platelet adhesion leads to platelet activation, invoking the release of stored granule contents. Cues from the wound environment such as hypoxia and acidosis enhance platelet degranulation [15]. Alpha-granules store growth factors such as platelet factor-4 (PF4), platelet derived-growth factor, fibronectin, vWF, and fibrinogen [16]. Many of these substances enhance platelet adhesion or activation. PF4 binds with high affinity to endothelial-derived heparin, which inactivates the molecule and promotes coagulation. Antibodies bind to the PF4-heparin complex on platelet membranes in the syndrome of heparin-induced thrombocytopenia (HIT), which can lead to dangerously low levels of platelets with a paradoxical increase in thrombosis [17].

Dense granules harbor smaller molecules involved in platelet activation such as ADP, ATP, calcium, and serotonin. Release of these molecules into the platelet cytosol initiates a G_q-linked protein receptor cascade, which results in an increased cytosolic calcium concentration.

The platelet glycoprotein IIb-IIIa receptor deserves mention because of its relevance to cardiovascular medicine and disease. The natural ligand of GPIIb-IIIa is fibrinogen, which links the coagulation cascade with platelet activation. Platelet activation leads to increasing its affinity to bind fibrinogen, which enhances platelet aggregation and clotting factor-mediated coagulation. The activated platelets change shape from spherical to stellate, and the fibrinogen cross-links with glycoprotein IIb-IIIa receptors in neighboring platelets to promote aggregation and eventual clot formation [18]. The GPIIb-IIIA receptor is the target of several antiplatelet agents including abciximab, eptifibatide, and tirofiban. Similarly, the drug clopidogrel is known to inhibit ADP binding to the GPIIb-IIIA receptor, which results in a reduced ability of platelets to aggregate and consequently form clots.

32.3.2 Inflammation

Vasoconstriction occurs at the wound site immediately after injury, which is the beginning of the second event in wound healing: inflammation. Vasoconstriction is primarily mediated by catecholamines (epinephrine and norepinephrine), prostaglandin $F_{2\alpha}$, and thromboxane A_2. The contraction of blood vessels aids platelet aggregation and hemostasis. Vasoconstriction is followed shortly by vasodilatation and increased vascular permeability, which allows access of inflammatory cells to the damaged tissue. Vasodilatation is mediated by prostaglandin E_2, prostacyclin, histamine, serotonin, and kinins [16]. Inflammatory cells undergo a three-stage process of rolling along the vascular endothelium, integrin-mediated adhesion to endothelial cells, and transmigration into the extracellular space [19].

Neutrophils are the first inflammatory cell to arrive at the wound and play a primary role in the phagocytosis of bacteria and tissue debris. A huge array of molecular signals are chemoattractant agents for neutrophils, including products of platelet degranulation, formyl methionyl peptides cleaved from bacterial proteins, and the degradation products of matrix proteins. Neutrophils are a major source of early cytokines in the systemic response to injury, including tumor necrosis factor (TNF)-α [20].

Oxygen delivery influences all stages of wound healing. In addition to providing a substrate for ATP synthesis in aerobic cell metabolism, large quantities of oxygen are used by neutrophils for superoxide radical generation in oxidative killing. Furthermore, molecular oxygen itself is toxic to anaerobic microorganisms, and reactive oxygen species are used as chemotactic and extracellular signaling including phyagocyte recruitment in the healing wound bed [21]. Wound oxygenation is determined by blood perfusion, hemoglobin dissociation, local oxygen consumption, fraction of inspired oxygen, hemoglobin content, arterial oxygen tension, circulating blood volume, cardiac output, arterial inflow, and venous drainage [22].

Another early cell to infiltrate the wound site are monocytes, which undergo phenotypic changes into macrophages. Macrophages can be regarded as a "master cell" involved in wound healing because of their central role in phagocytosis, inflammatory cell recruitment, and systemic inflammation. Macrophages release a variety of growth factors such as transforming growth factor-β (TGF-β), platelet-derived growth factor (PDGF), and fibroblast growth factor (FGF), which induce fibroblast proliferation and extracellular matrix production [23]. Macrophages express specific receptors for IgG (Fc receptor), complement C3b (CR1 and CR3), and fibronectin (integrins) that facilitate recognition and phagocytosis of opsonized pathogens. Importantly, macrophages also secrete cytokines such as IL-1 and TNF-α that modulate the systemic response to injury. Excessive production of TNF-α has been linked with multisystem organ failure as well as chronic non-healing ulcers [24]. As discussed later, both IL-1 and TNF-α appear to play crucial roles in early wound healing but may have an inhibitory effect on wound maturation if persistently elevated.

Emerging data suggest a role for nerve-derived neuropeptide in wound repair. Stimulation of efferent nerves is known to produce local vasodilation and plasma extravasation in skin, which contributes to the local inflammatory response. The neuropeptide substance P, released from terminal endings of sensory nerves in response to noxious stimuli, is known to influence inflammatory cell chemotaxis [25, 26], angiogenesis [27, 28], and keratinocyte proliferation [29]. We have previously suggested that the dysregulated neuroinflammation plays an important role in hypertrophic scarring, evident by increased levels of substance P and decreased levels of the regulating enzyme neutral endopeptidase [30], which is responsible for the exuberant matrix production, hyperemia, and pruritus seen in this condition [31].

A robust but appropriate inflammatory response is essential to prepare the wound bed for subsequent migration of proliferative cells. However, overzealous inflammation may inhibit the formation of granulation tissue and neovascularization. Experiments in mice constitutively expressing the chemotactic cytokine interferon-inducible protein 10 demonstrate that an intense inflammatory infiltrate inhibits angiogenesis and development of healthy granulation tissue [32]. Thus, as in all homeostatic systems, a careful balance of functionalized cellular and biochemical processes is essential to proper wound healing. Animal trials suggest a possible role for statins in wound healing in partial- and full-thickness burns. Whereas the combination of statins and angiotensin receptor antagonists have been demonstrated to reduce fibrosis in several organ systems, results in burn healing has been mixed. Atorvastatin has been shown to reduce inflammation and increase graft take in porcine wounds; however, in the same animal model, Losartan treatment resulted in decreased graft take, increased wound contraction and worse scarring [33, 34].

32.3.3 Proliferation

The proliferative phase is characterized by the formation of granulation tissue, which is a pink, soft, highly vascularized platform for tissue formation. Fibroblasts are evident at the wound site within 2–5 days and become the predominant cell type after the first week [35]. Macrophages drive the migration of fibroblasts by secreting a number of chemokines including TNF-α, PDGF, FGF, and TGF-β. Fibroblasts begin to deposit collagen and other extracellular matrix molecules that strengthen the wound bed. Macrophages stimulate fibroblasts to produce FGF-7 (keratinocyte growth factor) and IL-6, which promote keratinocyte migration and proliferation. IL-6 is also a potent stimulator of fibroblasts, which explains the decreased level found in aging fibroblasts and fetal wounds [36]. Unfortunately, granulation tissue also harbors high bacterial counts and proteolytic activity, so it may need to be excised before skin grafting. Granulation tissue in a burn wound prevents advancement of the epithelial tongue and epithelialization and likely leads to hypertrophic scar formation [37].

A number of other inflammatory cytokines may find clinical relevance in wound care. IL-8 secreted by macrophages and fibroblasts early in wound healing may have a stimulatory effect on keratinocytes and epithelialization. Topical application of IL-8 to human skin grafts in a chimeric mouse model enhanced keratinocyte proliferation and re-epithelialization [38]. Additionally, in both human and animal studies, topical application of PDGF improved wound strength and healing time [39]; unfortunately, clinical trials have demonstrated no significant difference in healing in chronic wounds [40].

TGF-β is expressed by platelets and fibroblasts in the wound bed and plays an important role in collagen deposition and turnover. TGF-β is the most potent known stimulator of fibroblast proliferation and can accelerate wound healing in steroid-treated and irradiated animals [41]. Overexpression of TGF-β mRNA has been found in keloid and hypertrophic scars, whereas fetal wounds contain relatively little TGF-β [42]. This contrast between the heavily fibrotic scars of keloid and the scarless repair observed in utero might underscore the importance of TGF-β in the fibrotic response to tissue injury. Gabriel [43] observed a similar phenomenon in burn injuries, where higher levels of TGF-β correlate with excessive wound contraction. Interestingly, exogenous application of TGF-β3 reduces monocyte and macrophage recruitment to the wound site, resulting in less deposition of collagen and fibronectin in the early stages of wound healing [44]. A formulation of TGF-β (Juvista) underwent phase III trials but failed to meet primary or secondary endpoints and was never widely released [45].

Coincident with fibroblast migration to the wound site is angiogenesis. Angiogenesis, or neovascularization, which has been thought to be a critical element of early wound healing for transport of metabolites to and from the regenerating tissue. More recent data suggest that normal healing can occur when angiogenesis is inhibited and that angiogenesis in the wound bed is not associated with increased blood flow to the wound. Vascular endothelial cells arise from both preexisting blood vessels and endothelial progenitor cells (EPCs) in bone marrow. The most important regulators of angiogenesis are vascular endothelial growth factor (VEGF) and FGF-2. Nissen et al. [46] observed a dose-dependent effect of both VEGF and FGF-2 in angiogenesis. VEGF is secreted as many different isoforms from a variety of stromal and mesenchymal cells, with the tyrosine kinase VEGF-receptor 2 emerging as the most preeminent in angiogenesis. VEGF/VEGFR2 signaling is involved in EPC migration from bone marrow, as well as promotion of endothelial cell proliferation and differentiation [47].

Hypoxia is a potent inducer of both angiogenesis and fibroblast proliferation. The major player in hypoxic gene expression is hypoxia-inducible factor 1 (HIF-1), a DNA-binding transcription factor that is known to alter gene transcription of a number of proteins involved in metabolism, angiogenesis, migration, and proliferation [48]. Cultured endothelial cells upregulate the expression of several pro-angiogenic molecules when cultured in hypoxia, including endothelin-1, VEGF, and PDGF-β chain [49]. Fibroblast replication and longevity are increased in low oxygen tension culture [50], as is TGF-β secretion [49]. These observations highlight the contribution of hypoxia in the wound bed in proliferative cell signaling.

Mechanotransduction or the translation of mechanical force into biochemical signaling represents one novel area of research [51]. Using matrix-integrin activation of signaling cascades, mechanical force is transmitted to targets including calcium-dependent signaling, nitric oxide signaling, mitogen-associated kinases, and Rho GTPases. The end product of these signals activate transcription factors that move to the nucleus and activate mechanoresponsive genes [51]. Silicone sheeting, a way of offloading skin tension in healing wounds, has shown promise in improving scaring. Further avenues to modulate the biochemical signaling and mechanotransduction networks have potential to reduce scar formation and promote skin regeneration [52, 53].

Recently, the role of immune cells, long ignored in wound healing research is under increased investigation. T cells migrate into the wound bed during the late proliferative and early remodeling phase. Mice deficient in T and B cells have a reduced capacity to scar [22], though contradictory reports exist concerning the beneficial effects of $CD4^+$ and $CD8^+$ lymphocytes on wound healing [54, 55]. Additionally, a unique type of T cell exists in the skin, known as dendritic epidermal T cells (DETC), which are thought to modulate many aspects of wound healing such as inflammation, host defense, and maintenance of tissue integrity. Mice lacking or defective in DETC show a delay in wound closure and a decrease in keratinocyte proliferation at the wound site [44, 56].

32.3.4 Epithelialization

Epithelialization is the third important response to cutaneous injury, critical because once the epithelial layer is regenerated the wound is often viewed as being "healed." Keratinocytes migrate from wound edges and dermal appendages such as hair follicles, sweat glands, and sebaceous glands. The role of the epidermal appendages is especially evident in partial-thickness burns. Since the advancing epithelial tongue at the wound edge can migrate no more than ~1 cm, wounds depend on epidermal sources at the center of the wound. Full-thickness wounds larger than 2 cm rarely heal other than by contraction. Subsequent proliferation of these cells at the wound site provides a neo-epidermal covering. Keratinocyte migration and proliferation follow a discrete sequence of events: disassembly of hemidesmosomes and desmosomes, retraction of intracellular tonofilaments and keratin filaments, and formation of focal contacts and cytoplasmic actin filaments [57]. Martin [58] has extensively studied the interplay between laminin, matrix metalloproteinases (MMPs), integrins, and soluble growth factors in this process.

Renewal of keratinocytes during normal homeostasis and wound repair is a defining feature of re-epithelialization. The upper region of hair follicles below the sebaceous gland (known as the bulge) contains multipotent progenitor cells that contribute to maintenance and renewal of epithelium [59, 60]. Additionally, epidermal cells migrate from neighboring unwounded epidermis or from the infundibulum, the portion of the hair follicle between the epidermis and the sebaceous gland [61].

The relative contributions of the follicular stem cells and epidermal stem cells to re-epithelialization is debated, although gentic analyses have confirmed that the epidermis has intrinsic capacity for self-renewal and does not depend on follicle-derived multipotent progenitor cells [62, 63]. Further evidence for this notion comes from reports of de novo hair follicle generation in healing skin of adult mice [64]. This phenomenon, which has never been observed in humans, is contingent upon WNT-mediated signaling which is also involved in pattern formation and the epithelial–mesenchymal transformation during embryogenesis [65]. Elucidation of the overlapping pathways in wound repair, and development is a central principle of efforts toward scarless repair and skin regeneration.

32.3.5 Remodeling

Remodeling is the replacement of granulation tissue with scar over months after "healing." A key feature of tissue remodeling that emerges during this stage of wound healing is the balance between extracellular matrix (ECM) synthesis and degradation. While fibrogenic growth factors such as PDGF and FGF stimulate fibroblast matrix deposition, resident cells induce continuous degradation by matrix metalloproteinases. MMPs are a family of zinc proteases that are capable of degrading a variety of ECM components such as collagen, fibronectin, proteoglycans, and laminin [66] which can improve wound healing through direct and indirect mechanisms [67].

Collagen composition of the wound appears to follow a similar pattern as embryogenesis. Granulation tissue is comprised of a large amount of collagen III, which is gradually replaced by collagen I. Collagen I provides a higher degree of tensile strength to the developing scar, although the final tensile strength approaches only 70% of uninjured skin [68]. A morphological change in fibroblasts ensues during wound contraction, in which fibroblasts begin to express alpha-smooth muscle actin and adapt functions of smooth muscle cells. The resulting cell is termed a myofibroblast and serves to enhance wound contraction.

32.3.6 Stem Cells

In addition to resident epidermal stem cells in the skin, bone marrow-derived stem cells may contribute substantially to cutaneous wound healing. Bone marrow contains both hematopoietic (CD34+) and non-hematopoietic (mesenchymal) stem cells which aid wound healing by direct contribution of cells as well as by paracrine signaling. A notable study, in which green fluorescent protein-labeled bone marrow stem cells were used to reconstitute the marrow of mice with cutaneous wounds, indicated that non-hematopoietic mesenchymal stem cells may contribute up to 15–20% of dermal fibroblasts in normal skin and healing cutaneous wounds. Fathke et al. [69] and Brittan et al. [70] have traced cells with a keratinocyte phenotype to bone marrow origin. Deng et al. [71] have shown evidence that bone marrow stem cells are involved in hair follicle regeneration. Bone marrow cells expand ex vivo to promote neovascularization [72], appendage regeneration [73], and accelerate wound closure [74].

Endothelial progenitor cells (EPCs) derive from CD34+ hematopoietic stem cells in the bone marrow and contribute some proportion of the endothelial cells to adult skin. Systemic transplantation of EPCs enhances wound healing in mice [75], as does topical application of EPCs to ischemic ulcers in diabetic mice [76]. The mechanism involves paracrine signaling from EPCs instead of direct contributions by endothelial cells [75].

Fibrocytes, a subpopulation of leukocytes that also arise in the bone marrow, were originally identified by their rapid recruitment from peripheral blood to wound sites in mice [77]. Fibrocytes are significantly increased in the blood of burned patients in comparison to normal individuals and appear to localize in the deeper papillary dermis [78]. These cells may contribute to the myofibroblast population in wounds and may be associated with hypertrophic scarring [79, 80].

32.4 Abnormal Wound Healing

32.4.1 Impaired Wound Healing

A variety of local and systemic factors are implicated in abnormal wound healing, which impair tissue regeneration by interrupting each of the stages of wound healing. Physical impediments (Table 32.2) to wound closure may delay or prevent healing, such as the presence of foreign bodies or neoplasms (for skin grafts, hematomas and seromas most commonly cause graft failure). Excessive tension on a wound or surrounding edema may compress the vascular supply and lead to ischemia; recent data also implicate mechanical tension as a leading cause for hypertrophic scar formation [81]. Therapeutic radiation and repetitive trauma are also well-known detriments to wound healing.

Table 32.2 Local and systemic factors that impair wound healing

Local factors	Systemic factors
Tension	Connective tissue disorders
Foreign bodies	Hypothermia
Infection	Oxygen
Ischemia	Tobacco smoking
Hematoma and seroma	Malnutrition
Trauma	Jaundice
Edema	Age
Irradiation	Diabetes mellitus
	Uremia
	Steroids
	Chemotherapeutic agents

Adapted from [82]

A variety of insults can disturb wound healing by evoking hypoxia in the evolving wound. Disruption of vascular supply and depletion of oxygen can lead to wound hypoxia, which is associated with systemic diseases such as connective tissue disorders and microvascular disease in diabetes mellitus. Tobacco smoking produces similar effects through nicotine-induced vasoconstriction and displacement of oxygen on hemoglobin with carbon monoxide [83].

Infection is another classic adversary of proper wound healing. Wounds with bacterial counts that exceeding 10^5 organisms per gram of tissue will generally not heal by any means, including flap closure, skin graft placement, or primary intention [84]. The introduction of early excision and grafting for burn wounds has significantly reduced the prevalence of burn wound sepsis—which was historically a leading cause of burn mortality. Endotoxin produced by gram-negative bacteria stimulates phagocytosis and collagenase expression, which contributes to matrix degradation and destruction of normal tissue. Bacteria also accelerate protease production in macrophages (such as MMPs) while inhibiting protease inhibitor expression. This effect leads to increased matrix destruction and degradation of growth factors, which are characteristics of chronic nonhealing wounds [85].

Nutritional status has a profound effect on wound healing as well. Serum albumin is one of the most accurate predictors of surgical morbidity and mortality, with levels below 2.1 g/dL associated with poorer outcomes [86]. Protein replacement enhances wound healing [87], as does supplementation with the amino acids arginine, taurine, and glutamine [88, 89]. Whereas patients with large burns characteristically have albumin levels below 1.0 g/dL, exogenous albumen has never been demonstrated to improve outcomes. Early introduction of nutrition is a critical component of acute burn care and wound healing, with micronutrients playing an important role [90, 91]. Data suggest that the catabolic state can be modulated by propranolol in children [92] and oxandrolone in children and adults [93, 94]. Propranolol, a nonselective β-blocker, improved wound healing and perioperative hemodynamics in severely burned adults by increasing vascular resistance in the burn beds by leaving α-adrenergic receptors unopposed and decreasing blood loss during operative interventions [95].

Vitamin C (ascorbic acid) is an essential cofactor in proline and lysine hydroxylation during collagen synthesis, and supplementation of 100–1000 g per day may improve wound healing [89]. Vitamin A (retinoic acid) is required for wound re-epithelialization, maintenance of normal epithelium, proteoglycan synthesis, and normal immune function. Oral retinoid therapy counteracts the detrimental effects of corticosteroids on wound healing, possibly through promotion of TGF-β and IL-1 signaling [96]. Vitamin K deficiency impedes clot formation and hemostasis, while vitamin D is required for bone healing and calcium metabolism. Finally, vitamin E supplementation may serve an important role as an antioxidant in trauma patients. Early administration of vitamin E reduces the incidence of organ failure and the average length of ICU stay in critically ill surgical patients and may be relevant for burn patients [97].

The dietary minerals associated with wound healing include zinc and iron. Zinc is an essential cofactor in RNA and DNA polymerases. Deficiency inhibits granulation tissue formation [98] and delays wound healing [99]. Desneves et al. [88] report that zinc supplementation improves wound healing. Iron, another cofactor in DNA synthesis, is also key to proline and lysine hydroxylation. Although the role of iron in normal hematopoiesis is well established, chronically anemic patients do not appear to suffer from delayed wound healing [100]. Whereas selenium deficiency causes hair and skin abnormalities in humans and selenoproteins have been implicated in keratinocyte function and cutaneous morphogenesis [101], but selenium deficiency is yet to be associated with abnormal wound healing.

32.4.2 Hypertrophic Scars and Keloids

Hypertrophic scar and keloids represent fibroproliferative scars, which are characterized by excessive collagen deposition. These two morphological aberrations are difficult to differentiate: keloids are defined as scars that grow beyond the periphery of the original wounds and hypertrophic scars represent raised scars that remain confined to the boundaries of the original wound. Keloids rarely regress with time; hypertrophic scars frequently regress spontaneously. Both scar types appear to have a strong genetic component, with more prevalence in dark-skinned patients of African, Asian, Native American, or Latin American descent. Hypertrophic scars, the result of prolonged inflammation, are influenced by wound depth, skin tension, and delayed wound healing with increased inflammatory response and enhanced fibroblast activity [102]. Though theoretically preventable, hypertrophic scars tend to occur in pigmented individuals [103], young people, and rarely in the aged. Interestingly, they often develop in highly contractible body sites and rarely form on the scalp or the lower leg [104]. Proposed therapies to control hypertrophic scars act to reduce inflammation including steroid injections, radiotherapies, compression, and surgical methods to reduce skin tension [105]. The single nucleotide polymorphism $p27^{kip1}$ decreases vascular restenosis due to fibrogenesis, but was not associated with hypertrophic scar severity [106]. Using a genome-wide association study of over 500 individuals with burn injuries, mutations in the CSMD1 gene have been associated with reduced hypertrophic scarring [107].

In light of its potent effect on fibroblast proliferation and collagen deposition, it is perhaps not surprising that TGF-β plays a central role in proliferative scarring. Colwell et al. [108] found increased levels of the TGF-β1 isoform in both keloids and hypertrophic scars. Likewise, antibodies to TGF-β isoforms reduce fibrosis in hypertrophic scars [109]. Novel therapies for hypertrophic and keloid scars are in development that target ECM synthesis and fibroblast proliferation [110].

32.4.3 Chronic Nonhealing Wounds

Dysfunction of normal wound healing processes leads to chronic wounds. In particular, chronic wounds appear to have sustained inflammation with less matrix production. Chronic wounds exhibit higher levels of cytokines such as IL-1, IL-6, and TNF-α, with reduced levels of essential growth factors such as EGF and PDGF. MMP-1, MMP-2, MMP-8, and MMP-9 are present at higher levels, with reduced levels of MMP inhibitors [111]. These nonhealing wounds are prone to developing squamous cell carcinoma, originally reported in burn wounds by Marjolin. Marjolin ulcers tend to be very aggressive and should be highly suspected with nonhealing burn wounds [112]. Therapy includes complete local extirpation of the cancer with negative margins and lymphatic mapping [113]. Other conditions such as osteomyelitis, pressure sores, venous stasis ulcers, and hidradenitis have also been associated with wound malignancies [114]; patients with impaired skin integrity due to burn injuries are at increased risk for decubitus ulcers, which constitute a closely monitored hospital acquired complication.

32.4.3.1 Wound Dressings

A variety of burn dressings and skin substitutes are employed in the treatments of burns and other wounds. One class of dressings is topical salves and ointments such as silver sulfadiazine, bacitracin, or mupirocin, which require daily dressing changes to minimize infection risks. Multi-day dressings such as Acticoat® (Smith & Nephew), or Mepilex® Ag (Molnlycke) can be used in wounds and partial-thickness burns, minimizing the need for dressing changes while having antimicrobial properties. Additionally, bioderived materials are being explored for wound healing properties as natural scaffolds including polysaccharide polymers such as cellulose, chitosan (similar to a glycosaminoglycan), and hyaluronic acid and natural proteins such as silk fibroin, fibrin glue, and collagen [115]. An ideal dressing should be antimicrobial, analgesic, long acting, easy to apply (transparent), and affordable. While no single product is a miracle cure, continued advancements and combinations show promise in complicated wound processes. Lupeol from the *Cassia fistula* fruit has shown some promise with antioxidative, antileukotriene, and antibacterial effects and can be released with a chitosan hydrogel mixture that may improve wound healing in some patients [116, 117]. Whereas the list of dressings and skin produces in Tables 32.3 and 32.4 is robust, it is by no means exhaustive, and new products are released regularly.

Table 32.3 Examples of burn dressings

Dressing type	Examples	Clinical use
Low adherence dressing	Jelonet® (Smith & Nephew) Atrauman® (Hartmann) Mepilex® (Molnlycke)	Superficial and partial-thickness burns with minimal exudate
Semi-permeable dressing	Opsite® (Smith & Nephew) Tegaderm® (3M)	Superficial and partial-thickness burns with minimal exudate
Hydrocolloids	Comfeel® (Coloplast) DuoDERM® (ConvaTec) Granuflex® (ConvaTec)	Superficial and partial thickness burns in high range of motion areas
Hydrofibers	Aquacel® (ConvaTec) Versiva® (ConvaTec)	Partial thickness burns with moderate exudate
Hydrogels	Aquafoam® (ConvaTec)	Small deep partial thickness burns with slough
Alginate	Kaltostat (ConvaTec)	Skin graft donor sites
Foam/hydrocellular	Allevyn® (Smith & Nephew) Biatain adhesive® (Coloplast)	Superficial and partial thickness burns with minimal exudate
Antimicrobials	Acticoat® (Smith & Nephew) Actisorb® (Johnson & Johnson) Aquacel Ag® (ConvaTec) Inadine® (Johnson & Johnson) Mepilex® Ag (Molnlycke)	Superficial and partial thickness burns with moderate exudate and or evidence of infection

Products are registered trademarks

Table 32.4 Examples of skin substitutes for burn wounds

Product	Composition	Clinical uses
Human allograft	Cadaveric epidermis and dermis	Temporary coverage of large excised burns
Porcine xenograft	Porcine dermis	Temporary coverage of large excised burns
Human amnion	Placental amniotic membrane	Temporary coverage of large excised burns
Oasis®	Porcine intestine submucosa	Superficial burns, skin graft donor sites, chronic wounds
Biobrane®	Silicone and collagen-nylon bilayer	Partial thickness burns, temporary coverage of excised burns
Transcyte®	Allogeneic dermis and silicone bilayer	Partial thickness burns, temporary coverage of excised burns
Apligraf	Collagen matrix with human neonatal fibroblasts and keratinocytes	Permanent coverage of excised burns, chronic wounds
OrCel®	Collagen matrix with human neonatal fibroblasts and keratinocytes	Skin graft donor sites, chronic wounds
Epicel®	Cultured autologous keratinocytes	Deep partial- and full-thickness burns
Alloderm®	Acellular human dermis	Soft tissue defects
Integra®	Silicone and collagen-glycosaminoglycan bilayer	Deep partial- and full-thickness burns

Oasis® (Healthpoint LTD, San Antonio, TX), Transcyte® (Advanced BioHealing, Westport, CT), Biobrane® (Smith & Nephew UK Limited, London, UK), Apligraf® (Organogenesis, Canton, MA), OrCel® (Forticel Bioscience, Englewood Cliffs, NJ), Epicel® (Genzyme, Cambridge, MA), Alloderm® (Lifecell, Brancburg, NJ), and Integra® (Integra Life Sciences, Plainsboro, NJ) are registered trademarks

32.5 Conclusions

Wound healing remains an integral element of modern surgical science, contributing to both the function and form of wounds in all surgical patients but especially those with burn injuries. The biology of wound healing entails many integrated, parallel processes that lead to decontamination and closure of a wound. Restoration of tissue integrity relies on a careful balance between inflammation, proliferation, and remodeling, which is tipped in pathologic states of insufficient or excessive wound repair. Efforts underway to unravel the pathways that can be modulated to improve wound regeneration may lead to novel treatments.

Summary Box

- Injuries can be caused by physical agents and classified into groups: mechanical trauma, thermal injury, chemical injury, electrical injury, and radiation injury each of which has multiple subtypes.
- Wound healing is divided into four phases: hemostasis, inflammation, proliferation, and remodeling. Hemostasis is characterized by the activation of platelets and the coagulation cascade. Inflammation consists of vasoconstriction and the presence of neutrophils and their inflammatory cytokines preparing the wound bed for proliferation. Proliferation forms highly vascularized granulation tissue and characterized by fibroblasts and the deposition of collagen. After the wound bed is created, epithelialization by migration of keratinocytes will determine when the wound is considered healed. Remodeling changes the granulation tissue into scar by using matrix metalloproteinases.
- Impaired wound healing can result from many local or systemic factors including tissue oxygenation, infection, and nutritional status.
- Hypertrophic scars and keloids form in the areas of injury with impaired wound healing.
- While injuries heal, there are a multitude of dressings including creams, ointments, and multi-day dressings that can be used to add moisture and antimicrobial properties to the wound.

References

1. Sipos P, Gyory H, Hagymasi K, Ondrejka P, Blazovics A. Special wound healing methods used in ancient Egypt and the mythological background. World J Surg. 2004;28(2):211–6. https://doi.org/10.1007/s00268-003-7073-x.
2. Forrest RD. Early history of wound treatment. J R Soc Med. 1982;75(3):198–205.
3. Markatos K, Tzivra A, Tsoutsos S, Tsouroufiis G, Karamanou M, Androutsos G. Ambroise Pare (1510-1590) and his innovative work on the treatment of war injuries. Surg Innov. 2018;25(2):183–6. https://doi.org/10.1177/1553350617744901.
4. Naylor IL, Curtis B, Kirkpatrick JJ. Treatment of burns scarsand contractures in the early seventeenth century: Wilhelm Fabry's approach. Med Hist. 1996;40:472–86.
5. Hattery E, Nguyen T, Baker A, Palmieri T. Burn care in the 1800s. J Burn Care Res. 2015;36(1):236–9. https://doi.org/10.1097/BCR.0000000000000112.
6. Lederberg J. Infectious history. Science. 2000;288(5464):287–93.
7. Jackson DM. [The diagnosis of the depth of burning]. Br J Surg. 1953;40(164):588–96.

8. Jackson DM. Second thoughts on the burn wound. J Trauma. 1969;9(10):839–62.
9. Lee RC. Injury by electrical forces: pathophysiology, manifestations, and therapy. Curr Probl Surg. 1997;34(9):677–764.
10. Tormoehlen LM, Tekulve KJ, Nanagas KA. Hydrocarbon toxicity: a review. Clin Toxicol (Phila). 2014;52(5):479–89. https://doi.org/10.3109/15563650.2014.923904.
11. Waselenko JK, MacVittie TJ, Blakely WF, Pesik N, Wiley AL, Dickerson WE, et al. Medical management of the acute radiation syndrome: recommendations of the strategic National Stockpile Radiation Working Group. Ann Intern Med. 2004;140(12):1037–51.
12. Macfarlane RG. An enzyme cascade in the blood clotting mechanism, and its function as a biochemical amplifier. Nature. 1964;202:498–9.
13. Foster K, Greenhalgh D, Gamelli RL, Mozingo D, Gibran N, Neumeister M, et al. Efficacy and safety of a fibrin sealant for adherence of autologous skin grafts to burn wounds: results of a phase 3 clinical study. J Burn Care Res. 2008;29(2):293–303. https://doi.org/10.1097/BCR.0b013e31816673f8.
14. Von Willebrand EA. Hereditary pseudohaemophilia. Haemophilia. 1999;5(3):223–31; discussion 2
15. Ramasastry SS. Acute wounds. Clin Plast Surg. 2005;32(2):195–208. https://doi.org/10.1016/j.cps.2004.12.001.
16. Singer AJ, Clark RA. Cutaneous wound healing. N Engl J Med. 1999;341(10):738–46. https://doi.org/10.1056/NEJM199909023411006.
17. Natelson EA, Lynch EC, Alfrey CP Jr, Gross JB. Heparin-induced thrombocytopenia. An unexpected response to treatment of consumption coagulopathy. Ann Intern Med. 1969;71(6):1121–5.
18. Calvete JJ. On the structure and function of platelet integrin alpha IIb beta 3, the fibrinogen receptor. Proc Soc Exp Biol Med. 1995;208(4):346–60.
19. Ley K. Leukocyte adhesion to vascular endothelium. J Reconstr Microsurg. 1992;8(6):495–503. https://doi.org/10.1055/s-2007-1006736.
20. Witko-Sarsat V, Rieu P, Descamps-Latscha B, Lesavre P, Halbwachs-Mecarelli L. Neutrophils: molecules, functions and pathophysiological aspects. Lab Invest. 2000;80(5):617–53.
21. Andre-Levigne D, Modarressi A, Pepper MS, Pittet-Cuenod B. Reactive oxygen species and NOX enzymes are emerging as key players in cutaneous wound repair. Int J Mol Sci. 2017;18(10). https://doi.org/10.3390/ijms18102149.
22. Gawronska-Kozak B, Bogacki M, Rim JS, Monroe WT, Manuel JA. Scarless skin repair in immunodeficient mice. Wound Repair Regen. 2006;14(3):265–76. https://doi.org/10.1111/j.1743-6109.2006.00121.x.
23. Leibovich SJ, Ross R. The role of the macrophage in wound repair. A study with hydrocortisone and antimacrophage serum. Am J Pathol. 1975;78(1):71–100.
24. Murphy MA, Joyce WP, Condron C, Bouchier-Hayes D. A reduction in serum cytokine levels parallels healing of venous ulcers in patients undergoing compression therapy. Eur J Vasc Endovasc Surg. 2002;23(4):349–52. https://doi.org/10.1053/ejvs.2002.1597.
25. Helme RD, Eglezos A, Hosking CS. Substance P induces chemotaxis of neutrophils in normal and capsaicin-treated rats. Immunol Cell Biol. 1987;65(Pt 3):267–9. https://doi.org/10.1038/icb.1987.30.
26. Kavelaars A, Jeurissen F, Heijnen CJ. Substance P receptors and signal transduction in leukocytes. Immunomethods. 1994;5(1):41–8.
27. Ziche M, Morbidelli L, Masini E, Amerini S, Granger HJ, Maggi CA, et al. Nitric oxide mediates angiogenesis in vivo and endothelial cell growth and migration in vitro promoted by substance P. J Clin Invest. 1994;94(5):2036–44. https://doi.org/10.1172/JCI117557.
28. Ziche M, Morbidelli L, Pacini M, Geppetti P, Alessandri G, Maggi CA. Substance P stimulates neovascularization in vivo and proliferation of cultured endothelial cells. Microvasc Res. 1990;40(2):264–78.
29. Paus R, Heinzelmann T, Robicsek S, Czarnetzki BM, Maurer M. Substance P stimulates murine epidermal keratinocyte proliferation and dermal mast cell degranulation in situ. Arch Dermatol Res. 1995;287(5):500–2.
30. Scott JR, Muangman PR, Tamura RN, Zhu KQ, Liang Z, Anthony J, et al. Substance P levels and neutral endopeptidase activity in acute burn wounds and hypertrophic scar. Plast Reconstr Surg. 2005;115(4):1095–102.
31. Scott JR, Muangman P, Gibran NS. Making sense of hypertrophic scar: a role for nerves. Wound Repair Regen. 2007;15(Suppl 1):S27–31. https://doi.org/10.1111/j.1524-475X.2007.00222.x.
32. Luster AD, Cardiff RD, MacLean JA, Crowe K, Granstein RD. Delayed wound healing and disorganized neovascularization in transgenic mice expressing the IP-10 chemokine. Proc Assoc Am Physicians. 1998;110(3):183–96.
33. Akershoek JJ, Brouwer KM, Vlig M, Boekema B, Beelen RHJ, Middelkoop E, et al. Differential effects of losartan and atorvastatin in partial and full thickness burn wounds. PLoS One. 2017;12(6):e0179350. https://doi.org/10.1371/journal.pone.0179350.
34. Akershoek JJJ, Brouwer KM, Vlig M, Boekema B, Beelen RHJ, Middelkoop E, et al. Early intervention by captopril does not improve wound healing of partial thickness burn wounds in a rat model. Burns. 2018;44(2):429–35. https://doi.org/10.1016/j.burns.2017.08.008.
35. Grinnell F. Fibroblasts, myofibroblasts, and wound contraction. J Cell Biol. 1994;124(4):401–4.
36. Liechty KW, Adzick NS, Crombleholme TM. Diminished interleukin 6 (IL-6) production during scarless human fetal wound repair. Cytokine. 2000;12(6):671–6. https://doi.org/10.1006/cyto.1999.0598.
37. Spyrou GE, Naylor IL. The effect of basic fibroblast growth factor on scarring. Br J Plast Surg. 2002;55(4):275–82.
38. Rennekampff HO, Hansbrough JF, Kiessig V, Dore C, Sticherling M, Schroder JM. Bioactive interleukin-8 is expressed in wounds and enhances wound healing. J Surg Res. 2000;93(1):41–54. https://doi.org/10.1006/jsre.2000.5892.
39. Smith PD, Kuhn MA, Franz MG, Wachtel TL, Wright TE, Robson MC. Initiating the inflammatory phase of incisional healing prior to tissue injury. J Surg Res. 2000;92(1):11–7. https://doi.org/10.1006/jsre.2000.5851.
40. Steed DL. Clinical evaluation of recombinant human platelet-derived growth factor for the treatment of lower extremity diabetic ulcers. Diabetic Ulcer Study Group. J Vasc Surg. 1995;21(1):71–8; discussion 9–81
41. Pierce GF, Mustoe TA, Lingelbach J, Masakowski VR, Gramates P, Deuel TF. Transforming growth factor beta reverses the glucocorticoid-induced wound-healing deficit in rats: possible regulation in macrophages by platelet-derived growth factor. Proc Natl Acad Sci U S A. 1989;86(7):2229–33.
42. Tredget EE, Wang R, Shen Q, Scott PG, Ghahary A. Transforming growth factor-beta mRNA and protein in hypertrophic scar tissues and fibroblasts: antagonism by IFN-alpha and IFN-gamma in vitro and in vivo. J Interferon Cytokine Res. 2000;20(2):143–51. https://doi.org/10.1089/107999000312540.
43. Gabriel VA. Transforming growth factor-beta and angiotensin in fibrosis and burn injuries. J Burn Care Res. 2009;30(3):471–81. https://doi.org/10.1097/BCR.0b013e3181a28ddb.
44. Mills RE, Taylor KR, Podshivalova K, McKay DB, Jameson JM. Defects in skin gamma delta T cell function contribute to delayed wound repair in rapamycin-treated mice. J Immunol. 2008;181(6):3974–83.
45. http://www.fiercebiotech.com/biotech/juvista-eu-phase-3-trial-results.
46. Nissen NN, Polverini PJ, Koch AE, Volin MV, Gamelli RL, DiPietro LA. Vascular endothelial growth factor mediates angiogenic activ-

ity during the proliferative phase of wound healing. Am J Pathol. 1998;152(6):1445–52.
47. Nagy JA, Dvorak AM, Dvorak HF. VEGF-A and the induction of pathological angiogenesis. Annu Rev Pathol. 2007;2:251–75. https://doi.org/10.1146/annurev.pathol.2.010506.134925.
48. Hopf HW, Gibson JJ, Angeles AP, Constant JS, Feng JJ, Rollins MD, et al. Hyperoxia and angiogenesis. Wound Repair Regen. 2005;13(6):558–64. https://doi.org/10.1111/j.1524-475X.2005.00078.x.
49. Shweiki D, Itin A, Soffer D, Keshet E. Vascular endothelial growth factor induced by hypoxia may mediate hypoxia-initiated angiogenesis. Nature. 1992;359(6398):843–5. https://doi.org/10.1038/359843a0.
50. Packer L, Fuehr K. Low oxygen concentration extends the lifespan of cultured human diploid cells. Nature. 1977;267(5610):423–5.
51. Wong VW, Akaishi S, Longaker MT, Gurtner GC. Pushing back: wound mechanotransduction in repair and regeneration. J Invest Dermatol. 2011;131(11):2186–96. https://doi.org/10.1038/jid.2011.212.
52. Wong VW, Longaker MT, Gurtner GC. Soft tissue mechanotransduction in wound healing and fibrosis. Semin Cell Dev Biol. 2012;23(9):981–6. https://doi.org/10.1016/j.semcdb.2012.09.010.
53. Ennis WJ, Meneses P, Borhani M. Push-pull theory: using mechanotransduction to achieve tissue perfusion and wound healing in complex cases. Gynecol Oncol. 2008;111(2 Suppl):S81–6. https://doi.org/10.1016/j.ygyno.2008.07.054.
54. Guo S, Dipietro LA. Factors affecting wound healing. J Dent Res. 2010;89(3):219–29. https://doi.org/10.1177/0022034509359125.
55. Park JE, Barbul A. Understanding the role of immune regulation in wound healing. Am J Surg. 2004;187(5A):11S–6S. https://doi.org/10.1016/S0002-9610(03)00296-4.
56. Jameson J, Ugarte K, Chen N, Yachi P, Fuchs E, Boismenu R, et al. A role for skin gammadelta T cells in wound repair. Science. 2002;296(5568):747–9. https://doi.org/10.1126/science.1069639.
57. Santoro MM, Gaudino G. Cellular and molecular facets of keratinocyte reepithelization during wound healing. Exp Cell Res. 2005;304(1):274–86. https://doi.org/10.1016/j.yexcr.2004.10.033.
58. Martin P. Wound healing—aiming for perfect skin regeneration. Science. 1997;276(5309):75–81.
59. Oshima H, Rochat A, Kedzia C, Kobayashi K, Barrandon Y. Morphogenesis and renewal of hair follicles from adult multipotent stem cells. Cell. 2001;104(2):233–45.
60. Taylor G, Lehrer MS, Jensen PJ, Sun TT, Lavker RM. Involvement of follicular stem cells in forming not only the follicle but also the epidermis. Cell. 2000;102(4):451–61.
61. Gurtner GC, Werner S, Barrandon Y, Longaker MT. Wound repair and regeneration. Nature. 2008;453(7193):314–21. https://doi.org/10.1038/nature07039.
62. Ito M, Liu Y, Yang Z, Nguyen J, Liang F, Morris RJ, et al. Stem cells in the hair follicle bulge contribute to wound repair but not to homeostasis of the epidermis. Nat Med. 2005;11(12):1351–4. https://doi.org/10.1038/nm1328.
63. Levy V, Lindon C, Harfe BD, Morgan BA. Distinct stem cell populations regenerate the follicle and interfollicular epidermis. Dev Cell. 2005;9(6):855–61. https://doi.org/10.1016/j.devcel.2005.11.003.
64. Ito M, Yang Z, Andl T, Cui C, Kim N, Millar SE, et al. Wnt-dependent de novo hair follicle regeneration in adult mouse skin after wounding. Nature. 2007;447(7142):316–20. https://doi.org/10.1038/nature05766.
65. Wodarz A, Nusse R. Mechanisms of Wnt signaling in development. Annu Rev Cell Dev Biol. 1998;14:59–88. https://doi.org/10.1146/annurev.cellbio.14.1.59.
66. Toy LW. Matrix metalloproteinases: their function in tissue repair. J Wound Care. 2005;14(1):20–2. https://doi.org/10.12968/jowc.2005.14.1.26720.
67. Meschiari CA, Jung M, Iyer RP, Yabluchanskiy A, Toba H, Garrett MR, et al. Macrophage overexpression of matrix metalloproteinase-9 in aged mice improves diastolic physiology and cardiac wound healing following myocardial infarction. Am J Physiol Heart Circ Physiol. 2018;314(2):H224–35. https://doi.org/10.1152/ajpheart.00453.2017.
68. Lawrence WT. Physiology of the acute wound. Clin Plast Surg. 1998;25(3):321–40.
69. Fathke C, Wilson L, Hutter J, Kapoor V, Smith A, Hocking A, et al. Contribution of bone marrow-derived cells to skin: collagen deposition and wound repair. Stem Cells. 2004;22(5):812–22. https://doi.org/10.1634/stemcells.22-5-812.
70. Brittan M, Braun KM, Reynolds LE, Conti FJ, Reynolds AR, Poulsom R, et al. Bone marrow cells engraft within the epidermis and proliferate in vivo with no evidence of cell fusion. J Pathol. 2005;205(1):1–13. https://doi.org/10.1002/path.1682.
71. Deng W, Han Q, Liao L, Li C, Ge W, Zhao Z, et al. Engrafted bone marrow-derived flk-(1+) mesenchymal stem cells regenerate skin tissue. Tissue Eng. 2005;11(1–2):110–9. https://doi.org/10.1089/ten.2005.11.110.
72. Wu Y, Chen L, Scott PG, Tredget EE. Mesenchymal stem cells enhance wound healing through differentiation and angiogenesis. Stem Cells. 2007;25(10):2648–59. https://doi.org/10.1634/stemcells.2007-0226.
73. Chen P, Hung WW. Geriatric orthopedic co-management of older adults with hip fracture: an emerging standard. Ann Transl Med. 2015;3(16):224. https://doi.org/10.3978/j.issn.2305-5839.2015.07.13.
74. Kwon DS, Gao X, Liu YB, Dulchavsky DS, Danyluk AL, Bansal M, et al. Treatment with bone marrow-derived stromal cells accelerates wound healing in diabetic rats. Int Wound J. 2008;5(3):453–63. https://doi.org/10.1111/j.1742-481X.2007.00408.x.
75. Suh W, Kim KL, Kim JM, Shin IS, Lee YS, Lee JY, et al. Transplantation of endothelial progenitor cells accelerates dermal wound healing with increased recruitment of monocytes/macrophages and neovascularization. Stem Cells. 2005;23(10):1571–8. https://doi.org/10.1634/stemcells.2004-0340.
76. Barcelos LS, Duplaa C, Krankel N, Graiani G, Invernici G, Katare R, et al. Human CD133+ progenitor cells promote the healing of diabetic ischemic ulcers by paracrine stimulation of angiogenesis and activation of Wnt signaling. Circ Res. 2009;104(9):1095–102. https://doi.org/10.1161/CIRCRESAHA.108.192138.
77. Bucala R, Spiegel LA, Chesney J, Hogan M, Cerami A. Circulating fibrocytes define a new leukocyte subpopulation that mediates tissue repair. Mol Med. 1994;1(1):71–81.
78. Yang L, Scott PG, Dodd C, Medina A, Jiao H, Shankowsky HA, et al. Identification of fibrocytes in postburn hypertrophic scar. Wound Repair Regen. 2005;13(4):398–404. https://doi.org/10.1111/j.1067-1927.2005.130407.x.
79. Wang J, Dodd C, Shankowsky HA, Scott PG, Tredget EE, Wound Healing Research Group. Deep dermal fibroblasts contribute to hypertrophic scarring. Lab Invest. 2008;88(12):1278–90. https://doi.org/10.1038/labinvest.2008.101.
80. Mori L, Bellini A, Stacey MA, Schmidt M, Mattoli S. Fibrocytes contribute to the myofibroblast population in wounded skin and originate from the bone marrow. Exp Cell Res. 2005;304(1):81–90. https://doi.org/10.1016/j.yexcr.2004.11.011.
81. Yagmur C, Akaishi S, Ogawa R, Guneren E. Mechanical receptor-related mechanisms in scar management: a review and hypothesis. Plast Reconstr Surg. 2010;126(2):426–34. https://doi.org/10.1097/PRS.0b013e3181df715d.
82. Souba WW, Fink MP, Jurkovic GJ. ACS surgery: principles and practice. BC Decker, Inc.; 2007.
83. Rinker B. The evils of nicotine: an evidence-based guide to smoking and plastic surgery. Ann Plast Surg. 2013;70(5):599–605. https://doi.org/10.1097/SAP.0b013e3182764fcd.

84. Robson MC. Wound infection. A failure of wound healing caused by an imbalance of bacteria. Surg Clin North Am. 1997;77(3):637–50.
85. Menke NB, Ward KR, Witten TM, Bonchev DG, Diegelmann RF. Impaired wound healing. Clin Dermatol. 2007;25(1):19–25. https://doi.org/10.1016/j.clindermatol.2006.12.005.
86. Gibbs J, Cull W, Henderson W, Daley J, Hur K, Khuri SF. Preoperative serum albumin level as a predictor of operative mortality and morbidity: results from the National VA Surgical Risk Study. Arch Surg. 1999;134(1):36–42.
87. Jeschke MG, Herndon DN, Ebener C, Barrow RE, Jauch KW. Nutritional intervention high in vitamins, protein, amino acids, and omega3 fatty acids improves protein metabolism during the hypermetabolic state after thermal injury. Arch Surg. 2001;136(11):1301–6.
88. Desneves KJ, Todorovic BE, Cassar A, Crowe TC. Treatment with supplementary arginine, vitamin C and zinc in patients with pressure ulcers: a randomised controlled trial. Clin Nutr. 2005;24(6):979–87. https://doi.org/10.1016/j.clnu.2005.06.011.
89. Williams JZ, Abumrad N, Barbul A. Effect of a specialized amino acid mixture on human collagen deposition. Ann Surg. 2002;236(3):369–74.; ; discussion 74–5. https://doi.org/10.1097/01.SLA.0000027527.01984.00.
90. Mandell SP, Gibran NS. Early enteral nutrition for burn injury. Adv Wound Care (New Rochelle). 2014;3(1):64–70. https://doi.org/10.1089/wound.2012.0382.
91. Nordlund MJ, Pham TN, Gibran NS. Micronutrients after burn injury: a review. J Burn Care Res. 2014;35(2):121–33. https://doi.org/10.1097/BCR.0b013e318290110b.
92. Williams FN, Herndon DN, Kulp GA, Jeschke MG. Propranolol decreases cardiac work in a dose-dependent manner in severely burned children. Surgery. 2011;149(2):231–9. https://doi.org/10.1016/j.surg.2010.05.015.
93. Demling RH, Orgill DP. The anticatabolic and wound healing effects of the testosterone analog oxandrolone after severe burn injury. J Crit Care. 2000;15(1):12–7. https://doi.org/10.1053/jcrc.2000.0150012.
94. Pham TN, Klein MB, Gibran NS, Arnoldo BD, Gamelli RL, Silver GM, et al. Impact of oxandrolone treatment on acute outcomes after severe burn injury. J Burn Care Res. 2008;29(6):902–6. https://doi.org/10.1097/BCR.0b013e31818ba14d.
95. Ali A, Herndon DN, Mamachen A, Hasan S, Andersen CR, Grogans RJ, et al. Propranolol attenuates hemorrhage and accelerates wound healing in severely burned adults. Crit Care. 2015;19:217. https://doi.org/10.1186/s13054-015-0913-x.
96. Wicke C, Halliday B, Allen D, Roche NS, Scheuenstuhl H, Spencer MM, et al. Effects of steroids and retinoids on wound healing. Arch Surg. 2000;135(11):1265–70.
97. Nathens AB, Neff MJ, Jurkovich GJ, Klotz P, Farver K, Ruzinski JT, et al. Randomized, prospective trial of antioxidant supplementation in critically ill surgical patients. Ann Surg. 2002;236(6):814–22.
98. Fernandez-Madrid F, Prasad AS, Oberleas D. Effect of zinc deficiency on nucleic acids, collagen, and noncollagenous protein of the connective tissue. J Lab Clin Med. 1973;82(6):951–61.
99. Andrews M, Gallagher-Allred C. The role of zinc in wound healing. Adv Wound Care. 1999;12(3):137–8.
100. Macon WL, Pories WJ. The effect of iron deficiency anemia on wound healing. Surgery. 1971;69(5):792–6.
101. Sengupta A, Lichti UF, Carlson BA, Ryscavage AO, Gladyshev VN, Yuspa SH, et al. Selenoproteins are essential for proper keratinocyte function and skin development. PLoS One. 2010;5(8):e12249. https://doi.org/10.1371/journal.pone.0012249.
102. Ogawa R, Akaishi S. Endothelial dysfunction may play a key role in keloid and hypertrophic scar pathogenesis—keloids and hypertrophic scars may be vascular disorders. Med Hypotheses. 2016;96:51–60. https://doi.org/10.1016/j.mehy.2016.09.024.
103. Allah KC, Yeo S, Kossoko H, Assi Dje Bi Dje V, Richard Kadio M. [Keloid scars on black skin: myth or reality]. Ann Chir Plast Esthet. 2013;58(2):115–22. https://doi.org/10.1016/j.anplas.2012.02.005.
104. Ogawa R, Okai K, Tokumura F, Mori K, Ohmori Y, Huang C, et al. The relationship between skin stretching/contraction and pathologic scarring: the important role of mechanical forces in keloid generation. Wound Repair Regen. 2012;20(2):149–57. https://doi.org/10.1111/j.1524-475X.2012.00766.x.
105. Ogawa R. Keloid and hypertrophic scars are the result of chronic inflammation in the reticular dermis. Int J Mol Sci. 2017;18(3). https://doi.org/10.3390/ijms18030606.
106. Thompson CM, Hocking AM, Honari S, Muffley LA, Ga M, Gibran NS. Genetic risk factors for hypertrophic scar development. J Burn Care Res. 2013;34(5):477–82. https://doi.org/10.1097/BCR.0b013e3182a2aa41.
107. Sood RF, Hocking AM, Muffley LA, Ga M, Honari S, Reiner AP, et al. Genome-wide association study of postburn scarring identifies a novel protective variant. Ann Surg. 2015;262(4):563–9. https://doi.org/10.1097/SLA.0000000000001439.
108. Colwell AS, Phan TT, Kong W, Longaker MT, Lorenz PH. Hypertrophic scar fibroblasts have increased connective tissue growth factor expression after transforming growth factor-beta stimulation. Plast Reconstr Surg. 2005;116(5):1387–90; discussion 91–2
109. Lu L, Saulis AS, Liu WR, Roy NK, Chao JD, Ledbetter S, et al. The temporal effects of anti-TGF-beta1, 2, and 3 monoclonal antibody on wound healing and hypertrophic scar formation. J Am Coll Surg. 2005;201(3):391–7. https://doi.org/10.1016/j.jamcollsurg.2005.03.032.
110. Tuan TL, Nichter LS. The molecular basis of keloid and hypertrophic scar formation. Mol Med Today. 1998;4(1):19–24. https://doi.org/10.1016/S1357-4310(97)80541-2.
111. Ladwig GP, Robson MC, Liu R, Kuhn MA, Muir DF, Schultz GS. Ratios of activated matrix metalloproteinase-9 to tissue inhibitor of matrix metalloproteinase-1 in wound fluids are inversely correlated with healing of pressure ulcers. Wound Repair Regen. 2002;10(1):26–37.
112. Bazalinski D, Przybek-Mita J, Baranska B, Wiech P. Marjolin's ulcer in chronic wounds—review of available literature. Contemp Oncol (Pozn). 2017;21(3):197–202. https://doi.org/10.5114/wo.2017.70109.
113. Copcu E. Marjolin's ulcer: a preventable complication of burns? Plast Reconstr Surg. 2009;124(1):156e–64e. https://doi.org/10.1097/PRS.0b013e3181a8082e.
114. Trent JT, Kirsner RS. Wounds and malignancy. Adv Skin Wound Care. 2003;16(1):31–4.
115. Da LC, Huang YZ, Xie HQ. Progress in development of bioderived materials for dermal wound healing. Regen Biomater. 2017;4(5):325–34. https://doi.org/10.1093/rb/rbx025.
116. Atarzadeh F, Kamalinejad M, Dastgheib L, Amin G, Jaladat AM, Nimrouzi M. Cassia fistula: a remedy from traditional Persian medicine for treatment of cutaneous lesions of pemphigus vulgaris. Avicenna J Phytomed. 2017;7(2):107–15.
117. Patel S, Srivastava S, Singh MR, Singh D. Preparation and optimization of chitosan-gelatin films for sustained delivery of lupeol for wound healing. Int J Biol Macromol. 2018;107(Pt B):1888–97. https://doi.org/10.1016/j.ijbiomac.2017.10.056.

Outpatient Burn Management 33

Charles J. Yowler and Tammy L. Coffee

33.1 Introduction

The majority of burn injuries are managed in the outpatient setting. Of the 450,000 burn injuries reported by the American Burn Association for the year 2012, only 40,000 were hospitalized. The remaining 91% of patients received immediate and follow-up care from emergency rooms, primary care physicians, and outpatient burn or plastic surgery clinics [1].

Due to limitations in outpatient epidemiologic studies and the National Burn Repository's focus on inpatient data, there is little data on the demographics of outpatient burn patients. Available studies suggest that the outpatient burn population is younger with burns more often caused by scald and contact injury than flames. The average total body surface area of outpatients is approximately 3%.

Historically, up to 33% of all burn center admissions were for pain control and wound care. Advances in pain management and new wound care products now make it possible to treat more victims entirely as outpatients [2]. Second-degree burns less than 15% in adults and 10% in children are now potential candidates for outpatient care. Advances in wound products also make it possible to more quickly transition from inpatient to outpatient care in patients with large burns [3].

33.2 Initial Evaluation and Selection of Patients

The success of outpatient management is dependent upon the selection of appropriate patients (Table 33.1). While the American Burn Association has established criteria for referral to a burn center (Table 33.2), these factors do not preclude outpatient management in the appropriate patient. Depending on size, burns of the face, hands, genitals, and feet may be managed in the ambulatory setting. The criteria for outpatient management vary based on the burn centers experience

Table 33.1 Factors to consider for outpatient management

Factors
• Size, depth, and location of burn
• Patient's age, comorbidities, and functional state
• Concern for abuse or neglect
• Home support including assistance in wound care and transportation

Table 33.2 Burn Center referral criteria

Burn injuries that should be referred to a burn center include:
1. Partial thickness burns greater than 10% total body surface area (TBSA)
2. Burns that involve face, hands, feet, genitalia, perineum, or major joints
3. Third-degree burns in any age group
4. Electrical burns, including lightning injury
5. Chemical burns
6. Inhalation injury
7. Burn injury in patients with preexisting medical disorders that could complicate management, prolong recovery, or affect mortality
8. Any patient with burns and concomitant trauma (such as fractures) in which the burn injury poses the greatest risk of morbidity or mortality. In such cases, if the trauma poses the greater immediate risk, the patient may be initially stabilized in a trauma center before being transferred to a burn unit. Physician judgment will be necessary in such situations and should be in concert with the regional medical control plan and triage protocols
9. Burned children in hospitals without qualified personnel or equipment for the care of children
10. Burn injury in patients who will require special social, emotional, or rehabilitative intervention

Excerpted from Guidelines for the Operation of Burn Centers (pp. 79–86), Resources for Optimal Care of the Injured Patient 2006, Committee on Trauma, American College of Surgeons

C. J. Yowler (✉)
MetroHealth Medical Center, Cleveland, OH, USA

Case Western Reserve University, Cleveland, OH, USA
e-mail: cyowler@metrohealth.org

T. L. Coffee
MetroHealth Medical Center, Cleveland, OH, USA
e-mail: tcoffee@metrohealth.org

M. G. Jeschke et al. (eds.), *Handbook of Burns Volume 1*, https://doi.org/10.1007/978-3-030-18940-2_33

and resources and include burns less than 15% total body surface area not requiring full resuscitation or operative procedures.

Comorbidities including cardiac disease, COPD, chronic kidney disease, dementia or psychological impairment, diabetes mellitus, and/or infirmity may complicate initial outpatient care. It may be necessary to admit these patients initially until a more in-depth assessment of their overall medical condition and home support system can be completed. Nevertheless, if the medical conditions are controlled and the patients' home support is acceptable or can be arranged, patients with comorbidities are excellent candidates for outpatient management.

Children are excellent candidates for outpatient care. One must ascertain the comfort of the family with outpatient care. The majority of parents clearly prefer outpatient care due to the decrease in family disruption. The child also often has less psychological stress in the home environment. However, dressing changes in children may require multiple caregivers, and the injured child who cannot return for dressing care may require admission.

Nonthermal injuries can also be treated on an outpatient basis. Low voltage household current (110–220 V) electrical injuries usually result in minor tissue damage. However, they may be associated with a syncopal event due to a concurrent dysrhythmia. Patients without syncope and with normal screening EKG may be treated as an outpatient without concern for subsequent cardiac complication. Patients with high voltage injuries (<1000 V), syncope, or EKG changes should be admitted for serial exams and telemetry.

Chemical burns involving less than 15% total body surface area may also be treated on an outpatient basis depending on the depth and location of the burn. Ocular involvement must be ruled out with an appropriate history and examination. Following appropriate lavage of the wound, an outpatient dressing may be applied. However, conversion to a deeper depth is common and patients selected for outpatient therapy must be able to return within 24–48 h for a repeat examination. Patients exposed to toxic chemicals such as hydrofluoric or chromic acid require admission.

Review of the patient's social situation is an essential component of the evaluation for outpatient care. Children and geriatric patients must have a safe home environment. There can be no suspicion of abuse or psychological conditions impairing the patient's safety. Family or friends must be available to support the patient who often has impairments in mobility and use of his limbs following a burn injury. Finally, there must be transportation available for return clinic visits. It is often necessary to admit a patient for a short period of time while the social support system is evaluated.

33.2.1 Initial Wound Management

The recommended immediate treatment of minor thermal burns is cool running water. Avoid the use of ice or ice water [4]. Cleaning the wound with a mild antibacterial soap and water is recommended. Careful debridement of ruptured blisters and other devitalized tissue should be performed. The patient's tetanus vaccination status must be assessed and tetanus toxoid administered if appropriate.

The management of intact blisters is controversial [5]. Blisters arise usually in the setting of superficial partial thickness injury by leakage of fluid from heat injured vessels deep in the zone of coagulation. Release of plasma protein and skin degradation products into the blister osmotically draws yet more fluid causing enlargement of a blister over a period of time.

Acceptable practices for managing blisters include leaving them intact, aspirating blister fluid and leaving the devitalized epidermis intact or unroofing the devitalized epidermis [6]. Clinicians who believe that the blisters should remain intact state that the blister indicates a superficial burn that will spontaneously heal in a few weeks. The intact blister creates its own biologic dressing, thereby keeping the wound clean, moist, and protected. The wound is protected from air making it less painful. Leaving burned blisters intact also reduces bacteria colonization of the wound. Burn blister fluid may stimulate the wound healing process since it contains multiple growth factors.

The case for debriding blisters is supported by studies that demonstrate that blister fluid depresses immune function by impairing neutrophil function. Inflammation is enhanced by the presence of metabolites of arachidonic acid in the blister fluid. Blister fluid may also provide a culture medium growth of any bacteria that enters that space.

The majority of evidence supports leaving blisters intact. Large blisters with thin walls should be debrided as they will likely rupture on their own, and it is beneficial from an infection standpoint to apply a dressing directly to the wound bed. Thicker blisters that interfere with proper range of motion of a joint should be aspirated leaving the blistered skin to protect to cover the wound. If the blister remains intact and the wound is a superficial partial thickness burn, spontaneous re-absorption of the fluid will begin within 1 week.

Intermediate and deep second degree burns may convert to full-thickness injury over 24–48 h. The outpatient management of these deeper partial thickness burns require repeat evaluation at 48–72 h. Patients unable to return within that time period may require admission.

33.2.2 Topical Burn Care and Dressings

The goal of topical burn care and dressings are to minimize pain, decrease the risk of infection, promote wound healing, minimize cosmetic deformity, and preserve function. Burn wounds heal best in a moist but not wet environment that promotes epithelialization and prevents cellular dehydration. This can best be accomplished by applying either a topical agent or an occlusive dressing to minimize fluid loss. There are a large number of excellent agents available, and all of them can be effectively employed when properly used by an experienced burn care provider (Table 33.3).

In general, one of two methods are used to treat partial thickness burns: an open method utilizing topical antimicro-

Table 33.3 Commonly used topical agents for burn wounds

Agent	Description	Action	Advantages	Disadvantages
Silver sulfadiazine (SSD)	Nontoxic salt of silver sulfadiazine in water-based cream	Binds to bacterial cell membranes and interferes with DNA synthesis	Painless Wide-spectrum antimicrobial action against gram-positive and gram-negative organisms Long shelf life Delays eschar separation to a lesser degree than do many other topical drugs Used for deep partial and full-thickness wounds	**Delays healing** **Stains tissue** **Contraindicated in sulfa allergy, pregnant women, newborns, and nursing mothers**
Mafenide acetate (Sulfamylon)	Soft white, non-staining cream, water-based topical cream	Bacteriostatic action against many gram-negative and gram-positive organisms	Effective against pseudomonas Penetrates thick eschar Used for deep burns and exposed cartilage	**Can be painful on application** **May delay healing or cause metabolic acidosis**
Bacitracin	Topical cream	Narrow antimicrobial coverage	Inexpensive Painless Can be used on face or near mucous membranes	**Requires frequent dressing changes** **May cause urticaria, burning** **Does not penetrate eschar**
Mupirocin (Bactroban)	Topical antibacterial cream	Bacteriostatic at low concentrations and bactericidal at high concentrations	Good gram-positive antimicrobial coverage Painless Can be used on face Active against most strains of methicillin-resistant *S. aureus*	**Expensive** **Requires frequent dressing changes**
Hydrocolloid (Duoderm)	Hydrophilic absorptive Dressing	Has a triple hydrocolloid matrix with a viral and bacterial barrier Forms a hydrophilic gel which facilitates autolytic debridement	Less pain Shorter time to wound closure than SSD Decrease dressing change and pain Inexpensive Keep underlying tissue moist	**Cannot be used with large exuding wounds**
Impregnated nonadherent gauze (Xeroform, Vaseline gauze, Adaptic)	Semi-occlusive Nonabsorptive dressing		Provides a nonadherent barrier over the burn Used for partial thickness burns Maintains a moist environment deodorizing agent Clings and conforms to all body contours	**No antimicrobial activity**
Silicone (Mepitel)	Nonabsorptive dressing	Conforms to shape of wound and allows for drainage of exudate to secondary bandage	Expensive Painless Decrease dressing changes Highly transparent May be left in place for 14 days Protect skin from additional trauma	**No antimicrobial activity** **Expensive**

(continued)

Table 33.3 (continued)

Agent	Description	Action	Advantages	Disadvantages
Silver-impregnated dressing				
Aquacel Ag	Nylon, silver-impregnated, antimicrobial, absorbent dressing	The silver in the dressing kills wound bacteria	Broad-spectrum antimicrobial coverage decreases dressing changes Reduces pain Decreases use of pain medications Faster wound closure than with standard therapies Decrease total cost compared with SSD	**Aquacel Ag is not compatible with oil-based products, such as petrolatum**
Mepilex Ag	Absorptive silicone dressing	Antimicrobial foam dressing that absorbs exudate and maintains a moist wound environment	Decrease pain Effects up to 7 days Nonadhering to the moist wound bed Easy application	**Do not use during MRI** **Do not use with hypochloride solutions or hydrogen peroxide** **Expensive**
Acticoat	Nonabsorptive dressing	Delivers low concentrations of silver when moisten with sterile water	Broad-spectrum antimicrobial coverage Nonadherent Reduces pain Decreases dressing changes	**Expensive** **May dry out and adhere to wound** **Do not use with oil-based products**
Collagenase (Santyl)	**Enzymatic debriding ointment**	**Digests collagen in necrotic tissue**	**Removes nonliving tissue without harming granulation tissue** **May be used with barrier dressing**	**Do not use dressings containing silver (Ag) or iodine (I_2)** **No antimicrobial activity**

bial agents covered by a nonadherent dressing or a closed method which uses occlusive dressings [7].

The purpose of the topical antimicrobial agent is to minimize bacterial and fungal colonization that may result in infection [8]. Limited randomized studies exist to support any particular agent. Topical silver sulfadiazine is a common agent used for partial thickness burns. However, it is contraindicated in patients with sulfa allergy. It should also be avoided in pregnancy, lactating women, or newborns [9]. Recent studies have demonstrated that silver sulfadiazine inhibits keratinocyte replication [10] and therefore delays healing of partial thickness burns and may result in increased scarring. A 2008 Cochrane review found that when compared to silver sulfadiazine, newer occlusive dressings resulted in faster healing, decreased pain, fewer dressing changes, and improved patient satisfaction.

Small studies have compared newer silver-based dressings with silver sulfadiazine. These have concluded that the use of these newer dressings should be considered because they result in faster healing, decreased pain, fewer dressing changes, and improved patient satisfaction. In the majority of studies, they were also more cost-effective. However, silver sulfadiazine may still be preferred in partial thickness burns with increased risk of infection such as contaminated wounds and burns of the perineum and diabetic foot.

Superficial second-degree wounds of the face are commonly treated with a clear antibacterial ointment such as bacitracin. Wounds around the eyes and ears can be treated with topical ophthalmic antibiotic ointments. Mupirocin may be used in patients known to be colonized with MRSA or if crusting of facial burns occur, suggesting the development of impetigo. Deeper burns to the external ear may require mafenide acetate as it penetrates the eschar and prevents purulent infection of the cartilage.

The closed method utilizes a biologic of synthetic dressing without topical application of an antimicrobial agent. Advocates of this method argue that occlusive dressings speed up wound healing. The moist environment enhances epithelial proliferation and collagen remodeling under the occlusive dressings. The occlusive dressings also provide protection and avoids damage to the newly found epithelium at the time of dressing changes.

If the occlusive dressing remains dry and intact, it may be left until wound healing is complete. It must however be used in caution with wounds that are not clearly clean and superficial. If an occlusive dressing is placed over devitalized tissue, infection can occur. Leakage of fluid from underneath the occlusive dressing requires aspiration or removal of the dressing.

Clinical trials have been unsuccessful in demonstrating a consistent advantage of occlusive dressing over standard topical open therapy for the management of most partial thickness burns. The tendency of fluid to accumulate under occlusive dressings necessitating early removal often limits their use to small burns with minor blistering. Large moist wounds which are more prone to infection are best treated with a topical antimicrobial agent and dressing or an absorbent dressing impregnated with silver.

33.2.3 Initial Pain Management

Control of pain in the outpatient setting can be difficult, and if pain and anxiety cannot be adequately managed at home, then hospitalization may be required. Narcotics are typically used as first-line treatment. Nonsteroidal anti-inflammatory drugs (NSAIDs) can be used alone or in conjunction with narcotics to assist in pain control. Studies have revealed 600 mg of ibuprofen is as efficacious as 15 mg of oxycodone hydrochloride [11]. NSAIDS should be avoided if there is a possibility of burn excision and grafting. Most patients will require additional dosing for pain during dressing changes and physical therapy. Pain management may be complicated by a history of alcohol or controlled substance abuse.

33.2.4 Instructions for Home Care

Instructions need to include information about pain management and the signs and symptoms of infection. The patient and/or caregivers must be taught how to perform any needed dressings. If necessary, discussions about potential scarring may be required.

Scheduling of follow-up visits during the acute care phase depend on the severity of the burn injury, the dressing used and social factors. If there are no caregivers at home to assist the patient with burn care and dressings, the patient may need to return to the clinic daily for dressing changes. The use of silver products reduces the need for this option. Finally, the patient must always be given a contact phone number that they may use to obtain further information and discuss problems that arise at home.

33.3 Outpatient Clinic Follow-Up

Follow-up clinic visits will vary from days to weeks depending on physician and institutional preferences. The key to the treatment plan, however, lies in the patient's physical, medical, and psychological conditions, along with wound care and therapy compliance.

In the acute burn setting, a superficial partial-thickness burn is expected to heal within 14 days, with a longer healing timeframe anticipated for diabetics, immunocompromised individuals, and the elderly. Areas of concern during this time are infection, edema, wound healing, pain control, and need for operative intervention. In general, weekly clinic visits suffice to ensure appropriate wound healing, pain control, and therapy compliance. This time interval also allows assurance of sufficient dressing and medication supplies and evaluation for the need of additional support services such as home health or outpatient therapy. Monitoring for edema during this time is crucial, since it can lead to immobility and joint stiffness. Use of compression bandages and elevation of affected extremities assist in decreasing edema. Inpatient admission may be necessary if issues arise with wound care, pain control, or therapy that cannot be appropriately managed in the outpatient setting. If the wound has failed to heal within 2 weeks, or a protracted time is anticipated, then surgical intervention can be discussed. Deep- to full-thickness burn injuries may be considered for surgery at any time.

For postoperative patients and those in the nonacute setting, outpatient clinic visits may initially be weekly to ensure therapy compliance and monitor wound healing. Once wound healing is complete, compression garments applied, and compliance demonstrated with physical and occupational therapy, clinic visits can be lengthened everyone to 3 months to evaluate for scar maturation, emergence of hypertrophic scar, and scar contractures. This time interval also allows for evaluating proper fit and utilization of compression garments. A multiteam approach addresses issues with scarring from both its physical (e.g., scar contractures, pruritus) and psychological implications. Work and school reentry programs can be initiated and patients introduced to social support groups such as SOAR (Survivors Offering Assistance in Recovery) and other support groups. Operative intervention during this time frame may be necessary for nonhealing wounds and scar contractures. Once scar maturation is completed, and compression garments are discontinued, follow-up clinic visits range from as needed to yearly visits.

33.4 Outpatient Management of Complications

Outpatient care can be complicated by multiple factors such as poor pain control, pruritus, wound infections, and scarring. All of these issues can be successfully managed in the vast majority of patients as an outpatient.

33.4.1 Pain

There are several tactics that can be utilized in the outpatient with unacceptable pain. Taking analgesics on a scheduled rather than as needed basis may improve pain control. If a short-acting agent requiring dosing every 4–6 h was initially prescribed, a change to a longer acting narcotic may improve pain control. Further questioning of the patient concerning timing of pain may also reveal that the pain is unacceptable during dressing changes and/or therapy sessions. Supplemental narcotic preparations given prior to these activities may improve pain control.

Questions concerning the nature of the pain may reveal that the perceived pain is due to inflammatory changes of the wound. This pain is often described as "throbbing pain" or "heat" and may respond to additional scheduled NSAIDs. Anxiety and/or acute stress disorders may also exaggerate the perception of pain. Low doses of scheduled anxiolytics may decrease the total dosage of narcotics required for comfort in patients with these symptoms. Sleep deprivation may also contribute to pain intolerance and may require treatment with appropriate bedtime dosing of narcotics and/or sleep medications. Diphenhydramine is useful if pruritus is interfering with sleep.

Finally, it must be appreciated that there is a subset of patients who will not tolerate any discomfort. Frank discussions about the ability of any drug regiment to completely eliminate pain and discomfort may result in improved patient satisfaction.

33.4.2 Pruritus

Pruritus, or itch, is a common occurrence following burn injury [12]. Pruritus occurs in over 90% of patients in the first month following a burn and may progress to a chronic condition. It is clear that multiple factors may contribute to its intensity.

Early pruritus is primarily due to histamine release from mast cells present in the wound during the phases of connective tissue proliferation and remodeling. Medications that block the histamine H-1 receptor such as cetirizine have been demonstrated to be superior to nonspecific antihistamines such a diphenhydramine. These should be dosed on a schedule basis and not on an as needed schedule.

The contribution of dry skin must also be appreciated. Initial treatment of pruritus must include frequent application and massage of moisturizers into the skin. The frequency of application is more important than the specific ingredient present in the lotion. However, it must also be appreciated that sensitivity to dermatological agents may occur over time. An increase in pruritus with inflammation of the wound may be secondary to the topical agent itself [13]. A combination of moisturizers and scheduled antihistamines will manage pruritus in the majority of patients with early symptoms. More severe pruritus may require application of topical doxepin, a tricyclic antidepressant with potent antihistamine properties. Multiple studies have demonstrated that topical corticosteroids do not reduce burn-related pruritus.

Long-term studies have noted the persistence of pruritus in 87% of patient at 3 months, 70% of patients at 12 months, and 60% of patients at 24 months. Another longitudinal study noted persistence in 40% at 7 years following the injury [14]. In this latter study, the pruritus interfered with sleep in 59% of symptomatic patients. Clinical factors that were associated with the persistence of pruritus included female sex, size of the burn, graft of burn, and size of grafted burn. Wound factors included dry skin and hypertrophic scar.

The contribution of neuropathic pathways in the persistence of pruritus has recently been delineated [15]. Itch-specific neurons in the burn wound are stimulated by neuroinflammatory transmitters present in the burn. This pathway responds to treatment with drugs commonly used in neuropathic pain such as gabapentin and pregabalin.

In summary, the treatment of pruritus requires the combination of adequate lubrication of the skin, anti-histamines, and occasionally agents specific for the neuropathic pathway. Once again improved results are seen when drugs are given on a scheduled basis rather than an as needed basis.

33.4.3 Infection

Infection is the most feared complication in a burn patient. Unfortunately, this results in the common prescription of prophylactic antibiotics and referral for inpatient care. Multiple studies demonstrate no reduction in burn wound infection with the use of prophylactic antibiotics, and this practice should be condemned [16].

A retrospective study of over 2200 outpatient burn patients treated without antibiotics reported an infection rate of 5% [17]. Age, etiology of burn, burn size, peripheral vascular disease, and even homelessness did not increase the risk of infection. Diabetics were found to have an increased infection rate of 15%. A subsequent prospective study of 72 diabetic patients treated initially as outpatients without antibiotics reported an infection rate of 11% [18]. The risk of infection in burns below the knee increased to 62%. However, 71/72 diabetic patients were successfully managed as outpatients including outpatient treatment of these infections.

Cellulitis that occurs during the initial 7–10 days following burn injury is effectively managed as an outpatient. The patient's own microbial flora is usually the bacterial source, and the infection responds to first-generation cephalosporins. Wound cultures have not been shown to be useful. Antibiotics may be altered for patients with known MRSA colonization or for patients with increased risk of gram-negative infections such as diabetics or patients with poor personal hygiene.

Infections occurring after 7–10 days are more likely to represent gram-negative infections. Ciprofloxacin may be added to the antibiotics listed above, and the results of the wound culture may provide useful information.

Outpatient treatment of burn infection is inappropriate if the patient demonstrates systemic toxicity such as weakness, chills, fevers, nausea, or vomiting. Successful outpatient management of wound infection requires frequent clinic visits to evaluate the response to treatment. Thus, outpatient management may not be appropriate if the burn center has limited outpatient availability or if the patient is unable to return for frequent visits.

33.4.4 Outpatient Therapy

A successful outpatient burn program must also provide access to physical and occupational therapy, nutritional support, and psychological services. These services must have clinic hours that parallel those of the outpatient burn clinic, thus reducing the number of trips to the center for the patient and his caretaker. While it may be necessary to arrange for the provision of these services at a medical facility closer to their homes, patients who must return on a frequent scheduled basis to the burn clinic will benefit from specialists familiar with burn patients.

33.4.5 Telemedicine

Finally, the use of telemedicine can serve as adjunct to outpatient burn care for those patients living outside of the specialty burn care region [19]. Acute and nonacute wound care, postoperative dressing changes, scar evaluation, and therapy compliance can be addressed either by interactive synchronous videoconference or by digital imagery. Medical prescriptions can be phoned or faxed to the pharmacy, supplies mailed, and compression garments evaluated for proper fit. In patient satisfaction surveys performed following telemedicine burn care, the satisfaction ratings have been similar to hospital burn clinic visits, with the added benefit of time and economic savings for the patient at the remote location.

Summary Box

- Over 90% of all burn patients may be treated entirely as outpatients.
- Selection for outpatient management must consider clinical factors such as location, size, and depth of burn.
- Patient factors to be considered include comorbidities, ability to care for the wound, social/economic support, and transportation.
- Thin-walled blisters should be aspirated or debrided while thick blisters may be aspirated and left in place.
- Use of silver-impregnated dressings decreases the need for clinic visits which decreases pain and overall cost.
- Early pruritus is treated with lotions and antihistamines while gabapentin or pregabalin is useful in chronic pruritus.
- There is no indication for use of prophylactic antibiotic in burn management.

References

1. American Burn Association. Burn incidence fact sheet, 2012. http://www.burn.org/resources_factsheet.php.
2. Brandt CP, Yurko L, et al. Complete integration of inpatient and outpatient burn care: evolution of an outpatient burn clinic. J Burn Care Rehabil. 1998;19:406–8.
3. Jansen LA, Hynes SL, et al. Reduced length of stay in hospital for burn patients following a change in practice guidelines: financial implications. J Burn Care Res. 2012;33:e275–9.
4. Cuttle L, Pearn J, et al. A review of first aid treatments for burn injuries. Burns. 2009;35:768–75.
5. Rockwell WB, Ehrlich HP. Should blister fluid be evacuated? J Burn Care Rehabil. 1990;11:93–5.
6. Sargent RL. Management of blisters in the partial thickness burn: an integrative research review. J Burn Care Res. 2006;27(1):66–81.
7. Wasiak J, Cleland H, Campbell F. Dressings for superficial and partial thickness burns. Cochrane Database Syst Rev. 2008;(4):CD002106.
8. Greenhalgh DG. Topical antimicrobial agents for burn wounds. Clin Plast Surg. 2009;36:597–606.
9. Fuller FW. The side effects of silver sulfadiazine. J Burns Care Res. 2009;30:464–70.
10. Heyneman A, Hocksema H, et al. The role of silver sulfadiazine in the conservative treatment of partial thickness bur wounds; a systematic review. Burns. 2016;42:1377–86.
11. Richards D. The Oxford Pain Group League table of analgesic efficacy. Evid Based Dent. 2004;5:22–3. https://doi.org/10.1038/sj.ebd.6400237.

12. Bell PL, Gabriel V. Evidence based review for the treatment of post-burn pruritis. J Burn Case Res. 2009;30(1):55–61.
13. Gehrig KA, Warshaw EM. Allergic contact dermatitis to topical antibiotics: epidemiology, responsible allergens and management. J Am Acad Dermatol. 2008;58:1–21.
14. Carrougher GJ, Martinez EM, et al. Pruritis in adult burn survivors: post-burn prevalence and risk factors associated with increased intensity. J Burn Care Res. 2013;34:94–101.
15. Wong L, Turner L. Treatment of post-burn neuropathic pain: evaluation of pregabalin. Burns. 2010;36(d):769–72.
16. Avni T, Levcovich A, et al. Prophylactic antibiotics for burn patients: systematic review and meta-analysis. BMJ. 2010;340:C241.
17. Coffee TL, Brandt CP, Yowler CJ. Risk factors for burn wound infections, in the outpatient burn patient. J Burn Care Res. 2007;28:S62.
18. Coffee TL, Brandt CP, Yowler CJ. Is there an indication for prophylactic antibiotics in the treatment of outpatient diabetic burn patients? J Burn Care Res. 2008;29:S77.
19. Holt B, Faraklas I, et al. Telemedicine use among burn centers in the United States: a survey. J Burn Care Res. 2012;33:157–62.

34 Surgical Management of Burn Patients

Jorge Leon-Villapalos

34.1 Introduction

Major burns greater than 20% Total Body Surface Area (TBSA) characteristically elicit not only a local response in the tissues but also a widespread inflammatory response affecting multiple body systems. Thermally damaged tissue perpetuates, through cytokine cascade, stimulation of this severe, sustained hypermetabolic response that appears to be much more intense than in any other forms of trauma.

It is then easy to understand that successful outcomes in burns surgery are linked to the understanding of several strategies performed in the acute period. These strategies highlight the importance of managing these patients according to recognized protocols of trauma resuscitation with emphasis in the accurate assessment of the burn wound in extent and depth. This assessment cannot be underestimated, as the TBSA determines the need for fluid resuscitation and the depth of the burn characteristically dictates the need for burn excision. Appropriate tissue perfusion, through judicious resuscitation, will ensure the viability of any potentially salvageable areas and avoid conversion to deeper patterns of injury.

Other determinants that impact on outcomes of surgery are an appropriate respiratory support, microbiological surveillance, control of infection, early enteral nutrition, and hypothermia control. Ultimately, the aim of surgery is safely performing early debridement of all devitalized tissue and complete wound closure. Burn debridement and wound cover remain as the pillars of the surgical management of burn patients as they ensure healing and functional and cosmetic recovery [1].

J. Leon-Villapalos (✉)
Chelsea and Westminster Hospital, London, UK

British Burns Association, London, UK

London and South East of England Burns Network, London, UK

Imperial College School of Medicine, London, UK
e-mail: Jorge.Leon-Villapalos@chelwest.nhs.uk

Recently published guidelines by the International Society for Burn injuries [2] provide structured recommendations for the management of the surgical wound with the contribution of an appropriately trained multidisciplinary team.

This international body addresses, in this landmark document, the standards for burns specialists over the world and recommends best practice in multiple aspects of the burns patient treatment. These include organization and delivery of burn care, initial assessment and stabilization, diagnosis and treatment of smoke inhalation injury, burn shock resuscitation, escharotomy and fasciotomy, infection control, nutrition, wound care, and the surgical management of the burn wound.

Specific recommendations for burn surgery include performing early debridement with a preferred technique of excision whenever a deep pattern of injury is present. The need for urgent excision is much more obvious and needs to be highlighted when the injuries are due to an electrical aetiology. Traditional sharp debridement techniques include tangential or fascial excision. New approaches supplementing the armamentarium of the burn surgeon include the use of hydro surgical devices [3] and very recently the choice of non-surgical options such as enzymatic debridement [4]. These techniques need to be performed with thorough preoperative preparation and a blood loss control approach to ensure successful full take skin cover. Ultimately, the aim is to restore the functional integrity of the patient and provide best cosmetic results with a prompt return to work and life; but this journey may involve a long and tortuous pathway. Initial stabilization is nearly always followed by a myriad of surgical procedures intercalated with a potentially long stay in the intensive care unit. Optimization strategies then follow in order to soften the effect of the hypermetabolic response to the burn injury. As in any form of trauma, catabolism is a constant companion in the recovery of the patient. Burns hypermetabolism may lead to organ dysfunction, impaired wound healing, increased infection rate, and even death. One of the life-saving strategies that will overturn this situation is

M. G. Jeschke et al. (eds.), *Handbook of Burns Volume 1*, https://doi.org/10.1007/978-3-030-18940-2_34

burns surgery with prompt, judicious removal of the devitalized tissues and cover of the defect with uninjured soft tissue over a fresh vascularized tissue layer.

The options for autologous skin grafting may be limited by the extent of the burn injury, as paucity of donor sites may not be sufficient to provide full cover and warrant healing. The decision-making process for the burn surgeon may require the involvement of temporizing options for the burn wounds such as deceased donor skin (allograft), skin substitutes, dermal templates, dressing techniques, or applying skin meshing expansion techniques to facilitate healing. These operations cannot be performed without preparation, multidisciplinary approach, technical skill, persistence, resilience, pastoral support, rehabilitation, and a positive mentality of the burns professional to overcome pessimism against slow recovery, graft failure and potential physiology setbacks.

It is necessary, then, to approach all the features of burns surgery that contribute to the successful and positive outcome of recovery of the severely burned patient.

34.2 Multidisciplinary Team Approach and Preparation for Surgery

34.2.1 Rationale for Multidisciplinary Team in Burn Surgical Management

There is no doubt that burn patients obtain better outcomes for their injuries if they are looked after in specialized burn centres. These institutions warrant focused, expert, round the clock patient treatment delivered by experienced burn professionals.

There are, characteristically, medical, surgical rehabilitative and psychosocial needs in the management of the burn patients. They need to be met from the initial admission to assure not only physiological stability and survival, but also to prepare the patient for the multiple surgical procedures required to restore functionality and aesthetic individuality.

The care of these extensively burned patients may be complex and require not only initial and ongoing fluid management, respiratory support, sedation and pain management, but also, —and in order to warrant recovery—, nutritional and microbiological surveillance, nursing and therapy input and surgical wound anatomical restoration.

The composition of the multidisciplinary burns team providing and supporting tissue healing includes characteristically a team leader, a core team and an allied team [5].

The burn team leader is often a clinician, characteristically an experienced burns surgeon with support of a senior nurse.

The core team includes medical, nursing and rehabilitation colleagues.

Plastic surgeons, intensive specialists, anaesthetists, paediatricians, microbiologists and pain team specialists are characteristically key components of the medical and surgical team.

The nursing team is characteristically skilled both in the surveillance of altered physiology and in the specialized care not only of acutely burned skin but also in that resurfaced post-surgery and requiring expert complex dressings.

Nutritionists, play specialists and burns psychologists are part of the allied time of burns professionals.

The rationale for the existence of the multidisciplinary team is mutual collaboration and support for the benefit of the burn victim, but specifically regarding surgical management, its importance is centred in the need for communication and interaction between the two teams mainly involved in surgery: the surgical and the anaesthesia and intensive care teams. This close interaction warrants survival by normalizing abnormal physiology prior to any surgical intervention. There are obvious advantages to this approach; the main one is to jointly decide optimum preparation and best timing for surgery in a patient with multiple rapidly changing physiological parameters. Distinctively, all the potential markers of tissue hypoperfusion in every single body system need to be corrected prior to the surgery. These involve adjustments to the airway and the mechanics of ventilation, best cardiovascular support to overcome hypovolemia caused by fluid loss and third-spacing, appropriate sedation and pain control, accurate assessment of the burn in depth and extent and appropriate environmental and patient temperature control. This decision-making guarantees that burn surgery remains multimodal in its techniques and multidisciplinary in its performance, with a clear dermal preservation approach.

This method of treatment requires early support of the nutrition team, part of the allied multidisciplinary team. Their early involvement softens the impact of catabolism in the loss of lean body mass. If this increased energy utilization as part of the body response to burn trauma is not ameliorated by appropriate enteral nourishment, the tissue loss will lead to loss of lean body mass, negative nitrogen balance, impaired immune function, impaired healing and potentially, death.

The psychology team, as part of the allied team, shares responsibility towards recovery by providing support towards the uncertainty in the outcome of the surgery, the potential alterations in body image, early appearance of scarring and disfigurement and ultimately, decreased capacity to work and social performance.

In summary, the multidisciplinary team admitting the burns victim to a specialized burn critical care service jointly provides a methodology of treatment that appears to significantly provide best outcomes and an obvious survival benefit [6].

34.2.2 Preparation for Surgery

There is agreement that early surgery and cover of the burn wound is the golden standard to aspire for the prompt recovery and rehabilitation of the burn patient [7, 8]. Reported positive outcomes include reduced healing time, length of stay, septic episodes and mortality [9].

These outcome measures are influenced by several factors that modulate the ultimate result of the surgery.

34.2.3 Temperature Control

Core temperature normothermia is recognized as one of the strategies that aim to modulate the metabolic response to burn injury [10]. Temperature homeostasis may be deranged from the very initial moment of the burn injury due to the loss of the thermoregulatory barrier that the intact skin provides. From here onwards, the journey of the burn patient from the scene of the injury to the burns unit or definitive care facility is burdened with adversities that affect smooth temperature control. The initial approaches that dictate the delivery of first aid, stopping the burning process and cooling the burn wound, may provoke hypothermia if they are delivered with excessively cold fluid or over an injudiciously long period of time. A recent study analysing factors at the scene and in transfer related to the development of hypothermia in major burns reported a 42% incidence of hypothermia in patients arriving at a major regional burns unit [11]. Other factors contributing to early hypothermia include the lack of wound cover in the early stages due to repeated wound inspection, soaked cold dressings with wet wound exudate and delayed transfer to the definite facility.

To ensure that the risk of hypothermia during transfer is minimized, accurately documented description of the wound and cover with a bio compatible dressing that facilitates wound assessment is recommended. On arrival to the burn unit, approaching the burn patient with reduction in wound exposure and an increase in room temperature will decrease heat loss, resting energy expenditure and hypermetabolism [12].

Hypothermia has a critical role in the safe performance of burns surgery. Surgical debridement of a large burn involves excision of the wound down to a vascularized layer of tissue. Blood losses can therefore be extensive. This blood loss will be accentuated if the coagulation cascade enzymes and platelet adhesion are affected by hypothermia. If clotting is unfavourably affected by continuous low core temperature, uncontrolled bleeding will follow, entering a potential lethal triad of hypothermia, coagulopathy and acidosis [13]. A recent study found a strong relationship between operative time longer than 4 h and the development of hypothermia. The onset of hypothermia itself led to higher rates of complications both infectious such as sepsis, pneumonia, UTI and wound infection; and non-infectious such as death, ARDS, DVT, arrhythmias, immunological and neurological dysfunction and pulmonary embolism [14].

In practical terms, burns patients undergoing surgery can be optimized for prevention of hypothermia using active external rewarming techniques or active core rewarming technique.

External rewarming techniques include the use of radiant heaters, space blankets and convective air re-warmers. Core rewarming techniques are more efficacious in raising body temperature and include the use of body cavity lavage techniques and continuous arteriovenous rewarming [15]. These approaches are undertaken in ascending order of complexity during the preparation for surgery, the intraoperative period and the postoperative recovery and transfer to the intensive care unit or burns unit ward.

Therefore, it is recommended that in order to avoid hypothermia-related coagulopathy, sustained acidosis and tissue hypoperfusion the following strategies are followed [16, 17]

- Avoidance of unnecessary or lengthy exposure of the burn wound if surgery is not directly or immediately performed on it.
- Hourly temperature checks during surgery.
- Consider limiting surgery to no more than 4 h.
- Resuscitation of the patient with warm intravenous fluids.
- Increase the temperature in the operating theatre or assessment room before and during the length of the surgery.
- Forced air technologies.
- Continuous radiant heating in the operating theatre.
- Use of intravascular temperature control devices to achieve normothermia.

34.2.4 Control of Blood Loss

Burns surgery aims to selectively debride devitalized tissue down to a vascularized dermal or fascial layer in which blood plexuses are intact and can act as a recipient site for a skin graft or other option of tissue cover. This surgery is radical in its approach, and despite its dermal preservation focus, may involve a large volume of blood loss. Control measures to prevent hypovolemia start preoperatively. In order to avoid lethal triad—hypovolemia, acidosis and hypothermia—and irreversible physiology derangement, accurate assessment and aggressive but judicious fluid resuscitation is mandatory [18]. This approach limits tissue hypoperfusion and acidosis and, together with the strategies for heat conservation described earlier, improves the chances of tissue salvage, avoiding the potential conversion of injured skin in the zone of stasis to a deeper, irreversible necrotic pattern of injury requiring debridement [19]. The implications for the burn patient are obvious; a lack of awareness towards avoidance of acidosis and burn shock will translate, at the time of operative management, into a more complex surgery incurring in blood loss, requiring potential transfusion, causing fluid shifts and closing dangerously on the risk of coagulopathy. Timing of burns surgery also influences the potential for blood loss. Early excision is defined as the debridement of the non-salvageable burn eschar within the first few days after injury, and certainly within the first week to 10 days. There is evidence that factors such as older age, male sex, larger body size, and a deep (full-thickness) pattern of burn injury correlate with blood loss, that increases with a delay in performing burn excision [20, 21]. These findings are echoed in more recent studies analysing the epidemiology and predictive factors of blood transfusions in severe burn patients [21]. It is stated that age, full-thickness TBSA and number of operations were independently associated with the number of red blood cells transfusion [22]. Once it has been ascertained that blood loss increases with delay in the primary burn excision and that haemostasis should be taken into consideration from the very beginning of the management of the burn wound, it is necessary to describe specific techniques that control blood loss during the process of burn debridement. In the operating theatre, best practice dictates that the multidisciplinary team needs to brief before surgery going through the surgical checklist. World Health Organization (WHO) checklists have been adopted in burns surgery to warrant patient safety, detect safety hazards, decrease complications and improve communication among the burns team [23] (Fig. 34.1).

With the patient surgically cleaned and draped, many techniques can be sequentially or concomitantly used to reduce blood loss [24]. The intraoperative measures available for the burns surgeons are multiple. The use of tourniquets in previously exsanguinated limbs has proved to be extremely useful in the control of blood loss whenever there is a need to use either tangential or fascial technique to achieve burn excision in the limbs [25]. To address control of dermal bleeding, the use of adrenaline infiltration and adrenaline soaks is one of the most widespread strategies. Characteristically, one ampoule of 1 cc of 1:1000 adrenaline is mixed with a litre of normal saline. The solution can be used topically soaking gauze material in order to control small bleeding points (Fig. 34.2). Tumescent adrenaline and saline infiltration can be used to pre-empty blood loss prior to excision by injecting in the dermal or subdermal planes appropriate volumes of a solution of 1:1000000 adrenaline [26]. The amount of fluid to be injected will depend on the size and depth of the area to treat. Infiltration characteristically produces local firmness, decrease in the capillary refill and swelling of the tissues (Fig. 34.3) and therefore contributes to control unnecessary bleeding from uninjured vascular plexuses. The infiltrated fluid also helps to create a firm convex skin grafting surface on top of which the harvesting of skin is facilitated. The benefits of fluid injection in the tissues can also be seen in the ease of dissection found whilst performing fascial excision, where the tissue planes become much more defined, facilitating surgery (Fig. 34.4). The use of monopolar and bipolar electrocautery with an attachment for smoke extraction is another recognized tool to limit bleeding whilst performing debridement [27]. Careful cautery control needs to be exercised whilst performing haemostasis with the diathermy. If a thorough and directed coagulation of the bleeding vessels is not performed, an extensive area of charring will be created which may leave areas of devitalization compromising the debridement and the success of any subsequent grafting.

An alternative approach to blood loss control during acute burns surgery is the use of topically applied or device delivered haemostatic agents that accelerate coagulation in tissue surfaces [28]. Fibrin sealants such as Artiss® and Tisseel® (Westlake Village, CA: Baxter Healthcare Corporation) are frequently used in acute burns surgery. These are slow-clotting mixtures of fibrin and prothrombin that act as alternatives to standard methods of graft fixation and donor and recipient site haemostasis. A recent admission to the armamentarium of fibrin sealants is Vivostat® System (Vivolution A/S, Allerod, Denmark). This is an autologous fibrin sealant and platelet rich fibrin (PRF) obtained through mechanical processing of a small sample of blood of the patient. This technique has so far shown promising results in promoting the healing of burn wounds, acting as a support for suspension of keratinocytes and as an enhancer in the successful take of micrografting techniques [29–31].

Sealant techniques can be complemented with systemic therapies such as the use of tranexamic acid. This is an antifibrinolytic agent that binds to plasminogen inhibiting breakdown of the fibrin clot. Even though there is limited evidence of its usefulness in acute burns surgery, the experience of its use in trauma suggests a reduction in the requirement for blood transfusion and a positive effect on graft take [32, 33].

34.2.5 Burns Surgery

Once stabilization of the burns patient is complete through prompt first aid, appropriate trauma management with accurate assessment of the burn wound in depth and extent, judicious resuscitation and physiology-protection measures to counterbalance the noxious multisystem effects of the hypermetabolic system, the need to restore anatomy and function becomes a priority. We have pointed out repeatedly how interlinked all these measures are and how their appropriate

SIGN IN

Brief Completed : Yes/ No

Time in the Anaesthetic room:

Patient has confirmed:
☐IDENTITY (NAME&DoB)
☐OPERATION SITE
☐IDBAND
☐PROCEDURE
☐CONSENT
☐ALLERGIES

Operation marked:

☐YES ☐ NO ☐ N/A

Anaesthesia machine and medication Check complete:

☐YES ☐ NO ☐ N/A

Difficult airway or aspiration risk:
☐YES (equipment/assistance available) ☐ NO

Has the availability of prosthesis/equipment been/ equipment been confirmed with scrub team?
☐YES ☐ NO ☐ N/A

Name of Anaesthetic Practitioner:

Name of responsible Anaesthetist:

PATIENT LABEL

Date & Time:
___/___/____ ___:___

TIME OUT

Have all team members introduced themselves by name and role: ☐YES ☐ NO

Surgeon, Anaesthetist and Scrub practitioner to confirm:
☐Patient Name, DoB & MRN
☐Patient ID Band
☐Procedure matches consent
☐Listed site/side matches skin marking
☐Allergies

Infection control issue:

Antibiotics required: ☐YES ☐ NO ☐ N/A

Anticipating > 500ml blood loss (7ml/kg in children) to share with the team:

Does patient have a valid group and save:

Patient specific concerns to share with the team:

Critical or unexpected steps to share with the team:

Essential images displayed:

VTE Prophylaxis undertaken:
☐YES ☐ NO ☐ N/A

Sterility of equipment confirmed (including indicator results):
☐YES ☐ NO ☐ N/A

Implants required:
☐YES ☐ NO ☐ N/A

Tourniquet used for IV cannulation removed:
☐YES ☐ NO ☐ N/A

Tourniquet Required: ☐YES ☐ NO

Warming devices applied:
☐YES ☐ NO ☐ N/A

Glycaemic control required: ☐YES ☐ NO ☐ N/A

Hair removal required: ☐YES ☐ NO ☐ N/A

Name of Surgeon:

Date & Time:
___/___/____ ___:___

SIGN OUT

Surgical Staff confirm:

Name of Procedure :

Instruments, swabs and sharps counts are complete:
☐YES ☐ NO ☐ N/A

Specimen labelled with name, site and side
☐YES ☐ NO ☐ N/A

IV Lines flushed ☐YES ☐ NO ☐ N/A

If throat pack has been used, has it been removed:
☐YES ☐ NO ☐ N/A

If any type of tourniquet has been used, has it been removed:
☐YES ☐ NO ☐ N/A
Tourniquet time:

Estimated blood loss recorded:
☐YES ☐ NO ☐ N/A

Surgical Staff Confirm:
Have any equipment problems been addressed:
☐YES ☐ NO ☐ N/A

Any concerns for recovery:
☐YES ☐ NO ☐ N/A

Senior responsible surgeon:

Date & Time:
___/___/____ ___:___

Fig. 34.1 WHO surgical safety checklist

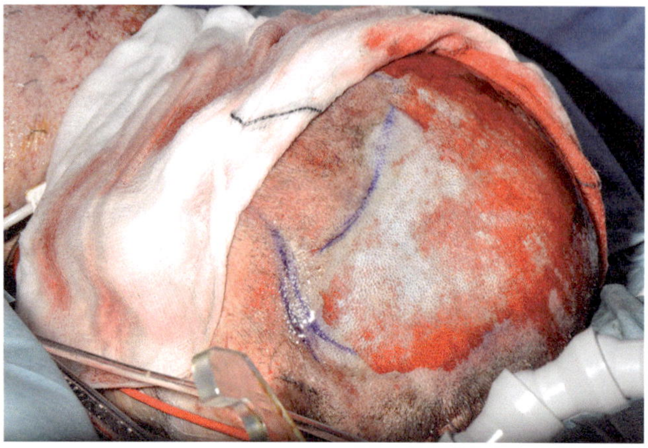

Fig. 34.2 Adrenaline soaks controlling the bleeding of a scalp donor site

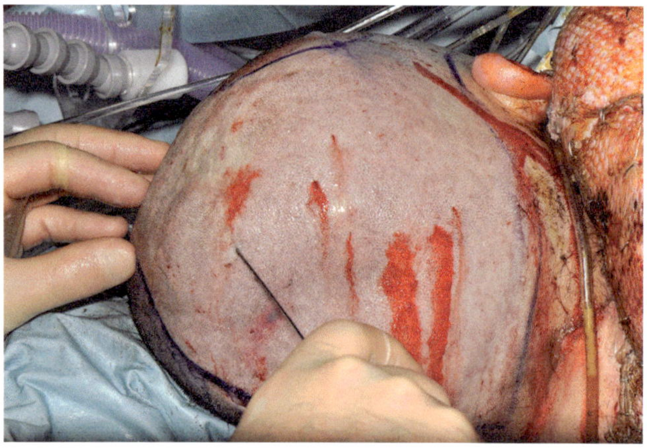

Fig. 34.3 Adrenaline tumescent infiltration of a scalp donor site

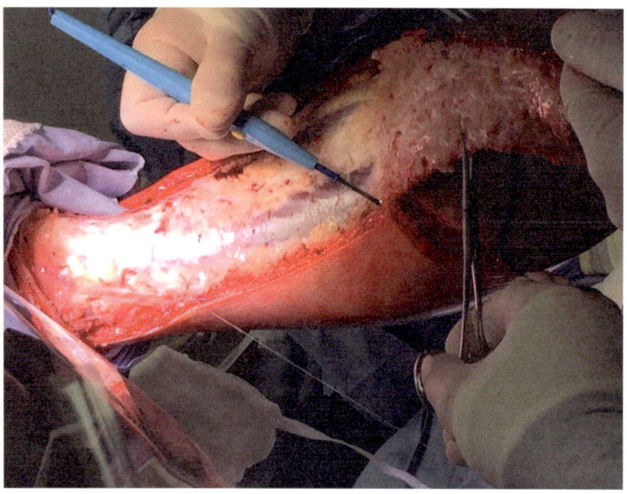

Fig. 34.4 Fascial excision facilitated by hydro dissection with tumescent infiltration

implementation decreases tissue damage and facilitates the debridement and soft tissue cover by instituting a dermal preservation approach. The practical translation of this approach is straightforward to understand.

The more judicious and contained the excision is, the less scarring and contracture will be an issue and the quicker the rehabilitation and social reintegration will become. Even though the restoration of body integrity through surgery ultimately reflects the role of the surgical team supported by other multidisciplinary members, burns surgeons intervene in the support of the burns victim in multiple other steps:

- Airway management and tracheostomy
- Escharotomy
- Early burn eschar excision
- Wound cover
- Urgent, essential and desirable burns reconstruction

34.2.6 Burns Surgery: Airway Management and Tracheostomy

The benefits of performing tracheostomy in burn patients include the ability to perform improved airway toilet and suctioning through a better tolerated and more secure airway, with improvement in the mechanics of ventilation [34]. Following tracheostomy, parameters of the work of breathing such as the airway resistance, peak inspiratory pressures and intrinsic positive end-expiratory pressure decrease facilitating comfort and weaning from mechanical ventilation [35]. Tracheostomy is, nevertheless, an invasive procedure that needs to be performed by experienced individuals either via a percutaneous or through a surgical approach. Clinically, whenever there are neck burns associated with the need for a lengthy period of mechanical ventilation, tracheostomy needs to be considered. To that effect, the burn surgeons perform a preferential debridement of the neck burned skin and resurface it with a sheet of skin graft as soon as possible with the aim of obtaining a healed surface for the tracheostomy site. Even though many studies have failed to show a definitive advantage of early tracheostomy on infection rates, ICU length of stay and hospital length of stay in the intensive care patient cohort [36, 37], burn patients tend to be considered for tracheostomy if there is no possibility of extubating or weaning the patient off the ventilator after 7–10 days of intubation. The options of surgical tracheostomy are reserved for patients with neck burns in which the percutaneous option is not feasible by the bedside, but in this case, the surgical approach is performed after 10 days of autografting of the neck. There does not appear to exist a clear difference in the complication rates for percutaneous vs. surgical tracheostomy [38]

In the paediatric burn population, tracheostomy is a safe method of airway management which appears to be related to the extent of burn injury, not to the age of the patient [39].

The surgical technique follows the steps of standard soft tissue dissection. Nevertheless, the tissue planes may be distorted due to swelling, tissue damage or the body habitus of the patient, which may be subjected to swelling and oedema. A thorough preparation and equipment check warrants lack of complications and a trouble-free insertion of the tracheostomy cannula.

34.2.7 Burns Surgery: Escharotomy

Prior to managing the burn wound with debridement and soft tissue cover, life and limb saving priorities need to be addressed. Unjustified assessment delay may result in catastrophic functional consequences and even death. On performing a structured protocol of assessment of the burn patient, inadequacy of the ventilation and compromise of circulation in the limbs may be ascertained. If circumferential deep burns of full-thickness pattern compromise the compliance of the chest and abdomen or the perfusion and viability of the distal perfusion of the limbs, the need for escharotomy needs to be considered. The consequences of not addressing these surgical alarms promptly, appropriately and by the most senior and experienced clinician, affect directly the viability of the soft tissues injured by the thermal injury and may have far-reaching fatal consequences.

When tissues are burned, the depth to which they do so depends on the intensity of the thermal injury. Deep injuries will not only damage the anatomical integrity of the skin, reducing its pliability and elasticity, but will also reduce the blood supply to its dermal component, making healing and self-regeneration unlikely. The clinical consequences of this scenario are a shift towards a deep pattern of injury and a migration towards tissue necrosis from the potentially salvageable zone of stasis. The resulting damage leaves the skin as a leathery, non-pliable structure that behaves as a tight restrain for deeper fascial layers, neurovascular bundles and muscular compartments. This alarming scenario will worsen when fluid shifts favoured by increased capillary permeability migrate towards the extracellular space. The tissue already damaged and hypoperfused will sustain further insult, potentially leading to interstitial oedema pain, hypoperfusion, vascular ischemia and hemodynamic and vascular compromise. Facing these concerns, not only escharotomies but also a full array of decompression strategies needs to be considered for chest, abdomen and limbs [40, 41]

There are recognized surgical approaches to performing escharotomies [42]:

- Perform under general anaesthesia, in a warm theatre, with full resources including back up of blood products.
- Use monopolar diathermy in cutting mode to perform initial incision from unburned skin to unburned skin. Do not advance in your incision unless you have full control of any bleeding points.
- Check with fingertip full release of the eschar down to subcutaneous tissue.
- Make a second pass along any tight unreleased areas by changing the mode of the diathermy to coagulation.
- In the case of extremities, the upper limbs need to be placed in the anatomical position, with the forearm supinated and palms facing up. The natural tendency of the oedematous burned upper limbs is to go into a pronation position. Failure to supinate the forearm will lead to potential misplacement of the escharotomy incisions in the antecubital fossa.
- Perform the escharotomies in upper and lower limbs along axial lines respecting anatomical structures of importance such as ulnar nerve in the upper limbs and (Fig. 34.5) the long saphenous vein and distal neurovascular bundles of the lower limb
- Perform chest escharotomy in response to poor ventilation compliance, anaesthetic concerns and high peak ventilation pressures along anterior axillary lines joining the incisions along costal margin and clavicle if necessary.
- Perform abdominal skin escharotomy to treat full-thickness burn of the abdominal wall but be ready to proceed to abdominal decompressing laparotomy, exploration and release together with general surgeons if abdominal compartment syndrome is suspected.
- Success of abdominal release for abdominal compartment syndrome will improve parameters of intraabdominal hypertension, respiratory function, hypoperfusion and acidosis [43, 44].

Complications of inadequate decompression escharotomy will lead to compartment syndrome muscle damage, neurovascular injury and potential amputation of the limb. Systemic complications include myoglobinuria, renal failure, metabolic acidosis and even death.

Burns surgeons recognize and accept that there is potential morbidity caused by escharotomy release. Nevertheless, certain mistakes should be avoided. Inadequate length or depth of the incisions will lead to unnecessary damage of underlying functional deep structures. Accurate assessment of the damaged tissue will stop unnecessary performing the procedure on likely-to heal skin and avoid complications such as unnecessary bleeding, infection and abnormal scarring.

The resulting escharotomy wounds are initially packed with a paraffin-impregnated dressing and loosely bandaged. They are eventually closed primarily once the tension of the tissues has subsided or split skin grafted.

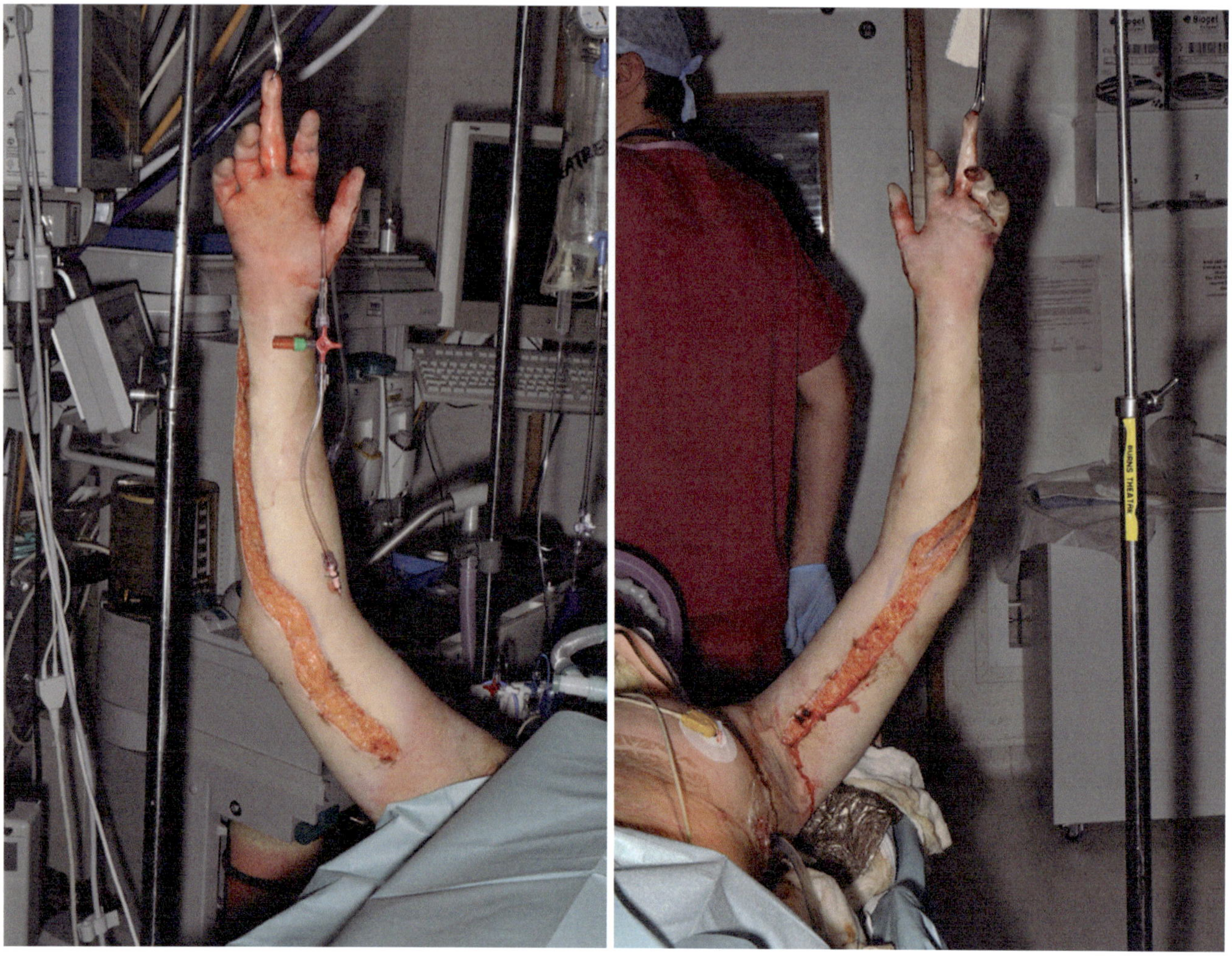

Fig. 34.5 Escharotomy of upper limbs

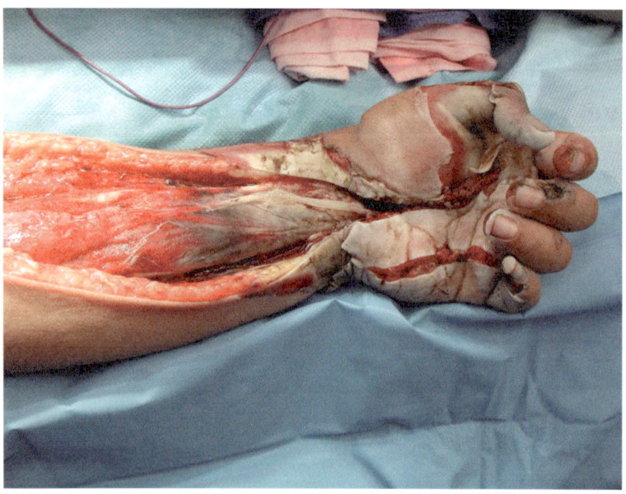

Fig. 34.6 Fasciotomy of the upper limb

Following electrical injuries, the escharotomy may not be sufficient to release the deep tissues. In these cases, performing fasciotomies may be required to salvage the viability of deep tissues (Fig. 34.6).

34.2.8 Burns Surgery: Wound Excision

Wound excision starts once the preparations for surgery have been completed and the optimization of the patient is appropriate. The operative team, with an experienced team of 4–6 surgeons supported by 2 anaesthetists, 2 scrub team members, intensivists and nursing team will work in a self-contained and fully staffed operating theatre with efficient climate control, and ready access to blood, fresh frozen plasma and allograft from a skin bank. They will have the backup of a full intensive care facility for ventilation and hemofiltration and on-site paediatricians, geriatricians, psychiatrists, dieticians, pharmacists, bacteriologists, haematologists and biochemists.

The excision techniques will be tailored to the depth and extent of the burn, but also to the ability of the patient due to age, physiology and comorbidities to withstand the trauma of the surgery, together with blood loss, hypothermia, acidosis and cardiorespiratory depression.

The excision techniques can be classified into sharp, hydro surgical and enzymatic. Sharp techniques can be subdivided into tangential and fascial.

A recent study designed to assess burn surgeons' preferences in excision and grafting to determine if surgical technique affects outcomes showed that clinical judgment is still the most likely method of assessment for excision. More than half of the surgeons perform excision as early as postburn day 1 and a clear majority of the surgeons surveyed would perform more than 20% TBSA in a single operation [45].

Tangential excision techniques follow the principles set by Janzekovic [46] and represent the most traditionally used technique to debride a burn wound. This technique will create a graftable surface by debriding sequentially layers of tissue of variable depth until finding either a glistening healthy dermis with punctate bleeding or a healthy fatty layer appropriately vascularized. It is performed with sharp, non-dermally selective tools (Fig. 34.7) that undoubtedly create abundant bleeding in the process. As we detailed previously, a combination of intraoperative techniques such as tourniquets and adrenaline solutions, either injected or applied topically in the tissues, greatly limits blood loss. Multiple reports suggest that blood loss under tourniquet control is less than after subcutaneous 1:1,000,000 adrenaline solution injection. Both reduce blood loss compared with using no haemostatic measures without dramatically causing abnormal cardiovascular rhythm changes [47]. Another challenge to haemostasis from tangential techniques is due to the fact that the diffuse and broad nature of the excision will create not only venous and arterial bleeding points that may well be controlled with diathermy, compression and vasoconstrictive solutions, but also blanket bleeding from capillary sources that can be problematic. The need for further haemostatic adjuncts such as thrombin and fibrin has been documented above [48]. Taking into consideration that it is possible to lose more than 4% of the total blood volume per % of burn excised [49], it is easy to understand then that appropriate use of tangential excision needs to be coupled with a zealous approach to blood loss reduction to avoid hematomas, unstable physiology and the need for transfusions. Sharp surgical excision techniques will therefore be characterized for blood loss and the creation of a defect of variable complexity that will need to be reconstructed. The comparison of tangential technique of excision with the other sharp excision technique, fascial excision (Fig. 34.8) exposes the contrast and impossible balance between blood loss, tissue excision, the creation of a non-reconstructable defect and the anatomical deficit created by it. Fascial excision is reserved for injuries of a full-thickness component and characteristically intense energy delivery to the tissues, such as electrical and flame burns. The excision runs with the deep fascia as the underlying boundary, with all tissue above this layer excised in a relatively bloodless plane with the help of a monopolar diathermy.

Hydro surgical techniques introduce an interesting element of addition to the armamentarium of the burns surgeon. The Versajet™ Hydro surgery System (Smith and Nephew Medical Ltd., Memphis TN, USA) is a debriding tool based on the Venturi effect that excises and removes necrotic tissue by emitting a pressurized saline stream acting like a scalpel.

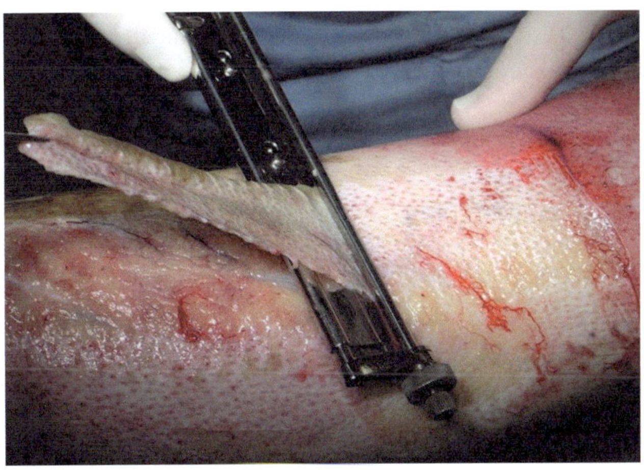

Fig. 34.7 Tangential excision

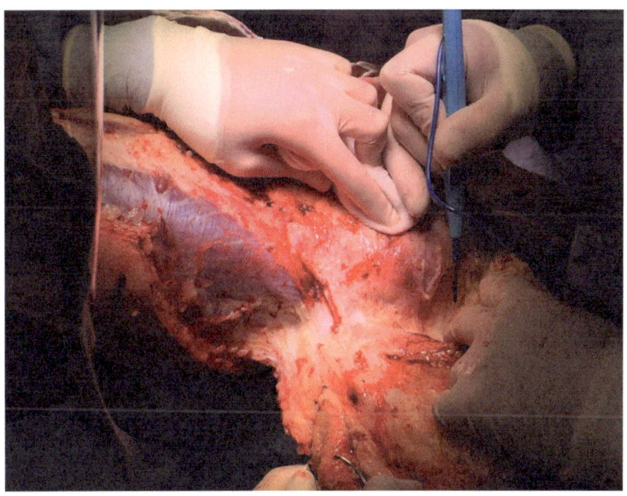

Fig. 34.8 Fascial excision

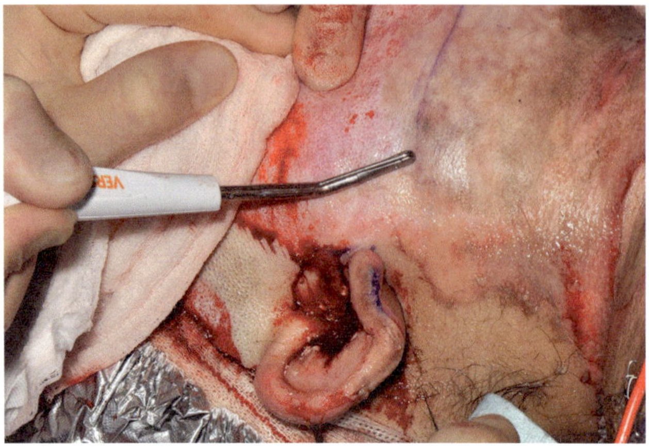

Fig. 34.9 Versajet debridement of the face

The debrided tissue is aspirated at high pressure into a cannister.

A recent study showed it to be safe, efficacious and cost-effective alternative for burned soft eschars, but not efficient in removal of leathery dry burn eschars [50], comparing well in results, efficacy and dermal preservation capabilities with classic escharectomy in difficult anatomical areas [51, 52]. Appropriate use of this technique allows careful dermal preservation debridement even in sensitive areas like the face (Fig. 34.9).

Enzymatic debridement represents an extra innovative debriding tool for deep burn injuries. It is important to state from the beginning that this Bromelain-based substance is not a substitute to skin grafting or soft tissue cover, as self-regeneration and healing will only occur if enough viable dermis remains in the wound after the process of application, removal and dressing care. The process for preparation and application is straightforward and involves a cleaning of all non-viable skin debris, a wet pre-soak of the wounds with saline and chlorhexidine of several hours, application of the product (Nexobrid®, Mediwound, Israel) for 4 h after appropriate analgesia, removal of the debris of the wound and the product and overnight post procedure soak of the area with saline. It is reported in several trials that this debriding option is a powerful tool to remove eschar in burn wounds, reducing blood loss, the need for autologous skin grafting and the number of wounds requiring surgical excision [53]. A recent European consensus established guidance over application guidance, timing of the procedure, blood loss, analgesia and dressing care [54]. A myriad of papers has been produced on this technique, expanding the indications for its usage and anatomical areas that can be treated [55, 56].

34.2.9 Burns Surgery: Wound Cover

Tissue cover is not the final step of burn care, but if successful, it is the first landmark towards definitive recovery, as it allows the patient to seal the wound, decrease infection and restore, even in a limited way, physical integrity and facilitate the pathway towards rehabilitation, recovery and social reintegration. The coverage of wounds nevertheless comes at the expense to create donor sites and new wounds, that are submitted, until healing to a potentially lengthy period of dressing changes supported by infection surveillance, nutrition and physical and emotional therapies. There will be situations in which due to the wound environment, the TBSA involved or the age, physiology or comorbidities of the patient, it will not be possible (the deep extensive wound) or necessary (the superficial extensive wound) to cover the wound immediately or in a single operation, and a staged temporizing approach with dressings, allograft or dermal replacements will be necessary.

When the wound is ready for definitive cover, skin grafts in variable regimes of meshing, supported or not by allograft or skin replacement materials, cell suspension techniques or flaps get the wound sealed and healed and represent the final process in anatomical and functional restitution.

34.2.10 Temporizing Options

The concept of burn wound temporizing cover involves two types of wounds, partial thickness with healing potential or deeper wounds requiring debridement that may need a period of alternative alloplastic cover before definitive autologous grafting.

The temporizing options for wound management can be synthetic (Biobrane®, Suprathel®, dressings, etc.) or biological (Allograft, Xenograft).

In the case of partial-thickness wounds with healing potential, the patient is taken to theatre for gentle debridement and assessment of the viability of the dermis. The wound will then be treated with a temporary layer of alloplastic material to ensure dermal protection, avoid desiccation and promote epithelialization.

In these cases, there is usually no need for sharp debridement and the wound is usually debrided with hydro surgical methods (Versajet®) and covered with either xenograft [52], or specialized dressing material such as Biobrane® (Smith and Nephew, UK) [57, 58], Suprathel® [59, 60] (PolyMedics Innovations, Germany), or dressings. The debridement with the hydro surgery tool is carried at low power in order to get a fine punctate bleeding indicative of dermal viability. The resulting fibrin layer from the clots acts as a gentle adhesive for these skin substitute materials.

The combination of hydro surgery and alloplastic cover is especially useful as a temporizing option due to the ability of Versajet® to debride soft eschars very efficiently even in anatomically sensitive areas like hands and faces. Biobrane®, a transparent, temporary wound cover familiar to the burn surgeon, promotes epithelialization due to its combination of nylon mesh and porcine collagen in partial-thickness burns, and it is easy to use and handle both in adults and paediatric patients.

Suprathel® is produced from a synthetic copolymer mainly based on DL-lactide (>70%), trimethylenecarbonate and ε-caprolactone. The material is presented as a desiccated thin layer which tends to become gently elastic with heat and that adheres well to the wound. It has significantly shown to reduce pain, it is easy to handle, comfortable for the patient and comparable to Biobrane® in indications and results.

In cases of burn wounds that require temporizing before autograft due to their deep pattern of injury, wound environment or to the paucity of donor sites, allograft [61] remains the main option for temporary cover. Allograft is usually obtained from tissue banks either as glycerol preserved or in freeze-dried sheet or pre-meshed packets. They need to be washed out and thawed and appropriately meshed (if not done so before) and then applied to the wound bed to temporize either as a watchful waiting option to prime the tissues for healing or to prepare the wound bed for autografting.

Healthy bleeding from the wound helps in the adhesion of the allograft sheets, which are regularly inspected for infection, hematomas, seromas, shearing or detachment. Allograft options reduce the possibility of fluid loss and act as indirect markers of the potential for autografting, as it already possesses many of the desirable properties of autologous skin. Following adhesion and neovascularization, the graft will characteristically exhibit rejection of its cellular elements and will eventually need to be changed or substituted by autografting [62, 63].

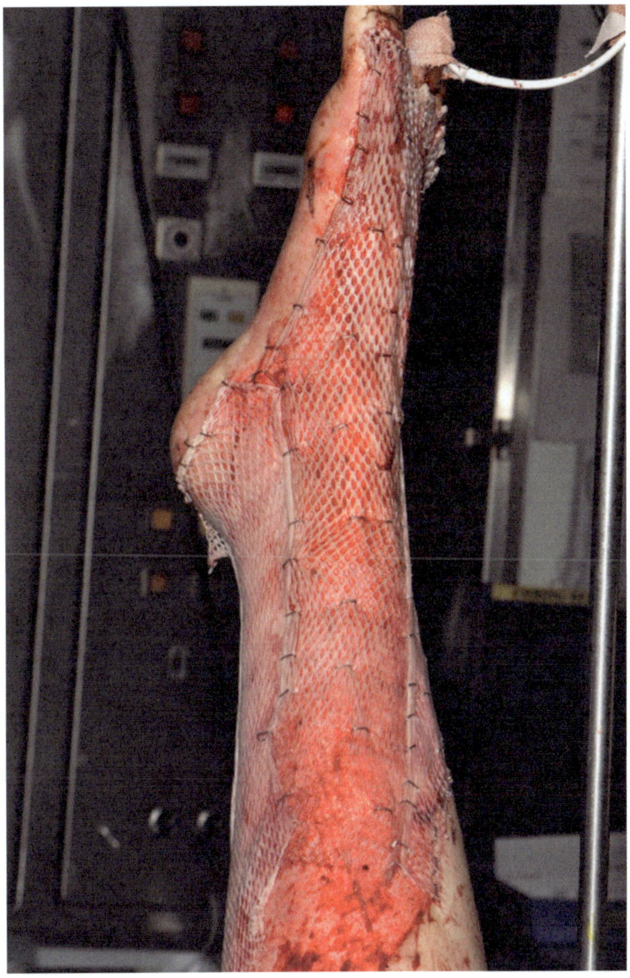

Fig. 34.10 2:1 Meshing split skin grafting regime of the lower limb

34.2.11 Definitive Soft Tissue Cover

The aim of permanent skin cover following debridement of the burn wound is to restore as much as possible the integrity of the damaged burn skin with tissue options that provide prompt healing, pliability, elasticity and a recovery of all skin functions. The reality is that this aspirational wish of the burn surgeon is met with cover strategies that may be limited in their quantities or anatomical integrity. Autologous donor skin will be limited if the burn is extensive. Even the provision of skin grafts represents the substitution of the full thickness of the skin for a thin layer of epidermis and papillary dermis that will obviously contract and scar to the point of limiting function. Definitive cover may need to be preceded, as detailed above, by a period of wound temporizing. The options for permanent cover reside then in manipulating the available donor skin and make it wider and larger by different meshing regimes, culture it to provide cover in situations of donor site paucity or a large burn or make it resemble as much as possible as the uninjured skin by combining it with a skin replacement or dermal template.

Full-thickness grafts contain all skin layers and constitute the best attempt to provide pliability, elasticity, colour and texture match in the reconstructed site, Unfortunately, their harvesting leaves a defect that needs to be closed primarily and the donor site areas may be limited (groin, supraclavicular, pre- and postauricular areas, flanks, abdomen). Their use is characteristically limited to cover anatomically sensitive areas like the face and the hands [64, 65].

Split thickness grafts constitute the most popular method of soft tissue cover for deep extensive burns. The paucity of donor sites and the need for the burn surgeon to be restrained and sensible in the amount of skin to be harvested makes skin meshing an excellent option to provide wide cover with reduced donor site morbidity, the options of meshing (Fig. 34.10) vary from 1:1 with minimal expansion to 6:1 expansion in combination with allograft for sandwich cover [66].

A recent study reported burn size in TBSA as the only consistent factor considered in the decision to use a 3:1 or higher split thickness skin graft meshing ratio. When treating a large burn, a 3:1 or higher meshing ratio should be considered once the burn TBSA approaches 30–50% or higher [67]. These grafts are fixed to the skin by a variety of methods including fibrin glue.

Suction blister epidermal grafts (SBEG) [68] using the KCI CelluTome™ epidermal harvesting system gives the surgeon an additional tool in the armamentarium of cover by obtaining thin epidermal blisters with a suction device under local anaesthesia and with minimal complications.

Cell suspension techniques like cultured epidermal autografts (CEA) [69, 70] provide a fragile permanent skin coverage for patients with extensive burns. Unfortunately, the long period of incubation necessary from the time of biopsy, the tendency to infection and the lack of dermal support limit their use on their own, and they are usually combined with the use of dermal templates or micrografting techniques (Fig. 34.11). Cell-spray autografting [71] is an innovative early treatment option for deep partial-thickness burns that can achieve rapid wound re-epithelialization, with a much smaller donor site. Non-confluent cell suspension techniques allow the delivery of sprayed cellular contents to the wound from a small thin biopsy taken intraoperatively that takes less than 20 min to transform into a cell solution. It appears to be very useful for the treatment and fast reepithelialization of superficial partial-thickness burns and for the management of hypopigmented healed areas [72, 73].

Micrografting techniques allow the delivery of stamps of skin expanded up to a 1:9 regime to cover large areas of burn wound when the donor sites are very sparse. This technique can be cumbersome and demanding in time and learning curve but provides the patient with an excellent quality reconstruction comparable to that of skin grafting and cosmetically more acceptable. With this technique burns of up to 75% TBSA can be treated with the remaining non-burned skin as sufficient donor tissue [74, 75].

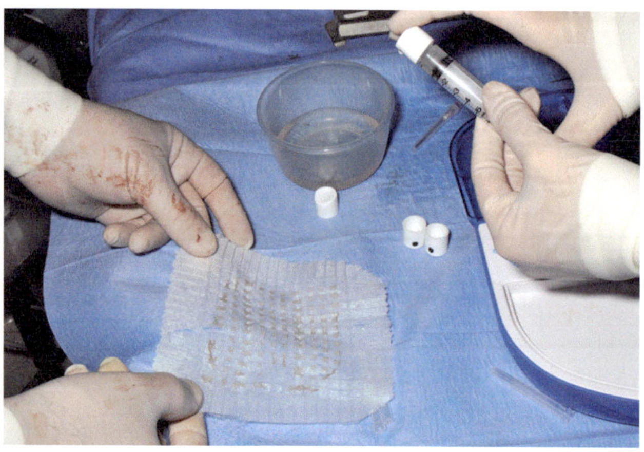

Fig. 34.11 Cultured epithelial autografts over a micrografting skin template

Skin replacements: Artificial dermal templates provide a stable, durable and flexible wound closure and they provide a scaffold for tissue repair. Their aim is to replicate the role of the dermis in the structure of the skin and restore pliability and elasticity in the reconstructed tissue. All dermal templates available require a split skin graft to complete healing of the wound after a period of neovascularization. Current most used options are Integra® (Fig. 34.12) (Integralife, USA), a two-staged reconstruction and Matriderm® (MedSkin Solutions Dr. Suwelack AG), a one-stage reconstruction. Integra® is composed of a crosslinked collagen and chondroitin-6-sulphate dermal replacement layer covered by a silicone temporary epidermal substitute to retard fluid loss and immediately close the wound bed [76, 77]. Matriderm® [78] (Fig. 34.13) is a one-stage extracellular tissue substitute made of a three-dimensional matrix that contains native collagen fibres along with elastin to support dermal regeneration. Both dermal matrices can be used for reconstruction and acute care and compare favourably to each other [79].

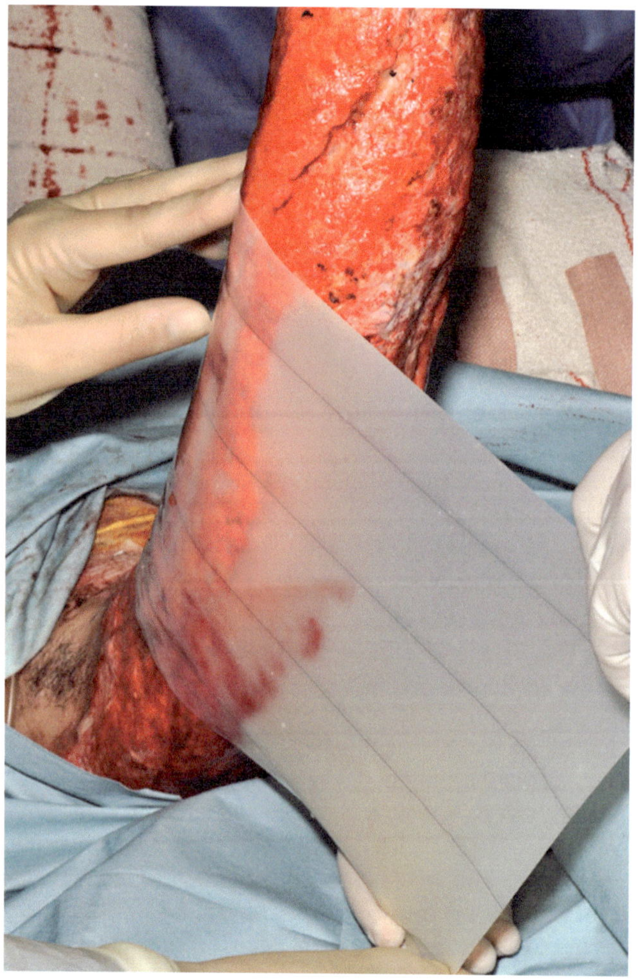

Fig. 34.12 Integra cover of a burned upper limb

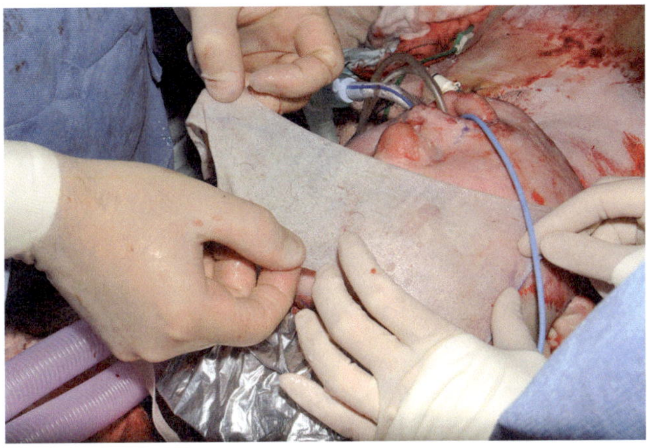

Fig. 34.13 Sheet grafting over dermal template following facial burn debridement

34.3 Conclusion

Burns surgery is multimodal, multidisciplinary and should be performed with a dermal preservation focus. It starts at prehospital level until reaching anatomical restoration with skin cover. Burns surgeons perform multiple tasks until that period to support the physiology of the patient and fight the hypermetabolic response.

Summary Box

- Following first aid, the acute management of the burn patient requires assessment according to recognized protocols of trauma resuscitation with specific attention to accurate recognition of the depth and the extent of the burn wound.
- Surgical management will be required when the burn wound is either extensive, deep in nature or complex in its presentation. Frequently, burn wounds present with these three attributes, making surgery unavoidable.
- Extensive burn wounds may require surgery to ensure patient comfort and appropriate wound management irrespective of their depth.
- Deep burn wounds will always require surgery due to their inability for self-healing and their potential for abnormal scarring with subsequent impact on function and cosmetic appearance.
- The pillars of burn surgery are early debridement and prompt soft tissue cover. These need to be supported by multidisciplinary team involvement to ensure successful outcomes, appropriate rehabilitation, and the return to society as an active member of the burns survivor.
- The extended competencies of the burn surgeon also involve airway management by providing surgical aids to ventilation, escharotomy if indicated, control of the different variables of the hypermetabolic response to burn injury such as temperature, infection, blood loss, nutrition and pharmacological modulation and further secondary procedures for contracture release, scar management and burns reconstruction.

References

1. Mohammadi AA, Mohammadi S. Early excision and grafting (EE&G): opportunity or threat? Burns. 2017;43(6):1358–9. https://doi.org/10.1016/j.burns.2017.03.021.
2. ISBI Practice Guidelines Committee. ISBI practice guidelines for burn care. Burns. 2016;42(1):953–1021.
3. Klein MB, et al. The Versajet™ water dissector: a new tool for tangential excision. J Burn Care Res. 2005;26(6):483–7. https://doi.org/10.1097/01.bcr.0000185398.13095.c5.
4. Rosenberg L, et al. A novel rapid and selective enzymatic debridement agent for burn wound management: a multi-center RCT. Burns. 2014;40(3):466–74.
5. Butler DP. The 21st century burn care team. Burns. 2013;39(3):375–9. https://doi.org/10.1016/j.burns.2013.01.004.
6. Win TS, et al. Relationship between multidisciplinary critical care and burn patients survival: a propensity-matched national cohort analysis. Burns. 2018;44(1):57–64.
7. Anzarut A, Chen M, Shankowsky H, Tredget EE. Quality-of-life and outcome predictors following massive burn injury. Plast Reconstr Surg. 2005;116:791–7.
8. Herndon DN, Barrow RE, Rutan RL, Rutan TC, Desai MH, Abston S. A comparison of conservative versus early excision. Therapies in severely burned patients. Ann Surg. 1989;209:547–52.
9. Ong YS, Samuel M, Song C. Meta-analysis of early excision of burns. Burns. 2006;32:145–50.
10. Williams FN, Herndon DN, Jeschke MG. The hypermetabolic response to burn injury and interventions to modify this response. Clin Plast Surg. 2009;36:583–96.
11. Steele JE, Atkins JL, Vizcaychipi MP. Factors at the scene and in transfer related to the development of hypothermia in major burns. Ann Burns Fire Disasters. 2016;29(2):103–7.
12. Rizzo JA, et al. Perioperative temperature management during burn care. J Burn Care Res. 2017;38:e277–83.
13. Keane M. Triad of death: the importance of temperature monitoring in trauma patients. Emerg Nurse. 2016;24(5):1354–5752.
14. Ziolkowski N, et al. The impact of operative time and hypothermia in acute burn surgery. Burns. 2017;43(8):1673–81.
15. Gentilello LM, Lawrence Reed R. Hypothermia and trauma. In: Asensio J, editor. Current therapy of trauma and surgical critical care. Amsterdam: Elsevier; 2016. p. 679–82.
16. Prunet B, Asencio Y, Lacroix G, et al. Maintenance of normothermia during burn surgery with an intravascular temperature control system: a non-randomised controlled trial. Injury. 2012;43:648–52.
17. Davis JS, Rodriguez LI, Quintana OD, et al. Use of a warming catheter to achieve normothermia in large burns. J Burn Care Res. 2013;34:191–5.
18. Latenser BA. Critical care of the burn patient: the first 48 h. Crit Care Med. 2009;37(10):2819–26.

19. Sherren PB, et al. Lethal triad in severe burns. Burns. 2014;40(8):1492–6.
20. Desai MH, Herndon DN, Broemeling L, Barrow RE, Nichols RJ Jr, Rutan RL. Early burn wound excision significantly reduces blood loss. Ann Surg. 1990;211:753–9; discussion 759–62
21. Hart DW, et al. Determinants of blood loss during primary burn excision. Surgery. 2001;130(2):396–402.
22. Wu G, Zhuang M, Fan X, Hong X, Wang K, Wang H, et al. Blood transfusions in severe burn patients: epidemiology and predictive factor. Burns. 2016;42(8):1721–7.
23. Treadwell JR, Lucas S, Tsou AY. Surgical checklists: a systematic review of impacts and implementation. BMJ Qual Saf. 2014;23(4):299–318.
24. Sterling JP, Heimbach DM. Hemostasis in burn surgery—a review. Burns. 2011;37(4):559–65.
25. Djurickovic S. Tourniquet and subcutaneous epinephrine reduce blood loss during burn excision and immediate autografting. J Burn Care Rehabil. 2001;22(1):1–5. https://doi.org/10.1097/00004630-200101000-00002.
26. Robertson RD, et al. The tumescent technique to significantly reduce blood loss during burn surgery. Burns. 2011;27(8):835–8.
27. Mitsukawa N, et al. Hemostasis by means of a cautery knife equipped with an air spray for burns over a large area. Burns. 2006;32:695–7.
28. Jeschke M, et al. Wound coverage technologies in burn care: novel techniques. J Burn Care Res. 2013;34(6):612–20.
29. Mittermayr R, Wassermann E, Thurnher M, Simunek M, Redl H. Skin graft fixation by slow clotting fibrin sealant applied as a thin layer. Burns. 2006;32:305–11.
30. Johnstone P, et al. Successful application of keratinocyte suspension using autologous fibrin spray. Burns. 2016;43(3):e27–30.
31. Chong SJ, et al. Technical tips to enhance micrografting results in burn surgery. Burns. 2017;43(5):983–6.
32. Tang YMJ. Use of tranexamic acid to reduce bleeding in burns surgery. J Plast Reconstr Aesthet Surg. 2011;65(5):684–6.
33. Walsh K, et al. What is the evidence for tranexamic acid in burns? Burns. 2014;40(5):1055–7.
34. Purdue GF. To trach or not to trach. J Burn Care Res. 2009;30(1):192–3. https://doi.org/10.1097/BCR.0b013e3181923ec6.
35. Diehl JL, et al. Changes in the work of breathing induced by tracheotomy in ventilator-dependent patients. Am J Respir Crit Care Med. 1999;159(2):383.
36. Terragni PP, et al. Early versus late tracheotomy for prevention of pneumonia in mechanically ventilated adult ICU patients: a randomized controlled trial. J Am Med Assoc. 2010;303(15):1483–9.
37. Young D, et al. Effect of early vs late tracheostomy placement on survival in patients receiving mechanical ventilation. J Am Med Assoc. 2013;309(20):2121–9.
38. Smailes ST, et al. Percutaneous dilational and surgical tracheostomy in burn patients: incidence of complications and dysphagia. Burns. 2014;40:436–42.
39. Sen S, et al. Tracheostomy in pediatric burn patients. Burns. 2014;41(2):248–51.
40. Burd A, et al. Decompression not escharotomy in acute burns. Burns. 2006;32(3):284–92.
41. Orgill DP, Piccolo N. Escharotomy and decompressive therapies in burns. J Burn Care Res. 2009;30(5):759–68. https://doi.org/10.1097/BCR.0b013e3181b47cd.
42. de Barros MEPM, et al. Revisiting escharotomy in patients with burns in extremities. J Burn Care Res. 2017;38(4):e691–8. https://doi.org/10.1097/BCR.0000000000000476.
43. Ruiz-Castilla M. Analysis of intra-abdominal hypertension in severe burned patients: the Vall d'Hebron experience. Burns. 2013;40(4):719–24.
44. Strang SG. A systematic review on intra-abdominal pressure in severely burned. Burns. 2013;40(1):9–16.
45. Israel JS, et al. Variations in burn excision and grafting: a survey of the American Burn Association. J Burn Care Res. 2017;38(1):e125–32. https://doi.org/10.1097/BCR.0000000000000475.
46. Janzekovic Z. A new concept in the early excision and immediate grafting of burns. J Trauma. 1970;10(12):1103–8.
47. Cartotto R. What are the acute cardiovascular effects of subcutaneous and topical epinephrine for Hemostasis during burn surgery? J Burn Care Rehabil. 2003;24:297–305.
48. Greenhalgh DG. Recombinant thrombin: safety and immunogenicity in burn wound excision and grafting. J Burn Care Res. 2009;30:371–9.
49. Housinger TA, Lang D, Warden GD. A prospective study of blood loss with excisional therapy in pediatric burn patients. J Trauma. 1993;34:262–3.
50. Kakagia DD, Karadimas EJ. The efficacy of Versajet™ Hydrosurgery system in burn surgery. A systematic review. J Burn Care Res. 2018;39(2):188–200.
51. Gravante G, et al. Versajet hydrosurgery versus classic escharectomy for burn de'bridment: a prospective randomized trial. J Burn Care Res. 2007;28:720–4.
52. Duteille F, Perrot P. Management of 2nd-degree facial burns using the Versajet® hydrosurgery system and xenograft: a prospective evaluation of 20 cases. Burns. 2012;38(5):724–9.
53. Rosenberg L, et al. Minimally invasive burn care: a review of seven clinical studies of rapid and selective debridement using a bromelain-based debriding enzyme (Nexobrid®). Ann Burns Fire Disasters. 2015;28(4):264–74.
54. Hirche C, et al. Eschar removal by bromelain based enzymatic debridement (Nexobrid®) in burns: an European consensus. Burns. 2017;43(8):1640–53. https://doi.org/10.1016/j.burns.2017.07.025.
55. Schulz A, et al. Enzymatic debridement of deeply burned faces: healing and early scarring based on tissue preservation compared to traditional surgical debridement. Burns. 2017;43(6):1233–43. https://doi.org/10.1016/j.burns.2017.02.016.
56. Rosenberg L, et al. Enzymatic debridement and care of 171 deeply burned hands with NexoBrid (NXB): single arm & controlled (RCT) studies. J Plast Reconstr Aesthet Surg. 2014;67(11):1605–6.
57. Schiefer JL, et al. A prospective intra-individual evaluation of silk compared to biobrane for the treatment of superficial burns of the hand and face. Burns. 2016;43(3):539–48.
58. Krezdorn N, et al. Biobrane versus topical agents in the treatment of adult scald burns. Burns. 2016;43(1):195–9.
59. Rahmanian-Schwarz A, et al. A clinical evaluation of Biobrane® and Suprathel® in acute burns and reconstructive surgery. Burns. 2011;37(8):1343–8.
60. Wahler S, et al. Cost-effectiveness comparison between biobrane and suprathel for partial thickness burn treatment. Value Health. 2017;20(9):A802.
61. Saffle JR. Closure of the excised burn wound: temporary skin substitutes. Clin Plast Surg. 2009;36(4):627–41.
62. Kagan R, et al. Surgical management of the burn wound and use of skin substitutes: an expert panel white paper. J Burn Care Res. 2013;34(2):e60–79.. https://doi.org/10.1097/BCR.0b013e31827039a6
63. Cleland H, et al. Clinical application and viability of cryopreserved cadaveric skin allografts in severe burn: a retrospective analysis. Burns. 2014;40(1):61–6.
64. Spence RJ. The application of full-thickness skin grafts in facial burn reconstruction. Management of facial burns. In: Geoffrey G, Peter N, editors. Plastic surgery, volume 1. Principles, vol. 21. Amsterdam: Elsevier; 2013. p. 468–99.
65. Park YS, et al. Algorithm for primary full-thickness skin grafting in pediatric hand burns. Arch Plast Surg. 2012;39(5):483–8.
66. Alexander JW, et al. Treatment of severe burns with widely meshed skin autograft and meshed skin allograft overlay. J Trauma. 1981;21:433–8.

67. Pripotnev S, et al. Split thickness skin graft meshing ratio indications and common practices. Burns. 2017;43(8):1775–81.
68. Howarth AL. A novel approach to graft loss in burn using the CelluTome™ epidermal harvesting system for spot grafting: a case report. Burns. 2015;41(6):e57–60.
69. Sood R, et al. Coverage of large pediatric wounds with cultured epithelial autografts in congenital nevi and burns: results and technique. J Burn Care Res. 2009;30(4):576–86. https://doi.org/10.1097/BCR.0b013e3181ac02de.
70. Chester DL, et al. A review of keratinocyte delivery to the wound bed. J Burn Care Res. 2004;25(3):266–75. https://doi.org/10.1097/01.BCR.0000124749.85552.CD.
71. Esteban-Vives R, et al. Cell-spray auto-grafting technology for deep partial thickness burns: problems and solutions during clinical implementation. Burns. 2018;44(3):549–59.
72. Busch KH, et al. Combination of medical needling and non-cultured autologous skin cell transplantation (ReNovaCell) for repigmentation of hypopigmented burn scars. Burns. 2016;42:1556–66.
73. Back C, et al. Noncultured keratinocyte/melanocyte cosuspension: effect on reepithelialization and repigmentation—a randomized, placebo-controlled study. J Burn Care Res. 2009;30:408–16. https://doi.org/10.1097/BCR.0b013e3181a28c4d.
74. Medina A, et al. Modified Meek micrografting technique for wound coverage in extensive burn injuries. J Burn Care Res. 2016;37(5):305–13. https://doi.org/10.1097/BCR.0000000000000244.
75. Ottomann C, et al. A tribute to Cicero Parker Meek. Burns. 2015;41:1660–3.
76. Heimbach DM. Multicenter postapproval clinical trial of Integra® dermal regeneration template for burn treatment. J Burn Care Rehabil. 2003;24(1):42–8. https://doi.org/10.1097/00004630-200301000-00009.
77. Ryan CM. Use of Integra® artificial skin is associated with decreased length of stay for severely injured adult burn survivors. J Burn Care Res. 2002;23(5):311–7.
78. Min JH. The use of matriderm and autologous skin graft in the treatment of full thickness skin defects. Arch Plast Surg. 2014;41(4):330–6.
79. Schneider J, et al. Matriderm® versus Integra®: a comparative experimental study. Burns. 2009;35(1):51–7.

Acute Management of Facial Burns, Acute Versus Long-Term, Surgical Versus Non-surgical Face Transplant

35

Juan P. Barret and Julia Barret-Joly

35.1 Introduction

Skin is the largest organ in the human body. Burn injury to the skin can range from being relatively trivial to one of the most severe injuries the human body can sustain. Major burn injury often requires multidisciplinary treatment in an intensive care setting, multiple surgical procedures to achieve wound healing followed by prolonged rehabilitation and possibly a lifetime of reconstructive procedures to achieve psychosocial, aesthetic and functional recovery. Burn injury is ubiquitous. Neanderthal cave paintings have been found depicting burn treatment. Hippocrates (400 years BC), Celsus (first century AD) and Galen (second century AD) all wrote on burn wound care. Ambrose Paré (1510–1590) described burn wound excision. Dupuytren (1832) described six degrees of burn depth that remain in use today. The twentieth century has brought great advances in burn care. These include the scientific understanding of fluid loss and resuscitation (Underhill 1920, Evans 1952), the hypermetabolic response to trauma (Sneve 1905, Wilmore 1974) and the control of infection with topical antimicrobial agents including silver sulfadiazine (Flamazine) (Moyer 1965, Fox 1969). In 1870, Pollock first described the skin grafting of a burn. In 1960, Jackson and colleagues pioneered excision and grafting. Janzekovic (1970) developed the technique of tangential excision of deep partial-thickness burns. Further advances in wound resurfacing such as the use of cultured skin and the development of integral artificial skin are more recent innovations [1, 2]. Ninety per cent of burn injuries are preventable. Prevention has traditionally been either via education or legislation. There have been numerous successful educational campaigns that have modified people's behaviour. Legislation has also been effective in the prevention of burn injuries. Examples include sprinkler systems and smoke detectors in public and commercial buildings, fireguards, transport and storage of flammable materials.

The management of a burn depends on many variables including the age of the patient, co-morbid factors and the size, depth and anatomical location of the injury. In general, the aims of burn care are to restore form, function and feeling. This involves early aesthetic wound closure, optimal rehabilitation to preinjury activities and psychosocial recovery [3, 4].

35.2 Modern Surgical Treatment

In general, burns that are deemed to be deep in nature are best excised, and the wounds are covered with autologous split skin grafts. The grafts usually require meshing, and the amount of wound that can be closed with autograft depends on the donor sites available and the mesh ratio used. Operative blood loss varies according to the post-burn time of excision and is preferably done as early as possible post injury [5, 6].

Cosmetically and functionally sensitive areas such as the face and hands need thicker sheet autograft for wound closure. In general, it is preferable to use sheet grafts in children as they give a better aesthetic result. If the burn size is large or if there is a lack of donor sites, then temporary wound closure with allograft, xenograft, other biological or semi-biological dressings and/or synthetic skin substitutes may be required while the donor sites heal. Patients with lager burns need to return to the operating room for further grafting when their donor sites are healed. This is usually done on a weekly basis [7].

J. P. Barret (✉)
Department of Plastic Surgery and Burns, University Hospital Vall d'Hebron, Universitat autonoma de Barcelona, Barcelona, Spain
e-mail: jpbarret@vhebron.net

J. Barret-Joly
SEK Catalunya International School, La Garriga, Spain

M. G. Jeschke et al. (eds.), *Handbook of Burns Volume 1*, https://doi.org/10.1007/978-3-030-18940-2_35

35.3 Surgical Treatment of Facial Burns

The goals of acute management of the burned face are similar to that of burns in other parts of the body. However, the outcome of facial burns has a significant social and functional implication. Patients whose face and hands have been spared present with excellent rates of social reintegration, whereas deep burns of the face and hands are devastating, requiring long-term physiotherapy, psychological intervention and reconstruction.

In general terms, unless gross destruction of skin and soft tissues is obvious, a delay in the excision of acute facial burns until day 10 allows better determination of tissue that will not heal within a 3-week period. Subsequent excision of deep partial- and full-thickness burns must be carefully planned and performed in a precise manner following strict principles. Still, the development of enzymatic debridement has produced a new prompt method for surgical (enzymatic) debridement of dead tissues of the face within hours from injury. This practice enhances wound healing and preserves living dermis, changing the paradigm of acute burn surgery.

Main principles of surgery and reconstruction include

- Respect for aesthetic units
- Sacrifice of less injured tissue to preserve aesthetic units
- Minimisation of blood loss
- Delayed coverage with autografts to minimise postoperative hematomas
- Early intervention of rehabilitation services

Daily hydrotherapy and topical antimicrobial cream application for 10 days is advised in face burns. This allows for viable tissue to heal and helps to determine which areas will not be healed without evident scarring and disfigurement. Face burns are debrided upon admission of loose blisters and dead skin. Burns are then treated conservatively with one of the following:

- Polysporin cream + Nystatin
- Silver sulfadiazine
- Cerium nitrate silver sulfadiazine
- Xenografts
- Amnion
- Bioactive creams/gels

Conservative treatment is then carried out until a definitive diagnosis and treatment plan is outlined.

The operation is performed in the supine position in the reverse Trendelemburg position under general anaesthesia. Extensive bleeding must be expected, and blood products should be available before the beginning of the operation. The endotracheal tube (ET) is fixed to the teeth, and a sterile endoscopic cover is inserted to allow full mobilisation and freedom of the anaesthesia tubing. The eyes should be protected with either protective contact lens or with temporary tarsorrhaphy stitches. Face burns are normally operated in a two-stage procedure. Burns are excised in the first operation and the wounds are closed with homografts or skin substitutes. A second-look operation is then performed within 4–7 days and wounds are closed with a definitive coverage. This allows for perfect haemostasis, preventing graft loss or artificial dermis loss due to hematomas, and it permits re-excision of non-viable tissue.

Patients are fed via an enteral tube that should be let in place until all grafts are stable, usually by day 7 post grafting. In non-ventilated patients, patients should be left intubated and ventilated for 48 h to preserve integrity of the grafted areas.

The aesthetic units that will not heal within 3 weeks of the injury are outlined with markers (Fig. 35.2). The excision must incorporate the whole aesthetic unit to render perfect outcomes. It is not uncommon to excise minor areas of normal skin or superficial wounds to comply with the aesthetic unit philosophy. When only a small area of an aesthetic unit is burned, it is either left unexcised or grafted preserving the rest of normal tissue. It is reconstructed at a later stage if the outcome is deemed unacceptable [8, 9].

35.3.1 Postoperative Care

Grafts are normally exposed unless an elastomer mould can be applied with interim pressure garments. If the use of elastomers is feasible (depending on rehabilitation services capabilities), a negative impression is made at the end of the excision and application of homografts (stage one). It allows the occupational and physical therapists to fabricate an elastomer that is applied under interim and permanent pressure garments.

In general, graft care includes the application of antimicrobial ointments on graft seams and Vaseline or antimicrobial creams on the graft surface to prevent desiccation. Grafts are inspected twice a day for seromas and hematomas. If they develop, they are drained through small incisions placed in the relaxed skin tension line. When hematomas are large, the patient is returned to theatre to lift the graft, remove the hematoma, and stitch the graft back under general anaesthesia.

Patients are kept NPO for 4 days, and they are fed via a nasogastric or naso-jejunal tube. Patients should refrain from talking for 5 days, and 48 h of ventilatory support should be considered in children and non-compliant adults. The head of bed should be elevated 45°, and all manoeuvres that may increase head and neck pressure and systemic pressure should be avoided. A calm and comfortable environment should be maintained to decrease the stress of patient and facilitate the postoperative care.

In case elastomers are not used during the immediate postoperative period, interim pressure garments followed by custom-made pressure garments, face masks and splints should be used as soon as the grafts are deemed to be stable [10–12].

35.4 Enzymatic Debridement of Facial Burn Wounds

The introduction of a new selective enzymatic debridement agent (Nexobrid®), in the armamentarium for burn wound management, has provided some new concepts in the initial management and wound healing. Patients with deep partial thickness burns treated with Nexobrid® experience great benefits in the reduction of the need for autografting compared with the standard of care. In major burns, besides the improvement in wound healing, an important improvement in their general state has been observed.

Deep burns to the face (ideally diagnosed with laser Doppler scanning, LDI, or similar) are treated with bromelain (enzymatic debridement) early after admission. The drug is applied on the surface with eye and normal skin protection (Vaseline or similar) for 4 h. The application is painful; thus, deep sedation or general anaesthesia is necessary. A fine layer of 3–5 mm is created. The area is then covered with a transparent plastic wrap. After 4 h the product is removed. All debris, necrotic tissue, exudate and bleeding are cleansed with intense brushing and irrigation. Next, a wet dressing is applied (0.9% saline solution) for 24 h. The area is irrigated and cleansed as needed.

Definitive treatment shall depend on the tissue remaining after enzymatic debridement. Areas with viable dermis that may heal spontaneously are best treated with homografts, xenografts, amnion, honey gel, etc. Any skin with fat exposure or areas that cannot heal in a reasonable period of time are autografted in aesthetic units. It is recommended that this definitive treatment is performed between 3 and 4 days after enzymatic debridement in order to enhance graft take (Figs. 35.1 and 35.2) [13].

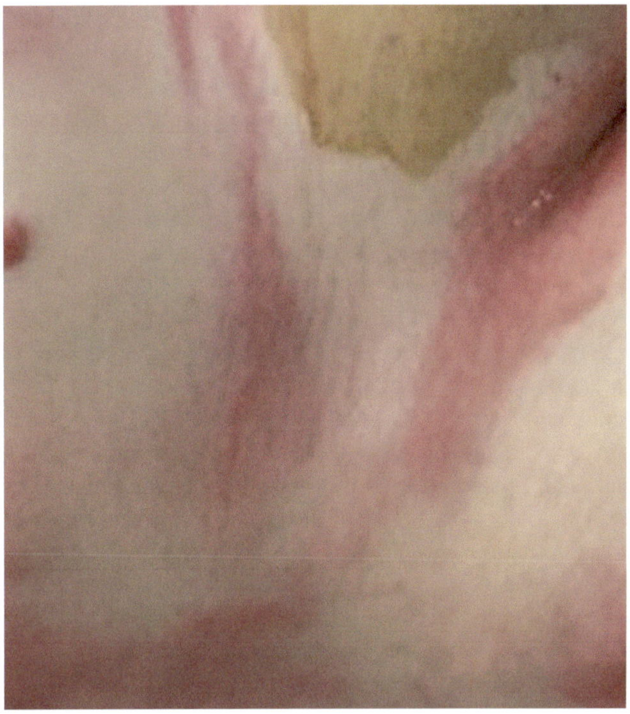

Fig. 35.1 Deep partial thickness burns. Aspect before enzymatic debridement

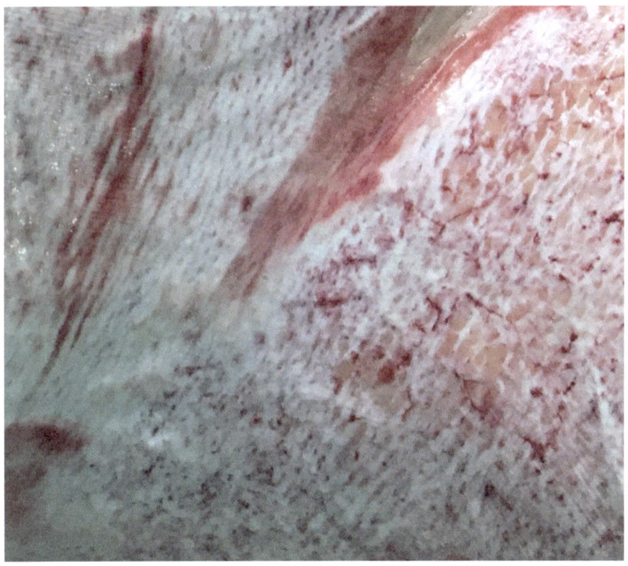

Fig. 35.2 Same wound after enzymatic debridement. Note that all dead tissues have been removed with the protection of living tissue

35.5 Face Transplantation

The modern history of vascularised composite tissue allotransplantation began in 1998, when the first human hand transplantation became a reality. Few years afterwards, in 2005, the first human face transplantation was attempted with success by Devauchelle and Dubernard in France [14].

Facial transplantation is a new achievement of transplantation medicine and microvascular reconstructive plastic surgery. During the past years, an important activity in the specialty of plastic and reconstructive surgery has been registered. In particular, a real revolution in reconstruction has occurred. The not-so-old dream of restorative surgery, namely the replacement of damaged parts of the body by new unharmed pre-formed tissues has become reality. The development of techniques aimed at the transplantation of vascularised composite tissues (VCA, composite vascularised allografts) has provided clinicians with a new robust tool for the reconstruction of deformities that were, no so long ago, impossible to achieve. History, development and classical attempts for VCA are not new. More than four decades ago, doctors in Ecuador attempted the transplantation of a hand limb. The transplant failed, but the dream survived. Pioneering laboratory work in experimental animals showed the path to clinicians for the achievement of human CVA. On the other hand, VCA has opened a new era not only in reconstructive surgery but also in transplant surgery. To date, there have been reports of successful transplantations of the knee joint, hand (unilateral and bilateral), arms (uni and bilateral), face (partial and total), abdominal wall, larynx, penis, digits and lower limbs; all recipients presented with deformities and/or amputations that were not amenable to be reconstructed by means of classical or traditional techniques. Such deformities affected non-vital parts and/or organs, and all of them had in common the impossibility to restore form, function, and cosmesis by means of conventional techniques and reconstructive surgery. The results of facial transplantation in humans demonstrate that facial transplantation is no longer an abstraction but a clinical reality. It has been implemented in the latest years with increasing interest and great success. The limits of indications are still, though, desperate catastrophic facial disfigurement. Today, we are in a position to say that it has been possible to perform facial transplantation both in animals and humans in a short period of time (Figs. 35.3 and 35.4).

Similar to that learnt in many other transplant and plastic surgery disciplines, the development of Facial Transplantation Programs calls for a strong team approach, building a multidisciplinary team that involves all necessary and diverse specialists to make a robust protocol and an experienced team that warrants excellency in outcomes. This multidisciplinary team is formed by all transplant disciplines usually involved in transplant medicine (surgeons, immunologists, infectious disease specialists and renal diseases specialists) but should include also experienced health professionals more involved in the plastic and reconstructive scenario, namely rehabilitation specialists, physiotherapists, occupational therapists, psychologists, psychiatrists and social workers. VCA procedures must be organised in tertiary centres with a strong commitment to transplant surgery and medicine. Such institutions have in common the required laboratory, clinical services and research units that are necessary to perform this new clinical discipline [15, 16].

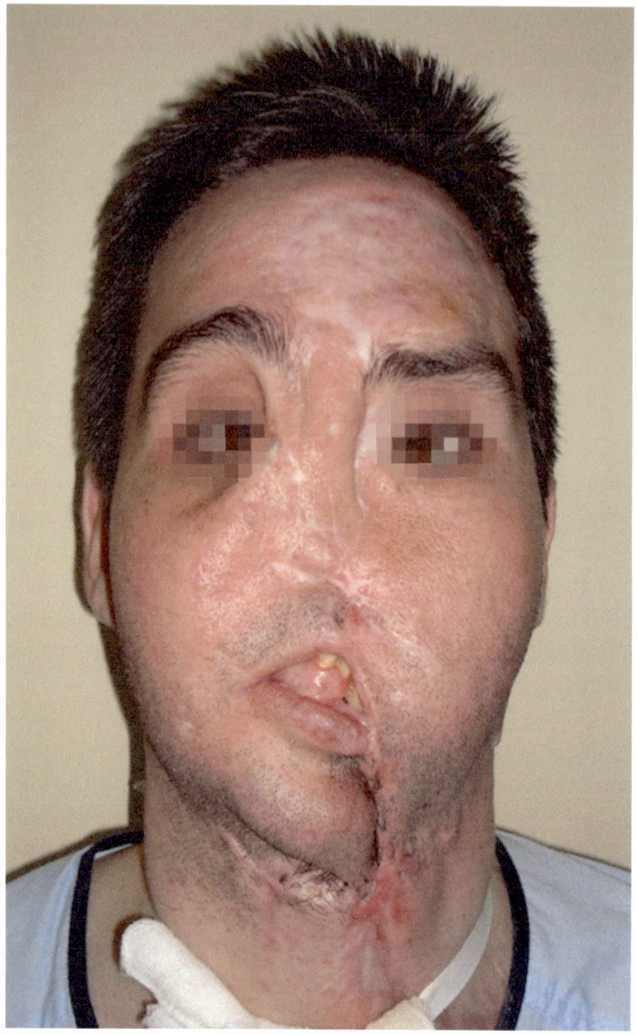

Fig. 35.3 Facial deformity after gun-shot injury to the face. Scarring, anatomic destruction including facial skeleton is common

35.5.1 Indications of Face Transplantation

The indication of facial transplantation resides on important deformities that affect different structures of the human face. They normally involve muscle sphincters (oral, ocular sphincter) and exhibit an important functional impact (impossibilities to speak, feed normally or breathe). The psychosocial impact of the deformity is extremely high, preventing them from functioning as normal human beings. Patients normally experience the facial deformity as health status worse than being death. The motivation of patients' concentrates on becoming "normal" again and being able to resume their pre-morbid lifestyle.

The usual aetiologies considered for facial transplantation include

1. Gun-shot injuries (ballistic trauma)
2. Other posttraumatic injuries
3. Burn deformity
4. Benign tumours (i.e. neurofibromatosis)
5. Postoncological deformities (tumour free and risk free)

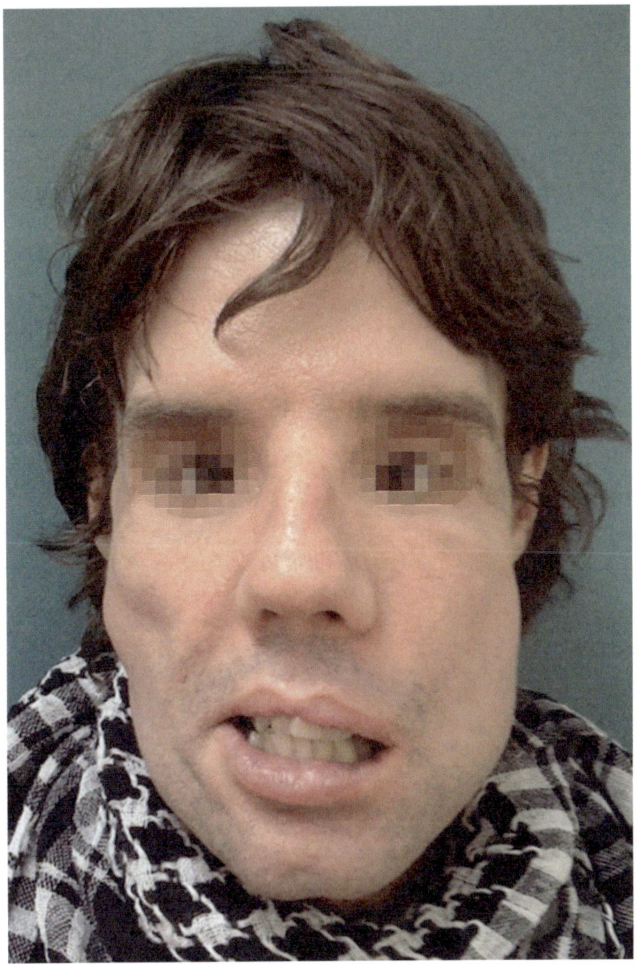

Fig. 35.4 Same patient after full-face transplantation including facial skeleton (type V-b face transplant)

However, when patients are considered for facial transplantation, benefits of the procedure should surpass the risks of the proposed treatment and the toxic and side effects of the immunosuppressant therapy.

Similarly, the expected result of the proposed technique must be superior to that obtained with traditional techniques. Functional and aesthetic outcomes of facial transplantation must be by far much better than those obtained with any other technique that is also available. Otherwise, the transplant should not be indicated, nor the reconstruction proceed without reconstructive allotransplantation [17, 18].

35.5.2 Facial Transplantation: Technical Aspects

Face transplantation consists in the extirpation of facial tissues of a donor with the diagnosis of brain death (solid organ donor) and its transplantation to a patient to reconstruct his/her facial defect. All deformed and scarred recipient facial tissues are removed and replaced by normal tissues, which restore anatomy and function. In general terms, facial CVA procedures utilise a two team technique approach: a donor's and a recipient's teams, similar to that employed in SOT, especially in heart and lung allotransplantation. The fabrication of a facial prosthesis must precede any CVA procedure (limbs, face, etc.). Maintaining the dignity of the patient during the whole donation process is mandatory, and bioethics during procurement call for excellency in the care of the donor. Similar to many other facial CVA transplantation teams, we recommend a heart-beating donation. It shortens the ischemia time, reduces the impact of ischemia-reperfusion injury and allows for correct haemostasis during the facial procurement operation. The donor operation starts securing a patent and safe airway. If tracheotomy is selected, it should be performed in the first tracheal rings to allow for a long tracheal segment if a double lung transplant is also planned. Major vessels are cannulated in the usual manner, which must include the carotid circulation to perfuse the graft when the in situ dissection is finished. The operation begins with the cervical incision and undermining under the platysma muscle. The external carotid artery is identified and dissected. Major external carotid artery branches are identified and preserved if necessary for the type of facial graft planned. In general terms, only the facial artery is necessary for nearly all facial transplants. Lingual artery is to be preserved if the tongue is included in the facial transplant. Similarly, the hypoglossal nerve is identified, dissected and included in the transplant (face and tongue transplantation). A bicoronal incision is performed next. Dissection proceeds in the subperiosteal plane up to the level of the orbit. The supraorbital nerve is identified and dissected inside the orbit in order to lengthen it and allow for a tension-free neurorrhaphy. Attention is directed to the lateral aspect of the face next. An incision is made at the appropriate level. If the ears are not included, a rhytidectomy incision is chosen. When the ears are transplanted, the incision is more posterior. The soft tissues are lifted and undermined. A deep dissection plane is employed, in order to include all facial muscles and nerves (a more superficial plane is employed if only skin and soft tissues are transplanted). All five facial nerve branches are identified at the anterior margin of the parotid gland, cut and included in the graft. The dissection approaches the infraorbital nerve, and it is freed of adhesions. It is severed at the appropriate level for each individual case. If necessary, the mucosa and submucosa layers of the cheek are included with a full-thickness dissection of the lips. Inferiorly, the dissection connects with the cervical flap. The dental nerve is identified at the mental foramen and severed and included in the flap. The final step during procurement consists of dissection and inclusion of the soft tissues and cartilages of the nose and section of the eyelids at the desired level. Current evidence supports good vascularization of an entire face graft by the facial vascular pedicle. However, the temporal vessels may be included in the flap if necessary, and they may be dissected in continuity with the facial arteries down to the external carotid. This procedure adds difficulty in the dissection with uncertain benefits in blood flow; however, it still is our first choice in full-face grafts. If a facial transplant including bone is planned, bone osteotomies are performed at this stage, leaving them attached to the soft tissues (good periosteal vascularization does exist). The entire face graft is then left pedicled on arteries and veins (retromandibular veins, facial veins and external jugular veins). The graft is simultaneously perfused with preservation fluid at 4 °C with the rest of solid organs.

After transportation to the recipient operation theatre, the second part of the operation starts. The recipient neck has been prepared and the major vessels dissected. Depending on the type of facial deformity, the deformed structures have been resected creating a defect on the recipient's face to be restored by the face transplant. Other teams prefer performing the resection of the recipient's face after revascularization. Arteries and veins are anastomosed in the standard fashion. Before reperfusion, 1 g of prednisone is infused i.v. to prevent any immunological reaction during this phase of the operation (immunosuppression induction therapy starts when the patient arrives at the operation theatre). The reconstructive phase of the operation begins with bone osteotomies and osteosynthesis with titanium miniplates, intraoral in-setting, nerve neurorrhaphies (dental nerve and infraorbital nerve are performed before the final miniplating), and the suture of soft tissues and skin [19].

Summary Box

1. Deep facial burns require early excision (either surgical or enzimatic).
2. Surgical treatment should follow strict principles.
3. The most relevant principles in facial burn treatment are: respect of aesthetic units, delayed definitive coverage, early rehabilitation.
4. Face transplantation is a novel technique that may be used to reconstruct in full facial defects.
5. Face transplantation should be reserved to patients with severe functional deficits, i.e. destruction of facial sphincters.

References

1. Thomas S, Barrow RE, Herndon DN. History of the treatment of burns. In: Herndon DN, editor. Total burn care. 5th ed. Amsterdam: Elsevier; 2017.
2. Heimbach DM, Warden GD, Luterman A, Jordan MH, Ozobia N, Ryan CM, Voigt DW, Hickerson WL, Saffle JR, DeClement FA, Sheridan RL, Dimick AR. Multicenter postapproval clinical trial of Integra dermal regeneration template for burn treatment. J Burn Care Rehabil. 2003;24(1):42–8.
3. National Burn Care Review. Standards and strategy for burn care; a review of burn care in the British Isles. In: Dunn KW. National Burn Care Review Committee; 2001.
4. Čapek KD, Culnan DM, Desai MH, Herndon DN. Fifty years of burn care at Shriners hospitals for children, Galveston. Ann Plast Surg. 2018;80(3 Suppl 2):S90–4.
5. Barret JP, Desai MH, Herndon DN. Massive transfusión of reconstituted whole blood is well tolerated in pediatric burn surgery. J Trauma. 1999;47(3):526–8.
6. Desai MH, Herndon DN, Broemeling L, Barrow RE, Nichols RJ Jr, Rutan RL. Early burn wound excision significantly reduces blood loss. Ann Surg. 1990;211(6):753–9; discussion 759–62.
7. Engrav LH, Donelan MB. Face burns: acute care and reconstruction. In: Operative techniques in plastic and reconstructive surgery. Vol. 4, No. 2. Philadelphia: W. B. Saunders; 1997.
8. Luce EA. Burn care and management. Clin Plast Surg. 2000;27(1). W. B. Saunders.
9. Remensynder JP, Donelan MB. Reconstruction of the head and neck. In: Herndon DN, editor. Total burn care. London: W. B. Saunders; 2002.
10. Achauer BM. Burn reconstruction. New York: Thieme; 1991.
11. Achauer BM. General reconstructive surgery. In: Plastic surgery, indications, operations, and outcomes. St. Louis: Mosby; 2000.
12. Barret JP, Herndon DN. The face. In: Principles and practice of burn surgery. New York: Marcel Dekker; 2005.
13. Palao R, Aguilera-Saez J, Serracanta J, Collado JM, Dos santos BP, Barret JP. Use of a selective enzymatic debridement agent (Nexobrid®) for wound management: learning curve. World J Dermatol. 2017;6(2):32–41.
14. Devauchelle B, Badet L, Lengelé B, Morelon E, Testelin S, Michallet M, D'Hauthuille C, Dubernard JM. First human face allograft: early report. Lancet. 2006;368(9531):203–9.
15. Barret JP, Gavaldà J, Bueno J, et al. Full face transplant: the first case report. Ann Surg. 2011;254(2):252–6.
16. Barret JP, Serracanta J, Collado JM, et al. Full face transplantation organization, development, and results—the Barcelona experience: a case report. Transplant Proc. 2011;43:3533–4.
17. Arno A, Barret JP, Harrison RA, Jeschke MG. Face allotransplantation and burns: a review. J Burn Care Res. 2012;33:561–76.
18. Barret JP, Tomasello V. Evaluation of candidates for face transplantation. In: Face transplantation: principles, techniques and artistry. Berlin: Springer; 2015.
19. Barret JP, Tomasello V. Face transplantation: surgical aspects. In: Face transplantation: principles, techniques and artistry. Berlin: Springer; 2015.

36 Hand Burns

Clifford C. Sheckter and Matthew B. Klein

36.1 Introduction

Loss of hand function is the leading cause of impairment following burn injury [1]. As the contact point for day-to-day activities, hand is both highly susceptible to injury and of paramount importance in preserving function. Over 80% of severe burn injuries include the hand [2], and even small burns localized to the hand can potentially impair function and quality of life.

Advances in acute burn care have made survival of previously fatal injuries possible and shifted the focus of burn care and research toward optimizing functional outcomes. Consequently, restoration of hand function has received increased attention with a multidisciplinary team of burn surgeons, plastic surgeons, rehabilitation physicians, physical therapists, and occupational therapists coordinating care at specialized burn centers. The complexity of hand anatomy and function necessitate thoughtful consideration by all burn team members.

36.2 Initial Evaluation and Hand Exam

All patients presenting with burn injuries should undergo an evaluation focusing on systemic illness and life-threatening injuries in accordance with standard trauma evaluation protocols. After life-threatening injuries have been evaluated, the burn injury can be addressed. In evaluating hand burns, a careful history, including handedness, prior injuries, occupation, and mechanism of acute injury should be obtained. The date of the patient's last tetanus vaccination or booster should be documented, and tetanus toxoid or immunoglobulin should be administered as necessary.

Physical examination should first establish the extent and depth of burns followed by a comprehensive hand exam. Starting with visual examination, the extent and depth of burns on all surfaces should be documented on a hand diagram with distinct markings for extent and depth of injury. Other injuries are assessed including crush, laceration, and avulsion. Any suspicion for fracture, dislocation, or foreign body should be further evaluated with x-ray imaging. Functional examination proceeds with active and passive range of motion for all joints, and any deficits should be documented and appropriately triaged by a hand surgeon. Note that functional examination may be limited by pain, mental status, or sedation.

Particular attention should be given to the neurovascular examination, as this dictates the need for emergent intervention. Any circumferential or full-thickness upper extremity burn is concerning for ischemia and deserves careful consideration. Decreased perfusion manifests in many forms including pain with passive motion, capillary refill greater than 2–3 s (or absent), diminished radial or ulnar pulses, and cold hand to touch. If ischemia is suspected, various tools can help confirm insufficient perfusion including Doppler ultrasound and pulse oximetry (reading <90%). In the event decreased perfusion is suspected, yet there is insufficient evidence for escharotomy, trending hand examinations (e.g., every hour) using Doppler ultrasound or pulse oximetry can demonstrate a trajectory toward watchful waiting or operative management. Arterial pressure monitoring catheters should never be placed in an extremity where there is concern for decreased perfusion.

Isolated nerve compression is rare, but can occur in electrical injuries. A nerve examination should be performed documenting the typical distributions of the median, ulnar, and radial nerves. Symptoms suggesting compression such as paresthesias, numbness, or decreased motor function should be considered for surgical release [3].

C. C. Sheckter
Division of Plastic and Reconstructive Surgery, Stanford School of Medicine, Stanford, CA, USA
e-mail: Sheckter@stanford.edu

M. B. Klein (✉)
Burn Center and Division of Plastic Surgery, Santa Clara Valley Medical Center, San Jose, CA, USA

M. G. Jeschke et al. (eds.), *Handbook of Burns Volume 1*, https://doi.org/10.1007/978-3-030-18940-2_36

36.3 Primary Management and Wound Care

During the initial burn wound evaluation, foreign material should be removed and thin or loose blisters debrided. An appropriate dressing is then applied, ensuring that burned digits are wrapped individually. The choice of dressing is dependent on the depth of the burn with the primary goals of preventing infection, promoting re-epithelialization, preventing desiccation, and maintaining euthermia. Additionally, the ideal dressing should be easy to apply, reduce pain, and allow for full range of motion. The affected hand(s) should be elevated as soon as feasible to limit edema. Commonly used means include securing band-net stocking to standing poles or gurney overhead rails.

Local wound care is the definitive treatment for superficial and superficial partial-thickness hand burns with the goal of optimizing re-epithelialization. We prefer an ointment with antimicrobial properties such as bacitracin and nonadherent gauze dressing (e.g., petroleum gauze or bismuth tribromophenate). For deeper burns that may form an eschar, we prefer silver sulfadiazine (Silvadene), which provides increased antibacterial protection and is soothing when applied. Silvadene forms a film or "pseudo-eschar" when applied necessitating daily cleansing prior to repeat application. Sulfamylon (mafenide) is preferred for infected burns due to sulfadiazine's poor eschar penetration. However, metabolic acidosis resulting from carbonic anhydrase inhibition is a potential side effect for which the treating physician must be vigilant. When epithelialization is imminent or occurring, the dressing may be switched to bacitracin and nonadherent gauze. There is no evidence supporting the use of prophylactic intravenous or oral antibiotics.

The ultimate goal in treating hand burns is return of function, which can be neglected by only focusing on wound care. Edema, especially on the dorsum of the hand and around joints, may lead to postures with decreased tension on the collateral ligaments. Corrective splinting in the position of safety and early motion minimizes the potential of future contractures. The position of safety also called "intrinsic plus" places the wrist in 5–10 degrees of extension, metacarpophalangeal joints in 70–90 degrees of flexion, and both interphalangeal joints in full extension. Occupational and physical therapists alike should be involved at the earliest opportunity. In the event the patient is sedated or unable to follow commands, allied therapists can passively range hand joints.

The hand and especially fingers have dense sensory nerve networks that lend to painful wound care, especially in partial-thickness burns. Placement of regional pain catheters by anesthesiologists can help facilitate more aggressive bedside debridement for patients requiring in-hospital wound management, and the catheters can also be used intraoperatively in cases requiring excision. In order to prevent immobility, the anesthetic infusions should be down-titrated between dressing changes to allow for full motor function and active range of motion exercises.

36.4 Escharotomy and Fasciotomy

Deep extremity burns—particularly those that are circumferential—must be closely monitored for distal vascular insufficiency. Patients who sustain extensive burn injuries require large volumes of intravenous fluid and will develop significant soft tissue edema under the tight shell-like eschar. Suspicion for compromised perfused should be addressed immediately with escharotomy to improve distal perfusion [4]. Escharotomy may be performed under general anesthesia in the operating room or, if necessary, at the bedside in the intensive care unit with appropriate analgesia and sedation. Eschar is insensate and pain should be minimal during the procedure. A full release of the forearm may be achieved using either electrocautery or a scalpel to incise the eschar through two longitudinal incisions (radially and ulnarly) down to the level of the first and fifth metacarpophalangeal joints. Further decompression of the hand itself is achieved through longitudinal incisions between the metacarpals from the base of the hand to the head of the metacarpal taking care not to expose any tendons (Fig. 36.1). Digital escharotomy is avoided at our institution; however, one small care

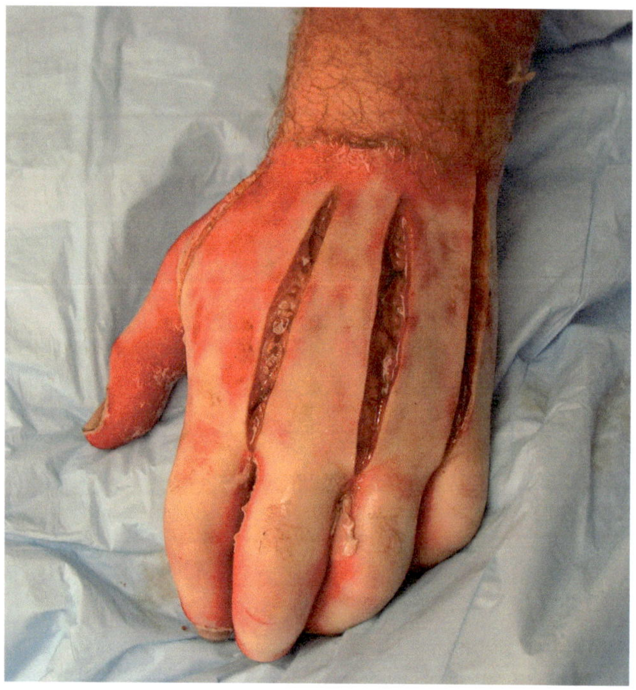

Fig. 36.1 Escharotomy of the hand is performed by incising the eschar in the intermetacarpal spaces. Care is taken not to unnecessarily sever or expose underlying extensor tendons

series suggests that it may decrease finger necrosis [5]. If digit escharotomy is performed, dorsal release avoids the volarly oriented neurovascular bundles. Digits 2–3 should be released on ulnar side to avoid future scar contact with the thumb during opposition. Similarly, digits 4–5 should be released radially to avoid scar contact with resting surfaces. Regardless of specific technique, escharotomy incisions should be limited to the eschar itself as unnecessary deep incisions can expose underlying vital structures.

Patients with circumferential forearm burns are at risk for compartment syndrome when edema collects deep to the unyielding eschar resulting in decreased arterial flow and venous congestion. If escharotomy is not performed as described above, ischemic tissues (i.e., skeletal muscle) will become edematous leading to compartment syndrome and permanent muscle death. Electrical injuries and burns with an associated crush injury are more likely to increase compartmental pressures, resulting in compartment syndrome due to muscle injury. Deep muscle compartments are often more injured than superficial after electrical burns due to bone's elevated resistance to current flow. Neuropraxia following electrical shock can also complicate the initial assessment. The diagnosis of compartment syndrome is generally clinical and heralded by the constellation of pain on passive stretch, paresthesias, pallor, paralysis, decreased pulses, and poikilothermia. Systemic signs, including myoglobin-induced metabolic acidosis, may be the only sign of compartment syndrome in an obtunded patient with myonecrosis. Compartmental pressures of >30 mmHg or within 10–20 mmHg of diastolic pressure are diagnostic of compartment syndrome [5]. In the setting of suspected compartment syndrome, or failure of escharotomy to restore distal perfusion, fasciotomy should be performed in the operating theater. Forearm incisions include a dorsally and volarly oriented release that targets all three compartments of the forearm (anterior, posterior, and mobile wad). Additionally, if compartment syndrome of the hand is suspected, a full release of all ten compartments and both peripheral nerve canals (carpal tunnel and Guyon's canal) should be performed [3, 6]. The compartment release is commonly achieved through four incisions: ulnar hand (hypothenar), thenar eminence, dorsal index finger metacarpal (interossei and adductor pollicis), and dorsal ring finger metacarpal (interossei). The carpal tunnel and Guyon's canal are released in a standard fashion.

36.5 Surgical Management

36.5.1 Early Excision and Grafting

Early excision and grafting have been shown to reduce hypertrophic scarring and subsequent contractures leading to a reduced need for later reconstructions [7–10]. Superficial and intermediate partial-thickness burns will often heal within 2 weeks and rarely require early excision. However, deeper wounds that are expected to take longer to heal (i.e., longer than 21 days) should be carefully monitored for healing potential. Burns should be excised and grafted once they demonstrate inability to heal. Given the relatively small surface area of the hand, timing of hand excision in a patient with extensive burns should be weighed against the need to remove large areas of eschar to prevent burn wound sepsis.

Excision and grafting are usually performed under general anesthesia, although limited debridements are possible with regional blocks (particularly when grafts are not harvested) [11]. Tourniquet use is recommended to limit blood loss, and tourniquet time should not exceed 2 h to avoid tissue ischemia. Excision is performed with the use of a Goulian knife to remove eschar to a depth of healthy, bleeding tissue. For excision of web spaces and other areas in which the Goulian knife is difficult to maneuver, the Versajet (Smith and Nephew, London, UK) is a high-pressure water jet system that navigates well [12, 13] (Fig. 36.2). Excision

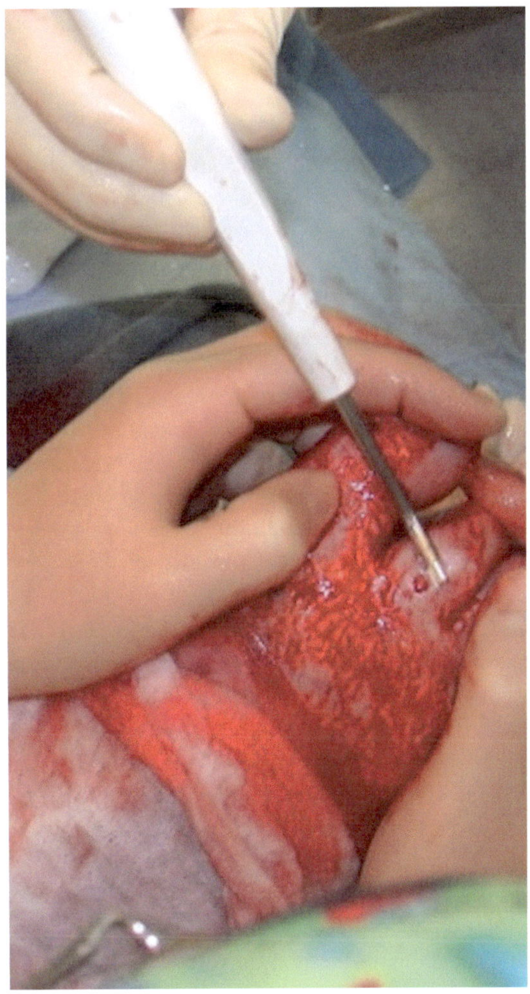

Fig. 36.2 The Versajet water dissector provides precise tissue excision and is particularly well suited for areas of convexity and concavity

on the dorsum of the hand should be performed carefully given the minimal subcutaneous tissue and the risk of exposing tendons. Small areas of exposed tendon may be covered with surrounding soft tissue to avoid the need for flap coverage; however, inevitable cases of tendon and joint exposure will require soft tissue flap coverage [14]. If tendon becomes exposed and soft tissue reconstruction is delayed, diligent moisture preserving measures are needed to prevent irreversible tendon desiccation and death. Once excision is complete, the tourniquet should be deflated to assess tissue viability by observing bleeding. Epinephrine (concentration 1:10,000) soaked Telfa (Mansfield, MA) and laparotomy pads should be applied for 10 min. The wound bed should then be assessed for hemostasis and epinephrine Telfa pads and laparotomy pads replaced as needed to achieve a bloodless field. Electrocautery should be used sparingly and only on small focal areas of bleeding. Unlike other areas of the body, over-excision of hand soft tissues can lead to permanent loss of critical structures that are difficult at best to reconstruct (joints, tendons, and neurovascular bundles). When depth of injury is in doubt, temporary placement of allograft is a reasonable approach to provide coverage and assess wound bed viability [15].

The majority of hand burns can be covered with split thickness skin grafts. In order to guide graft harvest, the wound bed should be templated and transposed to the planned donor site. The anterolateral thigh is a sufficient donor site for majority of patients. A dermatome with the widest guard appropriate for the amount of skin needed helps to minimize the number of graft junctions. For the majority of excised dorsal wounds, 0.012 inch thick grafts are sufficient while 0.015–0.018 inch thick grafts are necessary for the palm. Sheet grafts are preferred to mesh grafts in order to provide better functional and cosmetic results [16–18]. Full-thickness grafts harvested from the inguinal crease or the flank may be the most appropriate choice for small burns on both the dorsum and the palm. Grafts are affixed with absorbable sutures and fibrin glue in the wound bed. The edges of the graft are reinforced using with Hypafix (Smith and Nephew, London, UK) and Mastisol (Ferndale Laboratories, Ferndale, MI). A dressing of nonadherent material, fine-mesh gauze, Kerlix rolls, and a custom fabricated splint is applied. Of note, grafting should take place in the same position as splinting, attempting to maintain tension on the collateral ligaments (i.e., flexed metacarpophalangeal and extended interphalangeal) and abduct the first web space. The dressing is removed on post-operative day 1, and fluid collections are evacuated with a small incision in the graft. It is important to note that we do not make any piecrusting incisions in the graft at the time of placement but only over areas where fluid accumulates. The wound should be inspected daily until no fluid collections are noted. The dressing is then maintained until post-operative day 5 and then replaced with a lighter nonadherent dressing to allow for range of motion exercises [16]. Negative pressure therapy is an alternative postoperative dressing that provides bolstering and transudate evacuation with promising results compared to traditional methods [19]. The donor site, if properly harvested and dressed, should re-epithelialize spontaneously within 2 weeks. We prefer Mepilex Ag (Molnycke) a silver-impregnated dressing or absorbent Tegadem, although a nonadherent gauze and bacitracin are also acceptable.

36.5.2 Pediatric Hand Burns

The pediatric palm burn may be an exception to aggressive early excision. Palm burns are frequently encountered in the infant and toddler population after contacting a hot surface (e.g., stove, fireplace, or heater). These burns are usually deep partial-thickness injuries and, therefore, may heal without surgery; however, controversy remains over the timing of excision and choice of graft for indeterminate and deeper burns. While there are advocates for early excision and full-thickness grafting to prevent infection and limit future contractures [20], in the author's experience [21], a more conservative approach is warranted. There is no evidence to suggest that delay of the excision until week 2 or 3 prevents infection, and if the wound can heal within 3 weeks of time, avoiding excision may help to protect palmar sensation that is vital to overall hand function [22]. If excision is warranted, both split and full-thickness grafts are acceptable approaches to wound coverage. Typically, if the area of burn can be covered with a single full-thickness graft (i.e., harvested from a single site), then this will be performed; in other cases, a thick split thickness graft is used to minimize the need for multiple grafts with junctions on the palm. In the case of secondary reconstruction, full-thickness grafts are the preferred coverage following release.

Perhaps more important than the decision for surgery timing and choice of coverage is the need for aggressive hand range of motion therapy and splinting overnight. It is critical that children with palm burns undergo aggressive range of motion therapy immediately. Parents must be instructed on how to adequately range the hand and should do so at least 8–10 times daily. Splints should only be used at night or if early signs of contracture are noted.

36.5.3 Tissue Flaps

Severe burns, especially on the dorsum of the hand where the skin is thin with little underlying subcutaneous tissue, are often not amenable to skin grafting due to exposed bone or tendon and may require flap coverage. Digits sometimes require vascular soft tissue coverage to optimize function.

Numerous soft tissue flaps have been described to provide durable coverage for areas for which skin grafting would not be appropriate, and the most common coverage options are described below. It is important to keep in mind injuries to deeper hand structures may also require management prior to wound coverage. For example, in cases where the extensor tendon and joint are burned, one should consider early joint arthrodesis to stabilize joint positioning and allow for faster functional recovery.

Local flaps. The radial forearm fasciocutaneous or fascial flap, based on the radial artery, is an appropriate choice for local coverage when the donor site remains uninjured. An Allen's test, as well as Doppler examination of the superficial palmar arch, should be performed prior to raising the flap to ensure adequate ulnar perfusion of the hand. Skin grafting of the donor site in the case of a fasciocutaneous flap or recipient site in the case of a fascial flap will be necessary. The distally based posterior interosseus artery flap is a fasciocutaneous flap harvested from the dorsal aspect of the forearm and does not disrupt either of the major blood vessels perfusing the hand [23]. Although the flap's perfusing vessel is sometimes hypoplastic or absent, this flap is especially useful when there has been an injury to either the radial or ulnar artery.

Distant flaps. When local flaps are unavailable due to injury, distant flaps may be considered. The primary distant flaps used for hand coverage are the abdominal (random) or groin (pedicled) flaps [16]. In either case, a flap of Scarpa's fascia, subcutaneous tissue, and skin is templated, raised, and sutured onto the hand. The hand is left in situ for 2–3 weeks after which the flap is divided (Fig. 36.3). Vascularization of the flap can be determined, when in doubt, using indocyanine green fluorescence video angiography [21]. A variant of this procedure may be performed in which only Scarpa's fascia is transferred and skin grafted, leaving behind the abdominal or groin skin and subcutaneous tissue—the Crane procedure.

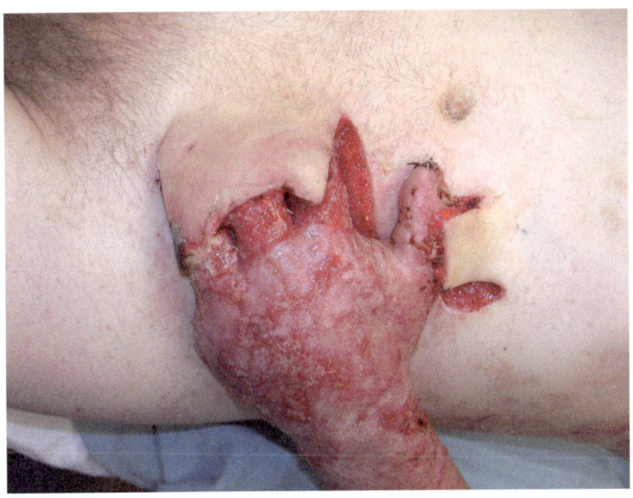

Fig. 36.3 A pedicled abdominal flap was used to provide soft tissue coverage over exposed joints and tendons of the hand. In this case two separate flaps were used—one for the thumb and one for digits

Free tissue transfer. Free tissue transfer is necessary when extensive burns preclude local or distant pedicled flaps. Numerous options exist and can be carefully selected following the principle of "replace like with like" [24]. For the dorsum of the hand, this calls for thinner tissue including fascial and fasciocutaneous flaps such as the contralateral radial forearm flap, temporoparietal fascial flap, lateral forearm flap, serratus fascial flap, dorsal thoracic fascial flap, and dorsalis pedis flap. For the palmar surface, the glabrous skin is more challenging to replace. The above flaps may all be considered with the addition of perforator flaps in a thin patient such as the anterolateral thigh (ALT) flap. Innervated palmar skin is essential for hand function; thus, sensate flaps should be considered first. Prior to considering a free tissue transfer, the viability of the recipient vessels must be evaluated to ensure that they have also not been damaged. In severe injuries where there is loss of all digits or the entire hand, muscle flaps can be utilized to provide wound closure and provide a foundation for subsequent reconstruction or prosthetic devices [14, 25].

36.5.4 Skin Substitutes

A full discussion of skin graft substitutes is beyond the scope of this chapter; however, products curtailed to the hand are important to note. Skin substitutes may be useful in cases of extensive burn injury where there is limited donor site for harvesting quality autografts. Skin substitutes are applied to the freshly excised wound bed, and just as in the case of autograft placement, it is essential that the wound bed is viable and hemostatic prior to placement. Broadly, substitutes are viewed in two categories: temporizing bridges to autografting and dermal regenerative matrices that are used in combination with autologous skin grafts. Multiple products exist in both categories with varying success [26]. Bridging coverage includes cadaveric human skin (allograft) and porcine skin (xenograft), which all must be removed prior to definitive autografting. These options are often utilized to test the viability of wound beds in addition to temporary coverage [15].

Dermal regenerative matrices are used in viable full-thickness wounds to promote the formation of dermis through ingrowth of scaffolds. For dorsal hand burns, these products provide bulk and coverage where skin grafts might otherwise not take or suffer significant contour deformities. Integra (Integra Life Sciences, Plainsboro, NJ) is shark- and bovine-derived acellular collagen matrix with a silicon pseudo-epidermis. The product is used in a two-stage manner, whereby initial placement on a vascular wound bed is followed by a 3-week delay to allow ingrowth and autografting (with removal of silicon sheet). This is an excellent option for dorsal defects where serial Integra stacking allows for tissue bulking prior to autografting. A similar product, Matriderm (Dr. Otto Suwelack Skin & Health Care AG, Billerbeck, Germany) is a single-stage bovine collagen matrix. Like Integra, it is placed in a viable full-thickness defect, but instead of staged autografting, a think skin graft is placed over the Matriderm at the time of initial surgery. Proponents of Matriderm cite its improved pliability over other products [27]. Though acellular dermal matrix is often used in bridging, others have described its success in definitive reconstruction when used with thin autografts [28].

36.5.5 Amputation

Severe burns of the hand may result in injuries for which salvage is either impossible or impractical. The ultimate goal of treatment of hand burns is optimizing function. The loss of a digit often provides the patient with a more favorable outcome when compared to an insensate, painful, and stiff digit. Delayed amputation may be required when all other treatment options have been exhausted or failed. Length should be preserved at all times. As is the case with all severe hand burns, realistic discussions about the goals of reconstruction should take place prior to embarking on a plan of treatment. In addition, an area of viable soft tissue on a digit that is to be amputated may be useful for coverage the hand elsewhere. For example, if the dorsal aspect of a digit is burned down through the tendon and joint, a filet flap from the volar aspect of the digit can be used to cover any exposed MP joints or tendons.

36.6 Postoperative Care and Long-Term Management

Hand therapy is an integral component in the treatment of any hand injury. Surgical management of hand burns without proper postoperative hand therapy, including splinting, edema management, and range-of-motion exercises, preferably led by an experienced burn therapist, is likely to result in suboptimal results. Hand therapy should begin within 24 h of injury. Edema management is initiated with elevation and proceeds to compressive wraps. Custom compressive gloves and sleeves should be fitted to the patient when there is no longer concern for a shear injury. Scar contractures of the hand typically result in a deformity known as the "burn claw," whereby proximal interphalangeal points are sharply flexed and the metacarpophalangeal joints are hyperextended [29] (Fig. 36.4). Any hand that assumes this posture should be aggressively splinted in the intrinsic plus position with the wrist in 30 degrees of extension, the metacarpophalangeal joints in 70–90 degrees of flexion, and the interphalangeal joint in full extension. The first web space should also be held in an abducted position. This posture will maintain the collateral ligaments in tension and help to avoid permanent fixed contractures. Palm burns, which are at significant risk of flexion contracture, should be splinted with all joints in full extension. Range of motion exercises should be withheld in the acute phase of graft or flap healing, but should be initiated as soon as possible thereafter, usually after 5 days in the case of split- or full-thickness skin grafting. If prolonged splinting is required, range of motion exercises out of the splint should occur several times a day, and nighttime only splinting should be considered. Independent therapy is also encouraged. Passive range of motion should be performed on intubated patients daily. Patients should not be discharged from the hospital until they have demonstrated that they are self-sufficient with both hand therapy and wound care [30, 31].

36.7 Secondary Reconstruction

Even optimal care of burned hands may result in scarring and contracture. In the largest review of all major burn survivors at one facility, nearly 23% suffered some form of contracture of the hand, with the wrist most commonly involved [32]. Contractures may be categorized as wrist, palmar, dorsal, digital, or syndactyly [33]. In select cases of severe early contracture, release and grafting may be considered within weeks after the injury; however, surgical treatment of contracted tissue more often occurs after the scar has fully matured—a period of 6–12 months. The patient must also be psychologically prepared to return to the operating room and participate in postoperative rehabilitation. In the case of pediatric patients, parental adherence must be assessed.

The approach to secondary reconstruction begins with defining the problem and functional deficit in light of realistic goals and expectations. Secondary reconstructions include scar rearrangement/lengthening and scar excision with soft tissue reconstruction using skin grafts, tissue flaps, or dermal regenerative matrices. Physical therapy should be initiated to both improve contracture and demonstrate future adherence. If two hands require surgery, only one should be addressed at a time. Surgeries with competing postoperative needs, such as prolonged immobilization and early motion, should also be performed separately and staged.

Regardless of location, scar lengthening and rearrangement techniques are often sufficient to treat single-scar contractures assuming adequate tissue laxity perpendicular to the scar. Plastic surgery techniques such as Z-plasty and V-to-Y flap release are commonly performed to release hand contractures. The Z-plasty is particularly well suited

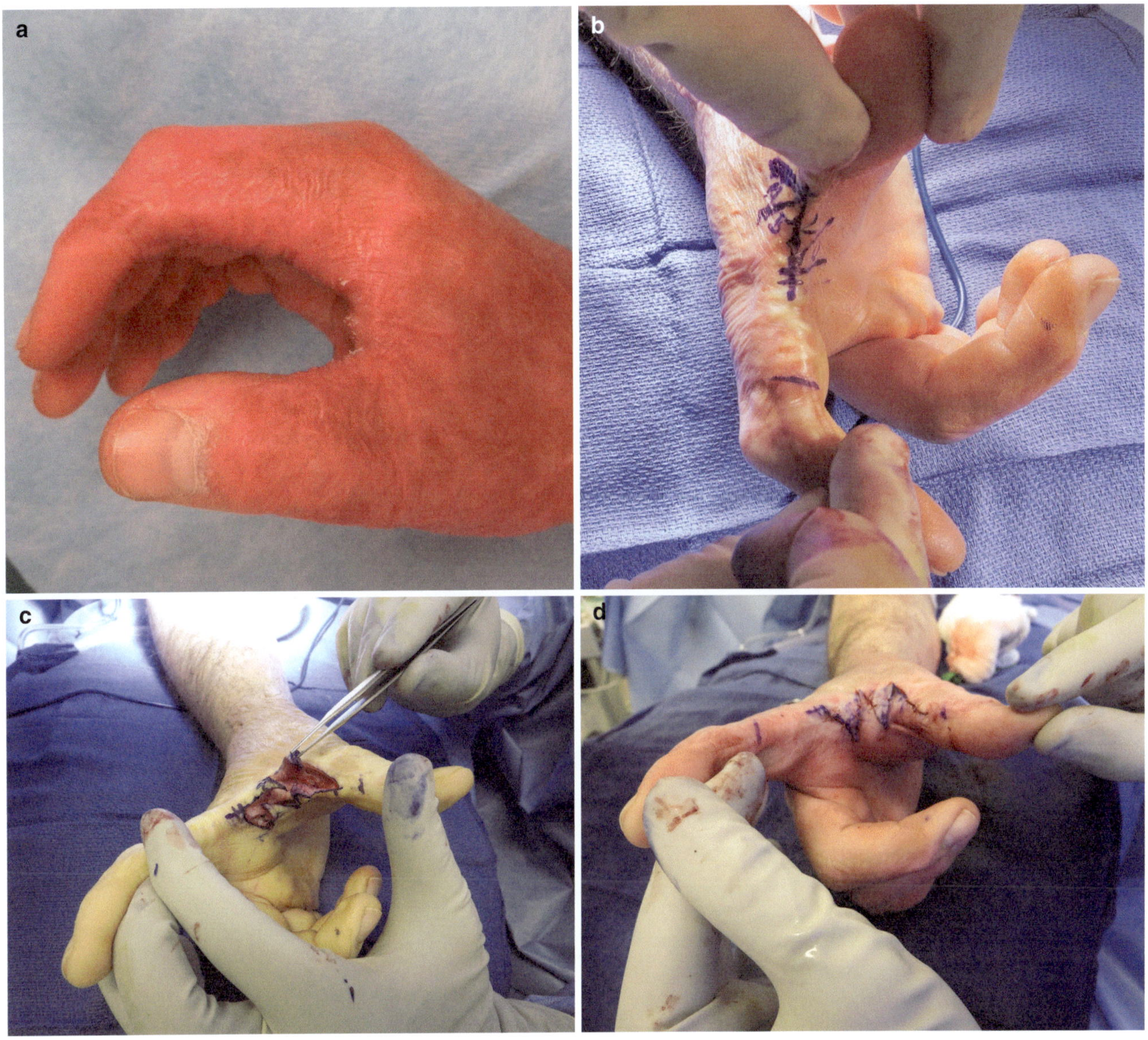

Fig. 36.4 A four-flap z-plasty was used for the correction of a first web space contracture to increase extension and abduction of the thumb (**a**). The central axis of the flap is designed directly over the thickest central scar (**b**). Each of the four limbs extends off the central limb at 60-degree angles. The four flaps are elevated and then transposed and advanced into place (**c** and **d**)

for web spaces (syndactyly), and the V-to-Y flap release is appropriate for small, linear contractures. For larger first web space contractures, the four-flap Z-plasty is an alternative [34] (Fig. 36.4).

When adjacent soft tissue is insufficient, scar excision with full-thickness skin grafts may be required to accommodate increased excursion. Local flaps as mentioned in the tissue flap section are also available. One smaller local option for first web space contractures includes the first dorsal metacarpal artery flap [35]. In cases of long-standing contracture, consideration of using Kirschner wire fixation in extension for 3 weeks to allow for optimal positioning should be made [29].

Fingernail scaring often occurs after burn injury due to contracture of skin leading to abnormal eponychium and exposed germinal matrix. The result can be a painful digit with reduced function. Treatment considerations include a dorsally based bipedicled advancement flap with full-thickness skin grafting to donor area [36].

Finger lengthening is a separate issue from contracture but is mentioned given the significance for hand function. Thumb function comprises nearly half of hand function, which is dependent on thumb length to accomplish opposition. Various techniques for thumb lengthening following burn injury have been described including pollicization of other fingers and toe-to-thumb transfer [37].

36.8 Outcomes and Horizons

Outcomes, both provider and patient reported, are increasingly important in a healthcare environment focused on quality and quality reporting. As mentioned in the introduction, significant burns are largely survivable today; however, they can lead to significant long-term morbidity. As the ambassador of daily activities, the hands are paramount in quality of life and are reflected as such in reporting metrics. There are a number of existing outcome measurement instruments developed for hand injuries (though not specifically burn injury). For provider-reported outcomes, measures in range of motion (ROM) and grip-pinch power are the foundation of gross hand function, while scoring metrics such as the Jebsen-Taylor Hand Function Test index the ability to perform multiple tasks. In regard to patient reported outcomes, two more frequently used tools are the Disabilities of the Arm, Shoulder, and Hand (DASH) and Michigan Hand Questionnaire (MHQ) [38]. Hand function is arguably the most important outcome in hand burns; thus, using objective metrics offers both providers and patients the opportunity to assess change and direct therapy.

There are a number of technological and scientific advances which may impact the management of extensive hand injuries in the future, particularly in the areas of prosthetics and composite tissue allotransplantation (CTA). There were a number of technological advances made as part of the experience of caring for soldiers with amputations injured during Operation Iraqi Freedom and Operating Enduring [39]. Advances in prosthetics, such as the direct brain wave control devices, are promising examples of future innovations that may more fully return function [40] in residual limbs. While still in its early stages, CTA may provide greater role in the future for persons with burn injuries. Successful hand transplants have been conducted around the world [41, 42]. The merits of CTA relative to the risks are still being debated, and thus, CTA is reserved for particular institutions and unique cases. A greater understanding of the potential benefits of CTA for burn patients as well as specific challenges such as sensitization from skin allograft exposure [43], are areas of active research.

Summary Box

Loss of hand function is the leading cause of impairment following burn injury. With majority of severe burns routinely survivable today, understanding the unique features of hand burn treatment is crucial for all burn surgeons. After trauma survey and resuscitation, evaluation for distal hand perfusion and upper extremity escharotomy + fasciotomy are the first steps in managing hand burns. As with all burns, the principle of early excision and grafting yields the best results in limiting scarring and contracture, although controversy surrounds the optimal timing of palm burns. Splinting and aggressive therapy are paramount in maintaining hand function. For inevitable contractures, tailored techniques with local and regional flaps can improve hand function. Careful consideration should always be given to the underlying osseous and ligamentous anatomy given the effects of scarring on joints of the hand.

References

1. Luce EA. The acute and subacute management of the burned hand. Clin Plast Surg. 2000;27(1):49–63.
2. Anzarut A, Chen M, Shankowsky H, Tredget EE. Quality-of-life and outcome predictors following massive burn injury. Plast Reconstr Surg. 2005;116(3):791–7.
3. Arnoldo B, Klein M, Gibran NS. Practice guidelines for the management of electrical injuries. J Burn Care Res. 2006;27(4):439–47.
4. Orgill DP, Piccolo N. Escharotomy and decompressive therapies in burns. J Burn Care Res. 2009;30(5):759–68.
5. Salisbury RE, Taylor JW, Levine NS. Evaluation of digital escharotomy in burned hands. Plast Reconstr Surg. 1976;58(4):440–3.
6. Burd A, Noronha FV, Ahmed K, Chan JYW, Ayyappan T, Ying SY, et al. Decompression not escharotomy in acute burns. Burns. 2006;32(3):284–92.
7. Tambuscio A, Governa M, Caputo G, Barisoni D. Deep burn of the hands: early surgical treatment avoids the need for late revisions? Burns. 2006;32(8):1000–4.
8. Goodwin CW, Maguire MS, McManus WF, Pruitt BA. Prospective study of burn wound excision of the hands. J Trauma. 1983;23(6):510–7.
9. van Zuijlen PP, Kreis RW, Vloemans AF, Groenevelt F, Mackie DP. The prognostic factors regarding long-term functional outcome of full-thickness hand burns. Burns. 1999;25(8):709–14.
10. Edstrom LE, Robson MC, Macchiaverna JR, Scala AD. Prospective randomized treatments for burned hands: nonoperative vs. operative. Preliminary report. Scand J Plast Reconstr Surg. 1979;13(1):131–5.
11. Albino FP, Fleury C, Higgins JP. Putting it all together: recommendations for improving pain management in plastic surgical procedures: hand surgery. Plast Reconstr Surg. 2014;134(4 Suppl 2):126S–30S.
12. Klein MB, Hunter S, Heimbach DM, Engrav LH, Honari S, Gallery E, et al. The Versajet water dissector: a new tool for tangential excision. J Burn Care Rehabil. 2005;26(6):483–7.
13. Rennekampff H-O, Schaller H-E, Wisser D, Tenenhaus M. Debridement of burn wounds with a water jet surgical tool. Burns. 2006;32(1):64–9.
14. Herter F, Ninkovic M, Ninkovic M. Rational flap selection and timing for coverage of complex upper extremity trauma. J Plast Reconstr Aesthet Surg. 2007;60(7):760–8.
15. Fletcher JL, Cancio LC, Sinha I, Leung KP, Renz EM, Chan RK. Inability to determine tissue health is main indication of allograft use in intermediate extent burns. Burns. 2015;41(8):1862–7.
16. Smith MA, Munster AM, Spence RJ. Burns of the hand and upper limb—a review. Burns. 1998;24(6):493–505.

17. Chandrasegaram MD, Harvey J. Full-thickness vs split-skin grafting in pediatric hand burns—a 10-year review of 174 cases. J Burn Care Res. 2009;30(5):867–71.
18. Schwanholt C, Greenhalgh DG, Warden GD. A comparison of full-thickness versus split-thickness autografts for the coverage of deep palm burns in the very young pediatric patient. J Burn Care Rehabil. 1993;14(1):29–33.
19. Moisidis E, Heath T, Boorer C, Ho K, Deva AK. A prospective, blinded, randomized, controlled clinical trial of topical negative pressure use in skin grafting. Plast Reconstr Surg. 2004;114(4):917–22.
20. Palmieri TL. Initial management of acute pediatric hand burns. Hand Clin. 2009;25(4):461–7.
21. Scott JR, Costa BA, Gibran NS, Engrav LH, Heimbach DH, Klein MB. Pediatric palm contact burns: a ten-year review. J Burn Care Res. 2008;29(4):614–8.
22. Mohammadi AA, Bakhshaeekia AR, Marzban S, Abbasi S, Ashraf AR, Mohammadi MK, et al. Early excision and skin grafting versus delayed skin grafting in deep hand burns (a randomised clinical controlled trial). Burns. 2011;37(1):36–41.
23. Agıı H, Sen C, Alagöz S, Onyedi M, Isil E. Distally based posterior interosseous flap: primary role in soft-tissue reconstruction of the hand. Ann Plast Surg. 2007;59(3):291–6.
24. Karanas YL, Buntic RF. Microsurgical reconstruction of the burned hand. Hand Clin. 2009;25(4):551–6.
25. Baumeister S, Köller M, Dragu A, Germann G, Sauerbier M. Principles of microvascular reconstruction in burn and electrical burn injuries. Burns. 2005;31(1):92–8.
26. Lou RB, Hickerson WL. The use of skin substitutes in hand burns. Hand Clin. 2009;25(4):497–509.
27. Haslik W, Kamolz L-P, Nathschläger G, Andel H, Meissl G, Frey M. First experiences with the collagen-elastin matrix matriderm as a dermal substitute in severe burn injuries of the hand. Burns. 2007;33(3):364–8.
28. Callcut RA, Schurr MJ, Sloan M, Faucher LD. Clinical experience with alloderm: a one-staged composite dermal/epidermal replacement utilizing processed cadaver dermis and thin autografts. Burns. 2006;32(5):583–8.
29. Fufa DT, Chuang S-S, Yang J-Y. Postburn contractures of the hand. J Hand Surg Am. 2014;39(9):1869–76.
30. Moore ML, Dewey WS, Richard RL. Rehabilitation of the burned hand. Hand Clin. 2009;25(4):529–41.
31. Lowell M, Pirc P, Ward RS, Lundy C, Wilhelm DA, Reddy R, et al. Effect of 3M coban self-adherent wraps on edema and function of the burned hand: a case study. J Burn Care Rehabil. 2003;24(4):253–8; discussion 252
32. Schneider JC, Holavanahalli R, Helm P, O'Neil C, Goldstein R, Kowalske K. Contractures in burn injury part II: investigating joints of the hand. J Burn Care Res. 2008;29(4):606–13.
33. Kamolz L-P, Kitzinger HB, Karle B, Frey M. The treatment of hand burns. Burns. 2009;35(3):327–37.
34. Woolf RM, Broadbent TR. The four-flap Z-plasty. Plast Reconstr Surg. 1972;49(1):48–51.
35. Eski M, Nisanci M, Sengezer M. Correction of thumb deformities after burn: versatility of first dorsal metacarpal artery flap. Burns. 2007;33(1):65–71.
36. Donelan MB, Garcia JA. Nailfold reconstruction for correction of burn fingernail deformity. Plast Reconstr Surg. 2006;117(7):2303–8; discussion 2309
37. Kurtzman LC, Stern PJ, Yakuboff KP. Reconstruction of the burned thumb. Hand Clin. 1992;8(1):107–19.
38. Lin S-Y, Chang J-K, Chen P-C, Mao H-F. Hand function measures for burn patients: a literature review. Burns. 2013;39(1):16–23.
39. Kauvar DS, Wolf SE, Wade CE, Cancio LC, Renz EM, Holcomb JB. Burns sustained in combat explosions in Operations Iraqi and Enduring Freedom (OIF/OEF explosion burns). Burns. 2006;32(7):853–7.
40. Zlotolow DA, Kozin SH. Advances in upper extremity prosthetics. Hand Clin. 2012;28(4):587–93.
41. Iglesias M, Butron P, Moran-Romero M, Cruz-Reyes A, Alberu-Gomez J, Leal-Villalpando P, et al. Bilateral forearm transplantation in Mexico: 2-year outcomes. Transplantation. 2016;100(1):233–8.
42. Eberlin KR, Leonard DA, Austen WG, Yaremchuk MJ, Mudgal CS, Winograd JM, et al. The volar forearm fasciocutaneous extension: a strategy to maximize vascular outflow in post-burn injury hand transplantation. Plast Reconstr Surg. 2014;134(4):731–5.
43. Garza RM, Press BH, Tyan DB, Karanas YL, Lee GK. Immunological effect of skin allograft in burn treatment: impact on future vascularized composite allotransplantation. J Burn Care Res. 2017;38(3):169–73.

Treatment of Burns: Established and Novel Technologies

37

Janos Cambiaso-Daniel, Stefanos Boukovalas, Alexis L. Boson, Ludwik K. Branski, and Lars-Peter Kamolz

37.1 Overview

Burns are one of the most devastating traumas, affecting more than two million individuals around the globe every year [1, 2]. The last few decades have been marked by several advances in the care of massive burns that have considerably diminished morbidity and improved survival [3]. These improvements are most notable in elderly individuals [4, 5] and children [6]. Burn care has seen advances in four major areas:

- Early patient management and fluid resuscitation
- Infection control
- Hypermetabolic response modulation
- Surgical techniques and wound care

Burn injury is associated with long-term exposure to inflammatory mediators and pathogens owing to the presence of extensive wounds. Immediate excision and coverage of the burn wound [7] have reduced the likelihood of critical systemic infection caused by burn wound infection [8]. Accordingly, early after burn injury, the preferred approach is to excise the full-thickness burn and cover the open wound with an autologous skin graft. A safe and effective reduction in blood loss can be achieved with early excision within the first 48 h [9–11]. When immediate permanent wound coverage is not feasible because burns cover large areas, these areas can be temporarily covered with allograft or xenograft. This protects the wound for several weeks until donor sites have sufficient time to generate autografts. Furthermore, overlaying widely meshed autografts with allograft or xenograft provide adequate coverage and permit repeat autografting within 1–2 weeks when donor sites are healed [9, 10, 12, 13]. Although this approach has not been widely implemented, some burn units around the world continue to use it, with minimal changes in the last few decades. Meanwhile, new approaches and devices are being introduced and studied, including fish-derived xenografts, synthetic membranes as PermeaDerm, and enzymatic debridement products. This chapter discusses some of these exciting developments and introduces new ideas in the treatment of burns.

J. Cambiaso-Daniel
Division of Plastic, Aesthetic and Reconstructive Surgery, Department of Surgery, Medical University of Graz, Graz, Austria

Department of Surgery, University of Texas Medical Branch, Shriners Hospitals for Children, Galveston, TX, USA

S. Boukovalas · A. L. Boson · L. K. Branski (✉)
Department of Surgery, University of Texas Medical Branch, Shriners Hospitals for Children, Galveston, TX, USA

Division of Plastic Surgery, University of Texas Medical Branch, Galveston, TX, USA
e-mail: lubransk@UTMB.EDU

L.-P. Kamolz
Division of Plastic, Aesthetic and Reconstructive Surgery, Department of Surgery, Medical University of Graz, Graz, Austria

37.2 Partial-Thickness Burns

Partial-thickness burns are considered superficial or deep depending on the extent of injury penetration. The former are painful, blanch with touch, erythematous, and often blister. Common causes include accidents such as immersion in an overheated bath tub containing water and flash flame burns. Epidermal structures that are present in rete ridges, hair follicles, and sweat glands enable spontaneous re-epithelialization within 1–2 weeks. After wound re-epithelialization, secondary scar maturation progresses and may lead to long life hyper- hypopigmentation.

If damage extends to the reticular dermis, the burns are considered deep dermal burns. These deep burns are painful to pinprick. They do not blanch with touch and have a pale and mottled appearance. Complete re-epithelialization from hair follicles and sweat glands may take up to 1 month, and significant scarring occurs on account of dermal loss.

Partial-thickness burns usually present with epidermal layer loss, leading to exposure of raw skin with nerve endings. Therefore, partial-thickness burns can be very painful

M. G. Jeschke et al. (eds.), *Handbook of Burns Volume 1*, https://doi.org/10.1007/978-3-030-18940-2_37

Table 37.1 Wound dressings commonly used for partial-thickness burns

Dressing agent	Active substance	Presentation	Main use	Advantages	Disadvantages
Bacitracin	Bacitracin	Ointment	Superficial burns, skin grafts	Gram + coverage	No Gram – or fungal coverage
Polymyxin	Polymyxin B	Ointment	Superficial burns, skin grafts	Gram – coverage	No Gram + or fungal coverage
Mycostatin	Nystatin	Ointment	Superficial burns, skin grafts	Good fungal coverage	No bacterial coverage
Silvadene	Silver sulfadiazine	Ointment	Deep burns	Good bacterial and fungal coverage, painless	Poor eschar penetration, sulfa moiety, leucopenia, pseudoeschar formation
Sulfamylon	Mafenide acetate	Ointment and liquid solution	Deep burns	Good bacterial coverage, good eschar penetration	Painful, poor fungal coverage, metabolic acidosis
Dakin's	Sodium hypochlorite	Liquid solution	Superficial and deep burns	Good bacterial coverage, inexpensive, and readily available	Very short half life
Silver	Silver nitrate, silver ion	Liquid solution, dressing sheets	Superficial burns	Good bacterial coverage, painless	Hyponatremia, dark staining of wounds and linens

Adapted with permission from *Jeschke et al., Wound coverage technologies in burn care: Established techniques. 2013, J Burn Care Res, Epub ahead of Print. DOI: 10.1097/BCR.0b013e3182920d29*

compared to other types of burns [14]. Historically, partial-thickness burns were treated in a conservative manner through removal of the damaged top layer of skin and then local administration of medications once or twice daily [15, 16]. Even with the use of opioids, this approach may cause considerable pain and distress.

37.2.1 Synthetic and Biosynthetic Membranes: Suprathel, Biobrane, and PermeaDerm

Alternative treatments for partial-thickness burns have been devised to increase patient comfort, protect against infection, and enhance skin regeneration. The most clinically applicable are the semi-occlusive and synthetic membranes. Re-epithelialization occurs under these dressings, and given that they are only partially occlusive, frequent dressing changes are not required, minimizing distress to the patient. Some are also occasionally utilized as skin substitutes for the temporary coverage of excised full-thickness burns. The most commonly used membranes are discussed below.

Suprathel, a product of Polymedics Innovations GmbH, (Denkendorf, Germany), is a copolymer membrane primarily consisting of DL-lactide as well as ε-caprolactone and trimethylene carbonate. This synthetic membrane is not only easily shaped, but also highly porous and permeable to water. It has an initial porosity over 80%, with interconnected pores between 2 and 50 μm. It is placed on the wound and overlaid with paraffin or non-adherent gauze. As wound re-epithelialization progresses, the membrane peels off, usually over the course of a couple of weeks [17]. Prospective randomized clinical studies have demonstrated that, compared to other commercially available membranes or dressing products, Suprathel decreases pain although it yields similar wound healing times and scar qualities over the long term [17–20].

Biobrane (Smith & Nephew, London, UK) consists of a semipermeable silicone film partially embedded with nylon fabric. In this biosynthetic wound dressing, collagen is chemically bound to a complex 3D structure of tri-filament thread and in this way, comes into contact with the wound bed. The dressing remains firmly attached to the wound, keeps the wound moist, and controls water vapor transfer, facilitating re-epithelialization. Since the 1980s, studies have demonstrated that Biobrane is efficacious in treating partial-thickness burns in children [21–27]. Biobrane can also be utilized for temporary coverage of partial-thickness burns and skin graft donor sites [28]. This product is versatile, relatively inexpensive, easy to store and apply, and safe with low infection rates when used according to the guidelines [29]. Recently, Biobrane has been proven effective for the temporary coverage of deep partial- or full-thickness wounds after debridement, as an alternative to allograft application [30]. Only a few studies have compared the outcomes of different skin substitutes, and no major differences in long-term scar quality have been detected [31]. Thus, burn wound characteristics and cost of treatment are critical factors in the selection of the appropriate skin substitute product.

PermeaDerm (PermeaDerm Inc., Carlsbad, California) is a biosynthetic product approved by the FDA in 2016.

This product was developed from Biobrane and designed to serve as a temporary skin substitute in excised full-thickness burns. PermeaDerm is composed of a monofilament nylon-knitted fabric bonded to a thin slitted silicone membrane. The nylon side of this dressing is coated with a mixture of hypoallergenic porcine gelatin and a pure fraction of aloe vera. Biobrane and PermeaDerm primarily differ with regard to pore size and regularity. PermeaDerm consists of numerous rows of slits with parallel orientation on the surface of the dressing for water vapor transmission. This product is unique in that the surgeon can decide how large the pore should be by the strength utilized in stretching the product before applying it. Preliminary studies have shown that PermeaDerm is an effective biologic dressing for the treatment of burns, having variable porosity, major flexibility, and better adherence than Biobrane. PermeaDerm is associated with an overall lower accumulation of fluid and inflammation. When grown on PermaDerm, cultured cells grown have uniform growth, increased migration, and decreased expression of alpha smooth muscle actin and fibronectin. Currently, no human studies have been reported [32].

37.3 Biological Membranes

For centuries, human amnion has been utilized to dress wounds, since the beginning of the last century in the western world. Davis performed skin transplantations utilizing amniotic membrane in 1910 [33]; however, it became apparent that amnion was more suitable as a temporary dressing than a permanent skin transplant. Amnion was first used in burn wounds in 1913. As temporary dressing, amnion has numerous advantages, including low infection rates [34–37], improved wound healing [33, 34, 38], ease of handling [39], and most notably, alleviation of pain. In 1952, amnion was first used of as a temporary skin substitute for burn wounds [40]. Since then, amnion has primarily become established as a treatment modality for partial-thickness burns [36, 38, 41–43].

The number of studies investigating the use of amnion in chronic wounds and burns has steadily increased over the past two decades. Safe and reliable production methods have been pursued to establish amnion as a standard dressing alternative. Several countries have established amnion banks alongside tissue banks in an effort to meet the need [44–46].

The advantages of amnion include its slender form, adhesiveness, pliability, and removability. These qualities are critically important, especially in pediatric populations. Branski et al. compared amnion with standard dressing regimens and found comparable rates of infection, equivalent wound healing, and similar long-term cosmetic results [47]. The authors concluded that temporary wound coverage with amniotic membranes can be safely implemented, with the main benefit being the need for significantly fewer full dressing changes. A recent drive towards the standardization and commercialization of amnion has led to the development of glycerol-preserved forms of amniotic membranes or fresh frozen amniotic membrane (Grafix™, Osiris Therapeutics, Inc.).

37.4 Xenograft

In 1880, Lee first described heterografts [48], now known as xenografts, which are used to provide temporary wound coverage and ensure wound homeostasis. Many species can serve as donors for xenografts although pigs are the most common. Porcine xenografts are typically distributed as a reconstituted product. Homogenized porcine dermis is harvested with dermatomes, fashioned into sheets and later meshed, sterilized via radiation, and finally frozen for storage [49]. Xenografts can be utilized as a stand-alone covering for partial-thickness burns or as an overlay for widely meshed autograft in the same manner as allograft. Porcine xenograft is an adequate substitute for cadaveric skin allograft owing to its structural and functional similarities to human skin, effectiveness in wound protection and pain reduction, ability to limit heat and fluid loss, and prevention of bacterial overgrowth [50–53].

Zawacki et al. showed that early treatment of the wound with a biologic dressing such as xenograft can block necrosis, which occurs in the zone of stasis (i.e., potentially salvageable areas adjacent to burned and irreversibly damaged sites) [54]. Application of xenograft on debrided mid-dermal burns can also sometimes supplant excision and autografting. Additionally, the combination of silver with porcine xenografts has been demonstrated to suppress wound colonization [55, 56]. This semi-occlusive wound dressing creates a moist environment, remains avascular, and can be applied on the wound for more than 7 days. Moreover, it can be supplemented with sulfamylon or silver nitrate soaks for local antimicrobial treatment. Finally, the most common complication of porcine xenografts is fever within 48–96 h after application. This complication generally responds well to antipyretics, cooling, and soaking of the wound.

In addition to pig xenograft, fish skin can be used as a temporary cover for burns and has appeared on the market in the last years. Fish skin is extremely similar to human skin [57] and thanks to the high concentrations of omega-3 fat; it has strong antiviral [58], antibacterial [59], and anti-inflammatory properties [60]. Currently, acellular fish skin is available in the USA and Europe under the commercial name Kerecis Omega3 (Kerecis, Isafjordur, Iceland). Studies support the potential utility of fish skin in treating chronic wounds [61, 62] and burns when compared to amnion/chorion. Magnusson et al. showed that fish skin is more porous and has superior 3D ingrown of cells compared to amnion/

chorion [63]. They also reported that bacterial invasion can be prevented up to 48–72 h from application and longer with application of additional omega-3.

37.5 Full-Thickness Burns

Full-thickness burns extend into the deep dermis. These so-called third-degree burn wounds rarely heal within 2–3 weeks. The preferred treatment is complete excision and either temporary coverage or permanent coverage, preferably with autograft. Early surgical treatment with excision of necrotic skin is paramount and has been the favored approach since the 1970s. In patients that have suffered extensive burns covering large areas of the total body surface area (TBSA), there may not be enough donor sites to provide coverage of the excised areas with autograft. In these cases, the burn surgeon should consider using homograft (or allograft) and dermal substitutes.

37.6 Dermal Analogs

For many years, burn research has focused on developing burn wound coverage methods that do not rely on autograft or homograft. That is, a readily available functional composite graft capable of dermal and epidermal replacement has been goal. The development of dermal analogs signifies progress towards this goal.

John Burke from Massachusetts General Hospital and Ioannis Yannas from Massachusetts Institute of Technology teamed to develop Integra (Integra LifeSciences Corporation, Plainsboro, NJ, USA). Integra is composed of bovine collagen and glycosaminoglycans, which permit fibrovascular ingrowth. After full-thickness excision, this dermal analog can be overlaid onto the wound bed, and the wound can then be covered with autograft 2–3 weeks later.

Alloderm is an alternative dermal analog composed of decellularized and de-epithelialized cadaveric dermis (LifeCell Corporation, The Woodlands, TX, USA). It is available for the treatment of full-thickness burns, is used in a way that is very comparable to other dermal analogs, and has exhibited favorable results [64, 65].

37.7 Non-surgical Debridement

Most enzymatic and chemical debridement products introduced thus far have been slow-acting and have been associated with an increased rate of infection because of maceration of necrotic tissue [66]. Recently, a new enzymatic debridement product known as Nexobrid has been introduced for burn wounds. This product incorporates partially purified and lyophilized bromelain into an inert carrier gel. The resultant gel dressing is able to debride burn wounds more rapidly than ever before [67]. Bromelain is a proteolytic enzyme derived from pineapple stems with specific enzymatic activity. Studies have shown that, at 4 h after application of Nexobrid, the burn eschar is removed and a clean wound bed is present [68]. Numerous studies have further shown that, when compared to standard of care for full-thickness burns, Nexobrid produces comparable long-term results and reduces the need for operations [68, 69]. Although Nexobrid is not intended to serve as a substitute for surgical debridement, it represents an extremely innovative and interesting product, especially under circumstances in which surgical procedures are not possible (e.g., on the battle field).

37.8 Negative Pressure Therapy

For almost two decades, negative pressure wound therapy has been used to treat acute and chronic wounds. This therapy is used also for burn wounds. It has been studied for the treatment of acute burn wounds, for bridging to skin graft, as bolster for autograft, as integration for dermal substitutes, and as a donor-site dressing [70]. Application of negative pressure in burns has recently led to the concept of total body wrap in patients with large burns. The idea of creating a total body dressing was first proposed by Genevoc et al., who argued that this approach would have the benefit of creating a sterile environment, securing skin grafts, promoting re-epithelization of donor sites, and removing inflammatory exudates from the burn areas [71]. The utility of this approach has recently been supported by two studies, which concluded that the total body negative pressure therapy is beneficial for healing and patient management and that it may enable one to monitor fluid loss for better resuscitation. However, both studies lacked objective endpoints and the number of patients included was very low [72, 73]. Despite the limitations of these recent studies, total body negative pressure is an interesting approach for patients suffering large burns and will require further investigation before it can be considered a consolidated therapy modality.

37.9 Keratinocyte Coverage

Cultured epithelial autografts (CEAs) are a sensible alternative under circumstances in which patients have massive burn injuries (e.g., >90% TBSA, full-thickness burns) and there is limited uninvolved skin available for coverage, even with the use of an expanding technique. In this approach, two full-thickness sections of unburned skin with a size of 2 × 6 cm are procured promptly upon admission. The samples then undergo processing and ex vivo culturing in the presence of murine fibroblasts, which promote growth (http://www.genzyme.com/business/biosurgery/burn/epicel_package_insert.pdf). Three weeks later, a CEA suitable for grafting is supplied as a 5 × 10 cm sheet of petrolatum gauze that is overlaid with keratinocytes 2–8 cells thick.

Special considerations must be taken into account when managing critically ill patients during manufacturing of the CEA. These include excision and temporary coverage with allograft or xenograft as well as aggressive treatment of complications such as wound infections and multiorgan failure. Execution of the above increases the prospects of survival and ultimately graft take.

CEAs are delicate and have been described as fragile wet tissue paper. Thus, they are difficult to apply. They are also susceptible to shearing and tend to be lost when applied to high stress areas such as the back, buttocks, and posterior lower extremities. Although CEAs are associated with longer hospitalization and the need for additional reconstruction, they provide better cosmetic outcomes than meshed autograft [74]. In recent studies, the outcomes of CEA application have been extraordinarily variable. In a retrospective cohort analysis, more than 30 patients with >75% TBSA burns had excellent survival, and CEAs were retained; however, this study lacked a control group [75]. A graft take exceeding 72% was reported with the combined use of allodermis base and CEA [76].

37.10 Keratinocyte Suspension

Variability in the effectiveness of CEA due to handling difficulties, fragility, and lack of standardized application, as noted by Wood et al. [77], have triggered interest in aerosolized delivery of a keratinocyte suspension. Aerosolized keratinocytes have proven to be an ingenious option in overcoming the limitations of CEAs. Reid et al. used a porcine model to investigate healing of split-thickness-grafted wounds in the presence or absence of aerosolized keratinocytes. They found that the addition of aerosolized keratinocytes significantly decreased contractures after healing ensued [78]. A subsequent clinical trial by James et al. revealed that the addition of aerosolized cultured autologous keratinocytes may assist in the reduction of meshed autograft contraction and decrease healing time [79]. In three-patient case report, Zweifel et al. described decreased hypertrophic scarring and faster healing time with an aerosol of non-cultured autologous keratinocytes, which were applied to split- and full-thickness burns at 2 days after admission [80].

Aerosolized keratinocytes are prepared by incubating a split-thickness skin graft in a 2% dispase solution on a shaking incubator until the epidermal layer is freed. The epidermal layer is then trypsinized to generate a single-cell suspension and expanded in culture over 3 weeks. This yields a final concentration of approximately 10^7 cells/mL, which can be used to create an aerosol capable of delivering 500,000 keratinocytes to every square centimeter of the wound. Nevertheless, a major shortcoming in the use of aerosolized keratinocytes is delayed application due to the amount of time required for cell expansion.

37.11 Facial Transplantation

Conventional treatment of severely disfiguring facial burns with various techniques and numerous reconstructive procedures typically produces mediocre aesthetic and functional results. In addition to experiencing physical distress and long-term disability, these patients can become socially isolated and may have psychological disorders and phobias. Composite tissue allo-transplantation may improve function and overall quality of life in patients with severe facial disfigurement after thermal, electrical, or chemical burn injuries. Facial transplants can be used to replace nonexistent facial tissue or reconstruct damaged tissue in these patients.

The first face transplantation took place in France in 2005 [81]. Twelve years and over 35 face transplants later, we can safely consider face transplantation an important medical milestone with promising application to the treatment of burn disfigurement. Current facial transplantation procedures have been refined over many years of use during reconstructive surgeries. Successful regimens developed to prevent organ rejection in solid organ transplantation are applicable to facial transplantations.

Clinical protocols for patient selection, procurement algorithms, and surgical techniques have been established, and several prospective studies are currently in progress [82, 83]. Current literature highlights the importance of proper recipient and donor selection. Recipients with a psychiatric history are at higher risk of adverse events. In the selection of the donor, it is critical to follow the established protocols to decrease the risk of rejection, especially in burn survivors who are often sensitized with numerous preformed antibodies [84, 85]. Life-long immunosuppression is a major commitment for patients, with associated risks having been well studied in solid organ transplantation. Pediatric patients are more challenging in this regard. Recent advances in immunomodulatory and immunosuppression agents hold potential for yielding more sustainable treatments. Even though considerable progress has been made in the last few years, facial transplantation is still at an experimental, trial-and-error stage, with many challenges yet to be addressed. Gaining a solid understanding of tolerance and rejection mechanisms, developing effective and safe therapies, monitoring long-term outcomes, assessing cost-benefit, and addressing existing ethical and psychosocial dilemmas are critical for the advancement of facial transplantation from an experimental modality to an established routine treatment for severe facial burns [86–90].

37.12 Tissue Engineering and Stem Cells

Current approaches to promoting wound healing, including skin grafting, are only partially successful. Drawbacks such as poor flexibility, elasticity, and scar production have fueled the search for a skin alternative that more closely recapitulates the histological characteristics of normal skin. A breakthrough innovation in this pursuit has been the combined dermal–epidermal replacement [91]. The combined product is produced by obtaining fibroblasts and keratinocytes from the patient, culturing them ex vivo, and inoculating them onto collagen-glycosaminoglycan substrates [92, 93]. The resulting cell–substrate sheet is cultured in a liquid medium at an air–liquid interface to provide nourishment to the dermal component and expose the epidermal component to air. This generates a keratinocyte layer that undergoes stratification and cornification [94, 95]. Moreover, a new autologous dermal matrix is created through fibroblast proliferation and expansion into collagen substrate and successive degradation within the dermal layer. In vitro production of collagen and formation of a basement membrane at the dermal–epidermal junction [96] increases junctional strength and decreases complications such as epidermolysis and blistering, which commonly occur with CEAs and split-thickness grafts.

Innovations in the engineering of these skin products has created replacements with improved color and cosmetic appearance through the addition of melanocytes and decreased hypopigmentation [97]. Introduction of angiogenic cytokines and vascular endothelial growth factors may assist in accelerating healing, averting graft loss, and overcoming the absence of a vascular plexus [98, 99].

As mentioned, Integra is one of the most commonly used dermal substitutes in the treatment of burns. This bilayer consisting of a shark chondroitin-6-sulfate and bovine collagen matrix covered by a synthetic silicone membrane offers an alternative for the coverage of deep partial or full-thickness burns. The silicone membrane is usually removed 3 weeks after initial application, with a thin split-thickness skin graft then being applied for definitive wound coverage. Integra has been shown to achieve more stable wound coverage with lower contracture rates, providing superior functional and aesthetic outcomes compared to split-thickness skin grafts alone [100, 101]. Surgical site infection remains the most common complication of Integra [102]. Meticulous wound debridement and appropriate wound care are critical; however, application of silver dressings with antibacterial properties or use of negative pressure dressing in combination with Integra has been shown to reduce the risk of infection and increase graft take [103–105]. Recently, early high levels of IL-4 and FGF-2 were shown to be predictors of the development of complications associated with Integra [106]. Despite the risks mentioned above, Integra provides good aesthetic and functional results when used for deep hand burns and thus, is a valid alternative to conventional treatments [47, 107, 108].

Stem cells participate in the wound healing process and hold potential in the treatment of burn injury. Several local and systematic mechanisms have been defined. Stem cells are present in human adipose tissue, umbilical cord blood, bone marrow, and embryonic blastocystic mass [115]. Use of human embryonic stem cells has raised ethical issues due to destruction of the human embryo. However, stem cells can be isolated from other tissue sources without damaging them, a capability that has propelled research in this field. Stem cells have a number of useful properties that can be exploited such as pluripotency, clonicity, and lack of immunogenicity. These characteristics would allow improved transplantation, re-epithelialization, and dermal regeneration [116, 117].

Studies of bone marrow stem cells have been shown that these cells migrate to injured tissue and facilitate the healing and regeneration process [118–120]. These stem cells are capable of blocking release of proinflammatory cytokines and stimulating expression of anti-inflammatory cytokines (e.g., IL-10) both while they are the bloodstream and after they have arrived at injured tissue [121].

Human embryonic stem cells can be forced to differentiate into keratinocytes while in culture and then stratified into an epithelial graft that is similar to human epidermis [122]. The resulting graft may be utilized as a temporary covering for wounds until an alternative or permanent coverage is possible. This method is currently undergoing initial experimental testing. Alternatively, stem cells can be co-delivered with skin composites or delivered in other ways [123].

Human epidermal stem cells and mesenchymal stem cells (MSCs) also hold promise for the treatment of severe burns. Epidermal stem cells can be used in the preparation of enriched cultured grafts to improve the properties and overall healing potential of these grafts [124]. They may also simulate the formation of fully functional skin, which includes dermal appendages including sebaceous glands and hair follicles [125]. However, creating a microenvironment that provides the appropriate molecular signals to stimulate stems cells so that they achieve the desired regeneration remains a challenge. MSCs offer another promising alternative for treating severe burns. They can be obtained from many different tissues, including amniotic membrane, adipose tissue, bone marrow, umbilical cord, cord blood, and the dermal papilla and sheath of the hair follicle [126–128]. Many animal and human studies have shown that cadaveric MSCs are safe and effective for skin regeneration after various types of injuries including burns [129–131]. The first clinical inves-

Table 37.2 Engineered skin substitutes

Model	Description	Indications
Acellular		
Biobrane (Bertek Pharmaceuticals, Morgantown, WV)	Very thin semipermeable silicone membrane bonded to nylon fabric	Temporary adherent wound covering for partial-thickness excised burns and donor sites
Integra (Integra Life Sciences, Plainsboro, NJ)	Bilayer structure; biodegradable dermal layer made of porous bovine collagen-chondroitin-6-sulfate matrix; temporary epidermal layer made of synthetic silicone polymer	Grafting of deep partial- or full-thickness burns; epidermal layer removed when donor sites available for autografting
Alloderm (LifeCell Corporation, Branchburg, NJ)	Structurally intact allogeneic acellular dermis; freeze-dried after cells were removed with detergent treatment; rehydrated before grafting	Dermal template for grafting to burns and other wounds; repair of soft tissue defects
Matriderm (Dr. Suwelack Skin & Health Care AG, Germany)	Non-cross-linked bovine collagen and elastin matrix that allows cellular ingrowth and neovascularization	Template for dermal reconstruction in the treatment of full-thickness burns
Cellular-allogeneic		
Dermagraft (Advanced Biohealing, Westport, CT)	Cryopreserved allogeneic neonatal foreskin fibroblasts seeded on bioabsorbable polyglactin mesh scaffold; cells are metabolically active at grafting	Treatment of full-thickness chronic diabetic foot ulcers
Apligraf (Organogenesis/Novartis, Canton, MA)	Bilayer; allogeneic neonatal foreskin fibroblasts and keratinocytes in bovine collagen gel	Treatment of chronic foot ulcers and venous leg ulcers; also used for burn wounds and EB
OrCel (Forticell Bioscience, Englewood Cliffs, NJ)	Bilayer; allogeneic neonatal foreskin fibroblasts and keratinocytes cultured in bovine collagen sponge	Treatment of split-thickness donor sites in patients with burn and surgical wounds in EB
Cellular-autologous		
Epicel (Genzyme Biosurgery, Cambridge, MA)	Autologous keratinocytes cultured from patient skin biopsy, transplanted as epidermal sheet using petrolatum gauze support	Permanent wound closure in patients with burn with greater than 30% TBSA injury and in patients with congenital nevus
Epidex (Modex Therapeutiques, Lausanne, Switzerland)	Autologous keratinocytes isolated from outer root sheath of scalp hair follicles; supplied as epidermal sheet discs with a silicone membrane support	Treatment of chronic leg ulcers
TranCell* (CellTran Limited, Sheffield, UK) [109]	Autologous keratinocytes cultured from patient skin biopsy, grown on acrylic acid polymer-coated surface; transplanted as epidermal sheets	Treatment of chronic diabetic foot ulcers
Cultured skin substitute* (University of Cincinnati/Shriners Hospitals, Cincinnati, OH) [110–114]	Bilayer; autologous keratinocytes and fibroblasts cultured from patient skin biopsy, combined with degradable bovine collagen matrix	Permanent wound closure in patients with burn with greater than 50% TBSA injury; also used in patients with congenital nevus and chronic wound

Adapted from *Lebeko, M. The use of* in vitro *co-culture models to determine the optimal keratinocyte:melanocyte ratio to be used in the development of pigmented 3D skin model. OpenUCT, July* 2015 and with permission from *Jeschke* et al., *Wound coverage technologies in burn care: Established techniques. 2013, J Burn Care Res, Epub ahead of Print. DOI: 10.1097/BCR.0b013e3182920d29*

tigation into the utility of allogenic bone marrow-derived MSCs in large burns is currently in progress in Argentina [132]. Preliminary results from the treatment of a patient with 60% total body surface burn are promising [133]. Additional clinical trials of stem cells are underway, highlighting the interest in this possible and innovative treatment modality.

37.13 Gene Therapy and Growth Factors

Gene therapy was first considered for only late-stage malignancy or congenital metabolic dysfunction [134]. Since this time, gene therapy research has targeted many other conditions, including disorders of the skin and may have potential benefits in the treatment of burns. Fibroblasts and keratinocytes are easy to harvest and cultivate, enabling the study of gene transfer in skin cells in vitro [135]. Skin is also easy to access, and the effects of any therapeutic interventions can be continually and reliably assessed, making it an ideal tissue for the study of gene transfer.

Viruses can be used for gene transfer, as they are able to efficiently transport and express their genes in host cells. Through genetic modification, they can be converted into appropriate gene therapy vectors. Viral replication can be lytic, destroying the host cell (as in the case of herpes simplex viruses, human adenoviruses, and adeno-associated viruses) or non-lytic, leaving the cell viable (retroviruses and lentiviruses). There is extensive literature describing the outcomes of viral gene transfer in the skin, including wounds [109–112, 136–146]. Viral vectors remain the best established gene transfer method. Despite the fact that there are many potential clinically applicable virus-mediated gene transfer

Table 37.3 Review of stem cell nomenclature

Cell	Source	Potency	Advantages	Disadvantages	Examples of utility
Embryonic stem cells	Inner cell mass of blastocyst	Pluripotent	Pluripotent Clonogenic	Teratogenic ethical controversy	Knockout mouse
Umbilical cord blood stem cells	Umbilical cord blood	Pluripotent	Pluripotent Non-immunogenic clonogenic	Limited supply with low yield	Bone marrow transplantation
Mesenchymal stem cells	Bone marrow stroma, blood	Multipotent	Autologous Accessible Clonogenic	Require time to culture Harvest invasive limited supply	Parkinson's, myocardial remodeling, wound healing
Adipose-derived stem cells	Adipose tissue	Multipotent	Non-immunogenic abundant supply accessible Clonogenic	Processing required	Wound healing, tissue engineering
Resident progenitor cells	Numerous tissues/organs	Unipotent	Accessible Potential for transdifferentiation	Limited potency and clonogenicity	Re-epithelialization of wounds from hair follicular cells

Adapted with permission from *Jeschke* et al., *Wound coverage technologies in burn care: Established techniques. 2013, J Burn Care Res, Epub ahead of Print. DOI: 10.1097/BCR.0b013e3182920d29*

models, transfection efficacy remains variable and the production of viral vectors is expensive and time-consuming. Additionally, there is risk of local or systemic infection, with potentially serious outcomes. This poses medical and ethical concerns for the use of viral gene transfer in the treatment of burns.

An alternative gene transfer method is direct injection of naked DNA. The first clinical application was in 1995, when Hengge and colleagues injected DNA encoding interleukin-8 into the skin [147]. Even though dermal neutrophils were recruited to the injection site, the transfection efficacy was low and the initial degradation rate was high. Naked DNA constructs are large, electrically charged, and fragile in the extracellular environment [148].

New injection techniques have been developed. "Microseeding," for instance, relies upon solid microneedles for the directly delivery of naked DNA into cells. Although initial results have been encouraging, penetration into deep tissues is minimal [114]. Another gene transfer device known as the "gene gun" relies on 1–5-micron, plasmid-carrying particles that are coated with gold or tungsten, which it propels into skin cells [112]. Expression of the introduced gene is mostly transient and peaks the first few days after injection. Although transfection rate and penetration depths vary, many studies have shown that wound healing is improved and that the injected DNA particles produce sustainable effects, suggesting that this approach may be clinically useful for the treatment of wounds and burns [109–112, 149–151].

Gene transfer can be facilitated by electroporation. The effects of gene transfer after application of an electric field has been investigated in several models [152–154]. Electroporation has been used to deliver genes encoding growth factors, including tissue growth factor-β1 and keratinocyte growth factor (KGF) [154, 155]. Many studies have shown that this approach increases the rate of re-epithelization and healing in chronic diabetic wounds compared to controls; however, the results were inconclusive when compared to growth factor or gene transfer alone. Thus, whether this approach may be of benefit is unclear.

A method of gene transfer that has yielded reliable and promising results in the skin involves the use of synthetic vesicles known as cationic liposomes (CLs). CLs have a positively charged surface, which allows them to loosely bind negatively charged DNA molecules as well as to negatively charged cell surfaces. The latter facilitates their endocytic uptake [156, 157]. CL-DNA complexes can be administered topically or through direct injection [155, 158, 159]. Moreover, CL-DNA complexes are resistant to degradation after injection into the wound environment. Several studies have been performed with CLs to investigate the effects of growth factor overexpression [112, 160, 161]. In a diabetic mouse model, fibroblast growth factor-1 (FGF-1) cDNA was administered in an injured area of skin via topical application and subcutaneous injection [161]. Analysis of the wounds showed that FGF-1 overexpression increased tensile strength. Jeschke et al. applied IGF-I cDNA constructs topically to rat skin after burn injury and found a transfection rate of 70–90% in macrophages, myofibroblasts, and endothelial cells [162]. In a similar rat model of thermal injury, application of liposomal IGF-I cDNA elevated body weight and muscle protein levels. When administration of naked IGF-I was compared to liposomal IGF-I, re-epithelialization was accelerated by nearly 15% [157]. Branski et al. found that transfection of liposomal PDGF cDNA in a porcine burn model [163] not only increased expression of PDGF mRNA and protein at 2–4 days after injection, but also hastened wound re-epithelialization and graft adherence at 9 days.

This investigation showed that CL-mediated gene delivery is possible in a large animal burn model and that PDGF may enhance wound healing as well as dermal and epidermal regeneration.

Wound healing has multiple phases, and different growth factors are involved in each. Thus, delivery and expression of a single growth factor may not be sufficient to stimulate all phases of wound healing. In a partial-thickness wound healing model, co-expression of PDGF and IGF-I was more beneficial than expression of either alone. In a rat wound healing model, PDGF and FGF-2 co-expression yielded higher DNA concentrations than either alone [164, 165]. Jeschke et al. found that, in an animal model, KGF and IGF-I co-expression diminished apoptosis of skin cells and increased proliferation and the rate of re-epithelization compared to either growth factor cDNA alone [162]. These findings suggest that sequential expression of a combination of genes at different stages of wound healing will simulate healing and maximize the benefits of gene transfer in treating burn wounds. Further investigations are needed to determine the precise timing of growth factor up- or down-regulation needed to promote wound healing and oppose scar formation.

Alternative routes of gene delivery have been investigated, including those relying on microbubble-enhanced ultrasound [166], calcium phosphate transfection [167], biomaterials [168], and diethylaminoethyl-dextran [113]. Moreover, both gene-delivering gel matrices [169] and slow-release matrices [170] have been used in clinical scenarios where prolonged transgenic expression is required. The concept of controlled transgenic expression, which can be activated through the presence of a stimulatory molecule in the wound environment, may allow for more targeted therapy via a "genetic switch" [171]. Biotechnological techniques such as the wound chamber technique [172] may also optimize gene delivery to wounds. These novel treatment modalities need to be investigated further to gauge their potential clinical benefit.

37.14 Conclusion

As the treatment of severe burns has evolved over the past decades, notable improvements have been seen in both short- and long-term survival. This has created new challenges in the burns field, including limiting hypertrophic scarring, translation of experimental techniques to clinically applicable wound healing therapies, and controlling treatment costs. New technologies from the bioengineering field may lead to the development of new clinically applicable products. Furthermore, development of effective treatment approaches will depend upon constant reappraisal of current methods for burn wound coverage as well as several other factors. These include gaining a more sophisticated understanding of the pathophysiological mechanisms underlying burn injury, taken with development of new molecular approaches and animal models to study these mechanisms; the conduct of integrated investigations including stem cell application; and validation of the efficacy and clinical utility of new products and approaches via randomized controlled multicenter clinical trials.

Summary Box

As the treatment of severe burns has evolved over the past decades, notable improvements have been seen in both short- and long-term survival. This has created new challenges in the burns field. Indeed new technologies from the bioengineering field may lead to the development of new clinically applicable products. Furthermore, development of effective treatment approaches will depend upon constant reappraisal of current methods for burn wound coverage as well as several other factors.

References

1. National Burn Repository. Chicago: American Burn Association; 2015.
2. Brigham PA, McLoughlin E. Burn incidence and medical care use in the United States: estimates, trends, and data sources. J Burn Care Rehabil. 1996;17(2):95–107. Epub 1996/03/01
3. Pereira C, Murphy K, Herndon D. Outcome measures in burn care. Is mortality dead? Burns. 2004;30(8):761–71.
4. National Burn Repository—2005 report. Chicago: American Burn Association; 2006.
5. Barrow RE, Herndon DN. Thermal burns, gender, and survival. Lancet. 1988;2(8619):1076–7. Epub 1988/11/05
6. Jeschke MG, Pinto R, Kraft R, Nathens AB, Finnerty CC, Gamelli RL, et al. Morbidity and survival probability in burn patients in modern burn care. Crit Care Med. 2015;43(4):808–15. Epub 2015/01/07
7. Janzekovic Z. A new concept in the early excision and immediate grafting of burns. J Trauma. 1970;10(12):1103–8. Epub 1970/12/01
8. Merrell SW, Saffle JR, Larson CM, Sullivan JJ. The declining incidence of fatal sepsis following thermal injury. J Trauma. 1989;29(10):1362–6. Epub 1989/10/01
9. Barret JP, Dziewulski P, Wolf SE, Desai MH, Nichols RJ 2nd, Herndon DN. Effect of topical and subcutaneous epinephrine in combination with topical thrombin in blood loss during immediate near-total burn wound excision in pediatric burned patients. Burns. 1999;25(6):509–13. Epub 1999/09/25
10. Barret JP, Wolf SE, Desai M, Herndon DN. Total burn wound excision of massive pediatric burns in the first 24 hours post burn injury. Ann Burns Fire Disasters. 1999;XIII(1):25–7.
11. Herndon DN, Barrow RE, Rutan RL, Rutan TC, Desai MH, Abston S. A comparison of conservative versus early excision. Therapies in severely burned patients. Ann Surg. 1989;209(5):547–52; discussion 552–3. Epub 1989/05/01

12. Herndon DN, Barrow RE, Kunkel KR, Broemeling L, Rutan RL. Effects of recombinant human growth hormone on donor-site healing in severely burned children. Ann Surg. 1990;212(4):424–9; discussion 430–1. Epub 1990/10/01
13. Herndon DN, Hawkins HK, Nguyen TT, Pierre E, Cox R, Barrow RE. Characterization of growth hormone enhanced donor site healing in patients with large cutaneous burns. Ann Surg. 1995;221(6):649–56; discussion 656–9. Epub 1995/06/01
14. Gallagher JJ, Wolf SE, Herndon DN. Burns. In: Townsend Jr CM, editor. Sabiston textbook of surgery. 18th ed. Philadelphia: Saunders Elsevier; 2007.
15. Dhennin C. [Methods of covering severe burns]. Soins. 2002;(669):45–7. Epub 2002/11/16. Methodes de recouvrement des brulures profondes.
16. Jones I, Currie L, Martin R. A guide to biological skin substitutes. Br J Plast Surg. 2002;55(3):185–93. Epub 2002/06/04
17. Uhlig C, Rapp M, Hartmann B, Hierlemann H, Planck H, Dittel KK. Suprathel-an innovative, resorbable skin substitute for the treatment of burn victims. Burns. 2007;33(2):221–9. Epub 2006/11/07
18. Hundeshagen G, Collins VN, Wurzer P, Sherman W, Voigt CD, Cambiaso-Daniel J, et al. A prospective, randomized, controlled trial comparing the outpatient treatment of pediatric and adult partial-thickness burns with Suprathel or Mepilex Ag. J Burn Care Res. 2018;39(2):261–7. Epub 2017/05/31
19. Schwarze H, Kuntscher M, Uhlig C, Hierlemann H, Prantl L, Noack N, et al. Suprathel, a new skin substitute, in the management of donor sites of split-thickness skin grafts: results of a clinical study. Burns. 2007;33(7):850–4. Epub 2007/05/12
20. Schwarze H, Kuntscher M, Uhlig C, Hierlemann H, Prantl L, Ottomann C, et al. Suprathel, a new skin substitute, in the management of partial-thickness burn wounds: results of a clinical study. Ann Plast Surg. 2008;60(2):181–5. Epub 2008/01/25
21. Bishop JF. Pediatric considerations in the use of Biobrane in burn wound management. J Burn Care Rehabil. 1995;16(3 Pt 1):331–3; discussion 3–4. Epub 1995/05/01
22. Cassidy C, St Peter SD, Lacey S, Beery M, Ward-Smith P, Sharp RJ, et al. Biobrane versus duoderm for the treatment of intermediate thickness burns in children: a prospective, randomized trial. Burns. 2005;31(7):890–3. Epub 2005/07/19
23. Demling RH. Use of Biobrane in management of scalds. J Burn Care Rehabil. 1995;16(3 Pt 1):329–30. Epub 1995/05/01
24. Lal S, Barrow RE, Wolf SE, Chinkes DL, Hart DW, Heggers JP, et al. Biobrane improves wound healing in burned children without increased risk of infection. Shock. 2000;14(3):314–8; discussion 318–9. Epub 2000/10/12
25. Lang EM, Eiberg CA, Brandis M, Stark GB. Biobrane in the treatment of burn and scald injuries in children. Ann Plast Surg. 2005;55(5):485–9. Epub 2005/11/01
26. Ou LF, Lee SY, Chen YC, Yang RS, Tang YW. Use of Biobrane in pediatric scald burns—experience in 106 children. Burns. 1998;24(1):49–53. Epub 1998/05/28
27. Whitaker IS, Prowse S, Potokar TS. A critical evaluation of the use of Biobrane as a biologic skin substitute: a versatile tool for the plastic and reconstructive surgeon. Ann Plast Surg. 2008;60(3):333–7. Epub 2008/04/30
28. Greenwood JE, Clausen J, Kavanagh S. Experience with biobrane: uses and caveats for success. Eplasty. 2009;9:e25. Epub 2009/07/28
29. Pham C, Greenwood J, Cleland H, Woodruff P, Maddern G. Bioengineered skin substitutes for the management of burns: a systematic review. Burns. 2007;33(8):946–57. Epub 2007/09/11
30. Tan H, Wasiak J, Paul E, Cleland H. Effective use of Biobrane as a temporary wound dressing prior to definitive split-skin graft in the treatment of severe burn: a retrospective analysis. Burns. 2015;41(5):969–76. Epub 2015/03/15
31. Philandrianos C, Andrac-Meyer L, Mordon S, Feuerstein JM, Sabatier F, Veran J, et al. Comparison of five dermal substitutes in full-thickness skin wound healing in a porcine model. Burns. 2012;38(6):820–9. Epub 2012/06/02
32. Woodroof A, Phipps R, Woeller C, Rodeheaver G, Naughton GK, Piney E, et al. Evolution of a biosynthetic temporary skin substitute: a preliminary study. Eplasty. 2015;15:e30. Epub 2015/08/01
33. Maral T, Borman H, Arslan H, Demirhan B, Akinbingol G, Haberal M. Effectiveness of human amnion preserved long-term in glycerol as a temporary biological dressing. Burns. 1999;25(7):625–35.
34. Ninman C, Shoemaker P. Human amniotic membranes for burns. Am J Nurs. 1975;75(9):1468–9.
35. Robson MC, Krizek TJ. The effect of human amniotic membranes on the bacteria population of infected rat burns. Ann Surg. 1973;177(2):144–9.
36. Robson MC, Krizek TJ, Koss N, Samburg JL. Amniotic membranes as a temporary wound dressing. Surg Gynecol Obstet. 1973;136(6):904–6.
37. Salisbury RE, Carnes R, McCarthy LR. Comparison of the bacterial clearing effects of different biologic dressings on granulating wounds following thermal injury. Plast Reconstr Surg. 1980;66(4):596–8.
38. Quinby WC Jr, Hoover HC, Scheflan M, Walters PT, Slavin SA, Bondoc CC. Clinical trials of amniotic membranes in burn wound care. Plast Reconstr Surg. 1982;70(6):711–7.
39. Gajiwala K, Gajiwala AL. Evaluation of lyophilised, gamma-irradiated amnion as a biological dressing. Cell Tissue Bank. 2004;5(2):73–80.
40. Douglas B. Homografts of fetal membranes as a covering for large wounds; especially those from burns; an experimental and clinical study. J Tn State Med Assoc. 1952;45(6):230–5.
41. Haberal M, Oner Z, Bayraktar U, Bilgin N. The use of silver nitrate-incorporated amniotic membrane as a temporary dressing. Burns Incl Therm Inj. 1987;13(2):159–63.
42. Ramakrishnan KM, Jayaraman V. Management of partial-thickness burn wounds by amniotic membrane: a cost-effective treatment in developing countries. Burns. 1997;23(Suppl 1):S33–6.
43. Branski LK, Herndon DN, Celis MM, Norbury WB, Masters OE, Jeschke MG. Amnion in the treatment of pediatric partial-thickness facial burns. Burns. 2008;34(3):393–9. Epub 2007/10/09
44. Hennerbichler S, Reichl B, Pleiner D, Gabriel C, Eibl J, Redl H. The influence of various storage conditions on cell viability in amniotic membrane. Cell Tissue Bank. 2007;8(1):1–8.
45. Ravishanker R, Bath AS, Roy R. "Amnion Bank"—the use of long term glycerol preserved amniotic membranes in the management of superficial and superficial partial thickness burns. Burns. 2003;29(4):369–74.
46. Tyszkiewicz JT, Uhrynowska-Tyszkiewicz IA, Kaminski A, Dziedzic-Goclawska A. Amnion allografts prepared in the Central Tissue Bank in Warsaw. Ann Transplant. 1999;4(3–4):85–90.
47. Branski LK, Herndon DN, Pereira C, Mlcak RP, Celis MM, Lee JO, et al. Longitudinal assessment of Integra in primary burn management: a randomized pediatric clinical trial. Crit Care Med. 2007;35(11):2615–23. Epub 2007/09/11
48. Lee EW. Zoografting in a burn case. Boston Med Surg. 1880;103:260.
49. Brennan D. Mediskin™ I. St. Paul: Brennan Medical LLC; 2010.
50. Bromberg BE, Song IC, Mohn MP. The use of pig skin as a temporary biological dressing. Plast Reconstr Surg. 1965;36:80–90. Epub 1965/07/01
51. Cohen IK, Diegelmann RF, Lindblad WJ. Wound healing: biochemical & clinical aspects, vol. xxv. Philadelphia: W.B. Saunders Co.; 1992. p. 630.

52. Fang Z. Application of skin and skin substitutes to burns wounds. In: Leung P, editor. Burns treatment and research. Singapore: World Scientific; 1991. p. 97–106.
53. Forbes P. Advances in the biology of skin hair growth. Oxford: Pergamon; 1969. p. 419–32.
54. Zawacki BE. Reversal of capillary stasis and prevention of necrosis in burns. Ann Surg. 1974;180(1):98–102. Epub 1974/07/01
55. Ersek RA, Denton DR. Silver-impregnated porcine xenografts for treatment of meshed autografts. Ann Plast Surg. 1984;13(6):482–7. Epub 1984/12/01
56. Ersek RA, Navarro JA. Maximizing wound healing with silver-impregnated porcine xenograft. Todays OR Nurse. 1990;12(12):4–9. Epub 1990/12/01
57. Rakers S, Gebert M, Uppalapati S, Meyer W, Maderson P, Sell AF, et al. 'Fish matters': the relevance of fish skin biology to investigative dermatology. Exp Dermatol. 2010;19(4):313–24. Epub 2010/02/18
58. Imai Y. Role of omega-3 PUFA-derived mediators, the protectins, in influenza virus infection. Biochim Biophys Acta. 2015;1851(4):496–502. Epub 2015/01/27
59. Mil-Homens D, Bernardes N, Fialho AM. The antibacterial properties of docosahexaenoic omega-3 fatty acid against the cystic fibrosis multiresistant pathogen Burkholderia cenocepacia. FEMS Microbiol Lett. 2012;328(1):61–9. Epub 2011/12/14
60. Serhan CN. Pro-resolving lipid mediators are leads for resolution physiology. Nature. 2014;510(7503):92–101. Epub 2014/06/06
61. Baldursson BT, Kjartansson H, Konradsdottir F, Gudnason P, Sigurjonsson GF, Lund SH. Healing rate and autoimmune safety of full-thickness wounds treated with fish skin acellular dermal matrix versus porcine small-intestine submucosa: a noninferiority study. Int J Low Extrem Wounds. 2015;14(1):37–43. Epub 2015/03/12
62. Yang CK, Polanco TO, Lantis JC 2nd. A prospective, postmarket, compassionate clinical evaluation of a novel acellular fish-skin graft which contains Omega-3 fatty acids for the closure of hard-to-heal lower extremity chronic ulcers. Wounds. 2016;28(4):112–8. Epub 2016/04/14
63. Magnusson S, Baldursson BT, Kjartansson H, Rolfsson O, Sigurjonsson GF. Regenerative and antibacterial properties of acellular fish skin grafts and human amnion/chorion membrane: implications for tissue preservation in combat casualty care. Mil Med. 2017;182(S1):383–8. Epub 2017/03/16
64. Sheridan RL, Choucair RJ. Acellular allogenic dermis does not hinder initial engraftment in burn wound resurfacing and reconstruction. J Burn Care Rehabil. 1997;18(6):496–9. Epub 1997/12/24
65. Wainwright DJ. Use of an acellular allograft dermal matrix (AlloDerm) in the management of full-thickness burns. Burns. 1995;21(4):243–8. Epub 1995/06/01
66. Klasen HJ. A review on the nonoperative removal of necrotic tissue from burn wounds. Burns. 2000;26(3):207–22. Epub 2000/03/31
67. Sheridan RL. Comprehensive treatment of burns. Curr Probl Surg. 2001;38(9):657–756. Epub 2001/09/25
68. Rosenberg L, Lapid O, Bogdanov-Berezovsky A, Glesinger R, Krieger Y, Silberstein E, et al. Safety and efficacy of a proteolytic enzyme for enzymatic burn debridement: a preliminary report. Burns. 2004;30(8):843–50. Epub 2004/11/24
69. Rosenberg L, Shoham Y, Krieger Y, Rubin G, Sander F, Koller J, et al. Minimally invasive burn care: a review of seven clinical studies of rapid and selective debridement using a bromelain-based debriding enzyme (Nexobrid(R)). Ann Burns Fire Disasters. 2015;28(4):264–74. Epub 2016/10/26
70. Kantak NA, Mistry R, Halvorson EG. A review of negative-pressure wound therapy in the management of burn wounds. Burns. 2016;42(8):1623–33. Epub 2016/07/06
71. Genecov DG, Schneider AM, Morykwas MJ, Parker D, White WL, Argenta LC. A controlled subatmospheric pressure dressing increases the rate of skin graft donor site reepithelialization. Ann Plast Surg. 1998;40(3):219–25. Epub 1998/04/02
72. Chong SJ, Liang WH, Tan BK. Use of multiple VAC devices in the management of extensive burns: the total body wrap concept. Burns. 2010;36(7):e127–9. Epub 2010/10/05
73. Low OW, Chong SJ, Tan BK. The enhanced total body wrap—the new frontier in dressing care for burns. Burns. 2013;39(7):1420–2. Epub 2013/06/08
74. Barret JP, Wolf SE, Desai MH, Herndon DN. Cost-efficacy of cultured epidermal autografts in massive pediatric burns. Ann Surg. 2000;231(6):869–76. Epub 2000/05/19
75. Carsin H, Ainaud P, Le Bever H, Rives J, Lakhel A, Stephanazzi J, et al. Cultured epithelial autografts in extensive burn coverage of severely traumatized patients: a five year single-center experience with 30 patients. Burns. 2000;26(4):379–87. Epub 2000/04/07
76. Sood R, Roggy D, Zieger M, Balledux J, Chaudhari S, Koumanis DJ, et al. Cultured epithelial autografts for coverage of large burn wounds in eighty-eight patients: the Indiana University experience. J Burn Care Res. 2010;31(4):559–68. Epub 2010/07/10
77. Wood FM, Kolybaba ML, Allen P. The use of cultured epithelial autograft in the treatment of major burn injuries: a critical review of the literature. Burns. 2006;32(4):395–401. Epub 2006/04/20
78. Reid MJ, Currie LJ, James SE, Sharpe JR. Effect of artificial dermal substitute, cultured keratinocytes and split thickness skin graft on wound contraction. Wound Repair Regen. 2007;15(6):889–96. Epub 2007/11/22
79. James SE, Booth S, Dheansa B, Mann DJ, Reid MJ, Shevchenko RV, et al. Sprayed cultured autologous keratinocytes used alone or in combination with meshed autografts to accelerate wound closure in difficult-to-heal burns patients. Burns. 2010;36(3):e10–20. Epub 2009/03/24
80. Zweifel CJ, Contaldo C, Kohler C, Jandali A, Kunzi W, Giovanoli P. Initial experiences using non-cultured autologous keratinocyte suspension for burn wound closure. J Plast Reconstr Aesthet Surg. 2008;61(11):e1–4. Epub 2007/09/18
81. Devauchelle B, Badet L, Lengele B, Morelon E, Testelin S, Michallet M, et al. First human face allograft: early report. Lancet. 2006;368(9531):203–9. Epub 2006/07/18
82. Brazio PS, Barth RN, Bojovic B, Dorafshar AH, Garcia JP, Brown EN, et al. Algorithm for total face and multiorgan procurement from a brain-dead donor. Am J Transplant. 2013;13(10):2743–9. Epub 2013/08/07
83. Mohan R, Borsuk DE, Dorafshar AH, Wang HD, Bojovic B, Christy MR, et al. Aesthetic and functional facial transplantation: a classification system and treatment algorithm. Plast Reconstr Surg. 2014;133(2):386–97. Epub 2014/01/29
84. Lantieri L, Grimbert P, Ortonne N, Suberbielle C, Bories D, Gil-Vernet S, et al. Face transplant: long-term follow-up and results of a prospective open study. Lancet. 2016;388(10052):1398–407. Epub 2016/08/29
85. Sosin M, Ceradini DJ, Levine JP, Hazen A, Staffenberg DA, Saadeh PB, et al. Total face, eyelids, ears, scalp, and skeletal subunit transplant: a reconstructive solution for the full face and Total scalp burn. Plast Reconstr Surg. 2016;138(1):205–19. Epub 2016/06/28
86. Aycart MA, Kiwanuka H, Krezdorn N, Alhefzi M, Bueno EM, Pomahac B, et al. Quality of life after face transplantation: outcomes, assessment tools, and future directions. Plast Reconstr Surg. 2017;139(1):194–203. Epub 2016/12/28
87. Giatsidis G, Sinha I, Pomahac B. Reflections on a decade of face transplantation. Ann Surg. 2017;265(4):841–6. Epub 2016/12/30
88. Nguyen LL, Naunheim MR, Hevelone ND, Diaz-Siso JR, Hogan JP, Bueno EM, et al. Cost analysis of conventional face recon-

struction versus face transplantation for large tissue defects. Plast Reconstr Surg. 2015;135(1):260–7. Epub 2014/12/30
89. Pomahac B, Pribaz J, Eriksson E, Bueno EM, Diaz-Siso JR, Rybicki FJ, et al. Three patients with full facial transplantation. N Engl J Med. 2012;366(8):715–22. Epub 2011/12/30
90. Pushpakumar SB, Barker JH, Soni CV, Joseph H, van Aalst VC, Banis JC, et al. Clinical considerations in face transplantation. Burns. 2010;36(7):951–8. Epub 2010/04/24
91. Boyce ST, Glatter R, Kitzmiller WJ. Treatment of chronic wounds with cultured cells and biopolymers: a pilot study. Wounds. 1995;7:24–9.
92. Boyce ST. Skin substitutes from cultured cells and collagen-GAG polymers. Med Biol Eng Comput. 1998;36(6):791–800. Epub 1999/06/15
93. Hansbrough JF, Boyce ST, Cooper ML, Foreman TJ. Burn wound closure with cultured autologous keratinocytes and fibroblasts attached to a collagen-glycosaminoglycan substrate. JAMA. 1989;262(15):2125–30. Epub 1989/10/20
94. Boyce ST, Williams ML. Lipid supplemented medium induces lamellar bodies and precursors of barrier lipids in cultured analogues of human skin. J Invest Dermatol. 1993;101(2):180–4. Epub 1993/08/01
95. Prunieras M, Regnier M, Woodley DT. Methods for cultivation of keratinocytes at the air-liquid interface. J Invest Dermatol. 1983;81:28S–33S.
96. Boyce ST, Supp AP, Swope VB. Vitamin C regulates keratinocyte viability, epidermal barrier, and basement membrane formation in vitro, and reduces wound contraction after grafting of cultured skin substitutes. J Invest Dermatol. 2002;118:565–72.
97. Swope VB, Supp AP, Cornelius JR. Regulation of pigmentation in cultured skin substitutes by cytometric sorting of melanocytes and keratinocytes. J Invest Dermatol. 1997;109:289–95.
98. Supp DM, Boyce ST. Overexpression of vascular endothelial growth factor accelerates early vascularization and improves healing of genetically modified cultured skin substitutes. J Burn Care Rehabil. 2002;23:10–20.
99. Supp DM, Supp AP, Bell SM. Enhanced vascularization of cultured skin substitutes genetically modified to overexpress vascular endothelial growth factor. J Invest Dermatol. 2000;114:5–13.
100. Dantzer E, Braye FM. Reconstructive surgery using an artificial dermis (Integra): results with 39 grafts. Br J Plast Surg. 2001;54(8):659–64. Epub 2001/12/01
101. Nguyen DQ, Potokar TS, Price P. An objective long-term evaluation of Integra (a dermal skin substitute) and split thickness skin grafts, in acute burns and reconstructive surgery. Burns. 2010;36(1):23–8. Epub 2009/10/30
102. Bargues L, Boyer S, Leclerc T, Duhamel P, Bey E. [Incidence and microbiology of infectious complications with the use of artificial skin Integra in burns]. Ann Chir Plast Esthet. 2009;54(6):533–9. Epub 2009/02/19. Incidence et microbiologie des complications infectieuses lors d'utilisation de la peau artificielle Integra chez le brule.
103. Leffler M, Horch RE, Dragu A, Bach AD. The use of the artificial dermis (Integra) in combination with vacuum assisted closure for reconstruction of an extensive burn scar—a case report. J Plast Reconstr Aesthet Surg. 2010;63(1):e32–5. Epub 2009/06/16
104. Moiemen NS, Yarrow J, Kamel D, Kearns D, Mendonca D. Topical negative pressure therapy: does it accelerate neovascularisation within the dermal regeneration template, Integra? A prospective histological in vivo study. Burns. 2010;36(6):764–8. Epub 2010/05/25
105. Shahrokhi S, Arno A, Jeschke MG. The use of dermal substitutes in burn surgery: acute phase. Wound Repair Regen. 2014;22(1):14–22. Epub 2014/01/08
106. Nessler M, Puchala J, Wood FM, Wallace HJ, Fear MW, Nessler K, et al. Changes in the plasma cytokine and growth factor profile are associated with impaired healing in pediatric patients treated with INTEGRA(R) for reconstructive procedures. Burns. 2013;39(4):667–73. Epub 2012/10/04
107. Danin A, Georgesco G, Touze AL, Penaud A, Quignon R, Zakine G. Assessment of burned hands reconstructed with Integra((R)) by ultrasonography and elastometry. Burns. 2012;38(7):998–1004. Epub 2012/06/15
108. Heimbach DM, Warden GD, Luterman A, Jordan MH, Ozobia N, Ryan CM, et al. Multicenter postapproval clinical trial of Integra dermal regeneration template for burn treatment. J Burn Care Rehabil. 2003;24(1):42–8. Epub 2003/01/25
109. Eming SA, Lee J, Snow RG, Tompkins RG, Yarmush ML, Morgan JR. Genetically modified human epidermis overexpressing PDGF-A directs the development of a cellular and vascular connective tissue stroma when transplanted to athymic mice—implications for the use of genetically modified keratinocytes to modulate dermal regeneration. J Invest Dermatol. 1995;105(6):756–63. Epub 1995/12/01
110. Eming SA, Medalie DA, Tompkins RG, Yarmush ML, Morgan JR. Genetically modified human keratinocytes overexpressing PDGF-A enhance the performance of a composite skin graft. Hum Gene Ther. 1998;9(4):529–39. Epub 1998/04/03
111. Eming SA, Snow RG, Yarmush ML, Morgan JR. Targeted expression of insulin-like growth factor to human keratinocytes: modification of the autocrine control of keratinocyte proliferation. J Invest Dermatol. 1996;107(1):113–20. Epub 1996/07/01
112. Eming SA, Whitsitt JS, He L, Krieg T, Morgan JR, Davidson JM. Particle-mediated gene transfer of PDGF isoforms promotes wound repair. J Invest Dermatol. 1999;112(3):297–302. Epub 1999/03/20
113. Eriksson E. Gene transfer in wound healing. Adv Skin Wound Care. 2000;13(2 Suppl):20–2. Epub 2000/11/15
114. Eriksson E, Yao F, Svensjo T, Winkler T, Slama J, Macklin MD, et al. In vivo gene transfer to skin and wound by microseeding. J Surg Res. 1998;78(2):85–91. Epub 1998/09/12
115. Butler KL, Goverman J, Ma H, Fischman A, Yu YM, Bilodeau M, et al. Stem cells and burns: review and therapeutic implications. J Burn Care Res. 2010;31(6):874–81. Epub 2010/09/23
116. Burd A, Ahmed K, Lam S, Ayyappan T, Huang L. Stem cell strategies in burns care. Burns. 2007;33(3):282–91. Epub 2007/03/03
117. Wu Y, Chen L, Scott PG, Tredget EE. Mesenchymal stem cells enhance wound healing through differentiation and angiogenesis. Stem Cells. 2007;25(10):2648–59. Epub 2007/07/07
118. Abe R, Donnelly SC, Peng T, Bucala R, Metz CN. Peripheral blood fibrocytes: differentiation pathway and migration to wound sites. J Immunol. 2001;166(12):7556–62. Epub 2001/06/08
119. Korbling M, Estrov Z, Champlin R. Adult stem cells and tissue repair. Bone Marrow Transplant. 2003;32(Suppl 1):S23–4. Epub 2003/08/22
120. Mansilla E, Marin GH, Drago H, Sturla F, Salas E, Gardiner C, et al. Bloodstream cells phenotypically identical to human mesenchymal bone marrow stem cells circulate in large amounts under the influence of acute large skin damage: new evidence for their use in regenerative medicine. Transplant Proc. 2006;38(3):967–9. Epub 2006/05/02
121. Weil BR, Markel TA, Herrmann JL, Abarbanell AM, Kelly ML, Meldrum DR. Stem cells in sepsis. Ann Surg. 2009;250(1):19–27. Epub 2009/06/30
122. Guenou H, Nissan X, Larcher F, Feteira J, Lemaitre G, Saidani M, et al. Human embryonic stem-cell derivatives for full reconstruction of the pluristratified epidermis: a preclinical study. Lancet. 2009;374(9703):1745–53. Epub 2009/11/26
123. Sun BK, Siprashvili Z, Khavari PA. Advances in skin grafting and treatment of cutaneous wounds. Science. 2014;346(6212):941–5. Epub 2014/11/22

124. Charruyer A, Ghadially R. Stem cells and tissue-engineered skin. Skin Pharmacol Physiol. 2009;22(2):55–62. Epub 2009/02/04
125. Oshima H, Rochat A, Kedzia C, Kobayashi K, Barrandon Y. Morphogenesis and renewal of hair follicles from adult multipotent stem cells. Cell. 2001;104(2):233–45. Epub 2001/02/24
126. Charbord P. Bone marrow mesenchymal stem cells: historical overview and concepts. Hum Gene Ther. 2010;21(9):1045–56. Epub 2010/06/23
127. Kita K, Gauglitz GG, Phan TT, Herndon DN, Jeschke MG. Isolation and characterization of mesenchymal stem cells from the sub-amniotic human umbilical cord lining membrane. Stem Cells Dev. 2010;19(4):491–502. Epub 2009/07/29
128. Miki T, Mitamura K, Ross MA, Stolz DB, Strom SC. Identification of stem cell marker-positive cells by immunofluorescence in term human amnion. J Reprod Immunol. 2007;75(2):91–6. Epub 2007/05/12
129. Bey E, Prat M, Duhamel P, Benderitter M, Brachet M, Trompier F, et al. Emerging therapy for improving wound repair of severe radiation burns using local bone marrow-derived stem cell administrations. Wound Repair Regen. 2010;18(1):50–8. Epub 2010/01/20
130. Lee KD. Applications of mesenchymal stem cells: an updated review. Chang Gung Med J. 2008;31(3):228–36. Epub 2008/09/12
131. Mansilla E, Drago H, Marin GH, Sturla F, Ibar R, Soratti C. Mesenchymal stem cells, could they be the link between tolerance and regeneration? Burns. 2007;33(2):137–8. Epub 2007/02/07
132. Mansilla E, Aquino VD, Roque G, Tau JM, Maceira A. Time and regeneration in burns treatment: heading into the first worldwide clinical trial with cadaveric mesenchymal stem cells. Burns. 2012;38(3):450–2. Epub 2011/11/02
133. Mansilla E, Marin GH, Berges M, Scafatti S, Rivas J, Nunez A, et al. Cadaveric bone marrow mesenchymal stem cells: first experience treating a patient with large severe burns. Burns Trauma. 2015;3:17. Epub 2015/01/01
134. Hernandez A, Evers BM. Functional genomics: clinical effect and the evolving role of the surgeon. Arch Surg. 1999;134(11):1209–15. Epub 1999/11/11
135. Khavari PA, Rollman O, Vahlquist A. Cutaneous gene transfer for skin and systemic diseases. J Intern Med. 2002;252(1):1–10. Epub 2002/06/21
136. Badillo AT, Chung S, Zhang L, Zoltick P, Liechty KW. Lentiviral gene transfer of SDF-1alpha to wounds improves diabetic wound healing. J Surg Res. 2007;143(1):35–42. Epub 2007/10/24
137. Bett AJ, Prevec L, Graham FL. Packaging capacity and stability of human adenovirus type 5 vectors. J Virol. 1993;67(10):5911–21.
138. Carretero M, Del Rio M, Garcia M, Escamez MJ, Mirones I, Rivas L, et al. A cutaneous gene therapy approach to treat infection through keratinocyte-targeted overexpression of antimicrobial peptides. FASEB J. 2004;18(15):1931–3. Epub 2004/10/01
139. Chen S, Kapturczak M, Loiler SA, Zolotukhin S, Glushakova OY, Madsen KM, et al. Efficient transduction of vascular endothelial cells with recombinant adeno-associated virus serotype 1 and 5 vectors. Hum Gene Ther. 2005;16(2):235–47.
140. Deodato B, Arsic N, Zentilin L, Galeano M, Santoro D, Torre V, et al. Recombinant AAV vector encoding human VEGF165 enhances wound healing. Gene Ther. 2002;9(12):777–85.
141. Galeano M, Deodato B, Altavilla D, Squadrito G, Seminara P, Marini H, et al. Effect of recombinant adeno-associated virus vector-mediated vascular endothelial growth factor gene transfer on wound healing after burn injury. Crit Care Med. 2003;31(4):1017–25.
142. Kozarsky KF, Wilson JM. Gene therapy: adenovirus vectors. Curr Opin Genet Dev. 1993;3(3):499–503.
143. Liechty KW, Nesbit M, Herlyn M, Radu A, Adzick NS, Crombleholme TM. Adenoviral-mediated overexpression of platelet-derived growth factor-B corrects ischemic impaired wound healing. J Invest Dermatol. 1999;113(3):375–83.
144. Lu B, Federoff HJ, Wang Y, Goldsmith LA, Scott G. Topical application of viral vectors for epidermal gene transfer. J Invest Dermatol. 1997;108(5):803–8.
145. Morgan JR, Barrandon Y, Green H, Mulligan RC. Expression of an exogenous growth hormone gene by transplantable human epidermal cells. Science. 1987;237(4821):1476–9.
146. Silman NJ, Fooks AR. Biophysical targeting of adenovirus vectors for gene therapy. Curr Opin Mol Ther. 2000;2(5):524–31.
147. Hengge UR, Chan EF, Foster RA, Walker PS, Vogel JC. Cytokine gene expression in epidermis with biological effects following injection of naked DNA. Nat Genet. 1995;10(2):161–6. Epub 1995/06/01
148. Vogel JC. Nonviral skin gene therapy. Hum Gene Ther. 2000;11(16):2253–9. Epub 2000/11/21
149. Dileo J, Miller TE Jr, Chesnoy S, Huang L. Gene transfer to subdermal tissues via a new gene gun design. Hum Gene Ther. 2003;14(1):79–87. Epub 2003/02/08
150. Nanney LB, Paulsen S, Davidson MK, Cardwell NL, Whitsitt JS, Davidson JM. Boosting epidermal growth factor receptor expression by gene gun transfection stimulates epidermal growth in vivo. Wound Repair Regen. 2000;8(2):117–27. Epub 2000/05/16
151. Yang NS, Sun WH. Gene gun and other non-viral approaches for cancer gene therapy. Nat Med. 1995;1(5):481–3. Epub 1995/05/01
152. Baker LL, Chambers R, DeMuth SK, Villar F. Effects of electrical stimulation on wound healing in patients with diabetic ulcers. Diabetes Care. 1997;20(3):405–12.
153. Gardner SE, Frantz RA, Schmidt FL. Effect of electrical stimulation on chronic wound healing: a meta-analysis. Wound Repair Regen. 1999;7(6):495–503.
154. Lee PY, Chesnoy S, Huang L. Electroporatic delivery of TGF-beta1 gene works synergistically with electric therapy to enhance diabetic wound healing in db/db mice. J Invest Dermatol. 2004;123(4):791–8. Epub 2004/09/18
155. Marti G, Ferguson M, Wang J, Byrnes C, Dieb R, Qaiser R, et al. Electroporative transfection with KGF-1 DNA improves wound healing in a diabetic mouse model. Gene Ther. 2004;11(24):1780–5. Epub 2004/10/08
156. Felgner PL, Ringold GM. Cationic liposome-mediated transfection. Nature. 1989;337(6205):387–8.
157. Jeschke MG, Barrow RE, Hawkins HK, Tao Z, Perez-Polo JR, Herndon DN. Biodistribution and feasibility of non-viral IGF-I gene transfers in thermally injured skin. Lab Invest. 2000;80(2):151–8.
158. Alexander MY, Akhurst RJ. Liposome-medicated gene transfer and expression via the skin. Hum Mol Genet. 1995;4(12):2279–85. Epub 1995/12/01
159. Slama J, Davidson JM, Eriksson E. Gene therapy of wounds. In: Falanga V, editor. Cutaneous wound healing. London: Taylor & Francis; 2001. p. 123–40.
160. Jeschke MG, Barrow RE, Hawkins HK, Yang K, Hayes RL, Lichtenbelt BJ, et al. IGF-I gene transfer in thermally injured rats. Gene Ther. 1999;6(6):1015–20.
161. Sun L, Xu L, Chang H, Henry FA, Miller RM, Harmon JM, et al. Transfection with aFGF cDNA improves wound healing. J Invest Dermatol. 1997;108(3):313–8.
162. Jeschke MG, Klein D. Liposomal gene transfer of multiple genes is more effective than gene transfer of a single gene. Gene Ther. 2004;11(10):847–55. Epub 2004/02/13
163. Branski LK, Masters OE, Herndon DN, Mittermayr R, Redl H, Traber DL, et al. Pre-clinical evaluation of liposomal gene transfer to improve dermal and epidermal regeneration. Gene Ther. 2010;17(6):770–8. Epub 2010/04/09
164. Lynch SE, Nixon JC, Colvin RB, Antoniades HN. Role of platelet-derived growth factor in wound healing: synergistic

effects with other growth factors. Proc Natl Acad Sci U S A. 1987;84(21):7696–700. Epub 1987/11/01

165. Sprugel KH, McPherson JM, Clowes AW, Ross R. Effects of growth factors in vivo. I. Cell ingrowth into porous subcutaneous chambers. Am J Pathol. 1987;129(3):601–13. Epub 1987/12/01
166. Lawrie A, Brisken AF, Francis SE, Cumberland DC, Crossman DC, Newman CM. Microbubble-enhanced ultrasound for vascular gene delivery. Gene Ther. 2000;7(23):2023–7. Epub 2001/02/15
167. Fu H, Hu Y, McNelis T, Hollinger JO. A calcium phosphate-based gene delivery system. J Biomed Mater Res A. 2005;74(1):40–8.
168. Shea LD, Smiley E, Bonadio J, Mooney DJ. DNA delivery from polymer matrices for tissue engineering. Nat Biotechnol. 1999;17(6):551–4. Epub 1999/06/29
169. Voigt M, Schauer M, Schaefer DJ, Andree C, Horch R, Stark GB. Cultured epidermal keratinocytes on a microspherical transport system are feasible to reconstitute the epidermis in full-thickness wounds. Tissue Eng. 1999;5(6):563–72. Epub 1999/12/28
170. Chandler LA, Gu DL, Ma C, Gonzalez AM, Doukas J, Nguyen T, et al. Matrix-enabled gene transfer for cutaneous wound repair. Wound Repair Regen. 2000;8(6):473–9. Epub 2001/02/24
171. Gossen M, Bujard H. Tight control of gene expression in mammalian cells by tetracycline-responsive promoters. Proc Natl Acad Sci U S A. 1992;89(12):5547–51. Epub 1992/06/15
172. Breuing K, Eriksson E, Liu P, Miller DR. Healing of partial thickness porcine skin wounds in a liquid environment. J Surg Res. 1992;52(1):50–8. Epub 1992/01/01

Scarring and Scar Management

38

Gerd G. Gauglitz and Julian Poetschke

38.1 Introduction

Scarring is the result of an injury of the deep portion of the dermis. It is commonly caused through elective or emergency surgery, accidental or deliberate trauma or through different dermatological afflictions. While most scars are inconspicuous, pathological forms of scarring can greatly influence the lives of affected patients. They are known for their aesthetically disfiguring properties, significant impairment of function, negative impact on quality of life as well as burdensome symptoms like pronounced pain and pruritus. To alleviate these bothersome symptoms and to improve the affected patients' physical and psychological well-being, physicians require in-depth knowledge about the pathophysiology of scarring as well as effective options for scar prophylaxis and treatment.

38.2 Clinical Aspects of Scarring

38.2.1 Scar Types

Scars come in a variety of shapes and forms. Some of them are benign and are part of the physiological wound healing cascade while others are the result of disturbed wound healing or a predisposition for excessive scarring.

The immature scar is the beginning of every scarring process. They are slightly raised and reddish in appearance and can go along with mild pruritus. Within a few months, usually within about half a year, immature scars usually develop into mature scars that appear flat, pale, and depigmented [1, 2].

G. G. Gauglitz (✉)
Department of Dermatology and Allergology, Ludwig Maximilians University, Munich, Germany
e-mail: gerd.gauglitz@med.uni-muenchen.de

J. Poetschke
Department of Plastic and Hand Surgery, Burn Center, Klinikum St. Georg gGmbH, Leipzig, Germany

Linear hypertrophic scars appear rope-like, show pronounced embossment and erythema, and commonly go along with symptoms like pruritus and pain. They develop 4–8 weeks after the causal trauma and continue to grow for up to 6 months before their development stagnates. This is usually followed by continuous scar regression which commonly lasts for over 1 year [3].

Widespread hypertrophic scarring is usually the result of widespread trauma like burn or scalding injuries. They are associated with irregular scar surface, rope-like scar strands, contractures, uneven skin pliability and indurations, erythema as well as symptoms like pain and pruritus. Depending on the scar localization, functional impairments are common and can lead to decreased range of motion, failure to open or close the eyes and mouth completely, thus leading to further complications. Aesthetic impairments and concurrent psychological strain are common, too. Like linear hypertrophic scars, scar involution can often be observed after an initial growth phase.

Keloids are often confused with hypertrophic scarring and vice versa. They appear round, plump, bulging and highly erythematous, the epithelium is often thinned exposing telangiectasia, and they are commonly associated with strong pruritus and pain, especially after irritation. Keloids exceed the margins of the original trauma, which oftentimes includes minor insect bites, and while they are commonly small, they can reach enormous dimensions in exceptional cases. Predilection sites include the chest, shoulders, and ear-lobes, and their appearance often occurs long after the underlying trauma or without apparent trauma [4].

38.2.2 Histology

Physiological scarring shows relaxed and randomly aligned collagen bundles which mostly consist of mature type I collagen. Hypertrophic scars show an overabundance of dermal collagen. Immature type III collagen is arranged parallel to the epidermis and the individual

M. G. Jeschke et al. (eds.), *Handbook of Burns Volume 1*, https://doi.org/10.1007/978-3-030-18940-2_38

bundles appear stretched and elongated. Nodules of myofibroblasts, extracellular collagen, mucopolysaccharides, and budding blood vessels can be found. While similar in their histologic make-up, keloids show thicker bundling of loosely arranged type I and III collagen. These bundles form acellular node-like structures not commonly found in hypertrophic scars [3, 5].

38.2.3 Epidemiology

Incidence rates of hypertrophic scarring vary throughout the literature with values reaching 70% for linear hypertrophic scar occurrence after surgery and 90% after burn injury. Patient age does not seem to be a contributing factor in hypertrophic scar occurrence [3, 6, 7]. Keloid scarring can be found in all races, though patients with darker skin are more susceptible to develop excessive scarring with research indicating incidence rates for keloids of up to 16% in the African population [3, 8]. Not unlike hypertrophic scarring, keloids occur with equal distribution in both sexes and are most common between the ages of 20 and 40 [3]. Keloids however are strongly associated with a genetic predisposition for excessive scarring and studies have shown that up to 50% of keloid patients have a positive family history regarding the affliction. A positive family history for keloid disease was also associated with keloid occurrence in multiple anatomical locations [9].

Studies found that up to 77% of burn patients experience pathologic scarring with hypertrophic scarring being one of the core problems. Even though widespread like linear hypertrophic scarring shows a distinct tendency for involution after initial growth, persisting aesthetic and functional impairments are common [10].

38.3 Physiological Scar Formation

The formation of scar tissue is the physiologic response to any insult extending to or beyond the deep dermis. Wound healing is a three-pronged process that can be divided into the phases of inflammation, proliferation, and remodeling [8].

Upon wounding, hemostasis sets in and a fibrin-rich bloodclot is formed that acts as a scaffold for the ensuing wound repair. Through the degranulation of thrombocytes, cytokines like insulin-like growth factor (IGF-I), platelet-derived growth factor (PDGF), epidermal growth factor (EGF), and transforming growth factor β (TGF-β) are released [2]. This attracts macrophages and neutrophils that dissolve necrotic tissue and create a clean wound ground while also stimulating fibroblasts and keratinocytes, thus aiding the transition into the proliferative phase, circa 48–72 h after the initial trauma. Activated fibroblasts create an extracellular matrix (ECM) scaffold formed by procollagen, elastin, proteoglycans, and hyaluronic acid. Stimulated by vascular endothelial growth factor (VEGF), vascular ingrowth into the granulation tissue is induced while activated myofibroblasts facilitate wound contraction and closure. This process commonly lasts 3–6 weeks [11]. Upon the achievement of full reepithelialization of the wound, the remodeling and maturation phase begins. There, immature procollagen is converted into mature type I collagen and excess scar tissue is degraded through the mediation of TGF-β3 and matrix metalloproteases. The process of scar maturation can take several months and is usually finished 1–1.5 years after trauma [3, 8, 12].

38.4 Pathological Scar Formation

During the wound healing process, a distinct balance between proliferative and regulatory processes is required. Upon disturbance, this concerted cascade is susceptible to aberrations resulting in the formation of excessive scarring like hypertrophic and keloid scars.

Commonly, an imbalance between the proliferation and degradation of extracellular matrix components leads to excessive scar formation. Risk factors for this include delayed epithelialization, wound infection, specific anatomic locations, or genetic predispositions [2].

On a molecular level, increased activity regarding scar proliferation is commonly mediated through inflammatory cells that secrete TGF-β1 and β2 which induce a fibrogenic response within the scar tissue. At the same time, scar remodeling stimulated through matrix metalloproteases and TGF-β3 is decreased [13–15]. Excessive scar formation is dependent on both the severity of the inflammation and the type of the immune response. While an immune environment dominated by a Th1-mediated response seems to result in decreased fibrogenesis, a primarily Th2-mediated inflammatory process is associated with significant fibrosis [2, 16].

Keloids commonly show a prolonged inflammatory phase as well as a pronounced immune cell presence [17]. This might explain their tendency to extend beyond the original wound's margins, while hypertrophic scarring, where the inflammatory process is less pronounced and slowly decreasing over time, adheres to the margins of the original trauma [17].

All in all, the exact molecular causal chain behind excessive scar formation in keloids and hypertrophic scarring remains to be fully elucidated. While advances in the understanding of the wound healing cascade have been made, deficits remain, especially when it comes to the differentiation of keloids and hypertrophic scars in regard to both their pathophysiology and their treatment.

38.5 Treatment Strategies

38.5.1 Prophylactic Options

38.5.1.1 Preventive Considerations During Surgery

To ensure undisturbed wound healing and to lay the groundwork to effective prevention of excessive scarring, scar prevention has to begin immediately after wounding. In traumatic injuries, this includes swift debridement of the wounds, sufficient hemostasis, and tension-free primary wound closure so as to ensure that epithelialization can progress rapidly and without delay as this presents a primary risk factor for hypertrophic scar development [3, 18]. In surgical wounds, physicians should consider placing surgical incision parallel to skin tension lines and to employ incision techniques that will result in minimal tensile forces on the wound margins after closure, especially in locations affected by the patient's movement. If tension-free skin closure is not possible, z-plasty, w-plasty, local flaps, or skin grafting should be considered to avoid pathological scar formation due to excessive stress on the wound margins [1]. Tension-free and aesthetic wound closure is ideally achieved by combining tension-relieving subcutaneous sutures with epidermal wound closure. Careful epidermal alignment that is neither too loose nor too tight should be observed and skin edges should be everted so as to achieve an even, level and thin scar [2]. While different recommendations regarding the optimum choice of suture material for both subcuticular and epidermal wound closure exist, there is currently no gold standard and standards will vary greatly between different departments, clinics, and countries. Care should be taken to choose a suture material that combines low tissue reactivity with tensile strength sufficient for the respective wound. Regarding subcuticular sutures, that retain most of the tensile forces on the wound margins, physicians should select their suture material with regard to the speed of absorption and the respective loss of tensile strength to ensure sufficient support throughout the wound healing process [19, 20].

38.5.1.2 Pressure Therapy

Pressure therapy is a well-established option for the prevention of excessive scarring and has been used successfully since the 1970s. Its use is most common in the prevention of excessive scarring after burn injury and consecutive split-thickness skin grafting, but it has also been used for the prevention of ear-keloids after surgical removal and for the treatment of younger children suffering from minor hypertrophic scarring or keloids.

The mechanism of action has not yet been completely elucidated though a decreased production of collagen through reduced capillary perfusion and resulting tissue hypoxia and an increase in the rate of fibroblast apoptosis are presumed [21, 22].

Pressure therapy can include the use of compression stockings, pants, sleeves, suits, gloves, bandages, masks, clip-on earrings, and special padding depending on the anatomical site requiring treatment. Pressure therapy is usually recommended to be applied for at least 23 h per day for 6–12 months. Pressure garments commonly loosen significantly over time and thus require replacement, in our experience usually every 3 months, to ensure sufficient compression [3, 23]. Studies suggest an improved efficacy of higher pressure (20–25 mmHg) when compared to lower pressure (10–15 mmHg) in pressure therapy for the treatment of hypertrophic scars, thus warranting additional attention regarding the proper fitting of the prescribed garments throughout the treatment process [24].

Pressure therapy is highly dependent on patient compliance. Achieving proper fitting of the garments is difficult and continuous wearing is often described as highly uncomfortable. Side effects include sweating, maceration, eczema, and strong odor especially during the summer months, thus further complicating patient compliance [2]. In addition, pressure garments are expensive and since an additional set for changing is usually required, the financial burden for patients not covered by comprehensive health insurance is significant.

While some meta-analyses, after analyzing the currently available data, could not elucidate a significant benefit of pressure therapy [25], it remains a well-established and clinically tested standard for hypertrophic scar prophylaxis in patients with severe burns and after split-thickness skin grafting [26]. It might also serve as an alternative to intralesional triamcinolone acetonide injections in children with hypertrophic scarring and keloids due to reduced side effects and significantly less treatment associated discomfort and pain while also showing better results in children than in adults [2]. Pressure therapy (through the application of pressure earrings) has also shown to significantly improve recurrence rates after the excision of earlobe keloids when applied postoperatively [27, 28].

38.5.1.3 Silicone Gel Sheeting

Silicone-based products are another option for the prevention of excessive scarring. Available as gels or wound dressings like patches or sheets, they have been a staple in scar therapy since the early 1980s. Their occlusive effect ensures sufficient skin hydration, thus normalizing the transepidermal water loss (TEWL) which has been identified as the most likely underlying mode of action, rather than the influence of inherent anti-scarring properties of silicone itself. Silicone patches or sheets should be applied for at least 12 h per day over a period of 12–24 weeks. Initial treatment can start as soon as complete reepithelialization of the wound has completed. Silicone gels are more apt for localizations under the influence of constant movement, where continuous adhesion of patches or sheets might prove insecure. Gels should be applied at least twice daily to achieve the desired effect [3].

So far, many studies have evaluated the therapeutic potential of silicone products and confirmed their efficacy [29–33]. A recent Cochrane review, however, stipulates that the overall research quality regarding silicone products for the prevention and treatment of hypertrophic scars and keloids is low and that uncertainties concerning the efficacy of this treatment paradigm remain [34]. Nevertheless, silicone gel and sheeting has been considered the first-line therapy for linear hypertrophic and widespread hypertrophic scars, as well as minor keloids, as noted in international and national guidelines on scar management from 2002, 2012, and 2014, and they have since been recommended as an option for the prevention of excessive scarring [18, 35–37].

38.5.1.4 Flavonoids

Scar creams and patches containing onion extract have become more and more popular in recent years. Their active components include flavonoids, among them quercetin, which is assumed to inhibit fibroblast proliferation and collagen synthesis through influence on TGF-β1, -2 and SMAD signaling pathways [38, 39]. While large parts of the supposed mode of action remain to be fully understood, studies suggest significant improvement of scar height and associated symptoms when comparing onion extract containing products with placebo compounds [40]. Current national and international guidelines support consideration of onion extract based creams and patches for the treatment of active hypertrophic scarring as well as for the post-surgical prevention of excessive scarring [35–37].

38.5.1.5 Imiquimod

Imiquimod is a toll-like receptor 7 ligand that can activate different immune pathways, thus modulating the immune systems response. It stimulates interferon and TNF-α, thus inducing the breakdown of collagen, reducing fibroblast-mediated collagen production, and influencing the expression of genes that induce apoptosis [41, 42]. So far, imiquimod 5% cream has been approved for the treatment of actinic keratosis, superficial basal cell carcinoma, and genital warts [3]. While different pilot studies confirmed the efficacy of imiquimod for the prevention of keloid recurrence after excision [43–46], others revealed no differences in recurrence rates when compared to placebo or extremely high recurrence rates that called into question the supposed treatment effect [47, 48]. Currently, the level of evidence of the available data on excessive scar prevention through the application of imiquimod remains low. Current guidelines on pathological scarring have thus so far omitted inclusion of this treatment option.

38.5.2 Treatment Options

38.5.2.1 Intralesional Corticosteroid Injections Combined with Cryotherapy

Hypertrophic and keloid scarring has been treated with intralesional steroid injections since the mid-1960s and has since then become a standard treatment option for both scar types [49]. Commonly, triamcinolone acetonide (TAC), a potent, crystalline synthetic steroid is used for intralesional injections. Its mode of action is largely routed in the anti-inflammatory properties of corticosteroids which results in decreased fibroblast proliferation, thus inhibiting collagen and glycosaminoglycan synthesis while upregulating dermal matrix remodeling [50–53].

Current therapeutic paradigms recommend three to four injections of TAC with concentrations between 10 and 40 mg/mL every 3–4 weeks. After starting treatment with lower doses of TAC, the dosage can be increased during subsequent treatment sessions to achieve sufficient results. While three to four sessions are usually enough to achieve satisfactory symptom control and flattening of hypertrophic and keloid scars, some cases might require prolonged treatment [36, 37]. To improve the efficacy of the TAC treatment, cryotherapy may be performed before the intralesional injection. Using liquid nitrogen and applying it on the scar in an open spray approach with two passes of 10–15 s each results in significant numbing as well as swelling of the treated area [54]. This edema then facilitates the subsequent injection as it separates the different anatomic layers, thus allowing for easier targeting of the appropriate injection site as well as for the injection of larger volumes of TAC. The hypothesized mode of action of cryotherapy as an enhancer of this therapeutic approach further includes local destruction of fibrotic tissue, vascular damage, tissue hypoxia and, as a result thereof, tissue necrosis [2, 3].

While injection of TAC alone has been described as an effective treatment method for keloids and hypertrophic scars with response rates varying between 50 and 100% and recurrence rates between 9 and 50%, the addition of cryotherapy has been reported to add further efficacy to this long proven treatment method (Fig. 38.1) [54–56].

Side effects of the TAC injection include dermal atrophy, telangiectasia, and pain at the injection site while cryotherapy is associated with permanent hypo- and hyperpigmentation, blistering, and postoperative pain [1].

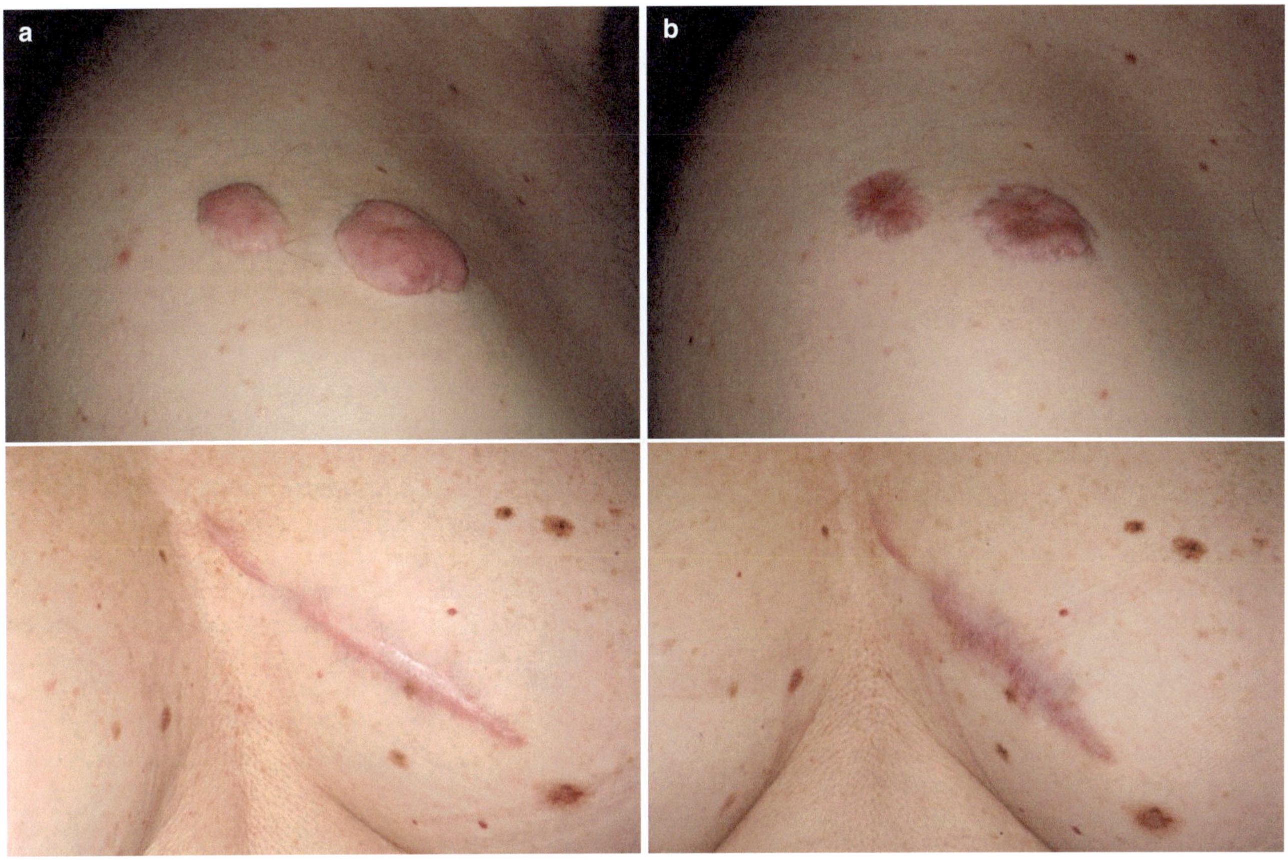

Fig. 38.1 Keloids (upper row) and hypertrophic scar (bottom row) before (**a**) and 6 months after (**b**) four sessions of open spray cryotherapy (two passes of 10 s each) followed by intralesional injection of triamcinolone acetonide (TAC) 40 mg/mL until a blanching effect was reached

38.5.2.2 Intralesional 5-Fluorouracil Injections

5-Fluorouracil (5-FU) has been used for the treatment of hypertrophic scars for decades and positive results were first reported by Fitzpatrick in 1999 after years of use [57]. It is a pyrimidine analog, which is commonly used as an antimetabolite for chemotherapy. In scar tissue, research showed that 5-FU directly increases fibroblast apoptosis by inhibiting the DNA synthesis in rapidly proliferating and metabolizing cells, thus drastically decreasing scar growth [3, 58].

Both high (40–50 mg/mL) and low dose (1.4–3.5 mg/mL) regimens showed positive results in studies evaluating the effects of 5-FU in keloid treatment [59–61]. 5-FU has also been evaluated in combination with TAC. One prospective study including 69 patients showed that a combination of TAC (40 mg/mL) and 5-FU (50 mg/mL) in a concentration of 1:9 injected intralesionally once per week over the course of 2 months, combined with pulsed dye laser treatment, resulted in greater improvements than intralesional TAC (40 mg/mL) alone [62].

Another double-blind, prospective study showed that the aforementioned intralesional regimen was more effective in reducing hypertrophic and keloid scar size and erythema [63]. A current meta-analysis compared the efficacy of combined intralesional 5-FU and TAC to TAC alone and found that 5-FU treatment for hypertrophic scars and keloids resulted in better treatment efficacy, as well as higher patient satisfaction and fewer side effects as TAC treatment alone [64].

Based on current research, intralesional therapy with 5-FU is a safe and effective approach for the treatment of hypertrophic scars and keloids and provides significant scar flattening and symptom control. Erythema and telangiectasia can be treated through adjuvant PDL treatment. Adverse effects include pain at the injection site, hyperpigmentation, skin irritation as well as ulceration, which is mostly seen in darker skin types and commonly resolves within weeks.

While systemic side effects are seldom observed, contraindications for intralesional 5-FU injections include anemia, leucopenia, thrombocytopenia, bone marrow depression, infections, and pregnancy [2, 3]. Women undergoing intralesional 5-FU treatment require a negative pregnancy test before treatment initiation and consequent contraception is mandatory. Current national and international guidelines for the therapy of pathological scarring recommend consideration of 5-FU as a treatment option in therapy-refractory keloids [36]. As hypertrophic scars commonly react well to intralesional TAC treatment, escalation of the treatment paradigm to intralesional 5-FU is rarely necessary. We commonly employ intralesional 5-FU treatment for therapy-refractory keloids in a ratio of 3:1 (5-FU 50 mg/dL: TAC 40 mg/mL) (Fig. 38.2) as well as for the prevention of recurrence in ear-keloids after surgical excision, where we inject small amounts of 5-FU (50 mg/mL) into the fresh scar tissue, beginning 2 weeks after surgery in bimonthly intervals.

38.5.2.3 Laser Therapy

A lot of different laser technologies are available for the treatment of pathological scarring. Nonablative lasers target physiological (hemoglobin, melanin) or artificial (tattoos) pigments while ablative lasers transfer a large part of their energy into water, thus vaporizing tissue and allowing for the controlled ablation of it [65]. Among nonablative lasers, the pulsed dye laser (PDL) has been around for years and its effects have been well researched for a variety of different applications. By targeting oxyhemoglobin, use of the PDL results in capillary destruction, thus inducing tissue hypoxemia which leads to a suppression of profibrotic processes and a supposed upregulation of dermal matrix remodeling through matrix metalloproteases [66, 67]. In a landmark study in 1995, Alster et al. described PDL treatment as an effective option to significantly improve color, height, pliability, and texture in keloids within two to six treatment sessions [68]. These results however could not be reproduced in subsequent studies and follow-up case control studies even reported no discernible differences between treated and untreated scars [69, 70]. Ultimately, further studies revealed that while PDL treatment might not be sufficient to achieve full scar remission, it can be a useful treatment option for fresh, severely erythematous and symptomatic scars or as an adjunct to primary treatment options like intralesional TAC and cryotherapy [35–37].

Side effects of PDL treatment are usually mild and include purpura that last for 1–2 weeks, vesicles, and crusting. Hyperpigmentation can sometimes be observed in darker skin types, but occurrence thereof is less likely with 595 nm wavelength PDL lasers than with units employing a wavelength of 585 nm [37, 65].

The 1064 nm neodymium-doped yttrium aluminum garnet (Nd:YAG) laser has also been suggested for the treatment of keloids and hypertrophic scars [71]. While its mode of action is similar to that of the PDL, the Nd:YAG's wavelength allows for deeper tissue penetration and its energy is less absorbed by melanin, thus suggesting greater efficacy in darker skin types [65]. In thicker lesions, however, the therapeutic effect might be reduced, as the efficacy decreases with the thickness of the scar [71]. Nevertheless, preliminary studies showed significant improvement pigmentation, vas-

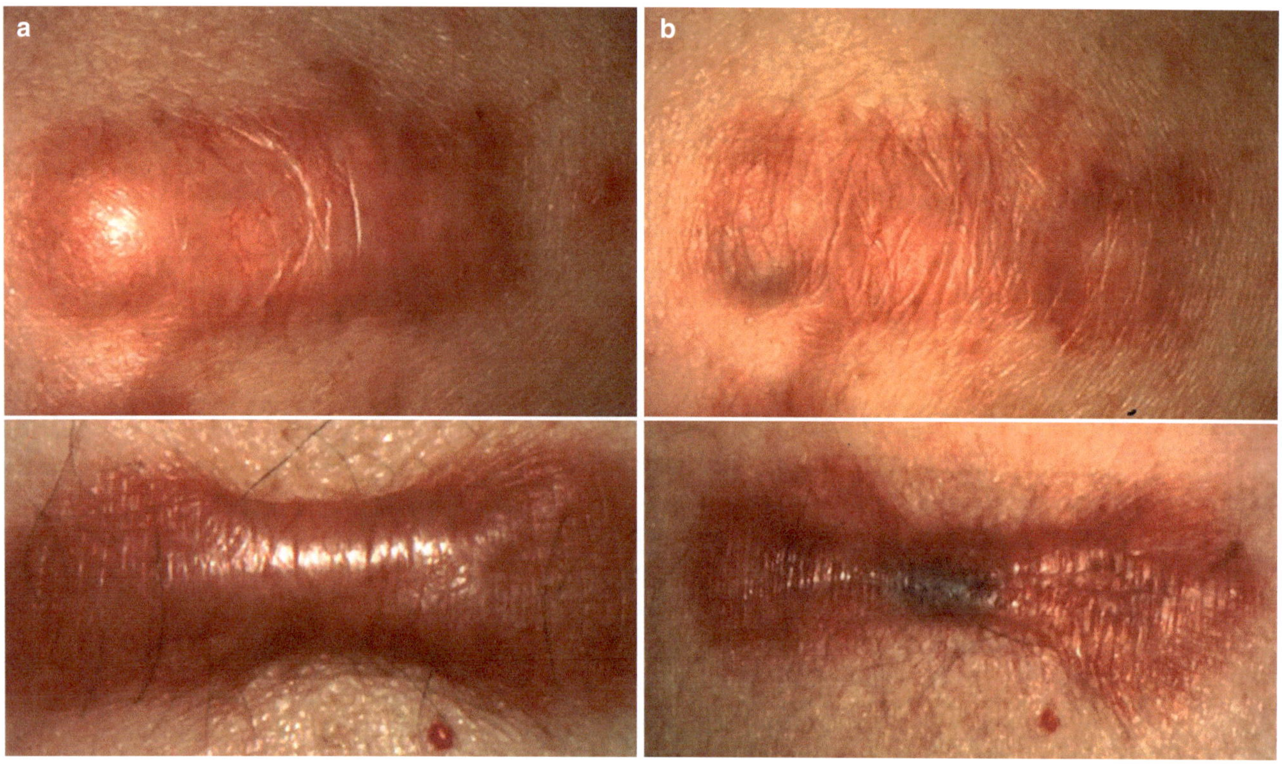

Fig. 38.2 Keloids before (**a**) and 12 months after (**b**) four sessions of 5-FU (50 mg/mL) and TAC (40 mg/mL), 3:1

cularity, pliability, and scar height in keloids and hypertrophic scars after five to ten treatments at 1–2 week intervals [72]. A study comparing PDL to Nd:YAG treatment regarding keloids and hypertrophic scars showed both options were effective. Significant differences between the two treatment modalities, however, could not be found [73]. Side effects were usually mild and included a prickling sensation within the treated area and post-treatment erythema [72]. Current research also showed that permanent hyper- and hypopigmentation were less likely with the 1064 nm Nd:YAG than with the PDL in darker skin types [74, 75]. Ultimately though, the effects of Nd:YAG laser treatment on hypertrophic scars and keloids are not well documented enough, yet, thus requiring further research to warrant guideline recommendations for the treatment of excessive scarring [2].

Ablative laser therapy allows for the controlled ablation, excision, and reshaping of tissue. The most common ablative laser is the carbon dioxide or CO_2 laser with a wavelength of 10,600 nm. Its energy is strongly absorbed by water and as skin cells are rich in water, the CO_2 laser can vaporize tissue in a controlled manner. During treatment, significant heat energy is also transferred into the surrounding tissue. This allows the treating physician to coagulate blood vessels, thus allowing for more extensive tissue ablation. The regeneration and remodeling of heat-damaged matrix proteins also leads to significant skin tightening [65].

Another ablative laser therapy option is the erbium-doped yttrium aluminum garnet laser, also known as the Er:YAG laser. It employs a wavelength of 2940 nm, which leads to significant energy absorption through water. This effect is much more pronounced than with the CO_2 laser which results in little to no heat transfer to the surrounding tissue. This effect is sometimes dubbed as "cold ablation." Thus, tissue ablation with the Er:YAG is less effective, as coagulation of blood vessels is not possible and the heat-induced effects on matrix regeneration and remodeling are much less pronounced [65, 76].

While originally most lasers employed continuous wave technology, that was later replaced in favor of pulsed devices that resulted in strongly reduced heat damage to surrounding tissue, recent modernization of laser technology has led to the development of fractional laser treatment [65]. In fractional laser treatment, the laser beam is divided into a large number of individual laser columns. This creates a pattern of so-called microthermal treatment zones (MTZs), which can reach depths of over 3 mm with the latest laser units. They are interspersed with untreated skin islets. While this results in slightly decreased treatment efficacy, downtime after laser treatment has been greatly decreased through fractional laser treatment [77, 78]. Deep fractional photothermolysis was also shown to significantly influence heat-shot proteins, TGF-β subtypes, and matrix metalloproteases, thus leading to regeneration of a physiological dermal matrix architecture and correction of pathological collagen profiles in scarred skin [79, 80].

Side effects of ablative laser treatment include swelling, erythema, skin infection, scarring, hypopigmentation as well as demarcation between treated and untreated skin.

In scar treatment, fractional ablative laser treatment can be considered as an option to ablate burnt-out linear hypertrophic scars as well as for the loosening of contractures [37, 81]. Studies suggest that the CO_2 laser provides superior results than the Er:YAG laser, possibly due to heat-derived effects on dermal matrix remodeling [65]. While this is not critical for the ablation of hypertrophic scar tissue, it significantly limits the lasers ability to improve contractures where modulation of dermal matrix architecture is vital to achieve the desired effects.

Widespread hypertrophic scarring, such as burn scarring, has become a new field for fractional ablative CO_2 laser treatment.

The molecular effects of fractional photothermolysis could be demonstrated in a variety of pilot studies. They showed that laser treatment resulted in the induction of heat-shock proteins, TGF-β isoforms, collagen subtypes I and III as well as different matrix metalloproteases. This led to significant changes in dermal matrix architecture amounting to a normalization of dermal and epidermal thickness as well as collagen arrangement and deposition levels [77–80, 82–84]. Applying these findings, different clinical studies showed significant scar improvement through fractional ablative CO_2 laser treatment. Levi et al. could demonstrate significant improvement in scar appearance, pliability, tightness, neuropathic pain, and pruritus after three treatment sessions in fourth month intervals [85]. A variety of other studies investigating the clinical effects of this treatment method reported significant scar improvement including scar texture and pliability as well as the ability to effectively loosen contractures through CO_2 laser treatment [86–92]. This resulted in both functional and aesthetic enhancements as well as significant patient satisfaction. Current guidelines therefore included fractional ablative CO_2 laser treatment as a promising treatment option for widespread hypertrophic scars and expert groups recommend extensive integration of fractional ablative laser treatment into existing treatment paradigms [36, 93]. Most studies thus far, however, relied on mainly subjective evaluation paradigms, employed unstandardized treatment settings as well as uncontrolled study designs. Our study group therefore tried to characterize the effects of one session of fractional ablative carbon dioxide laser (Lumenis Ultrapulse Encore, Lumenis Ltd., Yokneam, Israel) treatment in an in-patient controlled approach with standardized treatment settings. Both treated and untreated scars were repeatedly reevaluated over a 6-month follow-up period using both modern clinical imaging and elastometry as well as modern questionnaires for both scar and quality of life evaluation.

Scarred areas of 10 cm by 10 cm were treated using three passes with the fractional ablative CO_2 laser, each with different settings. During the first pass, the whole scarred area was treated using a high-energy, deep fractional mode (ScaarFX: 90–150 mJ/cm^2 (2–3.3 mm), density 1%, 250 Hz) to induce dermal remodeling. Secondly, fine scar strands were ablated using a small spot with a high density and medium intensity (ActiveFX (small spot): 40–90 mJ/cm^2, high density, 300 Hz). During the last pass, a large spot with a reduced density and high intensity was used for superficial smoothening of the whole scarred area (ActiveFX (large spot): 125 mJ/cm^2, low density, 125 Hz). Using this paradigm, we could establish significant improvements in the treated areas when compared to untreated scars (Fig. 38.3). Scar firmness could be reduced by over 30%, as could scar surface irregularities. Scar severity was significantly improved according to questionnaire scores and patients reported significantly improved quality of life scores [94].

Even though recent studies have helped establish the fractional CO_2 laser as a safe and efficacious option for the treatment of widespread hypertrophic scarring, further investigation into this method's potential is necessary to devise standardized treatment paradigms, to elucidate the optimal treatment settings and to determine the ideal point in time for laser intervention.

Keloid treatment with ablative lasers is rarely recommended. Not unlike surgery, monotherapy with ablative lasers results in high recurrence rates. Thus, ablative laser therapy is only recommended for the debulking of large lesions or for the treatment of therapy refractory scars, but only when combined with appropriate adjuvant measures such as intralesional TAC injections or pressure therapy [2].

38.5.2.4 Intralesional Cryotherapy

Intralesional cryotherapy is a relatively new approach for the treatment of hypertrophic scars and keloids. After making a small incision into the scar, the cryoneedle (CryoShape, Etgar Group Ltd., Kfar Saba, Israel) is inserted into the lesion and liquid nitrogen is pumped through the needle resulting in inside-out freezing of the scar tissue.

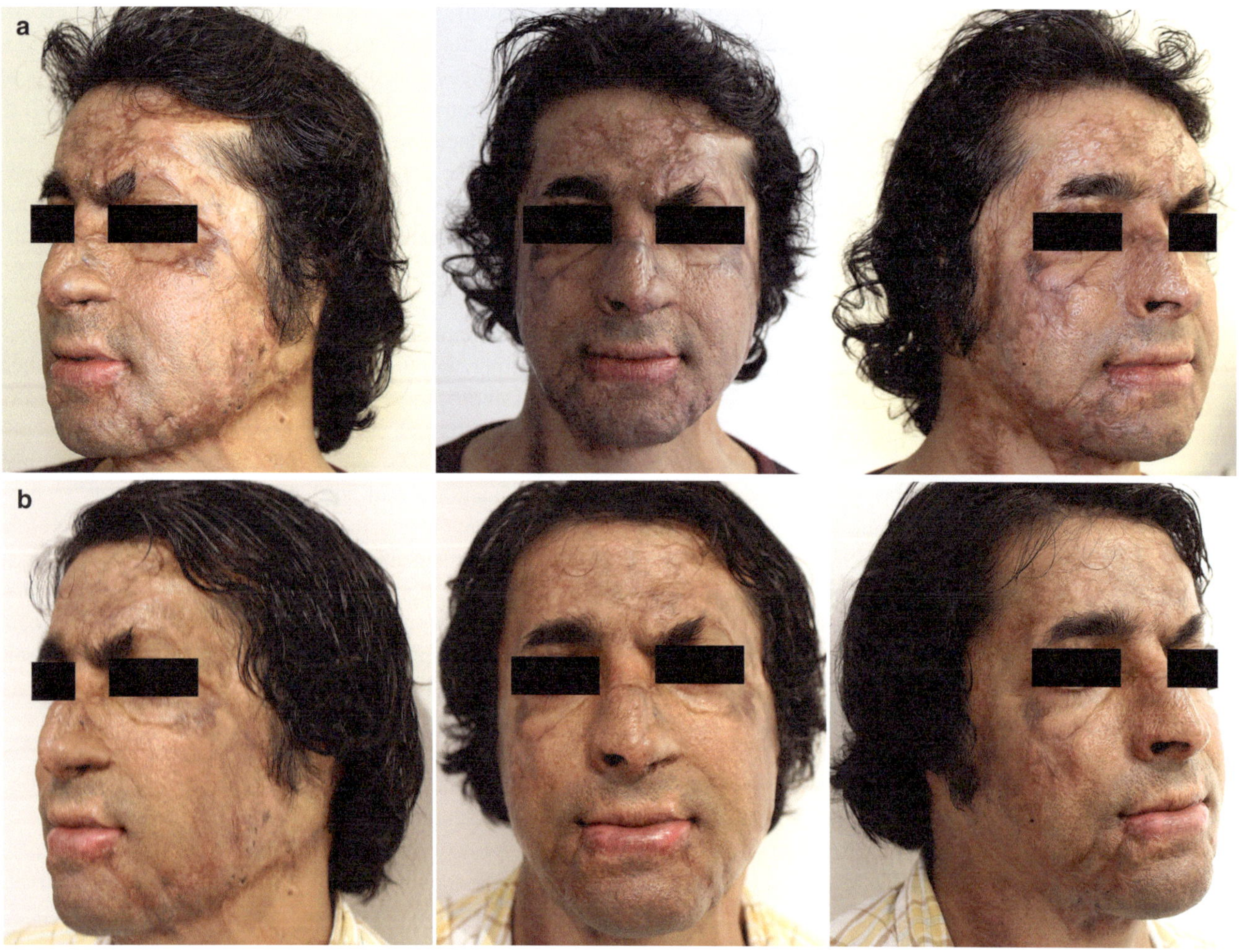

Fig. 38.3 Widespread facial hypertrophic burn scars, before (**a**) and after (**b**) three sessions of fractional ablative CO_2 laser treatment (Lumenis Ultrapulse Encore) using the aforementioned parameters

Initial studies demonstrated significant volume reduction of keloids on the ears, upper back, shoulders, and chest following a single treatment session while also alleviating symptoms like pain and pruritus [95–97]. Additionally, intralesional cryotherapy was reported to be superior to externally applied cryotherapy [98]. Van der Leeuwen et al. report favorable scar reduction and symptom relief, noting, however, that complete scar flattening could not be observed and that both recurrences as well as persistent hypopigmentation in darker skin types were observed [99]. Intralesional cryotherapy requires special equipment and the ability for sterilization of the needles after treatment, thus generating high costs. As its clinical efficacy still requires elucidation through further studies, no clear recommendations on its use for the treatment of hypertrophic scarring and keloids can be made thus far.

38.5.2.5 Surgery

Surgical excision remains a standard option for the treatment of hypertrophic scars and keloids. It should however be considered carefully. As hypertrophic scars often show spontaneous regression without further treatment, care should be taken to avoid unnecessary surgery [50]. On the other hand, hypertrophic scarring caused by excessive tension can be operated on early to treat the origin of the hypertrophy by employing tension-relieving techniques such as z-plasty, w-plasty, skin grafting, or local flaps [1, 2]. Hypertrophic scar recurrence after revision surgery is rarely observed [100, 101]. Keloids on the other hand should not be operated on without adjuvant therapy like intralesional TAC injections, pressure therapy, or radiotherapy, as recurrence rates for surgical monotherapy range from 50 to 100% [18]. Patients treated with keloid excision are at danger of developing an ever larger keloid post-surgery [55]. Therefore, surgery is usually only recommended as a last resort option or for the debulking of larger lesions when combined with proper adjuvant measures. Good results are generally reported for the surgical excision of ear-keloids when treated with pressure earrings immediately after full reepithelialization is reached. Cosmetic results are usually satisfying and recurrence rates are low [1, 3, 102].

38.5.2.6 Radiotherapy

Radiotherapy has mainly been used as an adjuvant treatment option after surgical removal of keloids. Its mode of action is based on the inhibition of vascular budding and fibroblast proliferation, which results in decreased collagen synthesis, thus limiting the growth of fresh scar tissue.

Employing X-rays, electron beam, low- or high-dose-rate brachytherapy after surgical excision, good results regarding recurrence rates could be observed in a number of studies [103–105]. Van der Kar et al. however concluded that surgical excision of keloids in combination with postoperative radiotherapy should be reserved as a last resort option as their prospective study observed a recurrence rate of over 70% [106]. A meta-analysis on the efficacy of radiotherapy treatment for keloids concluded that radiotherapy after surgery was more effective than radiotherapy alone, while brachytherapy resulted in the lowest recurrence rates (15%) when compared to electron-beam or X-ray radiotherapy [107].

Common side effects of radiotherapy include hypo- and hyperpigmentation as well as erythema, telangiectasia, and skin atrophy [108]. In regard to the potentially carcinogenic side effects of ionizing irradiation, radiotherapy should be considered carefully, especially in younger patients and in sensitive areas [101].

38.5.2.7 Bleomycin

Bleomycin sulfate is a glycopeptide and commonly used as a systemic chemotherapeutic agent. Since bleomycin inhibits collagen synthesis by decreasing TGF-β1 levels, it has been adapted for the intralesional treatment of excessive scarring.

A number of studies have since shown significant improvement of scar parameters like height, pliability, erythema as well as symptoms like pain and pruritus in hypertrophic scarring and keloids after three to five treatment sessions [109–111]. Combination of TAC and bleomycin for intralesional keloid and hypertrophic scar treatment also revealed significant effects in a small case series [112].

Side effects include long-term depigmentation and dermal atrophy and when applied systemically, its high toxicity may lead to serious effects on the pulmonary, renal, and hepatic organ systems among others. As with intralesional 5-Fluorouracil injections, however, systemic side effects have rarely been reported and are extremely unlikely in strictly intralesional use [101]. Overall, however, research data on bleomycin treatment for excessive scarring is still scarce, thus necessitating further investigation of its therapeutic efficacy to establish its role in the treatment of hypertrophic scars and keloids.

38.5.2.8 Interferon

Interferon (IFN) has been considered for the treatment of excessive scarring based on its antiproliferative effects that lead to decreased synthesis of collagen subtypes I and III. Interferon-α2b has been identified as the most promising compound for its properties that may help improve dermal fibrosis directly or by antagonizing the effects of TGF-β1, -β2 and histamine [113, 114].

Systemic administration of IFN-α2b could be shown to improve clinical appearance of hypertrophic burn scars and lowered serum levels of TGF-β were observed following treatment, while intralesionally applied IFN-α2b (1.5 million international units, injections twice per day over the course of 4 days) resulted in a 50% reduction of keloid size within 9 days in one study, with researchers claiming superior efficacy of IFN- α2b when compared to intralesional TAC [114, 115].

IFN treatment, however, goes along with frequent side effects including flu-like symptoms and injection site pain [101]. IFN therapy is also significantly more costly than other, more common forms of scar treatment. So far, while remaining a promising treatment option, guidelines for the treatment of pathological scarring have not yet included IFN treatment, as sufficient research data on its efficacy is currently not available.

38.5.2.9 Recombinant TGF-β3

Recombinant TGF-β3 was initially believed to be a potent upcoming option for the treatment of excessive scarring. While adult skin tissue is characterized by a balance of TGF-β isotypes with higher levels of fibrosis stimulating TGF-β1 and TGF-β2, fetal skin tissue shows heightened expression of TGF-β3 which induces anti-fibrotic changes during wound healing, as well as dermal matrix remodeling. This is assumed to play a pivotal role in the ability of fetal skin to heal almost scarlessly [116, 117]. But while initial results of placebo-controlled, double-blind phase I and phase II studies on the effects of recombinant TGF-β3 reported promising results, the subsequent phase III trial failed to hit its endpoints and development of the drug was ultimately halted [118]. While no treatment options based on recombinant TGF-β3 are available right now, research on this promising aspect of wound healing and its potential clinical applications continues [119–121].

Summary Box

Pathological scarring includes a variety of different subtypes that go along with tantalizing aesthetic and functional impairments and that remain difficult to treat successfully. As surgical interventions become more common in the developed world and trauma is ubiquitous, physiological as well as disturbed scarring is a global occurrence. Therefore, physicians require a basic understanding of the pathophysiology of scarring and knowledge about the most common therapeutic options, their potential as well as their side effects. While many of the most established interventional regimens like surgery and intralesional corticosteroid injections have been tried and tested throughout years of clinical application, a variety of once promising emerging options have now become established as standard forms of therapy and earned their place in treatment guidelines [36, 37]. Among them are the intralesional injection of 5-Fluorouracil for keloid treatment as well as the fractional ablative carbon dioxide laser treatment for widespread hypertrophic scarring. Undoubtedly, more options will follow, as researchers continue to evaluate new forms of scar treatment all the while reevaluating established treatment paradigms to reassess their role in current scar therapy. In this regard, the role of objective imaging and questionnaire based scar evaluation is becoming more and more important to ensure optimum treatment efficacy for every patient [122].

References

1. Poetschke J, Gauglitz GG. Current options for the treatment of pathological scarring. J Dtsch Dermatol Ges. 2016;14:467–77.
2. Gauglitz GG. Management of keloids and hypertrophic scars: current and emerging options. Clin Cosmet Investig Dermatol. 2013;6:103–14.
3. Gauglitz GG, Korting HC, Pavicic T, Ruzicka T, Jeschke MG. Hypertrophic scarring and keloids: pathomechanisms and current and emerging treatment strategies. Mol Med. 2011;17:113–25.
4. Reinholz M, Poetschke J, Schwaiger H, Epple A, Ruzicka T, Gauglitz GG. The dermatology life quality index as a means to assess life quality in patients with different scar types. J Eur Acad Dermatol Venereol. 2015;29:2112–9.
5. Tuan TL, Nichter LS. The molecular basis of keloid and hypertrophic scar formation. Mol Med Today. 1998;4:19–24.
6. Lewis WH, Sun KK. Hypertrophic scar: a genetic hypothesis. Burns. 1990;16:176–8.
7. Deitch EA, Wheelahan TM, Rose MP, Clothier J, Cotter J. Hypertrophic burn scars: analysis of variables. J Trauma. 1983;23:895–8.
8. Niessen FB, Spauwen PH, Schalkwijk J, Kon M. On the nature of hypertrophic scars and keloids: a review. Plast Reconstr Surg. 1999;104:1435–58.
9. Bayat A, Arscott G, Ollier WE, McGrouther DA, Ferguson MW. Keloid disease: clinical relevance of single versus multiple site scars. Br J Plast Surg. 2005;58:28–37.
10. Gangemi E, Gregori D, Berchialla P, et al. Epidemiology and risk factors for pathologic scarring after burn wounds. Arch Facial Plast Surg. 2008;10:93–102.
11. Slemp AE, Kirschner RE. Keloids and scars: a review of keloids and scars, their pathogenesis, risk factors, and management. Curr Opin Pediatr. 2006;18:396–402.
12. Tredget EE, Nedelec B, Scott PG, Ghahary A. Hypertrophic scars, keloids, and contractures. The cellular and molecular basis for therapy. Surg Clin North Am. 1997;77:701–30.
13. Szulgit G, Rudolph R, Wandel A, Tenenhaus M, Panos R, Gardner H. Alterations in fibroblast alpha1beta1 integrin collagen receptor expression in keloids and hypertrophic scars. J Invest Dermatol. 2002;118:409–15.
14. Kose O, Waseem A. Keloids and hypertrophic scars: are they two different sides of the same coin? Dermatol Surg. 2008;34:336–46.
15. Bock O, Yu H, Zitron S, Bayat A, Ferguson MW, Mrowietz U. Studies of transforming growth factors beta 1-3 and their receptors I and II in fibroblast of keloids and hypertrophic scars. Acta Derm Venereol. 2005;85:216–20.
16. Wynn TA. Fibrotic disease and the T(H)1/T(H)2 paradigm. Nat Rev Immunol. 2004;4:583–94.
17. Brown JJ, Bayat A. Genetic susceptibility to raised dermal scarring. Br J Dermatol. 2009;161:8–18.

18. Mustoe TA, Cooter RD, Gold MH, Hobbs FD, Ramelet AA, Shakespeare PG, et al. International clinical recommendations on scar management. Plast Reconstr Surg. 2002;110:560–71.
19. Tajirian AL, Goldberg DJ. A review of sutures and other skin closure materials. J Cosmet Laser Ther. 2010;12:296–302.
20. Regula CG, Yag-Howard C. Suture products and techniques: what to use, where, and why. Dermatol Surg. 2015;41(Suppl 10):S187–200.
21. Baur PS, Larson DL, Stacey TR, Barratt GF, Dobrkovsky M. Ultrastructural analysis of pressure-treated human hypertrophic scars. J Trauma. 1976;16:958–67.
22. Reno F, Sabbatini M, Lombardi F, Stella M, Pezzuto C, Magliacani G, et al. In vitro mechanical compression induces apoptosis and regulates cytokines release in hypertrophic scars. Wound Repair Regen. 2003;11:331–6.
23. Van den Kerckhove E, Stappaerts K, Fieuws S, Laperre J, Massage P, Flour M, et al. The assessment of erythema and thickness on burn related scars during pressure garment therapy as a preventive measure for hypertrophic scarring. Burns. 2005;31:696–702.
24. Candy LH, Cecilia LT, Ping ZY. Effect of different pressure magnitudes on hypertrophic scar in a Chinese population. Burns. 2010;36:1234–41.
25. Anzarut A, Olson J, Singh P, Rowe BH, Tredget EE. The effectiveness of pressure garment therapy for the prevention of abnormal scarring after burn injury: a meta-analysis. J Plast Reconstr Aesthet Surg. 2009;62:77–84.
26. Anthonissen M, Daly D, Janssens T, Van den Kerckhove E. The effects of conservative treatments on burn scars: a systematic review. Burns. 2016;42(3):508–18.
27. Kadouch DJ, van der Veer WM, Mahdavian Delavary B, Kerkdijk D, Niessen FB. Therapeutic hotline: an alternative adjuvant treatment after ear keloid excision using a custom-made methyl methacrylate stent. Dermatol Ther. 2010;23:686–92.
28. Park TH, Seo SW, Kim JK, Chang CH. Outcomes of surgical excision with pressure therapy using magnets and identification of risk factors for recurrent keloids. Plast Reconstr Surg. 2011;128:431–9.
29. Bianchi FA, Roccia F, Fiorini P, Berrone S. Use of patient and observer scar assessment scale for evaluation of facial scars treated with self-drying silicone gel. J Craniofac Surg. 2010;21:719–23.
30. Cassuto DA, Scrimali L, Sirago P. Treatment of hypertrophic scars and keloids with an LBO laser (532 nm) and silicone gel sheeting. J Cosmet Laser Ther. 2010;12:32–7.
31. Kwon SY, Park SD, Park K. Comparative effect of topical silicone gel and topical tretinoin cream for the prevention of hypertrophic scar and keloid formation and the improvement of scars. J Eur Acad Dermatol Venereol. 2014;28:1025–33.
32. Rhee SH, Koh SH, Lee DW, Park BY, Kim YO. Aesthetic effect of silicone gel on surgical scars in Asians. J Craniofac Surg. 2010;21:706–10.
33. Sakuraba M, Takahashi N, Akahoshi T, Miyasaka Y, Suzuki K. Use of silicone gel sheets for prevention of keloid scars after median sternotomy. Surg Today. 2011;41:496–9.
34. O'Brien L, Jones DJ. Silicone gel sheeting for preventing and treating hypertrophic and keloid scars. Cochrane Database Syst Rev. 2013; CD003826.
35. Gold MH, Berman B, Clementoni MT, Gauglitz GG, Nahai F, Murcia C. Updated international clinical recommendations on scar management: part 1-evaluating the evidence. Dermatol Surg. 2014;40:817–24.
36. Gold MH, McGuire M, Mustoe TA, Pusic A, Sachdev M, Waibel J, et al. Updated international clinical recommendations on scar management: part 2-algorithms for scar prevention and treatment. Dermatol Surg. 2014;40:825–31.
37. Nast A, Eming S, Fluhr J, Fritz K, Gauglitz G, Hohenleutner S, et al. German S2k guidelines for the therapy of pathological scars (hypertrophic scars and keloids). J Dtsch Dermatol Ges. 2012;10:747–62.
38. Phan TT, Lim IJ, Sun L, Chan SY, Bay BH, Tan EK, et al. Quercetin inhibits fibronectin production by keloid-derived fibroblasts. Implication for the treatment of excessive scars. J Dermatol Sci. 2003;33:192–4.
39. Phan TT, Lim IJ, Chan SY, Tan EK, Lee ST, Longaker MT. Suppression of transforming growth factor beta/smad signaling in keloid-derived fibroblasts by quercetin: implications for the treatment of excessive scars. J Trauma. 2004;57:1032–7.
40. Chanprapaph K, Tanrattanakorn S, Wattanakrai P, Wongkitisophon P, Vachiramon V. Effectiveness of onion extract gel on surgical scars in Asians. Dermatol Res Pract. 2012;2012:212945.
41. Zurada JM, Kriegel D, Davis IC. Topical treatments for hypertrophic scars. J Am Acad Dermatol. 2006;55:1024–31.
42. Arno AI, Gauglitz GG, Barret JP, Jeschke MG. Up-to-date approach to manage keloids and hypertrophic scars: a useful guide. Burns. 2014;40:1255–66.
43. Berman B, Kaufman J. Pilot study of the effect of postoperative imiquimod 5% cream on the recurrence rate of excised keloids. J Am Acad Dermatol. 2002;47:S209–11.
44. Chuangsuwanich A, Gunjittisomram S. The efficacy of 5% imiquimod cream in the prevention of recurrence of excised keloids. J Med Assoc Thai. 2007;90:1363–7.
45. Stashower ME. Successful treatment of earlobe keloids with imiquimod after tangential shave excision. Dermatol Surg. 2006;32:380–6.
46. Shin JY, Yun SK, Roh SG, Lee NH, Yang KM. Efficacy of 2 representative topical agents to prevent keloid recurrence after surgical excision. J Oral Maxillofac Surg. 2017;75:401.e401–6.
47. Berman B, Harrison-Balestra C, Perez OA, Viera M, Villa A, Zell D, et al. Treatment of keloid scars post-shave excision with imiquimod 5% cream: a prospective, double-blind, placebo-controlled pilot study. J Drugs Dermatol. 2009;8:455–8.
48. Cacao FM, Tanaka V, Messina MC. Failure of imiquimod 5% cream to prevent recurrence of surgically excised trunk keloids. Dermatol Surg. 2009;35:629–33.
49. Jalali M, Bayat A. Current use of steroids in management of abnormal raised skin scars. Surgeon. 2007;5:175–80.
50. Reish RG, Eriksson E. Scar treatments: preclinical and clinical studies. J Am Coll Surg. 2008;206:719–30.
51. Cruz NI, Korchin L. Inhibition of human keloid fibroblast growth by isotretinoin and triamcinolone acetonide in vitro. Ann Plast Surg. 1994;33:401–5.
52. Boyadjiev C, Popchristova E, Mazgalova J. Histomorphologic changes in keloids treated with Kenacort. J Trauma. 1995;38:299–302.
53. Poetschke J, Reinholz M, Schwaiger H, Epple A, Gauglitz GG. DLQI and POSAS scores in keloid patients. Facial Plast Surg. 2016;32:289–95.
54. Boutli-Kasapidou F, Tsakiri A, Anagnostou E, Mourellou O. Hypertrophic and keloidal scars: an approach to polytherapy. Int J Dermatol. 2005;44:324–7.
55. Robles DT, Berg D. Abnormal wound healing: keloids. Clin Dermatol. 2007;25:26–32.
56. Yosipovitch G, Widijanti Sugeng M, Goon A, Chan YH, Goh CL. A comparison of the combined effect of cryotherapy and corticosteroid injections versus corticosteroids and cryotherapy alone on keloids: a controlled study. J Dermatolog Treat. 2001;12:87–90.
57. Fitzpatrick RE. Treatment of inflamed hypertrophic scars using intralesional 5-FU. Dermatol Surg. 1999;25:224–32.
58. Apikian M, Goodman G. Intralesional 5-fluorouracil in the treatment of keloid scars. Australas J Dermatol. 2004;45:140–3.
59. Nanda S, Reddy BS. Intralesional 5-fluorouracil as a treatment modality of keloids. Dermatol Surg. 2004;30:54–6; discussion 56–57

60. Wu XL, Liu W, Cao YL. [Clinical study on keloid treatment with intralesional injection of low concentration 5-fluorouracil]. Zhonghua Zheng Xing Wai Ke Za Zhi. 2006;22:44–6.
61. Wu XL, Gao Z, Song N, Liu W. [Clinical study of auricular keloid treatment with both surgical excision and intralesional injection of low-dose 5-fluorouracil and corticosteroids]. Zhonghua Yi Xue Za Zhi. 2009;89:1102–5.
62. Asilian A, Darougheh A, Shariati F. New combination of triamcinolone, 5-fluorouracil, and pulsed-dye laser for treatment of keloid and hypertrophic scars. Dermatol Surg. 2006;32:907–15.
63. Darougheh A, Asilian A, Shariati F. Intralesional triamcinolone alone or in combination with 5-fluorouracil for the treatment of keloid and hypertrophic scars. Clin Exp Dermatol. 2009;34:219–23.
64. Kafka M, Collins V, Kamolz LP, Rappl T, Branski LK, Wurzer P. Evidence of invasive and noninvasive treatment modalities for hypertrophic scars: a systematic review. Wound Repair Regen. 2017;25:139–44.
65. Stewart N, Lim AC, Lowe PM, Goodman G. Lasers and laser-like devices: part one. Australas J Dermatol. 2013;54:173–83.
66. Alster T. Laser scar revision: comparison study of 585-nm pulsed dye laser with and without intralesional corticosteroids. Dermatol Surg. 2003;29:25–9.
67. Dierickx C, Goldman MP, Fitzpatrick RE. Laser treatment of erythematous/hypertrophic and pigmented scars in 26 patients. Plast Reconstr Surg. 1995;95:84–90; discussion 91–2
68. Alster TS, Williams CM. Treatment of keloid sternotomy scars with 585 nm flashlamp-pumped pulsed-dye laser. Lancet. 1995;345:1198–200.
69. Allison KP, Kiernan MN, Waters RA, Clement RM. Pulsed dye laser treatment of burn scars. Alleviation or irritation? Burns. 2003;29:207–13.
70. Wittenberg GP, Fabian BG, Bogomilsky JL, Schultz LR, Rudner EJ, Chaffins ML, et al. Prospective, single-blind, randomized, controlled study to assess the efficacy of the 585-nm flashlamp-pumped pulsed-dye laser and silicone gel sheeting in hypertrophic scar treatment. Arch Dermatol. 1999;135:1049–55.
71. Akaishi S, Koike S, Dohi T, Kobe K, Hyakusoku H, Ogawa R. Nd:YAG laser treatment of keloids and hypertrophic scars. Eplasty. 2012;12:e1.
72. Cho SB, Lee JH, Lee SH, Lee SJ, Bang D, Oh SH. Efficacy and safety of 1064-nm Q-switched Nd:YAG laser with low fluence for keloids and hypertrophic scars. J Eur Acad Dermatol Venereol. 2010;24:1070–4.
73. Al-Mohamady Ael S, Ibrahim SM, Muhammad MM. Pulsed dye laser versus long-pulsed Nd:YAG laser in the treatment of hypertrophic scars and keloid: a comparative randomized split-scar trial. J Cosmet Laser Ther. 2016;18:208–12.
74. Rossi A, Lu R, Frey MK, Kubota T, Smith LA, Perez M. The use of the 300 microsecond 1064 nm Nd:YAG laser in the treatment of keloids. J Drugs Dermatol. 2013;12:1256–62.
75. Sebaratnam DF, Lim AC, Lowe PM, Goodman GJ, Bekhor P, Richards S. Lasers and laser-like devices: part two. Australas J Dermatol. 2014;55:1–14.
76. Reinholz M, Schwaiger H, Heppt MV, Poetschke J, Tietze J, Epple A, et al. Comparison of two kinds of lasers in the treatment of acne scars. Facial Plast Surg. 2015;31:523–31.
77. Manstein D, Herron GS, Sink RK, Tanner H, Anderson RR. Fractional photothermolysis: a new concept for cutaneous remodeling using microscopic patterns of thermal injury. Lasers Surg Med. 2004;34:426–38.
78. Laubach HJ, Tannous Z, Anderson RR, Manstein D. Skin responses to fractional photothermolysis. Lasers Surg Med. 2006;38:142–9.
79. Dams SD, de Liefde-van Beest M, Nuijs AM, Oomens CW, Baaijens FP. Pulsed heat shocks enhance procollagen type I and procollagen type III expression in human dermal fibroblasts. Skin Res Technol. 2010;16:354–64.
80. Helbig D, Paasch U. Molecular changes during skin aging and wound healing after fractional ablative photothermolysis. Skin Res Technol. 2011;17:119–28.
81. Uebelhoer NS, Ross EV, Shumaker PR. Ablative fractional resurfacing for the treatment of traumatic scars and contractures. Semin Cutan Med Surg. 2012;31:110–20.
82. El-Zawahry BM, Sobhi RM, Bassiouny DA, Tabak SA. Ablative CO fractional resurfacing in treatment of thermal burn scars: an open-label controlled clinical and histopathological study. J Cosmet Dermatol. 2015;14(4):324–31.
83. Nicoletti G, De Francesco F, Mele CM, Cataldo C, Grella R, Brongo S, et al. Clinical and histologic effects from CO2 laser treatment of keloids. Lasers Med Sci. 2013;28:957–64.
84. Orringer JS, Kang S, Johnson TM, Karimipour DJ, Hamilton T, Hammerberg C, et al. Connective tissue remodeling induced by carbon dioxide laser resurfacing of photodamaged human skin. Arch Dermatol. 2004;140:1326–32.
85. Levi B, Ibrahim A, Mathews K, Wojcik B, Gomez J, Fagan S, et al. The use of CO2 fractional photothermolysis for the treatment of burn scars. J Burn Care Res. 2016;37:106–14.
86. Cervelli V, Gentile P, Spallone D, Nicoli F, Verardi S, Petrocelli M, et al. Ultrapulsed fractional CO2 laser for the treatment of post-traumatic and pathological scars. J Drugs Dermatol. 2010;9:1328–31.
87. Ho D, Jagdeo J. Excellent aesthetic and functional outcome after fractionated carbon dioxide laser skin graft revision surgery: case report and review of laser skin graft revision techniques. J Drugs Dermatol. 2015;14:1285–8.
88. Hultman CS, Edkins RE, Wu C, Calvert CT, Cairns BA. Prospective, before-after cohort study to assess the efficacy of laser therapy on hypertrophic burn scars. Ann Plast Surg. 2013;70:521–6.
89. Hultman CS, Friedstat JS, Edkins RE, Cairns BA, Meyer AA. Laser resurfacing and remodeling of hypertrophic burn scars: the results of a large, prospective, before-after cohort study, with long-term follow-up. Ann Surg. 2014;260:519–29; discussion 529–32
90. Krakowski AC, Goldenberg A, Eichenfield LF, Murray JP, Shumaker PR. Ablative fractional laser resurfacing helps treat restrictive pediatric scar contractures. Pediatrics. 2014;134:e1700–5.
91. Kwan JM, Wyatt M, Uebelhoer NS, Pyo J, Shumaker PR. Functional improvement after ablative fractional laser treatment of a scar contracture. PM R. 2011;3:986–7.
92. van Drooge AM, Vrijman C, van der Veen W, Wolkerstorfer A. A randomized controlled pilot study on ablative fractional CO2 laser for consecutive patients presenting with various scar types. Dermatol Surg. 2015;41:371–7.
93. Anderson RR, Donelan MB, Hivnor C, Greeson E, Ross EV, Shumaker PR, et al. Laser treatment of traumatic scars with an emphasis on ablative fractional laser resurfacing: consensus report. JAMA Dermatol. 2014;150:187–93.
94. Poetschke J, Dornseifer U, Clementoni MT, Reinholz M, Schwaiger H, Steckmeier S, et al. Ultrapulsed fractional ablative carbon dioxide laser treatment of hypertrophic burn scars: evaluation of an inpatient controlled, standardized treatment approach. Lasers Med Sci. 2017;32:1031–40.
95. Har-Shai Y, Amar M, Sabo E. Intralesional cryotherapy for enhancing the involution of hypertrophic scars and keloids. Plast Reconstr Surg. 2003;111:1841–52.
96. Har-Shai Y, Brown W, Labbe D, Dompmartin A, Goldine I, Gil T, et al. Intralesional cryosurgery for the treatment of hypertrophic scars and keloids following aesthetic surgery: the results of a prospective observational study. Int J Low Extrem Wounds. 2008;7:169–75.
97. Har-Shai Y, Sabo E, Rohde E, Hyams M, Assaf C, Zouboulis CC. Intralesional cryosurgery enhances the involution of recalcitrant auricular keloids: a new clinical approach supported by experimental studies. Wound Repair Regen. 2006;14:18–27.
98. Mourad B, Elfar N, Elsheikh S. Spray versus intralesional cryotherapy for keloids. J Dermatolog Treat. 2016;27:264–9.

99. van Leeuwen MC, Bulstra AE, Ket JC, Ritt MJ, van Leeuwen PA, Niessen FB. Intralesional cryotherapy for the treatment of keloid scars: evaluating effectiveness. Plast Reconstr Surg Glob Open. 2015;3:e437.
100. Muir IF. On the nature of keloid and hypertrophic scars. Br J Plast Surg. 1990;43:61–9.
101. Leventhal D, Furr M, Reiter D. Treatment of keloids and hypertrophic scars: a meta-analysis and review of the literature. Arch Facial Plast Surg. 2006;8:362–8.
102. Zuber TJ, DeWitt DE. Earlobe keloids. Am Fam Physician. 1994;49:1835–41.
103. Ragoowansi R, Cornes PG, Moss AL, Glees JP. Treatment of keloids by surgical excision and immediate postoperative single-fraction radiotherapy. Plast Reconstr Surg. 2003;111:1853–9.
104. Guix B, Henriquez I, Andres A, Finestres F, Tello JI, Martinez A. Treatment of keloids by high-dose-rate brachytherapy: a seven-year study. Int J Radiat Oncol Biol Phys. 2001;50:167–72.
105. Sallstrom KO, Larson O, Heden P, Eriksson G, Glas JE, Ringborg U. Treatment of keloids with surgical excision and postoperative X-ray radiation. Scand J Plast Reconstr Surg Hand Surg. 1989;23:211–5.
106. van de Kar AL, Kreulen M, van Zuijlen PP, Oldenburger F. The results of surgical excision and adjuvant irradiation for therapy-resistant keloids: a prospective clinical outcome study. Plast Reconstr Surg. 2007;119:2248–54.
107. Mankowski P, Kanevsky J, Tomlinson J, Dyachenko A, Luc M. Optimizing radiotherapy for keloids: a meta-analysis systematic review comparing recurrence rates between different radiation modalities. Ann Plast Surg. 2017;78:403–11.
108. Ogawa R, Mitsuhashi K, Hyakusoku H, Miyashita T. Postoperative electron-beam irradiation therapy for keloids and hypertrophic scars: retrospective study of 147 cases followed for more than 18 months. Plast Reconstr Surg. 2003;111:547–53; discussion 554–5
109. Espana A, Solano T, Quintanilla E. Bleomycin in the treatment of keloids and hypertrophic scars by multiple needle punctures. Dermatol Surg. 2001;27:23–7.
110. Naeini FF, Najafian J, Ahmadpour K. Bleomycin tattooing as a promising therapeutic modality in large keloids and hypertrophic scars. Dermatol Surg. 2006;32:1023–9; discussion 1029–30
111. Saray Y, Gulec AT. Treatment of keloids and hypertrophic scars with dermojet injections of bleomycin: a preliminary study. Int J Dermatol. 2005;44:777–84.
112. Camacho-Martinez FM, Rey ER, Serrano FC, Wagner A. Results of a combination of bleomycin and triamcinolone acetonide in the treatment of keloids and hypertrophic scars. An Bras Dermatol. 2013;88:387–94.
113. Jimenez SA, Freundlich B, Rosenbloom J. Selective inhibition of human diploid fibroblast collagen synthesis by interferons. J Clin Invest. 1984;74:1112–6.
114. Berman B, Duncan MR. Short-term keloid treatment in vivo with human interferon alfa-2b results in a selective and persistent normalization of keloidal fibroblast collagen, glycosaminoglycan, and collagenase production in vitro. J Am Acad Dermatol. 1989;21:694–702.
115. Tredget EE, Shankowsky HA, Pannu R, Nedelec B, Iwashina T, Ghahary A, et al. Transforming growth factor-beta in thermally injured patients with hypertrophic scars: effects of interferon alpha-2b. Plast Reconstr Surg. 1998;102:1317–28; discussion 1329–30
116. Young VL, Bush J, O'Kane S. A new approach for the prophylactic improvement of surgical scarring: avotermin (TGF beta 3). Clin Plast Surg. 2009;36:307–13, viii
117. Occleston NL, O'Kane S, Laverty HG, Cooper M, Fairlamb D, Mason T, et al. Discovery and development of avotermin (recombinant human transforming growth factor beta 3): a new class of prophylactic therapeutic for the improvement of scarring. Wound Repair Regen. 2011;19(Suppl 1):s38–48.
118. Ferguson MW, Duncan J, Bond J, Bush J, Durani P, So K, et al. Prophylactic administration of avotermin for improvement of skin scarring: three double-blind, placebo-controlled, phase I/II studies. Lancet. 2009;373:1264–74.
119. Samadikuchaksaraei A, Mehdipour A, Habibi Roudkenar M, Verdi J, Joghataei MT, As'adi K, et al. A dermal equivalent engineered with TGF-beta3 expressing bone marrow stromal cells and amniotic membrane: cosmetic healing of full-thickness skin wounds in rats. Artif Organs. 2016;40:E266–79.
120. Fang F, Huang RL, Zheng Y, Liu M, Huo R. Bone marrow derived mesenchymal stem cells inhibit the proliferative and profibrotic phenotype of hypertrophic scar fibroblasts and keloid fibroblasts through paracrine signaling. J Dermatol Sci. 2016;83:95–105.
121. Wu Y, Peng Y, Gao D, Feng C, Yuan X, Li H, et al. Mesenchymal stem cells suppress fibroblast proliferation and reduce skin fibrosis through a TGF-beta3-dependent activation. Int J Low Extrem Wounds. 2015;14:50–62.
122. Poetschke J, Schwaiger H, Gauglitz GG. Current and emerging options for documenting scars and evaluating therapeutic progress. Dermatol Surg. 2017;43(Suppl 1):S25–36.

Part V

Non-thermal Burns

Electrical Burn Injuries

39

Jessica Shih and Marc G. Jeschke

39.1 Epidemiology and Classification

Electrical injuries are relatively uncommon compared to thermal burn injuries; however, the short-term and long-term sequelae can be devastating. Unlike thermal injury, the morbidity and mortality of electrical injury can be disproportionately high relative to the amount of total body surface area affected [1–3], typically described as a "tip of the iceberg" phenomenon. Electrical injuries account for 4% of burn admission in the United States [4], approximately 0.04–5% of admissions to burn units in developed countries overall, and up to 27% in developing countries [5, 6]. The two most common populations susceptible to electrical injuries are adult male workers and young children. Electrical injury is the fourth leading cause of work-related traumatic death, with 75% of adult electrical injuries occurring in the workplace and the vast majority (94%) being male [7, 8]. Children are also susceptible to electrical injury at home with access to electrical outlets.

J. Shih
Faculty of Medicine, University of Toronto, Toronto, ON, Canada

Division of Plastic and Reconstructive Surgery, Department of Surgery, Faculty of Medicine, University of Toronto, Toronto, ON, Canada

M. G. Jeschke (✉)
Division of Plastic and Reconstructive Surgery, Department of Surgery, Faculty of Medicine, University of Toronto, Toronto, ON, Canada

Faculty of Medicine, Institute of Medical Science, University of Toronto, Toronto, ON, Canada

Biological Sciences, Sunnybrook Research Institute, Toronto, ON, Canada

Ross Tilley Burn Centre, Sunnybrook Health Sciences Centre, Sunnybrook Hospital, Toronto, ON, Canada

Department of Immunology, Faculty of Medicine, University of Toronto, Toronto, ON, Canada
e-mail: Marc.Jeschke@sunnybrook.ca

Classification of electrical injuries are typically divided into low-voltage (<1000 V) and high-voltage (>1000 V). Additional classifications include:power source (lighting vs. electrical), flow of electrical current—whether injury is caused by direct current flowing through the body (arc injury) or by indirect thermal heat (electrical flash injury), and current type—alternating current (AC) versus direct current (DC). Determining the type of electrical injury sustained will guide management and expectations of outcomes.

39.2 Pathophysiology

Electricity is a form of energy produced by the flow of electrons through a conductor. The type and extent of electrical injury is determined by voltage, current strength and type, duration of contact, pathway of current, and resistance of tissues. Ohm's Law, Current (I) = Voltage (V)/Resistance (R) describes the relationship between current being directly proportional to voltage, and inversely proportional to resistance. Higher voltage and amperage cause increased damage. The type of current and duration of contact are related to each other, as AC, the most common form of current in households that changes direction at a standardized frequency of 60 Hz, induces tetanic muscle contractions that prolong duration of contact with the source, often termed "no-let go" phenomenon. In contrast, a high-voltage DC current most often found in industrial settings will produce a single large muscle contraction that will throw the victim away from the source, decreasing duration of contact, but increasing the likelihood of traumatic and fall-related injuries. Organs and types of tissues most affected are determined by pathway of current and resistance of tissues. Often mistakenly termed "entry" and "exit" points, the presence of "contact points" may guide pathway of current, but this is not a reliable way to determine which internal organs and tissues may have been affected. Clinical correlation is the best guide

M. G. Jeschke et al. (eds.), *Handbook of Burns Volume 1*, https://doi.org/10.1007/978-3-030-18940-2_39

to determine whether tissues have been damaged. The resistance of tissues is related to the amount of electrical energy transformed into thermal energy. Therefore, more thermal damage will occur with high resistance tissues such as bone, tendon, and fat compared to tissues that are good conductors with low resistance such as nerve, blood vessels, and muscle. Skin has intermediate resistance. The severity of injury and resistance is also inversely proportional to cross-sectional area, which is also clinically evident with severe extent of injury associated with the wrists and ankles.

39.3 Initial Assessment and Acute Care

Initial assessment on the field requires ensuring the safety and protection of the field team and initial responders by disconnection from the electrical power source. Initial evaluation of the patient should always begin with ABLS protocols as well as ATLS protocols as there is higher likelihood of traumatic injury related to high-voltage electrical injury compared to isolated thermal burns. Once the patient has been stabilized and information has been gathered on the circumstances surrounding the injury (mechanism, type of injury, patient information), the patient should be transferred to the nearest specialized burn care center.

There are unique issues to be considered with resuscitation of the electrically injured patient. As mentioned, there is higher likelihood of traumatic brain, intra-abdominal, and extremity injuries with high-voltage injuries where the patient has been thrown away from the electrical source, especially from height. Estimating total body surface area (TBSA) is also especially difficult given deep unquantifiable damage. Therefore, fluid resuscitation should be based on adequate urine output per hour, with a goal of double the standard urine output of 50–100 cc/h. There is also the risk of myoglobinuria with electrical injury, and the goal of resuscitation of an individual with pigmented urine is to resuscitate until the urine is clear in an attempt to prevent acute tubular necrosis. Given the potential high requirement of fluids for resuscitation, at the same time, be wary of over-resuscitation and its related complications. More considerations of the electrically injured patient include determining who requires cardiac monitoring and for how long, as well as who requires emergency operative intervention, including the need for fasciotomy or emergent amputation.

39.4 Systems-Based Management of Electrical Injury

Given the unknown extent and depth of damage electrical injuries cause based on initial examination, it is especially important to be aware of potential systems involved with electrical injury and to involve multi-disciplinary care specialists for both short-term and long-term physical, mental, and rehabilitative sequelae.

39.4.1 Short-Term Outcomes

39.4.1.1 Skin and Soft Tissue

As with the management of thermal burns, appropriate management with dressings and serial debridement is indicated by depth and size of burn area. Electrical burns may have smaller average TBSA (14%) relative to extent of underlying injury; however, those with flash burns can have over 50% TBSA [7]. There was a statistically significant difference in the need for surgical intervention with high-voltage injuries (80%) compared to low-voltage injuries (54%) [7]. The basic principles of burn wound management apply to skin and soft tissue affected, with the goals of preventing infection, debriding non-viable tissue at regular intervals and eventual reconstruction at the appropriate time.

39.4.1.2 Musculoskeletal

Electrical injury can cause severe damage to muscles, especially in the distal extremities where cross-sectional area is smaller and resistance higher. Muscle compartment monitoring especially in the first 48 h is crucial, with the main method of monitoring being regular physical examination. Abnormal physical findings include pain of out proportion, pain on passive stretch, paresthesias, tenseness of compartment, and pulselessness. In addition to these physical findings, CK levels may be elevated and compartment pressure measurements will be higher than 30 mmHg for a diagnosis of compartment syndrome. Given high clinical suspicion of compartment syndrome, surgical exploration with fasciotomy is indicated to prevent further myonecrosis. According to Practice Guidelines for the Management of Electrical Injuries ([3] JBCR), indications for upper extremity surgical decompression include: progressive neurologic dysfunction, vascular compromise, increased compartment pressure, and systemic clinical deterioration from suspected ongoing myonecrosis. This includes forearm fasciotomy and assessment of muscle compartments, with carpal tunnel release determined on a case-by-case basis.

Decompression sites for upper extremity include: mobile wad, volar and dorsal compartments in the forearm, and carpal tunnel, Guyon's canal ± interosseous, thumb adductor, hypothenar and thenar compartments in the hand. Decompression sites of lower extremity include its four compartments: anterior, lateral, superficial posterior, and deep posterior compartments, most commonly performed with two longitudinal incisions. A second look is recommended 48–72 h post-initial decompression. Serial debridement may be needed prior to final closure or reconstruction, with moist dressings in the interim that can include VAC dressings.

There is no definitive data that immediate surgical decompression decreases amputation rate ([3] JBCR). Both fasciotomy and amputation rates are significantly higher in high-voltage injuries compared to low-voltage injuries (27% vs. 5% for fasciotomy and 30% vs. 7% amputation rate including digits and/or extremities, respectively) [7].

Rhabdomyolysis and muscle necrosis can also occur with electrical injury either through direct muscle injury or as a result of compartment syndrome. Leakage of intracellular contents such as myoglobin, creatine kinase, and lactate dehydrogenase occurs during rhabdomyolysis, which when entering the systemic circulation can be indicators as well as causes serious damage to organ systems such as the kidneys [9].

39.4.1.3 Renal

Electrical injury resulting in muscle destruction or rhabdomyolysis can lead to myoglobinuria and potential renal failure. Myoglobulin entering the systemic circulation can cause renal tubular destruction and renal failure as myoglobin precipitates in renal tubules. Clinical signs of high levels of myoglobin in urine are evident when myoglobin levels reach 100 mg/dL where urine appears darker, described as myoglobinuria [9]. Patients with high-voltage electrical injury are much more likely to sustain these injuries, with up to 40% of patients with myoglobinuria and 14% of patients developing renal failure [7]. In addition to high-voltage electrical injury, other high-risk factors for developing myoglobinuria include prehospital cardiac arrest, full-thickness burns, and compartment syndrome [10].

Identification of patients at risk and subsequent prevention of renal tubular destruction and potential renal failure is key by providing aggressive fluid replacement and diuresis until adequate urine output is achieved and urine color clears. This can be performed with calculated fluid resuscitation with avoidance of under- or over-resuscitation, use of loop diuretics, alkalinization of urine, and normalization of serum electrolytes [9].

39.4.1.4 Cardiac

Electrical injuries can result in an array of cardiac arrhythmias, ischemia, and possible cardiac arrest. An ECG should be performed as soon as possible to rule out an immediate dysrhythmia. If initial ECG is normal, guidelines can help determine the extent of cardiac monitoring needed. Cardiac arrhythmias occur in both low-voltage and high-voltage injuries, although high-voltage injuries have higher rates of ECG changes as high as 20% which may necessitate more extensive cardiac monitoring [3, 7]. The most common ECG changes include non-specific ST-T changes, atrial fibrillation, and ventricular fibrillation [3, 7]. In addition to cardiac monitoring through ECG or telemetry, further cardiac laboratory tests such as creatine kinase (CK) enzyme levels, including CK-MB fraction, are not reliable indicators of cardiac injury following electrical injury [3]. Troponin levels can be useful if suspicion of new onset cardiac ischemia.

Practical guidelines by Arnoldo et al. [3] suggest admission and cardiac monitoring in the form of telemetry for any patients with: history of loss of consciousness or documented dysrhythmia prior to or following presentation to hospital, and cardiac monitoring for patients with ECG evidence of ischemia. Not enough evidence is found in the literature to suggest duration of cardiac monitoring, although it appears that 24–48 h with no ECG changes is sufficient. With low-voltage injuries, both children and adults with no ECG abnormalities, no history of loss of consciousness, and no other indication for admission can be discharged from the emergency room without further cardiac monitoring [3].

39.4.1.5 Neuropathy

Peripheral neuropathies and spinal cord injuries can occur with electrical injury [11], therefore neuromuscular examination should be performed carefully at admission, and at regular intervals.

39.4.1.6 Trauma

Patients with high-voltage electrical injury can be thrown away from the electrical source. In the workplace, they may be at significant height relative to ground level, therefore traumatic-related injuries are not uncommon with high-voltage electrical injury. This includes injuries such as loss of consciousness, traumatic brain injury, cerebral dysfunction, traumatic intra-abdominal injury and associated fractures [7]. It is therefore important to be aware of these potential injuries related to trauma, and investigate and manage them appropriately with inclusion of neurosurgery, general surgery, and orthopedic colleagues as necessary.

39.4.2 Long-Term Outcomes

Electrical injuries are not only ridden with high immediate morbidity, but significant long-term morbidity, both physical and psychological. A small number of electrical injury patients develop cataracts and other ophthalmic injuries [12–20] with an incidence ranging between 0.03 and 20% [7, 21].

Of studies that track permanent disability as an outcome, a review of the literature has identified that almost 35% of electrical injury patients suffer from permanent disability [7], which has a profound outcome on return to work and psychological sense of well-being.

Neuropsychiatric sequelae are also prevalent following electric injury, with reports of post-traumatic stress disorder (PTSD), major depressive disorder, anxiety disorders, memory loss, neuropathic pain, insomnia, irritability, pruritus, and nerve compression syndromes [22, 23]. Although the incidence of PTSD following electrical injury has been estimated as high as 40–50% [23], and as low as 5.6% [7], it is clear that practitioners should be aware of long-term neuropsychiatric sequelae such as PTSD to identify those who suffer from such sequelae and offer appropriate treatment with neurorehabilitation. This involves a multi-disciplinary approach with psychological, neuropsychological, and psychiatric assessments, taking into account the patient's personal and work situation in the rehabilitation process [23].

39.4.3 Mortality

Mortality rates of high-voltage electrical injury worldwide are higher on-average than low-voltage electrical injury (5.2% vs. 2.6%, respectively) of patients that present to specialized burn care centers [7]. However, coroner's reports reveal higher mortality rates of patients with low-voltage electrical injury compared to high-voltage electrical injury, with a ratio of 2.4:1 [7]. This suggests that there may be a significant amount of immediate deaths associated with low-voltage injuries that do not make it to burn care centers.

The main causes of death reported in high-voltage electrical injuries that accounted for over 90% of mortality include TBSA >50%, and multi-organ failure and septicemia. The remainder of causes of mortality include pneumonia, ARDS, renal failure/acute tubular necrosis, ventricular fibrillation, myocardial infarction/cardiopulmonary arrest and hepatic failure [7].

39.5 Other Considerations

39.5.1 Lightning

Lightning strike is the second-leading cause of weather-related death, with worldwide mortality estimated to be 0.2–1.7 deaths/million people [24]. The United States National Weather Service reports a 11% average mortality rate, with an annual average of 279 lightning strike injuries, and 31 deaths between 2006 and 2015 [25]. Mortality is usually immediate, but can be delayed as a result of cardiopulmonary arrest following failed attempted resuscitation [24]. Morbidity from lightning strike includes cardiac manifestations, muscle injury, CNS abnormalities such as traumatic and hypoxic brain injury, loss of consciousness, confusion, amnesia, headaches, spinal cord injuries, paresthesias, and weakness, as well as otologic and ophthalmic findings. More specific to lightning strike includes Lichtenberg figures, an arborizing skin lesion consisting of extravasation of blood into the subcutaneous tissues, and keraunoparalysis—a self-limiting transient paralysis and loss of sensation as a result of massive catecholamine release [24].

Treatment of patients who have sustained lightning strike injuries should involve ATLS, ACLS, and ABLS principles, with emphasis on full spine immobilization. Subsequent care should revolve around basic principles of burn and electrical injury management.

39.5.2 Pediatric Electrical Injury

Electrical injuries occurring in pediatric patients occur more often at home, and often from low-voltage current through electrical outlets. Younger children can also sustain oral commissure burns. Less severe forms of oral commissure burns may heal with secondary intention; however, both functional and aesthetic concerns should be addressed. Primary or secondary reconstruction may be required to prevent or treat microstomia. Additional management of pediatric electrical injury should revolve around basic principles of burn and electrical injury management at a designated burn care center if possible.

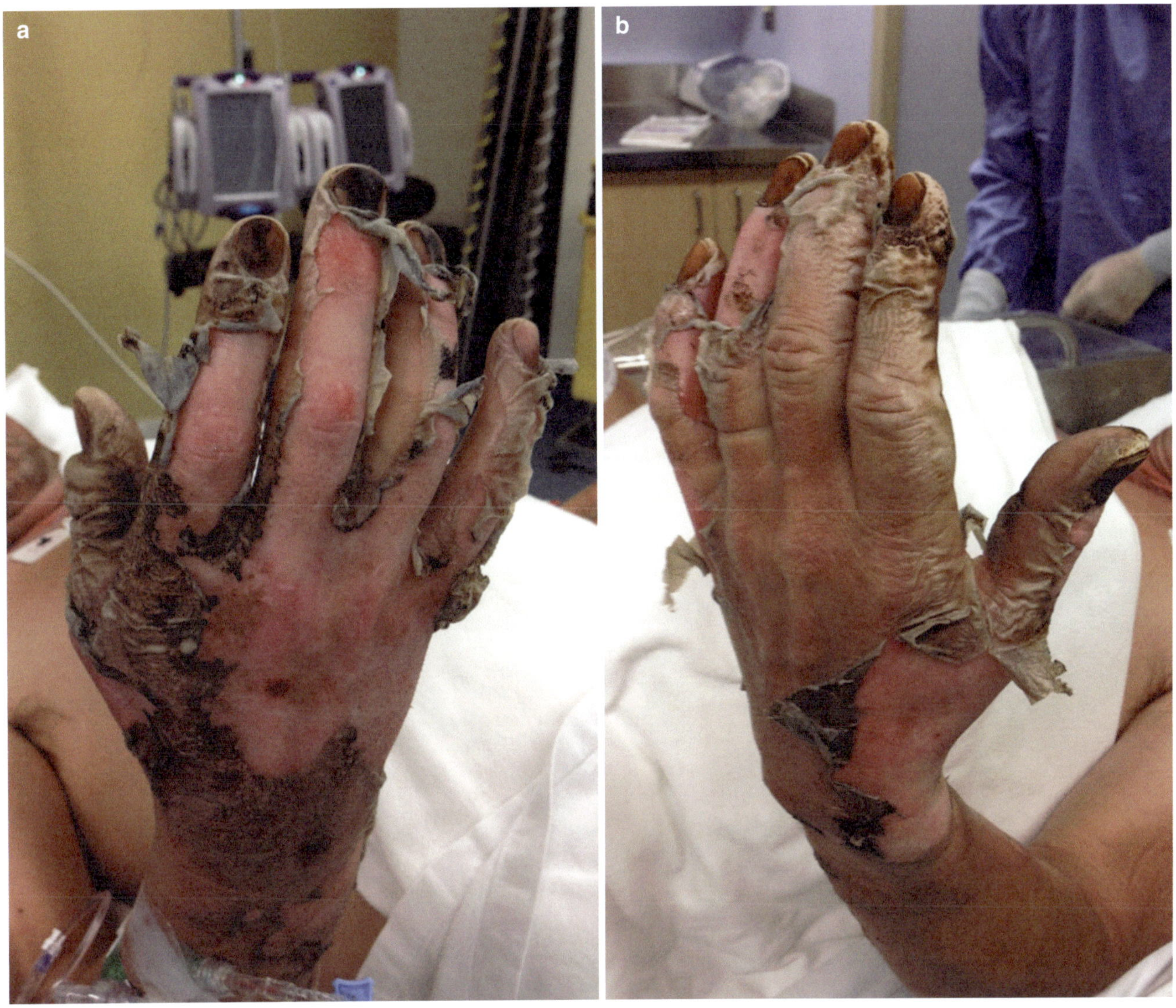

Fig. 39.1 Electrical-arch burn to bilateral hands. (**a**) Right hand; full-thickness component and skin degloving. (**b**) Full = thickness and degloving component of the left hand

Summary Box

- Electrical injuries are relatively uncommon compared to thermal injuries; however, they can have devastating short-term and long-term morbidity as well as significant mortality.
- Electrical injuries are typically classified by voltage (low-voltage <1000 V vs. high-voltage >1000 V), type of electrical current flow (direct arc injury vs. indirect electrical flash injury), and type of current (AC vs. DC).
- Initial assessment and acute care always begin with ABLS and ATLS protocol. Assess for any associated traumatic injuries.
- Electrical injuries require assessment, constant re-evaluation, and management of multi-system issues including skin and soft tissue, musculoskeletal, renal, cardiac, and nervous system.
- Electrical injuries can have a profound effect on psychological well-being and result in difficulties in returning to work. Electrical injury patients should be followed on a long-term basis for long-term ocular and neuropsychiatric sequelae such as post-traumatic stress disorder, depression, and anxiety.

Conflicts of Interest and Source of Funding This study was supported by National Institutes of Health R01-GM087285-01. CFI Leader's Opportunity Fund: Project #25407 and Canadian Institutes of Health Research (CIHR) grant #123336. Authors have no conflicts of interest to declare.

References

1. Vierhapper MF, Lumenta DB, Beck H, Keck M, Kamolz LP, Frey M. Electrical injury: a long-term analysis with review of regional differences. Ann Plast Surg. 2011;66(1):43–6.
2. Saracoglu A, Kuzucuoglu T, Yakupoglu S, et al. Prognostic factors in electrical burns: a review of 101 patients. Burns. 2014;40(4):702–7.
3. Arnoldo BA, Klein M, Gibran NS. Practice guidelines for the management of electrical injuries. J Burn Care Res. 2006;27(4):439–47.
4. American Burn Association. Burn incidence and treatment in the United States: 2016 fact sheet. [Online]. www.ameriburn.org/resources_factsheet.php. Accessed 4 Apr 2017.
5. Hunt JL, Sato RM, Baxter CR. Acute electric burns. Arch Surg. 1980;115:434–8.
6. Aggarwal S, Maitz P, Kennedy P. Electrical flash burns due to switchboard explosions in New South Wales—a 9-year experience. Burns. 2011;37(6):1038–43.
7. Shih JG, Shahrokhi S, Jeschke MG. Review of adult electrical burn injury outcomes worldwide: an analysis of low-voltage vs high-voltage electrical injury. J Burn Care Res. 2017;38(1):e293–8.
8. Koumbourlis AC. Electrical injuries. Crit Care Med. 2002;30(11 Suppl):S424–30.
9. Coban YK. Rhabdomyolysis, compartment syndrome and thermal injury. World J Crit Care Med. 2014;3(1):1–7.
10. Rosen CL, Adler JN, Rabban JT, Sethi RK, Arkoff L, Blair JA, Sheridan R. Early predictors of myoglobinuria and acute renal failure following electrical injury. J Emerg Med. 1999;17(5):783–9.
11. Lammertse DP. Neurorehabilitation of spinal cord injuries following lightning strike and electrical trauma. NeuroRehabilitation. 2005;20:9–14.
12. Arnoldo BA, Purdue GP, Kowalske K, et al. Electrical injuries: a 20-year review. J Burn Care Rehabil. 2004;25:479–84.
13. Norman ME, Albertson D, Younge B. Ophthalmic manifestations of lightning strike. Surv Ophthalmol. 2001;46(1):19–24.
14. Piotrowski A, Fillet AM, Perez P, et al. Outcome of occupational electrical injuries among French electric company workers: a retrospective report of 311 cases, 1996-2005. Burns. 2014;40(3):480–8.
15. Bae EJ, Hong IH, Park SP, Kim HK, Lee KW, Han JR. Overview of ocular complications in patients with electrical burns: an analysis of 102 cases across a 7-year period. Burns. 2013;39(7):1380–5.
16. Dega S, Gnaneswar SG, Rao PR, Ramani P, Krishna DM. Electrical burn injuries. Some unusual clinical situations and management. Burns. 2007;33(5):653–65.
17. Ferrerio I, Melendez J, Regalado J, Bejar FJ, Gabilondo FJ. Factors influencing the sequelae of high tension electrical injuries. Burns. 1998;24:649–53.
18. Cancio LC, Jimenez-Reyna JF, Barillo DJ, Walker SC, McManus AT, Vaughan GM. One hundred ninety-five cases of high-voltage electric injury. J Burn Care Res. 2005;26(4):331–40.
19. Butler E, Gant TD. Electrical injuries, with special reference to the upper extremities. Am J Surg. 1977;134:95–101.
20. DiVincenti FC, Moncrief JA, Pruitt BA. Electrical injuries: a review of 65 cases. J Trauma. 1969;9:497.
21. Sanford A, Gamelli RL. Chapter 65: lightning and thermal injuries. Handb Clin Neurol. 2014;120:981–6.
22. Chudasama S, Goverman J, Donaldson JH, van Aalst J, Cairns BA, Hultman CS. Does voltage predict return to work and neuropsychiatric sequelae following electrical burn injury? Ann Plast Surg. 2010;64(5):522–5.
23. Primeau M. Neurorehabilitation of behavioral disorders following lightning strike and electrical trauma. NeuroRehabilitation. 2005;20:25–33.
24. Ritenour AE, Morton MJ, McManus JG, et al. Lightning injury: a review. Burns. 2008;34:585–94.
25. National Weather Service, USA.gov. Lightning victims/medical: odds of being struck. [Online]. http://www.lightningsafety.noaa.gov/victims.shtml. Accessed 16 May 2017.

40 Chemical Burn: Diagnosis and Treatments

Ali Izadpanah

40.1 Chemical Burns

Chemical burns are caused by corrosive agents (acids or alkali) to the mucosa or skin. These injuries could be self-inflicted or occur secondary to work, school, and household accidents. There are over 65,000 chemicals available at any time on the market with 60,000 new chemicals being introduced annually and an approximate of 25,000 marketed chemicals capable of severe tissue damages. Thus, chemical burns could be quite common and lead to morbid injuries. In some studies, up to 10% of burn injuries could be caused by chemical materials.

Chemical burns mainly occur in men of working age, workers in industry and laboratories, and in the building industry.

The use of chemical materials as warfare has led to an advancement in the understanding and management of these injuries. These injuries have been reported up to the recent war between Iraq and Iran.

The Total Body Surface Area (TBSA) involved is usually lower than thermal injures with the face, trunk, and the extremities being mainly involved. Chemical burns are especially important when they involve the eyes. In addition, there may be associated severe digestive disorders when the substance is swallowed or inhaled.

40.2 Mechanism of Injury

Six main mechanisms have been suggested as the main inflicting causes of chemical injuries:

1. Reductive—the chemical will donate electrons, causing intermolecular bonds to become weak.
2. Oxidative—the chemical will gain electrons when in contact with the tissue and therefore denaturing the proteins and disrupt their covalent bonds. Their by-products are usually toxic and could continue to react.
3. Corrosive—these chemicals directly denature the proteins (alkalis).
4. Protoplasmic poisons—these chemicals bind to organic ions and inhibit their action (i.e., hydrofluoric acid).
5. Vesicants—these agents produce anoxic necrosis. These agents were popular agents in chemical warfare.
6. Desiccants—these agents produce exothermic reaction and hence leading to heating up the tissue and eventually cause dehydration (i.e., sulfuric acid).

It is also important to have in mind that some of the chemicals such as hydrofluoric acid could have systemic consequences which one should always consider when treating these patients.

40.3 Management

Like all injuries, the patient should be first assessed and cleared for any associated trauma according to the ATLS (Advanced Trauma Life Support) guidelines.

Upon the initial evaluation, it is imperative to find out the type of chemical causing the burn. There are certain chemicals that a through washout is contraindicated (i.e., sulfuric acid, phenol, hydrochloric acid, and dry lime).

Following specific steps pertaining to the ATLS should be considered when treating patients with chemical injuries:

1. ***Airway and C-spine***
   The airway might need special consideration in the case of ingestion of chemical material. Noxious fumes could cause delayed upper and lower airway swelling leading to life-threatening consequences. Upon the initial evaluation by laryngoscopy or bronchoscopy, the airway might not show much evidence of swelling; however, delayed

A. Izadpanah (✉)
Division of Plastic and Reconstructive Surgery, Department of Surgery, Regional Burn Unit, University of Montreal Health Centre, Montreal, QC, Canada

M. G. Jeschke et al. (eds.), *Handbook of Burns Volume 1*, https://doi.org/10.1007/978-3-030-18940-2_40

edema should be always suspected if pertinent history demonstrates such possibility [1, 2].

2. ***Breathing***
Inhalation of chemicals could lead to lung injuries and even systemic effects which might complicate the overall picture [3].
3. ***Circulation***
Deep burns could lead to circumferential injuries and subsequently requiring escharotomies. Majority of chemical burns lead to deep injuries however with low TBSA involvements (less than 10% TBSA). Fluid resuscitations should be done according to the TBSA involved [4].
4. ***Disability***
The ingestion of chemical materials could lead to altered Glasgow Coma Scores (GCS), mental status, or even seizure.
5. ***Exposure***
Systematic exposure of patient should be done. As with thermal counterparts, serial exposure of patient's body could lead to decreased potential of heat loss. Associated injuries are commonly seen with chemical injuries. Fractures are the most frequent associated injuries followed by inhalation injuries [1].
6. ***Decontamination***
Decontamination of an affected individual is one of the main steps in management of these injuries. As expected, the longer the exposure of the chemical remains, the greater the damage would be. Therefore, the caustic material should be removed as early as possible. Decontamination can be performed either specific or nonspecific. "Specific decontamination" involves the use of neutralizing agents, such as converting an acid into a salt, hydrolyzing toxic agents, or applying antidotes. On the other hand, "non-specific decontamination" uses mechanical debridement or extensive rinsing to dilute the offending agent.

40.4 Specific Organ System Approach

40.4.1 Respiratory Tract

Volatile gases can lead to direct injury to the upper and lower respiratory tracts. Symptoms such as coughing, burning sensation, dryness, and even chest pain could occur as the presenting symptoms. This could even lead to surfactant destruction, bronchoconstriction, and even pulmonary hypertension. These symptoms could occur in two phases, the immediate transient simulation followed by a delayed pulmonary edema occurring up to 72 h post exposure.

40.4.2 Ophthalmic

Chemical ocular injuries represent 7% of work-related eye injuries in the USA [5]. More than 60% of these injuries occur at work place, 30% at home, and 10% due to assaults [6]. Importantly, as many as 20% of chemical injuries could lead to significant visual deficits. The exposure of chemicals could lead to substantial damages necessitating urgent ophthalmological emergency. Many of chemical injuries could lead to irritation; however, strong alkali or acidic solutions could lead to serious ophthalmic damages with potential for long-term sequelae. Alkali burns usually can lead to a more severe ocular injury compared to the acidic solutions. The extent of damage is determined by the type of solution, the concentration and pH, the duration of exposure, and eventually to the degree of penetration. Acidic solutions damage the cornea through the release of protons while basic solutions are lipophilic and can penetrate the cell membrane.

Ocular injuries could be graded according to Thoft, Hughes, Roper-Hall, and Pfister. These injuries could be graded from 0 to 5 [7].

- Grade 0—Minimal epithelial defect, clear corneal stroma, no limbal ischemia
- Grade 1—Partial-complete epithelial defect, clear corneal stroma, no limbal ischemia, corneal epithelial involvement only
- Grade 2—Partial-complete epithelial defect, mild stromal haze, none or only mild limbal ischemia
- Grade 3—Complete epithelial defect, moderate stromal haze, less than one-third of the limbus is ischemic
- Grade 4—Complete epithelial defect, stromal haze blurring iris details, one-third to two-thirds of the limbus is ischemic
- Grade 5—Complete epithelial defect, stromal opacification, greater than two-thirds of the limbus is ischemic

Grades of 0–2 could heal with proper care and examinations. Grades 3–5 n the other hand may require further surgical care such as limbal stem cell transplantation. These cases have much poorer prognosis.

40.4.3 Gastrointestinal Tract

Ingestion of chemicals could lead to nausea, enteritis symptoms, burning sensation, and even hematemesis. Children compromise 80% of these injuries as expected by incidental ingestion [8]. Constrictions and even perforations could occur and lead to major complications after ingestion of these chemicals. As expected, the type of chemical, the durations of contact, and the concentration are the main players of the extent of injury. If the material has been ingested, inducing vomiting is contraindicated as it would re-expose the mucosa to the caustic agents. Administration of either charcoal or neutralizing agent is not recommended. Dilution with copious water ingestion is recommended.

While a 30% sodium hydroxide can cause full thickness injury, the acidic solution could lead to more systemic manifestations such as renal failure, liver dysfunction, disseminated intravascular coagulation, and hemolysis [9].

Esophageal injuries occur within minutes of the injury and they might persist for hours. Delayed vascular thrombosis and necrosis up to 7 days after these injuries is more important than the inflammation in the pathogenesis of these injuries [10]. Granulation tissue in these full-thickness injures could form between 4 and 7 days which could be covered by fibrin. If ulceration exceeds the muscular plane, perforation could occur. Since the tensile strength of these injuries is low, any endoscopic evaluation should be avoided between 5 and 15 days of injury [11]. In addition, after these injures, the lower esophageal sphincter becomes affected leading to gastroesophageal reflux (GER); therefore, motility agents are recommended to decrease structure formations [12]. Moreover, all caustic esophageal burn patients should be screened for GER periodically and it should be controlled aggressively.

Placement of stents and dilatation in the presence of strictures is recommended. Biodegradable stents (poly-*L*-lactide or polydioxanone) are under investigation for benign strictures [13]. Other modalities such as 5-fluorouracil (5-FU), antioxidant vitamins (vitamin E), H1 blockers, and mast cell stabilizers which could inhibit collagen production and eventual stricture formation have been shown to be useful in animal studies; however, up to this date, no human trials have been performed [14].

Dilatation and even surgical interventions could be necessary in the cases of substantial strictures. In cases of severe chemically induced injuries, use of nasogastric tubes (NGTs), especially in pediatric population, could be supported. However, long-standing use of NGTs could lead to structure formation by itself. However, gastrostomy is another safe option through which a safer retrograde dilatation of the structures could also be performed [15–17].

40.4.4 Hematological

The hematological manifestations of important chemical injuries including methemoglobinemia, hemolysis, and methemoglobinuria develop secondary to the formation of nitrous gas (NO). The clinical manifestations depending on the concentration could be gray-blue skin coloration, headache, fatigue, dizziness, tachycardia, bradycardia, respiratory depression, unconsciousness, or coma. It is recommended to administer vitamin C to accelerate the reduction of methemoglobinemia. Treatments such as positive end expiratory pressure (PEEP) and an exchange transfusion should be considered in life-threatening situations.

40.4.5 Nephrological

Acute renal failure due to acid-base imbalances could lead to tubular necrosis; therefore, extensive diuresis and addition of mannitol for osmotic diuresis is recommended.

40.5 Etiopathology

40.5.1 Inorganic Acids

Acids are considered proton donors that cause various injuries. They release hydrogen ions and cause the reduction of the physiologic pH from 7 down to as low as 0. Acids with pH less than 2 can cause coagulation necrosis upon contact with skin [18, 19]. A better method in assessing the effect of the involved acid is the amount of alkali that would be needed to raise the pH of an acid to neutral [20].

1. ***Hydrofluoric Acid***

   Hydrofluoric Acid (HF) is an agent commonly used in pottery, glass, or semiconductor industries. On the other hand, concentrations between 20% and 50% result in burns becoming apparent only hours after the exposure; when the concentration is less than 20%, the burn could only appear 24 hours or more after the exposure.

   Upon formation of the scab after the contact, the tissue damage continues until neutralized where it can be verified by the loss of pain. The systemic effect of this continuous damage could lead to hypocalcaemia and hypophosphatemia. These changes can cause cardiac arrhythmias which can even end in ventricular fibrillation resulting in shock and death. The calcium in the tissue is sequestered due to the fluoride ion forming an insoluble salt with calcium. In addition to the hypocalcaemia, the damage to the myocardium is caused by the interaction of adenylyl cyclase and adenosine phosphate.

   Inhalation of the HF gas can cause severe pneumonitis and the oral intake would lead to necrosis. The ocular injuries cause ulcers, corneal loss, loss of vision, and retractions. If calcium gluconate is not available, one should consider extreme water dilution to remove the substance completely [21].
2. ***Sulfuric Acid***

Injuries due to sulfuric acid and also nitric acids are usually caused by work, industrial, or laboratories accidents, although at times these injuries could be secondary to household accidents, criminal assaults, or even warfare acts. When sulfuric acid comes into contact with skin, there is protein coagulation and vascular thrombosis; a dark bronze scab can be formed that can be deepened until the substance is neutralized. Alkaline neutralization should not be considered as it can cause exothermic reaction and lead to further tissue damage due to heat. One should be aware that the absorption of the sulfuric acid can cause hemoglobinuria and ultimately could lead to acute tubular necrosis and acute kidney damage. Acute tubular necrosis is treated by aggressive fluid resuscitation in addition to the bicarbonate of soda according to the patient's weight. Forced hydration and even mannitol are beneficial to avoid renal damage [22].

3. ***Phosphorus***

Burns caused by phosphorus occur secondary to reacting with the oxygen and its derivatives. It is a frequent agent in wars and acts of terrorism. The injury continues as long as the agent is in contact with skin; therefore, it is imperative to remove the offending agent from skin using metal forceps. Use of Woods lamp could be beneficial in identifying the particles. The antidote for treatment of phosphorus contact is lavage with 1–2% copper sulfate. Excess copper sulfate must be removed, because absorption may cause hepatic and renal damage [19]. The systemic effect of phosphorus absorption could cause serious alterations in the concentration of body's phosphorus and calcium, leading to arrhythmias together with hemolysis, hematuria, and hemoglobinuria. This can cause kidney failure and even death. Therefore, alterations in EKG after exposure to phosphorus is important and the best course of action is to wash off the body with copious amount of soapy water immediately after the accident [2, 23, 24].

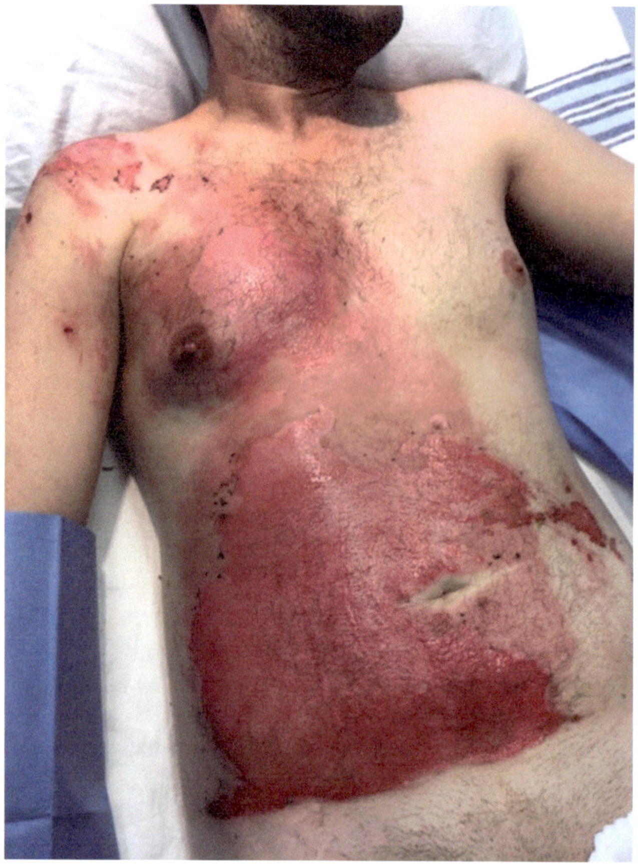

Fig. 40.2 Phosphorus burn

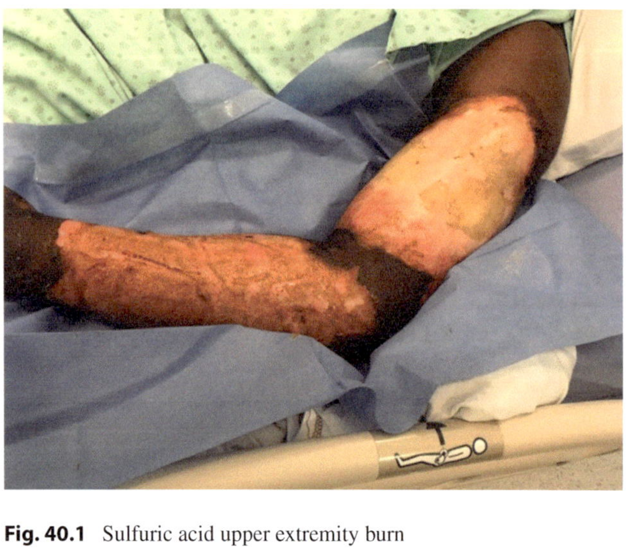

Fig. 40.1 Sulfuric acid upper extremity burn

40.5.2 Alkaline Agents

Alkalines are proton acceptors. They will strip the cells of their hydrogen ions mainly affecting the amine, and carboxylic groups. Alkalis with pH greater than 11.5 can produce severe tissue necrosis by means of liquefaction; this will loosen the tissue planes and allow deeper penetration of the agent. In other words, this mechanism will lead to much deeper burn injuries.

1. ***Cements***

Burns secondary to building cements usually do not have much pain. This is compared to hydroxides. The exact mechanism of burns secondary to cements is not clear. These compounds usually contain multiple metals such as chrome. Thus, a combination of high alkaline pH, contact, and allergic dermatitis could be in play [25].

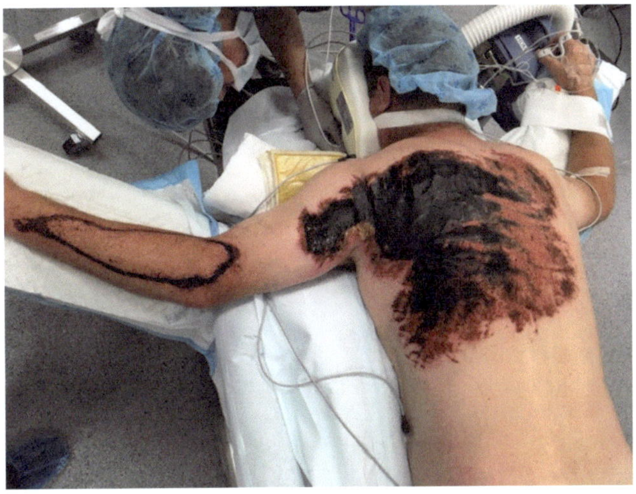

Fig. 40.3 Sodium hydroxide burn

2. ***Hydroxides***
   These chemicals have great penetrating and destructive potential. They usually cause extensive soft tissue damage until the chemical is inactivated and the pH is neutralized. Use of weak acid solutions such as 1% acetic acid has been proposed in some studies as neutralizing method of treating these injuries. One should always be considered of the exothermic reaction that these could cause. Copious irrigation with water until pH normalizes is also recommended. One exception to this is calcium hydroxide. This chemical has a very high hygroscopicity and causes a very exothermic reaction with water that could cause even a more severe injury [26].

3. ***Organic solutions***
   These materials act as dissolving agents for the lipid membrane of cells and causing the disruption of the cellular protein structure.

   Injuries due to these chemicals (petrol, kerosene, cresol, phenol, etc.) are as a result of direct contact with skin. Gasoline in a prolonged direct contact with skin can lead to full-thickness burns [27]. Its systemic effect could lead to paralysis, coma, hepatic damage, or motor-sensory neuropathies. Pulmonary lesions are the result of the chemical changing the production of surfactant. These organic materials could easily pass to the blood stream and cause cardiac or renal dysfunctions and even in severe cases, multiorgan failures. Kerosene is a lipid solvent and copious irrigation with soap is recommended to remove the offending material. Phenol and cresol on the other hand cause coagulation necrosis [28]. Following the exposure, dark thick scabs could form with minimal edema. The systemic effect could vary from hematuria and renal damage, digestive hemorrhages, increased liver transaminase with hepatic injuries, anemia, dyspnea, and hypotension.

4. ***Inorganic solutions***
   These chemicals damage the skin by direct binding and formation of salts. Many of these reactions are exothermic leading to thermal injuries.

40.6 Prevention

From a preventive point of view, proper legislations, and work-related regulations and trainings are mandatory to decrease these injuries. Compliance with safety regulations such as proper outfit, suitable clothing, boots, gloves, and protective goggles should be mandated. A product sheet should be available and correct labelling should be placed. Prevention is essential and in order to limit the damage, water points and showers should be placed next to the hazardous areas. Immediate washing and communication with the medical professionals upon transfer of the patient for proper treatment is recommended.

Summary Box

- Chemical burns are caused by corrosive materials to the skin or mucosa
- There are six mechanisms of injury after chemical burns: reductive, oxidative, corrosive, protoplasmic poisons, vesicants, and desiccants
- Upon these injuries, patients should be treated through the ATLS guidelines with specific attention and modifications according to the type of chemical
- Specific organ systems involved need to be treated differently
- Ocular injuries are medical emergencies and should be treated emergently according to the injury grading
- Inducing vomit or charcoal/neutralizing agents are not recommended for treatment of ingestion of chemical
- Acids lead to more frequent renal issues than alkaline
- Knowledge for treatment of specific chemical types in both acidic and alkaline burns are necessary
- Prevention is the main step in reducing the incidence of these injuries

References

1. Pruitt BA Jr. The burn patient: I. Initial care. Curr Probl Surg. 1979;16(4):1–55.
2. Kaufman T, Ullmann Y, Har-Shai Y. Phosphorus burns: a practical approach to local treatment. J Burn Care Rehabil. 1988;9(5):474–5.
3. Larson DL, Abston S. Acutely burned patient. Initial care and closure of burn wound. N Y State J Med. 1970;70(12):1626–33.
4. Sykes RA, Mani MM, Hiebert JM. Chemical burns: retrospective review. J Burn Care Rehabil. 1986;7(4):343–7.
5. Xiang H, et al. Work-related eye injuries treated in hospital emergency departments in the US. Am J Ind Med. 2005;48(1):57–62.
6. Morgan SJ. Chemical burns of the eye: causes and management. Br J Ophthalmol. 1987;71(11):854–7.
7. Dua HS, King AJ, Joseph A. A new classification of ocular surface burns. Br J Ophthalmol. 2001;85(11):1379–83.
8. Gumaste VV, Dave PB. Ingestion of corrosive substances by adults. Am J Gastroenterol. 1992;87(1):1–5.
9. Poley JW, et al. Ingestion of acid and alkaline agents: outcome and prognostic value of early upper endoscopy. Gastrointest Endosc. 2004;60(3):372–7.
10. Osman M, et al. Responses of the murine esophageal microcirculation to acute exposure to alkali, acid, or hypochlorite. J Pediatr Surg. 2008;43(9):1672–8.
11. Zargar SA, et al. The role of fiberoptic endoscopy in the management of corrosive ingestion and modified endoscopic classification of burns. Gastrointest Endosc. 1991;37(2):165–9.
12. Mutaf O, et al. Gastroesophageal reflux: a determinant in the outcome of caustic esophageal burns. J Pediatr Surg. 1996;31(11):1494–5.
13. ASGE Technology Committee, et al. Drug-eluting/biodegradable stents. Gastrointest Endosc. 2011;74(5):954–8.
14. Gunel E, et al. Effect of antioxidant therapy on collagen synthesis in corrosive esophageal burns. Pediatr Surg Int. 2002;18(1):24–7.
15. McGrath K, Brazer S. Combined antegrade and retrograde dilation: a new endoscopic technique in the management of complex esophageal obstruction. Gastrointest Endosc. 2002;56(1):163–4.
16. Bueno R, et al. Combined antegrade and retrograde dilation: a new endoscopic technique in the management of complex esophageal obstruction. Gastrointest Endosc. 2001;54(3):368–72.
17. Mukherjee K, et al. Antegrade and retrograde endoscopy for treatment of esophageal stricture. Am Surg. 2008;74(8):686–7; discussion 688
18. Jelenko C 3rd, Story J, Ellison RG Jr. Ingestion of mineral acid. Am Surg. 1974;40(2):97–104.
19. Jelenko C 3rd. Chemicals that "burn". J Trauma. 1974;14(1):65–72.
20. Palao R, et al. Chemical burns: pathophysiology and treatment. Burns. 2010;36(3):295–304.
21. Sheridan RL, et al. Emergency management of major hydrofluoric acid exposures. Burns. 1995;21(1):62–4.
22. Husain MT, Hasanain J, Kumar P. Sulphuric acid burns: report of a mass domestic accident. Burns. 1989;15(6):389–91.
23. Eldad A, et al. Phosphorous pentachloride chemical burn—a slowly healing injury. Burns. 1992;18(4):340–1.
24. Eldad A, Simon GA. The phosphorous burn—a preliminary comparative experimental study of various forms of treatment. Burns. 1991;17(3):198–200.
25. Solem LD. Emergent management of chemical burns. West J Med. 1987;147(3):308.
26. Benmeir P, et al. Chemical burn due to contact with soda lime on the playground: a potential hazard for football players. Burns. 1993;19(4):358–9.
27. Papini RP. 'Is all that's blistered burned?' … a case of kerosene contact burns. Burns. 1991;17(5):415–6.
28. Lin CH, Yang JY. Chemical burn with cresol intoxication and multiple organ failure. Burns. 1992;18(2):162–6.

Necrotizing Soft Tissue Infections

41

Helene Retrouvey and Shahriar Shahrokhi

Soft tissue infections have been classified as local or spreading, and as necrotizing or non-necrotizing by Smith and Lewis [1–3]. The Infectious Diseases Society of America (IDSA) and the U.S. Food and Drug Administration have further categorized soft tissue infections into: (1) uncomplicated infections and complicated infections; (2) acute and chronic infections; and (3) necrotizing and non-necrotizing infections [4, 5].

Necrotizing soft tissue infections (NSTIs) constitute a spectrum of diseases characterized by a necrotic infectious process primarily involving the fascia and the subcutaneous tissue with relative sparing of skin and underlying muscle [6, 7]. Necrotizing soft tissue infections (NSTIs) are the most severe among the spectrum of skin and soft tissue infections. In fact, the fulminant, widespread and rapidly progressive necrosis which occurs in NSTI is often associated with systemic toxicity and is usually fatal unless promptly recognized and aggressively treated [6–12]. The mortality rate of this life-threatening infection is often quoted at 30% [10].

41.1 History

Multiple terms have been used to refer to NSTI over the years, including hemolytic streptococcal gangrene, progressive synergistic bacterial gangrene, necrotizing erysipelas, suppurative fasciitis, acute dermal gangrene, hospital gangrene, necrotizing fasciitis, "flesh-eating disease," and Fournier's gangrene [6, 12–14].

H. Retrouvey
Division of Plastic and Reconstructive Surgery, University of Toronto, Toronto, ON, Canada

Department of Surgery, University of Toronto, Toronto, ON, Canada
e-mail: helene.retrouvey@mail.utoronto.ca

S. Shahrokhi (✉)
Ross Tilley Burn Centre, Sunnybrook Health Sciences Centre, Toronto, ON, Canada

Department of Surgery, University of Toronto, Toronto, ON, Canada
e-mail: shar.shahrokhi@sunnybrook.ca

Necrotizing infections were first described by Hippocrates in the fifth century BC [15]. These were then described as a complication of streptococcal infection known as "erysipelas" [6, 16]. Through the eighteenth and nineteenth century, European physicians described cases of NSTI, referring to them as phagedema gangrenosa, necrotizing or gangrenous erysipelas, nonclostridial gas gangrene, synergistic necrotizing cellulitis, hemolytic streptococcal gangrene, malignant ulcer, gangrenous ulcer, putrid ulcer, phagedena, phagedenic ulcer, phagedena gangraenosa, hospital gangrene, and bacterial synergistic gangrene [6, 10, 16]. By mid-nineteenth century, the preferred terms were hospital gangrene and phagedena [6]. The first American report of NSTI was in 1871 by Joseph Jones, a Confederate Army surgeon, whom described a case of hospital gangrene [6, 10, 17]. In 1883, a French venereologist Jean Alfred Fournier described five cases of necrotizing infection of the perineum and scrotum, giving rise to the term Fournier's gangrene [16, 18]. In 1952, the term necrotizing fasciitis was coined by Wilson; this term was created to encompass the most consistent feature of the infection, fascial necrosis [6, 7, 19, 20]. Recently, the term NSTI has been put forward to encompass all necrotizing infections [16].

41.2 Incidence

The true incidence of NSTIs is unknown, although it is thought to be uncommon with approximately 500–1500 cases per year in the United States or 0.04 cases per 1000 person-years. [6, 10, 13, 16, 20, 21]. In the United Kingdom, approximately 500 cases per year of NSTI are reported [12]. In Canada, approximately 90–200 cases of NSTI per year are reported [14].

41.3 Predisposing Factors

All age groups and genders can be affected by NSTIs, although higher rates of NSTI are observed in older patients (>60 years old) [6, 10, 16, 20, 22]. Malnutrition, comorbidities,

M. G. Jeschke et al. (eds.), *Handbook of Burns Volume 1*, https://doi.org/10.1007/978-3-030-18940-2_41

and intravenous drug use are also patient level risk factors for the development of NSTIs [16, 22–24]. Comorbidities associated with increased risk of NSTI include diabetes mellitus, peripheral vascular disease, obesity, alcoholism, liver disease, renal failure, immunosuppression, or malignancy [7, 12, 22, 23, 25]. Wong et al. reported that the majority of patients with NSTI presented with at least one comorbidity (86.5%), diabetes mellitus (70.8%) and peripheral vascular disease (22.5%) being the most common [7]. Tunovic et al. found that the most common predisposing factors were diabetes (33.8%), hypertension (33.1%), smoking (24.6%), obesity (13.1%), and substance abuse (23.1%) [14].

The microbes responsible for this infection can be introduced into the subcutaneous tissues: (1) via a break in the skin, (2) via hematogenous spread, or (3) via an unknown cause [1, 6, 10, 13, 16, 23, 25, 26]. First, introduction of the pathogen can occur through any mechanism that disrupts the skin, such as a cut, abrasion, burn, laceration, trauma, contusion, bite, injection, decubital ulcers, perirectal abscess, or surgical incision [6, 10, 23]. Wong et al. report that the portal of entry of infection was identified in 49.4% of patients, with causes including ulcers and bed sores (25.8%), trauma (13.5%), and postoperative infection (4.5%) [7]. Second, reports have described hematogenous spread of *Streptococcus pyogenes* from upper respiratory tract infections, presumed to be streptococcal pharyngitis, as the cause of NSTIs [6, 27, 28]. Lastly, the inciting event leading to NSTIs can be unknown [10]. Depending on the study, up to 31% of patients have no identifiable cause [6, 29].

41.4 Classification

Several classifications have been proposed for NSTIs, but none is universally accepted [4, 30]. NSTIs can be classified based on a specific characteristic, such as anatomical location, depth of invasion, and microbial source of infection [4, 6, 13, 16]. The anatomical location of the infection can be used to describe or label the infection, with Fournier's gangrene used to refer to NSTI of the perineum and/or scrotum [6, 13]. The abdominal wall, perineum, and extremities are the most common sites of infection [6, 10, 31]. In a cohort of 89 patients, Wong et al. found that the extremities were the most commonly involved site (79.8%) with majority being the lower extremity (69.7%), with the trunk as the second most common (20.2%). NSTI can also be classified based on the depth of the infection; the soft tissue layers include the epidermis; the dermis; the superficial fascia; the subcutaneous fat, nerves, arteries, or veins; the deep fascia; and the muscle. Terms such as cellulitis, adipositis, faciitis, and myositis are used to describe the exact depth of infection [16]. Necrotizing fasciitis primarily involves the superficial fascia, the subcutaneous fat, and the deep fascia, with sparing of the skin (epidermis and dermis) and the muscle [6, 10, 13]. Lastly, NSTIs can be classified based on the organism causing the infection: Type I—polymicrobial, Type II—monomicrobial (*Staphylococcus, Streptococcus), and Type III—Vibrio vulnificus* (Table 41.1) [13]. Of note, the classification of marine *Vibrios* as type III is not universally accepted [13].

The classification of NSTIs based on bacteriologic classes was first introduced by Giuliano in 1977 [10, 16, 32]. At the time, Giuliano et al. described two types: Type 1—anaerobic bacteria and facultative anaerobic bacteria and Type 2—Group A streptococcus alone or in combination with Staphylococcus aureus [32]. Later, Type III was introduced. This three type classification system is the most useful clinically as it describes populations at risk, potential microbiological organisms involved and relates to most effective treatment modalities [16]. But regardless of the type, in the acute period, NSTIs should be managed similarly with rapid diagnosis, supportive care, broad-spectrum antibiotics, and surgical debridement [6].

Table 41.1 Classification of NSTIs based on microbial source of infection

	Incidence	Microbiology	Anatomical location	Risk factors/population at risk
Type I	55–90%	– Polymicrobial (usually four to five different organisms per culture with at least one anaerobe) – Caused by enteric pathogens – Gram-positive cocci, Gram-negative rods, anaerobes	Perineum, abdomen, and trunk	Immunocompromised patients, older, diabetics, peripheral vascular disease, obesity, HIV, alcohol abuse, abscess, IV drug use, blunt or penetrating trauma, insect bites, surgical incisions, indwelling catheters, chicken pox, vesicles, and perforation of the gastrointestinal tract Postoperative wound
Type II	15–30%	– Monomicrobial – Due to skin flora – Group A β-hemolytic streptococcus alone or in combination with staphylococcus – May be associated with toxic shock syndrome or myonecrosis	Extremities Head/neck	Healthy, young, immunocompetent patients History of recent trauma or operation to the area
Type III		– Gram-negative rods – Marine vibrios	Extremities	Exposure to warm sea water with a break in the skin Ingestion of colonized foods by patients with moderate to severe liver disease

References for the table: [6, 10, 13, 16, 22, 23, 26, 30, 33]

Table 41.2 Microbiology of NSTIs

	Possible organisms
Gram-positive aerobic bacteria	*Group A, β-hemolytic streptococcus* *Group B streptococcus* *Enterococci* *Coagulase-negative staphylococci* *Staphylococcus aureus* *Bacillus* sp
Gram-negative aerobic bacteria	*Escherichia coli* *Pseudomonas aeruginosa* *Enterobacter cloacae* *Klebsiella* sp *Proteus* sp *Serratia* sp *Acinetobacter calcoaceticus* *Citrobacter freundii* *Pasteurella multocida*
Anaerobic bacteria	*Bacteroides* sp *Clostridium* sp *Peptostreptococcus* sp
Fungi	*Candida* sp *Aspergillus* sp *Rhizopus*
Marine Vibrio	*Vibrio vulnificus* *Vibrio parahemolyticus* *Vibrio damsela* *Vibrio alginolyticus*

References for the table: [6, 8]

41.5 Diagnosis

No investigation is diagnostic, but careful physical examination, abnormal laboratory values, and suspicious imaging can increase the suspicion for NSTI [12].

41.5.1 History and Physical Examination

High index of suspicion in the diagnosis of NSTIs is needed as the initial examination of the patient usually generates only nonspecific signs and symptoms [6, 7, 12, 34]. Wall et al. found that 61% of patients had no specific signs and symptoms on initial examination [34]. Conditions that may be confused with NSTI include cellulitis, adiposities, myonecrosis, non-infectious fasciitis, lymphedema, abscess, phlegmasia cerulea dolens, and myxedema [7, 10, 13]. Furthermore, the paucity of cutaneous findings on presentation can lead to a difficult diagnosis [6, 7]. If the diagnosis is in doubt, frequent and repeated examinations of the patient should be performed as patients with NSTI have a rapidly progressive infection that can lead to sudden deterioration with systemic toxicity [10, 13, 16, 30, 31].

The physical examination findings usually present within 7 days of the inciting event. Common signs and symptoms on presentation include erythematous, swollen, and warm skin, accompanied by pain and fever [6, 7, 13, 16, 23, 31]. Of all the findings on presentation, Wong et al. reported that the majority of patients presented with the triad of exquisite pain (97.8%), swelling (92.1%), and fever (79.8%) [7]. The lack of fever on presentation should not rule out NSTI as this finding is variable [31].

The most common finding upon initial evaluation is exquisite pain, specifically, pain out of proportion to what would be expected from the physical findings [1, 5–7, 10, 13, 29, 33, 34]. The pain not only exceeds what is expected, but it also extends beyond the margins of the infection [7, 16]. Swelling, warmth, and erythema of the infected area are also common findings on physical examination [6, 7, 10]. Swelling is diagnosed by observing smooth, tense and shiny skin in the area of concern [6, 10]. Erythema in NSTI differs from other pathological processes, as it is diffuse, lacks lymphangitis or lymphadenopathy as well as distinct borders [10].

Late signs and symptoms include crepitus, skin ecchymosis, skin necrosis, blistering and bullae formation, skin anesthesia, shock, and mental status change [13]. If bullae develop, they are initially filled with serous fluid, and with time become hemorrhagic [6, 13]. Several of these late findings are characteristic of NSTI and are considered "hard signs," specifically, presence of bullae, skin ecchymosis or necrosis, gas in the tissue (crepitus on examination or seen on imaging), cutaneous anesthesia, and hemodynamic instability [15, 16]. These signs are diagnostic of NSTI, but unfortunately, occur late in the course of the illness.

41.5.2 Laboratory Evaluation

Patients with NSTI have been found to have nonspecific abnormal laboratory values which include leukocytosis, acidosis, hyponatremia, hypocalcaemia, anemia and increased serum creatinine, C-reactive protein (CRP), blood urea nitrogen or glucose [5, 16, 23, 30].

Wall et al. found that white blood cell (WBC) count greater than 15.4 × 10^9/L and serum sodium concentration less than 135 μmol/L created a predictive model with a sensitivity of 90% and specificity of 76%, positive predictive value of 26%, and negative predictive value of 99% [34].

Wong et al. suggested a more comprehensive model, called the Laboratory Risk Indicator for Necrotizing Fasciitis (LRINEC) Score (Table 41.3), which incorporates WBC count, serum sodium, hemoglobin, serum creatinine, CRP and serum glucose, and stratifies the patients into risk categories (low, intermediate, or high) [13, 16, 36]. A score of 5 or less is categorized as low risk of NSTI (<50% probability), 6–7 points is intermediate (50–75% probability), and 8 and above is considered high risk (>75% probability). A LRINEC score above or equal to 6 points has high correlation

Table 41.3 Laboratory Risk Indicator for Necrotizing Fasciitis Score (LRINEC)

Laboratory marker	Scoring
C-reactive protein (CRP) (mg/L)	<150 = 0 points ≥150 = 4 points
WBC (cells per mm³)	<15 = 0 points 15–25 = 1 point >25 = 2 points
Hemoglobin (g/dL)	>13.5 = 0 points 11–13.5 = 1 point <11 = 2 points
Sodium (mmol/L)	≥135 = 0 points <135 = 2 points
Creatinine (μmol/L)	≤141 = 0 points >141 = 2 points
Glucose (mmol/L)	≤10 = 0 points >10 = 1 point

References for the table: [13, 15, 16, 36]

with NSTI, with a positive predictive value of 92% and a negative predictive value of 96% in the Singaporean population [36]. Sultan et al. found a sensitivity of 74% and specificity of 81% in the United Kingdom population using the same scoring technique [12].

These models and scoring systems have not been validated and should be used with caution as stated by the creators of these laboratory tools. The management of patients with suspicion for NSTI should therefore be driven by the broad clinical presentation of the patient, with the LRINEC or the Wall score used as one of the components in the decision-making [16, 36].

41.5.3 Imaging Evaluation

Plain radiography, computer tomography (CT) scan, magnetic resonance imaging (MRI), and ultrasonography are imaging modalities that can be and have been used in the diagnosis of NSTI. All modalities have low sensitivity and specificity to detect early NSTI and therefore have a limited role in the evaluation of suspected NSTI [16].

41.5.3.1 Plain Radiographs

Plain radiography can reveal subcutaneous gas or soft tissue swelling [13, 31]. Several studies have found that plain radiography was more sensitive than physical examination in detecting subcutaneous gas [6, 10, 37, 38]. As subcutaneous emphysema is rarely present in the early stages of the disease, and as prevalence at the time of presentation is variable (15–70%), pain radiography is a poor screening test for NSTI [10]. Furthermore, the absence of subcutaneous air does not rule out NSTI [13, 20]. Plain radiography should be used if needed as an imaging adjunct for patients with an unclear diagnosis.

41.5.3.2 Computer Tomography Scan

CT scan shows inflammatory changes through fascial edema or thickening, fluid collections such as abscess formation as well as subcutaneous gas [13, 39]. Wysoki et al. found that the majority of cases (80%) of NSTI that had CT scan imaging showed asymmetric fascial thickening with fat stranding [40]. CT scans have been compared to plain radiography and found to be more accurate in detecting soft tissue gas [6, 10]. Zacharias et al. report a sensitivity of 100%, specificity of 81%, positive predictive value of 76%, and negative predictive value of 100% using four criteria to diagnose NSTI, specifically (1) asymmetrical and diffuse areas of soft tissue inflammation and ischemia, (2) muscle necrosis, (3) gas across tissue planes, and (4) fluid collections [39]. CT scanning also allows for better delineation of the extent of spread of the infection, as compared to physical examination [6, 10]. CT scan imaging is therefore a rapid and reliable tool in the diagnosis of NSTI, and can be useful in surgical planning [39].

41.5.3.3 Magnetic Resonance Imaging

MRI can detect soft tissue or fascial thickening through hyperintense signal at the deep fascia level or within muscle [13]. Rahmouni et al. was able to differentiate NSTI from other pathological conditions by using MRI [41]. In fact, MRI has been found to have a high sensitivity (90–100%) and specificity (50–85%) in diagnosing NSTI [10, 13, 20]. Because the sensitivity exceeds specificity, MRI tends to overestimate the extent of deep fascial involvement [39, 42]. MRI interpretation should thus be combined with clinical findings in order to make an accurate diagnosis [39, 42]. As this imaging modality is costly, not readily available at all centers and may not be appropriate in critically ill patients, the use of MRI in NSTI diagnosis is limited [39].

41.5.3.4 Ultrasound

Lastly, ultrasonography can detect superficial fluid collections and aid in delineating the extent of disease [43]. Further, ultrasound can detect diffuse thickening of the subcutaneous tissue, fascial fluid collections, fascial irregularity, and subcutaneous air [20]. Ultrasonography has been suggested as a diagnostic aid for NSTI as it is a readily available, convenient and non-costly tool [43]. Yen et al. found a sensitivity of 88.2%, a specificity of 93.3%, a positive predictive value of 83.3%, negative predictive value of 95.4%, and an accuracy of 91.9% in NSTI of limbs [43]. For patients with perineal NSTI, Fournier's gangrene, ultrasonography can be useful to differentiate NSTI from other causes of acute scrotum [6, 44]. Other than these indications, ultrasound is generally not recommended for NSTI diagnosis due to its overall poor sensitivity and specificity, and the need for a skilled operator [13, 16, 20].

41.5.4 Operative Exploration

The gold standard for diagnosis of NSTI is operative exploration, with lack of resistance of the normally adherent fascia to blunt dissection, lack of bleeding of tissues, and foul-smelling "dishwater" discharge as ominous signs [6, 10, 13, 36].

Patients with high clinical suspicion of NSTI should undergo bedside surgical exploration with the "finger test" to confirm the diagnosis [13, 36]. A small (2 cm) incision through the patient's skin overlying the center of the disease process should be performed. Finger blunt dissection should be attempted; if the tissues lack resistance (the surgeon can easily slide their finger along the fascial planes) and/or foul-smelling "dishwater" discharge is found, NSTI diagnosis is confirmed [10, 13, 16].

Alternatively, a cutaneous biopsy of the tissue can be sent for urgent frozen section. This technique involves taking a tissue biopsy from the skin down to the deep fascia in the suspected area, and sending this specimen for prompt frozen section pathology [10, 45]. Studies have found that frozen-section soft tissue biopsy performed early can provide a definitive diagnosis at an early stage leading to improved patient outcomes [45]. However, as the biopsy specimens must be processed and interpreted immediately by an experienced dermato-pathologist. This technique is limited in its use for the diagnosis of NSTI [10].

41.6 Treatment

Early surgical debridement, broad-spectrum antibiotics, and supportive care are essential components of the treatment [1, 14]. Supportive care includes aggressive fluid resuscitation, analgesia, and early intensive care involvement [6, 46]. The most important determinant of mortality is early and adequate surgical debridement [6, 7, 13, 19, 31, 46–49]. Repeated surgical debridement, broad-spectrum antibiotics, supportive care, and adjuncts such as hyperbaric oxygen therapy also have major roles in survival [6, 10, 14, 31].

41.6.1 Medical Management

41.6.1.1 Antibiotic Therapy

Patients with suspected NSTI should be started on empiric broad-spectrum antibiotic therapy that covers both aerobic Gram-positive and Gram-negative organisms as well as anaerobes [6, 13, 20]. Coverage of methicillin-resistant Staphylococcus aureus (MRSA) should be considered [16]. Antibiotics are important in the management of NSTI, but do not replace the need for surgical debridement. The administration of antibiotics is to decrease systemic bacterial spread, and not for control of the local infection as they do not penetrate necrotic tissue [13].

Multiple different antibiotic regimens have been suggested with no consensus as to the optimal regimen [20]. Authors suggest a mix of specific antibiotics and subgroups of antibiotics to target the most likely pathogen causing NSTI, for example: (1) penicillin, carbapenem, and clindamycin [23]; (2) penicillin G, clindamycin, vancomycin, and gentamicin [16]; (3) ampicillin or penicillin, gentamicin and clindamycin [13]; and (4) a combination of a penicillin or cephalosporin, an aminoglycoside, and clindamycin or metronidazole [6]. Because of the emergence of penicillin-resistant staphylococci, some authors suggest an additional antibiotic such as vancomycin, linezolid, daptomycin, or quinupristin/dalfopristin for empiric coverage for MRSA [13, 23, 50]. Vancomycin remains the drug of choice in such a setting [10]. Clindamycin is recommended for group A streptococcus (GAS) infection because of its bacteriostatic abilities specifically, its ability to inhibit protein synthesis, to suppress production of GAS exotoxins and to enhance the phagocytosis of GAS by inhibiting M protein [10, 12, 13, 31]. Clindamycin can thus help control the inflammatory response [23]. Clinicians should tailor the antibiotic regimen to the suspected organisms, the likelihood of antibiotic resistance and of MRSA based on their geographic location and the patient's risk factors.

Antibiotics should be tailored to the causal organism once the wound cultures become available [25]. Duration of antibiotic treatment is variable, with no difference in mortality based on duration of antibiotic use [31]. The Infectious Disease Society of America (IDSA) recommends that antibiotics be continued until no signs of systemic toxicity are present, the patient is afebrile for 48 h, until no additional surgical debridement is needed and the patient's clinical condition is improving [13, 19]. The usual duration is 10–14 days [13].

41.6.1.2 Supportive Care

The treatment of NSTI requires multidisciplinary team efforts with coordination between the surgical and the intensive care team [13, 16, 51]. As soon as the diagnosis of NSTI is made, fluid resuscitation should be initiated to optimize the patient's physiological condition prior to surgery, without delaying the timing of the initial debridement [52]. Aggressive initial fluid resuscitation is aimed at restoring intravascular volume, maintaining adequate end-organ perfusion, and tissue oxygenation, and limiting the adverse effects of end-organ failure [52]. Aggressive fluid resuscitation and inotropic and/or vasoactive support are usually best achieved in an intensive care setting. Central venous access and arterial line may be needed to secure intravenous access and guide fluid resuscitation [52]. Endotracheal intubation and mechanical ventilation may also be necessary. Careful monitoring should be initiated to monitor for signs of coagulation derangements, cardiac and pulmonary dysfunction, and acute renal failure [51, 52].

Nutritional support should be initiated as soon it can be tolerated by the patient [52]. Early enteral nutritional support helps the catabolic response in NSTI patients [15]. Vitamins such as vitamins A, C, and D as well as minerals such as zinc should be supplemented for patients with large open wounds to optimize wound healing [15, 52].

41.6.2 Surgical Management

The cornerstone of treatment of NSTI is early and extensive debridement of all necrotic and devitalized tissue. [10, 13, 19]. The most important determinant of mortality for patients is early and adequate surgical debridement, hence the importance of this component in the management of NSTI [6, 7, 13, 19, 31, 46–49]. Specifically the time from admission to operation is predictive of mortality, with a shorter interval favoring survival [9, 19, 31]. Wong et al. found that a delay of more than 24 h from admission to surgery was significantly associated with increased mortality [7]. Furthermore, surgical delay or inadequate debridement increased fatal outcomes [31, 46].

Patients with suspected NSTI should therefore undergo wide resection of all necrotic tissue, identified as the tissue that can be easily elevated from the deep fascia with gentle finger dissection. Incision and drainage of the affected area is not sufficient for management of NSTI.

Patients should undergo initial debridement at the facility to which they first present and where the diagnosis is first suspected, in order to more rapidly achieve source control, provided an appropriately experienced surgeon is immediately available to perform the procedure [21]. Although immediate transfer to a center accustomed to managing severe soft tissue infections or injuries may seem appropriate, in a large observational study of 9958 patients, those debrided initially at the hospital to which they presented had a significantly reduced incidence of death compared to those transferred without debridement (15.5% vs. 8.7%) [21].

A circular pattern of debridement is advocated for the initial debridement, starting at the most severely involved region and progressively working outwards until healthy soft tissue is encountered [16]. No consideration for the subsequent reconstruction should be given, as doing so compromises a comprehensive surgical debridement. The debridement should extend beyond this into healthy tissue until normal bleeding is seen. The margin and depth of the wound should be thoroughly explored to ensure that there are no areas of extension of the infection.

Once the initial debridement has been performed, referral should ideally be initiated to a burn center for further debridement, subsequent soft tissue reconstruction, and rehabilitation. Burn centers are accustomed to managing patients with extensive wounds and are the optimal place to accommodate these patients [16, 35, 53–56].

Diverting colostomies may be needed for patients with abdominal and perineal wounds to reduce the risk of secondary wound contamination with enteric bacteria and optimize wound healing [6, 9, 10]. A less invasive but highly effective strategy for cases near the anal verge is to insert a rectal diversion device [57]. For maximal benefit, colostomy should be performed early in the surgical course.

In cases of NSTI of the extremity, amputation may be warranted to control the infection, particularly in patients at high risk of poor wound healing such as those with peripheral vascular disease, diabetes and above the age of 65 years [6, 9, 20]. Amputations are required in 11.7–26.3% of patients with NSTI [9, 20]. The timing of amputation depends on many patient factors. For some, primary amputation may be the more expeditious and potentially life-saving intervention reducing operative time and blood loss, compared with successive debridements [58–61].

Following the initial debridement, the surgical wound must be frequently reevaluated, usually every 24–48 h, and further debrided as needed to control the necrotizing process [6, 10, 31, 62]. An obligatory second-look surgery in the operating room should be scheduled and undertaken within 24 h after the initial debridement [20]. Physiologic deterioration within that time frame may necessitate earlier intervention. Procalcitonin level may also be monitored, with the postoperative procalcitonin ratio used as an indicator of successful surgical eradication of the infectious focus [63]. Subsequent debridements can be scheduled every 24–48 h. On average, between 2.3 and 5.6 debridements will be needed before definitive reconstruction can be initiated [16, 20, 56, 63, 64].

During the debridement process, appropriate wound dressings are needed to optimize the environment for wound healing. Despite surgical debridement, microbial pathogens remain present in the wound and contribute to delayed wound healing. To minimize the bacterial burden of the wound and mitigate their effects, antimicrobial dressings should be used. Available topical antimicrobials for reducing bioburden and surface contamination when treating NSTI include: dilute sodium hypochlorite 0.025% solution, polyhexamethylene biguanide/betadine (i.e., Prontosan), povidone iodine, acetic acid (0.5–2% concentration), mafenide acetate, and silver containing dressings. A favored silver dressings, Acticoat, is a nanocrystalline silver product that releases Ag^{1+} ions in a controlled manner.

Negative pressure wound therapy (NPWT), also called vacuum-assisted wound closure, is a dressing that can be used for ongoing antisepsis and wound bed preparation [16]. NPWT continuously or intermittently applies subatmospheric pressure to a filler substance (foam or gauze) placed on the surface of a wound.

NPWT maintains a moist, closed wound environment, manages excess exudate, and helps to prepare a wound bed for skin grafts or tissue flaps by stimulating granulation tissue [65–71].

Definitive wound closure can be initiated once necrosis has been controlled [19, 62]. Wound closure should be performed in conjunction with a plastic surgery team [52]. Split thickness skin grafts are often the modality used for wound closure [13, 52]. For patients with extensive loss of muscle or bone or with wounds in certain anatomic regions, full thickness skin grafts, free or rotational flaps may be needed [31].

41.6.3 Adjunct Therapy

41.6.3.1 Intravenous Immunoglobulin Therapy

Intravenous immunoglobulin (IVIg) therapy consists of a concentrated pooled product containing primarily immunoglobulin G isotypes derived from human donors [13, 72–74]. IVIg enhances the bactericidal activity of serum by facilitating bacterial opsonization, neutralizing super antigens and toxins [23]. IVIg also modulates leukocytes by exerting a generalized anti-inflammatory effect [23].

A recent meta-analysis demonstrated an overall reduction in mortality with the use of IVIg for patients with severe sepsis and septic shock in adults [73]. The use of IVIg in NSTI remains controversial [13, 23]. IVIg may be beneficial in the treatment of NSTI as it binds the exotoxins produced by staphylococcal and streptococcal bacterial infections, thereby limiting their systemic inflammatory response [13, 23].

Darenberg et al. attempted to evaluate the use of IVIg with a multicenter, randomized, double-blind, placebo-controlled trial, but unfortunately, the trial was prematurely terminated because of slow patient recruitment. From the 21 enrolled patients (10 IVIg and 11 placebo), a 3.6-fold non-statistically significant higher mortality rate was found in the placebo group [75]. Koch et al. reported a case that suggested that IVIg treatment of patients with necrotizing fasciitis may be beneficial in the context of critically ill patients with hemodynamic instability [23]. A cohort study of 21 patients by Kaul et al. revealed that IVIg increased the 30-day survival rates from 34% to 67% for patients suffering from streptococcal toxic shock syndrome [76]. Cawley et al. reported a case where IVIg had a beneficial effect in the management of a patient with streptococcal toxic shock syndrome associated with necrotizing fasciitis and multisystem organ failure [77].

With only small cohort studies and case reports, the use of IVIg in NSTI remains controversial [13, 23, 74–78]. The optimal dose and therapeutic window for its use are lacking. If used, IVIg should be restricted to critically ill patients with either staphylococcal or streptococcal NSTI [13]. Caution should be taken if used, as IVIg has potential serious risks, including anaphylaxis (in individuals with IgA deficiency) and renal failure [10].

41.6.3.2 Hyperbaric Oxygen Therapy

Hyperbaric oxygen (HBO) was first described in the early 1960s. HBO increases tissue oxygen tension thus enhancing local defense mechanisms [20]. HBO delivers 100% oxygen at two to three times atmospheric pressure resulting in arterial oxygen tension as high as 2000 mmHg and tissue oxygen tension of 300 mmHg. These values contrast with arterial oxygen tension of 300 mmHg and tissue oxygen tension of 75 mmHg with normobaric inhalation of 100% oxygen [13, 79]. HBO at the tissue level increases killing ability of leukocytes and killing of certain anaerobes, reduces tissue edema, stimulates fibroblast growth, preserves intracellular adenosine triphosphate and increases collagen formation [13, 46, 80]. Further, HBO may augment neutrophil microbicidal activity, impair the virulence of certain bacteria, promote angiogenesis and wound healing, increase red blood cell pliability, terminate lipid peroxidation and reduce local vasoconstriction [10]. Through these mechanisms, HBO is believed to provide some therapeutic benefit in NSTI patients [46, 80, 81].

Several authors noted benefits from HBO therapy, both from the perspective of improved mortality and morbidity. Riseman et al. evaluated the role of HBO in addition to surgery and antibiotics, and found that the addition of HBO significantly reduced mortality and number of debridements [82]. Elliott et al. found that non-survivors received fewer HBO treatments than survivors because of hemodynamic instability for transport [31]. Hollabaugh et al. found a mortality of 7% in the HBO group versus 42% in the non-HBO group for Fournier's gangrene [83]. Shupak et al. also found a reduced mortality rate among the HBO-treated patients (36%), as opposed to 25% in the non-treated group [84]. Escobar et al. found not only a reduced mortality (34% vs. 11.9%), but also reduced rate of amputations (50% vs. 0%) in the HBO-treated group [85]. Soh et al. found a significant lower mortality (4.5 vs. 9.4%, $p = 0.001$) in HBO-treated patients [86]. Shaw et al. found that patients who did not receive HBO therapy were less likely to survive their index hospitalization (odds ratio, 10.6; 95% CI 5.2–25.1) [87].

Other authors found no effect or a negative effect of HBO in the treatment of NSTI [84, 88, 89]. Brown et al. did not find a reduced mortality or a reduced number of debridements in the HBO group [90]. Mindrup et al. found a higher mortality in the HBO group, with 26.9% as compared to 12.5%. The authors highlight that the HBO group had higher morbidity, suggesting that the HBO treatment may have been given to patients who were more ill [91].

A systematic review of randomized clinical trials by Levett et al. in 2015 failed to locate relevant clinical evidence to support or refute the effectiveness of HBO in the management of necrotizing fasciitis [92]. Of note, no studies were included in the systematic review, indicating the lack of high level clinical evidence to guide the use of HBO.

Based on retrospective observational studies, most authors report mortality and morbidity benefits from HBO therapy in the context of NSTI, especially in patients with clostridial infections [1, 10, 13, 29, 31, 80, 93, 94]. At this time HBO therapy should not be considered as standard therapy, it can however provide benefit in a subgroup of patients with NSTI as an adjunct [6]. Its use should never delay early and definitive surgical debridement.

41.6.3.3 Activated Protein C

Activated protein C is believed to decrease inflammation, coagulation, and restore fibrinolysis in severe sepsis [25]. The Recombinant Human Activated Protein C Worldwide Evaluation in Severe Sepsis (PROWESS) trial found that recombinant human activated protein C significantly decreased mortality in patients with severe sepsis [25, 95]. In this trial, 24 of the 474 patients had surgeries classified as "skin," with unspecified number of cases of NSTI [95]. Due to the risk of serious bleeding with the use of activated protein C, the survival benefits of its use must always carefully be outweighed against this risk.

Two case reports have described benefits of activated protein C for patients with severe sepsis unresponsive to medical and surgical treatment [25, 95]. This evidence suggests a role for activated protein C for patients with severed sepsis and NSTI, but future evidence is needed to suggest incorporating this treatment modality as an adjunct for NSTI management.

41.6.3.4 Plasmapheresis

Plasmapheresis is a nonselective method by which plasma is separated from the blood and replaced with donor plasma and/or albumin [96]. Busund et al. observed significant reductions in APACHE II scores and a trend toward a reduced mortality rate (odds ratio 0.41, 95% confidence interval 0.15–1.19) for a cohort of patients with severe sepsis who received plasmapheresis. The authors suggested that plasmapheresis should be considered for fulminant Gram-negative septic shock [96]. Kyles et al. reported on a case of NSTI treated with both IVIg and plasmapheresis, and found that after both treatments, the patient required less vasopressor support and had decreased inflammation and normal coagulation and hemostasis [97]. The authors conclude that adjunctive plasmapheresis and IVIg may decrease mortality and improve outcomes when used for the treatment of severe sepsis related to NSTI [97]. Although these two case reports show promising effects of plasmapheresis, other investigators have not observed improvements in clinically relevant outcomes. The use of plasmapheresis is therefore not currently supported by evidence, as the effectiveness in reducing markers of inflammation and circulating cytokines has been inconsistent and promising effects have only been seen in a single case report.

41.7 Outcomes

Most patients (81.8%) experienced a complication during their hospitalization for NSTI [31]. Acute renal failure, respiratory distress syndrome, and multi-organ system dysfunction are among the most common [31]. Further, up to 30% of NSTI patients require amputations to control infection [9, 98, 99]. Independent predictors of limb loss included heart disease and shock (systolic blood pressure <90 mmHg) at hospital admission [98].

For patients whom survive their infection, up to 60% of patients have mild to severe functional limitations after discharge [62, 99, 100]. Causes of physical limitation included wound contraction before coverage procedures, peripheral nerve dysfunction, and deconditioning [62].

Involvement of an extremity, higher Acute Physiology and Chronic Health Evaluation score, longer intensive care unit days, and delay of therapy were associated with functional limitations [62, 101]. A number of therapies can be used to decrease functional limitations, including strength and flexibility training, splinting, scar management, occupational therapy, and training to perform activities of daily life.

Further, NSTI has an enormous impact on the lives of survivors, their family, and the patient's ability to interact with society [100]. The prolonged hospitalization and multiple procedures needed to treat NSTI, some of which may be disfiguring, are life-altering and place patients at risk of anxiety and depression [15, 102]. Further, patients experience relationship stresses, post-traumatic stress disorder (PTSD), and employment concerns after NSTI [16, 102].

Data has shown that survivors of NSTI not only have significant impairments in physical, emotional, and social functioning, but also have decreased health-related quality of life [16, 102].

Rehabilitation protocols should incorporate the physical, psychological, and social aspects into care of the patient. The aims of the rehabilitation team should therefore be to minimize the adverse effects caused by the injury, minimizing the development and effect of scarring, maximizing functional outcomes, and providing support to maximize psychological well-being and reintegration into society [16].

41.8 Mortality

Successful outcomes require early and aggressive debridement as well as a multidisciplinary critical care management strategy [33, 103]. Hospital mortality rates range from 6 to 76% in the literature for NSTI, although most studies quote mortality to be approximately 30% [14, 25, 31, 99]. Recent studies report even lower rates of mortality, at approximately 5–10% [20, 103]. Early deaths are related to septic shock, while late deaths are mostly secondary to multi-organ failure [20].

Poor prognostic factors included: extremes of age (<1 or >60 years), female gender, cardiac disease, renal disease, obesity, malnutrition, alcohol abuse, intravenous drug use, peripheral vascular disease, diabetes mellitus, greater number of comorbidities and chronic pulmonary disease [9, 10, 13, 20, 29, 31]. Elevated creatinine, higher base deficit, elevated blood lactate, increased days from admission to first debridement, increased body surface area, and higher number of organs failed on admission were also poor prognosticators [29, 31]. Clinical course which includes trunk or perineal involvement, delay in surgical debridement, positive blood cultures, and positive cultures for beta-streptococcus or anaerobic bacteria were associated with higher mortality [9, 29, 31]. Anaya et al. specifically found that white blood cell count greater than 30,000 × 10^3/μL, creatinine level greater than 2 mg/dL (176.8 μmol/L), and heart disease at hospital admission were independent predictors of mortality [98]. Delay in surgical debridement is the most significant factor, followed by advanced age [20].

Anaya et al. studied these prognostic factors and suggested the first clinical mortality score which includes: (1) patient age above 50 years, (2) heart rate >110 beats per minute, (3) body temperature less than 36 °C, (4) white blood cell count >40,000/μL, (5) serum creatinine >1.5 mg/dL, and (6) hematocrit >50% (Table 41.4) [104].

Patients with 0–2 points were grouped into the low risk category with 6% mortality, 3–5 points into the moderate risk category with 24% mortality, and greater or equal to 6 points into the high risk category with 88% mortality [15, 104]. The accuracy of this model is 86.8% [98, 104].

Faraklas et al. created another mortality risk calculator to address the limitations of the Anaya scoring system [105]. Elements included in the risk calculator were: age older than 60 years, partial or complete functional dependence, dialysis dependence, American Society of Anesthesiologists classification, need for emergent surgery, platelet count <150,000/mm^3, and presence of septic shock [105]. An online system calculates the risk of mortality, generating values between 1.8 and 85.5% depending on the presence of each of these factors [105].

Table 41.4 Score predictive of death in patients with NSTI

Factors on admission	Point
Heart rate >110 beats per minute	1
Body temperature less than 36 °C	1
Serum creatinine >1.5 mg/dL	1
White blood cell count >40,000/μL	3
Hematocrit >50%	3
Patient age above 50 years	3

References for the table [15, 104]

Summary Box

Prompt recognition and surgical treatment of NSTI are essential for survival [46, 49]. The cooperation of multiple specialists, including intensivists, general surgeons, plastic surgeons, and infectious disease specialists, and the involvement of a multidisciplinary team are crucial for optimal patient treatment and wound care [46].

The preferred management plan should include:

- Early surgical referral for patients with suspicious findings, particularly when pain is disproportionate to the physical findings.
- Prompt aggressive resuscitation with intravenous fluids, empiric broad-spectrum antibiotics, with intensive care involvement for monitoring.
- Diagnostic surgical exploration of the affected site for early diagnosis.
- Radical debridement of all the necrotic tissues if NSTI diagnosed on bedside surgical exploration.
- Frequent wound evaluation (every 24–48 h) to confirm the adequacy of debridement, and repeat debridements as needed.
- Reconstructive maneuvers and wound management once infection controlled.

References

1. Andreasen TJ, Green SD, Childers BJ. Massive infectious soft-tissue injury: diagnosis and management of necrotizing fasciitis and purpura fulminans. Plast Reconstr Surg. 2001;107(4):1025–35.
2. Lewis RT. Soft tissue infections. World J Surg. 1998;22(2):146–51.
3. Smith AJ, Daniels T, Bohnen JM. Soft tissue infections and the diabetic foot. Am J Surg. 1996;172(6A):7S–12S.
4. Esposito S, Bassetti M, Concia E, De Simone G, De Rosa FG, Grossi P, et al. Diagnosis and management of skin and soft-tissue infections (SSTI). A literature review and consensus statement: an update. J Chemother. 2017;29(4):197–214.
5. May AK, Stafford RE, Bulger EM, Heffernan D, Guillamondegui O, Bochicchio G, et al. Treatment of complicated skin and soft tissue infections. Surg Infect (Larchmt). 2009;10(5):467–99.
6. Green RJ, Dafoe DC, Raffin TA. Necrotizing fasciitis. Chest. 1996;110(1):219–29.
7. Wong CH, Chang HC, Pasupathy S, Khin LW, Tan JL, Low CO. Necrotizing fasciitis: clinical presentation, microbiology, and determinants of mortality. J Bone Joint Surg Am. 2003;85-A(8):1454–60.

8. Ciancio F, Parisi D, Portincasa A, Innocenti A. Erratum to: discussion: a new method of salvaging breast reconstruction after breast implant using negative-pressure wound therapy and instillation. Aesthetic Plast Surg. 2017;41(2):468.
9. McHenry CR, Piotrowski JJ, Petrinic D, Malangoni MA. Determinants of mortality for necrotizing soft-tissue infections. Ann Surg. 1995;221(5):558–63; discussion 63-5.
10. Young MH, Aronoff DM, Engleberg NC. Necrotizing fasciitis: pathogenesis and treatment. Expert Rev Anti Infect Ther. 2005;3(2):279–94.
11. Joshy S, Haidar SG, Iossifidis A. Necrotising fasciitis of the shoulder following muscular strain. Int J Clin Pract. 2006;60(7):856–7.
12. Sultan HY, Boyle AA, Sheppard N. Necrotising fasciitis. BMJ. 2012;345:e4274.
13. Sarani B, Strong M, Pascual J, Schwab CW. Necrotizing fasciitis: current concepts and review of the literature. J Am Coll Surg. 2009;208(2):279–88.
14. Tunovic E, Gawaziuk J, Bzura T, Embil J, Esmail A, Logsetty S. Necrotizing fasciitis: a six-year experience. J Burn Care Res. 2012;33(1):93–100.
15. Hussein QA, Anaya DA. Necrotizing soft tissue infections. Crit Care Clin. 2013;29(4):795–806.
16. Hakkarainen TW, Kopari NM, Pham TN, Evans HL. Necrotizing soft tissue infections: review and current concepts in treatment, systems of care, and outcomes. Curr Probl Surg. 2014;51(8):344–62.
17. Chapnick EK, Abter EI. Necrotizing soft-tissue infections. Infect Dis Clin North Am. 1996;10(4):835–55.
18. Korhonen K, Hirn M, Niinikoski J. Hyperbaric oxygen in the treatment of Fournier's gangrene. Eur J Surg. 1998;164(4):251–5.
19. Asfar SK, Baraka A, Juma T, Ma'Rafie A, Aladeen T, al Sayer H. Necrotizing fasciitis. Br J Surg. 1991;78(7):838–40.
20. Yeh DD, Velmahos G. Necrotizing soft tissue infections. In: Luchette FA, Yelon JA, editors. Geriatric trauma and critical care. Cham: Springer International; 2017. p. 187–200.
21. Holena DN, Mills AM, Carr BG, Wirtalla C, Sarani B, Kim PK, et al. Transfer status: a risk factor for mortality in patients with necrotizing fasciitis. Surgery. 2011;150(3):363–70.
22. O'Loughlin RE, Roberson A, Cieslak PR, Lynfield R, Gershman K, Craig A, et al. The epidemiology of invasive group A streptococcal infection and potential vaccine implications: United States, 2000-2004. Clin Infect Dis. 2007;45(7):853–62.
23. Koch C, Hecker A, Grau V, Padberg W, Wolff M, Henrich M. Intravenous immunoglobulin in necrotizing fasciitis—a case report and review of recent literature. Ann Med Surg (Lond). 2015;4(3):260–3.
24. Bosshardt TL, Henderson VJ, Organ CH Jr. Necrotizing soft-tissue infections. Arch Surg. 1996;131(8):846–52; discussion 52-4.
25. Purnell D, Hazlett T, Alexander SL. A new weapon against severe sepsis related to necrotizing fasciitis. Dimens Crit Care Nurs. 2004;23(1):18–23.
26. Bryant AE, Bayer CR, Huntington JD, Stevens DL. Group A streptococcal myonecrosis: increased vimentin expression after skeletal-muscle injury mediates the binding of Streptococcus pyogenes. J Infect Dis. 2006;193(12):1685–92.
27. Weinbren MJ, Perinpanayagam RM. Streptococcal necrotising fasciitis. J Infect. 1992;25(3):299–302.
28. Chelsom J, Halstensen A, Haga T, Hoiby EA. Necrotising fasciitis due to group A streptococci in western Norway: incidence and clinical features. Lancet. 1994;344(8930):1111–5.
29. Childers BJ, Potyondy LD, Nachreiner R, Rogers FR, Childers ER, Oberg KC, et al. Necrotizing fasciitis: a fourteen-year retrospective study of 163 consecutive patients. Am Surg. 2002;68(2):109–16.
30. Davies HD. Flesh-eating disease: a note on necrotizing fasciitis. Paediatr Child Health. 2001;6(5):243–7.
31. Elliott DC, Kufera JA, Myers RA. Necrotizing soft tissue infections. Risk factors for mortality and strategies for management. Ann Surg. 1996;224(5):672–83.
32. Giuliano A, Lewis F Jr, Hadley K, Blaisdell FW. Bacteriology of necrotizing fasciitis. Am J Surg. 1977;134(1):52–7.
33. Shiroff AM, Herlitz GN, Gracias VH. Necrotizing soft tissue infections. J Intensive Care Med. 2014;29(3):138–44.
34. Wall DB, Klein SR, Black S, de Virgilio C. A simple model to help distinguish necrotizing fasciitis from nonnecrotizing soft tissue infection. J Am Coll Surg. 2000;191(3):227–31.
35. Bernal NP, Latenser BA, Born JM, Liao J. Trends in 393 necrotizing acute soft tissue infection patients 2000-2008. Burns. 2012;38(2):252–60.
36. Wong CH, Khin LW, Heng KS, Tan KC, Low CO. The LRINEC (Laboratory Risk Indicator for Necrotizing Fasciitis) score: a tool for distinguishing necrotizing fasciitis from other soft tissue infections. Crit Care Med. 2004;32(7):1535–41.
37. Fisher JR, Conway MJ, Takeshita RT, Sandoval MR. Necrotizing fasciitis. Importance of roentgenographic studies for soft-tissue gas. JAMA. 1979;241(8):803–6.
38. Gozal D, Ziser A, Shupak A, Ariel A, Melamed Y. Necrotizing fasciitis. Arch Surg. 1986;121(2):233–5.
39. Zacharias N, Velmahos GC, Salama A, Alam HB, de Moya M, King DR, et al. Diagnosis of necrotizing soft tissue infections by computed tomography. Arch Surg. 2010;145(5):452–5.
40. Wysoki MG, Santora TA, Shah RM, Friedman AC. Necrotizing fasciitis: CT characteristics. Radiology. 1997;203(3):859–63.
41. Rahmouni A, Chosidow O, Mathieu D, Gueorguieva E, Jazaerli N, Radier C, et al. MR imaging in acute infectious cellulitis. Radiology. 1994;192(2):493–6.
42. Schmid MR, Kossmann T, Duewell S. Differentiation of necrotizing fasciitis and cellulitis using MR imaging. Am J Roentgenol. 1998;170(3):615–20.
43. Yen ZS, Wang HP, Ma HM, Chen SC, Chen WJ. Ultrasonographic screening of clinically-suspected necrotizing fasciitis. Acad Emerg Med. 2002;9(12):1448–51.
44. Begley MG, Shawker TH, Robertson CN, Bock SN, Wei JP, Lotze MT. Fournier gangrene: diagnosis with scrotal US. Radiology. 1988;169(2):387–9.
45. Stamenkovic I, Lew PD. Early recognition of potentially fatal necrotizing fasciitis. The use of frozen-section biopsy. N Engl J Med. 1984;310(26):1689–93.
46. Ward RG, Walsh MS. Necrotizing fasciitis: 10 years' experience in a district general hospital. Br J Surg. 1991;78(4):488–9.
47. Bilton BD, Zibari GB, McMillan RW, Aultman DF, Dunn G, McDonald JC. Aggressive surgical management of necrotizing fasciitis serves to decrease mortality: a retrospective study. Am Surg. 1998;64(5):397–400; discussion -1.
48. Voros D, Pissiotis C, Georgantas D, Katsaragakis S, Antoniou S, Papadimitriou J. Role of early and extensive surgery in the treatment of severe necrotizing soft tissue infection. Br J Surg. 1993;80(9):1190–1.
49. Rouse TM, Malangoni MA, Schulte WJ. Necrotizing fasciitis: a preventable disaster. Surgery. 1982;92(4):765–70.
50. Miller LG, Perdreau-Remington F, Rieg G, Mehdi S, Perlroth J, Bayer AS, et al. Necrotizing fasciitis caused by community-associated methicillin-resistant Staphylococcus aureus in Los Angeles. N Engl J Med. 2005;352(14):1445–53.
51. Cuschieri J. Necrotizing soft tissue infection. Surg Infect (Larchmt). 2008;9(6):559–62.
52. Phan HH, Cocanour CS. Necrotizing soft tissue infections in the intensive care unit. Crit Care Med. 2010;38(9 Suppl):S460–8.
53. Endorf FW, Cancio LC, Klein MB. Necrotizing soft-tissue infections: clinical guidelines. J Burn Care Res. 2009;30(5):769–75.

54. Endorf FW, Supple KG, Gamelli RL. The evolving characteristics and care of necrotizing soft-tissue infections. Burns. 2005;31(3):269–73.
55. Faucher LD, Morris SE, Edelman LS, Saffle JR. Burn center management of necrotizing soft-tissue surgical infections in unburned patients. Am J Surg. 2001;182(6):563–9.
56. Shah AK, Kumar NB, Gambhir RP, Chaudhry R. Integrated clinical care pathway for managing necrotising soft tissue infections. Indian J Surg. 2009;71(5):254–7.
57. Eray IC, Alabaz O, Akcam AT, Ulku A, Parsak CK, Sakman G, et al. Comparison of diverting colostomy and bowel management catheter applications in Fournier gangrene cases requiring fecal diversion. Indian J Surg. 2015;77(Suppl 2):438–41.
58. Busse JW, Jacobs CL, Swiontkowski MF, Bosse MJ, Bhandari M, Evidence-Based Orthopaedic Trauma Working Group. Complex limb salvage or early amputation for severe lower-limb injury: a meta-analysis of observational studies. J Orthop Trauma. 2007;21(1):70–6.
59. Stineman MG, Kwong PL, Xie D, Kurichi JE, Ripley DC, Brooks DM, et al. Prognostic differences for functional recovery after major lower limb amputation: effects of the timing and type of inpatient rehabilitation services in the Veterans Health Administration. PM R. 2010;2(4):232–43.
60. Uehara K, Yasunaga H, Morizaki Y, Horiguchi H, Fushimi K, Tanaka S. Necrotising soft-tissue infections of the upper limb: risk factors for amputation and death. Bone Joint J. 2014;96-B(11):1530–4.
61. Angoules AG, Kontakis G, Drakoulakis E, Vrentzos G, Granick MS, Giannoudis PV. Necrotising fasciitis of upper and lower limb: a systematic review. Injury. 2007;38(Suppl 5):S19–26.
62. Pham TN, Moore ML, Costa BA, Cuschieri J, Klein MB. Assessment of functional limitation after necrotizing soft tissue infection. J Burn Care Res. 2009;30(2):301–6.
63. Friederichs J, Hutter M, Hierholzer C, Novotny A, Friess H, Buhren V, et al. Procalcitonin ratio as a predictor of successful surgical treatment of severe necrotizing soft tissue infections. Am J Surg. 2013;206(3):368–73.
64. Glass GE, Sheil F, Ruston JC, Butler PE. Necrotising soft tissue infection in a UK metropolitan population. Ann R Coll Surg Engl. 2015;97(1):46–51.
65. Kim PJ, Attinger CE, Steinberg JS, Evans KK. Negative pressure wound therapy with instillation: past, present, and future. Surg Technol Int. 2015;26:51–6.
66. Wolvos T. The evolution of negative pressure wound therapy: negative pressure wound therapy with instillation. J Wound Care. 2015;24(4 Suppl):15–20.
67. Wolvos T. Wound instillation with negative pressure wound therapy. Ostomy Wound Manage. 2005;51(2A Suppl):21S–6S.
68. Huang WS, Hsieh SC, Hsieh CS, Schoung JY, Huang T. Use of vacuum-assisted wound closure to manage limb wounds in patients suffering from acute necrotizing fasciitis. Asian J Surg. 2006;29(3):135–9.
69. Ge K, Xu B, Wu JJ, Wu M, Lu S, Xie T. The use of negative pressure in critical necrotizing fasciitis treatment: a case presentation. Int J Low Extrem Wounds. 2014;13(3):230–2.
70. Birke-Sorensen H, Malmsjo M, Rome P, Hudson D, Krug E, Berg L, et al. Evidence-based recommendations for negative pressure wound therapy: treatment variables (pressure levels, wound filler and contact layer)—steps towards an international consensus. J Plast Reconstr Aesthet Surg. 2011;64(Suppl):S1–16.
71. Malmsjo M, Gustafsson L, Lindstedt S, Gesslein B, Ingemansson R. The effects of variable, intermittent, and continuous negative pressure wound therapy, using foam or gauze, on wound contraction, granulation tissue formation, and ingrowth into the wound filler. Eplasty. 2012;12:e5.
72. Darabi K, Abdel-Wahab O, Dzik WH. Current usage of intravenous immune globulin and the rationale behind it: the Massachusetts General Hospital data and a review of the literature. Transfusion. 2006;46(5):741–53.
73. Laupland KB, Kirkpatrick AW, Delaney A. Polyclonal intravenous immunoglobulin for the treatment of severe sepsis and septic shock in critically ill adults: a systematic review and meta-analysis. Crit Care Med. 2007;35(12):2686–92.
74. Norrby-Teglund A, Ihendyane N, Darenberg J. Intravenous immunoglobulin adjunctive therapy in sepsis, with special emphasis on severe invasive group A streptococcal infections. Scand J Infect Dis. 2003;35(9):683–9.
75. Darenberg J, Ihendyane N, Sjolin J, Aufwerber E, Haidl S, Follin P, et al. Intravenous immunoglobulin G therapy in streptococcal toxic shock syndrome: a European randomized, double-blind, placebo-controlled trial. Clin Infect Dis. 2003;37(3):333–40.
76. Kaul R, McGeer A, Norrby-Teglund A, Kotb M, Schwartz B, O'Rourke K, et al. Intravenous immunoglobulin therapy for streptococcal toxic shock syndrome—a comparative observational study. The Canadian Streptococcal Study Group. Clin Infect Dis. 1999;28(4):800–7.
77. Cawley MJ, Briggs M, Haith LR Jr, Reilly KJ, Guilday RE, Braxton GR, et al. Intravenous immunoglobulin as adjunctive treatment for streptococcal toxic shock syndrome associated with necrotizing fasciitis: case report and review. Pharmacotherapy. 1999;19(9):1094–8.
78. Norrby-Teglund A, Muller MP, McGeer A, Gan BS, Guru V, Bohnen J, et al. Successful management of severe group A streptococcal soft tissue infections using an aggressive medical regimen including intravenous polyspecific immunoglobulin together with a conservative surgical approach. Scand J Infect Dis. 2005;37(3):166–72.
79. Korhonen K, Kuttila K, Niinikoski J. Tissue gas tensions in patients with necrotising fasciitis and healthy controls during treatment with hyperbaric oxygen: a clinical study. Eur J Surg. 2000;166(7):530–4.
80. Kindwall EP. Uses of hyperbaric oxygen therapy in the 1990s. Cleve Clin J Med. 1992;59(5):517–28.
81. Cohn GH. Hyperbaric oxygen therapy. Promoting healing in difficult cases. Postgrad Med. 1986;79(2):89–92.
82. Riseman JA, Zamboni WA, Curtis A, Graham DR, Konrad HR, Ross DS. Hyperbaric oxygen therapy for necrotizing fasciitis reduces mortality and the need for debridements. Surgery. 1990;108(5):847–50.
83. Hollabaugh RS Jr, Dmochowski RR, Hickerson WL, Cox CE. Fournier's gangrene: therapeutic impact of hyperbaric oxygen. Plast Reconstr Surg. 1998;101(1):94–100.
84. Shupak A, Shoshani O, Goldenberg I, Barzilai A, Moskuna R, Bursztein S. Necrotizing fasciitis: an indication for hyperbaric oxygenation therapy? Surgery. 1995;118(5):873–8.
85. Escobar SJ, Slade JB Jr, Hunt TK, Cianci P. Adjuvant hyperbaric oxygen therapy (HBO2)for treatment of necrotizing fasciitis reduces mortality and amputation rate. Undersea Hyperb Med. 2005;32(6):437–43.
86. Soh CR, Pietrobon R, Freiberger JJ, Chew ST, Rajgor D, Gandhi M, et al. Hyperbaric oxygen therapy in necrotising soft tissue infections: a study of patients in the United States Nationwide Inpatient Sample. Intensive Care Med. 2012;38(7):1143–51.
87. Shaw JJ, Psoinos C, Emhoff TA, Shah SA, Santry HP. Not just full of hot air: hyperbaric oxygen therapy increases survival in cases of necrotizing soft tissue infections. Surg Infect (Larchmt). 2014;15(3):328–35.
88. Massey PR, Sakran JV, Mills AM, Sarani B, Aufhauser DD Jr, Sims CA, et al. Hyperbaric oxygen therapy in necrotizing soft tissue infections. J Surg Res. 2012;177(1):146–51.

89. George ME, Rueth NM, Skarda DE, Chipman JG, Quickel RR, Beilman GJ. Hyperbaric oxygen does not improve outcome in patients with necrotizing soft tissue infection. Surg Infect (Larchmt). 2009;10(1):21–8.
90. Brown DR, Davis NL, Lepawsky M, Cunningham J, Kortbeek J. A multicenter review of the treatment of major truncal necrotizing infections with and without hyperbaric oxygen therapy. Am J Surg. 1994;167(5):485–9.
91. Mindrup SR, Kealey GP, Fallon B. Hyperbaric oxygen for the treatment of Fournier's gangrene. J Urol. 2005;173(6):1975–7.
92. Levett D, Bennett MH, Millar I. Adjunctive hyperbaric oxygen for necrotizing fasciitis. Cochrane Database Syst Rev. 2015;1:CD007937.
93. Mulla ZD. Hyperbaric oxygen in necrotizing fasciitis. Plast Reconstr Surg. 2008;122(6):1984–5.
94. Hassan Z, Mullins RF, Friedman BC, Shaver JR, Brandigi C, Alam B, et al. Treating necrotizing fasciitis with or without hyperbaric oxygen therapy. Undersea Hyperb Med. 2010;37(2):115–23.
95. Bland CM, Frizzi JD, Reyes A. Use of drotrecogin alfa in necrotizing fasciitis: a case report and pharmacologic review. J Intensive Care Med. 2008;23(5):342–6.
96. Busund R. Plasmapheresis in the treatment of septic shock. Tidsskr Nor Laegeforen. 2004;124(6):776–8.
97. Kyles DM, Baltimore J. Adjunctive use of plasmapheresis and intravenous immunoglobulin therapy in sepsis: a case report. Am J Crit Care. 2005;14(2):109–12.
98. Anaya DA, McMahon K, Nathens AB, Sullivan SR, Foy H, Bulger E. Predictors of mortality and limb loss in necrotizing soft tissue infections. Arch Surg. 2005;140(2):151–7; discussion 8.
99. Kao LS, Lew DF, Arab SN, Todd SR, Awad SS, Carrick MM, et al. Local variations in the epidemiology, microbiology, and outcome of necrotizing soft-tissue infections: a multicenter study. Am J Surg. 2011;202(2):139–45.
100. Livingston DH, Tripp T, Biggs C, Lavery RF. A fate worse than death? Long-term outcome of trauma patients admitted to the surgical intensive care unit. J Trauma. 2009;67(2):341–8; discussion 8-9.
101. Light TD, Choi KC, Thomsen TA, Skeete DA, Latenser BA, Born JM, et al. Long-term outcomes of patients with necrotizing fasciitis. J Burn Care Res. 2010;31(1):93–9.
102. Hakkarainen TW, Burkette Ikebata N, Bulger E, Evans HL. Moving beyond survival as a measure of success: understanding the patient experience of necrotizing soft-tissue infections. J Surg Res. 2014;192(1):143–9.
103. Mills MK, Faraklas I, Davis C, Stoddard GJ, Saffle J. Outcomes from treatment of necrotizing soft-tissue infections: results from the National Surgical Quality Improvement Program database. Am J Surg. 2010;200(6):790–6; discussion 6-7.
104. Anaya DA, Bulger EM, Kwon YS, Kao LS, Evans H, Nathens AB. Predicting death in necrotizing soft tissue infections: a clinical score. Surg Infect (Larchmt). 2009;10(6):517–22.
105. Faraklas I, Stoddard GJ, Neumayer LA, Cochran A. Development and validation of a necrotizing soft-tissue infection mortality risk calculator using NSQIP. J Am Coll Surg. 2013;217(1):153–60 e3; discussion 60-1.

Frostbite

42

Christopher M. Nguyen, Rowan Chandler, Imran Ratanshi, and Sarvesh Logsetty

42.1 Introduction

Frostbite is a severe localized cold-induced injury caused by the freezing of soft tissue, secondary to exposure to temperatures below the freezing point of intact skin. It typically affects the peripheral upper and lower extremities but can also include areas of the face, such as the nose, cheeks, and ears. The sequelae of injury can be mild to severe, with treatment management ranging from watchful waiting to local wound care to major limb amputation. Intriguingly, it is a disease process that is unique in its vague initial presentation which can take a period of several months to determine the final demarcation of tissue damage. Given its nature of delayed presentation, a treatment guideline for early frostbite injuries remains elusive with no clear consensus of definitive intervention. As such, timely diagnosis, initial management, and patient education are vital in the prevention and provision of optimal treatment and tissue salvage in frostbite injuries [1].

This chapter will discuss and review the current understanding of epidemiology and risk factors, classifications and presentation, pathophysiology, diagnostic methods, and standard and developing management strategies for frostbite.

C. M. Nguyen · R. Chandler · I. Ratanshi
Manitoba Firefighters Burn Unit, Section of Plastic Surgery, Department of Surgery, Rady Faculty of Health Sciences, University of Manitoba, Winnipeg, MB, Canada
e-mail: nguyen33@myumanitoba.ca; chandler@myumanitoba.ca

S. Logsetty (✉)
Manitoba Firefighters Burn Unit, Section of Plastic Surgery, Department of Surgery, Rady Faculty of Health Sciences, University of Manitoba, Winnipeg, MB, Canada

Section of General surgery, Department of Surgery, University of Manitoba, Winnipeg, MB, Canada
e-mail: Sarvesh.Logsetty@umanitoba.ca

42.2 Epidemiology and Risk Factors

As most cases of frostbite injuries are rarely recorded and a national database or registry does not exist, there is no comprehensive statistical data in regard to prevalence of frostbite in the general population. Several studies have outlined statistics of incidence rates in specific regions of the world, race, and occupation. In general, frostbite is rather uncommon in North America with most reported cases in northern states, Alaska, and Canada, with studies reporting statistics in the military population. Other international statistics are limited to reported cases in Finland, British military, northern areas of Pakistan, and mountaineers in Iran.

The distribution and prevalence stratified by risk factors have been elucidated in current literature. The risk and predisposing factors that increase the incidence rates of frostbite can be categorized into (1) environmental, (2) socioeconomic and behavioral, (3) physiologic and genetic factors.

42.2.1 Environmental

Low temperature, high wind speeds, wetness, and high altitude are all factors that have a significant impact on frostbite rates. It is important to understand that cold air alone is a poor thermal conductor and that while it does have potential for frostbite at temperatures well below freezing, it has a much stronger effect on tissue heat loss in conjunction with high wind speeds. Wind chill is the measure of heat loss from the body due to wind speeds and cold air, and is thus reported as an index of skin surface temperature equivalent. At temperatures above −10° C, the risk of frostbite is minimal irrespective of the wind speed, but at temperatures below −25° C, there is a significant risk even at low wind speeds (7–10 km/h) [2, 3]. A wind chill equivalent temperature of less than −25 °C represents a mild risk of frostbite, while an index of below −45 °C represents a considerable risk of frostbite within minutes of exposure [2]. Low temperatures and high winds are not the only contributing factors to frostbite injury but the

M. G. Jeschke et al. (eds.), *Handbook of Burns Volume 1*, https://doi.org/10.1007/978-3-030-18940-2_42

hypoxic effect in high-altitude environments, where the partial pressure of oxygen is lower than at sea level, is also a determinant [4]. It has been reported in climbers of Mount Everest that the facial frostbite time dramatically decreases with wind chill equivalent temperatures, from less than 20 min in −30 °C to 5 min in −50 °C to less than 1 min in −60 °C temperatures. A study of 1500 cases of frostbite over a 10-year period in the Karakoram Mountains in Pakistan has described that the occurrence of frostbite becomes a very steep curve beyond 17,000 ft. This altitude was consequently deemed the “cut-off point” for high-altitude frostbite [5]. Apart from initial tissue hypoxia, prolonged exposure to altitudes greater than 17,000 ft triggers an adaptive physiologic response to increase blood packed-cell volume (polycythemia) due to decreased amounts of oxygen in the air, ultimately increasing blood viscosity [6, 7]. These physiologic responses in addition to vasoconstriction in the setting of severe cold are the main contributors to frostbite injuries [8]. Beyond these factors, it is important to recognize that water is known to have stronger thermal conduction properties than air, cooling the body surface rapidly upon contact approximately 25 times faster than air. Whether through direct submersion in cold water or simply having wet skin, the added element of heat transfer through conduction and evaporation causes accelerated heat loss [9]. More specifically, a small study found that at an air temperature of 5 °C, heat loss is doubled in wet clothes when compared in the setting of dry clothes [10]. Consequently, individuals in wet and windy environments, wet clothing, or submerged in water will be at higher risk of hypothermia and frostbite due to accelerated heat loss [11].

42.2.2 Socioeconomic and Behavioral

Homelessness, alcohol consumption, inadequate clothing, wet clothing, or tight constricting clothing to the extremities such as tight gloves or boots are strong predisposing factors for an increased susceptibility to frostbite [12, 13]. The lack of protective or fitted clothing, inadequate shelter, poor hygiene, propensity for substance abuse or alcoholism, substandard living conditions, and untreated psychiatric and medical comorbidities puts the homeless population at higher risk of frostbite as well [14, 15]. As frostbite injury progressively transpires when tissue heat loss overcomes tissue perfusion, constrictive and ill-fitted clothing, boots, and gloves restrict peripheral blood flow and subsequently decrease tissue temperature [16]. In children, although frostbite start at temperatures <−6 °C, amputations start below −23 °C. Two-thirds of frostbite in younger children is associated with lack of supervision, while frostbite in adolescents is related to intoxication [17]. Alcohol consumption is most notably the strongest contributor to frostbite as it causes the dual effect of heat loss from peripheral vasodilation and impaired judgment, which consequently inhibits self-protective instincts in the exposure to severe cold. It is the risk factor most associated with frostbite, with 45% of all urban frostbite cases involving alcohol intoxication [18]. Furthermore, occupations such as military, arctic explorers, and mountain climbers have been described to have a much higher incidence rate than the general civilian population given dehydration and association with high-altitude and cold environments [19]. In a 1995 Finish study, the mean annual incidence rate of frostbite in Finnish military population was 1.8 per 1000 recruits, with the hands, feet, and head being the areas most affected [20]. A more recent 2004 study of nearly 6000 Finnish young men aged 17–30 years further elucidates a high lifetime occurrence rate of 44 and 2.2% annual rate of frostbite during military service [21]. Skin emollients are widely used in mountain climbers, military conscripts, and those who venture in the arctic, however, their preventive effects of frostbite have been in question [22]. Several studies have found that the use of skin protective emollients doubled the incidence of facial frostbite where applied [23]. In vitro experiments testing different skin emollients yielded minimal thermal insulation and further correlation in in vivo subjects confirmed that emollient-treated skin cooled as quickly as non-medicated skin, yet subjective skin perception was a warming skin sensation [24]. As such the use of emollients have become a risk factor for facial frostbite and the increase in frostbite may be due to a false sense of security and through neglect of efficient protective measures [25]. Although the vast majority of frostbite injuries affect the feet, hands, and occasionally regions of the face, it has also been described to rarely involve the male genitalia in runners and Nordic skiers [13].

The occupational hazards of severe frostbite with the handling of refrigerant liquids and compressed gases, which are kept in liquid state at extremely low temperatures, such as chlorofluorocarbons (CFCs), liquid oxygen (−183 °C), liquid nitrogen (−196 °C), liquid helium (−296 °C), Freon (−40.5 °C) have been described [26–28]. In comparison with traditional frostbite from environmental cold exposure, these cryogenic burns from refrigerant agents are distinctive in their presentation in that they can induce through-and-through full thickness frostbite upon contact almost instantaneously given their extremely low boiling points. These injuries occur with direct contact to the liquid and the subsequent rapid intracellular ice crystal formation leading to cell death and potential involvement of severe deep soft tissue destruction.

42.2.3 Physiological and Genetic

Although the pediatric and elderly populations are highly susceptible to cold-induced injuries due to immature/impaired self-protective instincts to cold exposure, immobility, and frailty, frostbite is an injury most commonly observed in the middle-aged male population between 30 and 49 years with a mean age of 41 [15, 18]. This is likely from increased occupational hazard and exposure and increased risk-taking behavior [29, 30]. In regard to racial predisposition, current literature does suggest a genetic predisposition to cold-induced injury. Three studies conducted in military population report a higher risk of cold-induced injuries in African American and Pacific Islanders when compared to other races. These studies report that African American men and women were 4 times and 2.2 times, respectively, and Pacific Islanders are 2.6 times more likely to sustain cold-induced injuries as their Caucasian counterparts [31–33]. However, a previous military study in 1993 by Tek and Mackey opposed this notion, finding no difference in the prevalence of cold-induced injuries between African-American and other races [34]. Conversely, populations living in frigid environments, such as the Aboriginal people of Northern Canada (Inuit, Métis, First Nations), become acclimated to cold exposure with variant physiologic response, whereby transient peripheral vasoconstriction is followed by opening of arterio-venous communications in the forearm which maintains blood flow and warmth to the hand in cold climate. This protective physiologic phenomenon is known as the Hunting reflex or Lewis reaction and was first described in 1930. Intriguingly, it has been noted that through acclimatization, people originally residing in tropical environments can acquire this reflex which becomes indistinguishable from the cutaneous response seen in arctic residents. As such, the role and contribution of genetic factors is rather unclear as it becomes difficult to delineate genetic adaptation from environmental acclimatization [35]. Even though these studies investigated the correlation of race in cold-induced injury and not frostbite directly, it raises a strong case for the involvement of a racial component in the pathophysiology of the human vascular response to cold.

It is unclear whether prior injury of frostbite may increase the risk of sustaining future frostbite injury to the same affected limb. A 1974 study by Sumner et al. disclosed a 1.68 times increase in military personnel with a prior frostbite injury to sustain a repeat injury when compared to those without a prior frostbite history [16, 36]. Conversely, in a 2015 nonrandomized control study of 20 elite Alpinists who have and have not sustained prior freezing cold injuries were compared in terms of digit perfusion in cold water submersion tests showed that there was no significant difference of tissue rewarming rates and overall temperature in injured and uninjured finger and toes of the same individual [37]. Despite the study's small sample size, it suggests against the common belief that prior freezing injury may affect the vascular integrity and increase the risk of future frostbite injury to the same limb.

Additional vasoconstrictive factors secondary to diabetes, smoking, peripheral neuropathy, peripheral vascular disease, and cutaneous microvascular disorders such as Raynaud's disease, will further exacerbate frostbite in cold temperatures. Ervasti et al. in 2004 reported a significant synergistic increase in the rates of frostbite in Finnish young men with Raynaud's disease, regular smokers, and exposure to hand/arm vibration work [21]. The constituents in cigarette smoking reduces nitric oxide synthesis and potentiates thrombosis by increasing fibrinogen levels and platelet activity while absorbed nicotine elevate plasma catecholamine levels, thus all amplifying peripheral vasoconstriction and decreased blood flow in constricted areas leading to skin necrosis [38]. Raynaud's phenomenon affects 3–5% of the general population and is characterized by a hyperreactive vasoconstrictive response in the peripheral extremities during cold exposure, which can result in worsened cutaneous tissue ischemia-reperfusion injury. This pronounced reperfusion injury would further contribute to cell death in the setting of frostbite. Among other genetic factors, it has been reported that having the angiotensin-converting enzyme (ACE) DD allele and O group blood typing may increase risk as well [39]. The combination of these predisposing factors leads to a detrimental rapid loss of tissue heat and predisposes the body not only to frostbite but also to hypothermia.

42.3 Anatomy and Physiology

The normal core body temperature of a healthy adult human being at rest is 37 ° C while the average surface temperature of the skin is approximately 34 °C at an ambient room temperature of 15–20 °C [40–42]. As skin temperature steadily drops below 20 °C, the sensation of cutaneous pain is felt, and at a skin temperature below 10 °C, neurapraxia of the skin occurs. Human tissue begins to freeze between −0.53 and − 0.65 °C although it can be cooled to even lower temperatures [43].

42.3.1 The Skin and Its Structures

To fully understand the pathophysiologic mechanism of cold-induced injury, it is necessary to appreciate the skin structure, vascular layout, types of receptors, and physiologic feedback pathways involved. In brief, the skin is composed of two general layers, the epidermis and dermis. The epidermis can be further divided into five layers, from innermost (deepest) to outermost (superficial): stratum basale, stratum spinosum, stratum granulosum, stratum lucidum, and stratum corneum, while the dermis can be divided into the papillary and reticular layers. Within the layers of the epidermis and dermis reside the cutaneous receptors, which include mechanoreceptors, thermoreceptors, and nociceptors. These different types of receptors constitute the modalities of touch, pressure, vibration, temperature, and nociception (pain). In the context of frostbite, the focus will be primarily on the thermoreceptors and nociceptors. The cutaneous nociceptors are generally subdivided into several types according to the fibers supplying them, namely Aδ/β- or C fibers [44]. These fibers are further classified based on their conduction velocity and sensitivity to noxious mechanical (M), heat (H), and cold (C) stimuli [45]. Most notably in the setting of cold thermosensory perception are the Aδ and C fibers. Aδ fibers are thin (2–5 μm diameter) myelinated axons that elicit the sharp sensation of pain, while C fibers are unmyelinated axons that are responsible for the slow burning pain sensation [46]. It has been noted that at temperature range of 30–15° C, both types of fibers fire at an increased rate while warmer temperatures decrease the rate of firing. Clinically, this increase in firing rate as the skin reaches a temperature at or below 15° C is correlated with perception of cold and pain (burning, pricking, aching) is elicited [47, 48]. Below 10 °C, the rate of firing of Aδ and C fibers decrease and neurapraxia of the skin is exhibited. In regard to cutaneous circulation, the vast majority of blood vessels reside in the dermis with the exception of capillary loops that extend from the subpapillary plexus into the epidermis. Arterioles and venules form two important horizontal plexus networks at different tissue planes of the dermis, an upper plexus at the level of the papillary dermis and a lower plexus at the dermal subcutaneous level [49]. The upper and lower plexus networks are interconnected by branching vessels that provide perfusion to intermediate structures in the dermis such as hair bulbs and sweat glands. Vessels in the papillary dermis are primarily comprised of post-capillary venules which are physiologically the most reactive region of the microcirculation. In response to tissue damage and inflammation, endothelial cells develop intercellular gaps that increase vascular permeability and allow for leukocyte migration. Although similar in organizational structure, several differences exist between the papillary and deep dermal vessel morphology. At the deep dermal subcutaneous level, arterioles and venule vessel caliber seemingly double in diameter 50 μm vs. 25 μm, with thicker walls (10–16 μm vs. 4–5 μm) with more smooth muscle cells and pericytes (4–5 layers vs. 1–2 layers) [49]. This physiological difference explains the clinical difference in presentation seen in split thickness and full thickness thermal and frostbite injury, whereby clear-milky blister formation is seen in split-thickness involvement, while hemorrhagic blisters are seen in full thickness injury given larger vessel caliber.

42.3.2 Cutaneous Thermoregulatory Control

Due to an effective cutaneous vasoconstriction/vasodilation circulatory feedback system, the thermoregulatory control of human skin is strikingly robust in order to maintain thermal homeostasis. Of anatomical importance is the presence of arterio-venous anastomoses (AVAs) that are direct connections between small arteries and small veins. These vascular connections have a thick muscular wall composed of circular smooth muscle and inner lumen diameter lumen which ranges from 10 to 50 μm in size. As they do not possess a capillary segment, they are solely responsible for thermoregulatory control, providing warm core blood to more superficial regions [35, 49–53]. They are found abundantly in nail-beds of the fingers and toes (density 600 AVAs/cm^2) and glabrous skin of the hands and feet (100 AVAs/cm^2) [50]. In general, at ambient temperatures below thermoneutral state, these AVAs are closed for heat conservation towards the body core, whereas at higher temperatures, these AVAs are open for increased heat dissipation. However, as previously mentioned, there is a paradoxical protective phenomenon of cold-induced vasodilatation (CIVD), commonly referred to as the "hunting response," whereby a brief period of vasoconstriction in the setting of cold is followed by an increase in blood flow from vasodilatation and tissue rewarming occurs. Cycles of vasoconstriction-vasodilatation are seen approximately every 5–10 min and has been observed in the fingers, toes, face, and forearms [54, 55]. Since its description in 1930 by Sir Thomas Lewis, there have been many hypotheses on the mechanism of CIVD. Although the exact mechanism of CIVD remains unclear, the role of arterio-venous anastomoses (AVA) within the cutaneous microcirculation remains central in explaining CIVD. The most likely explanation surrounding paradoxical peripheral vasodilatation was proposed by Gardner and Webb in 1986 and supported by Daanen in 2003, whereby it was described that the local exposure to cold decreases the release of norepinephrine from adrenergic nerve endings due to a drastic decrease in sympathetic adrenergic neurotransmission to smooth muscle of AVAs [56]. Additionally, it has been shown that sensitivity of the α2-receptors for norepinephrine increases in the cold which may account for further decreasing tissue temperature to the point that nervous blockade occurs [35, 57]. This combination of decreased norepinephrine levels and decreased sympathetic drive ultimately induces vasodilation and shunting, temporarily rewarming the tissues and propagating the CIVD cycle. In regards to control of microcirculatory blood flow, the sympathetic nervous system plays a dual role of controlling noradrenergic vasoconstriction as well as sympathetic cholinergic active vasodilation in cutaneous vessels and AVAs [58]. In near hyperthermic environments, the vasodilatory effects can increase skin blood flow to nearly 6–8 L/min [59]. While in cold environments, thermoreceptors on the skin are activated and stimulate the sympathetic noradrenergic nervous system, which causes vasoconstriction in skin and the upper and lower extremities to reduce heat loss and favor central pooling of blood to the body core. Vasoconstriction occurs at 15 °C which can remarkably decrease the skin's blood flow to essentially zero [59, 60]. The typical pattern of frostbite injuries, whereby fingers, toes, nose, and ears are most affected, can be explained by the characteristic small-vessel vascular anatomy and the strong sympathetic innervated arterio-venous connections of these areas. As expected, with

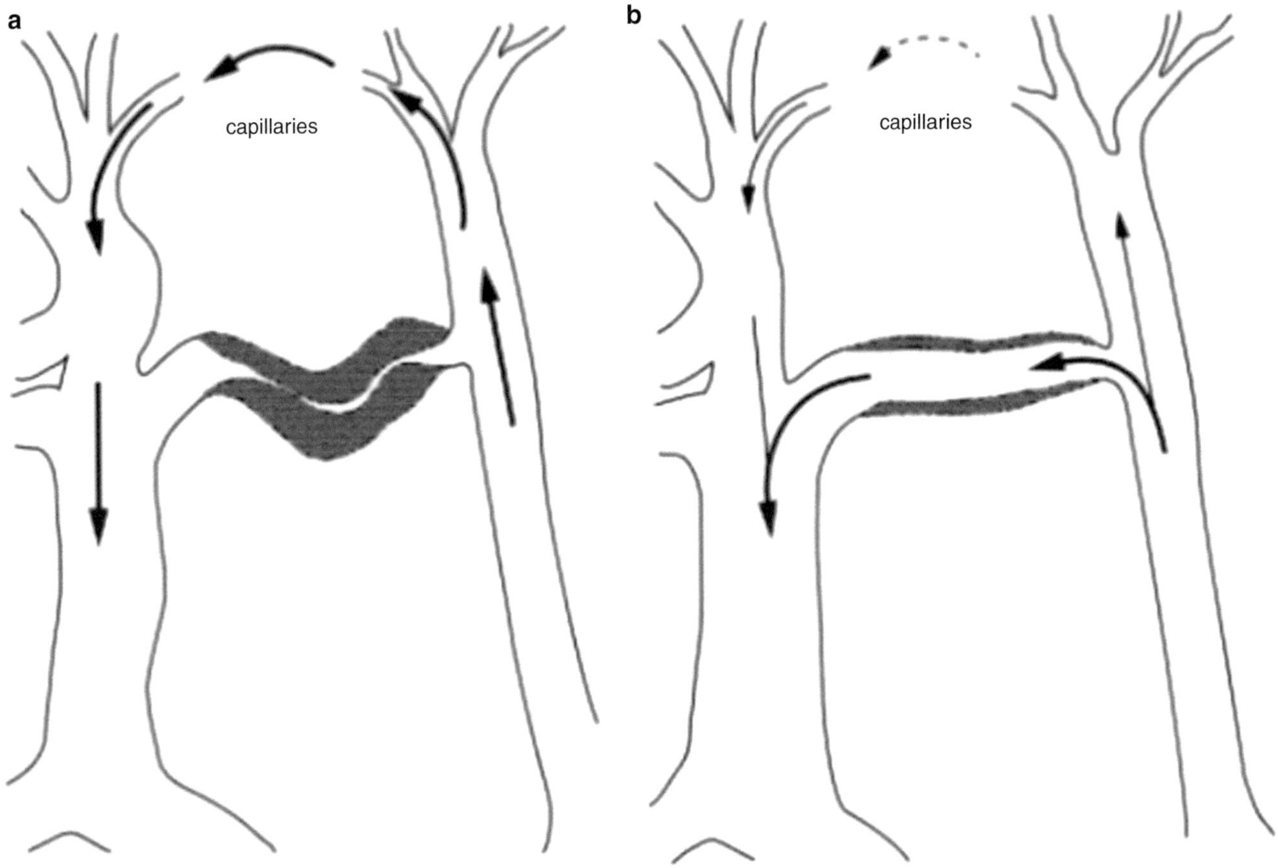

Fig. 42.1 Diagram showing the effect of a closed (a) and an open (b) arterio-venous anastomosis. From Boyd JD. Arterio-venous anastomoses. London Hospital Gazette 1939;42:2–8

increasing exposure time, frostbite injury extends more proximally from the initial affected distal extremities [61]. The risk of frostbite is linearly proportional to the skin surface temperature, such that as surface skin temperature decreases from −4.8 to −7.8 °C, the incidence of frostbite increases drastically from 5 to 95% [3].

42.4 Pathophysiology

The general frostbite sequence begins with complete tissue ischemia, followed by reperfusion, and ultimately tissue necrosis. Manson et al. defined a "double vascular lesion" phenomenon that occurs in cold injury: lack of tissue perfusion from large vessel vasoconstriction and loss microcirculatory control leading to stasis, vessel thrombosis, and tissue ischemia [62]. Three distinct mechanisms are central in understanding the pathophysiology of frostbite by which tissue damage can occur: direct cold-induced cell damage from cell crystallization, indirect cellular injury from local hypoxia from vasoconstriction and microvascular thrombosis, and release of inflammatory mediators post-thaw from reperfusion injury and cell death [15].

Further elucidating the mechanisms are four interconnected pathophysiological phases of the freezing cascade that depend on the temperature, conditions, and duration of cold exposure:

42.4.1 Phase I: Pre-freeze

As tissues begin to cool below 15 °C, vasospasms and eventual vasoconstriction occurs, blood viscosity increases, and tissue perfusion diminishes. Cold-induced vasodilation (CIVD) ceases at temperatures below 10 °C and ice crystal formation begins. This cycling of vasodilation and vasoconstriction is inherently protective to ice crystal formation.

42.4.2 Phase II: Freeze-Thaw Injury

As skin temperature reaches freezing point below −0.5 °C [16, 43], ice crystal formation occurs. There is a distinct difference in pathophysiologic effects with the rate of tissue cooling and absolute temperature to which the tissue is cooled. Rapid freezing of tissue below their freezing point through flash freeze or cold-contact mechanisms leads to the formation of large intracellular and extracellular ice crystals, leading to cell death and irreversible damage to skin [63]. Intracellular ice crystals denature cell membrane lipoproteins and can mechanically disrupt cell membrane integrity. The critical cellular freezing point occurs. With slow freezing, large ice crystals form in the extracellular space, increasing the osmotic pressure and subsequently drawing free water across the cell membrane into the extracellular space which leads to cellular dehydration and interstitial hyperosmolarity as the cell thaws. Cellular dehydration modifies protein structure, alters membrane lipids and cellular pH. Upon rewarming, the intracellular/extracellular ice melts, tissue ischemia is relieved, and reperfusion occurs. As vascular integrity remains grossly intact post-thaw, there is generally full restoration of circulatory reflow with increased vascular permeability due to endothelial damage. With an increase in fluid and protein leakage, blood viscosity further increases and platelet aggregation and coagulation cascade is initiated by the damage to the endothelium basement membrane [64, 65]. As such, despite near initial normal blood flow, within 3–5 min, disruption of flow is seen. Exposure to multiple freeze-thaw-refreeze cycles is detrimental to cell survival [66, 67].

42.4.3 Phase III: Vascular Stasis

As disruption of flow occurs and tissue ischemia persists from vasospasticity and increased blood viscosity secondary to transendothelial plasma leakage, arterio-venous shunting occurs more proximally as distal stasis occurs. These areas of stasis and ischemia lead to the buildup of inflammatory mediators (prostaglandins, histamine, thromboxane, bradykinin) which all propagate progressive tissue ischemia [68]. The combination of stasis and increased viscosity promotes thrombus formation.

42.4.4 Phase IV: Progressive or Late Ischemia

Thrombosis and proximal arterio-venous shunting lead to progressive dermal ischemia and loss of tissue. Final extent of demarcation and tissue necrosis is based most importantly on the degree of microvascular damage and vessel thrombosis. Gangrene eventually occurs from tissue necrosis and depending on degree of vascular compromise, mummification of the tissue can occur in severe cases.

Depending on the time of rewarming and therapeutic management for reperfusion, the increased cellular oxidative stress and inflammation associated with ischemia-reperfusion injury may contribute to further cellular damage and necrosis. The disruption of normal vascular flow due to microvascular thrombosis leads to cellular anaerobic metabolism and subsequent tissue hypoxia. These combined factors further stimulate the increased release of inflammatory mediators, prostaglandins PGF_2 and thromboxane A_2 (TXA_2). Robson and Heggers have reported elevated levels of prostaglandin F2α ($PGF_{2\alpha}$) and thromboxane B_2 (TXB_2), an inactive metabolite of TXA_2, in frostbite blister fluid. In addition, Özyazgan et al. reported increased prostaglandin I_2 and TXB_2 in frostbitten tissue by 188% and 249%, respectively. As PGI_2 and TXA_2 can be seen as physiologic antagonists of one another, it has been postulated that an increase in the ratio of TXA_2/PGI_2 could lead to increased platelet aggregation and thrombosis and thus the balance between physiologic levels of prostacyclin (prostaglandin I_2) and thromboxane A_2 is crucial for reducing further tissue necrosis in frostbite injury [69–71].

42.5 Classification

Frostbite ranges from the superficial freezing of the uppermost layers of skin, termed "frostnip," to severe frostbite which affects deeper tissues, such as muscles and bones. The severity of injury is related to the duration of exposure as well as the temperature in contact with the skin. As such, there are several frostbite injury classification systems (Tables 42.1, 42.2, and 42.3).

Table 42.1 Traditional classification

Degree of severity	Description and presentation	Clinical symptoms
First degree	Superficial partial thickness involvement of the epidermis that is characterized by erythema, edema, hyperemia with possible skin desquamation	Transient burning sensation with throbbing of the area
Second degree	Full thickness skin freezing that is characterized by erythema, marked edema characterized by vesicles of clear fluid. These blisters may desquamate and eschar formation may occur	Numbness of the affected area
Third degree	Full thickness skin with subcutaneous tissue involvement that is characterized by violaceous or hemorrhagic blisters with thickened areas of skin necrosis seen as bluish/gray discoloration	No sensation of the area but progresses to shooting burning pain that is throbbing and aching
Fourth degree	Full thickness skin, subcutaneous tissue, muscle, tendon, bone involvement characterized by little edema with initially mottled deep red or cyanotic area which eventually becomes dry mummified	May complain of joint pain

Table 42.2 Marsigny et al. Clinical Prediction Tool

Frostbite injury of extremities (hands and feet)	Grade 1	Grade 2	Grade 3	Grade 4
Extent of initial lesion at day 0 after rapid rewarming	Absence of initial lesion	Initial lesion on distal phalanx	Initial lesion on intermediary and proximal phalanx	Initial lesion on carpal/tarsal
Bone scanning results at day 2	Useless	Hypofixation of radiotracer uptake area	Absence of radiotracer uptake area on the digit	Absence of radiotracer uptake area on the carpal/tarsal
Blister presentation at day 2	Absence of blisters	Clear blisters	Hemorrhagic blisters on digit	Hemorrhagic blisters over carpal/tarsal
Prognosis at day 2	No amputation	Tissue amputation	Bone amputation of digit	Bone amputation of the limb ± systemic involvement ± sepsis
	No sequelae	Fingernail sequelae	Functional sequelae	Functional sequelae

Table 42.3 Wilderness Medical Society Practice Guideline

Degree of severity	Description and presentation
Superficial	There is none or minimal anticipated tissue loss, corresponding to first- and second-degree injury of the traditional scheme
Deep	Deeper injury and anticipated tissue loss, corresponding to third- and fourth-degree injury

Traditional classification follows the classic thermal burn scheme, which is based according to depth of injury, and is defined as follows (Table 42.1):

One criticism of the traditional classification scheme is that it does not take into consideration the unique delayed tissue necrosis demarcation in frostbite injuries and that treatment is directed as a typical burn injury resulting in sub-optimal care and patient expectations. As such, the clinical presentation and diagnosis of degree of frostbite injury in a patient who presents acutely in an urgent care setting may not be appropriate, as duration and time of frostbite onset may be unknown.

Of note, it is important to be able to recognize and differentiate "frostnip," a superficial non-freezing injury of exposed skin, from true frostbite. It is not to be confused with first-degree or superficial frostbite. Frostnip mostly presents as an exposed area with numbness, accompanied by palor or erythema, with potential ice crystal formation on the surface of the skin. By definition, there is no ice crystal formation in the dermis and there is thus no damage done beyond the epidermal layers. What further differentiates frostnip from frostbite is the rapid resolution of symptoms with no long-term sequelae through skin protection and rewarming [72].

Marsigny et al. Clinical Prediction Tool developed in 2001 to classify frostbite injuries of the hands and feet mainly based on locations of lesions and early bone scan results from initial presentation (day 0) (Table 42.2):

Wilderness Medical Society Practice Guideline recommends a simple two-tier classification scheme that can be employed after rewarming but before imaging [72] (Table 42.3):

This system is highly practical and used clinically as most long-term sequelae and tissue viability are unknown until several months from injury. As such, descriptive diagnosis of frostbite degree from the traditional system becomes inaccurate as previously described.

42.5.1 Hennepin Score

Beyond clinical classification schemes, this quantification scoring system also exists which is currently used for research purposes to investigate the treatment outcomes of frostbite injuries. Developed in 2016, the tool is used to quantify the similar to the Total Body Surface Area (TBSA) calculators in burn injuries [1, 61] (Table 42.4):

Table 42.4 Radiography (Limb X-Ray)

Stage and time frame	Radiographic findings
Early: immediate to weeks after injury	– May be normal, depending on injury severity – Soft tissue swelling – Tissue atrophy and distortion in severely affected areas – Subcutaneous emphysema – No bone or joint changes
Intermediate: weeks to months after injury	– Bone demineralization – Periostitis
Late: months to years after injury	– Acro-osteolysis – Sclerosis at ends of involved bone – Asymmetric early osteoarthrosis of the affected limb – Small periartibular erosion – In children, epiphyseal fragmentation and/or premature fusion with resulting deformities

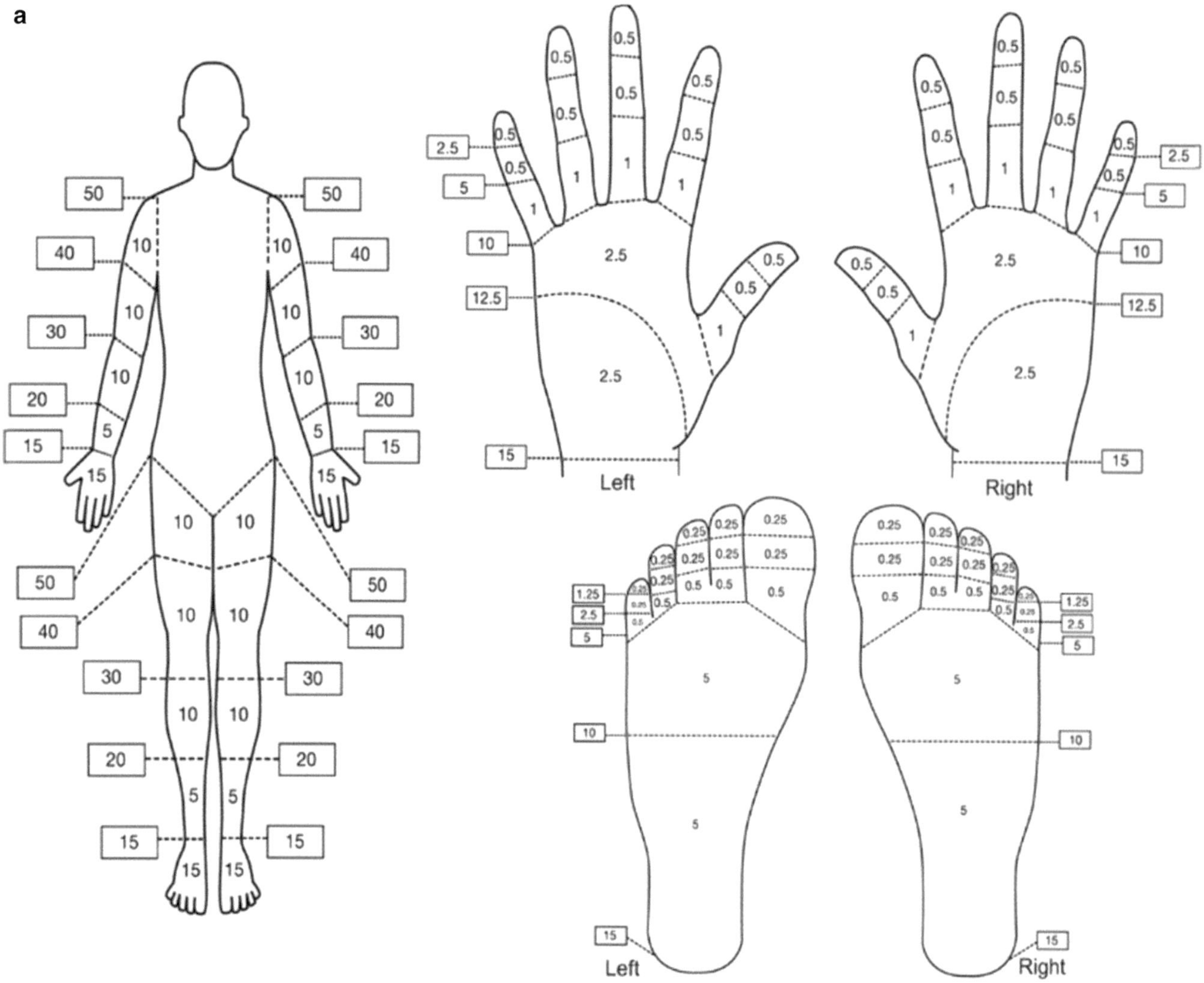

The purpose of the Hennepin score is to devise a standardized rating scale for researchers across academic centers to accurately measure injury and salvage rate outcomes to evaluate treatment efficacy. Imaging modalities that are included in the scale are Doppler ultrasound, magnetic resonance imaging, angiography, and bone scanning [61]. However as we will discuss below, currently there are no accurate means for diagnosis at the early stages of frostbite.

42.6 Diagnostic Methods

Most frostbite injuries are diagnosed clinically in the context of symptoms, physical examination, detailed history. In the setting to determine the extent of soft tissue injury and long-term tissue viability, diagnostic radiologic imaging modalities that aim to determine tissue perfusion and vessel patency have proven valuable. The main objective of imaging in the context of frostbite is to assess depth of involvement, severity, and to direct treatment based on surgical or non-surgical indications. It also allows for objective determination of frostbite treatment response and efficacy.

42.6.1 Radiography (Limb X-Ray)

In general, X-ray is not useful in the initial context except to rule out a trauma-related fracture. It is however, a rapid and inexpensive imaging modality in the late context that can show bone demineralization changes as soon as 1 week after frostbite injury, and bone artifacts and/or epiphyseal arrest after 6 weeks of injury in children [12]. Millet et al. have described the radiographic findings in relation to the stages of frostbite.

In summary, these radiographic findings can range from a normal X-ray with evidence of soft tissue swelling to severe bone destruction and demineralization depending on the severity of frostbite and the duration of time since the injury. Early radiographic evidence of mild injury can demonstrate osteopenia or show no prominent pathology. However most notable is the evidence of acro-osteolysis, sclerotic areas at terminal ends of affected bones, as well as early osteoarthritis, months to years after injury. All of which are indicative of previous deep frostbite injury that involve the tips of fingers or joints [73]. In children, epiphyseal fractures and premature fusion of the growth plates have been reported to occur, often months to years after injury. This can result in finger malformation and debilitating chronic joint problems. As a clinical tool, radiography can be a useful modality to follow the progression of injury but there may be discrepancies in clinical correlation as radiographic evidence is nonspecific and has no predictive value in determining the level of tissue necrosis. Management would indeed be based on clinical examination.

42.6.2 Digital Subtraction Angiography (DSA)

The main goal of using DSA is to identify potential targets for thrombolysis in patients presenting within 24 h with deep frostbite injury. Initial DSA will demonstrate lack of perfusion in affected digit and may show areas of impaired perfusion that do not appear affected on physical examination. Patients undergoing thrombolytic therapy can be followed with repeat DSA imaging at 12 h increments for up to 48 h to assess response to thrombolytics. By reversing the microvascular thrombosis present in frostbite injury, flow can be restored and prevent further tissue ischemia [74, 75].

42.6.3 Magnetic Resonance Imaging

Magnetic resonance angiography (MRA) has been suggested as a noninvasive alternative to DSA for evaluating the patency of vessels in frostbite injuries [76]. However, this modality lacks the benefit of being both diagnostic and therapeutic, unlike DSA. There is limited evidence suggesting that MRA might be able to define occluded vessels and demarcate soft tissue injury after more than 24 h of injury [77, 78].

42.6.4 Technetium (Tc)-99 m Scintigraphy

Also known as triple-phase bone scanning, Technetium-99 m (Tc-99m) has been in use for the past two decades for evaluating frostbite wounds. It involves a nuclear isotope that is taken up by osteoblasts. If the bone's blood supply has been compromised secondary to frostbite, the tracer will not be present in the bone. There are 3 phases in scanning: flow phase, blood pool image, and delayed phase. The first phase (seconds after the injection of the isotope) illustrates perfusion to an area. The blood pool phase occurs 5 min after injection and this shows the vascularity of the region. Finally, the delayed phase occurs about 3 h after injection. By this time, most of the isotope will have been metabolized and bone turnover can be better assessed.

Tc-99m scintigraphy is indicated in patients who present with deep (second, third, and fourth degree) frostbite injuries and is recommended to have bone scanning performed within 2–4 days after frostbite injury [79, 80]. The scan should not be performed immediately after cold exposure, as microvascular thrombosis can progress over time and what is defined on imaging may not be the level of tissue necrosis. Cauchy et al. in 2000, report that the level of amputation can be closely predicted in approximately 84% of cases at the initial scan, many weeks before the nonviable tissue declares itself on physical exam. Moreover, it has been suggested that any blisters should be debrided before the scans are performed to prevent accumulation of tracer in the blister fluid and lead to false-positive interpretation [80]. Again, larger prospective randomized studies are warranted to evaluate the reliability of such an imaging modality to predict the level of tissue demarcation and subsequent amputation, which would ultimately limit patient morbidity.

42.6.5 Single-Photon Emission Computed Tomography + CT (SPECT/CT)

By combining both the functional information from scintigraphy (bone perfusion) and uptake with the anatomic information derived from CT, a more specific image can be rendered than a conventional bone scan alone. More specifically, a CT scan is sequentially performed immediately after the delayed phase of nuclear bone scan and the images are merged, allowing for more exact delineation of the level at which the bone loses perfusion. It becomes particularly useful in assessment of the distal ends of digits as conventionally these regions can be difficult to properly visualize on bone scintigraphy alone. Most recently in a retrospective case series ($N = 7$), Kraft et al. describe the effectiveness of SPECT-CT in determining level of more distal amputation, allowing for preservation of digit length [81]. Six patients were able to undergo more distal amputation based on SPECT-CT imaging correlation. Although suggesting that SPECT-CT has a favorable predictive capacity, this is early evidence and further comparative and prospective studies are warranted for validation. It may be an important modality for surgical planning and minimizing the amount of tissue that is excised and limit patient morbidity.

42.6.6 Microangiography

Recently, Masters et al. describe a case report indocyanine green fluorescence microangiography to monitor clinical progression of perfusion in severe frostbite in hyperbaric oxygen therapy and propose its potential role in frostbite monitoring [82]. The benefits of indocyanine green microangiography are that it can be administered through a peripheral intravenous line; it is hepatically cleared and is thus safe in renally impaired patients and has a short half-life. On a technical and operator standpoint, it also does not require the consultation of a radiologist or dedicated imaging department, but rather can be done in the office or clinic. The dye travels to areas where there is perfusion and with a near-infrared laser and camera, blood flow is visualized by brightness. Given the potential benefits and portability of this imaging modality, further studies are required to determine its efficacy and practicality in the setting of frostbite.

42.7 Management

As initially indicated, the key factor that will determine the type of management is duration of exposure to subzero temperatures. The classic management of frostbite has been resuscitation, rewarming, and watchful waiting. Over the past 50 years, the adage "Frostbite in January, amputation in July" remains relevant despite advancements in the understanding of frostbite pathogenesis and advancements in thrombolytic therapy. The main goal of treatment is to prevent further tissue damage and to limit limb morbidity. As such, rapid triage and initiation of proper treatment for frostbite can lead to remarkable improvements in outcome and prognosis.

42.7.1 Clinical

The initial clinical manifestations of frostbite injury are similar for superficial and deep tissue damage, thus early treatment is identical for all injuries.

42.7.1.1 Rewarming

The mainstay of treatment is to ensure that core body temperature is raised to near physiologic 37 °C and that rewarming of the affected area is quickly initiated. Rapid rewarming ideally occurs through total immersion of the affected area in a warm whirlpool water bath between 37 and 44 °C [15]. Given that it has been shown that anoxic reperfusion injury occurs from slow thawing, rapid rewarming is recommended [15, 63, 83]. Rewarming time can vary from 15 to 30 min and up to an hour and can be stopped based on clinical judgment of tissue color with the goal of a red/purple color and good tissue pliability [29, 72].

42.7.1.2 Blister Debridement

Rewarming of skin in cases of superficial frostbite may result in the formation of clear blisters while cases of deep frostbite results in hemorrhagic blisters [2]. It has been shown that blisters filled with clear or milky fluid contain elevated levels of inflammatory mediators prostaglandin F2α (PGF2α) and thromboxane B2, an inactive metabolite/product of thromboxane A2 (TXA_2), which both propagate platelet aggregation, thrombosis, and vasoconstriction. As such, in order to prevent further damage to the sub-dermal plexus, most evidence in literature supports superficial debridement of white or clear blisters. It is however not recommended to debride blisters in the field to prevent infection [84]. It is also an indication to debride blisters if they are on joint surfaces and restrict movement [85]. Should blisters be debrided, the wound is to be covered with topical antimicrobial and possibly aloe cream, which has properties that inhibit the arachidonic acid cascade and thromboxane synthesis [15]. There is no evidence supporting either debriding or leaving intact hemorrhagic blisters.

42.7.1.3 Tetanus Prophylaxis

The administration of tetanus toxoid is based on standard guidelines. Frostbitten tissues are not especially prone to tetanus infection [29, 86].

42.7.1.4 Systemic Antibiotics

The call for systemic antibiotic administration is based on the presence of infection or open trauma. The role and benefits of prophylactic antibiotics in frostbite has not been proven and is not recommended unless signs of infection develop [29, 87, 88]. Antibiotics should be considered for prophylactic administration in severe frostbite injuries (second or third degree) where there is presence of an open wound [84, 88].

42.7.1.5 Wound Care

Unsalvageable tissue will eventually necrose and potentially become gangrenous without proper wound care. Tissue gangrene and mummification requires daily wound care to ensure that the wound stays dry to prevent wet gangrene infection. Use of topical antimicrobial dressings similar to burn dressings are recommended until mummification occurs after which dry dressings can be used. Furthermore, tissue protection through removable protective splinting, interdigit padding, or orthotics is also important considerations during the demarcation period to prevent further tissue tear and infection [29].

42.7.2 Therapeutic

As of current literature, there are no human randomized controlled trials with an objective reproducible method to assess the change in demarcation level from the intervention, making the recommendation of therapeutic interventions difficult. There are several emerging treatment options being increasingly studied in cases of severe frostbite within the first 24 h of injury.

42.7.2.1 Topical Aloe Vera

As elevated levels of prostaglandin production contribute to the pathogenesis of frostbite, early prevention with anti-thromboxanes such as topical aloe vera gel has suggested as treatment adjuncts. Aloe vera has been shown to inhibit TXA_2 synthetase and maintain PGE_2 and $PGF_{2\alpha}$ levels to maintain vasodilation in both thermal and frostbite injuries [89, 90]. An early animal study using frostbitten rabbit ear models showed that tissue survival can be improved with the administration of topical aloe vera and that its effects are comparable to the therapeutic effects of systemic pentoxifylline, a phosphodiesterase inhibitor [91]. Clinically, it is to be applied to all frostbitten areas every 6 h until wound healing is completed.

42.7.2.2 Non-steroidal Anti-inflammatory (NSAID) Medication

Most commonly used NSAIDs are ibuprofen and aspirin (ASA) which hold the dual purpose of providing anti-inflammatory activity and analgesia. This medication work by inhibiting cyclooxygenase enzymes (COX) that converts arachidonic acid to prostaglandin H_2 (PGH_2), which is ultimately converted to other prostaglandins (PGD_2, PGE, PGF_2, PGI_2) involved in inflammation, as well as TXA_2. Ibuprofen is a nonspecific COX inhibitor, reversibly blocking both COX-1 and COX-2, but has higher inhibition of thromboxanes than other prostanoids [87, 92]. Early oral administration of ibuprofen at a dose of 12 mg/kg/d to a maximum of 2400 mg/d provides early systemic anti-prostaglandin activity, limiting inflammatory damage [86]. Similarly, aspirin is also an effective analgesic and suppresses prostaglandins and thromboxanes through irreversible inactivation of COX-1 and COX-2, thus having a prolonged anti-platelet property. ASA may also inhibit endothelial cell synthesis of PGI_2, a prostaglandin involved in platelet aggregation inhibition. Although, in terms of pathophysiology, the use of either aspirin or ibuprofen in initial supportive frostbite treatment would be reasonable, there is insufficient evidence to support the benefits of aspirin in preventing tissue loss secondary to frostbite. The only study in humans supporting aspirin dates to 1983, whereby 38 patients with first- and second-degree frostbite upon presentation were treated with ASA and aloe vera showing no major tissue loss. However, there was no control group, 2 patients with acute second-degree progressed to third degree, and no mention of the time to treatment post-injury [68]. Conversely, ibuprofen has shown stronger evidence to support its efficacy in frostbite. A nonrandomized control trial by Heggers et al. in 1987 reported that patients treated with ibuprofen and aloe vera had a significant reduction in morbidity, whereby in all degrees of frostbite 67.9% healed without tissue loss vs. 32.7% in the control group, and 7% in the ibuprofen treatment group vs. 32.7% in the control group required amputation. As such, evidence thus far has suggested that ibuprofen should be considered as adjuvant therapy for the management of frostbite [12, 29, 93]. There remains no study that compare directly aspirin and NSAID for frostbite treatment, and there is no study that compares the different types of anti-inflammatory agents in frostbite therapy.

42.7.2.3 Tissue Plasminogen Activator (tPA)

A protease enzyme involved in fibrinolytic pathway in the breakdown of blood clots, tPA has been used as a mainstay treatment in the setting of acute ischemic stroke and is postulated to resolve microvascular thrombosis and ultimately restore perfusion in severe frostbite injury. The mechanism of thrombolysis is through the activation of plasminogen conversion to plasmin, which is capable of cleaving cross-links between fibrin molecules that form thrombi. Historically, evidence to support the effectiveness of thrombolytics in frostbite dates back to the 1980s where antithrombotic agents (streptokinase, urokinase) were proposed in rabbit and rat animal models, showing positive results [94, 95]. The earliest clinical data of tPA use in frostbite was in 1992, whereby 14 patients with severe frostbite, confirmed through triple-phase bone scanning, were treated conservatively with supportive measures ($N = 10$) and tPA ($N = 4$). It was seen that all 10 patients treated with supportive therapy required amputations while 3 out of 4 (75%) of those treated with tPA required no amputation [65].

More recently, two studies have reported significant limb salvage rates in severe frostbites following tissue plasminogen activator (tPA) therapy. In 2005, Twomey et al. published a nonrandomized prospective trial with historical controls, reporting an 18.9% rate of amputation in 19 patients with severe frostbite with a total of 174 digits at risk, 33 of which required amputation, that were treated with intravenous tPA ($N = 13$), intra-arterial tPA ($N = 6$), and subsequent intravenous heparin. Those who did not respond to therapy were more than 24 h post-injury, warm ischemia time of greater than 6 h, or evidence of multiple freeze-thaw cycles [74]. Furthermore, this study supported that tPA and heparin administration concurrently are safe and tPA administration, whether intravenous or intra-arterial, shows similar therapeutic effect in terms of digital limb salvage. In 2007, Bruen et al. published results from a single-center, retrospective review, comparing 32 patients recruited from 2001 to 2007 who were treated with intra-arterial tPA to historical controls from 1995 to 2001 presenting more than 24 h post-injury. It was found that those with severe frostbite treated with tPA within 24 h of injury and found the incidence of digital amputation was reduced from a potential amputation rate of 97 out of 234 digits (40%) at risk to 6 out of 59 digits (10%) at risk [75]. Similar to Twomey et al., it was noted that the patients who failed to improve blood flow and required amputations were those who presented to hospital post 24 h from injury. Both studies suggested that early tPA administration can result in digital salvage rate of 85–90% [75]. However, both studies use nonrandomized controls without an objective means of assessing the demarcation level.

In regard to thrombolytic therapy in general, Gonzaga et al. in 2016 published a retrospective observational cohort study of 69 patients from 1994 to 2007 with severe frostbite confirmed by angiography, 62 of whom underwent thrombolytic therapy which included Urokinase (N = 19), tPA (N = 18), Reteplase (N = 14), and TNKase (N = 11). Of these groups, there was no significant difference in response to different thrombolytic agents. They report a combined 68.6% digit salvage rate with 148 digits requiring amputation out of 472 digits at risk. Similar to both studies by Twomey and Bruen, Gonzaga et al. also describe the scenario in which 7 patients were given intra-arterial thrombolytic therapy post-24 h and none of the patients responded, all requiring digit amputations [63].

The dosage and duration of tPA administered in these studies varied per patient, ranging from an infusion of 0.25–1 mg/h with an overall duration of 8–42 h of treatment time. Bruen et al. initiated therapy with intra-arterial tPA bolus of 2–4 mg followed by a constant infusion 1 mg/h with heparin infusion of 500 units/h (Fig. 42.2). The duration of therapy was based on angiographical improvements at 12 h post-infusion and subsequently 24 h. Twomey et al. recommends a bolus of 0.15 mg/kg followed by a constant 0.15 mg/kg/h. infusion over 6 h up to a maximum of 100 mg with a therapeutic heparin infusion for 3–5 days titrated to double

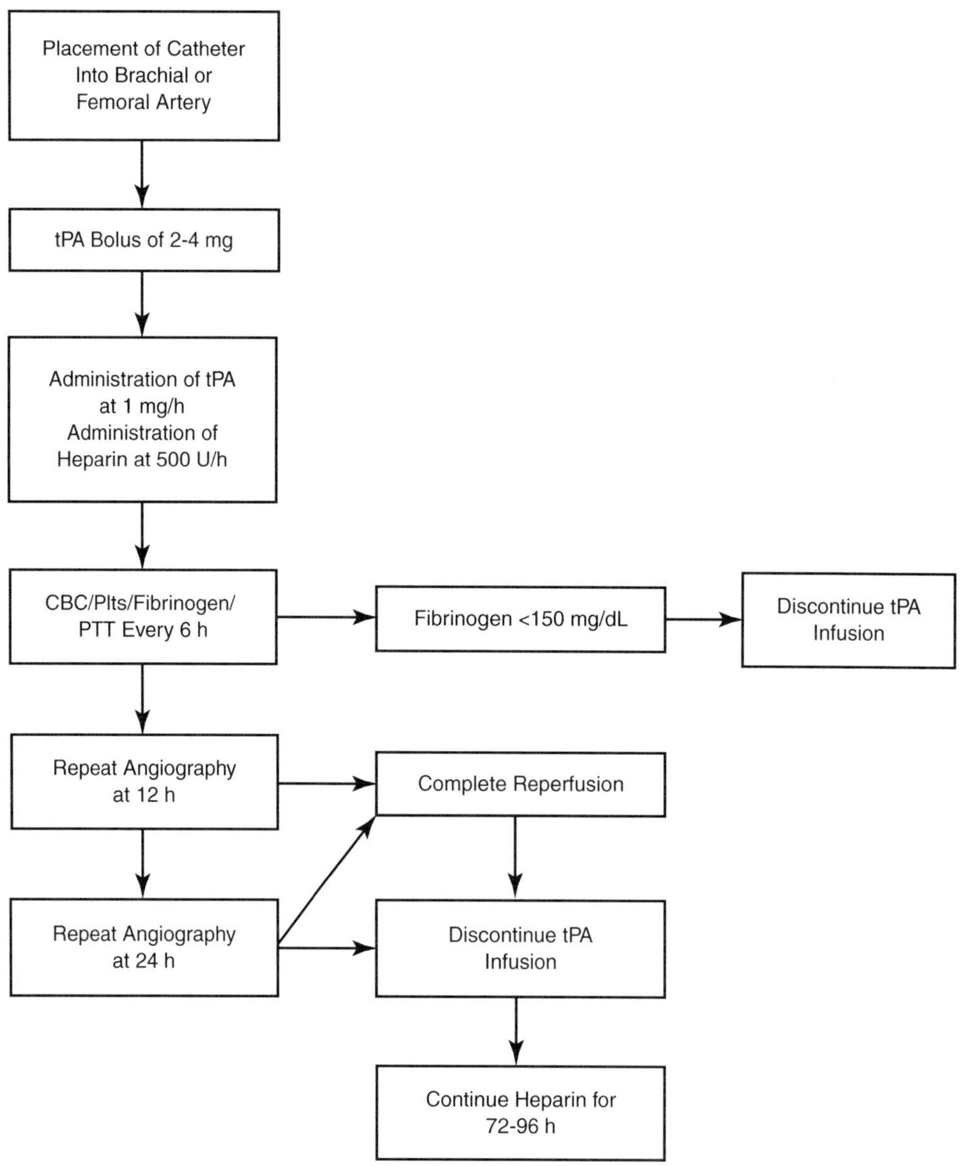

Fig. 42.2 The University of Utah frostbite treatment algorithm. *CBC* complete blood cell count; *Plts* platelets; *PTT* partial thromboplastin time; *tPA* tissue plasminogen activator. From Bruen KJ, Ballard JR, Morris SE, Cochran A, Edelman LS, Saffle JR. Reduction of the incidence of amputation in frostbite injury with thrombolytic therapy. Arch Surg. 2007;142(6):546–53

PTT control values. In cases of post 24 h of cold exposure, warm ischemia time of greater than 6 h, or evidence of multiple freeze-thaw cycles, administration of tPA showed little benefit to limb salvage [74]. Furthermore, the call to administer tPA also is based on eligibility of the patient for thrombolytic therapy. Criteria of contraindications include evidence or possibility of internal bleeding, history of intracranial hemorrhage, recent surgery, neurological impairment, or bleeding diathesis.

Early evidence suggests that tPA use in frostbite is that, when used within the first 24 h of injury, it significantly reduces tissue death and ultimately the need for amputation [74, 75, 84]. Although both Twomey et al. and Bruen et al. report convincingly remarkable results, it is important to note the limitations of these studies. Both studies use historical control groups that date back to more than a decade. It can be argued that medical management and wound care has improved over the years and there was no mention of whether the included patients were administered aspirin or nonsteroidal anti-inflammatory drugs during the initial triage. Thus, it may have been possible that patients who received tPA might have improved without thrombolytic therapy. Furthermore, as many patient comorbidities can affect tissue perfusion and subsequent recovery, it is unclear of the patient factors in these control groups. The administration of tPA is also not without risk, Twomey et al. describe 2 patients who developed retroperitoneal bleeding as a complication of tPA therapy. As such, the decision to initiate thrombolytic therapy should have all these factors considered, and the appropriate risks and complications should be explained to patient prior to administration.

42.7.2.4 Iloprost

A synthetic analogue of prostacyclin PGI_2, Iloprost produces vasodilation, inhibits platelet aggregation, and enhances fibrinolytic activity [64, 76, 96, 97]. Given its properties, it has been used clinically for pulmonary hypertension, healing of digital ulcers secondary to systemic sclerosis and Raynaud's phenomenon, and peripheral arterial disease ineligible for revascularization [98–100]. In vitro animal studies have shown evidence to suggest that it exhibits cytoprotective properties to vascular endothelium in the hypoxic environments [97]. It is primarily hepatically metabolized and possesses a half-life of 20–30 min. Mechanistically, Iloprost binds to G protein coupled prostacyclin (IP) and prostaglandin EP1 receptors which act to stimulate adenylate cyclase producing cyclic AMP (cAMP). This increase in cAMP results in the relaxation of vascular smooth muscle through the activation of protein kinase A (PKA) to promote phosphorylation of myosin light chains [101]. cAMP also results in the inhibition of platelet aggregation through the inhibition of TXA_2-induced cytosolic calcium increase [102]. In a similar setting of progressive tissue ischemia, Musial et al. studied the effects of Iloprost in patients with peripheral arterial disease and demonstrated an enhanced profibrinolytic activity with increased levels of intrinsic tissue plasminogen activator (tPA) in those administered Iloprost 5 h a day for 3 days, suggesting that PGI_2 facilitates the release of thrombolytic activity via tissue plasminogen activator (tPA) from the vessel wall [76]. Furthermore, PGI_2 has also been shown to inhibit arachidonic acid-induced platelet shape change and prevent sphering that is associated with platelet aggregation [96]. All these effects are beneficial in reducing further progression of tissue ischemia secondary to microcirculatory thrombosis post freeze-thaw phase in frostbite injury. Currently, it is not commercially available in an intravenous form in Canada nor the United States but has been used in Europe since the 1990s.

Iloprost has been a medication of much interest in the treatment of frostbite. The first report of its efficacy in severe frostbite was in 1994 where Groechenig described the treatment potential of iloprost after noting full recovery in 5 patients with grade 2 and 3 frostbite injuries that were treated for 14 days at a dose of 2 ng/kg [64]. More recently in 2011, Cauchy et al. published a randomized control trial comparing the efficacy of aspirin + buflomedil, aspirin + iloprost, and aspirin + iloprost + recombinant tissue plasminogen activator (rt-PA) in rates of digit amputation. In 47 patients with severe (grade 3 or grade 4) frostbite, they report a significant difference in the amputation rate of 60% (9/15 patients) in the group treated with buflomedil, 0% (0/16 patients) in the group treated with iloprost, and 19% (3/16 patients) in the group treated with iloprost plus rt-PA [103]. Most recently in 2017, Lindford et al. published a small retrospective observation cohort study involving 14 patients with severe frostbite, nine of whom underwent fibrinolytic therapy with tPA, three underwent iloprost therapy, and two patients received neither treatments due to contraindications. Despite the large discrepancy in sample sizes between test groups, they report an overall digital salvage rate of 75% in the tPA group, and a 78% salvage rate in the patients treated with iloprost. It was also noted that the digital salvage rate in one patient after iloprost infusion was 11% as they were treated more than 24 h from injury [104].

The benefits of iloprost compared to tPA therapy are fourfold: it does not require angiographic evaluation every 24 h to titrate therapy, it can be administered on a general ward, it does not have contraindications in the setting of trauma, and early evidence has shown efficacy in even after 24 h post frostbite injury [84, 105]. Cauchy et al. recommend iloprost administration within 48 h after rewarming [106]. Although iloprost is not currently, available in the United States or Canada, Poole and Gauthier published a recent case series in 2016, reporting favorable results in 2 patients in Northern Canada with full recovery from grade 3 frostbite injury and supporting the feasibility and efficacy of iloprost therapy in a community hospital setting [107]. Heil et al. have described an early suggestive algorithm (Fig. 42.3).

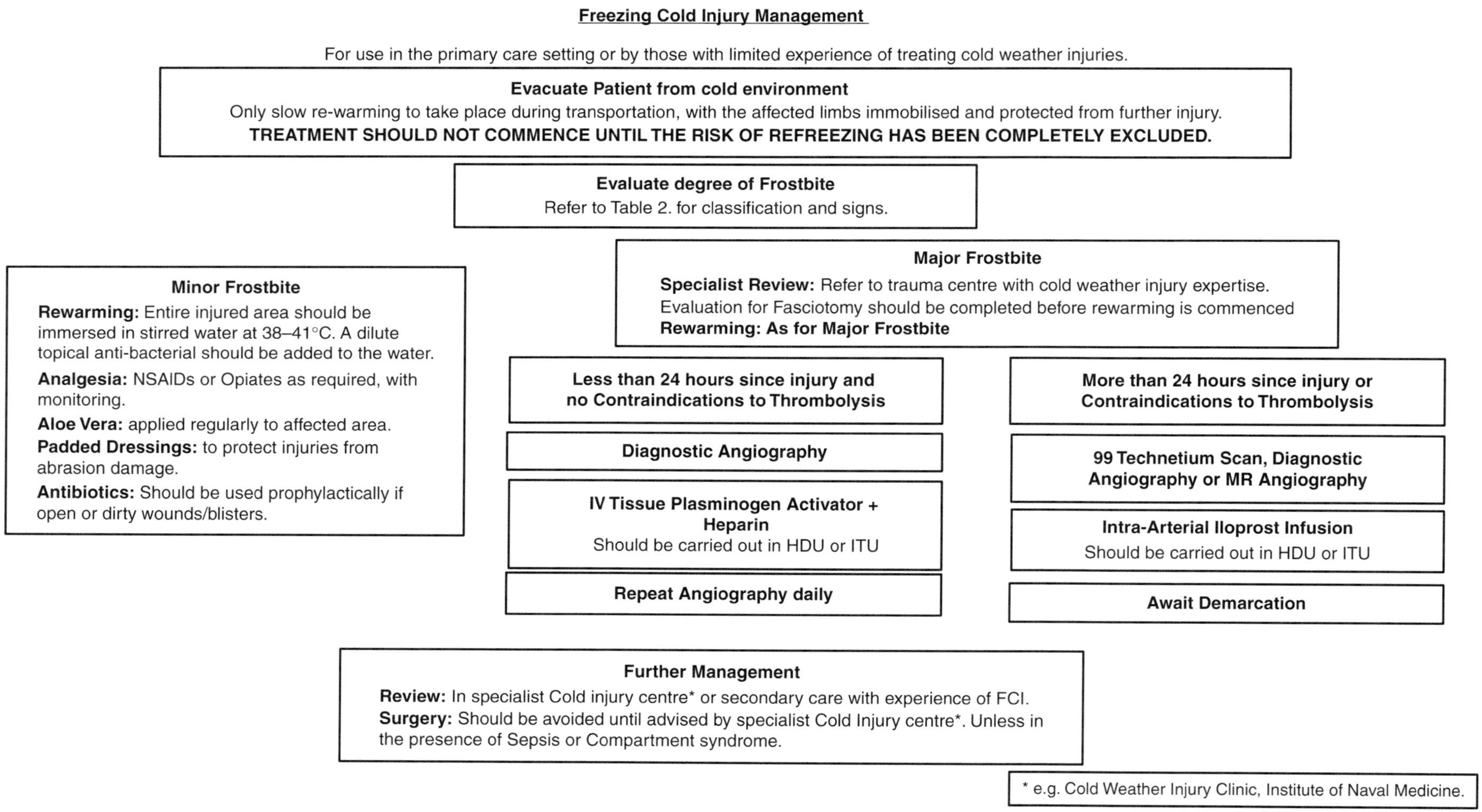

Fig. 42.3 Freezing cold injury management. From Heil K, Thomas R, Robertson G, Porter A, Milner R, Wood A. Freezing and non-freezing cold weather injuries: a systematic review. Br Med Bull. 2016;117(1):79–93

The dosage and duration of iloprost therapy has ranged from a low (0.5 ng/kg/min) dose increasing to the standard (2 ng/kg/min) for 6 h a day for 5–8 days. The infusion rate is increased gradually to avoid adverse effects such as headaches or hypotension. In the similar context of cold vasospasm, Torley et al. showed that both the low and standard doses were equally as effective in reducing severity of Raynaud's phenomenon secondary to connective tissue disease and improve ulcer and ischemic lesion healing in these patients [108].

42.7.3 Potential Adjunctive Therapies

The following therapeutic options have only been described in case reports/series. As such, there is currently insufficient evidence to determine their efficacy and further prospective randomized control trials are warranted.

42.7.3.1 Hyperbaric Oxygen

The goal of hyperbaric oxygen (HBO_2) is to correct tissue ischemia by increasing arterial PO_2 and subsequent the diffusion radius of oxygen. Physiologically, HBO_2 therapy has been shown to reduce reperfusion injury by decreasing hypoxia-inducible factor 1 (HIF-1) and subsequent inflammation by inhibiting neutrophil β2 integrin function, reducing pro-inflammatory cytokine production from monocyte-macrophages, and increasing the synthesis of wound healing mediators (FGF, TGF-β_1, PDGF) [109]. HBO_2 in severe frostbite was initially studied in 1963 with further case reports reporting favorable results in the following years [110–112]. This was further studied in depth through experimental animal studies in 1970 and 1972 using mouse and rabbit models showing no difference in tissue survival [113, 114]. It has also been elucidated that HBO_2 therapy at 2.5 atmospheres absolute (ATA) of 100% O_2 for 28 treatments of 90 min each over 14 days decreased tissue levels of inflammatory cells, increased PGI_2 levels, and did not change TXA_2 levels in frostbitten rabbit ears [115].

Although unconvincing animal study results, several case reports in human patients have reported remarkable results [116, 117]. In terms of duration and settings of treatment, Lansdorp et al. describe two patients treated with HBO_2 at 2.5 ATA for 80 min/session for a total of 30 sessions after 4 weeks of injury with deep frostbite injury showing quick demarcation and some tissue preservation [118]. Similarly, it has been reported in one case that the density of nutritive capillaries increases immediately after HBO_2 therapy in a patient 2 weeks from frostbite injury [117]. Dwivedi et al. describe a case report of grade 3 frostbite treated with HBO_2 in addition to aloe vera gel, pentoxifylline, and ibuprofen. Treatment duration was 2.0 ATA, total time of 90 min/session, twice/day for a total of 20 sessions with remarkable recovery [119].

Apart from several case reports, there have been no prospective control trials formally addressing the effectiveness of HBO_2 therapy in frostbite. As previously noted, early case reports have suggested physiologic effects and earlier demarcation in cases presenting more than 2 weeks after frostbite injury. As such evidence and indications for use as an adjunctive therapy clinically for frostbite injury remain unclear and unsupported.

42.7.3.2 Sympathectomy

As the sympathetic noradrenergic system controls vasoconstriction, eliminating input from the sympathetic nervous system would theoretically increase perfusion and alleviate tissue ischemia. Sympathectomy also aims to address late complications of frostbite and may have a role in alleviating long-term sequelae such as Raynaud's syndrome, hyperhidrosis, and chronic pain secondary to vasomotor dysfunction.

It has been shown that early sympathectomy done within the first few hours of injury has been found to increase tissue edema and subsequent tissue loss. However, if performed after 24–48 h post-thaw, it has been shown to decrease tissue edema and expedite ulcer healing [120]. As such, it is not recommended to perform sympathectomy as part of acute frostbite management [29]. Cervico-thoracic sympathectomy has shown relief in cases of debilitating Raynaud's syndrome in the upper extremities while lumbar sympathectomy alleviates pain and paresthesia after frostbite [120, 121]. It is most important to consider that the surgical procedure is irreversible and invasive.

Moreover, sympathectomy has been achieved using intra-arterial sympathetic blocking medication reserpine and tolazoline in animal models with frostbite showing reduced tissue loss similar to rapid rewarming [122]. Medical sympathectomy with guanethidine block has shown no significant result in treating acute frostbite [123]. There is no evidence showing that either surgical or medical sympathectomy improves the rate of tissue salvage after frostbite injury in humans. With the advent of intravenous vasodilators such as iloprost, the indications for surgical sympathectomy remain unsupported and, thus, are not recommended [13].

42.7.4 Surgical

In the acute setting, fasciotomies may be required given tissue edema post-thaw with evidence of compartment syndrome

[29, 124]. In the more chronic setting of gangrenous or mummified regions, surgical debridement and amputation for necrotic areas should be delayed at least 60–90 days (2–3 months) unless infection supervenes and overwhelming sepsis is present. This allows adequate timing to allow tissue to mummify, eschar to separate, and gangrenous area to clearly demarcate the borders of viable tissue. After adequate time for demarcation has passed, the mummified tissue is to be debrided or amputated as it may serve as a nidus for infection.

42.8 Conclusion

Frostbite is a common injury of morbidity that can lead to severe consequences. Its presentation and clinical sequelae is unique with an aspect of reperfusion injury and subsequent long time of demarcation. As discussed, seemingly benign initial presentation of frostbite may indeed lead to critical limb ischemia and gangrene requiring invasive surgical intervention of amputation over a period of months. Diagnostic methods are continuously being studied and are aimed at predictive value for being able to predict the extent of demarcation or degree of injury for early intervention and improvement of morbidity. Current standards include Technetium (Tc)-99m scintigraphy (triple-phase bone scanning), SPECT-CT, and digital subtractive angiography in regard to estimating the extent of injury. Management is based on degree of injury and duration since initial injury. Early reported evidence has suggested favorable effects of thrombolysis and Iloprost administration in regard to remarkable tissue salvage within the first 24 h of injury although high-quality randomized controlled trials are lacking. After 24–48 h post-thaw in severe frostbite or if the tissue endured several cycles of freeze-thaw injury, the definitive options for salvage are usually limited to surgical intervention. As most published studies that report remarkable recovery are case series, there are very limited randomized control trials that objectively define the superiority and efficacy of therapeutic agents. Most importantly, there is currently no reliable predictor of level of limb amputation. Imaging modalities such as angiography or triple-phase bone scan have been routinely used for evaluating efficacy of treatments but no studies have shown reliability in predicting the level of demarcation. In order to further understand and determine the optimal therapeutic frostbite management options, larger multi-center, high-quality trials are warranted. Despite the current limitations in evidence, Frostbite continues to be an intriguing topic with new emerging therapeutic options and imaging modalities becoming available to reduce morbidity of injury.

Summary Box

- Frostbite is a cold-induced injury to the skin and deeper tissues that can lead to significant morbidity.
- What is visible on initial presentation may not be what the final extent of injury is as demarcation of tissue necrosis occurs over a period of months.
- There are three distinct mechanisms for frostbite: (1) direct cold-induced cell damage from cell crystallization; (2) indirect cellular injury from local hypoxia from vasoconstriction and microvascular thrombosis; (3) release of inflammatory mediators post-thaw from reperfusion injury and cell death.
- Four phases of frostbite pathophysiology: (1) Prefreeze; (2) Freeze-Thaw injury; (3) Vascular stasis, (4) Progressive/late ischemia
- Classification systems: Traditional (first-Superficial partial, second-Full thickness, third-Full Thickness + subcutaneous involvement, fourth degree—Full Thickness + muscles/bone involvement); Marsigny et al. Clinical Prediction Tool for hands and feet (Grade 1–4).
- Management options should be taken to stabilize, rewarm, and optimize the environment for both the patient and wounds with Aloe Vera and NSAID to prevent further inflammatory injury.
- Current diagnostic standards include Technetium (Tc)-99m scintigraphy (triple-phase bone scanning), SPECT-CT, and digital subtractive angiography in regard to estimating the extent of injury. No diagnostic modality has been adequately correlated and validated with final demarcation.
- Surgical intervention for amputation is indicated when wet gangrene is present or when wound necrosis is fully demarcated.
- Early reported anecdotal evidence has suggested favorable effects of thrombolysis and Iloprost administration in regard to tissue salvage and possibly reduction in amputation level and rate. Further comparative clinical trials are needed before these interventions can be advocated.
- There is currently no reliable modality for predicting the level of tissue demarcation that would be able to guide early amputation.

References

1. Nygaard RM, Lacey AM, Lemere A, et al. Time matters in severe Frostbite: assessment of limb/digit salvage on the individual patient level. J Burn Care Res. 2017;38(1):53–9.

2. Biem J, Koehncke N, Classen D, Dosman J. Out of the cold: management of hypothermia and frostbite. Can Med Assoc J. 2003;168(3):305–11.
3. Danielsson U. Windchill and the risk of tissue freezing. J Appl Physiol. 1996;81(6):2666–73.
4. Moore GW, Semple JL. Freezing and frostbite on Mount Everest: new insights into wind chill and freezing times at extreme altitude. High Alt Med Biol. 2011;12(3):271–5.
5. Hashmi MA, Rashid M, Haleem A, Bokhari SA, Hussain T. Frostbite: epidemiology at high altitude in the Karakoram mountains. Ann R Coll Surg Engl. 1998;80(2):91–5.
6. Friedman NB, Kritzler RA. The pathology of high-altitude Frostbite. Am J Pathol. 1947;23(2):173–87.
7. Durand J, Varene P, Jacquemin C. Cardiac output and regional blood flows in altitude residents. In: Brendel W, Zink RA, editors. High altitude physiology and medicine. New York, NY: Springer; 1982. p. 129–41.
8. Hu J, Li H, Geng X, et al. Pathophysiologic determination of Frostbite under high altitude environment simulation in Sprague-Dawley rats. Wilderness Environ Med. 2016;27(3):355–63.
9. Molnar GW, Hughes AL, Wilson O, Goldman RF. Effect of skin wetting on finger cooling and freezing. J Appl Physiol. 1973;35(2):205–7.
10. Castellani JW, Young AJ, Ducharme MB, Giesbrecht GG, Glickman E, Sallis RE. American College of Sports Medicine position stand: prevention of cold injuries during exercise. Med Sci Sports Exerc. 2006;38(11):2012–29.
11. Giesbrecht GG, Wilkerson JA. Hypothermia, Frostbite and other cold injuries: prevention, survival, rescue, and treatment. Seattle, WA: Mountaineers Books; 2006.
12. Murphy JV, Banwell PE, Roberts AH, McGrouther DA. Frostbite: pathogenesis and treatment. J Trauma. 2000;48(1):171–8.
13. Imray C, Grieve A, Dhillon S. Cold damage to the extremities: frostbite and non-freezing cold injuries. Postgrad Med J. 2009;85(1007):481–8.
14. Wrenn K. Foot problems in homeless persons. Ann Intern Med. 1990;113(8):567–9.
15. Reamy BV. Frostbite: review and current concepts. J Am Board Fam Pract. 1998;11(1):34–40.
16. Fudge J. Exercise in the cold: preventing and managing hypothermia and Frostbite injury. Sports Health. 2016;8(2):133–9.
17. Boles R, Gawaziuk JP, Cristall N, Logsetty S. Pediatric frostbite: a 10-year single center retrospective study. Burns. 2018;44(7):1844–50. https://doi.org/10.1016/j.burns.2018.04.002. Epub 2018 Jul 30.
18. Valnicek SM, Chasmar LR, Clapson JB. Frostbite in the prairies: a 12-year review. Plast Reconstr Surg. 1993;92(4):633–41.
19. Harirchi I, Arvin A, Vash JH, Zafarmand V. Frostbite: incidence and predisposing factors in mountaineers. Br J Sports Med. 2005;39(12):898–901; discussion 901.
20. Lehmuskallio E, Lindholm H, Koskenvuo K, Sarna S, Friberg O, Viljanen A. Frostbite of the face and ears: epidemiological study of risk factors in Finnish conscripts. BMJ. 1995;311(7021):1661–3.
21. Ervasti O, Juopperi K, Kettunen P, et al. The occurrence of frostbite and its risk factors in young men. Int J Circumpolar Health. 2004;63(1):71–80.
22. Lehmuskallio E, Anttonen H. Thermophysical effects of ointments in cold: an experimental study with a skin model. Acta Derm Venereol. 1999;79(1):33–6.
23. Lehmuskallio E. Cold protecting ointments and frostbite. A questionnaire study of 830 conscripts in Finland. Acta Derm Venereol. 1999;79(1):67–70.
24. Lehmuskallio E, Rintamaki H, Anttonen H. Thermal effects of emollients on facial skin in the cold. Acta Dermato Venereol. 2000;80(3):203–7.
25. Lehmuskallio E. Emollients in the prevention of frostbite. Int J Circumpolar Health. 2000;59(2):122–30.
26. Wegener EE, Barraza KR, Das SK. Severe frostbite caused by Freon gas. South Med J. 1991;84(9):1143–6.
27. Sever C, Kulahci Y, Acar A, Karabacak E. Unusual hand frostbite caused by refrigerant liquids and gases. Ulus Travma Acil Cerrahi Derg. 2010;16(5):433–8.
28. Uygur F, Sever C, Noyan N. Frostbite burns caused by liquid oxygen. J Burn Care Res. 2009;30(2):358–61.
29. Handford C, Buxton P, Russell K, et al. Frostbite: a practical approach to hospital management. Extreme Physiol Med. 2014;3:7.
30. Millet JD, Brown RKJ, Levi B, et al. Frostbite: spectrum of imaging findings and guidelines for management. Radiographics. 2016;36(7):2154–69.
31. DeGroot DW, Castellani JW, Williams JO, Amoroso PJ. Epidemiology of U.S. Army cold weather injuries, 1980-1999. Aviat Space Environ Med. 2003;74(5):564–70.
32. Burgess JE, Macfarlane F. Retrospective analysis of the ethnic origins of male British army soldiers with peripheral cold weather injury. J R Army Med Corps. 2009;155(1):11–5.
33. Candler WH, Ivey H. Cold weather injuries among U.S. soldiers in Alaska: a five-year review. Mil Med. 1997;162(12):788–91.
34. Tek D, Mackey S. Non-freezing cold injury in a marine infantry battalion. J Wilderness Med. 1993;4(4):353–7.
35. Daanen HA. Finger cold-induced vasodilation: a review. Eur J Appl Physiol. 2003;89(5):411–26.
36. Sumner DS, Criblez TL, Doolittle WH. Host factors in human frostbite. Mil Med. 1974;141(6):454–61.
37. Morrison SA, Gorjanc J, Eiken O, Mekjavic IB. Finger and toe temperature responses to cold after freezing cold injury in elite alpinists. Wilderness Environ Med. 2015;26(3):295–304.
38. Black CE, Huang N, Neligan PC, et al. Effect of nicotine on vasoconstrictor and vasodilator responses in human skin vasculature. Am J Physiol Regul Integr Comp Physiol. 2001;281(4):R1097–104.
39. Kamikomaki N. A climber with the DD ACE allele developed frostbite despite taking more than adequate measures against cold on Mount Everest. High Alt Med Biol. 2007;8(2):167–8.
40. Blatteis CM. Physiology and pathophysiology of temperature regulation. Singapore: World Scientific; 1998.
41. Rintamaki H. Human responses to cold. Alaska Med. 2007;49(2 Suppl):29–31.
42. Darby SA, Frysztak RJ. Chapter 9—Neuroanatomy of the spinal cord. Clinical anatomy of the spine, spinal cord, and ANS. 3rd ed. Saint Louis: Mosby; 2014. p. 341–412.
43. Keatinge WR, Cannon P. Freezing-point of human skin. Lancet. 1960;1(7114):11–4.
44. Mense S. 5.03—Anatomy of Nociceptors A2—Masland, Richard H. In: Albright TD, Albright TD, Masland RH, et al., editors. The senses: a comprehensive reference. New York: Academic; 2008. p. 11–41.
45. Dubin AE, Patapoutian A. Nociceptors: the sensors of the pain pathway. J Clin Invest. 2010;120(11):3760–72.
46. Hanninen OOP, Atalay M. Physiology and maintenance—volume I: general physiology. Oxford: Eolss; 2009.
47. Park B, Kim SJ. Cooling the skin: understanding a specific cutaneous thermosensation. J Lifestyle Med. 2013;3(2):91–7.
48. Voets T, Droogmans G, Wissenbach U, Janssens A, Flockerzi V, Nilius B. The principle of temperature-dependent gating in cold- and heat-sensitive TRP channels. Nature. 2004;430(7001):748–54.
49. Braverman IM. The cutaneous microcirculation. J Investig Dermatol Symp Proc. 2000;5(1):3–9.
50. Walløe L. Arterio-venous anastomoses in the human skin and their role in temperature control. Temperature. 2016;3(1):92–103.
51. Sherman JL Jr. Normal arteriovenous anastomoses. Medicine. 1963;42(4):247–68.

52. Gray H, Lewis W. Anatomy of the human body. Philadelphia: Lea & Febiger.
53. Roddie IC. Circulation to skin and adipose tissue. In: Terjung R (ed) Comprehensive physiology; 2011. Wiley. https://doi.org/10.1002/cphy.cp020310.
54. Brajkovic D, Ducharme MB. Facial cold-induced vasodilation and skin temperature during exposure to cold wind. Eur J Appl Physiol. 2006;96(6):711–21.
55. Ducharme MB, VanHelder WP, Radomski MW. Cyclic intramuscular temperature fluctuations in the human forearm during cold-water immersion. Eur J Appl Physiol Occup Physiol. 1991;63(3–4):188–93.
56. Gardner CA, Webb RC. Cold-induced vasodilatation in isolated, perfused rat tail artery. Am J Physiol. 1986;251(1 Pt 2):H176–81.
57. Freedman RR, Sabharwal SC, Moten M, Migaly P. Local temperature modulates alpha 1- and alpha 2-adrenergic vasoconstriction in men. Am J Physiol. 1992;263(4 Pt 2):H1197–200.
58. Wong BJ, Hollowed CG. Current concepts of active vasodilation in human skin. Temperature. 2017;4(1):41–59.
59. Charkoudian N. Skin blood flow in adult human thermoregulation: how it works, when it does not, and why. Mayo Clin Proc. 2003;78(5):603–12.
60. Cheng MDC, Matsukawa MDT, Sessler MD, Daniel I, et al. Increasing mean skin temperature linearly reduces the core-temperature thresholds for vasoconstriction and shivering in humans. Anesthesiology. 1995;82(5):1160–8.
61. Nygaard RM, Whitley AB, Fey RM, Wagner AL. The Hennepin score: quantification of Frostbite management efficacy. J Burn Care Res. 2016;37(4):e317–22.
62. Manson PN, Jesudass R, Marzella L, Bulkley GB, Im MJ, Narayan KK. Evidence for an early free radical-mediated reperfusion injury in frostbite. Free Radic Biol Med. 1991;10(1):7–11.
63. Gonzaga T, Jenabzadeh K, Anderson CP, Mohr WJ, Endorf FW, Ahrenholz DH. Use of intra-arterial thrombolytic therapy for acute treatment of frostbite in 62 patients with review of thrombolytic therapy in frostbite. J Burn Care Res. 2016;37(4):e323–34.
64. Groechenig E. Treatment of frostbite with iloprost. Lancet. 1994;344(8930):1152–3.
65. Skolnick AA. Early data suggest clot-dissolving drug may help save frostbitten limbs from amputation. JAMA. 1992;267(15):2008–10.
66. Nagpal BM, Sharma R. Cold injuries: the chill within. Med J Armed Forces India. 2004;60(2):165–71.
67. Gross EA, Moore JC. Using thrombolytics in frostbite injury. J Emerg Trauma Shock. 2012;5(3):267–71.
68. McCauley RL, Hing DN, Robson MC, Heggers JP. Frostbite injuries: a rational approach based on the pathophysiology. J Trauma. 1983;23(2):143–7.
69. Waris T, Kyosola K. Cold injury of the rat skin. A fluorescence histochemical study of adrenergic nerves, mast cells and patency of cutaneous blood vessels. Scand J Plast Reconstr Surg. 1982;16(1):1–9.
70. Ozyazgan I, Tercan M, Melli M, Bekerecioglu M, Ustun H, Gunay GK. Eicosanoids and inflammatory cells in frostbitten tissue: prostacyclin, thromboxane, polymorphonuclear leukocytes, and mast cells. Plast Reconstr Surg. 1998;101(7):1881–6.
71. Cheng Y, Austin SC, Rocca B, et al. Role of prostacyclin in the cardiovascular response to thromboxane A2. Science. 2002;296(5567):539–41.
72. McIntosh SE, Opacic M, Freer L, et al. Wilderness Medical Society practice guidelines for the prevention and treatment of frostbite: 2014 update. Wilderness Environ Med. 2014;25(4 Suppl):S43–54.
73. Kemp SS, Dalinka MK, Schumacher H. Acro-osteolysis: etiologic and radiological considerations. JAMA. 1986;255(15):2058–61.
74. Twomey JA, Peltier GL, Zera RT. An open-label study to evaluate the safety and efficacy of tissue plasminogen activator in treatment of severe frostbite. J Trauma. 2005;59(6):1350–4; discussion 1354-1355.
75. Bruen KJ, Ballard JR, Morris SE, Cochran A, Edelman LS, Saffle JR. Reduction of the incidence of amputation in frostbite injury with thrombolytic therapy. Arch Surg. 2007;142(6):546–53.
76. Musiał J, Wilczyńska M, Sładek K, Cierniewski CS, Nizankowski R, Szczeklik A. Fibrinolytic activity of prostacyclin and iloprost in patients with peripheral arterial disease. Prostaglandins. 1986;31(1):61–70.
77. Raman SR, Jamil Z, Cosgrove J. Magnetic resonance angiography unmasks frostbite injury. Emerg Med J. 2011;28(5):450.
78. Barker JR, Haws MJ, Brown RE, Kucan JO, Moore WD. Magnetic resonance imaging of severe frostbite injuries. Ann Plast Surg. 1997;38(3):275–9.
79. Cauchy E, Marsigny B, Allamel G, Verhellen R, Chetaille E. The value of technetium 99 scintigraphy in the prognosis of amputation in severe frostbite injuries of the extremities: a retrospective study of 92 severe frostbite injuries. J Hand Surg Am. 2000;25(5):969–78.
80. Ikawa G, dos Santos PA, Yamaguchi KT, Stroh-Recor C, Ibello R. Frostbite and bone scanning: the use of 99m-labeled phosphates in demarcating the line of viability in frostbite victims. Orthopedics. 1986;9(9):1257–61.
81. Kraft C, Millet JD, Agarwal S, et al. SPECT/CT in the evaluation of Frostbite. J Burn Care Res. 2017;38(1):e227–34.
82. Masters T, Omodt S, Gayken J, et al. Microangiography to monitor treatment outcomes following severe Frostbite injury to the hands. J Burn Care Res. 2017;39:162–7.
83. Su CW, Lohman R, Gottlieb LJ. Frostbite of the upper extremity. Hand Clin. 2000;16(2):235–47.
84. Heil K, Thomas R, Robertson G, Porter A, Milner R, Wood A. Freezing and non-freezing cold weather injuries: a systematic review. Br Med Bull. 2016;117(1):79–93.
85. Robson MC, Heggers JP. Evaluation of hand frostbite blister fluid as a clue to pathogenesis. J Hand Surg Am. 1981;6(1):43–7.
86. Handford C, Thomas O, Imray CHE. Frostbite. Emerg Med Clin North Am. 2017;35(2):281–99.
87. Heggers JP, Robson MC, Manavalen K, et al. Experimental and clinical observations on frostbite. Ann Emerg Med. 1987;16(9):1056–62.
88. Bilgiç S, Özkan H, Özenç S, Safaz I, Yildiz C. Treating frostbite. Can Fam Physician. 2008;54(3):361–3.
89. Heggers JP, Pelley RP, Robson MC. Beneficial effects of aloe in wound healing. Phytother Res. 1993;7(7):S48–52.
90. Obeng MK, Motykie GD, Dastgir A, McCauley RL, Heggers JP. Aloe vera in thermal and frostbite injuries. Aloes. 2004;11:251–64.
91. Miller MB, Koltai PJ. Treatment of experimental frostbite with pentoxifylline and aloe vera cream. Arch Otolaryngol Head Neck Surg. 1995;121(6):678–80.
92. Parks WM, Hoak JC, Czervionke RL. Comparative effect of ibuprofen on endothelial and platelet prostaglandin synthesis. J Pharmacol Exp Ther. Nov 1981;219(2):415–9.
93. Hallam MJ, Cubison T, Dheansa B, Imray C. Managing frostbite. BMJ. 2010;341:c5864.
94. Salimi Z, Wolverson MK, Herbold DR, Vas W, Salimi A. Treatment of frostbite with i.v. streptokinase: an experimental study in rabbits. Am J Roentgenol. 1987;149(4):773–6.
95. Zdeblick TA, Field GA, Shaffer JW. Treatment of experimental frostbite with urokinase. J Hand Surg Am. 1988;13(6):948–53.
96. Ehrman ML, Jaffe EA. Prostacyclin (PGI2) inhibits the development in human platelets of ADP and arachidonic acid-induced shape change and procoagulant activity. Prostaglandins. 1980;20(6):1103–16.

97. Turker RK, Demirel E. Iloprost maintains acetylcholine relaxations of isolated rabbit aortic strips submitted to hypoxia. Pharmacology. 1988;36(3):151–5.
98. Kawald A, Burmester GR, Huscher D, Sunderkotter C, Riemekasten G. Low versus high-dose iloprost therapy over 21 days in patients with secondary Raynaud's phenomenon and systemic sclerosis: a randomized, open, single-center study. J Rheumatol. 2008;35(9):1830–7.
99. Piaggesi A, Vallini V, Iacopi E, et al. Iloprost in the management of peripheral arterial disease in patients with diabetes mellitus. Minerva Cardioangiol. 2011;59(1):101–8.
100. Whittle BJ, Silverstein AM, Mottola DM, Clapp LH. Binding and activity of the prostacyclin receptor (IP) agonists, treprostinil and iloprost, at human prostanoid receptors: treprostinil is a potent DP1 and EP2 agonist. Biochem Pharmacol. 2012;84(1):68–75.
101. Fetalvero KM, Shyu M, Nomikos AP, et al. The prostacyclin receptor induces human vascular smooth muscle cell differentiation via the protein kinase A pathway. Am J Physiol Heart Circ Physiol. 2006;290(4):H1337–46.
102. Zavoico GB, Feinstein MB. Cytoplasmic Ca2+ in platelets is controlled by cyclic AMP: antagonism between stimulators and inhibitors of adenylate cyclase. Biochem Biophys Res Commun. 1984;120(2):579–85.
103. Cauchy E, Cheguillaume B, Chetaille E. A controlled trial of a prostacyclin and rt-PA in the treatment of severe frostbite. N Engl J Med. 2011;364(2):189–90.
104. Lindford A, Valtonen J, Hult M, et al. The evolution of the Helsinki frostbite management protocol. Burns. 2017;43:1455–63.
105. Roche-Nagle G, Murphy D, Collins A, Sheehan S. Frostbite: management options. Eur J Emerg Med. 2008;15(3):173–5.
106. Cauchy E, Davis CB, Pasquier M, Meyer EF, Hackett PH. A new proposal for management of severe frostbite in the Austere environment. Wilderness Environ Med. 2016;27(1):92–9.
107. Poole A, Gauthier J. Treatment of severe frostbite with iloprost in northern Canada. Can Med Assoc J. 2016;188(17–18):1255–8.
108. Torley HI, Madhok R, Capell HA, et al. A double blind, randomised, multicentre comparison of two doses of intravenous iloprost in the treatment of Raynaud's phenomenon secondary to connective tissue diseases. Ann Rheum Dis. 1991;50(11):800–4.
109. Thom SR. Hyperbaric oxygen—its mechanisms and efficacy. Plast Reconstr Surg. 2011;127(Suppl 1):131S–41S.
110. Ward MP, Garnham JR, Simpson BR, Morley GH, Winter JS. Frostbite: general observations and report of cases treated by hyperbaric oxygen. Proc R Soc Med. 1968;61(8):787–9.
111. Cooke JN. Hyperbaric oxygen treatment in the Royal Air Force. Proc R Soc Med. 1971;64(9):881–2.
112. Ledingham IM. Some clinical and experimental applications of high pressure oxygen. Proc R Soc Med. 1963;56:999–1002.
113. Gage AA, Ishikawa H, Winter PM. Experimental frostbite. The effect of hyperbaric oxygenation on tissue survival. Cryobiology. 1970;7(1):1–8.
114. Hardenbergh E. Hyperbaric oxygen treatment of experimental frostbite in the mouse. J Surg Res. 1972;12(1):34–40.
115. Uygur F, Noyan N, Sever C, Gümüş T. The current analysis of the effect of hyperbaric oxygen therapy on the frostbitten tissue: experimental study in rabbits. Central Eur J Med. 2009;4(2):198–202.
116. von Heimburg D, Noah EM, Sieckmann UP, Pallua N. Hyperbaric oxygen treatment in deep frostbite of both hands in a boy. Burns. 2001;27(4):404–8.
117. Finderle Z, Cankar K. Delayed treatment of frostbite injury with hyperbaric oxygen therapy: a case report. Aviat Space Environ Med. 2002;73(4):392–4. PMID 11 952 063. Vol 732002.
118. Lansdorp CA, Roukema GR, Boonstra O, Dokter J. Delayed treatment of frostbite with hyperbaric oxygen: a report of two cases. Undersea Hyperbaric Med. 2017;44(4):365–9.
119. Dwivedi DA, Alasinga S, Singhal S, Malhotra VK, Kotwal A. Successful treatment of frostbite with hyperbaric oxygen treatment. Indian J Occup Environ Med. 2015;19(2):121–2.
120. Taylor MS. Lumbar epidural sympathectomy for frostbite injuries of the feet. Mil Med. Aug 1999;164(8):566–7.
121. Khan MI, Tariq M, Rehman A, Zafar A, Sheen SN. Efficacy of cervicothoracic sympathectomy versus conservative management in patients suffering from incapacitating Raynaud's syndrome after frost bite. JAMC. 2008;20(2):21–4.
122. Snider RL, Porter JM. Treatment of experimental frostbite with intra-arterial sympathetic blocking drugs. Surgery. 1975;77(4):557–61.
123. Engkvist O. The effect of regional intravenous guanethidine block in acute frostbite. Case report. Scand J Plast Reconstr Surg. 1986;20(2):243–5.
124. Mills WJ, Frostbite J. A discussion of the problem and a review of the Alaskan experience. 1973. Alaska Med. 1993;35(1):29–40.

Epidermal Necrolysis Spectrum from Basic Theory to Practice Essentials

43

Neil Shear and Abrar Bukhari

43.1 Introduction

Stevens–Johnson syndrome (SJS) and toxic epidermolysis necrosis (TEN) are rare, severe adverse cutaneous reactions that are often due to drugs with high morbidity and mortality. In the past, erythema multiforme (EM) was considered as part of epidermal necrolysis spectrum including Stevens–Johnson syndrome (SJS) and TEN. Since the SCAR study, most authors have agreed on using the SCAR study classification to separate EM from epidermal necrolysis (EN) (Table 43.1). SJS-TEN is used to describe a spectrum [2]. SJS is characterized by less than 10% total body surface area of detached or detachable skin and SJS-TEN overlap has 10–30%, while TEN has more than 30% body surface area detachment.

Table 43.1 SCAR study classification of EMM and EN

Classification	Type of lesions	Distribution	%BSA
EMM	Typical target	Acral	–
SJS	Spots atypical target	Widespread	<10
SJS–TEN overlap	Spots atypical target	Widespread	10–30%
TEN with spots	Spots atypical target	Widespread	≥30%
TEN without spots	Diffuse erythema, no spots or target	Widespread	≥30%

Adopted from Jean-Claude Roujeau [1]
SCAR Severe Cutaneous Adverse Reactions study, *BSA* body surface area

N. Shear (✉)
Sunnybrook and Women's College Health Science Center, Toronto, ON, Canada
e-mail: Neil.Shear@sunnybrook.ca

A. Bukhari
Department of Dermatology, College of Medicine, Al Imam Mohammad Ibn Saud Islamic University (IMSIU), Riyadh, Saudi Arabia
e-mail: aebukhari@imamu.edu.sa

43.2 Epidemiology

The incidence is 2–7 cases per million people per year [3]. It is well known that this rare drug reaction affects women at a slightly higher rate than men. SJS/TEN can occur at any age group, but it appears to affect adults more than children [4]. Mortality rates of SJS, SJS-TEN, and TEN were 5–10%, 30%, and 50%, respectively [5, 6].

Certain risk factors make patients at higher risk of this disorder such as being a slow acetylator, immunocompromised hosts, concurrent use of radiotherapy and anticonvulsants, specific human leukocyte antigen (HLA) alleles, and ethnicity. Racial disparities in SJS/TEN incidence was reported by a large population-based study, which found that SJS/TEN is more strongly associated with people of non-white ethnicities, particularly Asians and Blacks [7]. Asian patients have twofold higher risk when compared to Caucasian patients [8]. Thus, FDA recently recommended genotyping of Asians for the allele HLA-B∗15:02 prior to the administration of carbamazepine (Table 43.2).

Use of medication is the most common cause of EN. Other rare causes reported in literature include infection and vaccination, and collagen vascular diseases have been found to account for a small number of cases [10–13]. This is most likely due to confusion regarding diagnostic consideration among SJS, EM, and *Mycoplasma pneumoniae*-induced rash and mucositis (MIRM).

Hundreds of medications have been reported as being associated with EN. Commonly implicated medications are allopurinol, aromatic anticonvulsants, antimicrobial sulfonamides, lamotrigine, nevirapine, and oxicam nonsteroidal anti-inflammatory drugs (Table 43.3). Other low-risk medication includes sertraline, acetic acid nonsteroidal anti-inflammatory drugs, macrolides, quinolones, cephalosporins, and aminopenicillins [14]. Newer drugs such as nivolumab and ipilimumab have likewise been reported to cause SJS/TEN [15, 16].

M. G. Jeschke et al. (eds.), *Handbook of Burns Volume 1*, https://doi.org/10.1007/978-3-030-18940-2_43

Table 43.2 HLA association in different population

Associated drug	HLA allele	Specific eruption	Ethnicity
Aromatic convulsant	B*15:02	SJS/TEN	Han Chinese, Indian, Malaysian, Vietnamese, Singaporean, Hong Kongese
Carbamazepine	A*31:01	DRESS/SJS/TEN	Northern European, Japanese, Korean
	B*15:11	SJS/TEN	Han Chinese, Japanese, Korean
	B*59:01	SJS/TEN	Japanese
	B*38:01	SJS/TEN	Spanish
	B*15:02	SJS/TEN	Han Chinese, Thai
	B*51:01	SJS/TEN	Han Chinese, Japanese, Malaysian
Oxcarbazepine	A*33:03, B*38:02, B*51:01, B*56:02, B*58:01, C*14:02	SJS/TEN	Thai
Phenytoin	B*15:13	DRESS/SJS/TEN	Malaysian
	CYP2C9*3	DRESS/SJS/TEN	Han Chinese, Japanese, Malaysian
	CYP2C9*3	SJS/TEN	Thai
	B*15:02	SJS/TEN	Han Chinese
	B*38; B*58:01, A*68:01, Cw*07:18	SJS/TEN	European
Phenobarbital	B*38:01	SJS/TEN	Spanish
Lamotrigine	A*31:01	SJS/TEN	Korean
	A*24:02	DRESS/SJS/TEN	Spanish
Allopurinol	B*58:01	DRESS/SJS/TEN	Han Chinese, Thai, Japanese, Korean, European
Nevirapine	C*04:01	DRESS/SJS/TEN	Malawian
Cotrimoxazole	B*15:02, C*06:02, C*08:01	SJS/TEN	Thai
Sulfamethoxazole	B*38:02	SJS/TEN	European
Sulfonamide	A*29, B*12, DR*7	TEN	European
Oxicam NSAIDs	B*73:01	SJS/TEN	European
Methazolamide	B*59:01, CW*01:02	SJS/TEN	Korean, Japanese

Adopted with modification from Chun-Bing Chen et al. [9]

Table 43.3 High-risk drug causing epidermal necrolysis

Allopurinol
Aromatic anticonvulsants: carbamazepine, phenobarbital, phenytoin
Antibacterial sulfonamides: sulfamethoxazole, sulfasalazine
Lamotrigine
Nevirapine
Oxicam nonsteroidal anti-inflammatory drugs

43.3 Pathogenesis

Several theories have been proposed for the pathogenesis of epidermolytic necrolysis, but molecular sequencing and cellular events are not fully understood. In susceptible individuals, upon exposure to a certain drug or one of its metabolite, a series of reactions occur that lead to keratinocytes apoptosis and subsequent epidermal necrosis and detachment [9].

43.3.1 Antigen Presentation

Drugs are considered as foreign body material that are too small on their own to be immunogenic. But when they bind to hapten-carrier complex, they are presented to HLA molecules, and then are recognized by T-cell receptors (TCR). This recognition results in the induction of drug-specific immune response by CD8+ cytotoxic T cell (CTL).

43.3.2 Fas-FasL Interaction

Fas ligands (FasL) are transmembrane protein molecules expressed on target cells that belong to tumor necrosis factor (TNF) family. Upon their interaction, Fas-associated death domain proteins (FAAD) is recruited and bind to Fas-FasL complex. Subsequently, FAAD recruits procaspase 8, turning it into caspase 8 and triggering it into caspase cascade which result in DNA degranulation. However, the molecular events leading to the upregulation of surface keratinocyte FasL during TEN remain unknown [17].

43.3.3 Perforin/Granzyme B

Other research suggests that perforin and granzyme B play more important role in keratinocytes apoptosis in EN than does Fas–FasL interaction. Granzyme B is a serine protease released by cytoplasmic granules that induce apoptosis. Upon activation, CTL and natural killer cells (NK) produce perforin, which in turn delineates the entry of granzyme B into the target cells [18–20].

43.3.4 Granulysin

Granulysin is a cytolytic protein produced mainly by CTL, NK cells, and NK T cells. This molecule participates in programmed cellular death by creating holes in cellular membrane and thereby cellular destruction. In 2008, Chung et al. provided evidence that granulysin is the key mediator for disseminated keratinocyte apoptosis in SJS/TEN. This study found that the granulysin level in blister fluids of SJS/TEN patient was much higher than other cytotoxic proteins, such as Fas-FasL, perforin, and granzyme B [21].

43.3.5 Delayed-Type Drug Hypersensitivity

Specific T lymphocytes or NK cells are activated upon antigen recognition. Soon afterwards, various cytokines/chemokines are released to attack keratinocytes or promote trafficking, proliferation, regulation, or activation of T cells and other leukocytes.

43.3.6 Other Cytokines and Chemokines Are Involved in EN Pathogenesis Such as TNF-α, IFN-γ and IL-15 & IL-36

TNF-α is a major proinflammatory cytokine and is produced by macrophages, T lymphocytes, NK cells, neutrophils, mast cells and eosinophils. This molecule is highly expressed in plasma and blister fluids of SJS/TEN and appear to be a significant inducer of keratinocyte apoptosis [22].

IFN-γ is a significant cytokine for innate and adaptive immunity that is mainly produced by CD4+ T-helper cells, CD8+ CTL, and NK cells. IFN-γ was found to be elevated in skin tissue, blister, and plasma of SJS/TEN patients. In 2013, Viard-Leveugle et al. suggested a link between two path mechanism modalities of EN, delayed-type drug hypersensitivity and target cellular death. This study demonstrated that activated T cells secrete high amount of TNF-α and IFN-γ which lead to an increased expression and activity of inducible nitric oxide synthetase (iNOS). The resulting increase in nitric oxide significantly upregulates keratinocyte FasL expression and eventually keratinocyte apoptosis.

IL-15 and IL-36 participate in the immune reaction of EN by regulating trafficking, proliferation, and activation of T lymphocytes. Moreover, IL-15 has also been shown to enhance the cytotoxicity of cultured NK cells and blister cells from TEN [5]. Thereby IL-15 has been found to be associated with disease severity and mortality of SJS/TEN.

43.4 Clinical Presentation

EN presentation starts typically within 4–28 days of exposure to medication, with a prodrome of malaise, fatigue, anorexia, cough, and fever. Three days later, skin lesions appear on the trunk or face and progress to the extremities; with painful ill-defined erythematous coalescing macules and patches and central purpura (Fig. 43.1). These lesions could be confused with the targetoid lesions of erythema multiforme. A clinical clue that could differentiate between these two entities is that in SJS the rash is macular and flat in nature, while in EM it is more popular and raised which is also associated with more classic target lesions.

These lesions will evolve into extensive areas of detached epidermis (Fig. 43.2). If spontaneous detachment was absent at clinical presentation, Nicolsky sign must be sought by exerting tangential force by a thumb to several macules. This sign is considered positive if dermo-epidermal shearing was induced. Ocular stinging, photophobia, conjunctival itching, bleeding of lips, epistaxis, dysphagia, odynophagia, dysuria, hematuria, and genital pain are early signs and symptoms of mucosal involvement. Systemic manifestation include fever, lymphadenopathy, transaminitis and cellular cytopenia.

When necrotic epidermis detaches from underlying dermis, fluid fills in this gap, giving rise to flaccid bullae. These blisters will spread laterally if a slight pressure was applied "Asboe-Hansen sign, Nikolsky II sign or Indirect Nikolsky sign." Tense bullae are rare findings that could appear on palmoplantar surfaces where epidermis is thicker. Sloughing of

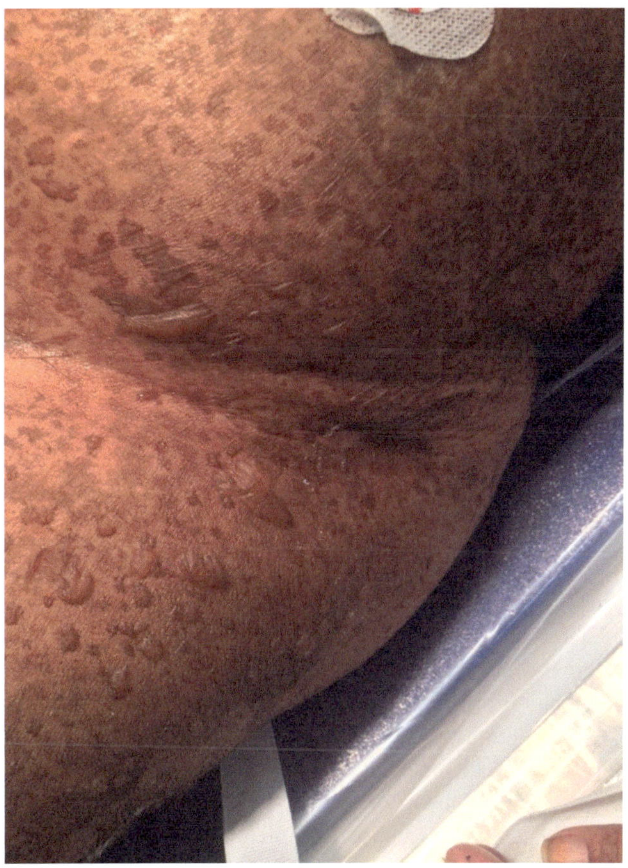

Fig. 43.1 Multiple coalescing dusky erythematous patches. Some of these patches have central purpura and or bullae

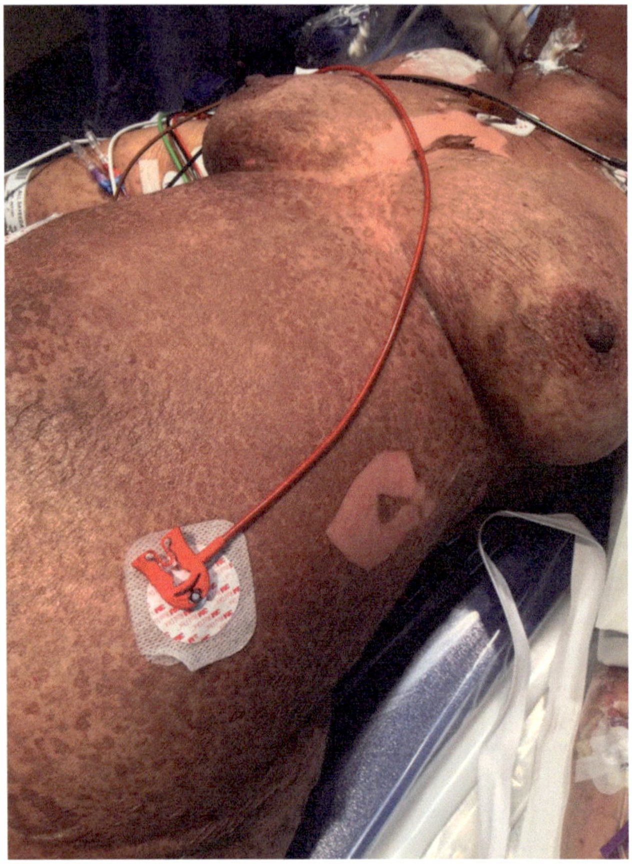

Fig. 43.2 Extensive large epidermal sheet detachment

large sheets of epidermis leaves exposed weepy denuded bleeding dermis and threat of infection, dehydration, hypothermia, and high cardiac output failure [23].

Erosive mucosal lesions are described in 97% of patients with the involvement of oral mucosa present in almost all patients, eyes in 75% and genital lesions in 50% [24]. Any mucosal surface could be affected, and consequently, stomatitis, conjunctivitis, adhesions, vision loss, urethritis, proctitis, vaginitis, tracheo-bronchitis, pneumonia, and enteritis will take place.

Epidermal detachment may progress for 7 days. Followed by re-epithelialization over 3 weeks. Mucosal re-epithelialization except oral mucosa may require several months to be completed. Unfortunately, healing can be imperfect, and patients suffer from the consequences of scarring including but not limited to symblepharon, ankyloblepharon, entropion, subsequent trichiasis, phimosis, and vaginal synechiae, cutaneous scarring, eruptive melanocytic nevi, nail dystrophy, and diffuse hair loss.

When admitting such a patient, the exact percentage of epidermal detachment should be documented accurately as it constitutes a major prognostic factor. Usually, epidermal necrolysis is overestimated; hence, clinicians should include detached and detachable patches without purely

Table 43.4 SCORTEN calculation and predicted mortality

Calculation	Age > 40 years Presence of malignancy Heart rate >120 beats/min Epidermal detachment >10% at admission Serum urea >10 mmol/L Serum glucose >14 mmol/L Bicarbonate <20 mmol/L
Number of parameters	Predicted mortality (%)
0	1
1	4
2	12
3	32
4	62
5	85
6	95
7	99

Adopted with modification from D. Creamer et al. [25]

erythematous patches. Extent of detachment helps define three categories of EN:

$$< 10\% : \text{SJS}$$

$$10 - 30\% : \text{SJS} - \text{TEN overlap}$$

$$> 30\% : \text{TEN}$$

Unfortunately, there are no clear criteria to predict which SJS patient will progress to TEN.

SCORTEN is a system used on day 0 and day 3 to predict mortality risk in TEN patients. It is calculated based on seven parameters: age, malignancy, heart rate more than 120, body surface area of more than 10% at admission, and certain blood chemistries (serum urea, bicarbonate, and glucose) (Table 43.4). Some studies have confirmed SCORTEN as an accurate predictor of TEN-related mortality [26, 27]. One third of TEN patients die with the most common cause of death is infection. The most common infective organism is *Staphylococcus aureus* followed by *Pseudomonas aeruginosa* after prolonged admission. Other causes of mortality include pulmonary embolism, respiratory distress syndrome, gastrointestinal hemorrhage, and multiorgan failure secondary to massive trans-epidermal fluid loss associated with electrolyte imbalance, inhibition of insulin secretion, insulin resistance, and onset of a hypercatabolic state.

43.5 Differential Diagnosis

Conditions that can mimic SJS/TEN include erythema multiforme, mycoplasma pneumoniae-induced rash and mucositis (MIRM), generalized fixed drug eruption, drug reaction with eosinophilia and systemic symptoms (DRESS), acute generalized exanthematous pustulosis (AGEP), linear IgA bullous disease, pemphigus vulgaris, paraneoplastic pemphigus,

TEN-like acute cutaneous lupus, TEN -like bullous Pemphigoid, staphylococcal scalded skin syndrome, Kawasaki disease, toxic erythema of chemotherapy, and acute graft versus host disease (GVHD). It is crucially important to involve dermatology as early as possible to confirm the diagnosis.

43.6 Approach

The diagnosis of SJS/TEN is based on three clinical elements: cutaneous and mucous membrane involvement and histological findings. Drug causality is best to be assessed using the Algorithm of Drug causality for epidermal necrolysis (ALDEN). This algorithm takes into consideration duration from drug intake to onset of rash, presence of drug in body on index day, rechallenge, dechallenge, and other alternative causes [28]. If EN is suspected, the most important initial step is discontinuing any potential culprit drug immediately. Studies have estimated that prompt withdrawal of any probable offending drug reduces the risk of death by 30% per day [29]. Patients must be assessed by a dermatologist as soon as possible and immediate processing of frozen cryostat section for confirmation of diagnosis (Table 43.5).

Table 43.5 Initial approach

Immediate discontinuation of any potential drug	Use ALDEN score to assess causality. Over the counter, herbal and alternative medication must be included as well
History	Detailed chronological order of medications and symptoms
Physical examination	Vital signs, extent of epidermal involvement, all mucosal membrane
Investigations	– CBC, CRP, liver function, electrolytes, serum urea nitrogen, creatinine, glucose level, bicarbonate, mycoplasma serology, HSV serology, DFA and chest X-ray – HLA typing patients' ethnicity – Multiple skin biopsies from most representative lesions, one of which should be a perilesional skin biopsy and sent for DIF – If prednisone, cyclosporine or etanercept was considered: add the following investigations: hepatitis B immune status, hepatitis C, HIV, quantiferon gold, uric acid, and pregnancy test – If IVIG is considered for the treatment, add the IgA level
Assessment of SCORTEN	Calculate the score at admission (day 0) and repeat in day 3
Assessment of multiorgan failure	Blood and wound cultures every 48 h Use sepsis score No need for prophylactic antibiotic Discontinue any existing antibiotic in the absence of documented infection
Urgent consultation	Ophthalmology ENT GYN/urology Pain management specialist

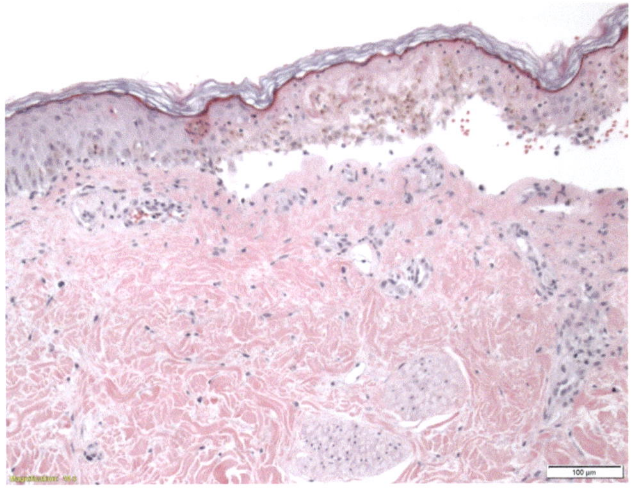

Fig. 43.3 Histopathological features of epidermal necrolysis. Partial intact epidermis transitioning to confluent epidermal necrosis with sloughing, subtle background interface dermatitis, and paucicellular lymphocytic infiltrate. Courtesy of *Shachar Sade, MD*

Histological findings depend on the age of the skin lesions. In early lesions, apoptotic keratinocytes are observed at basal and suprabasilar epidermal layers which correlate clinically with dusky erythematous macules. Later on, subepidermal blister with panepidermal necrosis is observed with sparse perivascular lymphocytic infiltrate (CD8+) and macrophages (Fig. 43.3). Patients should be shifted to intensive care unit for better observation and management. However, as epidermal detachment approaches 20%, transferring the patient to a burn unit with expertise in dealing with EN cases is preferable due to complexity of wound care and pain management. The most important point to keep in mind while managing EN patient is that it needs a multidisciplinary team approach and meticulous assessment and follow-up to improve prognosis as it is a rapidly progressive disease.

43.7 Management

43.7.1 Supportive Care

Supportive care is an essential primary step in managing this complex multisystemic disease which is similar to that performed for severe thermal burns, and it is aimed at limiting associated complications mentioned earlier. Ambient room temperature should be increased to 30–32 °C. Instead of regular bed and sheets, use of a controlled pressure, thermoregulated bed and an aluminum survival sheet is recommended. The patient should be handled in a sterile environment with the least manipulation possible as each and every movement is a potential trigger of epidermal detachment. Peripheral venous access should ideally be established in intact skin and should be changed every 48 h if possible. Initial fluid replacement is calculated by the formula

$$2\text{mL} / \text{kg} \times \text{percentage of body skin area skin detachment}$$

which is then titrated based on the patients' response to prevent organ hypoperfusion and shock [30]. The target point is to maintain mean arterial pressure >65 mmHg and urine output of 0.5–1 mL/kg/h. A urinary catheter is a good accurate tool to monitor urine out and assist fluid replacement. In case of urogenital involvement, it also helps managing micturition associated dysuria and retention. Cutaneous pain is very common in SJS/TEN especially at detached areas. Until now, there is no disease-specific evidence for pain management in SJS/TEN, and it is managed similarly to burn patients. Thus, pain management should be based upon patient's assessment at least once a day using a numerical scale and managed based on World Health Organization's (WHO) analgesic ladder [31]. Nonsteroidal anti-inflammatory drugs should be avoided because of the potential renal and gastric injury. Several pharmacological agents can be considered including nonopioid analgesics, anxiolytics, and anesthetics. Opioids such as morphine and fentanyl are the most commonly used agents for acute pain relief. Nonopioid analgesics (e.g., dexmedetomidine and ketamine) could also be considered for short period analgesia and sedation during debridement and/or dressing. Anxiolytic drugs such as benzodiazepines can be useful in premediating patients for wound care [32].

As patient will be bed bound for a prolonged time, thromboprophylaxis is a must unless contraindicated. In such a hypercatabolic state, feeding and accurate calorie intake is vital for patients' recovery, e.g., deliver up to 20–25 kcal/kg daily during the early, catabolic phase of SJS/TEN. During the anabolic, recovery phase, the aim should be to provide between 25 and 30 kcal/kg daily [25].

43.7.2 Dressing

As mentioned earlier, due to severe pain, handling skin should be done under conscious sedation, once daily with least manipulation possible. Although there is controversy between debridement and avoiding debridement, avoiding debridement is preferable to keep detached epidermis as a biological dressing and reduce the risk of infection. Despite all the similarities between burn injury and EN, injury in EN is from an endogenous versus an exogenous source in burn.

Bullae and larger vesicles should be aspirated followed by allowing roof to settle onto underlying dermis. Bland emollient such as soft paraffin should be applied generously to skin affected areas after cleaning with warm sterile isotonic sodium chloride solution. Denuded dermis exudes serum and hemorrhagic crust which serve a rich environment for microbial biofilms, which in turn will impair healing and predispose to systemic sepsis.

Topical antimicrobial ointment such as mupirocin or less preferably silver containing dressing/products due to potential risk of argyria when these products are applied over large body surface area.

Skin re-epithelialization start from adjacent intact hair follicles, which is impaired when large body surface area is affected. Hence, if TBSA >40%, use of skin substitute should be considered such as Biobrane (Smith & Nephew, London, UK, allograft, xenograft). The dressing over the graft should have some antimicrobial agent and changed every 1–3 days. Other option is silicon dressing which could be left in place till re-epithelialization occurs, but it needs to be cleansed every day.

Multiple swabs for bacterial and candidal from different sites particularly the sloughy or crusted areas must be taken every other day throughout the acute phase of SJS/TEN. Herpes activation should be considered when vesicular lesions become more painful or healing slows down particularly in genital and oral sites.

43.7.3 Special Care to Specific Mucosal Surfaces

43.7.3.1 Ocular

Ocular involvement in EN is evolved rapidly, and hence, ophthalmology should be involved urgently at initial assessment and followed up daily afterwards. Preservative-free artificial tears and ointment should be applied every 2 h. Removal of inflammatory debris and break down of conjunctival adhesion should be carried out by an ophthalmologist. Blind sweeping of fornices should be avoided as it might cause damage. Topical corticosteroid drops will reduce ocular surface damage in acute phase of SJS/TEN. Broad spectrum topical antibiotic prophylaxis is recommended in the presence of corneal fluorescein staining or frank ulceration. In patients with ocular epithelial loss, amniotic membrane transplant (AMT) can be used as research has shown that AMT could improve ocular outcome.

Patients with chronic eye involvement require lifelong follow-up for dryness, conjunctival inflammation, and ocular discomfort.

43.7.3.2 Oral

White oral soft paraffin should be applied to lips every 2 h. Mouth should be cleaned daily with warm sterile saline mouthwash and oral sponges to reduce fibrotic scar formation. Antiseptic oral rinse such as hydrogen peroxide or diluted 0.2% chlorhexidine mouthwash should be used twice to reduce bacterial colonization. Better local pain management can be achieved by using viscous lidocaine application or similar products. Topical corticosteroid should be applied four times a day. If there is profound bleeding, topical epinephrine or tranexamic acid can be used.

Long-term squeal of oral involvement can appear as sicca syndrome secondary to salivary gland involvement or intra-oral scarring which may result in difficulty in speaking or eating.

43.7.3.3 Genital

Early assessment by a gynecologist is a must for full vaginal examination and prevention of scarring. White soft paraffin should be reapplied every 2–4 h. A clinician should have a low threshold for diagnosing infection such as bacterial or yeast infection or herpes reactivation. A dilator/tampon warped in Mepitel and catheter should be inserted into vagina and urethra, respectively, to prevent syncchiae formation which will result in long-term sexual and urethral dysfunction. A potent topical steroid "Clobetasol propionate ointment"can be applied once on the involved uneroded surfaces.

43.7.4 Sepsis Detection and Management

Clinical presentation of SJS/TEN could include fever, neutrophilia/neutropenia as well as elevated inflammatory markers (ESR and CRP), which makes diagnosis of sepsis as trickier. Hence, patient should be observed for clinical signs of systemic infection such as confusion, hypotension, reduced oxygen saturation, reduced urinary output, and most importantly positive bacterial culture from blood, urine, or sputum. TEN/DRESS overlap syndrome must be considered as it mimics sepsis in the absence of positive microbial culture. Indiscriminate prophylactic systemic antibiotic may increase cutaneous colonization in particular with *Candida albicans*; therefore, antibiotics should be restricted for patients with confirmed infection.

43.7.5 Medications

Recently a randomized controlled study concluded by Chuang WW et al. was published. This study compared the efficacy of TNA-α inhibitor etanercept versus systemic corticosteroids [22]. Etanercept improved SCORTEN-based predicted mortality rate (17.7% and 8.3%, respectively). Etanercept should be given at 50 mg upon arrival as soon as possible on day 0. Based on patient evolution, a second dose can be given on day 4 [3].

A study by Valeyrie-Allanore et al. compared SCORTEN-predicted mortality between 29 patients received cyclosporine and six patients treated with systemic steroids and demonstrated a benefit of cyclosporine over corticosteroids [26]. A concomitant intravenous administration of cyclosporine at a dose of 5 mg/kg/day is divided into twice daily for 10 days. Followed by switching to oral dosing once re-epithelialization is started, oral intake is possible and tapering over 30 days.

If cyclosporine was contraindicated due to renal impairment or if there were suggesting clinical features of DRESS syndrome or TEN/DRESS overlap such as fever, eosinophilia, facial edema, adenopathy, or atypical lymphocytes, a short course of intravenous corticosteroid (methylprednisolone) serves a good alternative therapeutic option. Solumedrol 125–250 mg can be given intravenously twice a day for 3 days and then tapered over 7 days.

Intravenous immunoglobulin (IVIG) is still popular in many centers in North America. However, there is no high-quality evidence to support the use of IVIG in EN.

43.7.6 Discharge and Follow-Up

Before discharge, patients must be provided with information about culprit drug and cross reactors and the need for strict avoidance as re-exposure might be fatal. Drug sensitivity must be documented in patient's chart and a detailed letter should be sent to the patient's family doctor. SJS awareness and support group can be accessed by patients (http://www.sjscanada.org/).

Psychological disorders including depression and anxiety are common among survivors [33]. In fact, psychological impact has been compared to that of posttraumatic stress disorder [34]. Dodiuk-Gad et al. conducted a cohort study that included 17 survivors post EN to assess long-term psychological complications of this disease using psychometric, validated scales [35]. She found that 65% of participants had symptoms of posttraumatic stress, 29% had total scores in keeping with clinical signs of possible posttrauma stress disorder and 71% had scores indicating clinically significant psychological distress.

EN patients suffer from long-term multisystemic complications. The most common complications are post-inflammatory dyschromia, cutaneous scars, dry eyes, symblepharon, and chronic ocular surface inflammation [36]. Other complications included chronic fatigue and pruritus. Thus, follow-up in dermatology, ophthalmology, and gynecology/urology is mandatory to monitor and manage chronic complications.

Patch testing can be used to confirm the identification of culprit medication. Despite its low sensitivity, it is a much safer alternative to intradermal injection or re-challenge test. If a genetic predisposition is identified in the patient for allopurinol, phenytoin, or carbamazepine, counseling should be provided for family members to undergo specific HLA typing. Moreover, in genetically susceptible group, HLA typing should be ordered prior to initiating a high-risk medication.

Summary Box

TEN is a complex and challenging disease process that requires attention to detail in terms of not only care but also the cause of the disease. A positive biopsy is an essential part of admission to a center specialized in treating TEN and should be conducted as soon as TEN is suspected. Treatment is geared toward organ support and induction of wound healing while eyes and genitals are being protected. Immunosuppression and blockade of the hyperinflammatory autoimmune response are integral part of therapy. Once wounds are closing, the likelihood of surviving is high. TEN usually does not heal as a scar, and follow-up is more focused on eyes, genitals, mental health, and prevention.

References

1. Roujeau J-C. Epidermal necrolysis (Stevens Johnson syndrome and toxic epidermal necrolysis): historical considerations. Dermatol Sin. 2013;31(4):169–74.
2. Bastuji-Garin S, Rzany B, Stern RS, Shear NH, Naldi L, Roujeau J-C. A clinical classification of cases of toxic epidermal necrolysis, Stevens-Johnson syndrome and erythema multiforme. Arch Dermatol. 1993;129:92–6.
3. Mereniuk A, Jaque A, Jeschke M, Shear NH. Toxic epidermal necrolysis spectrum management at Sunnybrook Health Sciences Centre: our multidisciplinary approach after review of the current evidence. J Cutan Med Surg. 2018;22(2):213–9.
4. Hsu DY, et al. Pediatric Stevens-Johnson syndrome and toxic epidermal necrolysis in the United States. J Am Acad Dermatol. 2017;76(5):811–7.
5. Su SC, Mockenhaupt M, Wolkenstein P, et al. Interleukin-15 is associated with severity and mortality in Stevens-Johnson syndrome/toxic epidermal necrolysis. J Invest Dermatol. 2017;137(5):1065–73.
6. Chung WH, Wang CW, Dao RL. Severe cutaneous adverse drug reactions. J Dermatol. 2016;43(7):758–66.
7. Hsu DY, Brieva J, Silverberg NB, Silverberg JI. Morbidity and mortality of Stevens-Johnson syndrome and toxic epidermal necrolysis in United States adults. J Invest Dermatol. 2016;136(7):1387–97.
8. Frey N, Jossi J, Bodmer M, et al. The epidemiology of Stevens-Johnson syndrome and toxic epidermal necrolysis in the UK. J Invest Dermatol. 2017;137(6):1240–7.
9. Chin CB, et al. An updated review of the molecular mechanisms in drug hypersensitivity. J Immunol Res. 2018;2018:6431694.
10. Auquier-Dunant A, Mockenhaupt M, Naldi L, et al. Correlations between clinical patterns and causes of erythema multiforme majus, Stevens-Johnson syndrome, and toxic epidermal necrolysis—results of an international prospective study. Arch Dermatol. 2002;138(8):1019–24.
11. Yildirim Cetin G, Sayar H, Ozkan F, Kurtulus S, Kesici F, Sayarlioglu M. A case of toxic epidermal necrolysis like skin lesions with systemic lupus erythematosus and review of the literature. Lupus. 2013;22(8):839–46.
12. Olson D, Watkins LK, Demirjian A, et al. Outbreak of mycoplasma pneumoniae associated Stevens-Johnson syndrome. Pediatrics. 2015;136(2):386–94.
13. Chung WH, Shih SR, Chang CF, et al. Clinicopathologic analysis of coxsackievirus a6 new variant induced widespread mucocutaneous bullous reactions mimicking severe cutaneous adverse reactions. J Infect Dis. 2013;208(12):1968–78.
14. Mockenhaupt M, Viboud C, Dunant N, Naidi L, Halevy S, Bouwes Bavinck JN, et al. Stevens–Johnson syndrome and toxic epidermal necrolysis: assessment of medication risks with emphasis on recently marketed drugs. The EuroSCAR-study. J Invest Dermatol. 2007;128(1):35–44.
15. Dika E, Ravaioli GM, Fanti PA, et al. Cutaneous adverse effects during ipilimumab treatment for metastatic melanoma: a prospective study. Eur J Dermatol. 2017;27(3):266–70.
16. Vivar KL, Deschaine M, Messina J, et al. Epidermal programmed cell death-ligand 1 expression in TEN associated with nivolumab therapy. J Cutan Pathol. 2017;44(4):381–4.
17. Viard-Leveugle I, Gaide O, et al. TNF-α and IFN-γ are potential inducers of Fas-mediated keratinocyte apoptosis through activation of inducible nitric oxide synthase in toxic epidermal necrolysis. J Invest Dermatol. 2013;133(2):489–98.
18. Posadas SJ, Padial A, Torres MJ, et al. Delayed reactions to drugs show levels of perforin, granzyme B, and Fas-L to be related to disease severity. J Allergy Clin Immunol. 2002;109(1):155–61.
19. Nassif A, Bensussan A, Dorothee G, et al. Drug specific cytotoxic T-cells in the skin lesions of a patient with toxic epidermal necrolysis. J Invest Dermatol. 2002;118(4):728–33.
20. Voskoboinik I, Whisstock JC, Trapani JA. Perforin and granzymes: function, dysfunction and human pathology. Nat Rev Immunol. 2015;15(6):388–400.
21. Chung WH, Hung SI, Yang JY, et al. Granulysin is a key mediator for disseminated keratinocyte death in Stevens-Johnson syndrome and toxic epidermal necrolysis. Nat Med. 2008;14(12):1343–50.
22. Wang C-W, Yang L-Y, et al. Randomized, controlled trial of TNF-α antagonist in CTL-mediated severe cutaneous adverse reactions. J Clin Invest. 2018;128(3):985–96.
23. Papp A, Sikora S, Evans M, Song D, Kirchhof M, Miliszewski M, Dutz J. Treatment of toxic epidermal necrolysis by a multidisciplinary team. A review of literature and treatment results. Burns. 2018;44(4):807–15.. S0305-4179(17)30590–9
24. Boorboor P, Vogt PM, Bechara FG, Alkandari Q, Aust M, Gohritz A, et al. Toxic epidermal necrolysis: use of Biobrane1 for skin coverage reduces pain, improves mobilization and decreases infection in elderly patients. Burns. 2008;34(4):487–92.
25. Creamer D, Walsh SA, et al. U.K. guidelines for the management of Stevens–Johnson syndrome/toxic epidermal necrolysis in adults 2016. Br J Dermatol. 2016;174(6):1194–227.
26. Valeyrie-Allanore L, Wolkenstein P, Brochard L, et al. Open trial of ciclosporin treatment for Stevens-Johnson syndrome and toxic epidermal necrolysis. Br J Dermatol. 2010;163:847–53.
27. Firoz BF, Henning JS, Zarzabal LA, Pollock BH. Toxic epidermal necrolysis: five years of treatment experience from a burn unit. J Am Acad Dermatol. 2012;67:630–5.
28. Sassolas B, Haddad C, Mockenhaupt M, et al. ALDEN, an algorithm for assessment of drug causality in Stevens-Johnson syndrome and toxic epidermal necrolysis: comparison with case-control analysis. Clin Pharmacol Ther. 2010;88(1):60–8.
29. Garcia-Doval I, LeCleach L, Bocquet H, et al. Toxic epidermal necrolysis and Stevens-Johnson syndrome: does early withdrawal of causative drugs decrease the risk of death? Arch Dermatol. 2000;136:323–7.
30. Shiga S, Cartotto R. What are the fluid requirements in toxic epidermal necrolysis? J Burn Care Res. 2010;31(1):100–4.
31. World Health Organization. WHO's pain relief ladder. 2009. http://www.who.int/cancer/palliative/painladder/en/.
32. Mendoza A, Santoyo FL, Agulló A, Fenández-Cañamaque JL, Vivó C. The management of pain associated with wound care in severe burn patients in Spain. Int J Burns Trauma. 2016;6(1):1–10.

33. Butt TF, Cox AR, Lewis H, et al. Patient experiences of serious adverse drug reactions and their attitudes to medicines: a qualitative study of survivors of Stevens-Johnson syndrome and toxic epidermal necrolysis in the UK. Drug Saf. 2011;34:319–28.
34. Dodiuk-Gad RP, Olteanu C. Major emotional and physical complications among survivors of Stevens-Johnson syndrome and toxic epidermal necrolysis. J Am Acad Dermatol. 2016;74(5):AB61.
35. Dodiuk-Gad RP, Olteanu C, Feinstein A, Hashimoto R, Alhusayen R, Whyte-Croasdaile S, Finkelstein Y, Burnett M, Sade S, Cartotto R, Jeschke M, Shear NH. Major psychological complications and decreased health-related quality of life among survivors of Stevens-Johnson syndrome and toxic epidermal necrolysis. Br J Dermatol. 2016;175(2):422–4.
36. Olteanu C, Shear NH, Chew HF, Hashimoto R, Alhusayen R, Whyte-Croasdaile S, Finkelstein Y, Burnett M, Ziv M, Sade S, Jeschke MG, Dodiuk-Gad RP. Severe physical complications among survivors of Stevens-Johnson syndrome and toxic epidermal necrolysis. Drug Saf. 2018;41(3):277–84.

Part VI

Challenging Burn Cases Examples

44 Burn Reconstruction: The Role of Integra in the Dorsum Hand and Wrist Reconstruction

Anthony Papp

A male in his 60s sustained flame burns to the dorsum of both hands and wrist. Initially, the burn injuries were treated accordingly with early excision and STSG (split thickness skin graft).

He developed chronic folliculitis on the dorsum of his hands, along with inability to flex metacarpo-phalangeal joints due to scar tightness on the dorsum of the hand (Fig. 44.1).

Decision was taken to completely excise all the scarred tissue and previous skin grafts and reconstruct with Integra as dermal substitute (Fig. 44.2). Skin grafting was performed as part of the second-stage Integra application 3 weeks later (Fig. 44.3).

After the reconstruction with Integra, the patient was able to make a full fist (Fig. 44.4).

The long-term follow-up has shown a good pliability of the area reconstructed with Integra and the gain of full range of movement in both hands (Fig. 44.5).

A. Papp (✉)
Vancouver General Hospital, Vancouver, BC, Canada

M. G. Jeschke et al. (eds.), *Handbook of Burns Volume 1*, https://doi.org/10.1007/978-3-030-18940-2_44

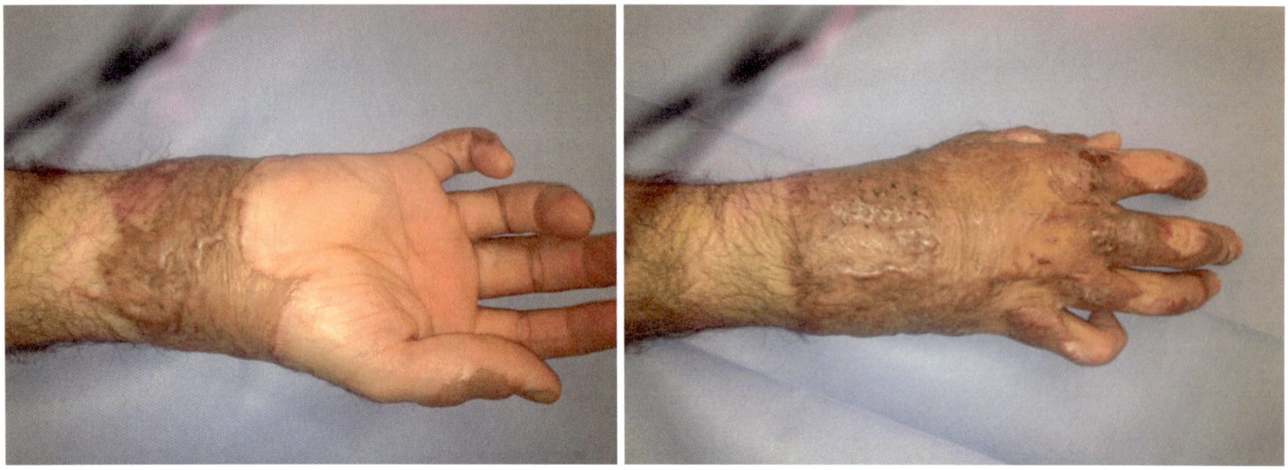

Fig. 44.1 Folliculitis, both dorsum hands

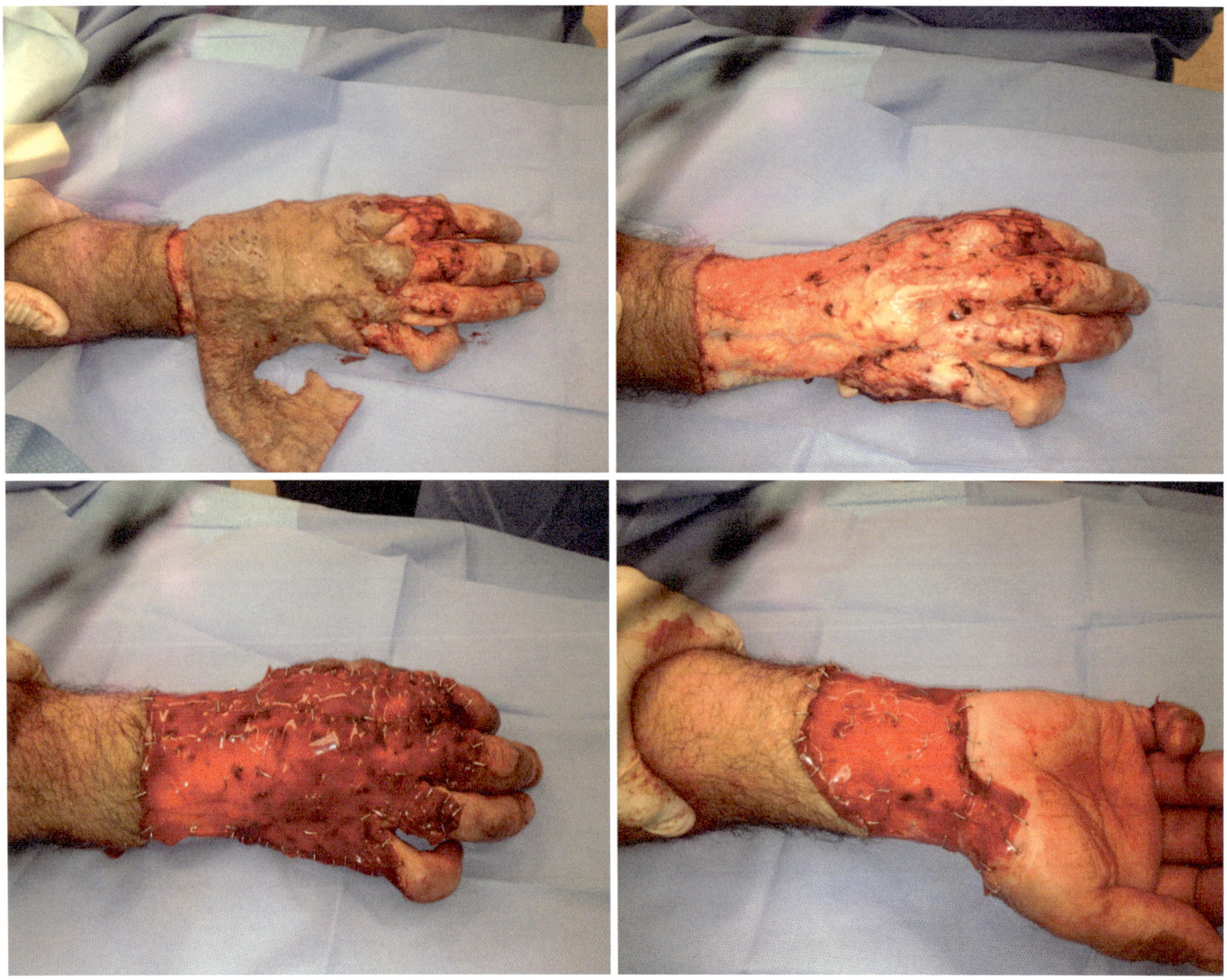

Fig. 44.2 Excision scar tissue and Integra application

Fig. 44.3 Integra application and skin graft to dorsum both hands

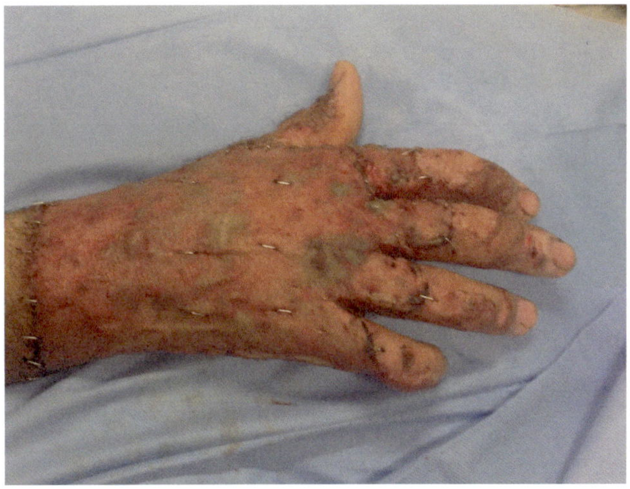

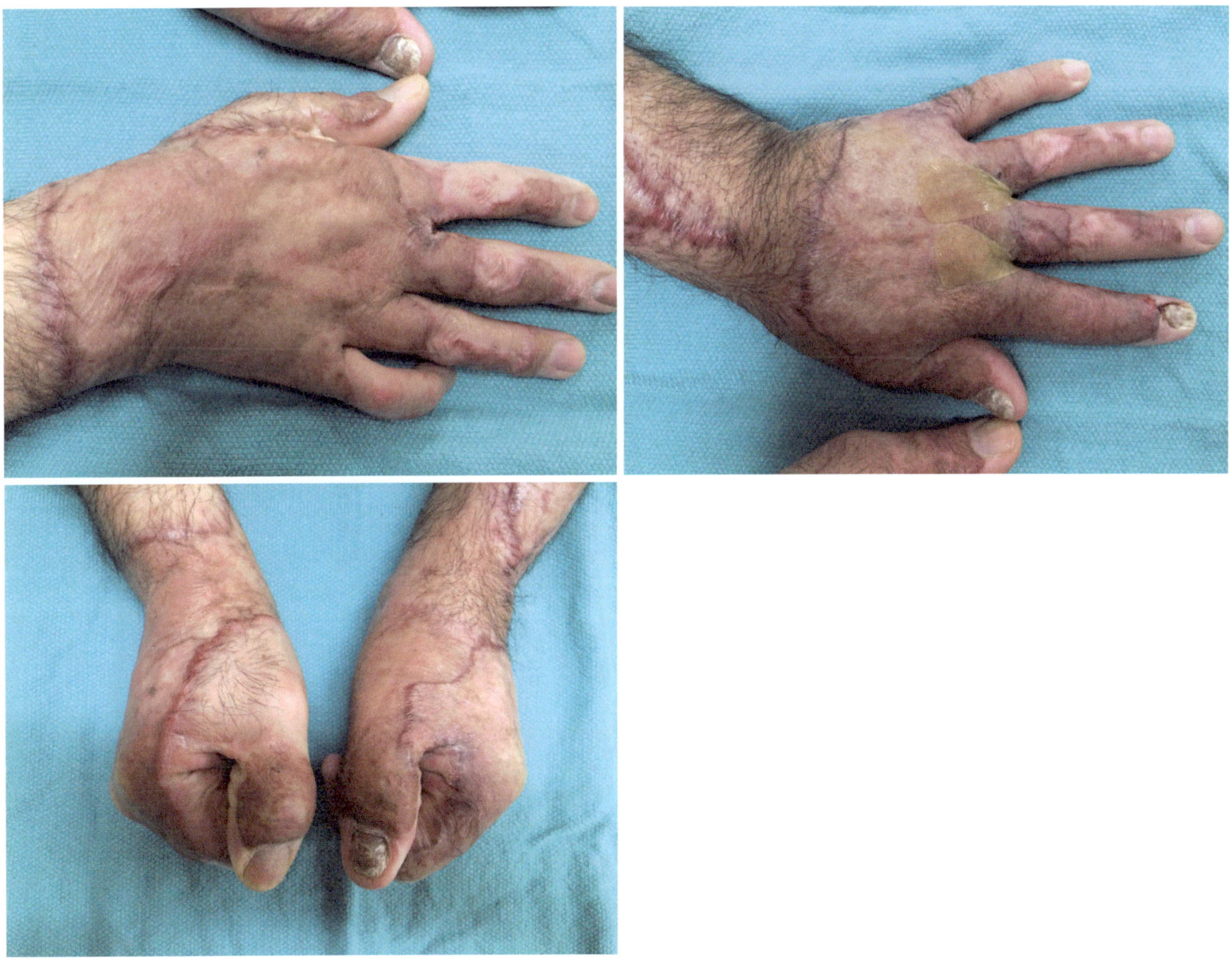

Fig. 44.4 Early results of Integra application

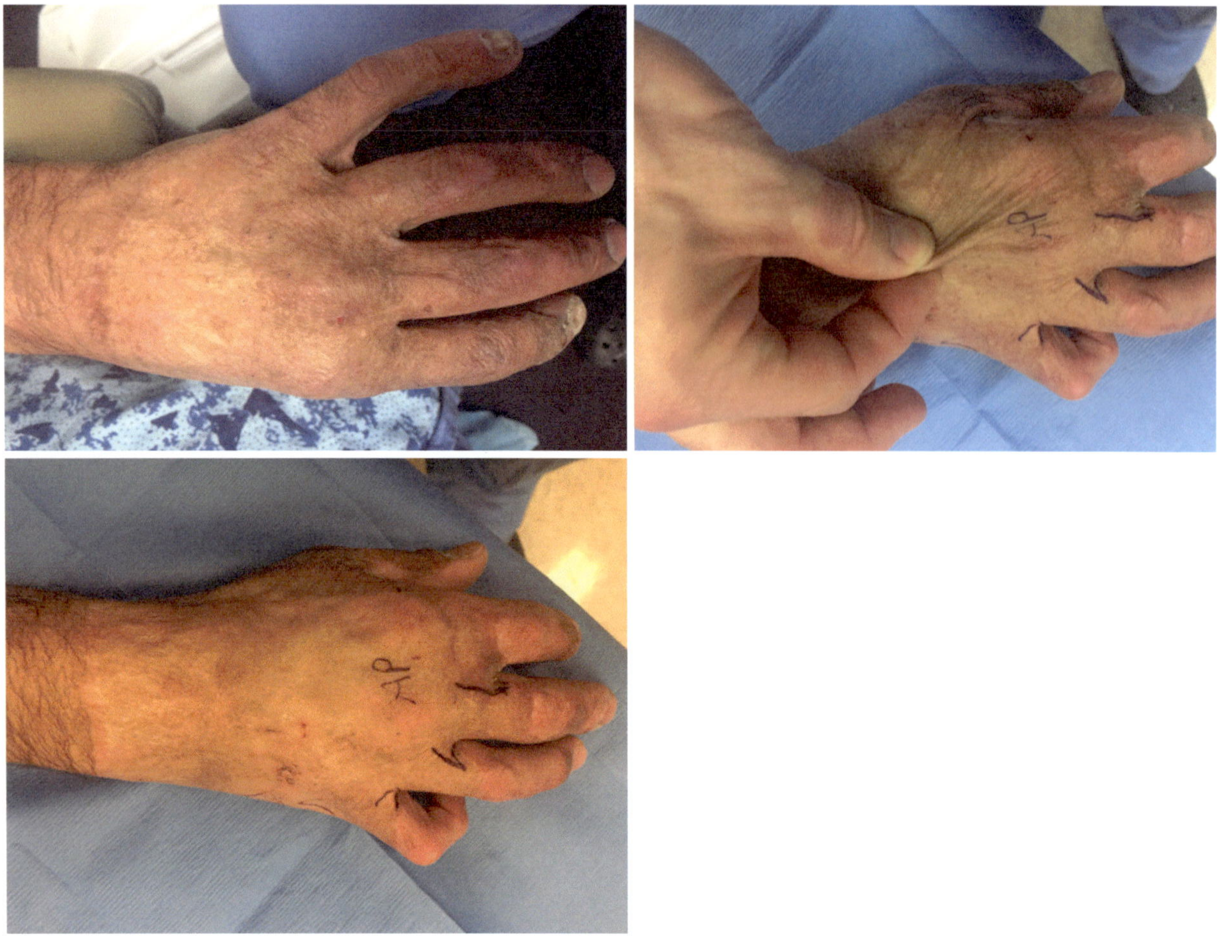

Fig. 44.5 Long-term results of Integra application

45 Innovative Autologous Coverage for a 90% TBSA Full-Thickness Burns

Isabelle Perreault and Patricia Bortoluzzi

This young patient of 10 years of age sustained an extensive full-thickness burn injury when his pyjamas caught on fire. He presented with a 90% full-thickness burn and a Grade 2 moderate inhalation injury without any concomitant trauma. Unaffected areas were the right scalp, right upper and mid-face, and feet. ABSI burn outcome prediction score was 12 with a predicted mortality rate of ≥80%. The mortality rate as per reported in the NBR for a population of similar age (5–15, 9 years) and %TBSA (≥90% TBSA) was 68% [1, 2].

The patient was transferred to the ICU for initial fluid resuscitation and critical care management according to our institution standardized burn protocols. Multiple escharotomies were done upon admission. The patient received 6, 56 mL/kg/%TBSA of fluid resuscitation during the initial 24 h after injury, maintained urine outputs above 1 mL/kg/h and maintained good hemodynamic stability as demonstrated by extended hemodynamic monitoring during burn shock resuscitation. Early debridement of this very deep burn injury down to the fascia was completed in 5 days. Allografts were used for temporary coverage.

The main challenge with this case was autologous coverage. The ultimate goals of the treatment plan were survival and prevention of significant scarring and donor site morbidity to assure this young patient's future quality of life. Usual treatment options involve multiple and repeated very thin STSG harvesting at the few available donor sites (scalp and feet). In this case, donor site availabilities were extremely limited and located in cosmetic and functional body areas, where repeated harvesting would, if at all feasible, create significant sequelae. Innovative burn wound treatment was paramount for this particular patient [3, 4].

Given the extent to the surface area of the burn, all autologous reconstituted options for coverage were explored in order to expedite definitive coverage [5–7]. Hence, both ADM with CEA and a bi-layer autologous self-assembled skin substitutes (SASSs) (LOEX Tissue Engineering Laboratory, Quebec City, Canada) were used [8, 9]. This latter substitute is available through Health Canada's Special Access Program, which allows extensive burn injuries to be acutely treated with SASSs. This autologous skin substitute is a construct from keratinocytes and fibroblast cultures, allowing the replacement of both dermis and epidermis in a single surgical procedure, using a 5 cm^2 biopsy of native skin. The main drawbacks of SASSs are pigmentation flaws precluding its use in aesthetic areas and the required production time of several weeks.

Early autograft coverage of some instrumentation areas, as well as dorsum of hands, face, and neck (PBD 4), was done with thick split thickness autologous scalp skin grafts. Palmar aspects of hands were reconstructed using plantar and dorsal aspect of the feet as donor. Because the cultured epithelial cells took less production time relative to SASS, CEA coverage was first initiated. In preparation for CEAs, the anterior and posterior trunk was first covered with ADM (Integra) meshed in a 1 to 1 ratio (PBD 8). The Integra did not show any signs of infection and revascularized appropriately. Two weeks later, cultured epithelial cells (CEA) were put in place to substitute the silicone membrane. Between 7 and 12 POD, patches of the construct showed unstable epithelial coverage in some areas. Despite appropriate wound care and a second procedure with CEA grafting, those areas did not heal and required thin STSG harvested on feet, in conjunction with SASSs.

Once the SASSs where available, knowing their heightened capacity for minimal hypertrophic scarring and contractures, they were used to reconstruct the remaining functional areas. These bilayer substitutes where placed on the upper and lower limbs, excluding posterior axilla, hands, and groins at the eighth week postburn. Five procedures with an interval of 1 week between each were required for this autologous substitute covering 29% TBSA. This bilayer substitute demonstrated a constant engraftment rate with no graft loss and no wound infection.

I. Perreault (✉) · P. Bortoluzzi
Sainte-Justine Mother and Child University Hospital Center at University of Montreal, Montreal, QC, Canada

M. G. Jeschke et al. (eds.), *Handbook of Burns Volume 1*, https://doi.org/10.1007/978-3-030-18940-2_45

The patient survived this massive burn injury with a good quality of life. SASS showed a permanent stable coverage throughout time, and a biopsy done 1 year later showed similar histology to native skin. Interestingly, contractures were documented in the sites of previous split thickness skin grafts and ADM, but no contractures occurred with the bilayer skin substitute. Later, SASSs were used for reconstructive purposes as an interpositional skin graft when doing a scar releasing surgery with good long-term results and no recurrence of contracture.

Fig. 45.1 Patient at admission, presenting a 90% TBSA full-thickness burn injury

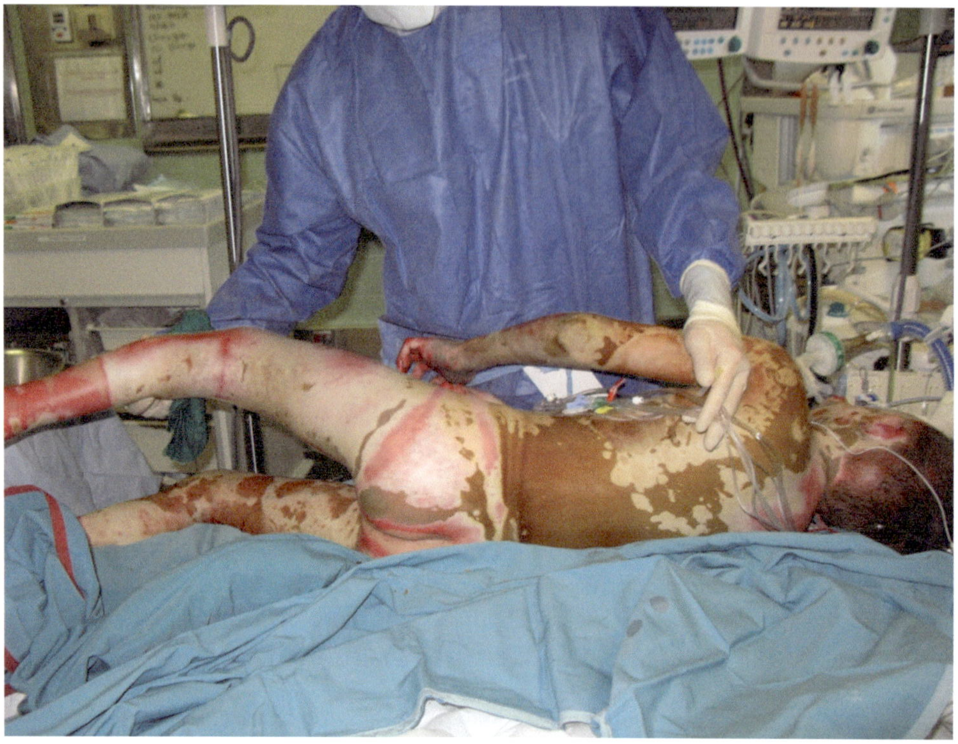

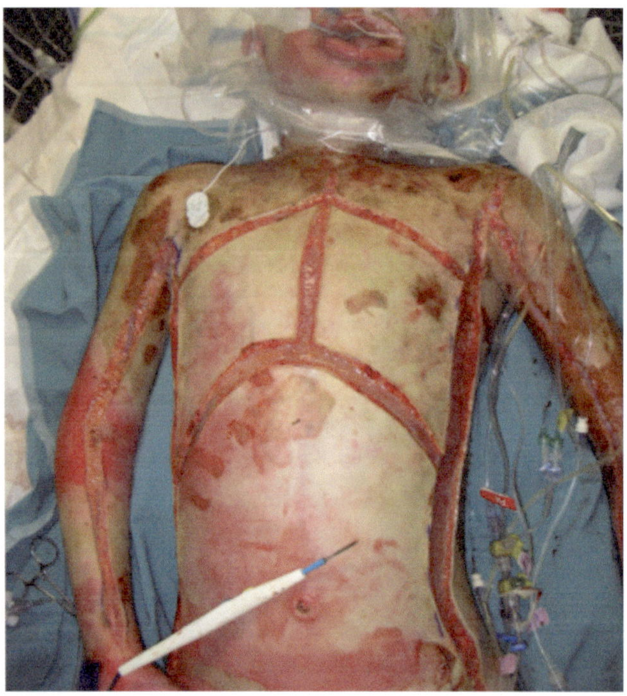

Fig. 45.2 Multiple escharotomies were done upon admission

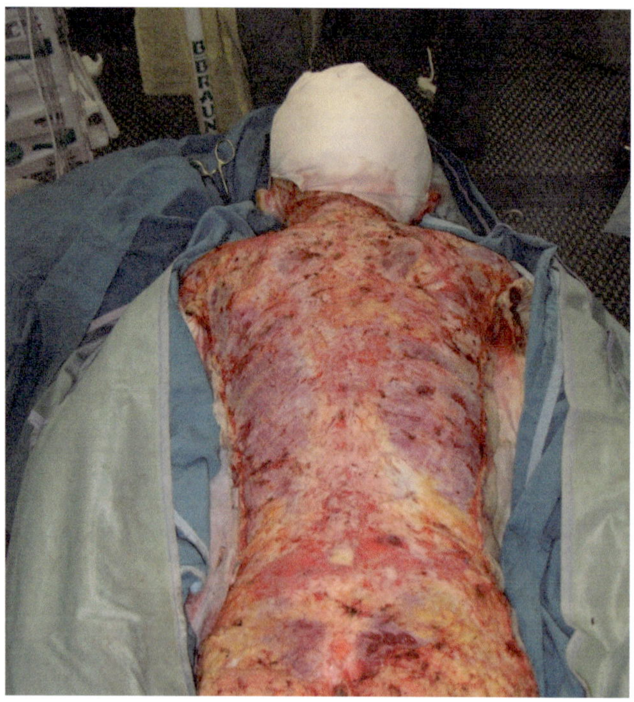

Fig. 45.3 Early debridement of this very deep burn injury down to the fascia

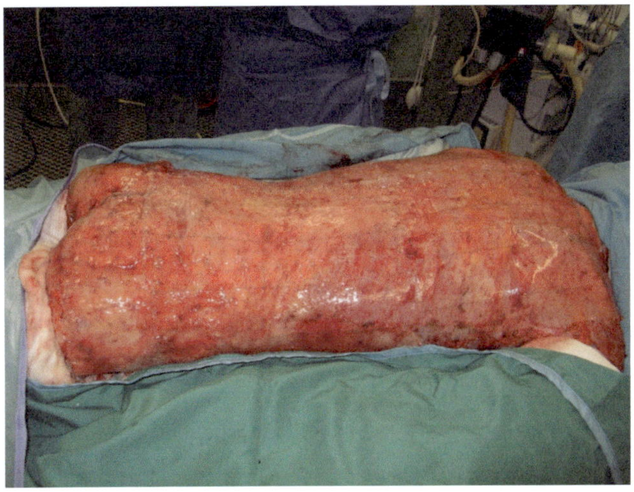

Fig. 45.4 Posterior trunk was first covered with ADM (Integra) meshed in a 1 to 1 ratio (PBD 8)

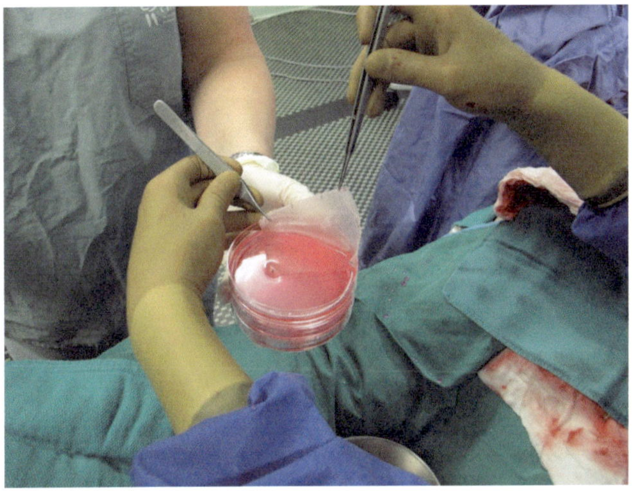

Fig. 45.5 CEA

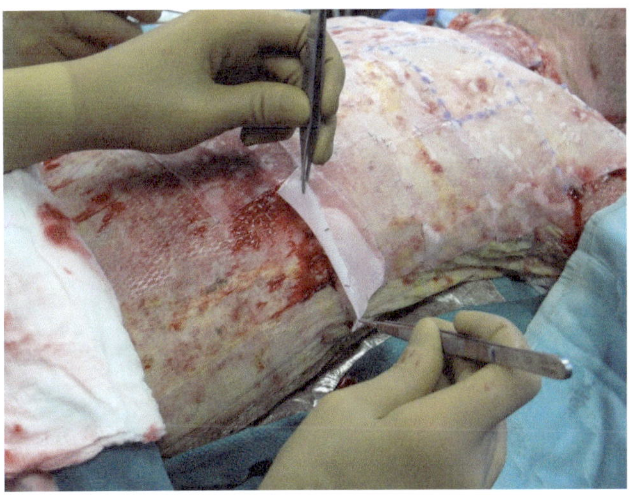

Fig. 45.6 Cultured epithelial cells (CEA) were put in place to substitute the silicone membrane (PBD22)

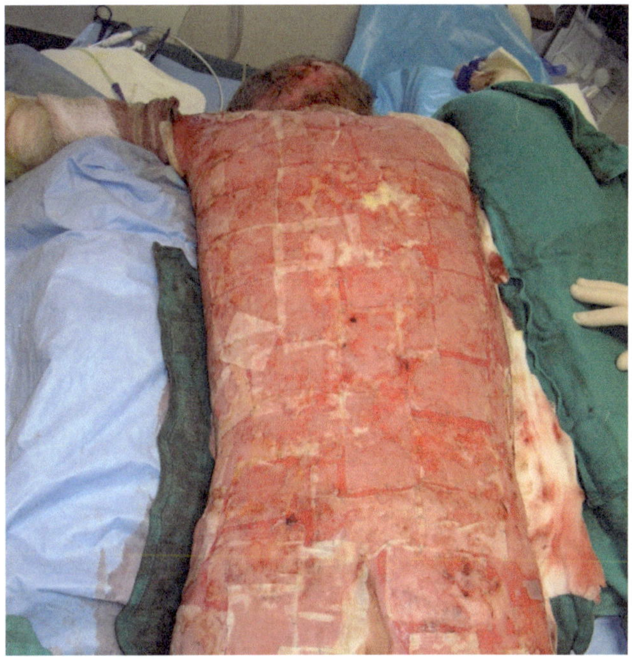

Fig. 45.7 Patches of the ADM-CEA construct showed unstable epithelial coverage in some areas

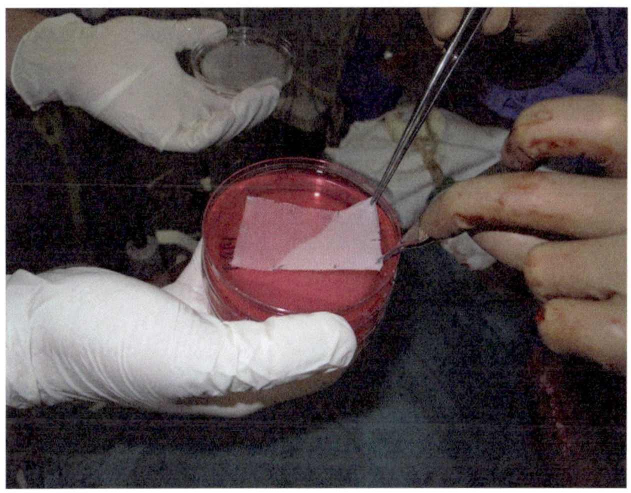

Fig. 45.8 SASSs

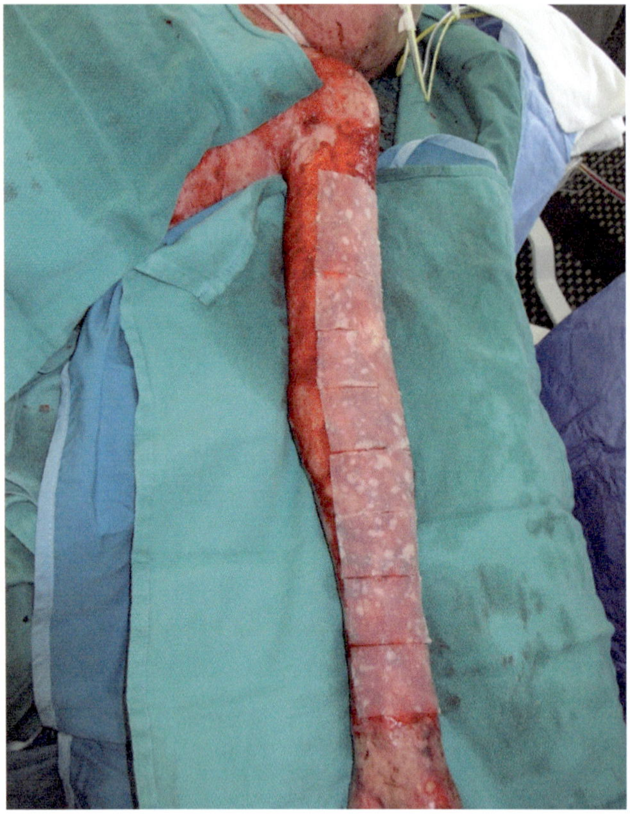

Fig. 45.9 SASSs applied on the debrided burn wound

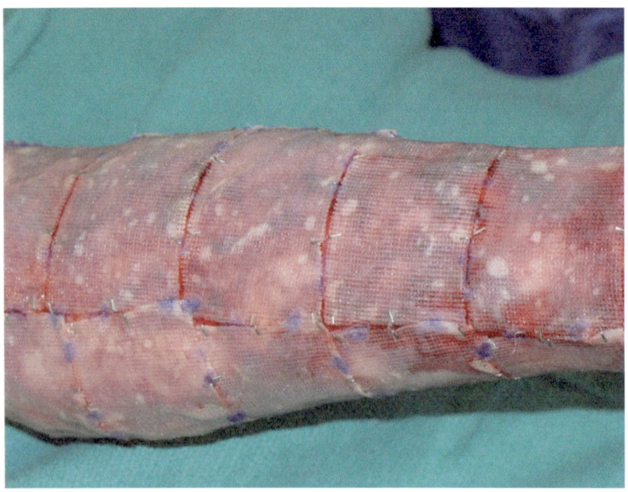

Fig. 45.10 Fixation of the SASSs

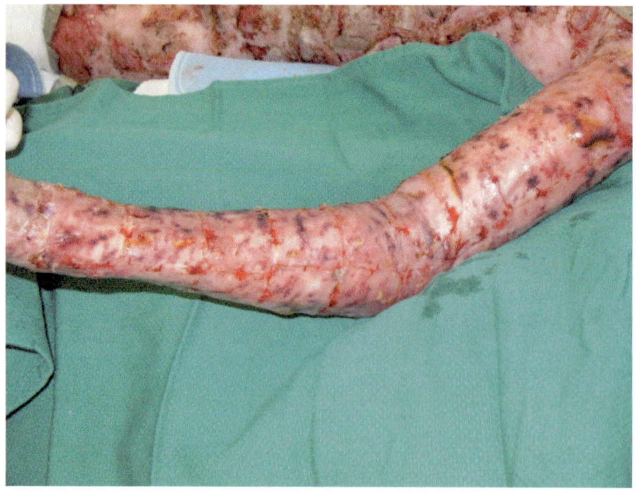

Fig. 45.11 SASSs grafted to the left upper limb after 1 week (POD 7)

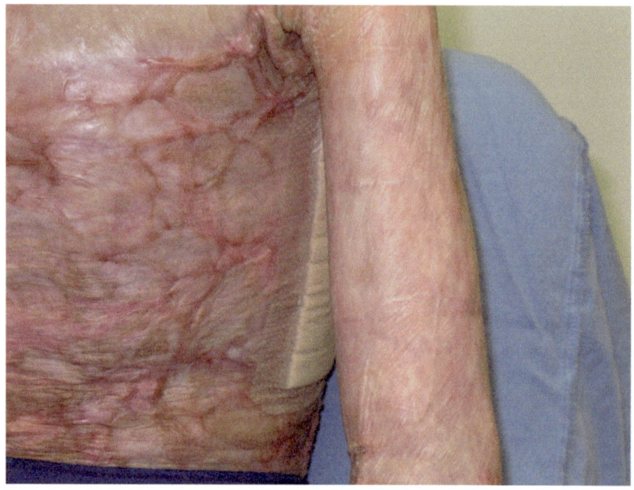

Fig. 45.12 Comparison of the trunk grafted with STSG and left upper limb grafted with SASSs

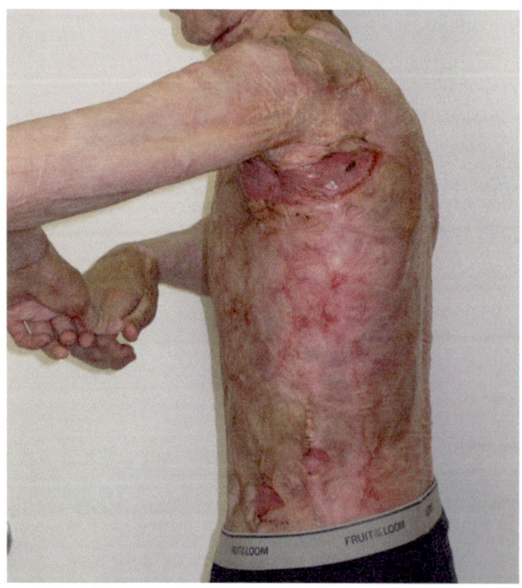

Fig. 45.13 SASSs used as an interpositional skin graft when doing a scar releasing surgery of the left axilla

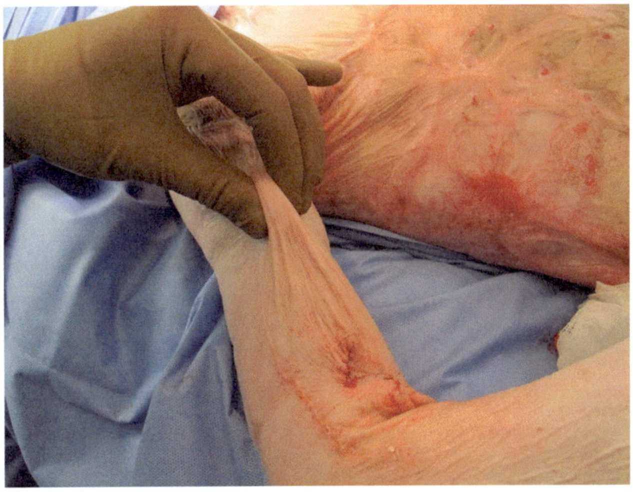

Fig. 45.14 Skin of the left upper limb reconstructed with SASSs showing good elasticity

Acknowledgments Dr. Lucie Germain PhD, Dr. Véronique Moulin PhD, Dr. François Auger, LOEX Tissue Engineering Laboratory, Quebec City, Canada.

References

1. Kraft R, Herndon DN, Al-Mousawi AM, Williams FN, Finnerty CC, Jeschke MG. Burn size and survival probability in paediatric patients in modern burn care: a prospective observational cohort study. Lancet. 2012;379:1013–21.
2. 2016 National Burn Repository. Report of data from 2006-2015. Version 12.0. Chicago: American Burn Association; 2016.
3. Finnerty CC, Jeschke MG, Branski LK, Dziewulski P, Herndon DN. Hypertrophic scarring: the greatest unmet challenge after burn injury. Lancet. 2016;388:1427–36.
4. Varkey M, Ding J, Tredget EE. Advances in skin substitutes potential of tissue engineered skin for facilitating anti-fibrotic healing. J Funct Biomater. 2015;6(3):547–63.
5. Boyce ST, Kagan RJ, Meyer NA, Yakuboff KP, Warden GD. Cultured skin substitutes combined with Integra artificial skin to replace native skin autograft and allograft for the closure of excised full-thickness burns. J Burn Care Rehabil. 1999;20:453–61.
6. Boyce ST, Kagan RJ, Yakuboff KP, et al. Cultured skin substitutes reduce donor skin harvesting for closure of excised, full-thickness burns. Ann Surg. 2002;235:269–79.
7. Boyce ST, Kagan RJ, Greenhalgh DG, et al. Cultured skin substitutes reduce requirements for harvesting of skin autograft for closure of excised, full-thickness burns. J Trauma. 2006;60:821–9.
8. Larouche D, Cantin-Warren L, Desgagne M, Guignard R, Martel I, Ayoub A, et al. Improved methods to produce tissue-engineered skin substitutes suitable for the permanent closure of full-thickness skin injuries. Biores Open Access. 2016;5(1):320–9.
9. Lavoie A, Fugere C, Beauparlant A, Goyer B, Larouche D, Paquet C, et al. Human epithelial stem cells persist within tissue-engineered skin produced by the self-assembly approach. Tissue Eng Part A. 2013;19(7-8):1023–38.

Delayed Management of Acute Burn Wounds in Rural Areas of Low-Income Countries: Global Burn Surgery

46

Claudia C. Malic

Inadequate acute management of burn injuries (debridement, skin grafting, physiotherapy, long-term splinting, and scar management) is the main source of morbidity, leading to burn contractures and significant functional deficit.

The inadequate management is multifactorial, but it could be the result of insufficient or lack of local resources with burn expertise, the socioeconomic status of the patient, with direct impact on the access to specialized care.

Burn contractures in the head and neck areas as well as around major joints could have significant impact on patients' life and their close family.

During the surgical camps in the low-income countries, burn contractures could represent a significant load of the cases. With minimal resources, but with a close follow-up, some of the burn contractures could be managed with a small armamentarium of surgical skills: thick split thickness graft, Z plasty and variants, local advancement, or transpositional flaps.

Here are some examples of burn contracture management of such situations:

46.1 Patient 1: Long-Term Lower Face and Neck Contracture

During one of our surgical camp at Deendayal Research Institute and Arogyadam, Chitrakoot, India, an 18-year-old male patient presented with significant contracture of distal third of the face, as well as the neck (Fig. 46.1a–c). He sustained a flame burn injury at age 10 and was treated conservatively. He had difficulties eating and drinking due to lower lip incontinence. Due to its pull on the lower lip, the teeth were affected as well (Fig. 46.1).

Under general anesthesia, the burn contractures were released at the base of the neck contracture. When released, the soft tissues above incision managed to cover the lower face till marginal mandibular area. A thicker split thickness skin graft was applied on the anterior aspect of the neck and in the submental area. Quilting was required, and grafts were checked at 1 week (Fig. 46.2). Some epidermolysis and around 20% of the skin graft were lost after surgery. Regular dressings were carried out, and no further surgical intervention was required.

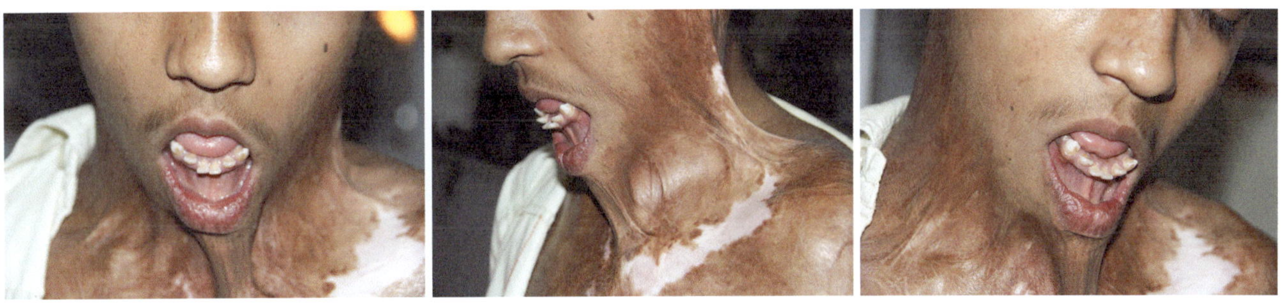

Fig. 46.1 Lower face and neck contracture with oral incontinence—preoperative photos

C. C. Malic (✉)
University of Ottawa, Ottawa, ON, Canada
e-mail: cmalic@cheo.on.ca

M. G. Jeschke et al. (eds.), *Handbook of Burns Volume 1*, https://doi.org/10.1007/978-3-030-18940-2_46

The patient was fitted with a soft collar for the next 6 months, and no pillows were allowed during the sleep. No orthodontic treatment was carried out.

He presented 6 years later to our surgical camp for release of his left axilla. At that time, we assessed the results of the neck contracture release (Fig. 46.3). Donor site had a good healing and no hypertrophic scars (Fig. 46.4).

46.2 Patient 2: Long-Term Right Side Lower Face and Neck Contracture Along with Right Axillary Contracture

During one of our surgical camp in India, a 17-year-old female presented with significant burn contracture affecting the right side of her lower face, neck, chest, and right axilla (Fig. 46.5). This was the result of a flame burn at the age 7 while helping her mother to cook on the open fire. The burn wounds were treated conservatively with regular dressings. The scar contracture was pulling significantly on the right corner of the mouth, and there was significant axillary contracture.

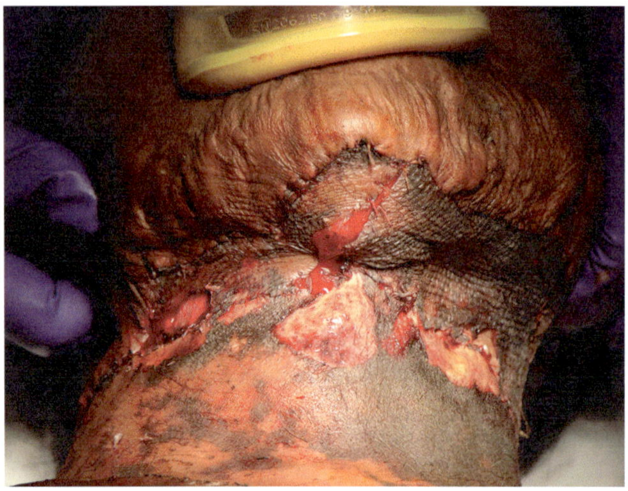

Fig. 46.2 One week after neck contracture release: wound check with some epidermolysis

Under general anesthesia, the burn contractures from the lower face and right side neck were released from the chest on its most caudal zone. When released, the soft tissues above incision covered the lower part of the face and the upper third of the neck. A thicker split thickness skin graft was applied on the defect created after the contracture release. Release of the axilla was carried out in the same procedure, and further skin graft was used for reconstruction, along with jumping man plasty and multiple Z plasties.

She was fitted with a soft collar for the next 6 months, and no pillows were allowed during the sleep. For the axilla, an airplane cast was created, and the patient used it for 3 months.

She presented 6 years later to our surgical camp for follow-up. We assessed the results of the neck contracture release, as well as axillary release (Fig. 46.6).

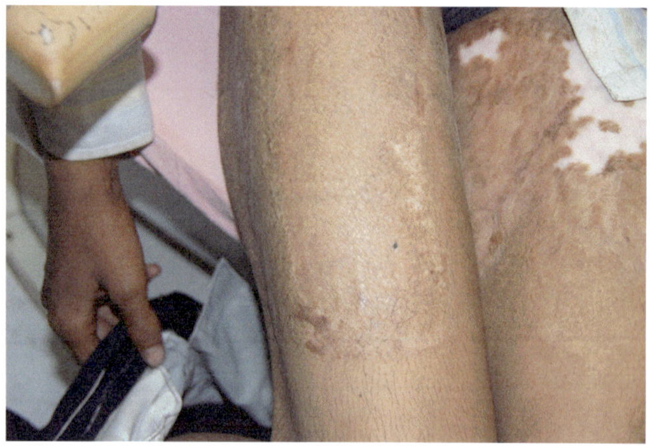

Fig. 46.4 Donor site: right thigh

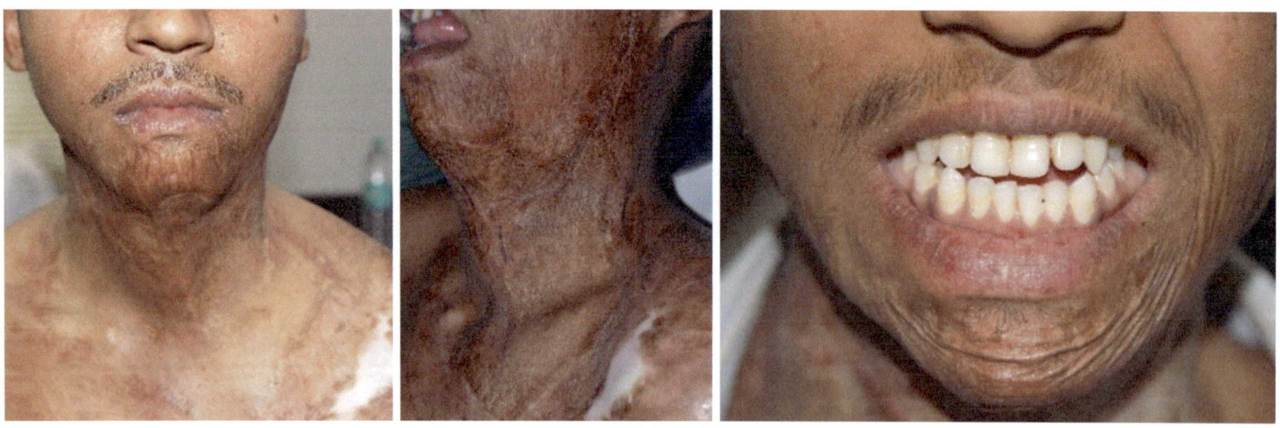

Fig. 46.3 Follow-up 6 years after initial release

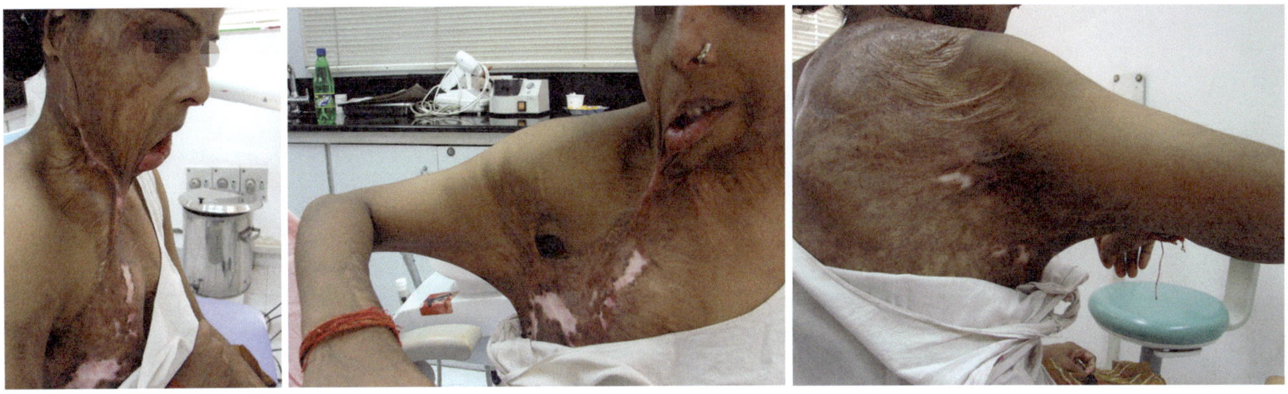

Fig. 46.5 Lower face, neck, chest, and axillary contracture—preoperative photos

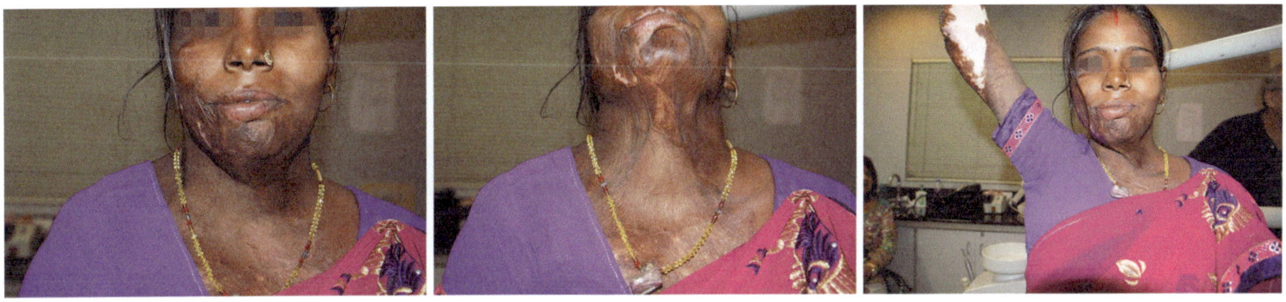

Fig. 46.6 Follow-up 6 years after initial release of the lower face, neck, chest, and right axilla

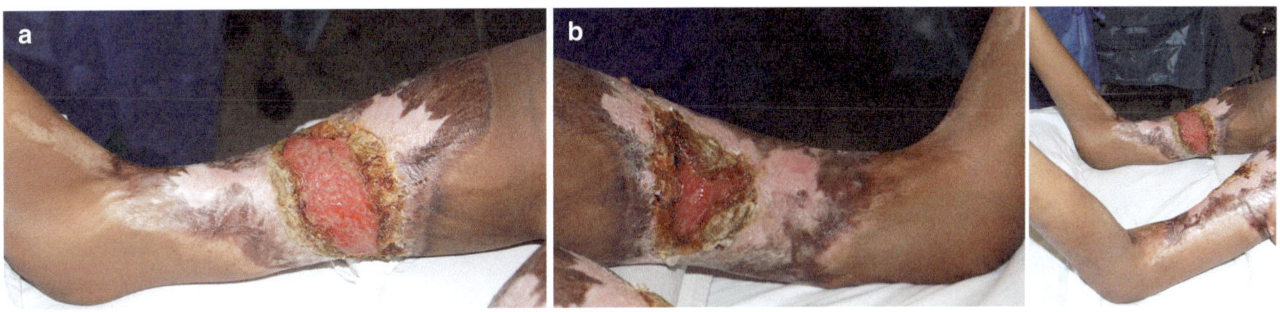

Fig. 46.7 Chronic wounds in bilateral thighs, posterior aspect—preoperative photos. (**a**) left thihg posterior, (**b**) right thigh postero-medial aspect

46.3 Patient 3: Short-Term Bilateral Knee Contractures After Full-Thickness Burns to Thighs Treated Conservatively for 3 Months

During our surgical camp at Deendayal Research Institute and Arogyadam, Chitrakoot, India, a 10-year-old female presented with inability to walk after burn wounds on the posterior thigh more than 3 months ago. She was treated with conservative dressings and no splints or physiotherapy. The burn injuries occurred in home settings while cooking. On examination of posterior aspect of both thighs, there were chronic granulating wounds, surrounded by the indurated scarred area (Fig. 46.7). She had 90 degrees flexion contracture of both knees.

Under general anesthesia, the patient was placed prone and the chronic wounds were excised. Transpositional flaps and Z plasties were performed along with skin grafting. Due to cultural beliefs and traditional clothing, the skin grafts were harvested from buttocks and lateral aspect of the thighs. In this way she could wear a sari. During the procedure, continuous stretching of the soft tissue was performed till full extension of the knees was achieved. Splints were made of plaster of Paris. The graft take and flap viability were checked at 1 week post release, and there was minimal slough of the skin grafts and a loss of around 10% (Fig. 46.8).

Regular dressings lead to complete healing. She ambulated 1 week post surgery with Zimmer frame. At present she is able to walk now with no aides or limping and pain free.

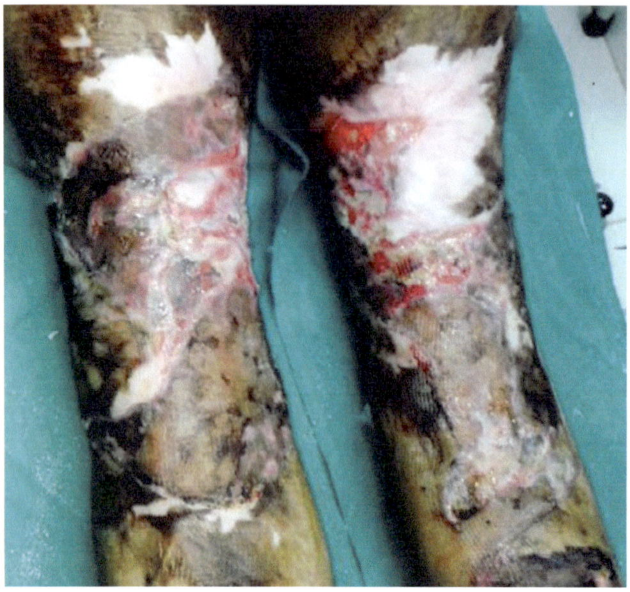

Fig. 46.8 Partial loss of the skin graft and some epidermolysis at 1 week post release burn contractures

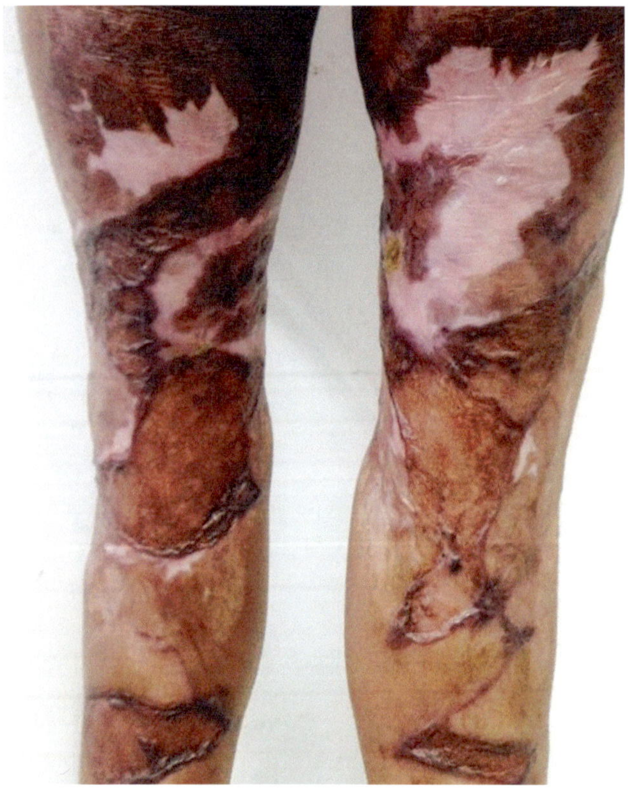

Fig. 46.9 Scars and appearance 3 months post surgery

Scar massage and splints were carried out for 3 months (Fig. 46.9).

She returned for follow-up 6 months post surgery, and there is no relapse of the contracture (Fig. 46.10).

The difficulties of these cases were as follows:

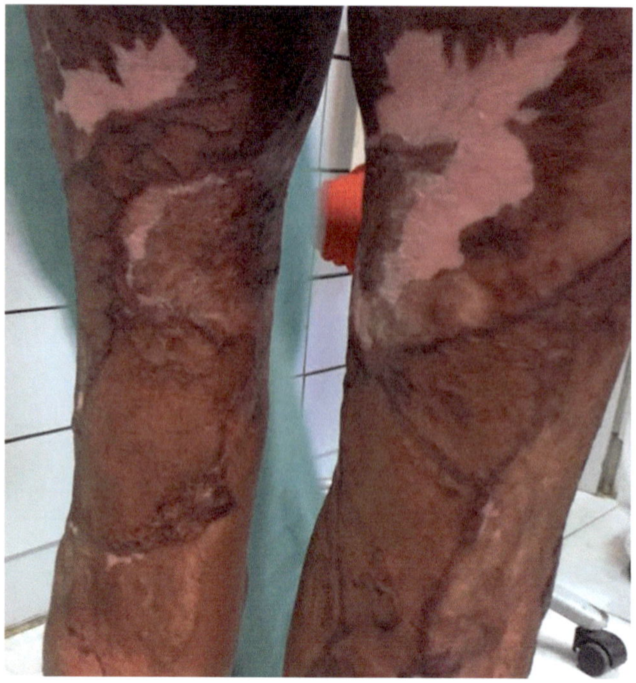

Fig. 46.10 Scar appearance 6 months after release of the knee contracture and wound excision

1. Limited resources for reconstruction (no sources for a pedicled flap).
2. The placement of the incisions to release contracture in order to avoid skin grafts on the lower part of the face and perioral.
3. The aftercare and maintenance of the contracture release, as no hard collars or other rigid splint was available for the neck.

Tips

1. If the soft tissues along the burn contracture are mature and supple, it should be brought cephalad as much as possible by placing the releasing incisions at the base of the contracture with the neck in extension or the contracture band in maximum tension. In this way, the skin grafting will be performed on the base of the neck and chest for better aesthetic outcome (Fig. 46.7a preoperatively, Fig. 46.7b 1 year postoperatively).
2. Do not excise the scar tissue if it is supple and scars are mature.
3. If the settings are very basic, difficult procedure which requires intensive aftercare should be avoided or choose wisely.

Summary Box

This chapter is a series of difficult and complex cases during the acute and reconstruction phases.

47 Levamisole: Adulterated Cocaine-Induced Soft Tissue Necrosis

Sarvesh Logsetty and Shahriar Shahrokhi

A male in his 30s presented with 1 week history of fever, arthralgia, and purpuric rash after inhalation of cocaine. Medical history was significant for hypertension, gastroesophageal reflux disease, sleep apnea, biliary colic, and type II diabetes.

Four years prior to this event, the patient had developed a similar purpuric rash on the ears after exposure to levamisole-adulterated crack cocaine that resulted in the admission for membranous nephropathy, which resolved with medical management.

This time, the purpuric rash began on the left ear and progressed to involve the chest, back, and all extremities. At the time of presentation, the patient was in profound shock requiring emergent intubation and subsequent critical care. His medical issues included renal failure and decreased level of consciousness, with associated diffuse purpuric rash associated with bullae and foul discharge covering all extremities.

Urine toxicology screen was positive for levamisole; further immunological testing revealed pANCA-myeloperoxidase (MPO+) (97, normal 0–20), cACNA-proteinase 3− (12, normal 0–20). The patient's WBC count was elevated initially and subsequently developed profound neutropenia. The areas of purpura subsequently progressed to full-thickness skin necrosis in all affected areas. By admission on day 7, all areas of purpura had progressed to full-thickness necrosis with final %TBSA involvement being 70%.

Surgical debridement included excision of all necrotic soft tissue down to muscular fascia in most areas. These areas required staged skin grafting (allograft followed by autograft).

Tissue biopsies obtained intra-operatively showed evidence of isolated thrombotic vasculopathy. Direct immunofluorescence findings were negative for IgG and positive for IgA, IgM, and C3 localizing to the lumen and walls of the superficial and deep dermal blood vessels.

In total, the patient required six operations for debridement and grafting of all affected areas. The grafts achieved 100% incorporation throughout with a good result, and the patient was discharged to a rehabilitation facility. The length of hospital admission was 120 days.

S. Logsetty (✉)
Manitoba Firefighters Burn Unit, Sections of Plastic and General Surgery, Department of Surgery, University of Manitoba, Health Science Centre, Winnipeg, MB, Canada
e-mail: Sarvesh.Logsetty@umanitoba.ca

S. Shahrokhi
Ross Tilley Burn Centre, Sunnybrook Health Sciences Centre, Toronto, ON, Canada

M. G. Jeschke et al. (eds.), *Handbook of Burns Volume 1*, https://doi.org/10.1007/978-3-030-18940-2_47

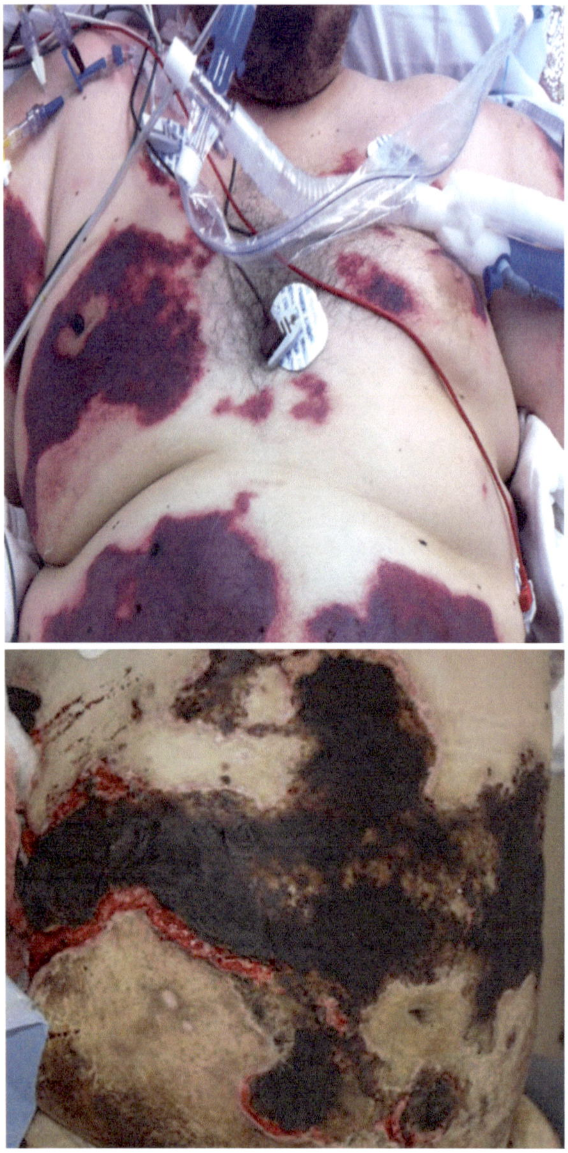

Figs. 47.1 and 47.2 Extensive purpura visible on abdomen on presentation and the final full-thickness eschar prior to debridement

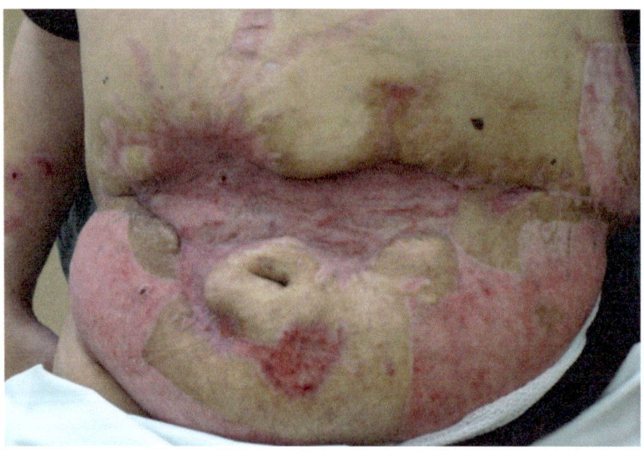

Fig. 47.3 Appearance of healed wounds on abdomen

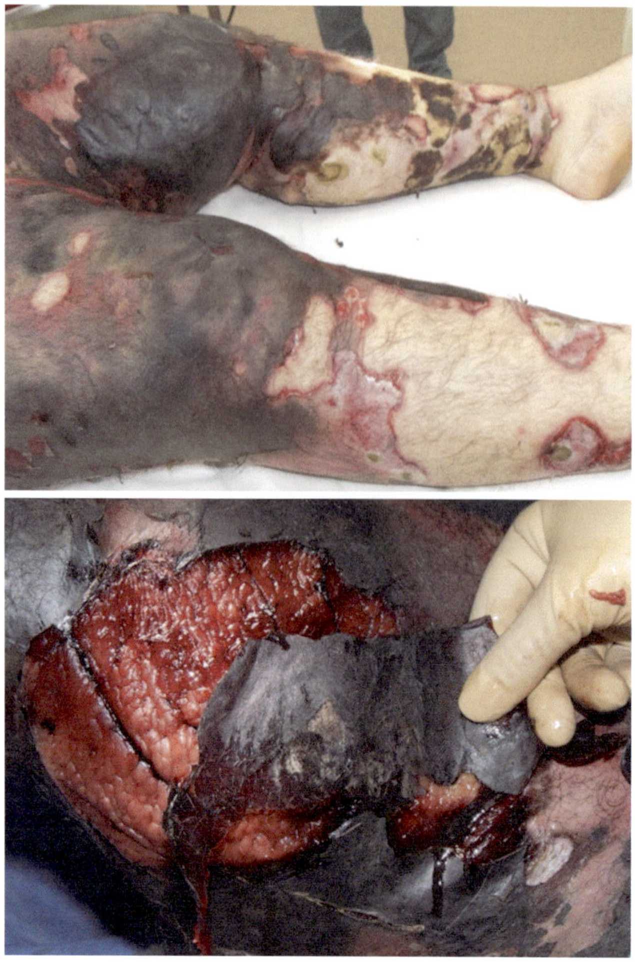

Figs. 47.4 and 47.5 Full-thickness wounds on lower legs and intraoperative debridement of full-thickness eschar

Reference

1. McEvenue G, Brichacek M, Logsetty S, Shahrokhi S. Surgical management of levamisole-adulterated cocaine induced soft tissue necrosis: case study and treatment algorithm. J Burn Care Res. 2017;38:e638–46.

48 Outcome of an Extensive Cold Injury with a Burn Injury Component

Claudia C. Malic, Marc G. Jeschke, and Shahriar Shahrokhi

She was from the northern community of Canada, and she was exposed outside to a temperature of −40 °C for possibly 2 h while under the influence of alcohol.

Her temperature was 32 °C prior to rewarming. After resuscitation with 10 L of fluids and prophylactic intubation, the patient was transferred first to an ICU in Ottawa. Her injuries spared the hands and feet, as well as her face, trunk, and FOUR limb distribution.

A tissue biopsy has shown frostbite with no elements of necrotizing fasciitis. She was transferred to RTBC 4 days later sedated, ventilated, on vasopressors, and broad-spectrum antibiotics.

The wounds were initially treated with Aloe Vera and subsequently dressed with silver sulfadiazine as they appeared to be full-thickness.

There were queries in regard to the wounds being due to a thermal injury rather frostbite vs. combination of the two, given the distribution.

The indirect calorimetry has shown a caloric requirement similar to a burn injury (149%, week 1) along with hypoalbuminemia.

The patient requires multiple debridements and allograft application. Complete closure of the wounds was achieved on day 53 since her initial injury. The patient also required a tracheostomy given the prolonged need for intubation.

During admission, the patient was also diagnosed with Ogilvie syndrome, which resolved with nonsurgical management. She required psychiatric input for her anxiety, as well as ENT consult for a CT-documented subglottic stenosis.

At the time of discharge, the patient still had the tracheostomy in place, was mobilizing, and her BMI dropped to 30. Since discharge, the patient has been followed up, her BMI normalized, and she is recovering well with no PTSD symptoms.

This is an unusual presentation of an extensive freezing injury documented by tissue biopsy diagnosis, which presented with hypercatabolic state and a picture similar to a burn injury that was treated by a multidisciplinary team at Ross Tilley Burn Centre.

C. C. Malic (✉)
Children's Hospital of Eastern Ontario, Ottawa, ON, Canada
e-mail: cmalic@cheo.on.ca

M. G. Jeschke
Faculty of Medicine, Institute of Medical Science, University of Toronto, Toronto, ON, Canada

Biological Sciences, Sunnybrook Research Institute, Toronto, ON, Canada

Ross Tilley Burn Centre, Sunnybrook Health Sciences Centre, Sunnybrook Hospital, Toronto, ON, Canada

Division of Plastic and Reconstructive Surgery, Department of Surgery, Faculty of Medicine, University of Toronto, Toronto, ON, Canada

Department of Immunology, Faculty of Medicine, University of Toronto, Toronto, ON, Canada
e-mail: Marc.Jeschke@sunnybrook.ca

S. Shahrokhi
Ross Tilley Burn Centre, Sunnybrook Health Sciences Centre, Toronto, ON, Canada

M. G. Jeschke et al. (eds.), *Handbook of Burns Volume 1*, https://doi.org/10.1007/978-3-030-18940-2_48

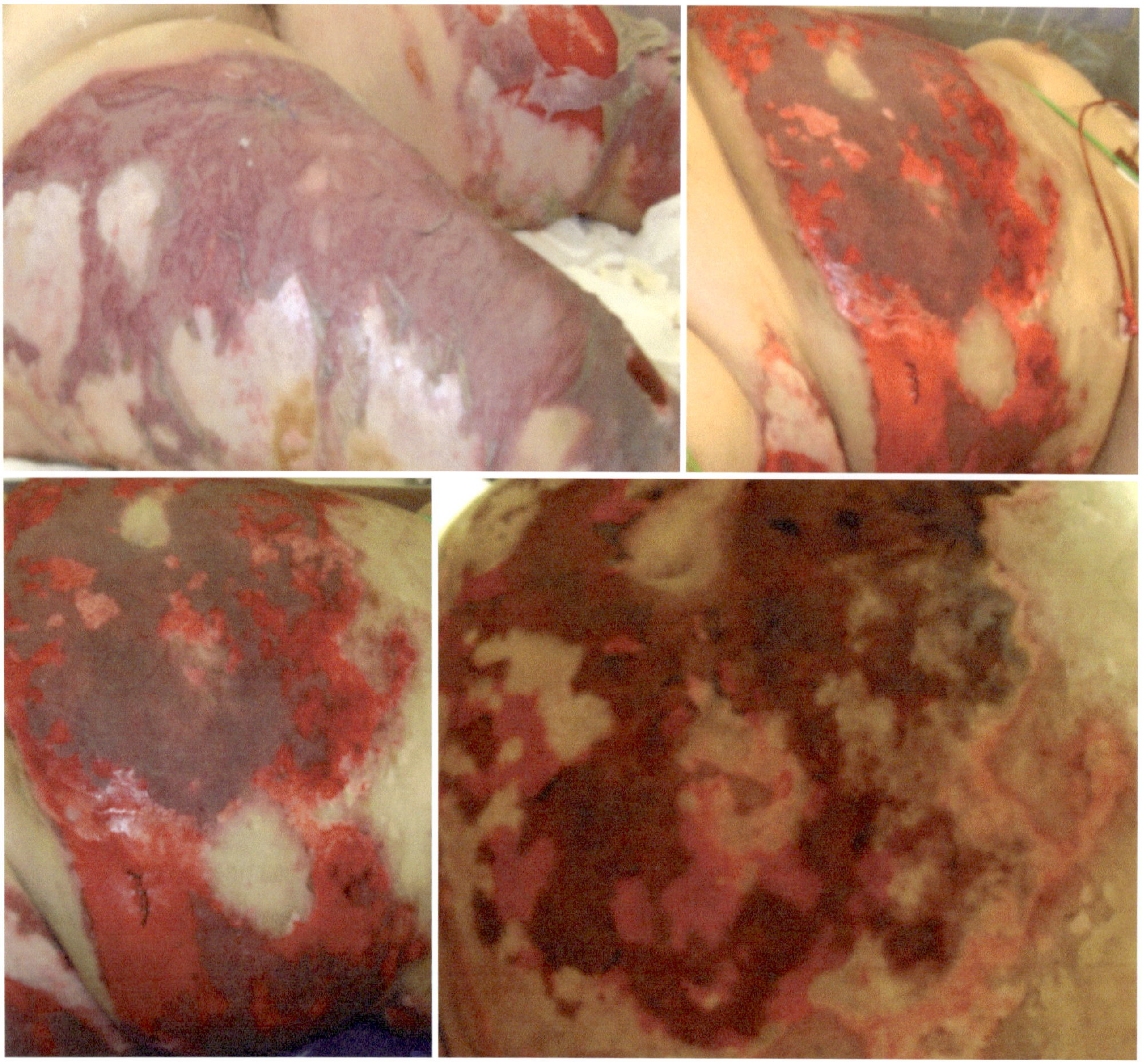

Fig. 48.1 Images from the wounds of various body locations

Index

M. G. Jeschke et al. (eds.), *Handbook of Burns Volume 1*, https://doi.org/10.1007/978-3-030-18940-2

D

E

O

P

Q

R

MIX
Papier aus verantwortungsvollen Quellen
Paper from responsible sources
FSC® C105338

If you have any concerns about our products,
you can contact us on
ProductSafety@springernature.com

In case Publisher is established outside the EU,
the EU authorized representative is:
Springer Nature Customer Service Center GmbH
Europaplatz 3, 69115 Heidelberg, Germany

Printed by Libri Plureos GmbH
in Hamburg, Germany